CROHN'S DISEASE
The Complete Guide to Medical Management

CROHN'S DISEASE

The Complete Guide to Medical Management

EDITED BY

GARY R. LICHTENSTEIN, MD, FACP, FACG, AGAF

PROFESSOR OF MEDICINE

UNIVERSITY OF PENNSYLVANIA SCHOOL OF MEDICINE
DIRECTOR, CENTER FOR INFLAMMATORY BOWEL DISEASE
DEPARTMENT OF MEDICINE, DIVISION OF GASTROENTEROLOGY
PHILADELPHIA, PENNSYLVANIA

ASSOCIATE EDITOR

ELLEN J. SCHERL, MD, FACP, AGAF

DIRECTOR, JILL ROBERTS CENTER FOR INFLAMMMMATORY BOWEL DISEASE
NEW YORK-PRESBYTERIAN HOSPITAL
JILL ROBERTS ASSOCIATE PROFESSOR OF CLINICAL MEDICINE
WEILL MEDICAL COLLEGE OF CORNELL UNIVERSITY
ADJUNCT PROFESSOR OF MEDICINE
COLUMBIA UNIVERSITY MEDICAL CENTER
NEW YORK, NEW YORK

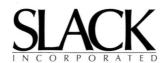

SLACK
INCORPORATED

A companion to this book, *Ulcerative Colitis: The Complete Guide to Medical Management*, by Dr. Gary R. Lichtenstein, MD, FACP, FACG, AGAF is also available for purchase from SLACK Incorporated (ISBN 978-1-55642-945-3). Additional details and order information can be found at www.slackbooks.com.

ISBN: 978-1-55642-944-6

The procedures and practices described in this book should be implemented in a manner consistent with the professional standards set for the circumstances that apply in each specific situation. Every effort has been made to confirm the accuracy of the information presented and to correctly relate generally accepted practices. The authors, editor, and publishers cannot accept responsibility for errors or exclusions or for the outcome of the material presented herein. There is no expressed or implied warranty of this book or information imparted by it. Care has been taken to ensure that drug selection and dosages are in accordance with currently accepted/recommended practice. Off-label uses of drugs may be discussed. Due to continuing research, changes in government policy and regulations, and various effects of drug reactions and interactions, it is recommended that the reader carefully review all materials and literature provided for each drug, especially those that are new or not frequently used. Any review or mention of specific companies or products is not intended as an endorsement by the authors or publishers.

SLACK Incorporated uses a review process to evaluate submitted material. Prior to publication, educators or clinicians provide important feedback on the content that we publish. We welcome feedback on this work.

www.slackbooks.com

Published by: SLACK Incorporated
                   6900 Grove Road
                   Thorofare, NJ 08086 USA
                   Telephone: 856-848-1000
                   Fax: 856-848-6091
                   www.slackbooks.com

Contact SLACK Incorporated for more information about other books in this field or about the availability of our books from distributors outside the United States.

Library of Congress Cataloging-in-Publication Data

Crohn's disease : the complete guide to medical management / edited by Gary R. Lichtenstein, associate editor, Ellen J. Scherl.
      p. ; cm.
  Includes bibliographical references and index.
  ISBN 978-1-55642-944-6 (alk. paper)
  1. Crohn's disease. I. Lichtenstein, Gary R., II. Scherl, Ellen J.
  [DNLM: 1. Crohn Disease. WI 512 C556 2010]
  RC862.E52C783 2010
  616.3'44--dc22

                      2010007950

Printed in the United States of America.

Last digit is print number: 10 9 8 7 6 5 4 3 2 1

DEDICATION

I dedicate this book to my wife, Nancy, and my children, Danielle and Julie, whose unwavering support has permitted me the opportunity to pursue my aspirations.

I also acknowledge my patients who are victims of ulcerative colitis and Crohn's disease.

My mentors have supported me and guided me throughout my career. They have enabled me to continually learn with goals of improving the lives of patients for whom I have had the privilege of caring.

I would also like to dedicate this book to my mother, Joan Lichtenstein, and in memory of my father, Abraham Lichtenstein.

CONTENTS

ACKNOWLEDGMENTS

We would like to acknowledge many individuals who have contributed in many different ways to allow this book to become a reality.

- The contributing authors
- The staff at SLACK Incorporated (including Carrie Kotlar, Senior Acquisitions Editor and April Billick, Managing Editor) and Kristin Della Volpe, Freelance Editor. Without their dedication and tireless and endless effort, this production would not have occurred
- The Crohn's and Colitis Foundation of America
- Our respective institutions: The University of Pennsylvania School of Medicine and the University of Pennsylvania Health System and Weill Medical College of Cornell University
- Dr. Anil Rustgi, for his support and friendship

ABOUT THE EDITOR AND ASSOCIATE EDITOR

Gary R. Lichtenstein, MD, FACP, FACG, AGAF is the Director of the Inflammatory Bowel Disease Center and a Professor of Medicine in the Gastrointestinal Division of the Department of Medicine at the Hospital of the University of Pennsylvania and the University of Pennsylvania School of Medicine in Philadelphia, Pennsylvania.

Dr. Lichtenstein earned his medical degree from the Mount Sinai School of Medicine in New York, New York. He then completed his internship and residency in Internal Medicine at Duke University Medical Center in Durham, North Carolina. He also served a fellowship in Gastroenterology at the Hospital of the University of Pennsylvania of the University Of Pennsylvania School of Medicine. His current research interests encompass investigational therapies for the treatment of ulcerative colitis and Crohn's disease. Dr. Lichtenstein has received numerous research grants focusing on these areas and has served as the national/international principal investigator evaluating novel agents for therapeutic trials in the treatment of ulcerative colitis and Crohn's disease.

A Fellow of the American Gastroenterological Association, the American College of Physicians, and the American College of Gastroenterology, Dr. Lichtenstein has served as Medical Secretary for the American Board of Internal Medicine, Gastroenterology Section. He holds membership and committee positions in many professional societies at a national level, including the American Gastroenterological Association, where he has served as the vice-chair of the Clinical Practice Committee and Practice Economics Committee and where he has served as chair of the Clinical Practice Committee; the American Society for Gastrointestinal Endoscopy, where he has served on the Committee on Training; and the American College of Gastroenterology, where he has served on the Education Committee, Programs Committee, and the Nominations Committee. He recently served as a member of the Research Committee. He has been the chair of the Abstract Review Committee for Inflammatory Bowel Disease for the American College of Gastroenterology. He is also a member of the Crohn's and Colitis Foundation of America, where he serves at the national level as the chair of the Membership Committee of the Clinical Research Alliance; he has served on the National Grants Review Committee and the National Physician Education Committee as well. Additionally, Dr. Lichtenstein is a longstanding member of the American College of Physicians and the American Medical Association.

Dr. Lichtenstein has received numerous awards. including the award for the top specialist in the University of Pennsylvania Health System—the Louis A. Duhring Award. He is the recipient of the Christina and Marie Lindback award, which is the top teaching award in the entire University of Pennsylvania. He has received Penn Pearls Award for medical school teaching. He has received the Donald B. Martin Teaching Award for the Department of Medicine Housestaff. He has received the Sidney Cohen Teaching Award for the Gastroenterology Division. He is listed in "The Best Doctors in America" for Inflammatory Bowel Disease, and was listed among the Top Gastroenterologists for the Elderly in Philadelphia and Top Gastroenterologists in Philadelphia (Special Focus: Inflammatory Bowel Disease) by *Philadelphia Magazine*. He is the recipient of the CCFA Physician of the Year Award, Philadelphia and Delaware Valley Chapters.

In addition to having served on the Editorial Board of *Gastroenterology, American Journal of Gastroenterology, Inflammatory Bowel Diseases, World Journal of Gastroenterology*, and *Digestive Diseases and Sciences*, Dr. Lichtenstein is the current section editor of Selected Summaries and the section editor of Print and Media Review in *Gastroenterology*. He has served as a reviewer for such journals as *The New England Journal of Medicine, Gastroenterology, The Lancet*, the *Annals of Internal Medicine, Gut, Journal of Parenteral and Enteral Nutrition*, the *American Journal of Gastroenterology*, the *World Journal of Gastroenterology* and the *Journal of Clinical Gastroenterology*. He is the executive editor of the newly indexed journal *Gastroenterology and Hepatology*, and serves as Associate Editor of *Therapeutic Advances in Gastroenterology, The Physician and Sportsmedicine*, and *Clinical Investigation*, and is currently Assistant Editor-in-Chief of the *World Journal of Gastroenterology*. An invited lecturer at the local, national, and international levels, Dr. Lichtenstein is the author or co-author of more than 250 peer-reviewed primary articles, chapters, letters, and editorials, and he has presented over 250 abstracts and edited 18 books. He has lectured at over 300 invited conferences, symposiums, and institutional grand rounds.

Ellen J. Scherl, MD, FACP, AGAF, is the Jill Roberts Associate Professor of Clinical Medicine and Director of The Jill Roberts Center for Inflammatory Bowel Disease at Weill Medical College of Cornell University/New York-Presbyterian Hospital. She holds a bachelor's degree in English from Barnard College, Columbia University, and a medical degree from New York Medical College. She is a fellow of the American College of Physicians and the American Gastroenterological Association (AGA), a member of the American Society of Gastrointestinal Endoscopy, and a past president of the New York Society for Gastrointestinal Endoscopy (NYSGE). She is currently Vice President of the New York Academy of Gastroenterology.

Dr. Scherl is Chairperson of the New York Chapter of the Crohn's and Colitis Foundation of America and is involved in the New York Crohn's Foundation. She received the 2008 AGA Outstanding Women in Science award and the 2006 NYSGE Florence Lefcourt Distinguished Service Award, and has been awarded by the Crohn's and Colitis Foundation of America. She is an American Society of Gastrointestinal Endoscopy Circle of Life Member and a member of the AGA Legacy Society. She is board certified in medicine and gastroenterology.

Dr. Scherl is an editorial reviewer for *IBD Journal, Journal of Clinical Gastroenterology, Gastrointestinal Endoscopy, Digestive Diseases and Sciences,* and *Journal of Gastroenterology and Hepatology.* She is co-author of the chapter "Crohn's Disease of the Small Intestine" in *Gastroenterology and Hepatology: The Comprehensive Visual Reference,* associate editor of *Inflammatory Bowel Disease: The Complete Guide to Medical Management,* and coauthor of *An Interactive Dialogue on IBD.*

Dr. Scherl established the first IBD tissue bank in New York City at Weill Medical College of Cornell University/New York-Presbyterian Hospital. She has extensive experience as an investigator in clinical trials and is currently participating in national multicenter trials and in investigator-initiated trials focusing on ulcerative colitis and Crohn's disease.

CONTRIBUTING AUTHORS

Faten Aberra, MD, MSCE (Chapter 37)
Division of Gastroenterology
University of Pennsylvania School of Medicine
Hospital of the University of Pennsylvania
Philadelphia, Pennsylvania

Maria T. Abreu, MD (Chapter 20)
Director, Inflammatory Bowel Disease Center
Associate Professor of Medicine
Mount Sinai School of Medicine
New York, New York

Pietro G. Andres, MD (Chapter 1)
Assistant Adjunct Professor of Medicine
Division of Gastroenterology
University of California, San Francisco
San Francisco, California

Robert N. Baldassano, MD (Chapter 5)
Colman Family Chair in Pediatric Inflammatory Bowel
Disease
Professor, University of Pennsylvania, School of Medicine
Director, Center for Pediatric Inflammatory Bowel Disease
The Children's Hospital of Philadelphia
Philadelphia, Pennsylvania

Theodore M. Bayless, MD (Chapter 23)
Sherlock Hibbs Professor of IBD
Meyerhoff IBD Center
Johns Hopkins Hospital
Baltimore, Maryland

Charles N. Bernstein, MD (Chapter 24)
University of Manitoba Section of Gastroenterology
University of Manitoba IBD Clinical and Research Centre
Winnipeg, Manitoba, Canada

Stephen J. Bickston, MD, AGAF (Chapter 17)
Professor of Internal Medicine
Director, Inflammatory Bowel Disease Center
Associate Chair of Gastroenterology
Virginia Commonwealth University Health Center
Richmond, Virginia

Henry J. Binder, MD (Chapter 34)
Department of Internal Medicine
Yale University School of Medicine
New Haven, Connecticut

Alain Bitton, MD, FRCP(C) (Chapter 21)
Associate Professor
Director, Division of Gastroenterology
McGill University & McGill University Health Centre
Montreal, Quebec, Canada

Wojciech Blonski, MD, PhD (Prologue, Chapters 11, 37)
Division of Gastroenterology
University of Pennsylvania
Philadelphia, Pennsylvania
Department of Gastroenterology
Medical University
Wroclaw, Poland

Brian P. Bosworth, MD (Chapter 32)
Assistant Professor of Medicine
Weill Cornell Medical College
Anne and Ken Estabrook Clinical Scholar in
Gastroenterology
Roberts IBD Center Associate Director, Gastroenterology
and Hepatology Fellowship Program
New York Presbyterian Hospital—Weill Cornell Center
New York, New York

Aaron Brzezinski, MD, FRCP(C) (Chapter 36)
Staff Gastroenterologist
Digestive Disease Institute
Cleveland Clinic Foundation
Cleveland, Ohio

Alan L. Buchman, MD, MSPH (Chapters 30, 31)
Division of Gastroenterology
Feinberg School of Medicine
Northwestern University
Chicago, Illinois

Robert Burakoff, MD, MPH, FACG, FACP (Chapter 27)
Associate Professor of Medicine
Harvard Medical School
Division of Gastroenterology
Brigham and Women's Hospital
Boston, Massachusetts

Ashish Chawla, MD (Chapter 4)
Department of Hepatology and Gastroenterology
The Cleveland Clinic
Cleveland, Ohio

Adam Cheifetz, MD (Chapter 3)
Clinical Director, Center for Inflammatory Bowel Disease
Beth Israel Deaconess Medical Center
Harvard Medical School
Boston, Massachusetts

Lawrence W. Comerford, MD (Chapter 17)
Assistant Professor of Medicine, Gastroenterology and Hepatology
Digestive Health Center of Excellence
University of Virginia
Charlottesville, Virginia

Themistocles Dassopoulos, MD (Chapter 23)
Associate Professor
Director, Inflammatory Bowel Diseases
Gastroenterology Division
Washington University School of Medicine
St. Louis, Missouri

Geert D'Haens, MD, PhD (Chapter 26)
Imelda GI Clinical Research Center
Department of Medicine, Division of Gastroenterology
University of Leuven
Leuven, Belgium

Iris Dotan, MD (Chapter 19)
Head, IBD Center
Department of Gastroenterology and Liver Diseases
Tel Aviv Sourasky Medical Center
Tel Aviv, Israel

Francis A. Farraye, MD, MSc, FACP, FACG (Chapter 7)
Section of Gastroenterology
Boston University School of Medicine
Boston, Massachusetts

Richard N. Fedorak, MD, FRCP(C) (Chapters 28, 33)
Division of Gastroenterology
University of Alberta
Edmonton, Alberta, Canada

Denis Franchimont, MD, PhD (Chapter 22)
Division of Gastroenterology
Erasme University Hospital
Free University of Brussels
Brussels, Belgium

Lawrence S. Friedman, MD (Chapter 1)
Professor of Medicine, Harvard Medical School
Professor of Medicine
Tufts University School of Medicine
Assistant Chief of Medicine
Massachusetts General Hospital
Boston, Massachusetts
Chair, Department of Medicine
Newton-Wellesley Hospital
Newton, Massachusetts

Masayuki Fukata, MD, PhD (Chapter 20)
Assistant Professor of Clinical Medicine
Division of Gastroenterology
University of Miami Miller School of Medicine
Miami, Florida

Louis R. Ghanem, MD, PhD (Chapter 5)
Fellow
Division of Gastroenterology, Hepatology and Nutrition
The Children's Hospital of Philadelphia
Philadelphia, Pennsylvania

Peter H.R. Green, MD (Chapter 32)
Celiac Disease Center
Columbia University College of Physicians and Surgeons
New York, New York

Gordon R. Greenberg, MD, FRCP(C) (Chapter 13)
Professor of Medicine, University of Toronto
Division of Gastoenterology, Mt. Sinai Hospital
Toronto, Ontario, Canada

Stephen B. Hanauer, MD (Chapter 10)
Professor of Medicine and Clinical Pharmacology
Director
Section of Gastroenterology and Nutrition
University of Chicago Medical Center
Chicago, Illinois

Vinita Elizabeth Jacob, MD (Chapter 8)
Assistant Clinical Professor of Medicine
Division of Gastroenterology and Hepatology
Weill Medical College of Cornell University
New York Presbyterian Hospital—Weill Cornell Center
New York, New York

Sunanda V. Kane, MD, MSPH, FACG, FACP, AGAF
(Chapter 9)
Mayo Clinic College of Medicine
Rochester, Minnesota

Gilaad G. Kaplan, MD, FRCP(C) (Chapter 29)
University of Calgary
Calgary, Alberta, Canada

Arthur Kaser, MD (Chapter 25)
Department of Medicine
Division of Gastroenterology and Hepatology
Innsbruck Medical University
Innsbruck, Tyrol, Austria

Jeffry A. Katz, MD (Chapter 8)
Associate Professor of Medicine
Case Western Reserve University School of Medicine
University Hospitals of Cleveland
Cleveland, Ohio

Joshua R. Korzenik, MD (Chapter 6)
Gastrointestinal Unit and MGH Crohn's and Colitis Center
Massachusetts General Hospital and Harvard Medical School
Boston, Massachusetts

David Kotlyar, MD (Prologue, Chapter 11)
Division of Gastroenterology
University of Pennsylvania
Philadelphia, Pennsylvania
Department of Medicine
Montefiore Medical Center/Albert Einstein College of Medicine
Bronx, New York

Harrison Lakehomer, BA (Chapter 15)
Amherst College
Researcher, Jill Roberts Center for Inflammatory Bowel Disease
Weill Medical College of Cornell University/New York Presbyterian Hospital
New York, New York

James D. Lewis, MD, MSCE (Chapter 2)
Division of Gastroenterology
Center for Clinical Epidemiology and Biostatistics
University of Pennsylvania
Philadelphia, Pennsylvania

Wee-Chian Lim, MD, MBBS, MMed, MRCP (Chapter 10)
Section of Gastroenterology and Nutrition
University of Chicago Medical Center
Chicago, Illinois

Ming V. Lin, MD (Prologue)
Department of Medicine
Pennsylvania Hospital
Philadelphia, Pennsylvania

Karen L. Madsen, PhD (Chapter 28)
Division of Gastroenterology
University of Alberta
Alberta, Canada

Gerassimos J. Mantzaris, MD, PhD, AGAF (Chapter 16)
Consultant Gastroenterologist
Head, 1st Department of Gastroenterology
Evangelismos Hospital
Athens, Greece

Manuel Mendizabal, MD (Chapter 11)
Division of Gastroenterology
University of Pennsylvania
Philadelphia, Pennsylvania
Department of Medicine
Hospital Universitario Austral
Pilar, Argentina

Tarun Misra, MD, FRCP(C) (Chapter 33)
Division of Gastroenterology
University of Alberta
Alberta, Canada

David N. Moskovitz, MD, FRCP(C) (Chapter 26)
Imelda GI Clinical Research Center
Department of Medicine, Division of Gastroenterology
University of Leuven
Leuven, Belgium

Alan C. Moss, MD (Chapter 3)
Center for Inflammatory Bowel Disease
Beth Israel Deaconess Medical Center
Harvard Medical School
Boston, Massachusetts

Pia Munkholm, MD, DMSCi (Chapter 12)
Herlev University Hospital
Copenhagen, Denmark

Jane E. Onken, MD, MHS (Chapter 35)
Associate Professor of Medicine, Division of Gastroenterology
Director, Inflammatory Bowel Disease Clinic
Duke University Medical Center
Durham, North Carolina

Mark T. Osterman, MD (Chapter 14)
Assistant Professor of Medicine
Hospital of the University of Pennsylvania and the Presbyterian Medical Center of Philadelphia
Philadelphia, Pennsylvania

Jaime A. Oviedo, MD (Chapter 7)
Section of Gastroenterology
Boston University School of Medicine
Boston, Massachusetts

Remo Panaccione, MD, FRCP(C) (Chapter 29)
Associate Professor of Medicine
Director, Inflammatory Bowel Disease Clinic
University of Calgary
Calgary, Alberta, Canada

Robert M. Penner, BSc, MD, FRCP(C), MSc (Chapter 28)
Assistant Clinical Professor
University of British Columbia
Vancouver, British Columbia, Canada
Assistant Clinical Professor
University of Alberta
Edmonton, Alberta, Canada

Daniel Rachmilewitz, MD (Chapter 19)
Professor of Medicine
Division of Gastroenterology
Tel Aviv Sourasky Medical Center
Tel Aviv, Israel

Mamoon Raza, MD (Chapter 24)
University of Manitoba Section of Gastroenterology
University of Manitoba IBD Clinical and Research Centre
Winnipeg, Manitoba, Canada

Sarathchandra I. Reddy, MD, MPH (Chapter 27)
Instructor in Medicine
Harvard Medical School
Division of Gastroenterology
Brigham and Women's Hospital
Boston, Massachusetts

Lene Riis, MD (Chapter 12)
Herlev University Hospital
Cophenhagen, Denmark

Felice H. Schnoll-Sussman, MD (Chapter 32)
Director of Research, The Jay Monahan Center for Gastrointestinal Health
Assistant Attending Physician, New York-Presbyterian Hospital/Weill Cornell Medical Center
Assistant Professor of Medicine, Weill Medical College of Cornell University
New York, New York

Corey A. Siegel, MD (Chapter 6)
Gastrointestinal Unit and MGH Crohn's and Colitis Center
Massachusetts General Hospital and Harvard Medical School
Boston, Massachusetts

Kenneth Simpson, BVM&S, PhD (Chapter 4)
Professor of Medicine
College of Veterinary Medicine
Cornell University
Ithaca, New York

Miles P. Sparrow, MD, MBBS, FRACP (Chapter 10)
Section of Gastroenterology and Nutrition
University of Chicago Medical Center
Chicago, Illinois

Chinyu Su, MD (Chapter 2)
Division of Gastroenterology
University of Pennsylvania
Philadelphia, Pennsylvania

Arun Swaminath, MD (Chapter 15)
Assistant Professor in Clinical Medicine
Department of Medicine, Division of Digestive and Liver
Diseases
Columbia University Presbyterian Hospital
New York, New York

Herbert Tilg, MD (Chapter 25)
Department of Medicine
Division of Gastroenterology and Hepatology
Innsbruck Medical University
Innsbruck, Austria

Ryan Urquhart Warren, MD (Chapter 15)
Brown University
Researcher, Jill Roberts Center for Inflammatory
Bowel Disease
Weill Medical College of Cornell University/New York-
Presbyterian Hospital
New York, New York

Douglas M. Weine, MD (Chapter 32)
Clinical Fellow in Gastroenterology and Hepatology
Weill Medical College of Cornell University/New York-
Presbyterian Hospital
New York, New York

Gary Wild, MD (Chapter 22)
Division of Gastroenterology
Montreal General Hospital
McGill University Health Centre
Montreal, Quebec, Canada

INTRODUCTION

Since the historical description of Crohn's disease by Drs. Burrill Crohn, Leon Ginzburg, and Gordon Oppenheimer in 1932 and the historical description of ulcerative colitis by Dr. Samuel Wilks and Dr. Walter Moxon in 1859, much has been learned about the etiology, pathogenesis, and treatment of these 2 idiopathic inflammatory bowel disorders. These disorders occur at any age, spare no socioeconomic class, and have the potential to significantly impair patient's quality of life. Significant progress has been made in the past decade related to Crohn's disease and ulcerative colitis; however, the medical therapy of inflammatory bowel disease has had the greatest impact on patients' lives. Although these disorders are remarkably similar in many ways, they have vast differences when comparing response to specific medical therapies. As a consequence, it was elected to separately focus on medical therapy of ulcerative colitis and distinguish this from medical therapy of Crohn's disease.

The authors who have contributed to this textbook are regionally and internationally recognized experts in inflammatory bowel disease. The mainstay of literature in the past decade focusing on medical therapy of inflammatory bowel disease has emanated from the work of these distinguished authors. In this book, the authors discuss the current medical therapies and review the clinical trial data that established the foundation for their use. The individual chapters in this book not only review the current medical therapy in use for treatment of patients with inflammatory bowel disease but they also review the basic pathophysiologic principles supporting the use of these and future therapeutics. Additionally, novel therapeutics that have potential impact and significance to the practicing physician are highlighted.

I am indebted to my contributors for providing superb, detailed, critical chapters amid their already busy schedules. I would also like to thank Dr. Ellen Scherl for her expertise and the countless hours she has spent in making this textbook a reality. Additionally, I am most appreciative and extend thanks to all my colleagues, patients, and those who have supported research in the field who have helped me uncover and extend the boundaries of my knowledge in inflammatory bowel disease. Lastly, I am most appreciative of my wife Nancy and my children Julie and Danielle for allowing me to spend countless hours doing what I thoroughly enjoy: patient care, research, and education.

Gary R. Lichtenstein, MD, FACP, FACG, AGAF

PROLOGUE
HISTORICAL PERSPECTIVE OF CROHN'S DISEASE

Wojciech Blonski, MD, PhD; David Kotlyar, MD; Ming V. Lin, MD; and Gary R. Lichtenstein, MD, FACP, FACG, AGAF

It has been suggested that the symptoms of Crohn's disease (CD) were reported for the first time more than 1000 years ago when the English king, Alfred (849 to 899 AD), had a disease presenting with symptoms of pain during eating and abdominal discomfort, with much embarrassment, plaguing the king without remission.[1] The disease was thought to be caused by witchcraft or the king's infidelities.[1] Ulcerated and fibrous cecum was observed by the German physician Wilhelm Fabry (1560 to 1634) during the autopsy of a boy complaining of persistent "subhepatic pain," and that "the cecum (was) contracted and invaginated into the ileum ... such that it was not possible for anything to pass from the proximal intestine into the colon."[2] An autopsy of King Louis XIII in 1643 revealed the presence of ulceration of both the small and large bowels along with abscesses and fistulas consistent with either ileocecal tuberculosis or regional enteritis.[3]

Giovanni Battista Morgagni (1682 to 1771), in his book *De Sedibus et Causis Morborum*, wrote a section based on the results of an autopsy of a 20-year-old man who died due to perforation of the terminal ileum and provided a macroscopic description[4] of the disease that has been considered consistent with contemporary CD.[5] The observed case featured ulcerations and erosions in the terminal ileum and enlarged massive mesenteric lymph nodes.[4] Combe and Saunders in 1813 described a patient who presented with strictures and thickening of the ileum.[6] Subsequently, Abercombie in 1828 published a case of a patient with thickening of the ileum and involvement of ulceration of the cecum and a short part of the ascending colon.[7]

Several studies describing features of CD (abdominal inflammatory masses) were published in the medical literature in the 20th century prior to the landmark article by Crohn et al in 1932,[8] including reports by Braun (1901),[9] Koch (1903),[10] Lesniowski (1903),[11] Wilmanns (1905),[12] Moynihan (1907),[13] Proust (1907),[14] Monsarrat (1907),[15] Lejars (1908),[16] von Bergmann (1911),[17] Dalziel (1913),[18] and Moschowitz and Wilensky[19] (1923, cited by Crohn et al in their landmark paper).[8] These masses resembled tumors and were considered "malignant" and "untreatable" due to limited abdominal surgery.[20]

The report by Sir T. Kennedy Dalziel (1913)[18] is to be distinguished. Dalziel (1861 to 1924), a Glasgow surgeon, described 13 cases of "chronic interstitial enteritis."[18] The first described case was a physician presenting with bowel obstruction preceded by attacks of colic abdominal pain and diarrhea.[18] The autopsy revealed chronically inflamed and narrowed small and large intestines with enlarged mesenteric lymph nodes.[18] The jejunum, mid-ileum, transverse, and sigmoid colon were involved by the disease in other patients.[18] Histologic examination of the bowel revealed that the earliest change was acute congestion with dilated vessels and edema of the submucosa with infiltration of polymorphs and mononuclear cells.[18] Subsequently, the infiltration and necrosis of muscularis mucosa were observed.[18] An increased number of eosinophils and the presence of a few giant cells in the granulation tissue replacing mucosa were also described.[18] Dalziel excluded tuberculosis in his reported patients and hypothesized that the observed disease resembled chronic bacterial enteritis of cattle (Johne's disease), called at that time *pseudotuberculous.*[18] Of note, this hypothesis was rejected 87 years later by Van Kruiningen.[21] Despite the fact that Dalziel's manuscript was published in the *British Medical Journal* in 1913, it did not have an impact comparable to that of Crohn's paper published nearly 20 years later.[8]

Moschcowitz and Wilensky from Mount Sinai Hospital in New York City in 1923 described 4 cases of nonspecific granulomata of the intestine that were observed in young patients with a history of appendicitis and appendectomy.[19] They described "a firm, dense, uncircumscribed tumor involving all the coats of the large intestine causing stricture of the lumen."[19] The striking pathologic finding was a massive presence of giant cells.[19] The authors initially thought that the observed lesion had a predilection primarily to the colon, but in the follow-up article published in 1927, they acknowledged that the described lesion might also be localized in the small intestine as they described the young patient with granuloma exclusively within the small intestine.[22]

CD has been named after Dr. Burrill Crohn (1884 to 1983) who, along with Drs. Leon Ginzburg and Gordon Oppenheimer, published a landmark article entitled "Regional Ileitis: A Pathologic and Clinical Entity" in the *Journal of the American Medical Association* (*JAMA*) in October 1932.[8] The authors from Mount Sinai Hospital in New York City described pathological and clinical features of the disease of terminal ileum in 14 young adult patients (age range was 17 to 52 years and only 2 patients exceeding 40 years of age).[8] The new entity was "characterized by a subacute or chronic necrotizing and cicatrizing inflammation."[8] Ginzburg and Oppenheimer studied 12 patients, whereas Crohn studied 2 patients.[3] The authors used the term *segmental hypertrophic ulcerative stenosis of the distal ileum.*[23] Crohn himself named this new entity *terminal ileitis.*[23] The authors also observed that "the ulceration of the mucosa is accompanied by a disproportionate connective tissue reaction of the remaining walls of the involved intestine, a process which frequently leads to stenosis of the lumen of the intestine, associated with the formation of multiple fistulas."[8] The clinical course of the disease, named by the authors as *regional ileitis*, was divided into either "(1) acute intra abdominal disease with peritoneal irritation, (2) symptoms of ulcerative enteritis, (3) symptoms of chronic obstruction of the small intestine or (4) persistent and intractable fistulas in the right lower quadrant following previous drainage for ulcer or abdominal abscess."[8] All patients underwent surgical treatment performed by Dr. Berg, which resulted in restitution of health in 13 patients.[8] Macroscopic evaluation of resected specimens revealed a thickened, soggy, and edematous wall of terminal ileum with markedly thickened mesentery.[8] Microscopic examination of the terminal ileum demonstrated the presence of acute, subacute, or chronic inflammation with a striking presence of giant cells in some cases.[8] The authors noticed that lesions at early stages were diffused, whereas the inflammatory process had a focal character at later stages.[8]

Upon further questioning, the authors claimed that they excluded every etiologic factor known at that time such as tuberculosis, amebiasis, syphilis, actinomycosis, Hodgkin's disease, or lymphosarcoma that might have caused this disease.[8] All the authors agreed that their names would appear in the manuscript in alphabetical order. Of note, Dr. Berg rejected the suggestion that he should also be included as an author of the manuscript due to the fact that he had a custom of not putting his name on manuscripts he had not written himself.[23]

During the American Gastroenterological Association meeting in Atlantic City, New Jersey on May 2-3, 1932, Ginzburg and Oppenheimer presented the study entitled, "Non-specific Granulomata of the Intestine (Inflammatory Tumors and Strictures of Bowel)."[3] Ginzburg and Oppenheimer acknowledged that part of the study regarding localized ileitis was performed in cooperation with Crohn.[3] The study was subsequently published in *Transactions of the American Gastroenterological Association*, the journal of the American Gastroenterological Association.[24] They presented the detailed description of 52 patients with inflammatory tumors or strictures of the large or small intestine who were observed and treated surgically at Mount Sinai Hospital.[24] The work was a result of retrospective and prospective research initiated in 1925 and dated back to 1920.[24,25] Patients with sigmoid diverticulitis were not included.[24,25] This study was subsequently published in a national medical journal, *Annals of Surgery*, in 1933 with the addition of radiologic and pathologic images.[25] Studied patients were divided into the following 6 groups: "(1) extra- or peri-intestinal granulomata secondary to sealed-off perforations of the bowel, (2) granulomata secondary to known vascular disturbances of the gut, (3) localized hypertrophic ulcerative stenosis of the terminal ileum, (4) localized hypertrophic colitis with or without low-grade generalized colitis, (5) simple penetrating ulcers of the colon, and (6) lesions secondary to inflammation of the appendages of the bowel, such as appendicitis, diverticulitis, typhlitis."[24,25] At the same time, on May 13, 1932, Crohn presented the study on 14 patients with regional ileitis at the meeting of the Gastroenterology and Proctology section of the American Medical Association held in New Orleans,[3] which was subsequently published in *JAMA* in October 1932.[8] The 14 patients with regional ileitis presented by Crohn were also included in the presentation by Ginzburg and Oppenheimer.[24,25] However, Crohn did not acknowledge the contribution of Ginzburg and Oppenheimer in his presentation.[3] Crohn's presentation was listed in the meeting program as "Terminal Ileitis: Its Clinical Manifestations (Lantern Demonstration). Burrill B. Crohn, New York. Discussion to be opened by John E. Jennings, Brooklyn."[26] The reason the presentation given by Crohn gained much more attention than the one given by Ginzburg and Oppenheimer is that Crohn addressed a larger audience than Ginzburg and Oppenheimer,[3] and subsequent publication in *JAMA*[8] was available earlier than manuscripts by Ginzburg and Oppenheimer.[24,25]

The term *Crohn's disease* was introduced in the United States by Harris et al in 1933 in the paper entitled, "Chronic Cicatrizing Enteritis: Regional Ileitis (Crohn). A New Surgical Entity."[27] A similar title was used by Cushway in a case report entitled, "Chronic Cicatrizing Enteritis-Regional Ileitis (Crohn)."[28] Researchers in England started using the term Crohn's disease as early as 1937[29] and 1938.[30] In 1939, Armitage and Wilson stated that the term Crohn's disease "avoids confusion" and "conveys an exact meaning, is easily remembered by students, and pays a well deserved tribute."[31] Various names of the new entity have been implemented, such as *Lesniowski-Crohn's disease* in Poland,[32] *Crohn-Dalziel's disease* in Scotland,[33] or *Saunders-Abercombie-Crohn's disease* in England.[34] Armitage and Wilson, in their review of the literature regarding CD, noted that the term *cicatrizing enteritis* was suggested by Warren and Sommers.[31] In 1968, the term Crohn's disease was coined at the 8th International Congress of Gastroenterology in Prague (Czechoslovakia at that time, Czech Republic at present).[20] It is commonly known that studies by Crohn, Ginzburg, and Oppenheimer describing regional enteritis caused increased attention to this new entity.[20] Crohn in turn devoted a long-term commitment to popularization, publication, lecturing, spreading knowledge,[23] and further investigating this new disease.[5]

There were substantial controversies surrounding Crohn's contribution to the original description of regional enteritis. In 1986, Ginzburg published a letter to the editor of *Gastroenterology* in which he criticized "some extravagant claims made by Dr. Crohn in his discussion of IBD" in his published memoirs that completely excluded a significant contribution to the discovery of regional enteritis by Oppenheimer and Ginzburg.[23] Crohn claimed that he himself discovered a new clinical entity, terminal ileitis, that was not detected by pathologists or surgeons.[23] Ginzburg wrote that in 1931 during a conversation with Crohn, they discussed 2 cases of his patients who were operated on by Dr. Berg due to unusual lesions in the terminal ileum.[23] Crohn was informed by the pathology laboratory that similar cases were previously described by Ginzburg and Oppenheimer.[23] Subsequently, Crohn talked to Dr. Berg, who requested that Ginzburg should give his identified studies and written article to Crohn.[23] In 1932, a group of Mount Sinai Medical Staff investigated why the names of Ginzburg and Oppenheimer did not appear in the presentation given by Crohn on terminal ileitis at the American Medical Association meeting in New Orleans.[23] The investigation resulted in the decision to put the names of Ginzburg and Oppenheimer in the published article.[23] Ginzburg also recalled that Crohn claimed that the study describing

regional ileitis included 14 of Crohn's patients, whereas in reality Crohn contributed 2 patients to 12 patients already studied by Ginzburg and Oppenheimer.[23] Crohn also claimed that Ginzburg and Oppenheimer were added as coauthors only because it was suggested by Dr. Berg.[23] It is unquestionable that both Ginzburg and Oppenheimer initiated and published their research regarding granulomatous bowel disease before Crohn showed his interest in this matter.[23] Ginzburg published his first articles regarding this problem in 1927[35] and 1928.[36]

In 1934, Colp[37] described cecal involvement in CD, and in 1938 Penner and Crohn[38] reported perianal fistulae complicating CD. In 1939, Ginzburg et al described the results of ileocolostomy with exclusion of diseased bowel from the fecal stream in 19 patients with regional ileitis as a successful treatment of lesions localized in the terminal ileum.[39] In 1945 and 1951, Garlock and Crohn[40] and Garlock et al[41] published the results of surgical treatment of terminal ileitis, including resection of the bowel or ileocolostomy with exclusion. In October 1952, Charles Wells, a surgeon from the University of Liverpool, delivered a lecture at the Royal College of Surgeons of England regarding differentiation between ulcerative colitis and CD.[42] Wells introduced the term *segmental colitis*, an entity that he considered a form of Crohn's colitis, observed in patients without small bowel lesions characteristic of CD.[42] Wells defined Crohn's colitis as "thickening and fibrosis of bowel wall, patchy ulceration of the mucosa and a tendency to spread by 'skips.'"[42] Wells wrote, "I am prepared to believe that although the same glandular involvement is not evident, this 'segmental colitis' is a colonic form of CD. Crohn himself, however, does not sanction this extension of the entity to which we give this name. I am therefore content to describe it as separate entity."[42] In 1962, Wolf and Marshak published an important article describing radiologic features of Crohn's colitis.[43] Not only was CD observed in various parts of the gastrointestinal tract (eg, duodenum, stomach, gallbladder, and pancreas[44-47]) but also in other parts of the human body. Lesions consistent with CD were observed in the mouth,[48] skin,[49-51] umbilicus,[52] urine bladder,[53] bone,[54] muscles,[55] and lungs.[56,57]

In 1996, a French group led by Hugot identified the susceptibility locus for CD on chromosome 16 using a wide-genome search on 2 consecutive and independent panels of families with multiple affected members.[58] In 2001, 2 groups of researchers, Hugot et al from France[59] and Ogura et al from the United States,[60] independently described the NOD2/CARD15 gene, the first susceptibility gene for CD localized on chromosome 16. It has been proposed that the NOD2 gene induces activation of nuclear factor (NF)-κB, thus making it responsive to bacterial lipopolysaccharides.[61] On the other hand, such activation does not occur in mutant NOD2, implicating an association between an innate immune response to bacterial components and development of CD.[60]

TREATMENT

Surgery initially was considered the main treatment of CD and was infrequently performed as abdominal exploration due to diagnosis of "malignant tumor" up to 1930 and after 1930 more frequently for acute appendicitis.[62] In 1941, Crohn himself wrote that there was no specific conservative treatment of regional enteritis and that the course of the disease could not be altered by any method available at that time.[62] In 1978, an editorial published in the *British Medical Journal* presented a 40-year summary of treatment of CD.[63] At that time, supporting medical treatment providing adequate nutrition was considered the mainstay of treatment.[63] A surgical approach (resection of the affected part of the bowel) was recommended only in patients with disabling symptoms.[63] The authors also reviewed the surgical treatment of CD from a historical perspective. From 1939 to 1972, ileocolostomy with exclusion of the diseased part of the bowel was considered ideal surgical treatment.[39-41] This approach changed in 1972, and at that time resection was considered the proper treatment.[64] A retrospective analysis of the results of surgery performed between 1932 and 1975 demonstrated high recurrence rates (65% for resection, 82% for bypass with exclusion, and 94% for simple bypass) during 15 years of follow-up.[65] The authors of an editorial concluded that as of 1978, "Crohn's disease will remain a life-sentence until a specific treatment is found."[63]

CORTICOSTEROIDS

Medical treatment of CD was initiated in the 1950s. In 1951, Stanley et al suggested that therapy with corticotrophin or cortisone might be an ideal maintenance treatment of CD in patients resistant to the usual methods of treatment.[66] At the same time, Gray et al, based on the rapid improvement of 2 patients treated with corticotrophin, considered long-term maintenance therapy with corticotrophin an ideal treatment.[67] In 1952, Kirsner et al suggested that although treatment with corticotrophin of chronic regional enteritis was beneficial to patients, its effect was less pronounced than that in those with ulcerative colitis.[68] In their analysis of 54 patients with CD, Sparberg and Kirsner observed that "the response is variable and unpredictable."[69] At the same time, Jones and Lennard-Jones recommended the use of corticosteroids and corticotrophin in patients presenting either with extensive small bowel CD or after postoperative recurrence.[70] In 1994, Munkholm et al introduced the term *corticosteroid dependency* in CD based on the observation that up to 36% of patients with CD receiving corticosteroids were corticosteroid dependent (ie, such patients relapsed either after complete cessation of treatment or dose reduction).[71] A new-generation corticosteroid, controlled-release budesonide, was found to have a comparable efficacy and significantly less systemic adverse events than traditional corticosteroids in treatment of CD,[72] particularly of the terminal ileum and right colon.[73] Budesonide given at 9 mg daily was also found to be superior to placebo in treatment of active Crohn's disease of the ileum and proximal colon.[74] The maintenance effect of budesonide was found not to exceed 1 year of treatment.[75]

AMINOSALICYLATES

Aminosalicylates (sulfasalazine: sulfapyridine linked by azo-bond with 5-aminosalicylic acid [5-ASA]) were introduced to CD treatment in the 1970s.[76,77] Large clinical trials demonstrated superiority of sulfasalazine over placebo in treating CD.[76,77] Due to systemic side effects associated with the presence of the sulfapyridine moiety in sulfalazine, preparations consisting of 5-ASA alone (mesalamine) were initiated in the treatment of CD.[78]

ANTIBIOTICS

Due to the concept of bacterial involvement in the pathogenesis of CD, antibiotics have been studied in the treatment of this entity since the 1970s.[79] An initial randomized controlled trial published in 1985 did not show any therapeutic benefit of metronidazole or co-trimoxazole in treatment of CD.[80] It was subsequently suggested that metronidazole might be effective in treating CD with large bowel involvement.[81] The later results of studies of metronidazole or ciprofloxacin showed its efficacy in treatment of CD comparable with steroids or mesalamine.[82-85] It was recently suggested that bacterial overgrowth, which frequently accompanies CD, might be effectively treated with ciprofloxacin or metronidazole.[86]

IMMUNOMODULATORS

Azathioprine was introduced as a CD treatment in the early 1970s.[87-90] The drug was considered effective in the treatment of CD, allowing for discontinuation of corticosteroids in patients requiring them to control their symptoms. A pilot open label study of methotrexate in inflammatory bowel disease was published in 1989 by Kozarek et al.[91] In 1995, the North American Crohn's Study Group Investigators published the results of the first randomized placebo controlled trial of weekly injections of methotrexate (25 mg) in patients with chronic active CD despite a minimum of 3 months of prednisone therapy.[92] The results of a subsequent trial published in 2000 demonstrated the efficacy of methotrexate in the lower dose of 15 mg.[93] The use of cyclosporine in the treatment of CD was studied in the 1990s, but the studies did not demonstrate efficacy.[94-96]

Biologic Therapy

It has been recently demonstrated that CD is a chronic recurrent gastrointestinal disorder with involvement of proinflammatory cytokines and chemokines. Several biologic agents targeting specific disease mechanisms have been considered potentially efficacious in the treatment of inflammatory bowel disease (IBD). The first pilot study of a chimeric, monoclonal anti-tumor necrosis factor alpha (TNFα) antibody for CD, infliximab, was published in 1995.[97] Subsequently, several randomized placebo-controlled clinical trials, including the ACCENT I and ACCENT II trials, have shown the efficacy of this new agent in inducing and maintaining remission in CD.[98-101] In 1998, the US Food and Drug Administration (FDA) approved infliximab for the treatment of moderately to severely active CD in patients with an inadequate response to conventional therapy as well as a treatment for patients with fistulizing CD for reduction in the number of draining enterocutaneous fistulas. In 2007, the FDA approved a fully human monoclonal antibody to TNFα, adalimumab, as a treatment of active CD in patients unresponsive to conventional therapy. Patients with CD who are intolerant to infliximab or lost response to infliximab are also recommended to be treated with adalimumab. The efficacy of adalimumab was demonstrated in the CLASSIC I[102] and CHARM trials.[102] Most recently, in 2008, the FDA approved the third anti-TNFα biologic agent, polyethylene glycolated Fab' fragment of humanized anti-TNFα monoclonal antibody, certolizumab, in the treatment of CD following the results of a randomized placebo-controlled clinical trial.[103] In 2008, another biologic agent, a humanized immunoglobulin G (IgG)4 monoclonal antibody against alpha4beta1 integrin-mediated leukocyte migration, natalizumab, was approved by the FDA for the treatment of CD wherein efficacy was shown in several clinical trials.[104-107] This drug had been used in patients with multiple sclerosis since 2004, was withdrawn from the market by the manufacturer in 2005 due to reports of progressive multifocal leukoencephalopathy,[108] and was then reintroduced to the market in 2006. Several other agents have also been evaluated for the treatment of CD such as etanercept (fully human anti-TNFα fusion protein),[109] CNI-1493 (a small molecule-blocking TNFα gene expression by inhibiting mitogen-activated protein kinase),[110] onercept (genetically engineered recombinant human TNFα-receptor p55 monomer neutralizing TNFα),[111] ustekinumab (a human interleukin-12/23 monoclonal antibody),[112] an antisense oligonucleotide to intracellular adhesion molecule-1,[113-117] anti-human CD40 Mab ch5D12,[118] recombinant human interleukin 10,[119-122] recombinant human interleukin-11,[123,124] anti-interleukin-12 antibody,[125] anti-interferon-γ antibodies,[126] human growth hormone,[127] interferon-α-2b,[128] granulocyte colony- and granulocyte macrophage colony-stimulating factors,[129-131] or antibody to interleukin-6 receptor.[132]

Several known historical figures suffered from CD. It has been suggested that President Eisenhower suffered from CD of the small intestine, which caused acute obstruction necessitating immediate surgeries in June 1956[53] and February 1969.[133,134] Unfortunately, cardiac complications after the latter surgery led to the death of the president on March 28, 1969.[133,134] However, some authors question the accuracy of diagnosis of CD in this case.[135] Ludwig Van Beethoven's deafness is now believed to have been caused by immunopathy associated with either CD or ulcerative colitis.[136] A recent publication by Orrego and Quintana claims that Charles Darwin suffered from CD.[137]

CONCLUSION

CD has been recognized as a distinct entity since the dawn of human history, and new treatments have revolutionized the understanding of the pathogenesis of the disease and has enormously helped the many thousands of patients with the disease.

REFERENCES

1. Simon C. Inflammatory bowel disease. *InnovAiT.* 2008;9:615-622.
2. Fabry W. Ex scirro et ulcere cancioso in intestino cocco exorta iliaca passio. In: *Opera, Observatio LXI.* Vol. 31. Frankfort: J.L. Dufour, 1682:49. Cited by: Fielding JF. Crohn's disease and Dalziel's syndrome. A history. *J Clin Gastroenterol.* 1988;10:279-285.
3. Baron JH. Inflammatory bowel disease up to 1932. *Mt Sinai J Med.* 2000;67:174-189.
4. Morgagni G. The seats and causes of disease investigated by anatomy. In: Johnson A, Payne B, eds. *Five Books Containing a Great Variety of Dissections With Remarks.* London: A. Millar and T. Cadell; 1769:200-204.
5. Kirsner JB. Historical aspects of inflammatory bowel disease. *J Clin Gastroenterol.* 1988;10:286-297.
6. Combe C, Saunders W. A singular case of stricture and thickening of the ileum. *Medical Transactions of the Royal College of Physicians London.* 1813;4:16-21.
7. Abercombie J. *Pathological and Practical Researches on Disease of the Stomach, the Intestinal Tract and Other Viscera of the Abdomen.* Waugh and Innes; 1828.
8. Crohn BB, Ginzburg L, Oppenheimer GD. Regional ileitis: a pathologic and clinical entity. 1932. *Mt Sinai J Med.* 2000;67:263-268.
9. Braun H. Uber entzundliche geschwulste es netzes. *Arch Klin Chir.* 1901;63:378-381.
10. Koch J. Ueber einfach entzundliche stricturen des dickdarms. *Arch Klin Chir.* 1903;70:876-896.
11. Lesniowski A. Przyczynek do chirurgii kiszek. *Medycyna.* 1903; 31:460-518.
12. Wilmanns R. Ein fall von darmstenose infolge cronisch etzundlicher vrdickung der ieocacal kappe. *Beit z Klin Chir.* 1905;46:221-232.
13. Moynihan B. The mimickry of malignant disease in the large bowel. *Edinburgh Med J.* 1907;21:203-228.
14. Proust R. Tumeur paraintestinale. *Bull Mem Soc Chir Paris.* 1907; 33:1158-1160.

15. Monsarrat K. A clinical lecture on the stimulation of malignant disease by chronic inflammatory affections of the sigmoid flexure. *Br Med J (Clin Res)*. 1907;2:65-67.

16. Lejars F. Des tumeurs inflammatories paraintestinal. *Bull Mem Soc Chir Paris*. 1908;34:9-11.

17. von Bergmann A. Tumorbildung bei appendicitis und ihre radikale behandlung. *St. Petersburger Med Wochschr*. 1911;36:512-523.

18. Dalziel T. Chronic intestinal enteritis. *Br Med J (Clin Res)*. 1913;2:1068-1070.

19. Moschowitz E, Wilensky A. Non-specific granulomata of the intestine. *Am J Med Sci*. 1923;166:48-66.

20. Kirsner JB. Crohn's disease. In: Kirsner JB, ed. *Origins and Directions of Inflammatory Bowel Disease. Early Studies of the "Nonspecific" Inflammatory Bowel Diseases*. London: Kluwer Academic Publishers; 2001:55-101.

21. Van Kruiningen HJ. Lack of support for a common etiology in Johne's disease of animals and Crohn's disease in humans. *Inflamm Bowel Dis*. 1999;5:183-191.

22. Moschowitz E, Wilensky A. Non-specific granulomata of the intestine. *Am J Med Sci*. 1927;173:374-380.

23. Ginzburg L. Regional enteritis: historical perspective (B. Crohn and L. Ginzburg). *Gastroenterology*. 1986;90:1310-1311.

24. Ginzburg L, Oppenheimer GD. Non-specific granulomata of the intestine (inflammatory tumors and strictures of bowel). 1932. *Mt Sinai J Med*. 2000;67:246-262.

25. Ginzburg L, Oppenheimer GD. Non-specific granulomata of the intestines: inflammatory tumors and strictures of the bowel. *Ann Surg*. 1933;98:1046-1062.

26. Program of the Section on Gastroenterology and Proctology of the American Medical Association, Friday, May 3, 1932. *J Am Med Assoc*. 1932;98:1297.

27. Harris F, Bell G, Brunn H. Chronic cicatrizing enteritis: regional ileitis (Crohn): a new surgical entity. *Surg Gynecol Obstet*. 1933;57:637-645.

28. Cushway B. Chronic cicatrizing enteritis-regional ileitis (Crohn). *Illinois Med J*. 1934:525-533.

29. Hodgson J. Regional ileitis—Crohn's disease. *Lancet*. 1937;1:926-927.

30. Barrington-Ward L, Norrish R. Crohn's disease or regional ileitis. *Br J Surg*. 1938;25:530-537.

31. Armitage G, Wilson M. Crohn's disease: a survey of the literature and a report on 34 cases. *Br J Surg*. 1950;38:182-193.

32. Lichtarowicz AM, Mayberry JF. Antoni Lesniowski and his contribution to regional enteritis (Crohn's disease). *J R Soc Med*. 1988;81:468-470.

33. Harmer M. Crohn's disease: a misnomer? *Bristol Med Chir J*. 1988;103:9-10.

34. Goldstein H. The history of regional enteritis (Saunders-Abercrombie-Crohn ileitis). In: Kagan S, ed. *Victor Robinson Memorial Essays on History of Medicine*. New York: Froben Press; 1948:99-104.

35. Ginzburg L, Beller AJ. The clinical manifestations of non-metallic perforating intestinal foreign bodies. *Ann Surg*. 1927;86:928-939.

36. Ginzburg L, Klein E. Late intestinal stenosis following strangulated hernia. *Ann Surg*. 1928;88:204-211.

37. Colp R. A case of nonspecific granuloma of the terminal ileum and the cecum. *Surg Clin N Am*. 1934;14:443-449.

38. Penner A, Crohn BB. Perianal fistulae as a complication of regional ileitis. *Ann Surg*. 1938;108:867-873.

39. Ginzburg L, Colp R, Sussman M. Ileocolostomy with exclusion. *Ann Surg*. 1939;110:648-658.

40. Garlock JH, Crohn BB. An appraisal of the results of surgery in the treatment of regional ileitis. *J Am Med Assoc*. 1945;127:205-208.

41. Garlock JH, Crohn BB, Klein SH, Yarnis H. An appraisal of the long-term results of surgical treatment of regional ileitis. *Gastroenterology*. 1951;19:414-423.

42. Wells C. Ulcerative colitis and Crohn's disease. *Ann R Coll Surg Engl*. 1952;11:105-120.

43. Wolf BS, Marshak RH. Granulomatous colitis (Crohn's disease of the colon). Roentgen features. *Am J Roentgenol Radium Ther Nucl Med*. 1962;88:662-670.

44. Rutgeerts P, Onette E, Vantrappen G, Geboes K, Broeckaert L, Talloen L. Crohn's disease of the stomach and duodenum: a clinical study with emphasis on the value of endoscopy and endoscopic biopsies. *Endoscopy*. 1980;12:288-294.

45. Post AB, van Stolk R, Broughan TA, Tuthill RJ. Crohn's disease of the gallbladder. *J Clin Gastroenterol*. 1993;16:139-142.

46. Gschwantler M, Kogelbauer G, Klose W, Bibus B, Tscholakoff D, Weiss W. The pancreas as a site of granulomatous inflammation in Crohn's disease. *Gastroenterology*. 1995;108:1246-1249.

47. Reynaert H, Peters O, Van der Auwera J, Vanstapel MJ, Urbain D. Jaundice caused by a pancreatic mass: an exceptional presentation of Crohn's disease. *J Clin Gastroenterol*. 2001;32:255-258.

48. Sircus W, Church R, Kelleher J. Recurrent aphthous ulceration of the mouth; a study of the natural history, aetiology, and treatment. *Q J Med*. 1957;26:235-239.

49. McCallum DI, Gray WM. Metastatic Crohn's disease. *Br J Dermatol*. 1976;95:551-554.

50. Tweedie JH, McCann BG. Metastatic Crohn's disease of thigh and forearm. *Gut*. 1984;25:213-214.

51. Phillips SS, Baird DB, Joshi VV, Rosenberg AJ, Janosko EO. Crohn's disease of the prepuce in a 12-year-old boy: a case report and review of the literature. *Pediatr Pathol Lab Med*. 1997;17:497-502.

52. Veloso FT, Cardoso V, Fraga J, Carvalho J, Dias LM. Spontaneous umbilical fistula in Crohn's disease. *J Clin Gastroenterol*. 1989;11:197-200.

53. Davidson ED. Crohn's disease with spontaneous cutaneous-urachovesicoenteric fistula. *Dig Dis Sci*. 1980;25:460-463.

54. Nugent FW, Glaser D, Fernandez-Herlihy L. Crohn's colitis associated with granulomatous bone disease. *N Engl J Med*. 1976;294:262-263.

55. Menard DB, Haddad H, Blain JG, Beaudry R, Devroede G, Masse S. Granulomatous myositis and myopathy associated with Crohn's colitis. *N Engl J Med*. 1976;295:818-819.

56. Puntis JW, Tarlow MJ, Raafat F, Booth IW. Crohn's disease of the lung. *Arch Dis Child*. 1990;65:1270-1271.

57. Shah SM, Texter EC Jr, White HJ. Inflammatory bowel disease associated with granulomatous lung disease: report of a case with endoscopic findings. *Gastrointest Endosc*. 1976;23:98-99.

58. Hugot JP, Laurent-Puig P, Gower-Rousseau C, et al. Mapping of a susceptibility locus for Crohn's disease on chromosome 16. *Nature*. 1996;379:821-823.

59. Hugot JP, Chamaillard M, Zouali H, et al. Association of NOD2 leucine-rich repeat variants with susceptibility to Crohn's disease. *Nature*. 2001;411:599-603.

60. Ogura Y, Bonen DK, Inohara N, et al. A frameshift mutation in NOD2 associated with susceptibility to Crohn's disease. *Nature*. 2001;411:603-606.

61. Ogura Y, Inohara N, Benito A, Chen FF, Yamaoka S, Nunez G. Nod2, a Nod1/Apaf-1 family member that is restricted to monocytes and activates NF-kappaB. *J Biol Chem*. 2001;276:4812-4818.

62. Kirsner JB. The early treatment of inflammatory bowel disease. In: Kirsner JB, ed. *Origins and Directions of Inflammatory Bowel Disease: Early Studies of the "Nonspecific" Inflammatory Bowel Diseases*. London: Kluwer Academic Publishers; 2001:207-225.

63. Crohn's disease—40 years on. *Br Med J*. 1978;2:1106-1107.

64. Alexander-Williams J, Fielding JF, Cooke WT. A comparison of results of excision and bypass for ileal Crohn's disease. *Gut.* 1972;13:973-975.

65. Homan WP, Dineen P. Comparison of the results of resection, bypass, and bypass with exclusion for ileocecal Crohn's disease. *Ann Surg.* 1978;187:530-535.

66. Stanley MM, Rosenberg IN, Cleroux AP. The use of corticotropin (ACTH) in the treatment of chronic regional enteritis. *Med Clin North Am.* 1951;35:1255-1265.

67. Gray SJ, Reifenstein RW, Benson JA Jr, Young JC. Treatment of ulcerative colitis and regional enteritis with ACTH; significance of fecal lysozyme. *AMA Arch Intern Med.* 1951;87:646-662.

68. Kirsner JB, Palmer WL, Klotz AP. ACTH in severe chronic regional enteritis: observations in four patients. *Gastroenterology.* 1952;20:229-233.

69. Sparberg M, Kirsner JB. Long-term corticosteroid therapy for regional enteritis: an analysis of 58 courses in 54 patients. *Am J Dig Dis.* 1966;11:865-880.

70. Jones JH, Lennard-Jones JE. Corticosteroids and corticotrophin in the treatment of Crohn's disease. *Gut.* 1966;7:181-187.

71. Munkholm P, Langholz E, Davidsen M, Binder V. Frequency of glucocorticoid resistance and dependency in Crohn's disease. *Gut.* 1994;35:360-362.

72. Rutgeerts P, Lofberg R, Malchow H, et al. A comparison of budesonide with prednisolone for active Crohn's disease. *N Engl J Med.* 1994;331:842-845.

73. Bar-Meir S, Chowers Y, Lavy A, et al. Budesonide versus prednisone in the treatment of active Crohn's disease. The Israeli Budesonide Study Group. *Gastroenterology.* 1998;115:835-840.

74. Greenberg GR, Feagan BG, Martin F, et al. Oral budesonide for active Crohn's disease. Canadian Inflammatory Bowel Disease Study Group. *N Engl J Med.* 1994;331:836-841.

75. Greenberg GR, Feagan BG, Martin F, et al. Oral budesonide as maintenance treatment for Crohn's disease: a placebo-controlled, dose-ranging study. Canadian Inflammatory Bowel Disease Study Group. *Gastroenterology.* 1996;110:45-51.

76. Summers RW, Switz DM, Sessions JT Jr, et al. National Cooperative Crohn's Disease Study: results of drug treatment. *Gastroenterology.* 1979;77:847-869.

77. Malchow H, Ewe K, Brandes JW, et al. European Cooperative Crohn's Disease Study (ECCDS): results of drug treatment. *Gastroenterology.* 1984;86:249-266.

78. Singleton JW, Hanauer SB, Gitnick GL, et al. Mesalamine capsules for the treatment of active Crohn's disease: results of a 16-week trial. Pentasa Crohn's Disease Study Group. *Gastroenterology.* 1993;104:1293-1301.

79. Paulley JW. Crohn's disease: treatment by corticosteroids, antibiotics and psychotherapy. *Psychother Psychosom.* 1971;19:111-117.

80. Ambrose NS, Allan RN, Keighley MR, et al. Antibiotic therapy for treatment in relapse of intestinal Crohn's disease: a prospective randomized study. *Dis Colon Rectum.* 1985;28:81-85.

81. Sutherland L, Singleton J, Sessions J, et al. Double blind, placebo controlled trial of metronidazole in Crohn's disease. *Gut.* 1991;32:1071-1075.

82. Prantera C, Zannoni F, Scribano ML, et al. An antibiotic regimen for the treatment of active Crohn's disease: a randomized, controlled clinical trial of metronidazole plus ciprofloxacin. *Am J Gastroenterol.* 1996;91:328-332.

83. Colombel JF, Lemann M, Cassagnou M, et al. A controlled trial comparing ciprofloxacin with mesalazine for the treatment of active Crohn's disease. Groupe d'Etudes Therapeutiques des Affections Inflammatoires Digestives (GETAID). *Am J Gastroenterol.* 1999;94:674-678.

84. Arnold GL, Beaves MR, Pryjdun VO, Mook WJ. Preliminary study of ciprofloxacin in active Crohn's disease. *Inflamm Bowel Dis.* 2002;8:10-15.

85. Steinhart AH, Feagan BG, Wong CJ, et al. Combined budesonide and antibiotic therapy for active Crohn's disease: a randomized controlled trial. *Gastroenterology.* 2002;123:33-40.

86. Castiglione F, Rispo A, Di Girolamo E, et al. Antibiotic treatment of small bowel bacterial overgrowth in patients with Crohn's disease. *Aliment Pharmacol Ther.* 2003;18:1107-1112.

87. Brooke BN, Javett SL, Davison OW. Further experience with azathioprine for Crohn's disease. *Lancet.* 1970;2:1050-1053.

88. Rhodes J, Bainton D, Beck P. Azathioprine in Crohn's disease. *Lancet.* 1970;2:1142.

89. Rhodes J, Bainton D, Beck P, Campbell H. Controlled trial of azathioprine in Crohn's disease. *Lancet.* 1971;2:1273-1276.

90. Rosenberg JL, Levin B, Wall AJ, Kirsner JB. A controlled trial of azathioprine in Crohn's disease. *Am J Dig Dis.* 1975;20:721-726.

91. Kozarek RA, Patterson DJ, Gelfand MD, Botoman VA, Ball TJ, Wilske KR. Methotrexate induces clinical and histologic remission in patients with refractory inflammatory bowel disease. *Ann Intern Med.* 1989;110:353-356.

92. Feagan BG, Rochon J, Fedorak RN, et al. Methotrexate for the treatment of Crohn's disease. The North American Crohn's Study Group Investigators. *N Engl J Med.* 1995;332:292-297.

93. Feagan BG, Fedorak RN, Irvine EJ, et al. A comparison of methotrexate with placebo for the maintenance of remission in Crohn's disease. North American Crohn's Study Group Investigators. *N Engl J Med.* 2000;342:1627-1632.

94. Brynskov J, Freund L, Norby Rasmussen S, et al. Final report on a placebo-controlled, double-blind, randomized, multicentre trial of cyclosporin treatment in active chronic Crohn's disease. *Scand J Gastroenterol.* 1991;26:689-695.

95. Nicholls S, Domizio P, Williams CB, et al. Cyclosporin as initial treatment for Crohn's disease. *Arch Dis Child.* 1994;71:243-247.

96. Stange EF, Modigliani R, Pena AS, Wood AJ, Feutren G, Smith PR. European trial of cyclosporine in chronic active Crohn's disease: a 12-month study. The European Study Group. *Gastroenterology.* 1995;109:774-782.

97. van Dullemen HM, van Deventer SJ, Hommes DW, et al. Treatment of Crohn's disease with anti-tumor necrosis factor chimeric monoclonal antibody (cA2). *Gastroenterology.* 1995;109:129-135.

98. Targan SR, Hanauer SB, van Deventer SJ, et al. A short-term study of chimeric monoclonal antibody cA2 to tumor necrosis factor alpha for Crohn's disease. Crohn's Disease cA2 Study Group. *N Engl J Med.* 1997;337:1029-1035.

99. Present DH, Rutgeerts P, Targan S, et al. Infliximab for the treatment of fistulas in patients with Crohn's disease. *N Engl J Med.* 1999;340:1398-1405.

100. Hanauer SB, Feagan BG, Lichtenstein GR, et al. Maintenance infliximab for Crohn's disease: the ACCENT I randomised trial. *Lancet.* 2002;359:1541-1549.

101. Sands BE, Anderson FH, Bernstein CN, et al. Infliximab maintenance therapy for fistulizing Crohn's disease. *N Engl J Med.* 2004;350:876-885.

102. Colombel JF, Sandborn WJ, Rutgeerts P, et al. Adalimumab for maintenance of clinical response and remission in patients with Crohn's disease: the CHARM trial. *Gastroenterology.* 2007;132:52-65.

103. Schreiber S, Rutgeerts P, Fedorak RN, et al. A randomized, placebo-controlled trial of certolizumab pegol (CDP870) for treatment of Crohn's disease. *Gastroenterology.* 2005;129:807-818.

104. Gordon FH, Lai CW, Hamilton MI, et al. A randomized placebo-controlled trial of a humanized monoclonal antibody to alpha4 integrin in active Crohn's disease. *Gastroenterology.* 2001;121:268-274.

105. Ghosh S, Goldin E, Gordon FH, et al. Natalizumab for active Crohn's disease. *N Engl J Med*. 2003;348:24-32.

106. Sandborn WJ, Colombel JF, Enns R, et al. Natalizumab induction and maintenance therapy for Crohn's disease. *N Engl J Med*. 2005;353:1912-1925.

107. Targan SR, Feagan BG, Fedorak RN, et al. Natalizumab for the treatment of active Crohn's disease: results of the ENCORE Trial. *Gastroenterology*. 2007;132:1672-1683.

108. Adelman B, Sandrock A, Panzara MA. Natalizumab and progressive multifocal leukoencephalopathy. *N Engl J Med*. 2005;353:432-433.

109. Sandborn WJ, Hanauer SB, Katz S, et al. Etanercept for active Crohn's disease: a randomized, double-blind, placebo-controlled trial. *Gastroenterology*. 2001;121:1088-1094.

110. Hommes D, van den Blink B, Plasse T, et al. Inhibition of stress-activated MAP kinases induces clinical improvement in moderate to severe Crohn's disease. *Gastroenterology*. 2002;122:7-14.

111. Rutgeerts P, Sandborn WJ, Fedorak RN, et al. Onercept for moderate-to-severe Crohn's disease: a randomized, double-blind, placebo-controlled trial. *Clin Gastroenterol Hepatol*. 2006;4:888-893.

112. Sandborn WJ, Feagan BG, Fedorak RN, et al. A randomized trial of ustekinumab, a human interleukin-12/23 monoclonal antibody, in patients with moderate-to-severe Crohn's disease. *Gastroenterology*. 2008;135:1130-1141.

113. Schreiber S, Nikolaus S, Malchow H, et al. Absence of efficacy of subcutaneous antisense ICAM-1 treatment of chronic active Crohn's disease. *Gastroenterology*. 2001;120:1339-1346.

114. Yacyshyn BR, Barish C, Goff J, et al. Dose ranging pharmacokinetic trial of high-dose alicaforsen (intercellular adhesion molecule-1 antisense oligodeoxynucleotide) (ISIS 2302) in active Crohn's disease. *Aliment Pharmacol Ther*. 2002;16:1761-1770.

115. Yacyshyn BR, Bowen-Yacyshyn MB, Jewell L, et al. A placebo-controlled trial of ICAM-1 antisense oligonucleotide in the treatment of Crohn's disease. *Gastroenterology*. 1998;114:1133-1142.

116. Yacyshyn BR, Chey WY, Goff J, et al. Double blind, placebo controlled trial of the remission inducing and steroid sparing properties of an ICAM-1 antisense oligodeoxynucleotide, alicaforsen (ISIS 2302), in active steroid dependent Crohn's disease. *Gut*. 2002;51:30-36.

117. Yacyshyn B, Chey WY, Wedel MK, Yu RZ, Paul D, Chuang E. A randomized, double-masked, placebo-controlled study of alicaforsen, an antisense inhibitor of intercellular adhesion molecule 1, for the treatment of subjects with active Crohn's disease. *Clin Gastroenterol Hepatol*. 2007;5:215-220.

118. Kasran A, Boon L, Wortel CH, et al. Safety and tolerability of antagonist anti-human CD40 Mab ch5D12 in patients with moderate to severe Crohn's disease. *Aliment Pharmacol Ther*. 2005;22:111-122.

119. van Deventer SJ, Elson CO, Fedorak RN. Multiple doses of intravenous interleukin 10 in steroid-refractory Crohn's disease. Crohn's Disease Study Group. *Gastroenterology*. 1997;113:383-389.

120. Schreiber S, Fedorak RN, Nielsen OH, et al. Safety and efficacy of recombinant human interleukin 10 in chronic active Crohn's disease. Crohn's Disease IL-10 Cooperative Study Group. *Gastroenterology*. 2000;119:1461-1472.

121. Fedorak RN, Gangl A, Elson CO, et al. Recombinant human interleukin 10 in the treatment of patients with mild to moderately active Crohn's disease. The Interleukin 10 Inflammatory Bowel Disease Cooperative Study Group. *Gastroenterology*. 2000;119:1473-1482.

122. Colombel JF, Rutgeerts P, Malchow H, et al. Interleukin 10 (Tenovil) in the prevention of postoperative recurrence of Crohn's disease. *Gut*. 2001;49:42-46.

123. Sands BE, Bank S, Sninsky CA, et al. Preliminary evaluation of safety and activity of recombinant human interleukin 11 in patients with active Crohn's disease. *Gastroenterology*. 1999;117:58-64.

124. Sands BE, Winston BD, Salzberg B, et al. Randomized, controlled trial of recombinant human interleukin-11 in patients with active Crohn's disease. *Aliment Pharmacol Ther*. 2002;16:399-406.

125. Mannon PJ, Fuss IJ, Mayer L, et al. Anti-interleukin-12 antibody for active Crohn's disease. *N Engl J Med*. 2004;351:2069-2079.

126. Reinisch W, Hommes DW, Van Assche G, et al. A dose escalating, placebo controlled, double blind, single dose and multidose, safety and tolerability study of fontolizumab, a humanised anti-interferon gamma antibody, in patients with moderate to severe Crohn's disease. *Gut*. 2006;55:1138-1144.

127. Slonim AE, Bulone L, Damore MB, Goldberg T, Wingertzahn MA, McKinley MJ. A preliminary study of growth hormone therapy for Crohn's disease. *N Engl J Med*. 2000;342:1633-1637.

128. Gasche C, Reinisch W, Vogelsang H, et al. Prospective evaluation of interferon-alpha in treatment of chronic active Crohn's disease. *Dig Dis Sci*. 1995;40:800-804.

129. Dieckgraefe BK, Korzenik JR. Treatment of active Crohn's disease with recombinant human granulocyte-macrophage colony-stimulating factor. *Lancet*. 2002;360:1478-1480.

130. Korzenik JR, Dieckgraefe BK. An open-labeled study of granulocyte colony-stimulating factor in the treatment of active Crohn's disease. *Aliment Pharmacol Ther*. 2005;21:391-400.

131. Korzenik JR, Dieckgraefe BK, Valentine JF, Hausman DF, Gilbert MJ. Sargramostim for active Crohn's disease. *N Engl J Med*. 2005;352:2193-2201.

132. Ito H, Takazoe M, Fukuda Y, et al. A pilot randomized trial of a human anti-interleukin-6 receptor monoclonal antibody in active Crohn's disease. *Gastroenterology*. 2004;126:989-996; discussion 947.

133. Heaton LD, Ravdin IS, Blades B, Whelan TJ. President Eisenhower's operation for regional enteritis: a footnote to history. *Ann Surg*. 1964;159:661-666.

134. Hughes CW, Baugh JH, Mologne LA, Heaton LD. A review of the late General Eisenhower's operations: epilog to a footnote to history. *Ann Surg*. 1971;173:793-799.

135. Marston A. Did President Eisenhower have Crohn's disease? *J Med Biogr*. 2002;10:237-239.

136. Karmody CS, Bachor ES. The deafness of Ludwig van Beethoven: an immunopathy. *Otol Neurotol*. 2005;26:809-814.

137. Orrego F, Quintana C. Darwin's illness: a final diagnosis. *Notes Rec R Soc Lond*. 2007;61:23-29.

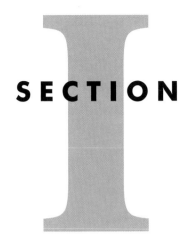

SECTION

I

GENERAL

THE NATURAL HISTORY OF INFLAMMATORY BOWEL DISEASE

Pietro G. Andres, MD and Lawrence S. Friedman, MD

Inflammatory bowel disease (IBD) encompasses at least two forms of idiopathic intestinal inflammation: ulcerative colitis (UC) and Crohn's disease (CD). The latter is also called *regional enteritis, regional ileitis, Crohn's ileitis,* and *granulomatous colitis.* Although other inflammatory disorders affect the gastrointestinal tract, they can be distinguished from IBD by the presence of a specific underlying agent or by the character and manifestations of the inflammatory activity. In contrast, the causes of IBD are unknown.

UC and CD are at least partially distinct in their initial pathogenic events, but they may have key pathophysiologic processes in common. Moreover, UC and CD each may encompass several variants, which are at least partially distinct. For example, patients with CD may manifest different complications (fistulas or stenoses) and may express different inflammatory mediators, perhaps due to underlying genetic differences or environmental exposures between the two groups. Thus, patient subgroups defined by disease location, specific pathologic findings (the presence or absence of granulomas in patients with CD), or disease complications may reflect a multiplicity of diseases with some shared features. In the absence of identifiable causative agents, UC and CD are defined by their typical clinical, pathologic, endoscopic, and laboratory features. In some patients, it is impossible to distinguish with confidence UC from CD affecting the colon using any of the conventional diagnostic criteria. Such cases are labeled *indeterminate colitis.*

Study of the natural history of UC and CD is challenging, in part because of the intrinsic nature of the disorders.[1,2] The clinical presentation of IBD may be insidious, and the time interval between the initial etiologic event and diagnosis of the disease may be quite long, thereby making it difficult to identify and study the inciting events. Because IBD is relatively uncommon, it is also difficult to find a population of adequate size from which deductions about natural history can be drawn.[2] Moreover, many affected persons may be asymptomatic or have only mild symptoms and may either not seek medical attention or escape detection.[3]

Performance of natural history studies of IBD that are similar and easily compared has been hampered by the lack of universally adopted diagnostic criteria for these disorders. Published diagnostic criteria[4-6] have been difficult to apply in many studies, because the criteria include endoscopic and radiologic techniques that require skill and expertise and that are not easily performed on a large scale. To compensate, investigators have often selected patients from specialized medical centers, a practice associated with a risk of bias toward more severely ill patients.[1] The problems created by a lack of universally adopted diagnostic criteria are further compounded by a high rate of misdiagnosis in patients with inflammatory colitis. Not only are infectious processes often difficult to differentiate from idiopathic IBD, but (as noted previously) in up to 10% of patients it may also be impossible to distinguish UC from CD at the time of initial presentation.[7]

Lichtenstein GR, ed.
Crohn's Disease: The Complete Guide to Medical Management (pp 11-24).
© 2011 SLACK Incorporated

ULCERATIVE COLITIS

EXTENT AND SEVERITY OF DISEASE

At the time of diagnosis, a majority of patients with UC have disease limited to the rectum, rectosigmoid, or left colon (ie, from the rectum to the splenic flexure). Assessing the precise frequencies of the extent of colonic involvement is difficult to determine from the literature, because different investigators have not used the same definitions of disease extent consistently. Various studies have found that 14% to 36.7% of patients have pancolitis, 36% to 41% have disease extending beyond the rectum (but not to the cecum), and 44% to 49% have proctitis (defined as mucosal changes in the rectum on sigmoidoscopy with a normal colonic appearance) in more proximal segments as determined by barium enema (BE).[8-11] Because the extent of disease in these studies was determined by flexible sigmoidoscopy and BE, rather than colonoscopy, the extent of involvement was probably underestimated.

In general, the clinical severity of disease at presentation correlates with the extent of colonic involvement. Patients with pancolitis tend to have more severe clinical symptoms than do those with disease limited to the rectum. In a population-based study from Copenhagen, Langholz et al found that of all patients diagnosed with UC between 1962 and 1987, 20.2% experienced mild symptoms (defined as less than 4 stools per day, no systemic disturbances, and a normal erythrocyte sedimentation rate [ESR]); 70.7% had moderate disease (defined as more than 4 stools per day but minimal systemic effects); and 9.1% had severe disease (defined as 6 or more bowel movements per day with bloody stools, fever, tachycardia, anemia, or an ESR > 30 mm/hr).[12]

DISEASE COURSE

Most patients with UC experience a chronic, intermittent clinical course. Less commonly, patients have either continuous, unrelenting symptoms or a single episode of colitis. Among 1161 patients with UC from Copenhagen who did not require colectomy and were followed for up to 25 years by Langholz et al, the cumulative probability of a relapsing course (defined as "clinical remission longer than 1 month without corticosteroid or immunosuppressive therapy within 1 year or years without disease activity in between years with disease activity") was 90%.[9] The probability of a completely relapse-free course was 10.6% at 25 years, whereas that of a continuously active course was only 0.1%. By using a Markov chain analysis, the authors calculated that the probability that a patient with clinically inactive disease would remain in remission the following year was 80% to 90%, whereas the risk of relapse in the following year was only 10% to 20%. By contrast, those patients with clinically active disease had a 70% probability

of having a relapse during the following year. Overall, as the number of years in which a patient had active disease increased, so did the probability of relapse during the following year. However, the probability of having active disease every year after a relapse fell from 50% at 2 years to 10% to 15% at 10 years.

In this study,[9] the clinical course over the 25-year follow-up was not influenced by the age or sex of the patient, anatomic extent of disease at the time of diagnosis, presenting symptoms, length of time between onset of symptoms and diagnosis, initial treatment, use of systemic corticosteroids, or occurrence of extraintestinal manifestations. Only three factors influenced the course of the disease in these patients. First, the number of years in relapse since diagnosis correlated directly with the subsequent chance of disease flares. Second, the occurrence of systemic symptoms (fever and weight loss) at diagnosis correlated inversely with subsequent disease activity. (That is, patients presenting initially with severe disease that subsequently responded to medical therapy, and thus did not require surgery, had a high probability of a subsequent long-term remission.) Lastly, development of disease later in the study period correlated with a greater chance of a prolonged remission, an indication that medical management had improved over the 25 years of the study.[9]

When patients who require colectomy are included in the analysis of disease course, investigators have found that, at least in the short term, the extent of colonic involvement at the time of diagnosis influences both the frequency of subsequent anatomic extension and the clinical severity of the disease.[13,14] For example, patients with proctitis are unlikely to develop extension past the splenic flexure. In two case-control studies by Meucci et al[13] and Powell-Tuck et al,[14] 60% to 70% of patients who presented with proctitis continued to have disease limited to the rectosigmoid colon after 20 years. Moreover, the majority of patients who developed more extensive disease did so within the first 5 years. The overall prognosis of patients diagnosed with proctitis is good, with only 4% to 5% requiring surgery for their disease within 20 years of diagnosis.[14]

By contrast, Langholz et al found that patients with proctosigmoiditis had a greater than 50% chance of developing more extensive disease and a 12% frequency of colectomy within 25 years of diagnosis. Similarly, these investigators observed that patients with radiological evidence of colitis proximal to the rectum had a 9% chance of progression to pancolitis and a 23% frequency of colectomy. As one would expect, the probability of colectomy was highest in patients with pancolitis (40%)[8] (Figure 1-1). Hendriksen et al also found that one third of patients with pancolitis required colectomy within the first year of diagnosis, compared with less than 8% of those with more limited disease.[10]

Patients with total colonic involvement are more likely to experience complications of UC than are patients with more limited disease. In a cohort study of 1116 patients

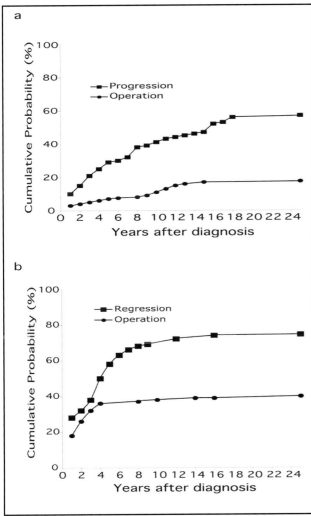

FIGURE 1-1. (A) Cumulative probability of progression and colectomy in patients with ulcerative colitis (UC) who present with proctosigmoiditis. (B) Cumulative probability of regression and colectomy in patients with UC who present with pancolitis. (Reprinted with permission from Langholz E, Munkholm P, Davidsen M, Nielsen OH, Binder V. Changes in extent of ulcerative colitis: a study on the course and prognostic factors. *Scand J Gastroenterol.* 1996;31:260-266.)

diagnosed with UC at the Cleveland Clinic Foundation between 1960 and 1983, Farmer et al found that in patients with pancolitis, toxic dilatation developed in 21%, bleeding developed in 25%, and surgery was required in 60%.[11] By contrast, in patients with proctitis, the frequency of toxic dilatation and bleeding was 3% and 9.5%, respectively, and only 14% required surgery. However, once the first year after diagnosis had passed, the clinical course of the disease became similar for all patients regardless of initial extent at the time of presentation. Thus, after the first year, the annual colectomy rate was 1% for all patients.[11]

COMPLICATIONS

ACUTE LOCAL COMPLICATIONS

As discussed above, the frequency of acute colonic complications of UC is generally related to the anatomic extent and clinical severity of the disease. Massive hemorrhage occurs in up to 3.5% of patients and may be an indication for colectomy if bleeding persists despite blood transfusions and immunosuppressive therapy. Acute colonic dilatation can occur in up to 5% of patients with severe attacks of UC. One half of these patients may respond to medical therapy alone, whereas those who fail to respond to therapy or show signs of deterioration require colectomy.[15] Colonic perforation is the most dangerous local complication and is an indication for urgent colectomy. Greenstein and Aufses reported a mortality rate of 16% in UC patients with colonic perforation,[16] a finding that underscores the need for aggressive medical and surgical management in these patients.

EXTRAINTESTINAL COMPLICATIONS

Many extraintestinal manifestations are associated with UC (Table 1-1). The most common is an acute arthropathy, which can affect up to 20% of patients[17] and can present as either a large joint pauciarticular arthritis or as a small joint symmetrical polyarthropathy reminiscent of rheumatoid arthritis. Orchard et al found pauciarticular arthritis in 3.6% of patients with UC and observed that the clinical flares of arthritis generally paralleled the activity of the bowel disease. By contrast, the vast majority of the 2.5% of UC patients with small joint polyarthropathy experienced persistent articular symptoms independent of the clinical activity of colitis.[18]

Sacroiliitis and ankylosing spondylitis are less common than peripheral arthropathy, with frequencies of 11% to 15% and 1% to 2% of UC patients, respectively. The frequency is higher if asymptomatic patients with radiologic evidence of axial arthropathy are included in the analysis. For example, 11% of patients with UC have evidence of sacroiliitis by plain radiography, but 70% have evidence of the disease by technetium bone scan.[17] The majority of patients with sacroiliitis are HLA-B27-negative and do not progress to ankylosing spondylitis. By contrast, 80% of UC patients with ankylosing spondylitis are HLA-B27-positive. The course of the spondylitis is independent of the activity of the bowel disease; in fact, spinal symptoms may develop prior to the onset of colitis.[15]

Ocular complications of UC include anterior uveitis and episcleritis and occur in 5% to 15% of patients with UC. The course of these complications tends to parallel that of the underlying bowel disease.[19]

TABLE 1-1

EXTRAINTESTINAL COMPLICATIONS OF INFLAMMATORY BOWEL DISEASE

COMPLICATION	ULCERATIVE COLITIS (%)	CROHN'S DISEASE (%)
Acute arthropathy	10 to 20	15 to 20
Sacroiliitis	9 to 11	9 to 11
Ankylosing spondylitis	1 to 3	3 to 5
Ocular complications	5 to 15	5 to 15
Erythema nodosum	10 to 15	15
Pyoderma gangrenosum	1 to 2	1 to 2
Primary sclerosing cholangitis	2 to 7.6	1
Choledocholithiasis	–	15 to 30 (patients with small bowel disease)
Nephrolithiasis	–	5 to 10
Amyloidosis	–	Rare

The most common dermatologic complication of UC is erythema nodosum, arising in up to 15% of UC patients, often in association with peripheral arthropathy or ankylosing spondylitis.[17,20] Both uveitis and erythema nodosum are associated with HLA-B27, -B58, and -DRB1*0103.[20] Other less common cutaneous manifestations of UC include pyoderma gangrenosum (1% to 2% of patients with UC) and Sweet's syndrome, or neutrophilic dermatosis (rare).[21] The activity of these dermatologic complications tends to parallel the activity of the bowel disease,[15] although pyoderma gangrenosum may persist despite resolution of colitis or even colectomy.

Hepatobiliary disease is common in patients with UC. Elevations of serum aminotransferase levels may be found in over 50% of patients with active colitis,[22] usually as a consequence of malnutrition, sepsis, fatty liver, or administration of total parenteral nutrition. The elevated enzyme levels usually return to normal with treatment of the underlying colitis. Primary sclerosing cholangitis (PSC) is a chronic hepatobiliary disease found in 2% to 7.6% of patients with UC. The converse association is stronger, with 70% of patients with PSC having IBD, usually UC. In most of these patients (60%), the diagnosis of IBD is made before that of PSC.[23] Persons with PSC are usually diagnosed in the fourth decade of life, although liver biochemical abnormalities may be noted up to 10 years earlier.[24-26] Two thirds of patients are men. The disease is progressive, eventually causing cirrhosis and liver failure. Five- and 10-year survival rates are 85% and 75%, respectively. The 5-year survival rate after liver transplantation for PSC has been reported to be 85%.[27-30] PSC is also associated with a risk of cholangiocarcinoma, with a frequency of 8% to 10% over 6 years, although the risk is much lower in patients with the intrahepatic small-duct variant of PSC.[31]

Several reports have linked UC with an increased risk of lymphoma[32]; however, a large population-based cohort study did not confirm this association.[33]

COLON CANCER

The association between UC and colon cancer is well established. The exact risk of colon cancer associated with UC has varied among epidemiologic studies, but most indicate that the risk is highest in patients with extensive colonic involvement and a duration of disease of more than 10 years.[15] Other risk factors for colon cancer include a family history of colon cancer and possibly young age at diagnosis of UC and presence of backwash ileitis.[34]

For unclear reasons, the risk of colon cancer in patients with UC has declined, and in some populations an elevated risk of colon cancer relative to the general population can no longer be demonstrated.[34] Possible reasons for the decline in incidence of colon cancer in this population are widespread use of surveillance colonoscopy and maintenance drug therapy.

Ekbom et al followed a cohort of 3117 patients with UC for up to 35 years and found that the incidence of colorectal cancer was 5.7 times the expected rate for an age-matched cohort.[35] The risk was proportional to the extent of colonic disease: patients with proctitis had a standardized incidence ratio of 1.7 (95% confidence interval [CI] 0.8-3.2), those with left-sided colitis had a ratio of 2.8 (95% CI 1.6-4.4), and those with pancolitis had a ratio of 14.8 (95% CI 11.4-18.9). The cumulative incidence of colorectal cancer was also found to depend on the age at diagnosis (Figure 1-2). Patients with pancolitis diagnosed after age 40 had a 20-year frequency of colon cancer of 16%, compared to 5% in those diagnosed before age 14. With longer follow-up,

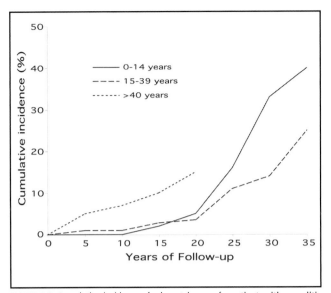

FIGURE 1-2. Cumulative incidence of colorectal cancer for patients with pancolitis according to age at diagnosis. (Reprinted with permission from Ekbom A, Helmick C, Zack M, Adami HO. Ulcerative colitis and colorectal cancer: a population-based study. *N Engl J Med.* 1990;323:1228-1233. Copyright © 1990 Massachusetts Medical Society. All rights reserved, used with permission.)

however, those with pancolitis diagnosed at a younger age were found to have a higher absolute risk of colon cancer than patients who were older at the time of diagnosis.[35] By contrast, Jess et al found that in Olmsted County, Minnesota, the risk of colon cancer was increased among patients with extensive UC but not among UC patients overall.[36] Although greater clinical severity and frequency of attacks of colitis do not seem to increase the risk of colorectal cancer,[37] there is a direct correlation with the severity of colonic inflammation.[38]

Overall, the annual incidence of colon cancer in patients with UC of more than 10 years duration may be as low as 1 in 500 to 1 in 1600.[34] The prognosis of colon cancer is poorer in patients with UC than in those without UC, despite a similar distribution of stages at diagnosis.[39]

It has been recognized that colonic malignancies in patients with IBD originate from mucosal dysplasia. Up to 19% of patients with low-grade dysplasia (LGD) have associated cancer found on examination of colectomy specimens.[40] Moreover, in patients who initially had a negative colonoscopy and were later diagnosed with LGD, 16% to 53% progressed to high-grade dysplasia (HGD), dysplasia-associated lesion or mass (DALM), or cancer.[40-42] However, because 50% of patients with LGD do not have dysplasia on follow-up surveillance,[43] optimal therapy for LGD remains controversial. Because HGD and DALM are associated with the presence of cancer in 32% to 53% of cases,[40,44] colectomy rather than continued surveillance is recommended for these lesions.

The risk of colorectal cancer appears to be especially high in patients with both UC and PSC. Several population

and cohort studies have estimated that these patients have a 3- to 10-fold increased risk for developing colonic neoplasia as compared to patients with UC alone.[45-48] The cancers in these patients tend to occur in the right colon, supporting the concept that secondary bile acids are carcinogenic and increase the likelihood of cancer in the proximal colon.[47] Further support for this hypothesis comes from data demonstrating that oral administration of ursodeoxycholic acid (UDCA), which decreases fecal levels of deoxycholic acid,[49,50] significantly reduces the risk of colonic neoplasia (risk ratio # [RR] = 0.26; CI 0.07 to 0.99).[51]

Retrospective matched case-control studies have generated optimism that mesalamine (5-aminosalicylic acid, 5-ASA) therapy may protect against the development of colonic neoplasia in patients with UC.[52-54] Using a conditional logistic regression analysis, Eaden et al found that regular use of these agents has a profound protective effect (up to a 91% risk reduction with mesalamine use).[52] Prospective trials designed to confirm this effect are ongoing.[55,56] A meta-analysis has suggested that use of mesalamine reduces the risk of colorectal carcinoma by 50%.[56] A case-control study suggested that the risk of colorectal carcinoma is higher in patients who have pseudopolyps and lower in those who take anti-inflammatory medications.[57]

MORTALITY

Mortality as a consequence of UC has decreased dramatically since the introduction of corticosteroids, and studies indicate that long-term survival rates for patients with UC do not differ from that of the general population.[6,19,58,59] Ekbom et al, however, found that the 10-year survival rate of patients with UC was slightly (but significantly) less than that of the general Swedish population. The slightly increased mortality rate in patients with UC was attributable to patients with extensive colonic involvement. The prognosis was slightly worse in patients with pancolitis than in those with left-sided colitis, with 10-year survival rates of 92.8% and 96.0%, respectively. Moreover, patients with ulcerative proctitis had a 10-year survival rate of 97.9%, which was not significantly lower than that of the control population.[60]

In a large, population-based cohort study, Persson et al found a similar pattern, with a standardized 15-year mortality ratio of 1.37 for patients with UC.[61] The increase in mortality may be most prominent in patients in whom colitis develops after age 60: Persson et al found the 15-year relative survival rate for this cohort was 24%; however, this rate was not significantly different from that of the general population.[61] Using a similar study design, Winther et al found a significantly increased mortality risk in men and women diagnosed with extensive ulcerative colitis after age 50 (Figure 1-3).[59] Jess et al found that in Olmsted County, Minnesota, overall survival in patients with UC was actually slightly greater than expected because of decreased mortality from cardiovascular disease.[62] Sonnenberg has

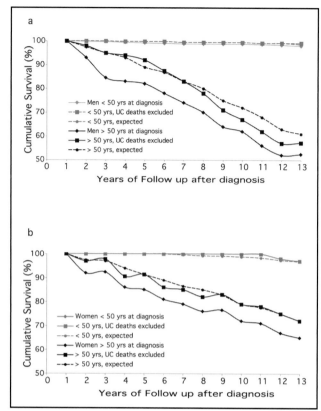

FIGURES 1-3. Cumulative survival (%) of (A) men and (B) women with extensive colitis at diagnosis and aged <50 years and >50 years at diagnosis, respectively. (Reprinted with permission from Winther KV, Jess T, Langholz E, Munkholm P, Binder V. Survival and cause-specific mortality in ulcerative colitis: follow-up of a population-based cohort in Copenhagen County. *Gastroenterology.* 2003;125:1576-1582.)

cautioned that data from cohort studies may underestimate the actual mortality risk from UC, which generally affects populations of higher socioeconomic strata, a subgroup characterized by low death rates for other diagnoses.[63]

As discussed earlier, the occurrence of acute, local complications of UC is associated with a significant increase in 1-year mortality rates in patients with newly diagnosed UC. In this group of patients, the mortality rate is 2.4- to 2.78-fold higher than that of age-matched controls.[59,64] The mortality rate for patients with complications in the setting of pancolitis is greater than that for patients with complications in the setting of less extensive disease.[59,60]

QUALITY OF LIFE

UC is a chronic disease with a significant lifelong impact on a patient's quality of life. Nevertheless, many studies have demonstrated that more than 90% of affected persons are fully capable of working effectively after successful treatment of an initial attack of UC.[9,10] Despite the tendency for intermittent disease activity, UC does not appear to affect the capacity of patients in the workplace

substantially. These data do not, however, provide information about the impact of UC on other aspects of a patient's lifestyle.

Several questionnaire-based tools designed to determine health-related quality of life (HRQOL) have been developed and applied to IBD.[65] The results suggest that patients with UC experience moderate impairment in social and emotional functioning and that these impairments are more severe than the cumulative physical obstacles patients endure. This impairment may be more pronounced in women than men.[66,67] The emotional concerns of patients with IBD were examined by Hjortswang et al, who found that patients with UC worried most frequently about the impact that an ostomy bag would have on their lives. Their other concerns (in order of decreasing frequency) were having surgery, cancer, losing bowel control, uncertainty about the course of the disease, and effects of medication.[68] The degree of a patient's concerns correlates inversely with his or her knowledge of the disease.[69] This observation underscores the important role of the physician in not only treating a patient's medical symptoms but also instructing the patient about the natural history of the disease to alleviate some of the associated emotional concerns.

CROHN'S DISEASE

EXTENT AND SEVERITY OF DISEASE

Unlike UC, CD can involve any or multiple segments of the gastrointestinal tract. Of 615 new patients diagnosed consecutively at the Cleveland Clinic, Farmer et al found that 40.9% had ileocolonic disease, 28.6% had disease limited to the small intestine, and 30.4% had disease involving only the colon or anorectal area.[70] Of patients with disease limited to the colon, only 25% have inflammation affecting the entire colon. In the remaining 75%, any area of the colon may be affected, with the distal colon affected most commonly. In the vast majority of patients with small intestinal disease, the terminal ileum is involved.[71]

Because of the variable nature of CD, the severity of disease does not correlate directly with the extent of bowel involvement. Instead, patients generally present with one of three patterns of disease: predominantly inflammatory, stricturing, or fistulizing. These disease patterns, rather than the extent of inflammation, determine the disease course and the nature of associated complications.

DISEASE COURSE

The clinical course of CD is often erratic. Years of frequent relapses may be followed by years of virtually complete remission. Munkolm et al followed 373 patients with CD in Copenhagen for a mean of 8.5 years and found that the number of patients with a relapse-free course decreased

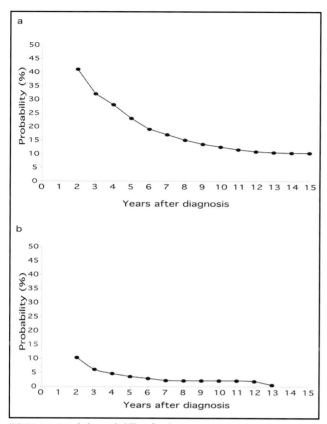

FIGURE 1-4. Cumulative probability of patients experiencing: (A) only one attack of Crohn's Disease (CD), and (B) a chronic persistent course of CD over a 15-year period. (Reprinted with permission from Munkholm P, Langholz E, Davidsen M, Binder V. Disease activity courses in a regional cohort of Crohn's disease patients. *Scand J Gastroenterol.* 1995;30:699-706.)

rapidly, from 42% at 2 years to 12% after 10 years.[72] The probability of a continuously active course was also low, declining from 10% at 2 years to 1% after 10 years (Figure 1-4). By Markov chain analysis, the investigators determined that a patient with clinically active disease has a 70% to 80% chance of having clinically active disease the following year. Similarly, 80% of patients in remission will remain so the following year. Over a 4-year period, 25% of patients had persistently active disease, 22% were in remission, and 53% had a course that fluctuated between years of remission and years with clinically active disease. The disease course was not affected by the patient's age, sex, time between onset of symptoms and diagnosis, anatomic location of disease, nature of the symptoms at the time of diagnosis, or initial mode of treatment (medical versus surgical).[72]

Although the clinical activity of CD is independent of the anatomic location and extent of the disease, the clinical manifestations and need for surgery are not. Several studies have shown that patients with small intestinal disease are more likely to have an obstructive disease pattern characterized by symptomatic fixed narrowing (fibrostenosis) of the bowel.[70,73,74] In contrast, those with colonic disease

are more likely to have symptoms resulting from inflammation, including bleeding.[73] In addition, 16% to 35% of all patients with CD develop fistulas or abscesses regardless of the anatomic location of the intestinal inflammation.[70,73,75] In one population-based study, 46% of patients with fistulizing disease developed a fistula before or at the time of diagnosis.[75]

The frequency of indications for surgery parallels the frequency of local intestinal complications of CD. Up to 74% of all patients will eventually require surgical intervention for their disease,[70,76] and more than 80% of patients with fistulizing disease will require an operation.[75] In one half of patients, surgery is required within 6 months of diagnosis.[76] Not surprisingly, surgery to relieve obstruction is required most often in patients with small bowel disease, whereas surgery for toxic dilatation and perineal disease is required most often in those with colonic disease (Table 1-2).[70] As observed by Polito et al, patients diagnosed before age 20 are at higher risk of small bowel disease than are patients diagnosed after age 20 and have an almost 2-fold relative risk of requiring surgery. Moreover, patients diagnosed before age 20 have a nearly 2-fold relative risk of requiring surgery for intractable disease. Because younger patients are more likely to have a positive family history of CD, Polito et al speculated that an inherited form of CD may exist that has a younger age of onset and is associated with a more severe course than later-onset CD.[73] An association between mutations in the NOD2/CARD15 gene and ileal and fibrostenotic disease is consistent with this observation.[77,78] An association between the TC haplotype of the organic cation transporter genes (OCTN1 and OCTN2) and nonfistulizing, nonfibrostenotic colonic disease has been suggested.[79]

One of the greatest challenges in managing patients with CD is the high frequency of recurrent disease following surgery. The anatomic distribution of recurrent disease correlates with the original pattern of disease: patients who undergo ileal resection typically develop recurrent disease just proximal to the ileocolonic anastomosis, whereas in those with colonic disease the site of recurrence can be on either or both sides of the anastomosis.[71] Ascertaining the exact frequency of recurrence after surgical resection depends on how recurrence is defined. If recurrence is defined as the need for another surgical intervention, 25% to 38% of CD patients treated surgically will have a recurrence by 5 years, and 40% to 70% will have a recurrence by 15 years.[80,81] Of those who undergo a second operation, 37% will require a third operation.[80] By contrast, endoscopic evidence of recurrence can be found in up to 93% of patients 1 year after surgery.[82] Overall, the data suggest that patients should be advised that disease recurrence following surgery for CD is likely. Nevertheless, surgery is an important therapeutic modality that, at least in the short term, can provide substantial improvement in clinical symptoms and quality of life.

TABLE 1-2

INDICATION FOR INITIAL SURGERY IN PATIENTS WITH CROHN'S DISEASE, WITH RESPECT TO CLINICAL PATTERN OF PRESENTATION*

	CLINICAL PATTERN		
INDICATION FOR SURGERY[†]	ILEOCOLONIC (N = 199)	COLONIC OR ANORECTAL (N = 97)	SMALL INTESTINAL (N = 100)
Intestinal obstruction	96 (48.2%)	21 (22.3%)	56 (61.1%)
Internal fistula	53 (26.8%)	16 (17.0%)	21 (22.1%)
Toxic dilatation	10 (5%)	25 (26.6%)	2 (2.1%)
Perianal disease	63 (31.7%)	36 (37.9%)	15 (15.8%)
Perforation or abscess	43 (21.6%)	13 (13.8%)	15 (15.8%)

*Reprinted with permission from Farmer RG, Whelan G, Fazio VW. Long-term follow-up of patients with Crohn's disease. *Gastroenterology.* 1985;88:1818-1825.

[†]At times, more than one indication was present (internal fistula and perforation with abscess was the most frequent combination).

Treatment with biologic agents, such as infliximab, a chimeric monoclonal antibody against tumor necrosis factor-alpha, may alter the natural history of CD. Within 2 weeks of starting therapy, nearly 60% of patients have a clinical response, and, of these, approximately 40% can be maintained in remission for 54 weeks with infusions of the drug every 8 weeks, as compared to 21% of those receiving infusions of placebo.[83] Similarly, maintenance therapy with infliximab maintains closure of fistulas in 36% of treated patients compared to 19% of those treated with placebo.[84] Although more than 50% of patients treated with infliximab for fistulas will still require surgery,[85] the ability of this agent to promote endoscopic healing in parallel with clinical improvement suggests that the drug has the potential to alter the natural history of the disease.[86]

EXTRAINTESTINAL MANIFESTATIONS

Patients with CD are at risk of developing many of the same extraintestinal complications seen in patients with UC (see Table 1-2). Indeed, the frequencies of dermatologic, arthritic, and ocular complications are similar in both forms of IBD,[21] although the frequency of erythema nodosum is slightly higher in patients with CD than in those with UC.[71] Several additional complications are unique to CD patients as a consequence of either the ulcerating nature of CD or involvement of the small intestine.

Although patients with either UC or CD are at risk of osteoporosis as a consequence of corticosteroid use, patients with CD and extensive small bowel involvement are at additional risk of vitamin D and calcium malabsorption.[87] As a result, these patients have an excess risk of fracture of both vertebra and hip (odds ratio [OR] of 2.5 and 1.8, respectively), and the risk is proportional to the severity of the bowel disease, as assessed by the number of symptoms.[88] Therefore, these patients should start on a medical regimen to preserve bone density, including combined calcium and vitamin D and possibly estrogen therapy for women. Perhaps most effective are bisphosphonates, which can increase bone density in patients with IBD.[89]

Patients with terminal ileal disease or resection are also at risk of bile acid malabsorption that may result in formation of gallstones. In addition, interruption of the enterohepatic circulation may lead to oxalate kidney stones because of both an increase in oxalate absorption in the colon as a result of increased mucosal permeability and a reduction in luminal calcium concentrations as a result of increased binding to long-chain free fatty acids. Gallstones develop in 15% to 30% of patients with small bowel CD, whereas oxalate nephrolithiasis occurs in 5% to 10%.[71] Folate absorption may also be reduced because of small bowel disease as well as treatment with sulfasalazine, and folate supplementation should be considered.

Less frequent complications of CD include amyloidosis and hepatobiliary dysfunction. Amyloidosis is rare in patients with CD. Farmer et al found only one case of amyloidosis in 615 CD patients followed prospectively.[70] This complication generally presents several years after the diagnosis of CD has been made, most frequently in patients with longstanding fistulizing disease, and may involve almost any organ, most often the kidneys.[71] As in UC, abnormal liver biochemical tests are common in patients with CD, occurring in up to 30% of patients.[90] However, PSC is less common in CD than in UC. PSC has been reported as a complication in 1% to 2% of CD cases, and of the 70% of patients with PSC who have IBD, only 6% have CD.[91]

INTESTINAL AND EXTRAINTESTINAL CANCER

Patients with CD are at increased risk of cancer of both the small and large intestines. Compared to sporadic small intestinal adenocarcinomas, small bowel adenocarcinomas in patients with CD tend to occur at a younger age and have a different anatomic distribution. The mean age at diagnosis in patients with CD is 46, compared to 64 in the general population.[92] Whereas sporadic small intestinal carcinomas occur most commonly in the duodenum and proximal jejunum, those in patients with CD tend to arise in areas of longstanding inflammation, often the distal jejunum and ileum.[93] Although patients with CD are up to 40 times as likely as the general population to develop small bowel carcinoma,[36,94,95] the absolute risk is exceedingly small.

It is now clear that patients with CD, like those with UC, are at increased risk of colon cancer.[95-97] The risk is especially high in patients with extensive colonic involvement. In this group, the overall risk of colorectal cancer is increased as much as 18-fold, and the cumulative risk is 8% at 22 years. The relative risk is especially high in patients in whom CD is diagnosed before age 25. The risk of colon cancer in patients with extensive colonic CD is equal to that of patients with ulcerative pancolitis,[95,96] a finding that suggests that the extent and duration of the inflammation, not the form of IBD, predisposes to cancer.

The risk of colon cancer in CD patients with less extensive colonic inflammation is not well defined but appears to be small.[94,95] For patients with ileal disease, the risk of colon cancer does not appear to be increased above that of the general population.[94] Perhaps because the symptoms of CD may resemble those of rectal cancer, rectal tumors tend to be diagnosed at a later stage than those in patients without CD and thus have a poorer prognosis.[98]

There is evidence that patients with CD have a higher relative risk of developing certain extraintestinal malignancies. Both Hodgkin's and non-Hodgkin's lymphomas have been reported to occur with increased frequency in patients with CD,[95,99,100] although this association has been put into question by results of a large population-based cohort study.[33] In addition, squamous cell cancer of the anus and vulva occur with a frequency up to 5-fold of that of the general population.[101] The risk is especially high in patients with longstanding perineal disease.[102,103]

MORTALITY

Crohn's disease is associated with an increased mortality rate relative to the general population and independent of whether the small intestine, large intestine, or both are affected.[19,60-62,70] The excess mortality is most notable in the first few years after diagnosis and is most often attributable to complications of CD, including gastrointestinal cancer,[60-62] as well as a number of comorbid conditions or complications, such as shock, volume depletion, protein/calorie malnutrition, and anemia.[104] Most population-based studies have found an overall standardized mortality ratio (SMR) of 1.3 to 1.5 for patients with CD.[61,105] In a population-based study from Copenhagen, Jess et al found that the highest mortality risk was in women younger than 50 years of age at diagnosis (SMR 3.42; 95% CI 2.21 to 5.04). In this study, the higher mortality risk in women with disease onset before age 50 was attributed to a more aggressive disease course[105]; other studies have found a similar association between female sex and increased mortality.[60,61,106] On the other hand, a population-based study from 7 European countries and Israel reported an increased overall mortality risk in patients with CD 10 years after diagnosis, with an age greater than 40 years at diagnosis as the sole factor associated with increased mortality.[107] Which concurrent medications patients were using in many of these studies is uncertain. Certain medications (ie, corticosteroids) have been recognized to augment the risk of severe infectious complications and even the risk of mortality in this patient population.[108]

QUALITY OF LIFE

Like UC, CD is a lifelong disease that causes symptoms that may interfere with social activities, interpersonal relationships, and employment. Several questionnaire-based studies have found that patients with CD have worse HRQOL scores than healthy controls or patients with UC (standardized IBD questionnaire [IBDQ] scores of 6.66 for healthy subjects, 5.90 for inactive UC, and 5.25 for patients with stable CD; range: 1 = poor to 7 = optimum).[69,109-111] Not surprisingly, patients with active ileocolonic disease and ileocecal disease have an even worse quality of life than the overall CD population (HRQOL scores of 4.09 and 3.97, respectively).[65] The reduction in quality of life is attributable, in part, to stress that patients experience because of concerns about their disease. Blondel-Kucharski et al found that patients' principal concern was having an ostomy bag, followed in frequency by the uncertain prognosis associated with their disease, reduced energy level, and possibility of needing surgery. Factors associated with a reduced HRQOL include female gender, tobacco use, involvement of the colon, hospitalization, corticosteroid treatment, and recent surgery.[112] Use of immunomodulators,[112] including infliximab,[113,114] was associated with a better HRQOL. As in patients with UC, patients' concerns were best allayed when physicians instructed them about what to expect from their disease.[69]

Despite an impaired quality of life, several studies have found that patients with CD can lead lives that are as productive as those of healthy subjects. Although younger patients with CD miss a greater number of school days than healthy controls, they achieve similar academic success.[115] Similarly, unemployment rates are not higher among patients with CD than among age-matched controls.[71]

SPECIAL POPULATIONS

IBD in the Pediatric Population

IBD often has its onset in adolescence; however, the incidence of IBD in children remains lower than in adults. Langholz et al found the incidence of UC in children below age 15 to be 2.0 per 10^5 and that for CD to be 0.2 per 10^5.[116] In this age group, up to 15% of patients change diagnosis from UC to CD or CD to UC during the course of the illness,[117] and 23% to 50% may be diagnosed with indeterminate colitis at initial presentation.[117-119] In the pediatric population, however, the incidence of CD has increased since the 1950s, whereas that of UC has remained relatively constant.[120] In fact, the incidence of CD in children is approaching, and in some areas has overtaken, that of UC.

ULCERATIVE COLITIS

Although the clinical features and natural history of IBD in children are similar to those of adults, several important differences exist. In a study comparing the natural history of UC in adults and children, Langholz et al found that children tended to have more extensive disease (29% had pancolitis and 25% had proctitis, compared to 14% and 46% in adults, respectively). In addition, pediatric patients presented more frequently with abdominal pain as a chief complaint.[116] In another series of 171 children with UC, 22% had proctosigmoiditis, 36% left-sided colitis, and 43% pancolitis. Forty-three percent were initially diagnosed with mild disease, and, of these, more than 90% had their symptoms resolve after 6 months. After 1 year of follow-up, 55% were symptom free, 38% had intermittent symptoms, and 7% had persistent symptoms. Of the 57% initially diagnosed with moderate to severe disease, 81% were symptom free at 6 months. The outcome was independent of the disease extent, and the overall 5-year rate of surgery was 19%.[121]

CROHN'S DISEASE

Comprehensive studies of the natural history of Crohn's disease in children are lacking.[119] Growth retardation has been found to be an important clue to the diagnosis of CD in children, and growth rates are less than expected in up to 40% of children with CD.[122] In a study of 100 consecutive pediatric patients with CD, Griffiths et al found that 33% had mild disease and never required corticosteroids, whereas 33% had at least one flare that required the use of these agents. In addition, 19% had chronically active disease that required immunomodulatory or surgical therapy to induce remission, and 10% had corticosteroid-dependent or refractory disease.[122] The use of infliximab has been shown, at least in the short term, to be safe in children with CD.[123] It is not yet clear how this agent will alter the natural history of the disease in this population.

IBD in the Elderly

ULCERATIVE COLITIS

The clinical features of UC in the elderly are generally similar to those in younger patients. However, at the time of presentation, patients older than age 60 tend to have less extensive, predominantly distal disease. Watts et al found that 42% of older patients presented with proctitis, and 12% presented with pancolitis; the corresponding rates for patients younger than age 60 were 33% and 26.5%, respectively.[124] Surprisingly, the higher frequency of distal colonic disease in the older group does not translate into less clinical severity. In a retrospective population-based study of patients from Scotland, Sinclair et al found that 14% of patients presenting after age 70 had a severe initial attack, compared to only 7% of those under age 30 and 3% of those between ages 30 and 69. Severe attacks carried a mortality rate of 23%, and in this study, the overall mortality rate was higher in elderly patients than in younger patients.[125]

Not all studies have demonstrated a worse prognosis for elderly patients. In fact, most have shown that patients over age 60 respond well to medical management, have lower rates of relapse than younger patients, and have mortality rates that are comparable to that of age-matched controls.[126] Hendriksen et al followed 783 Dutch patients with UC over an 18-year period and found only a slight increase in mortality in patients diagnosed after age 40. The increase in mortality was confined to the first 2 years after presentation; the subsequent survival rate was equal to that of the younger population.[10]

CROHN'S DISEASE

Compared to younger populations, older patients with CD tend to develop disease involving the colon and obstructive and inflammatory (rather than fistulizing) complications. Despite these differences, young and elderly patients present with similar symptoms, although on initial presentation elderly patients are more likely to be misdiagnosed as having diverticulitis or colon cancer.[127] Elderly patients respond as well as younger patients to medical and surgical therapy.[126,128] Moreover, postoperative recurrence rates are up to 5 times higher in younger patients.[126,129] In fact, the onset of CD later in life does not appear to affect mortality adversely, and mortality rates for elderly patients with CD are no different from those for the general population.[72]

REFERENCES

1. Sandler R, Loftus EV Jr. The epidemiology of idiopathic inflammatory bowel disease. In: Sartor R, Sanborn W, eds. *Kirsner's Inflammatory Bowel Disease.* Baltimore, MD: Saunders; 2004:259-268.

2. Panaccione R, Sutherland L. Clinical course and complications of ulcerative colitis. In: Targan S, Sharahan F, Karp L, eds. *Inflammatory Bowel Disease: From Bench to Bedside*. Baltimore, MD: Kluwer Academic Publishers; 2003:269-290.

3. Mayberry JF, Ballantyne KC, Hardcastle JD, Mangham C, Pye G. Epidemiological study of asymptomatic inflammatory bowel disease: the identification of cases during a screening programme for colorectal cancer. *Gut*. 1989;30:481-483.

4. Garland CF, Lilienfeld AM, Mendeloff AI, Markowitz JA, Terrell KB, Garland FC. Incidence rates of ulcerative colitis and Crohn's disease in fifteen areas of the United States. *Gastroenterology*. 1981;81:1115-1124.

5. Stowe SP, Redmond SR, Stormont JM, et al. An epidemiologic study of inflammatory bowel disease in Rochester, New York. Hospital incidence. *Gastroenterology*. 1990;98:104-110.

6. Hiatt RA, Kaufman L. Epidemiology of inflammatory bowel disease in a defined Northern California population. *West J Med*. 1988;149:541-546.

7. Podolsky DK. Inflammatory bowel disease. *N Engl J Med*. 2002; 347:417-429.

8. Langholz E, Munkholm P, Davidsen M, Nielsen OH, Binder V. Changes in extent of ulcerative colitis: a study on the course and prognostic factors. *Scand J Gastroenterol*. 1996;31:260-266.

9. Langholz E, Munkholm P, Davidsen M, Binder V. Course of ulcerative colitis: analysis of changes in disease activity over years. *Gastroenterology*. 1994;107:3-11.

10. Hendriksen C, Kreiner S, Binder V. Long term prognosis in ulcerative colitis—based on results from a regional patient group from the county of Copenhagen. *Gut*. 1985;26:158-163.

11. Farmer RG, Easley KA, Rankin GB. Clinical patterns, natural history, and progression of ulcerative colitis. A long-term follow-up of 1116 patients. *Dig Dis Sci*. 1993;38:1137-1146.

12. Langholz E, Munkholm P, Nielsen OH, Kreiner S, Binder V. Incidence and prevalence of ulcerative colitis in Copenhagen county from 1962 to 1987. *Scand J Gastroenterol*. 1991;26:1247-1256.

13. Meucci G, Vecchi M, Astegiano M, et al. The natural history of ulcerative proctitis: a multicenter, retrospective study. Gruppo di Studio per le Malattie Infiammatorie Intestinali (GSMII). *Am J Gastroenterol*. 2000;95:469-473.

14. Powell-Tuck J, Ritchie JK, Lennard-Jones JE. The prognosis of idiopathic proctitis. *Scand J Gastroenterol*. 1977;12:727-732.

15. Jewell D. Ulcerative colitis. In: Feldman M, Friedman LS, Sleisenger MH, eds. *Sleisenger and Fordtran's Gastrointestinal and Liver Disease*. Vol. 2. Philadelphia, PA: WB Saunders; 2002:2039-2067.

16. Greenstein AJ, Aufses AH Jr. Differences in pathogenesis, incidence and outcome of perforation in inflammatory bowel disease. *Surg Gynecol Obstet*. 1985;160:63-69.

17. Levine JB, Lukawski-Trubish D. Extraintestinal considerations in inflammatory bowel disease. *Gastroenterol Clin North Am*. 1995;24:633-646.

18. Orchard TR, Wordsworth BP, Jewell DP. Peripheral arthropathies in inflammatory bowel disease: their articular distribution and natural history. *Gut*. 1998;42:387-391.

19. Palli D, Trallori G, Saieva C, et al. General and cancer specific mortality of a population based cohort of patients with inflammatory bowel disease: the Florence Study. *Gut*. 1998;42:175-179.

20. Orchard TR, Chua CN, Ahmad T, Cheng H, Welsh KI, Jewell DP. Uveitis and erythema nodosum in inflammatory bowel disease: clinical features and the role of HLA genes. *Gastroenterology*. 2002;123:714-718.

21. Bernstein CN. Extraintestinal manifestations of inflammatory bowel disease. *Curr Gastroenterol Rep*. 2001;3:477-483.

22. Raj V, Lichtenstein DR. Hepatobiliary manifestations of inflammatory bowel disease. *Gastroenterol Clin North Am*. 1999;28:491-513.

23. MacLean AR, Lilly L, Cohen Z, O'Connor B, McLeod RS. Outcome of patients undergoing liver transplantation for primary sclerosing cholangitis. *Dis Colon Rectum*. 2003;46:1124-1128.

24. Chapman RW, Arborgh BA, Rhodes JM, et al. Primary sclerosing cholangitis: a review of its clinical features, cholangiography, and hepatic histology. *Gut*. 1980;21:870-877.

25. Wiesner RH, LaRusso NF. Clinicopathologic features of the syndrome of primary sclerosing cholangitis. *Gastroenterology*. 1980; 79:200-206.

26. Lee YM, Kaplan MM. Primary sclerosing cholangitis. *N Engl J Med*. 1995;332:924-933.

27. Gow PJ, Chapman RW. Liver transplantation for primary sclerosing cholangitis. *Liver*. 2000;20:97-103.

28. Feith MP, Klompmaker IJ, Maring JK, et al. Biliary reconstruction during liver transplantation in patients with primary sclerosing cholangitis. *Transplant Proc*. 1997;29:560-561.

29. Harrison RF, Davies MH, Neuberger JM, Hubscher SG. Fibrous and obliterative cholangitis in liver allografts: evidence of recurrent primary sclerosing cholangitis? *Hepatology*. 1994;20:356-361.

30. Abu-Elmagd KM, Malinchoc M, Dickson ER, et al. Efficacy of hepatic transplantation in patients with primary sclerosing cholangitis. *Surg Gynecol Obstet*. 1993;177:335-344.

31. Broome U, Glaumann H, Lindstom E, et al. Natural history and outcome in 32 Swedish patients with small duct primary sclerosing cholangitis (PSC). *J Hepatol*. 2002;36:586-589.

32. Loftus EV Jr, Sandborn WJ. Lymphoma risk in inflammatory bowel disease: influences of referral bias and therapy. *Gastroenterology*. 2001;121:1239-1242.

33. Lewis JD, Bilker WB, Brensinger C, Deren JJ, Vaughn DJ, Strom BL. Inflammatory bowel disease is not associated with an increased risk of lymphoma. *Gastroenterology*. 2001;121:1080-1087.

34. Loftus EV Jr. Epidemiology and risk factors for colorectal dysplasia and cancer in ulcerative colitis. *Gastroenterol Clin North Am*. 2006:517-531.

35. Ekbom A, Helmick C, Zack M, Adami HO. Ulcerative colitis and colorectal cancer. A population-based study. *N Engl J Med*. 1990; 323:1228-1233.

36. Jess T, Loftus EV Jr, Velayos FS, et al. Risk of intestinal cancer in inflammatory bowel disease: a population-based study from Olmsted County, Minnesota. *Gastroenterology*. 2006:1039-1046.

37. Choi PM, Kim WH. Colon cancer surveillance. *Gastroenterol Clin North Am*. 1995;24:671-687.

38. Rutter M, Saunders B, Wilkinson K, et al. Severity of inflammation is a risk factor for colorectal neoplasia in ulcerative colitis. *Gastroenterology*. 2004;126:451-459.

39. Jensen AB, Larsen M, Gislum M, et al. Survival after colorectal cancer in patients with ulcerative colitis: a nationwide population-based Danish study. *Am J Gastroenterol*. 2006:1283-1287.

40. Bernstein CN, Shanahan F, Weinstein WM. Are we telling patients the truth about surveillance colonoscopy in ulcerative colitis? *Lancet*. 1994;343:71-74.

41. Ullman TA, Loftus EV Jr, Kakar S, Burgart LJ, Sandborn WJ, Tremaine WJ. The fate of low grade dysplasia in ulcerative colitis. *Am J Gastroenterol*. 2002;97:922-927.

42. Ullman T, Croog V, Harpaz N, Sachar D, Itzkowitz S. Progression of flat low-grade dysplasia to advanced neoplasia in patients with ulcerative colitis. *Gastroenterology*. 2003;125:1311-1319.

43. Lynch DA, Lobo AJ, Sobala GM, Dixon MF, Axon AT. Failure of colonoscopic surveillance in ulcerative colitis. *Gut*. 1993;34:1075-1080.

44. Blackstone MO, Riddell RH, Rogers BH, Levin B. Dysplasia-associated lesion or mass (DALM) detected by colonoscopy in long-standing ulcerative colitis: an indication for colectomy. *Gastroenterology*. 1981;80:366-374.

45. Broome U, Lofberg R, Veress B, Eriksson LS. Primary sclerosing cholangitis and ulcerative colitis: evidence for increased neoplastic potential. *Hepatology*. 1995;22:1404-1408.

46. Kornfeld D, Ekbom A, Ihre T. Is there an excess risk for colorectal cancer in patients with ulcerative colitis and concomitant primary sclerosing cholangitis? A population based study. *Gut*. 1997;41:522-525.

47. Marchesa P, Lashner BA, Lavery IC, et al. The risk of cancer and dysplasia among ulcerative colitis patients with primary sclerosing cholangitis. *Am J Gastroenterol*. 1997;92:1285-1288.

48. Leidenius MH, Farkkila MA, Karkkainen P, Taskinen EI, Kellokumpu IH, Hockerstedt KA. Colorectal dysplasia and carcinoma in patients with ulcerative colitis and primary sclerosing cholangitis. *Scand J Gastroenterol*. 1997;32:706-711.

49. Rodrigues CM, Kren BT, Steer CJ, Setchell KD. The site-specific delivery of ursodeoxycholic acid to the rat colon by sulfate conjugation. *Gastroenterology*. 1995;109:1835-1844.

50. Batta AK, Salen G, Holubec H, Brasitus TA, Alberts D, Earnest DL. Enrichment of the more hydrophilic bile acid ursodeoxycholic acid in the fecal water-soluble fraction after feeding to rats with colon polyps. *Cancer Res*. 1998;58:1684-1687.

51. Pardi DS, Loftus EV Jr, Kremers WK, Keach J, Lindor KD. Ursodeoxycholic acid as a chemopreventive agent in patients with ulcerative colitis and primary sclerosing cholangitis. *Gastroenterology*. 2003;124:889-893.

52. Eaden J, Abrams K, Ekbom A, Jackson E, Mayberry J. Colorectal cancer prevention in ulcerative colitis: a case-control study. *Aliment Pharmacol Ther*. 2000;14:145-153.

53. van Staa TP, Card T, Logan RF, Leufkens HGM. 5-Aminosalicylate use and colorectal cancer risk in inflammatory bowel disease: a large epidemiologic study. *Gut*. 2005:1573-1578.

54. Rubin DT, LoSavio A, Yadron N, et al. Aminosalicylate therapy in the prevention of dysplasia and colorectal cancer in ulcerative colitis. *Clin Gastroenterol Hepatol*. 2006:1346-1350.

55. Bernstein CN, Eaden J, Steinhart AH, Munkholm P, Gordon PH. Cancer prevention in inflammatory bowel disease and the chemoprophylactic potential of 5-aminosalicylic acid. *Inflamm Bowel Dis*. 2002;8:356-361.

56. Velayos FS, Terdiman JP, Walsh JM. Effect of 5-aminosalicylate use on colorectal cancer and dysplasia risk: a systematic review and metaanalysis of observational studies. *Am J Gastroenterol*. 2005;100:1345-1353.

57. Velayos FS, Loftus EV Jr, Jess T, et al. Predictive and protective factors associated with colorectal cancer in ulcerative colitis: a case-control study. *Gastroenterology*. 2006;130:1941-1949.

58. Selby W. The natural history of ulcerative colitis. *Bailliers Clin Gastroenterol*. 1997;11:53-64.

59. Winther KV, Jess T, Langholz E, Munkholm P, Binder V. Survival and cause-specific mortality in ulcerative colitis: follow-up of a population-based cohort in Copenhagen County. *Gastroenterology*. 2003;125:1576-1582.

60. Ekbom A, Helmick CG, Zack M, Holmberg L, Adami HO. Survival and causes of death in patients with inflammatory bowel disease: a population-based study. *Gastroenterology*. 1992;103:954-960.

61. Persson PG, Bernell O, Leijonmarck CE, Farahmand BY, Hellers G, Ahlbom A. Survival and cause-specific mortality in inflammatory bowel disease: a population-based cohort study. *Gastroenterology*. 1996;110:1339-1345.

62. Jess T, Loftus EV Jr, Harmsen WS, et al. Survival and cause specific mortality in patients with inflammatory bowel disease: a long term outcome study in Olmsted County, Minnesota, 1940-2004. *Gut*. 2006;55:1248-1254.

63. Sonnenberg A. Deadly IBD. *Inflamm Bowel Dis*. 2006;3:246.

64. Langholz E, Munkholm P, Davidsen M, Binder V. Colorectal cancer risk and mortality in patients with ulcerative colitis. *Gastroenterology*. 1992;103:1444-1451.

65. Irvine EJ. Quality of life issues in patients with inflammatory bowel disease. *Am J Gastroenterol*. 1997;92(12 suppl):18S-24S.

66. Hjortswang H, Jarnerot G, Curman B, et al. The influence of demographic and disease-related factors on health-related quality of life in patients with ulcerative colitis. *Eur J Gastroenterol Hepatol*. 2003;15:1011-1020.

67. Rubin GP, Hungin AP, Chinn DJ, Dwarakanath D. Quality of life in patients with established inflammatory bowel disease: a UK general practice survey. *Aliment Pharmacol Ther*. 2004;19:529-535.

68. Hjortswang H, Strom M, Almer S. Health-related quality of life in Swedish patients with ulcerative colitis. *Am J Gastroenterol*. 1998;93:2203-2211.

69. Drossman DA, Patrick DL, Mitchell CM, Zagami EA, Appelbaum MI. Health-related quality of life in inflammatory bowel disease. Functional status and patient worries and concerns. *Dig Dis Sci*. 1989;34:1379-1386.

70. Farmer RG, Whelan G, Fazio VW. Long-term follow-up of patients with Crohn's disease. Relationship between the clinical pattern and prognosis. *Gastroenterology*. 1985;88:1818-1825.

71. Sands BE. Crohn's disease. In: Feldman M, Friedman LS, Sleisenger MH, eds. *Sleisenger and Fordtran's Gastrointestinal and Liver Disease*. Vol. 2. Philadelphia, PA: WB Saunders; 2002:2005-2038.

72. Munkholm P, Langholz E, Davidsen M, Binder V. Disease activity courses in a regional cohort of Crohn's disease patients. *Scand J Gastroenterol*. 1995;30:699-706.

73. Polito JM II, Childs B, Mellits ED, Tokayer AZ, Harris ML, Bayless TM. Crohn's disease: influence of age at diagnosis on site and clinical type of disease. *Gastroenterology*. 1996;111:580-586.

74. Lichtenstein GR, Olson A, Travers S, et al. Factors associated with the development of intestinal strictures or obstructions in patients with Crohn's disease. *Am J Gastroenterol*. 2006:1030-1038.

75. Schwartz DA, Loftus EV Jr, Tremaine WJ, et al. The natural history of fistulizing Crohn's disease in Olmsted County, Minnesota. *Gastroenterology*. 2002;122:875-880.

76. Sands BE, Arsenault JE, Rosen MJ, et al. Risk of early surgery for Crohn's disease: implications for early treatment strategies. *Am J Gastroenterol*. 2003;98:2712-2718.

77. Cuthbert AP, Fisher SA, Mirza MM, et al. The contribution of NOD2 gene mutations to the risk and site of disease in inflammatory bowel disease. *Gastroenterology*. 2002;122:867-874.

78. Abreu MT, Taylor KD, Lin YC, et al. Mutations in NOD2 are associated with fibrostenosing disease in patients with Crohn's disease. *Gastroenterology*. 2002;123:679-688.

79. Torok HP, Glas J, Tonenchi L, et al. Polymorphisms in the DLG5 and OCTN cation transporter genes in Crohn's disease. *Gut*. 2005;54:1421-1427.

80. Whelan G, Farmer RG, Fazio VW, Goormastic M. Recurrence after surgery in Crohn's disease. Relationship to location of disease (clinical pattern) and surgical indication. *Gastroenterology*. 1985;88:1826-1833.

81. Sachar DB. The problem of postoperative recurrence of Crohn's disease. *Med Clin North Am*. 1990;74:183-188.

82. Olaison G, Smedh K, Sjodahl R. Natural course of Crohn's disease after ileocolic resection: endoscopically visualised ileal ulcers preceding symptoms. *Gut*. 1992;33:331-335.

83. Hanauer SB, Feagan BG, Lichtenstein GR, et al. Maintenance infliximab for Crohn's disease: the ACCENT I randomised trial. *Lancet.* 2002;359:1541-1549.

84. Sands BE, Anderson FH, Bernstein CN, et al. Infliximab maintenance therapy for fistulizing Crohn's disease. *N Engl J Med.* 2004; 350:876-885.

85. Poritz LS, Rowe WA, Koltun WA. Remicade does not abolish the need for surgery in fistulizing Crohn's disease. *Dis Colon Rectum.* 2002;45:771-775.

86. Sninsky CA. Altering the natural history of Crohn's disease? *Inflamm Bowel Dis.* 2001;7(suppl 1):S34-S39.

87. Vestergaard P, Krogh K, Rejnmark L, Laurberg S, Mosekilde L. Fracture risk is increased in Crohn's disease, but not in ulcerative colitis. *Gut.* 2000;46:176-181.

88. van Staa TP, Cooper C, Brusse LS, Leufkens H, Javaid MK, Arden NK. Inflammatory bowel disease and the risk of fracture. *Gastroenterology.* 2003;125:1591-1597.

89. Haderslev KV, Tjellesen L, Sorensen HA, Staun M. Alendronate increases lumbar spine bone mineral density in patients with Crohn's disease. *Gastroenterology.* 2000;119:639-646.

90. Heikius B, Niemela S, Lehtola J, Karttunen T, Lahde S. Hepatobiliary and coexisting pancreatic duct abnormalities in patients with inflammatory bowel disease. *Scand J Gastroenterol.* 1997;32:153-161.

91. Rasmussen HH, Fallingborg JF, Mortensen PB, Vyberg M, Tage-Jensen U, Rasmussen SN. Hepatobiliary dysfunction and primary sclerosing cholangitis in patients with Crohn's disease. *Scand J Gastroenterol.* 1997;32:604-610.

92. Collier PE, Turowski P, Diamond DL. Small intestinal adenocarcinoma complicating regional enteritis. *Cancer.* 1985;55:516-521.

93. Bernstein D, Rogers A. Malignancy in Crohn's disease. *Am J Gastroenterol.* 1996;91:434-440.

94. Canavan C, Abrams KR, Mayberry J. Meta-analysis: colorectal and small bowel cancer risk in patients with Crohn's disease. *Aliment Pharmacol Ther.* 2006;23:1097-1104.

95. Bernstein CN, Blanchard JF, Kliewer E, Wajda A. Cancer risk in patients with inflammatory bowel disease: a population-based study. *Cancer.* 2001;91:854-862.

96. Gillen CD, Walmsley RS, Prior P, Andrews HA, Allan RN. Ulcerative colitis and Crohn's disease: a comparison of the colorectal cancer risk in extensive colitis. *Gut.* 1994;35:1590-1592.

97. Gillen CD, Andrews HA, Prior P, Allan RN. Crohn's disease and colorectal cancer. *Gut.* 1994;35:651-655.

98. Sjodahl RI, Myrelid P, Soderholm JD. Anal and rectal cancer in Crohn's disease. *Colorectal Dis.* 2003;5:490-495.

99. Loftus EV Jr, Tremaine WJ, Habermann TM, Harmsen WS, Zinsmeister AR, Sandborn WJ. Risk of lymphoma in inflammatory bowel disease. *Am J Gastroenterol.* 2000;95:2308-2312.

100. Greenstein AJ, Mullin GE, Strauchen JA, et al. Lymphoma in inflammatory bowel disease. *Cancer.* 1992;69:1119-1123.

101. Ekbom A, Helmick C, Zack M, Adami HO. Extracolonic malignancies in inflammatory bowel disease. *Cancer.* 1991;67:2015-2019.

102. Ky A, Sohn N, Weinstein MA, Korelitz BI. Carcinoma arising in anorectal fistulas of Crohn's disease. *Dis Colon Rectum.* 1998; 41:992-996.

103. Buchman AL, Ament ME, Doty J. Development of squamous cell carcinoma in chronic perineal sinus and wounds in Crohn's disease. *Am J Gastroenterol.* 1991;86:1829-1832.

104. Cucino C, Sonnenberg A. Cause of death in patients with inflammatory bowel disease. *Inflamm Bowel Dis.* 2001;7:250-255.

105. Jess T, Winther KV, Munkholm P, Langholz E, Binder V. Mortality and causes of death in Crohn's disease: follow-up of a population-based cohort in Copenhagen County, Denmark. *Gastroenterology.* 2002;122:1808-1814.

106. Card T, Hubbard R, Logan RF. Mortality in inflammatory bowel disease: a population-based cohort study. *Gastroenterology.* 2003;125:1583-1590.

107. Wolters FL, Russel MG, Sijbrandij J, et al. Crohn's disease: increased mortality 10 years after diagnosis in a Europe-wide population based cohort. *Gut.* 2006;55:510-518.

108. Lichtenstein GR, Feagan BG, Cohen RD, et al. Serious infections and mortality in association with therapies for Crohn's disease: TREAT registry. *Clin Gastroenterol Hepatol.* 2006;4:621-630.

109. Farmer RG, Easley KA, Farmer JM. Quality of life assessment by patients with inflammatory bowel disease. *Cleve Clin J Med.* 1992; 59:35-42.

110. Drossman DA, Leserman J, Li ZM, Mitchell CM, Zagami EA, Patrick DL. The rating form of IBD patient concerns: a new measure of health status. *Psychosom Med.* 1991;53:701-712.

111. Cohen RD. The quality of life in patients with Crohn's disease. *Aliment Pharmacol Ther.* 2002;16:1603-1609.

112. Blondel-Kucharski F, Chircop C, Marquis P, et al. Health-related quality of life in Crohn's disease: a prospective longitudinal study in 231 patients. *Am J Gastroenterol.* 2001;96:2915-2920.

113. Lichtenstein GR, Yan S, Bala M, Hanauer S. Remission in patients with Crohn's disease is associated with improvement in employment and quality of life and a decrease in hospitalizations and surgeries. *Am J Gastroenterol.* 2004;99:91-96.

114. Feagan BG, Yan S, Bala M, Bao W, Lichtenstein GR. The effects of infliximab maintenance therapy on health-related quality of life. *Am J Gastroenterol.* 2003;98:2232-2238.

115. Mayberry MK, Probert C, Srivastava E, Rhodes J, Mayberry JF. Perceived discrimination in education and employment by people with Crohn's disease: a case control study of educational achievement and employment. *Gut.* 1992;33:312-314.

116. Langholz E, Munkholm P, Krasilnikoff PA, Binder V. Inflammatory bowel diseases with onset in childhood. Clinical features, morbidity, and mortality in a regional cohort. *Scand J Gastroenterol.* 1997; 32:139-147.

117. Mamula P, Telega GW, Markowitz JE, et al. Inflammatory bowel disease in children 5 years of age and younger. *Am J Gastroenterol.* 2002;97:2005-2010.

118. Lindberg E, Lindquist B, Holmquist L, Hildebrand H. Inflammatory bowel disease in children and adolescents in Sweden, 1984-1995. *J Pediatr Gastroenterol Nutr.* 2000;30:259-264.

119. Mamula P, Markowitz JE, Baldassano RN. Inflammatory bowel disease in early childhood and adolescence: special considerations. *Gastroenterol Clin North Am.* 2003;32:967-995, viii.

120. Kirschner BS. Ulcerative colitis in children. *Pediatr Clin North Am.* 1996;43:235-254.

121. Hyams JS, Davis P, Grancher K, Lerer T, Justinich CJ, Markowitz J. Clinical outcome of ulcerative colitis in children. *J Pediatr.* 1996; 129:81-88.

122. Griffiths AM, Nguyen P, Smith C, MacMillan JH, Sherman PM. Growth and clinical course of children with Crohn's disease. *Gut.* 1993;34:939-943.

123. Stephens MC, Shepanski MA, Mamula P, Markowitz JE, Brown KA, Baldassano RN. Safety and steroid-sparing experience using infliximab for Crohn's disease at a pediatric inflammatory bowel disease center. *Am J Gastroenterol.* 2003;98:104-111.

124. Watts JM, De Dombal FT, Watkinson G, Goligher JC. Long-term prognosis of ulcerative colitis. *Br Med J.* 1966;5501:1447-1453.

125. Sinclair TS, Brunt PW, Mowat NA. Nonspecific proctocolitis in northeastern Scotland: a community study. *Gastroenterology.* 1983; 85:1-11.

126. Fleischer DE, Grimm IS, Friedman LS. Inflammatory bowel disease in older patients. *Med Clin North Am.* 1994;78:1303-1319.

127. Wagtmans MJ, Verspaget HW, Lamers CB, van Hogezand RA. Crohn's disease in the elderly: a comparison with young adults. *J Clin Gastroenterol*. 1998;27:129-133.

128. Shivananda S, Lennard-Jones J, Logan R, et al. Incidence of inflammatory bowel disease across Europe: is there a difference between north and south? Results of the European Collaborative Study on Inflammatory Bowel Disease (EC-IBD). *Gut*. 1996;39:690-697.

129. Softley A, Myren J, Clamp SE, Bouchier IA, Watkinson G, de Dombal FT. Inflammatory bowel disease in the elderly patient. *Scand J Gastroenterol Suppl*. 1988;144:27-30.

CLINICAL RESEARCH IN INFLAMMATORY BOWEL DISEASE

PLACEBO RESPONSE IN CLINICAL TRIALS

Chinyu Su, MD and James D. Lewis, MD, MSCE

A major goal of clinical research is to identify new therapies for the treatment of disease. In addition, research is used to define the potential risks of therapeutic interventions. In the realm of inflammatory bowel disease (IBD), there has been an enormous explosion in our knowledge of the underlying cause of these diseases and in development of therapeutic interventions. This chapter will provide a brief overview of the design and interpretation of clinical trials, with a focus on the role of placebos.

OVERVIEW OF CLINICAL RESEARCH DESIGNS

Clinical research can be divided into descriptive and analytic studies. Descriptive studies include case reports, case series, and analyses of secular trends. The feature that most distinguishes descriptive studies from analytic studies is the lack of a control group. Because there is no control group for comparison, descriptive studies are generally viewed as useful for hypothesis generation but play a small role in proving causality. As will be discussed later in this chapter, uncontrolled studies of drug therapies for IBD (ie, case series) play an important role in selecting medications for further investigation. By themselves, however, these studies cannot be used to determine efficacy.

In contrast to descriptive studies, analytic studies are characterized by the inclusion of a control group, thereby allowing the investigator to test a hypothesis. Analytic studies can be further divided into observational studies and experimental studies. The prototypical classification of observational analytic studies includes case-control studies and cohort studies. In case-control studies, the investigator identifies subjects with the outcome of interest and control subjects without the outcome. One then examines the subjects' prior exposures to determine whether there is an association between the outcome and the exposure. An example would include studies comparing patients with ulcerative colitis and colon cancer to others with ulcerative colitis and no colon cancer to determine whether prior use of mesalamine is associated with a reduced risk of colon cancer.

Cohort studies use the opposite design, starting with subjects who are exposed to medication and others who are not. These subjects are then followed over time to determine which subjects develop the outcome of interest. For example, one could follow a group of patients with ulcerative colitis, some of whom are receiving mesalamine therapy and others who are not. The investigator could then determine whether the incidence of colon cancer differed between these two groups.

In broad terms, major potential limitations of observational analytic studies include information bias, selection bias, and confounding. Information bias (ie, bias resulting from inaccurate or incomplete data collection) can often be prevented or minimized through appropriate design of the study. Selection bias can lead to incorrect conclusions from observational studies when the probability of selection is related to both the exposure under study and the outcome of interest. Appropriate measures can minimize the probability of selection bias, although in practical terms, it is often difficult to know for certain how well this has been accomplished. *Confounding* refers to a mixing of effects. If the exposure of interest is associated with a third factor that is also associated with the outcome of interest, failure to account for this third factor in the design or analysis of the study can lead to a biased result. Unfortunately, one can only account for confounding factors that are known or suspected prior to the start of the study. Thus, all observational analytic studies have the potential limitation of bias from unknown (and/or unmeasured) confounders.

Experimental analytic studies include clinical trials. The key feature that distinguishes experimental studies from observational studies is that the investigator assigns the treatment to subjects. The randomized clinical trial design is considered the gold standard for proving efficacy of an intervention. In the case of IBD, the intervention is typically medical therapy. Nearly all clinical trials use random allocation to assign the treatment categories. In the prototypical randomized clinical trial, patients are randomly assigned to receive 1 of the 2 or more exposures or interventions to be tested. They are then followed over a predetermined study period to measure the incidence of the outcome of interest. The main reason that the randomized clinical trial is afforded such accolades is that with a large enough sample size, the use of randomization prevents bias from unequal distribution of known and unknown confounders. In addition, because assignment of exposure status is random, selection bias is not a problem. For these reasons, the randomized clinical trial usually provides the strongest evidence of efficacy of any of the analytic designs.

Not all clinical trials are randomized controlled trials. Phase 1 drug studies are used to examine the safety of compounds that have not been previously given to humans. These studies typically treat a small number of subjects with the new medication. The study begins with very low doses and gradually increases the dose either between subjects or within subjects to establish a maximum tolerated dose. There is no control group in phase 1 studies. Phase 2 studies are designed to gain additional safety data, to begin to collect evidence of efficacy, and to select the optimal dose for use in phase 3 studies. Phase 2 studies will often include several different doses of the medications. While traditionally phase 2 studies did not include a placebo arm, in recent years it has been common to see placebo arms in phase 2 trials. Phase 3 trials are designed to prove efficacy. These are generally large randomized controlled trials that typically include a placebo arm but could also compare the new therapy to an existing alternative.

INTERPRETATION OF CLINICAL TRIAL RESULTS

Clinical trials generally report their results as incidence rates in the different treatment arms, relative risks, risk differences, and/or the number needed to treat. For studies with 2 treatment arms, the investigators may report relative risks (or relative rates for longer studies). Relative risks are a proportion of incidence rates. Thus, a relative risk of 2 implies that the exposed group is twice as likely as the control group to experience the outcome of interest. Results may also be reported as risk differences. This is the absolute difference in the incidence rates between the 2 groups. For example, if the incidence of remission in the group treated with mesalamine was 50% and it was 10% in the control group, the risk difference would be 40%. This provides a measure of the absolute benefit one might expect from the therapy. It is important to realize that 2 interventions can have the same relative risk and yet have very different risk differences, or vice versa. For example, if arm A had a 20% remission rate and arm B had a 40% remission rate, the relative risk of arm B versus arm A would be 2 with a risk difference of 20%. In contrast, if arm A had a 10% remission rate and arm B had a 20% remission rate, the relative risk of arm B versus arm A would again be 2, but with a risk difference of only 10%. To help place these into context, investigators often report the number needed to treat in order to achieve 1 additional outcome with 1 therapy versus the alternative. This is calculated as the inverse of the risk difference. Thus, in these examples, in the first study, the number needed to treat with B compared to A to achieve 1 additional remission would be 5, whereas in the second study it would be 10. Thus, for a fixed relative risk, one must look at the risk difference to understand the number needed to treat.

CHOICE OF CONTROL GROUPS FOR RANDOMIZED CLINICAL TRIALS

When designing a randomized clinical trial, investigators must choose between an active control or a placebo (ie, an inert substance). There are several advantages and disadvantages to each option. Let's consider an example of a new therapy for severe steroid refractory ulcerative colitis. If one compares the new therapy to placebo therapy, the results will provide strong evidence of whether the new therapy is biologically active. It will not provide information on whether the intervention is as good or better than the currently available therapies, however. In addition, patients with severe disease may be reluctant to enroll in a study where they may receive a placebo. Finally, some people might argue that enrolling patients into a trial with a placebo arm when there are known efficacious alternatives is unethical. Though discussion of the ethics of the use of placebo is beyond the scope of this chapter, there are nearly always at least some subgroups of patients for whom no reasonable alternative therapy exists, thus making placebo an option.

It is this concern over the ethics of the use of placebo that often leads people to suggest the use of an active comparator arm. Use of active comparator arms is also fraught with problems of interpretation, particularly if studies do not prove superior or equivalent efficacy of the new therapy. When designing a study using an active comparator, it is critical that the active comparator be proven to be efficacious. Even if this criterion is met, use of an active comparator can still result in difficulties with interpretation. Imagine a scenario where the standard therapy is known to induce remission in 60% of patients. In a clinical trial of a new therapy versus the standard therapy, the remission rates are 40% and 60%, respectively. After the study, one concludes that the new therapy is not superior or even equivalent to the standard therapy. However, it is still possible that the new therapy is efficacious, albeit less so than the standard therapy. Without a placebo control arm, this cannot be known. As such, a potentially beneficial therapy may be wrongly discarded. Patients who do not respond to the standard therapy or who have a contraindication to the standard therapy may have been wrongly deprived of potentially helpful therapy because no placebo arm was used. Thus, even in the 21st century, the use of placebo in randomized controlled trials remains important and is often preferred to active comparators for initial studies of efficacy. Once an intervention is proven efficacious, head-to-head comparisons to alternative therapies are incredibly helpful in designing appropriate treatment algorithms. Bypassing the placebo-controlled studies, however, is potentially fraught with error. Placebo control is particularly important in diseases such as IBD that are characterized by spontaneous periods of acute exacerbation and quiescence.

PLACEBO VERSUS BLINDING

One might ask whether it is necessary to use a placebo versus randomizing patients to no therapy. To understand this, one must understand the concept of *blinding* (also referred to as *masking*). Blinding refers to concealing the treatment assignment in such a manner that the subject and/or the investigator do not know who is receiving which treatment. The importance of blinding is to prevent detection bias. From the perspective of the patient, he or she may be more likely to report a side effect or to report improvement in symptoms if he knows that he is receiving the active therapy. Likewise, the investigator may be biased in his or her assessment of efficacy or adverse events if he knows which patients are receiving which therapy. Blinding can prevent such bias. One role of placebo is to facilitate blinding in medication studies. By using an inactive substance designed to be indistinguishable from the active therapy, one can achieve blinding of both patients and physicians.

Not all placebos are able to achieve blinding. Many medications have known side effect profiles or other characteristics that can result in unblinding. For example, if a medication has a unique taste or odor, this may be difficult to mimic in the placebo. Thus, use of a placebo does not assure effective blinding of subjects or investigators.

IS THE USE OF PLACEBO REALLY INERT?

Although the goal of a placebo-controlled trial is to determine whether a new therapy is better than no therapy, one might suspect that the use of placebo is not entirely inert. In fact, placebo can be defined as "any therapeutic procedure, without any specific activity, given deliberately to have an effect, or unknowingly has an effect on a patient, symptom, syndrome or disease, but which is objectively without specific activity for the condition being treated."[1] There is ample evidence in the medical literature that placebo therapy may not be inert. A systematic review of clinical trials comparing placebo to no treatment documented superiority of placebo in several conditions.[2] In general, placebo appeared superior to no treatment when the outcome was subjective and was measured on a continuous scale.[2]

Better outcomes with placebo compared to no treatment could occur for several reasons. First, the magnitude of the "placebo effect" may depend on the type of patient, the personality of the physician and health-care providers involved in the care, and their interactions. Patients who enroll in a clinical trial do not receive standard care. Rather, they usually receive much closer follow-up and frequent questioning about their medication adherence and are asked to pay closer attention to their symptoms, etc. All of these could potentially affect the outcome of the disease. For these reasons, the outcomes observed in clinical trials do not always mirror those observed in actual practice (ie, efficacy does not always equate to effectiveness). Another important factor is the patient's expectation regarding the therapy. Placebo effect is unlikely to be present if the patient knows that the treatment is ineffective. In addition, it is possible that there are true biological effects resulting from treatment with a substance that the patient believes to be effective, even if it is not. Thus, the placebo effect likely has no single specific mechanism of action whereby clinical and/or physiological changes take place.

It is also important to note that response or improvement observed in placebo-treated patients is in reality the result of the sum of the true placebo effect and the natural history of the disease. Importantly, patients tend to enroll in clinical trials when their disease is near its worst. In this case, there is greater opportunity for improvement than for further worsening. This is often referred to as *regression to the mean*.

TABLE 2-1

FACTORS ASSOCIATED WITH REMISSION OUTCOMES IN PLACEBO-TREATED GROUPS IN SYSTEMATIC REVIEWS OF CLINICAL TRIALS FOR ACTIVE CROHN'S DISEASE[7,8]*

POSITIVE ASSOCIATION	NEGATIVE ASSOCIATION
Study duration	Baseline CDAI scores
Number of study visits	Baseline CRP levels

* CDAI indicates Crohn's Disease Activity Index; CRP, c-reactive protein.

Adapted from Su C, Lichtenstein GR, Krok K, Brensinger CM, Lewis JD. A meta-analysis of the placebo rates of remission and response in clinical trials of active Crohn's disease. *Gastroenterology.* 2004;126:1257-1269 and Will M, Nikolaus S, Freitag S, Arpe N, Krawczak M, Schreiber S. Placebo response in the therapy of Crohn's disease: A comprehensive analysis of primary data from 733 patients from 13 randomized controlled trials. *Gastroenterology.* 2005;128:A-48.

WHAT FACTORS INFLUENCE THE OUTCOMES IN THE PLACEBO GROUP

Several studies have examined the outcomes of patients treated with placebo in both ulcerative colitis and Crohn's disease trials. Systematic reviews of the literature in this regard have generally focused on patients with active disease. Much less is known about patients who receive placebo in maintenance trials. Furthermore, these trials are more difficult to interpret because many studies allowed all patients to be on some form of therapy with or without the medication under study. The discussion in this chapter will therefore focus predominantly on trials of therapies for active IBD.

CROHN'S DISEASE

One major difficulty in interpreting the placebo outcomes in randomized controlled trials for IBD is the variability in the definition of outcomes among studies. In trials for Crohn's disease, the Crohn's Disease Activity Index (CDAI) is the most commonly employed disease activity measure.[3] This measure incorporates both objective and subjective measures of disease activity. The summary score can range from 0 to approximately 600 with higher scores reflecting more severe disease. A CDAI of less than 150 is generally used to define remission, and a decrease of more than 70 or 100 points is often used to define a clinical response.

Meyers and Janowitz reviewed the outcomes of patients receiving placebo for active Crohn's disease in 3 early clinical trials.[4] Their qualitative review highlighted several important observations. First, some patients treated with placebo will enter clinical remission. They noted that remission rates were relatively similar in the National Cooperative Crohn's Disease Study (NCCDS) (26% at 17

weeks)[5] and the European Cooperative Crohn's Disease Study (ECCDS) (42% at 100 days).[6] In addition, Meyers and Janowitz noted that there were a few features that seemed to identify which patients treated with placebo were more likely to improve. In the NCCDS study, patients not previously treated with steroids, with lower initial CDAI scores, with postsurgical recurrence, and without perianal disease appeared to fare better.[5] In the ECCDS, patients treated with placebo were more likely to enter remission if they had not received prior therapy for Crohn's disease or if they had small bowel disease.[6]

More recently, we examined the outcome of patients randomized to placebo in a systematic review and meta-analysis.[7] Our meta-analysis included 23 studies that used the CDAI to measure disease activity. All studies were randomized controlled trials of therapies for active Crohn's disease. We observed a pooled estimate of remission among placebo-treated patients of 18%, although there was wide variability between studies. The median remission rate was 19% with a range from 0% to 50%. The pooled estimate of placebo response was 19%, with similarly wide variability among studies (range, 0%-46%).

Several factors were identified that appeared to contribute to the remission rate among placebo-treated patients (Table 2-1). The most important factor appeared to be the study duration. The pooled estimate of the remission rate was 12% for studies less than 2 months in duration, 19% for studies 2 to 4 months in duration, and 32% for studies more than 4 months in duration. Other factors that were also positively associated with remission included increasing number of study visits and lower CDAI scores at entry into the study. The positive association between the placebo remission rate and duration of follow-up was unlikely a sustaining phenomenon over time. Few placebo, randomized controlled trials provided outcomes at multiple time points beyond 4 months. In the NCCDS, 18% and 12% of patients remained in remission on placebo therapy at 1 year and 2 years, respectively.[5] Similar findings were reported in

TABLE 2-2

SUMMARY OF PLACEBO OUTCOMES IN PUBLISHED META-ANALYSES OF CLINICAL TRIALS FOR ACTIVE ULCERATIVE COLITIS

STUDIES	REMISSION			RESPONSE		
	CLINICAL	ENDOSCOPIC	HISTOLOGIC	CLINICAL	ENDOSCOPIC	HISTOLOGIC
Su[7]	13%	18%	8%	28%	–	–
Sutherland[15]	–	–	–	21.6%	–	–
Kornbluth[16]	–	–	–	31.4%	–	–
Ilnyckyj[18]	9.1%	13.5%	8.6%	26.7%	30.3%	25.2%

ECCDS, where the remission rates among placebo-treated patients were 18% at 300 days and 9% at 700 days.[6]

We also examined factors associated with a clinical response among the placebo-treated patients. In general, the relationship between factors present at randomization and the probability of response were the same as those that were associated with remission. The major exception was that patients with a higher CDAI score at entry appeared more likely to have a response and less likely to achieve remission.

Both of the systematic reviews described above focused on clinical factors. Several investigators have also looked at biochemical predictors of outcome among placebo-treated patients. C-reactive protein (CRP) levels have been the most widely studied. Will and colleagues performed a pooled analysis of response to placebo therapy using primary data from 13 clinical trials.[8] In both acute disease and maintenance trials, mean CRP levels at randomization were lower in placebo responders than non-responders. In another trial, Schreiber et al demonstrated a strongly negative correlation between baseline CRP levels and the placebo response rate, providing further evidence that CRP levels are related to outcomes among placebo-treated patients.[9]

There are several potential explanations for the relation between CRP levels and outcomes among placebo-treated patients. Despite symptoms suggestive of active Crohn's disease, some patients with low CRP likely do not have active disease despite an elevated CDAI score. For example, some patients may have concomitant irritable bowel syndrome (IBS). The natural history of IBS would project that some patients would have improved symptoms over the time course of a study.[10,11] Alternatively, patients with a low CRP may represent those with milder Crohn's disease.[12-14] This population may be more likely to experience spontaneous improvement in their disease.

ULCERATIVE COLITIS

A few investigators have also explored the outcomes of patients treated with placebo in ulcerative colitis trials (Table 2-2). Sutherland and colleagues performed a meta-analysis of randomized clinical trials of sulfasalazine and mesalamine for ulcerative colitis. From among 8 clinical trials for active disease, the median placebo response rate was 21.6%.[15] In reviews of the early literature on placebo-controlled trials for active ulcerative colitis, clinical response was reported in a mean of approximately 32% of patients.[16,17] Ilnyckyj et al subsequently performed a systematic review of placebo-controlled trials for active ulcerative colitis that included 38 studies.[18] In these studies, the pooled estimates of response were 9.1% for clinical remission, 26.7% for clinical response, 13.5% for endoscopic remission, 30.3% for endoscopic response, 8.6% for histological remission, and 25.2% for histological improvement. These investigators noted that placebo-treated patients with 3 or more study visits had higher rates of clinical response, endoscopic remission, and histological remission but not clinical remission. They did not observe differences in remission or response rates according to the route of administration of the drug, type of drug, or duration of treatment.

We have also examined this question by performing a meta-analysis of 22 studies that examined the remission rate in active treatment studies.[19] In our analysis, the pooled estimate of remission rate was 13%. Secondary analyses were also performed limiting the studies using a common metric, the Disease Activity Index[20] or slight modifications of this index. This 12-point scale is widely used in ulcerative colitis clinical trials, although no consensus exists for defining remission. Six studies used a definition of remission of a score less than 3 and 6 used a score of 0 to define remission. The pooled estimate of the placebo remission rate in these studies was 17% and

5%, respectively. Both follow-up duration and number of study visits were positively associated with a final Disease Activity Index score of 0 in the placebo-treated patients, whereas the baseline Disease Activity Index score was negatively associated with the placebo remission rate. The estimated rates of endoscopic and histological remission in placebo-treated patients were 18% and 8%, respectively.

CONCLUSION

There are a wide range of clinical research studies, each bearing respective advantages and limitations. Randomized placebo-controlled trials remain the gold standard for proving efficacy of a new or existing therapy in IBD. Placebo outcomes in published clinical trials for active Crohn's disease varied among studies, with an estimated remission rate of 18%. Study duration and number of study visits appeared to be positively associated with achieving remission in placebo-treated patients, whereas the CDAI scores and CRP levels at study entry were inversely associated with such an outcome. Systematic reviews of placebo outcomes in clinical trials for active ulcerative colitis were hampered by the inconsistency of definition of outcomes. Similar to clinical trials for active Crohn's disease, the number of study visits, study duration, and baseline disease severity have all been identified to influence the remission rate in placebo-treated groups. Further studies are clearly necessary to examine factors, both clinical and biochemical, influencing the placebo outcomes in clinical trials for active and quiescent IBD.

REFERENCES

1. Shapiro AK. Factors contributing to the placebo effect. *Am J Psychother.* 1961;18:73-88.

2. Hrobjartsson A, Gotzsche PC. Is the placebo powerless? An analysis of clinical trials comparing placebo with no treatment. [erratum appears in *N Engl J Med.* 2001;345:304]. *N Engl J Med.* 2001;344:1594-1602.

3. Best WR, Becktel JM, Singleton JW, Kern F Jr. Development of a Crohn's disease activity index. National Cooperative Crohn's Disease Study. *Gastroenterology.* 1976;70:439-444.

4. Meyers S, Janowitz HD. "Natural history" of Crohn's disease. An analytic review of the placebo lesson. *Gastroenterology.* 1984;87:1189-1192.

5. Summers RW, Switz DM, Sessions JT Jr, et al. National Cooperative Crohn's Disease Study: results of drug treatment. *Gastroenterology.* 1979;77:847-869.

6. Malchow H, Ewe K, Brandes JW, et al. European Cooperative Crohn's Disease Study (ECCDS): results of drug treatment. *Gastroenterology.* 1984;86:249-266.

7. Su C, Lichtenstein GR, Krok K, Brensinger CM, Lewis JD. A meta-analysis of the placebo rates of remission and response in clinical trials of active Crohn's disease. *Gastroenterology.* 2004;126:1257-1269.

8. Will M, Nikolaus S, Freitag S, Arpe N, Krawczak M, Schreiber S. Placebo response in the therapy of Crohn's disease: A comprehensive analysis of primary data from 733 patients from 13 randomized controlled trials. *Gastroenterology.* 2005;128:A-48.

9. Schreiber S, Rutgeerts P, Fedorak RN, et al. Certolizumab pegol (CDP870) appears effective and is well tolerated in Crohn's disease: A randomized, placebo-controlled trial. *Gastroenterology.* 2005;129:807-818.

10. Camilleri M, Northcutt AR, Kong S, Dukes GE, McSorley D, Mangel AW. Efficacy and safety of alosetron in women with irritable bowel syndrome: A randomised, placebo-controlled trial. *Lancet.* 2000;355:1035-1040.

11. Camilleri M, Chey WY, Mayer EA, et al. A randomized controlled clinical trial of the serotonin type 3 receptor antagonist alosetron in women with diarrhea-predominant irritable bowel syndrome. *Arch Intern Med.* 2001;161:1733-1740.

12. Fagan EA, Dyck RF, Maton PN, et al. Serum levels of C-reactive protein in Crohn's disease and ulcerative colitis. *Eur Clin Invest.* 1982;12:351-359.

13. Chambers RE, Stross P, Barry RE, Whicher JT. Serum amyloid A protein compared with C-reactive protein, alpha 1-antichymotrypsin and alpha 1-acid glycoprotein as a monitor of inflammatory bowel disease. *Eur Clin Invest.* 1987;17:460-467.

14. Solem CA, Loftus EV, Tremaine WJ, Harmsen S, Zinsmeister AR, Sandborn WJ. Correlation of C-reactive protein (CRP) with clinical, radiographic, and endoscopic activity in inflammatory bowel disease. *Gastroenterology.* 2004;126:A-477.

15. Sutherland LR, May GR, Shaffer EA. Sulfasalazine revisited: a meta-analysis of 5-aminosalicylic acid in the treatment of ulcerative colitis. *Ann of Intern Med.* 1993;118:540-549.

16. Kornbluth AA, Salomon P, Sacks HS, Mitty R, Janowitz HD. Meta-analysis of the effectiveness of current drug therapy of ulcerative colitis. *J Clin Gastroenterol.* 1993;16:215-218.

17. Meyers S, Janowitz HD. The "natural history" of ulcerative colitis: an analysis of the placebo response. *J Clin Gastroenterol.* 1989;11:33-37.

18. Ilnyckyj A, Shanahan F, Anton PA, Cheang M, Bernstein CN. Quantification of the placebo response in ulcerative colitis. *Gastroenterology.* 1997;112:1854-1858.

19. Su C, Lewis J, Goldberg B, Brensinger C, Lichtenstein G. A meta-analysis of the placebo rates of remission and response in clinical trials of active ulcerative colitis. *Gastroenterology.* 2007;132:516-526.

20. Sutherland LR, Martin F. 5-Aminosalicylic acid enemas in treatment of distal ulcerative colitis and proctitis in Canada. *Dig Dis Sci.* 1987;32:64S-66S.

THE ROLE OF THE FDA IN DRUG DEVELOPMENT IN INFLAMMATORY BOWEL DISEASE

Alan C. Moss, MD and Adam Cheifetz, MD

Inflammatory bowel disease (IBD) affects approximately 1 million individuals in the United States and 4 million people worldwide, the majority of whom are prescribed medication for induction or maintenance of remission. At any point in time, more than 75% of patients with IBD are taking prescription medication, which is 3 times higher than the non-IBD population.[1] In addition to standard therapies, developments in molecular biology have identified many novel therapeutic targets that will add to the patient's options. Currently, 24 new drugs are registered in development for ulcerative colitis, and 36 for Crohn's disease, in the United States.[2] As a consequence, the market for drugs for IBD patients is valued at $1 to $2 billion in the United States, a number that is expected to rise with increasing use of biologics.[3] The Food and Drug Administration (FDA) has the responsibility to ensure the safety and efficacy of all drugs used in the "cure, mitigation, treatment, or prevention of disease in man." In IBD, a major role for the FDA is its assessment of new therapeutic agents as they navigate the drug development pipeline.

A BRIEF HISTORY OF THE FDA

The FDA has the broad oversight responsibility for all medical products in the United States.[4] Its legislative basis originated in the Federal Food, Drug and Cosmetic Act of 1938, which required that new drugs be tested for safety before they could be marketed and the results submitted to the FDA. This act arose out of the sulfanilamide elixir disaster of 1937, when more than 100 people died from poisoning by diethylene glycol contained in the elixir. The FDA's role was further expanded with the Kefauver-Harris Amendments in 1962, after the harmful effects of thalidomide on the fetus became known. These amendments required drug manufacturers to prove to the FDA that their products were both safe *and* effective prior to marketing. They also included control over prescription drug advertising and the requirement of informed consent for clinical trials. Biologic agents, medical products derived from living sources, came under the FDA's control in 1972 and later the Center for Biologics Evaluation and Research (CBER).

The Prescription Drug User Fee Act (PDUFA) of 1992 authorized the FDA to levy user fees on manufacturers who submit applications to the agency. This is a method of funding additional staff positions from fees collected directly from drug companies, in order to reduce new drug approval times. The Food and Drug Administration Modernization Act of 1997 expanded the legislation to include accelerated review of drugs and medical devices, as well as regulation of advertising of unapproved uses (off-label) of approved drugs. In 2003, the FDA transferred jurisdiction of many biologics, including monoclonal antibodies, cytokines, novel proteins, immunomodulators, and growth factors, to the Center for Drug Evaluation and Research (CDER), which regulates the approval process for most drugs. CBER maintained jurisdiction over other biologics, such as vaccines, blood products, and gene therapy.

Lichtenstein GR, ed.
Crohn's Disease: The Complete Guide to Medical Management (pp 31-38).
© 2011 SLACK Incorporated

TABLE 3-1

CENTERS OF THE FOOD AND DRUG ADMINISTRATION PERTINENT TO MEDICAL THERAPY

	CENTER	RESPONSIBILITY FOR
CDER	Center for Drug Evaluation & Research	Drugs, biologics
CBER	Center for Biologics Evaluation & Research	Vaccines, blood, gene therapy
CDRH	Center for Devices & Radiological Health	Medical devices
NCTR	National Center for Toxicological Research	Toxicology research
ORA	Office of Regulatory Affairs	Enforcement

FDA ORGANIZATION

The FDA is supervised by the Commissioner of Food and Drugs, who is appointed by the president of the United States. The Office of the Commissioner (OC) oversees all the agency's workings and is responsible for implementing the FDA's mission. There are 7 centers within the FDA, each with a different product responsibility (Table 3-1). The CDER has oversight for all drugs and most biologic therapeutic products. CDER is responsible for regulating the manufacturing, labeling, and advertising of drug products. Its main objective is to ensure "safe and effective agents are available to improve the health of consumers."[4] The CDER has 4 functional areas: new drug development and review, post-market drug surveillance, generic drug review, and over-the-counter drug review. New drug development constitutes a major function of the CDER, as it takes approximately 8 years to study and test a new drug before it is approved for use by the public.

FDA PROCESS OF DRUG APPROVAL

The Code of Federal Regulations governs the supervision of new drug development by the FDA. There are 3 key stages: an investigational new drug application, a new drug application, and postmarketing surveillance. This process (Figure 3-1) starts with the filing of an Investigational New Drug (IND) application, a requirement before any clinical trials can take place in humans.[5] The IND is not an application for marketing approval but actually a request for an exemption from the federal statute that prohibits an unapproved drug from being shipped in interstate commerce. Commercial INDs are applications that are submitted primarily by companies whose ultimate goal is to obtain marketing approval for a new product. However, the vast majority of INDs are in fact filed for noncommercial research, including Investigator INDs for research

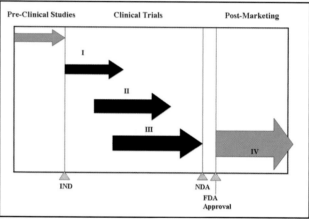

FIGURE 3-1. Overview of drug development process in relation to Food and Drug Administration (FDA) requirements.

proposals and Emergency Use INDs and Treatment INDs in cases where no other treatments are available for a condition. Once the IND application has been approved, the drug sponsor can undertake clinical trials in humans. This clinical studies process typically takes months to years to complete and involves hundreds to thousands of patients (Table 3-2). At its completion, the drug sponsor can submit a New Drug Application (NDA) to the FDA. Once the division director for that therapeutic area signs an approval action letter, the product can be legally marketed starting that day in the United States.

PRECLINICAL TESTING

Prior to submission of a commercial IND, the sponsor will have compiled evidence of extensive preclinical testing in vitro and in vivo in animals to test the safety of any potential therapeutic agent. The FDA requires a minimum information profile on the drug's pharmacological profile (pharmacokinetics and pharmacodynamics), acute toxicity in at least 2 animal species, and short-term toxicity studies from 2 weeks to 3 months' duration.[6] Genotoxicity (DNA mutations) screening is performed, as well as investigations

TABLE 3-2

PHASES OF DRUG TESTING REQUIRED FOR FDA ASSESSMENT*

PHASE	PARTICIPANTS	PURPOSE	TIMELINE (APPROX)
Preclinical	Cell lines	Pharmacokinetics	18 months
	≥2 Animal models	Pharmacodynamics	1 to 3 years
		Toxicology	
I	<100 Healthy volunteers	Safety	12 to 18 months
		Dose escalation	
		Pharmacokinetics	
II	<500 Affected patients & controls in trial setting	Safety	1 to 2 years
		Effectiveness	
III	100s to 1000s of affected patients and controls in trial setting	Safety	~3 years
		Effectiveness	
		Dosing	
IV	1000s of affected patients in actual practice setting (after FDA approval)	Safety	Indefinite
		Long-term effects	
		Expanded variety of recipients	

*FDA indicates Food and Drug Administration.

on drug absorption and metabolism, the toxicity of the drug's metabolites, and the speed with which the drug and its metabolites are excreted from the body.[7] This process can take up to 3 years, but in most cases it can be completed in 18 months. With some agents, long-term animal studies may continue in parallel with human clinical trials, particularly if the drug is to be used for chronic or recurrent conditions. A sponsor can also demonstrate that a drug is safe by providing data from previous clinical testing or marketing of the drug in the United States or another country. The FDA encourages meetings with the sponsor at this stage to review plans for further testing.

Comprehensive preclinical testing alone does not entirely predict safety of new agents in humans. The starkest example of this was with the drug TGN1412, a monoclonal antibody against the CD28 receptor in T-cells approved by the European Medicines Agency in 2005. TGN1412's role as an activator of regulatory T-cells would have made it attractive for IBD studies. Although preclinical testing in macaques caused mild lymphadenopathy, phase I studies in healthy human volunteers caused multi-organ failure in 4 subjects within hours of receiving the drug by infusion.[8] Systemic allergic reactions such as these are difficult to predict in preclinical models. A study of more than 400 new drugs identified 14 that elicited systemic hypersensi-

tivity in guinea pigs in preclinical testing, of which only 3 caused immune-related adverse reactions in humans.[9] Similarly, preclinical studies of immunosuppressive effects are limited to conventional measurements of myelosuppression, or increased incidence of tumors or infections in animal models.[6] These studies may not detect functional alterations in immune function not apparent in morphological testing, which involves immune function testing as required by European regulators.[10]

INVESTIGATIONAL NEW DRUG APPLICATION

Once the preclinical data collection is completed, the sponsor submits an IND application, which includes manufacturing information, pharmacological data, and toxicology results. The manufacturing data detail production processes to ensure consistent and untainted drug product. The sponsor also provides names of the principal investigators (PIs) who will undertake the clinical trials if the IND is approved. Once the IND is received by the FDA, it has 30 days in which to notify the sponsor of concerns that may lead it to place a "hold" on the process or permit the sponsor to proceed with clinical trials while addressing deficiencies in the IND. If the sponsor receives no communication from the FDA, it can proceed with the proposed clinical trials at the end of the 30-day period.

CLINICAL TRIALS

The process of organizing clinical trials, recruiting healthy volunteers and patients, and compiling outcomes constitutes the most expensive and time-consuming component of the FDA approval process. Each center that intends to recruit participants will be headed by a PI, who has responsibility for ensuring that the study has local institutional review board (IRB) approval and that the safety and rights of participants are protected during the clinical trial.[11] The PIs must maintain adequate records and submit timely reports that contain relevant features of enrolled patients, outcomes, and adverse events during the study process. The local IRB is mandated by the federal Office of Human Research Protection to oversee the implementation of the trial in a manner that protects the safety, rights, and privacy of participants. The IRB reviews reports of adverse events, as well as reports from the data and safety monitoring committee for each study, to decide whether the study may continue based on interim safety reports. Once the IRB approves the design and implementation of a study and its consent form, the investigator may recruit patients. In practice, industry-sponsored trials for new agents, such as biologics, will often involve contract research organizations to assist the investigator in compliance with local and federal regulations pertinent to clinical trials.

PHASE I STUDIES

The purpose of phase I studies is to determine a drug's safety and side effects at different doses. This involves pharmacokinetics, metabolism and excretion, and toxicity by administering the agent starting at subclinical doses in healthy human volunteers. Typically, up to 100 volunteers are recruited over 6 to 18 months until sufficient pharmacological data are available to plan valid phase II studies. Occasionally, phase I studies may involve those with advanced malignancies for whom no other therapies are available. Only about 70% of all INDs proceed from phase I to phase II studies.[12]

PHASE II STUDIES

The next step in the development process assesses the drug's efficacy and safety in a well-defined cohort of patients with the disease of interest. This may include open trials (IIA) followed by randomized controlled trials (IIB) or randomized trials alone. The primary aim here is proof-of-concept that the drug is effective in treating a specific illness. A few hundred patients with strict eligibility criteria are enrolled and followed over a few years, usually at least 2 years. Further evidence of safety is also obtained from these studies, as a larger number of participants are involved, and adverse events particular to patients with the disease of interest may be highlighted. If the efficacy and safety data from a phase II trial are positive and robust,

the next step is a large, expensive phase III study. Examples of phase II trials include the original infliximab trial in Crohn's disease, the CLASSIC trial of adalimumab, and the anti-interleukin-12 and ustekinumab trials.[13,14]

PHASE III STUDIES

These are the pivotal, large randomized controlled trials that validate the results of phase II studies and further assess safety and dosing schedules in a defined population with the disease and controls. Most such studies include hundreds or thousands of patients over a number of years and contain sufficient statistical power to detect differences between the agent and placebo. The results from phase III studies are the cornerstone of a sponsor's NDA to the FDA and are the basis of the prescribing and package insert information if the drug is approved for marketing. Only about 30% of INDs submitted will complete phase III studies.[12] Examples of phase III include the ACCENT, CHARM, PRECISE, ENACT-1, and ENACT-2 trials.[15-18]

NEW DRUG APPLICATION

The endpoint of this massive undertaking is the accumulation of sufficient data to submit an application to the FDA for approval to market the drug. The NDA includes a comprehensive evaluation of the drug's characteristics, including physical composition, manufacturing process, pharmacological effects, toxicology, clinical efficacy, and case report data. Such case reports are required for all study participants. The NDA is reviewed by CDER expert panels in each of the areas of interest, and external advisory committees (FDA Advisory Committees) provide further input. In recent years, the composition and potential conflicts of interest of these committees has been the subject of scrutiny, particularly in light of cardiovascular safety concerns with the coxibs.[19]

The key questions the FDA has to answer are:

1. Is this drug effective in treating the condition it purports to treat?

2. Do the results support an acceptable benefit-to-risk ratio?

The FDA's evaluation may include inspection of the manufacturing facilities and clinical trial sites to verify the details in the submitted application. If the information supplied by the sponsor is insufficient to answer these questions, then further data are sought. The FDA is required to provide an interim evaluation within 6 months, and the average time to final decision is around 24 months. During this time, the FDA is in regular contact with the drug's sponsor to ensure that all additional information (or data) required by the expert panels is provided. The final decision of the CDER panel is either "approval," "approvable with minor changes," or "not approvable." The majority of NDAs are approved, allowing the sponsor to begin manufacturing and distribution. Those considered not approvable can request an appeal hearing or retract the application and re-apply with adjustments.

POSTMARKETING SURVEILLANCE

Once an agent is approved for general use, it is really the first time it is tested in individuals who were ineligible for controlled trials, which may include women of child-bearing age, children, the elderly, and patients with comorbid conditions. Ironically, the elderly, who constitute about 70% of medication recipients, only make up about 30% of clinical trial participants. In addition, the numbers of people exposed to the drug expands significantly beyond the confines of clinical studies to general practice. As a consequence, rare side effects or adverse events in special situations and long-term morbidity may only become apparent at this point. The CDER's Office of Drug Safety (ODS) thus monitors a drug's safety profile even after it has been approved for use. This is undertaken via a requirement of pharmaceutical companies to report all adverse events associated with a new drug and the voluntary system of reporting by health-care workers (MedWatch). The ODS is responsible for updating labeling, public notification of new risks, implementing risk management programs, and (rarely) drug withdrawal. So-called phase IV studies incorporate such postmarketing surveillance. For example, the risk of progressive multifocal leukoencephalopathy (PML) was detected during postmarketing surveillance of natalizumab in 1 patient with Crohn's disease and 2 with multiple sclerosis.[20] This led the sponsors to voluntarily withdraw the drug for a period of time, although it was eventually brought back to the market for multiple sclerosis with certain stipulations.

Similarly, an increased number of cases of tuberculosis (TB) were identified with early use of infliximab through MedWatch.[21] More recently, histoplasmosis and lymphomas have been recognized with both infliximab and adalimumab.[22,23] Such instances may lead the FDA to revise a drug's package inserts, warn the public and health-care providers, or (rarely) withdraw approval of a drug. The postmarketing surveillance "net" has its flaws also, as it is dependent on either health-care providers or pharmaceutical companies to notify the FDA of adverse events.

Though the Prescription Drug User Fee Act (PDUFA) deadlines have favorably changed approval decisions of the FDA, discovery of unanticipated postmarketing safety problems is more likely to occur among drugs approved immediately before a deadline. Relying more on increased staffing and less on deadlines may result in greater efficiency without increasing cost and the risk of postmarketing drug safety problems.[24] The renewal and reauthorization of PDUFA may improve the way FDA regulation responds to the risk and benefits of drugs and may allow Congress to provide increased funding for postapproval drug safety.[25]

ALTERNATIVE PATHWAYS

The process outlined above is obviously a time-consuming and expensive process; the estimated time for development of a new drug is 15 years and $900 million from drug discovery to market launch.[26] There are many cases where such an undertaking may impede access to potential therapy for life-threatening conditions or be commercially unattractive for rare diseases. A number of pathways exist in such circumstances, but those that are relevant to IBD include the following.

ORPHAN DRUGS

A condition that affects less than 200,000 patients in the United States, or one whose prevalence exceeds 200,000 but there is "no reasonable expectation" that the costs of developing and making the drug available will be recovered from sales in the United States, is considered a rare disease.[27] In these circumstances, drugs used to treat these diseases are called *orphan drugs*, and their development is promoted by tax incentives, FDA assistance in study design, phase I/II funding, and 7 years of marketing exclusivity. More than 200 such agents have been approved, and a number of agents used in IBD have received FDA grant funding from this program, including infliximab, rifabutin, and 4-aminosalicylic acid.[28] A number of biotech companies have specialized in such markets.

TREATMENT IND

A treatment IND allows expanded access to promising drugs in serious or life-threatening diseases where there is preliminary evidence of efficacy or diseases where no comparable treatment exists. This was originally developed for new cancer agents in the 1970s but later became prominent in the treatment of acquired immunodeficiency syndrome (AIDS) in the 1980s. The sponsor still has to seek IRB approval, and the recipient may be charged by the sponsor for the costs of the agent with the FDA's knowledge.

ACCELERATED REVIEW

Accelerated review process was introduced in 1992 to expedite development of promising agents for serious or life-threatening diseases without existing treatments. In this situation, the FDA can grant approval of a drug based on a surrogate endpoint that predicted therapeutic benefit, rather than "hard" endpoints such as survival. Once approved, the sponsor must continue postmarketing studies to confirm the safety and efficacy using clinical endpoints. An example would be reduction in C-reactive protein (CRP), or improved endoscopic appearance, rather than long-term remission rates. Natalizumab was initially approved for multiple sclerosis in this manner in 2004.

CURRENT ISSUES IN DRUG DEVELOPMENT IN IBD

The drug development process is a major undertaking for any drug sponsor. Challenges exist in providing safe, effective, and affordable therapies to patients with IBD in a timely manner, as the regulatory and clinical research environment becomes more complex.[29] For clinicians and hospitals enrolling patients, and their IRBs, the increasing emphasis on training and regulatory compliance places a significant time burden on research-associated staff.[30] The FDA expects principal investigators to personally supervise the trials for which they are responsible, in addition to their other clinical and research responsibilities. The increasing number of trainees opting for private practice rather than academic medicine has limited the number of gastroenterologists willing or able to undertake the mantle of PI for clinical trials.[31] For the FDA, there are opposing pressures to approve therapies as rapidly as possible, while comprehensively assessing for potential adverse effects and protecting the public.

In IBD, there are a number of issues in the drug development process that present challenges. We have yet to see agents that incorporate advances in genomic medicine into effective therapies for CD or UC. The majority of agents in development target late events in the inflammatory cascade, as a consequence of our lack of understanding of the key factors that "trigger" the process in susceptible individuals. A number of disease phenotypes, such as pouchitis, irritable pouch syndrome, prevention of postoperative CD, perianal disease, and structuring disease would benefit from targeted therapies beyond conventional agents. The heterogeneous nature of patients with IBD and the wide variation of some clinical markers such as the Crohn's Disease Activity Index (CDAI) have invariably produced high placebo response rates in clinical trials in CD. More objective, minimally invasive markers of disease activity would strengthen the statistical analysis in phase II and III trials in patients with IBD. Finally, the many exclusion criteria of sponsored trials have limited the numbers of eligible patients, leading to increased recruitment in South America and Eastern Europe for these studies. The ethical issues arising from clinical trials in settings where other therapeutic options are limited for financial or supply reasons are complex.

The past 10 years have seen a major expansion in the available biologic agents to treat active IBD, agents whose mechanism of action we still, in some cases, do not understand and that have been associated with rare but serious adverse effects. The current FDA system is effective at requiring sponsors to provide evidence of safety in a contained setting and superiority to placebo but has limitations in terms of rare side effects and the effects in a variety of patient phenotypes. This knowledge should encourage physicians treating patients with IBD to be vigilant as these agents reach their patient population, while taking advantage of their efficacy.

REFERENCES

1. Longobardi T, Jacobs P, Bernstein CN. Utilization of health care resources by individuals with inflammatory bowel disease in the United States: a profile of time since diagnosis. *Am J Gastroenterol.* 2004;99:650-655.

2. The Pharmaceutical Research and Manufacturers of America. New medicines database. 2007. Available at: http://www.phrma.org/medicines_in_development. Accessed November 1, 2010.

3. Lead Discovery. Emerging treatments for inflammatory bowel disease (IBD). 2005. Available at: http://www.leaddiscovery.co.uk/PharmaReport%20Alert-Emerging%20treatments%20for%20inflammatory%20bowel%20disease%20(IBD).html#feature. Accessed May 21, 2007.

4. Center for Drug Evaluation and Research. A brief history of the Center for Drug Evaluation and Research. 2007. Available at: http://www.fda.gov/AboutFDA/WhatWeDo/History/FOrgsHistory/CDER/default.htm. Accessed November 1, 2010.

5. Meadows M. The FDA's drug review process: Ensuring drugs are safe and effective. *FDA Consum.* 2002;36:19-24.

6. Center for Drug Evaluation and Research. *Immunotoxicology Evaluation of Investigational New Drugs.* US Department of Health and Human Services, Food and Drug Administration; 2002.

7. Lesko LJ, Salerno RA, Spear BB, et al. Pharmacogenetics and pharmacogenomics in drug development and regulatory decision making: report of the first FDA-PWG-PhRMA-DruSafe Workshop. *J Clin Pharmacol.* 2003;43:342-358.

8. Suntharalingam G, Perry MR, Ward S, et al. Cytokine storm in a phase 1 trial of the anti-CD28 monoclonal antibody TGN1412. *N Engl J Med.* 2006;355:1018-1028.

9. Weaver JL, Staten D, Swann J, Armstrong G, Bates M, Hastings KL. Detection of systemic hypersensitivity to drugs using standard guinea pig assays. *Toxicology.* 2003;193:203-217.

10. Vos JG, Van Loveren H. Markers for immunotoxic effects in rodents and man. *Toxicol Lett.* 1995;82-83:385-394.

11. Department of Health and Human Services. *The CDER Handbook.* 2007. Available at: http://www.fda.gov/downloads/AboutFDA/CentersOffices/CDER/UCM198415.pdf. Accessed November 1, 2010.

12. Flieger K. FDA finds new ways to speed treatment to patients. *FDA Consum.* 1993;27:14-18.

13. Mannon PJ, Fuss IJ, Mayer L, et al. Anti-interleukin-12 antibody for active Crohn's disease. *N Engl J Med.* 2004;351:2069-2079.

14. Sandborn WJ, Feagan BG, Fedorak RN, et al. A randomized trial of ustekinumab, a human interleukin-12/23 monoclonal antibody, in patients with moderate-to-severe Crohn's disease. *Gastroenterology.* 2008;135:1130-1141.

15. Hanauer SB, Feagan BG, Lichtenstein GR, et al. Maintenance infliximab for Crohn's disease: the ACCENT I randomised trial. *Lancet.* 2002;359:1541-1549.

16. Colombel JF, Sandborn WJ, Rutgeerts P, et al. Adalimumab for maintenance of clinical response and remission in patients with Crohn's disease: the CHARM trial. *Gastroenterology.* 2007;132:52-65.

17. Schreiber S, Khaliq-Kareemi M, Lawrance IC, et al. Maintenance therapy with certolizumab pegol for Crohn's disease. *N Engl J Med.* 2007;357:239-250.

18. Sandborn WJ, Colombel JF, Enns R, et al. Natalizumab induction and maintenance therapy for Crohn's disease. *N Engl J Med.* 2005;353:1912-1925.

19. Okie S. Raising the safety bar—the FDA's coxib meeting. *N Engl J Med.* 2005;352:1283-1285.

20. Van Assche G, Van Ranst M, Sciot R, et al. Progressive multifocal leukoencephalopathy after natalizumab therapy for Crohn's disease. *N Engl J Med.* 2005;353:362-368.

21. Keane J, Gershon S, Wise RP, et al. Tuberculosis associated with infliximab, a tumor necrosis factor alpha-neutralizing agent. *N Engl J Med.* 2001;345:1098-1104.

22. Infliximab [package insert]. Malvern, PA: Centocor, Inc; 2008.

23. Adalimumab [package insert]. Abbott Park, IL: Abbott Laboratories; 2008.

24. Carpenter D, Zucker EJ, Avorn J. Drug-review deadlines and safety problems. *N Engl J Med.* 2008;358:1354-1361.

25. Hennessy S, Strom BL. PDUFA reauthorization—drug safety's golden moment of opportunity? *N Engl J Med.* 2007;356:1703-1704.

26. DiMasi JA, Hansen RW, Grabowski HG. The price of innovation: new estimates of drug development costs. *J Health Econ.* 2003; 22:151-185.

27. Department of Health and Human Services. Orphan drugs. 2007. Available at: http://www.fda.gov/cder/handbook/orphan.htm. Accessed

28. Office of Orphan Products Development. Orphan Products Grants Program. 2007. Available at: http://www.fda.gov/orphan/grants/previous.htm. Accessed November 1, 2010.

29. DeMets D, Califf R, Dixon D, et al. Issues in regulatory guidelines for data monitoring committees. *Clin Trials.* 2004;1:162-169.

30. Department of Health and Human Services. *Institutional Review Boards: A Time for Reform.* Washington, DC. 1998.

31. Hanauer SB. Another one bites the dust. *Nat Clin Pract Gastroenterol Hepatol.* 2005;2:435.

UTILITY OF ANIMAL MODELS FOR THE STUDY AND TREATMENT OF INFLAMMATORY BOWEL DISEASE

Ashish Chawla, MD and Kenneth Simpson, BVM&S, PhD

Inflammatory bowel disease (IBD) is a chronic inflammatory disorder of the intestine that is characterized by exaggerated adaptive and acquired immune responses. Since the exact pathogenesis of IBD is unknown, murine models of colitis have been developed to investigate disease pathogenesis and novel treatment modalities. These model systems suggest that either an excessive Th1 or Th2 T cell response mediates mucosal inflammation. This dysregulated cytokine response results from defects in peripheral T cell responses and plays a critical role in colitis. The models of murine colitis can be divided up into 5 categories: chemically induced models, immune cell transfer models, colitis due to gene knockout, colitis via introduction of a transgene, and spontaneous colitis models. Each model has unique advantages for studying the pathway of mucosal inflammation. The spontaneous colitis models and gene knockout models have been particularly influential in current human immune therapies. The objective of this review is to give an overview of the colitis models and to highlight potential novel therapies based on specific models. Limitations of each model and applicability towards human disease are also discussed.

IBD develops in approximately 0.1% of the Western population, but the etiology and pathogenesis of the disease is unknown. During the past decade, UC and CD have gained increased importance because of increased incidence and prevalence. Older treatment modalities are largely nonspecific and just alleviate the symptoms without altering the natural history of the disease. Therefore, murine models of colitis have been developed to study the pathogenesis, genetics, and treatment of colitis. These models have increased our knowledge of mucosal inflammation and have led to the development of alternative therapies. In order to better understand murine colitis models, it is first

important to understand the key players in the intestinal immune response.

T CELL DIFFERENTIATION AND THE INTESTINAL IMMUNE SYSTEM

The intestinal mucosa serves as an interface for the interaction of the host with its environment. Due to its large surface area, the intestinal mucosa is constantly exposed to bacterial flora and exogenous antigens. In general, the intestinal immune system displays a state of hypo-responsiveness and "tolerance" towards commensal bacteria and some foreign antigens. Oral tolerance results from a complex interplay between the intestinal immune system and the mucosal flora, such that most mucosal responses are self-limited and do not result in inflammation. This homeostatic balance is functionally disturbed in human IBD. Many components in the intestinal immune response have been evaluated as a source for human IBD. These include T cells, antigen presenting cells (APCs), epithelial cells, and cytokines. Though distinct alterations in these components have been noted in human CD and ulcerative colitis, most evidence suggests that mucosal inflammation is almost always mediated by exaggeration of 1 of 2 pathways: either an excessive T helper 1 (Th1) T cell response or an excessive T helper 2 (Th2) T cell response.

CD4+ T cells are pivotal in mediating and controlling mucosal immune responses. Upon exposure to an antigen, naïve CD4+ T cells can differentiate into 3 distinct subsets of T cells: Th1, Th2, and T regulatory cells (Tr1, Th3, and CD4+ CD25+) (Figure 4-1). These cells can be distinguished from

Lichtenstein GR, ed.
Crohn's Disease: The Complete Guide to Medical Management (pp 39-50).
© 2011 SLACK Incorporated

FIGURE 4-1. Peripheral T cell differentiation. Upon antigen exposure, naïve T cells can differentiate into 3 functionally distinct subsets: T helper 1 (Th1), T helper 2 (Th2), and T regulatory cells. Differentiation to a specific effector type is based on the stimulus and cytokine milieu. The specific cell fate is driven by transcription factors (Tbet, GATA-3, and Foxp3), which serve as master regulators of lineage commitment. Th1 type T cells secrete IL-12, interferon gamma (IFN-γ), tumor necrosis factor-α (TNFα), and IL-2, whereas Th2 cells secrete IL-4, IL-5, and IL-13. T regulatory cells can secrete transforming growth factor-β (TGFβ) and/or IL-10.

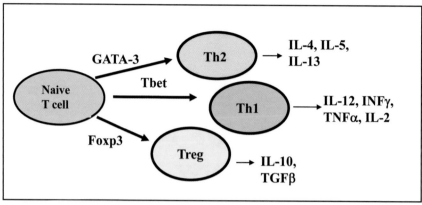

each other based on functional cytokine production, cell surface phenotypes, and survival requirements.[1] The Th1 cells are critical for macrophage activation and help secrete IL-2, IL-12, interferon gamma (IFN-γ), and tumor necrosis factor-α (TNFα). Unlike the Th1 response, Th2-mediated inflammation occurs secondary to IL-4, IL-5, and IL-13. In addition, Th2 responses aid in the production of antibodies. In recent years, it has become evident that there is another set of effector cells involved in post-thymic tolerance. These regulatory T cells are able to suppress responder T cells via the production of transforming growth factor-β (TGF-β), IL-10, or both.[2] One such T regulatory subset (CD4+ CD25+) is present in 5% to 10% of peripheral CD4+ T cells, and elimination of this subset leads to autoimmune diseases in mice (eg, gastritis, colitis, orchitis, and thyroiditis).[3] This balance between Th1/Th2 effector versus T regulatory cell responses plays a key role in the production of mucosal inflammation.

ANIMAL MODELS OF COLITIS

Despite the varying nature and source of inflammation in these models, most murine models of colitis support the notion that IBD results from an inappropriate and exaggerated immune response to normal constituents of intestinal microflora in genetically susceptible hosts. These models can be broadly characterized into 5 groups: chemically induced models, immune cell transfer models, colitis due to gene knockout, colitis via introduction of a transgene, and spontaneous colitis models (Table 4-1).

CHEMICALLY INDUCED COLITIS

Several important murine models utilize the exposure of exogenous chemical (haptenizing) agents in order to instigate colitis. Chemically induced models of colitis are produced by either rectal installation or oral consumption of different agents including trinitrobenzene sulphonic acid (TNBS), oxazolone, and dextran sodium sulfate (DSS).

TNBS COLITIS

Murine colitis due to TNBS installation occurs after destruction of the mucosal barrier with an ethanol enema. The extent of colitis can vary with mouse strain, but some strains develop an acute colitis, which eventually leads to a Th1 mediated chronic colitis. There is transmural inflammation present in the intestine often associated with granulomas, thus mimicking CD. Exposure to TNBS leads to a hapten-induced delayed hypersensitivity reaction with production of IL-12 by macrophages and IFN-γ and IL-2 by lymphocytes.[4] This simple model has been particularly useful in the development and testing of novel therapeutic molecules (including antibodies to IL-12 that abrogate the colitis). Monoclonal antibody neutralization of IL-12/23 via the shared p40 subunit has reversed active colitis in T cell–mediated mouse models.[5] Recently, genome-wide association studies have identified genes that encode a subunit for the receptor of IL-23 in CD.[6] Ustekinumab is a monoclonal antibody against the p40 subunit of IL-12/23 and has induced clinical response in a subgroup of patients with moderate-to-severe CD who are nonresponsive to infliximab.[7]

OXAZOLONE COLITIS

Similar to TNBS colitis, the rectal installation of oxazolone with ethanol has been shown to induce murine colitis.[8] Unlike the TNBS colitis, the colitis induced by oxazolone occurs earlier and is characterized by superficial ulceration and inflammation predominantly localized to the distal colon, features that mimic human ulcerative colitis. Recent studies have shown that oxazolone-induced colitis results from the induction of natural killer T cells (NKT) that produce IL-13 and subsequently IL-4 (Th2-mediated cytokines). In fact, elimination of NKT cells or suppression of IL-13 can prevent the development of colitis. These data suggest that oxazolone colitis is mediated by an excessive Th2 effector response.[9]

The dichotomy of mucosal inflammation (Th1 or Th2) by TNBS and oxazolone-mediated colitis is also suggested

TABLE 4-1

MOUSE MODELS OF IBD*

ANIMAL MODELS	TYPE OF INFLAMMATION	UTILITY TOWARD IBD
CHEMICALLY INDUCED		
TNBS colitis	Chronic Th1 type	Models identify the role of Th1 (Crohn's) versus Th2 (UC) responses in IBD. Useful models for investigation for potential therapies for IBD.
Oxazolone colitis	Chronic Th2 type	
DSS colitis	Superficial acute, Th1/Th2 (chronic)	
IMMUNE TRANSFER		
Adoptive transfer colitis	Chronic Th1 type	Stress the importance of T regulatory cells in prevention and amelioration of IBD. Suggest a role for TGFβ and IL-10 for inhibition of Th1 cytokine response.
GENE KNOCKOUT		
IL-2 KO	Th1/Th2	Gene KO models have identified the specific cytokines important in pathogenesis of IBD. Proof of concept for anti-TNFα therapy for CD. Suggest possible roles for other therapy (anti-IL-6).
IL-10 KO	Th1 early/Th2 late	
TNFα ΔARE mice	Th1, ileocolitis/granulomas	
TCRα KO	Th2 colitis	
Trefoil factor KO	Th1	
TRANSGENIC MODELS		
IL-7 Transgenic	Th2 colitis	Demonstrate role of specific bacteria in development/treatment of colitis. Role of defects in innate immunity (APCs, macrophages, NK cells) in IBD. Exciting as no exogenous manipulation required for development of colitis.
HLA-B27	Th1 colitis	
Myeloid specific STAT3 deficiency	Th1 colitis due to loss of IL-10 signaling	
SPONTANEOUS COLITIS		
C3H/HejBir mice	Th1 colitis	These models have been described to develop colitis and are also prone to developing colonic carcinoma and sclerosing cholangitis.
Cotton top tamarins	Colitis	Histiocytic ulcerative/granulomatous colitis in Boxer dogs represents an inability to kill a subset of resident *Escherichia coli* that selectively exploit a genetically susceptible individual.
Boxer dogs	Granulomatous colitis	First mouse model to demonstrate ileitis with perianal disease and fistulas.
SPONTANEOUS ILEITIS		
SAMP1/Yit	Th1 ileitis	
SAMP1/YitFc	Perianal disease (fistulas)	

*IBD indicates inflammatory bowel disease; TNBS, trinitrobenzene sulphonic acid; Th1, T helper 1; Th2, T helper 2; DSS, dextran sodium sulfate; TGF, transforming growth factor; KO, knockout; TNFα, tumor necrosis factor alpha; ARE, AU-rich element; TCR, T cell antigen receptor; APC, antigen presenting cell; NK, natural killer.

in human IBD. There is considerable evidence that T cells derived from ulcerations in human CD produce IFN-γ and IL-12 (Th1 cytokines) but little evidence exists that T cells from UC lesions produce excess IL-4. However, recent findings support the role of Th2-mediated inflammation in the pathogenesis of ulcerative colitis. The presence of increased levels of autoantibodies and increased secretion of IL-5 and IL-13 seen in UC are both features of Th2-mediated response.[10] Through the development of these 2 mouse models, we have been able to elucidate the inflam-

FIGURE 4-2. Adoptive transfer colitis model.

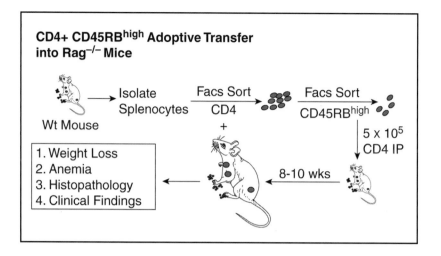

matory mediators (lymphocytes, macrophages, and cytokines) important in chronic colitis. The use of these models also helps demonstrate the differential cytokine response that can be seen in human CD and ulcerative colitis.

DSS COLITIS

Colitis occurs after DSS is dissolved in the water given to mice or rats and leads to progressive weight loss, diarrhea, hematochezia, and shortening of the intestine in a few weeks. The acute colitis results from epithelial disruption, which results in luminal bacterial translocation and subsequent infiltration of neutrophils. This response is induced by the innate immune system, because severe combined immunodeficiency mice (SCID mice, who lack B and T cells) also develop acute colitis upon exposure to DSS.[11] Unlike acute colitis, the chronic colitis seen with DSS is caused by the activation of lymphocytes and release of cytokines (both Th1 and Th2).[12] The DSS colitis model has led to increased understanding in the pathogenic role of activated lymphocytes and the secreted cytokines. Others have used this model to evaluate the role of leukocyte adhesion molecules in the prevention of colitis. Soriano et al demonstrated that blockade of adhesion molecules that prevent leukocyte adhesion and migration on endothelial cells could represent a novel approach to treatment of IBD. This study demonstrated that immunoneutralization of VCAM-1 can lead to amelioration of DSS colitis and possible treatment of human IBD.[13]

LIMITATIONS

Although the chemical colitis models help us understand the pathways of inflammation, a major limitation is that they do not represent the initiating events in human IBD. The models rely on the chemical destruction of the epithelial barrier. This allows for evaluation of the acute colitic process but makes it difficult to analyze chronic colitis. For example, acute DSS colitis occurs in the absence of the acquired immune system (SCID mice that lack lymphocytes). Unlike DSS colitis, human IBD clearly involves a complex interplay between defective T cell and innate immune response to host mucosal antigens.

IMMUNE TRANSFER MODEL OF COLITIS

The adoptive transfer model of colitis results from a change in the number of naïve versus regulatory T cells that are usually required to maintain oral tolerance. This model involves the transfer of CD4$^+$ T cells expressing CD45RB^{high} (naïve) from immunocompetent mice into immunodeficient SCID or Rag$^{-/-}$ mice, resulting in Th1-mediated colitis.[14] The recipient mice develop a chronic and terminal wasting disease, accompanied by anemia and diarrhea within 6 to 8 weeks. The mice generally die after 16 weeks (Figure 4-2). On histopathology, the entire colon is involved with almost complete sparing of the small intestine. During the course of 6 to 8 weeks, the CD4$^+$ CD45RB^{high} T cells expand and proliferate in the peripheral compartment of the recipient mice. These naïve cells are primed and develop into Th1 effector cells via exposure to commensal bacteria in the recipient mice. The pathogenic potential of these cells, which is normally controlled by CD4$^+$ CD45RB^{low} T regulatory lymphocytes, is left unchecked. This allows for T effector cells to proliferate and secrete TNFα and IFN-γ in the lamina propria of the intestine.[15]

The CD4$^+$ CD45RB^{low} T cell pool is composed of T regulatory cells (CD4$^+$ CD25$^+$) and recent thymic emigrants. Transfer of the CD4$^+$ CD45RB^{low} T lymphocytes into immunodeficient mice does not lead to the induction of colitis. In fact, cotransfer of CD4$^+$ CD45RB^{low} with the CD45RB^{high} cells inhibits the development of colitis.[16,17] Recent data also indicate that transfer of CD45RB^{low} cells (CD4$^+$ CD25$^+$) into a mouse with preexisting colitis leads to resolution of both the colitis and the terminal wasting.[18] Interestingly, control of the immune pathology is regulated by the expression of TGF-β. This observation is based on experiments where cotransfer of both CD4+ CD45RB subsets along with intraperineal (IP) injection of anti-TGF-β antibody resulted in the development of colitis.[19] These findings suggest that deficiencies in regulatory T cell responses play a critical role in mucosal inflammation. Whether patients with IBD have underlying defects in regulatory T cells has not been clearly determined. It is known that T cells isolated from patients with IBD can proliferate and produce cytokines in vitro in response to their own microflora (whereas cells from control patients do not). These findings suggest either an excessive effector or defective regulatory T cell response. At present, it is not possible to measure human regulatory T cell response with any degree of confidence. Despite these limitations, it is clear that activation of T regulatory cells could serve as novel therapy for IBD.

LIMITATIONS

The adoptive transfer colitis model highlights the importance of T regulatory cells in the prevention of murine colitis. This model also emphasizes the role of IL-10 and TGF-β for the amelioration of already developed colitis. However, the profound immune abnormalities in the recipient mice (lack of B and T cells) make this model unsuitable for investigating the complex interplay of the acquired immune response in human IBD.

GENE KNOCKOUT MOUSE MODELS OF COLITIS

Gene knockout models of colitis have increased our understanding of IBD and have led to the development of novel therapies (anti-TNFα therapy). Through the deletion of genes critically involved in inflammatory cascade, researchers have been able to dissect the sequence and pathogenesis of chronic intestinal inflammation.

INTERLEUKIN-2 KNOCKOUT/IL-2 RECEPTOR (R) A KNOCKOUT MICE

IL-2 is an indispensable cytokine that is important in the regulation and activation of T cells, macrophages, natural killer cells, and NKT cells. It also plays a key role in B cell differentiation and in the induction of apoptosis of T cells (activation-induced cell death). In 1993, Sadlack et al[20] demonstrated that mice with a disrupted IL-2 gene developed autoimmune hemolytic anemia, lymphadenopathy, and splenomegaly. Half of these mice died at 4 to 9 weeks of age, whereas the rest of the animals developed chronic colitis with inflammation, ulcers, and wall thickening from

cecum to the rectum. The colitis occurred between 6 and 15 weeks and seemed to spare the small intestine. Histology confirmed crypt abscesses, mucin depletion, and dysplasia of epithelial cells, features that are consistent with human IBD.[20] Other studies crossbred the IL-2 knockout mice with deletion of other genes including RAG-2-/-, JH-/-, and β2 microglobulin-/-. These studies confirmed that CD4+ T cells but not B cells or CD8+ T cells were essential for the activation of colitis. Colitis in the IL-2 knockout model is considered secondary to lack of T cell apoptosis and thymic agenesis, which leads to incomplete depletion of activated T cells.[21] Loss of activation-induced cell death may explain the presence of pathogenic T effector cells found in human chronic colitis. In fact, evidence suggests that human IBD is caused by a loss of oral tolerance, which could be caused by defective deletion of pathogenic T cells.

IL-10 KNOCKOUT MICE

IL-10, which is produced by T cells, B cells, macrophages, thymic cells, and keratinocytes, plays a critical role in down-regulating the function of Th1 cells and macrophages. IL-10 knockout mice develop colitis in the entire intestine with significant inflammation in the duodenum, jejunum, and ascending colon. As with the IL-2 knockout mice, the source of inflammation is felt to be secondary to the presence of activated CD4+ Th1 cells and depletion of regulatory T cells.[22] IL-10 knockout mice have also been used to evaluate the role of anti-TNFα antibodies in treatment of murine colitis. IL-10 knockout mice injected intraperitoneally with anti-TNFα antibodies showed significant improvement in inflammation with resolution of diarrhea and bleeding.[23] However, treatment of patients with CD with IL-10 has been more variable. Patients with mild to moderate colitis (not on steroids) had a beneficial effect with subcutaneous IL-10. However, patients with severe CD had clinical improvement in Crohn's disease activity index (CDAI) (decrease to 100 or less) but remission was not seen. A major problem of human IL-10 therapy has been its side effects, including fever, arthralgias, headaches, lymphopenia, and thrombocytopenia.[24] Also, discontinuation of IL-10 therapy results in recurrence of disease.

TNF ΔARE MICE

A large body of data is emerging in regards to the role of TNFα in the pathogenesis of CD. TNFα is an inflammatory cytokine produced by T cells and macrophages. It is secreted in an inactive form and is activated by a metalloproteinase, TNFα-activating enzyme. The TNFα mRNA contains a repeated AU-rich element (ARE) consisting of AUUUA repeats in its 3' untranslated region that is implicated in post-transcriptional and translational regulation of TNFα synthesis. Mice that have a 69 bp deletion of the ARE region (ΔARE) have high circulating levels of TNFα and develop severe wasting syndrome, chronic inflammatory arthritis, and inflammation of the terminal ileum and proximal colon. This phenotype is similar to CD and occurs between 2 and 4 weeks of age.[25] Studies have demonstrated that intestinal inflammation in the ΔARE mouse depends on Th1-type cytokines, IL-12, and IFN-γ and requires the function of CD8+ T cells.[26] Although no mutation in the 3′ AU-rich region of the TNFα gene has been isolated in patients with CD, anti-TNFα therapy has become the mainstay in the treatment of CD. Infliximab, a monoclonal mouse–human chimeric antibody against TNFα, has been shown to improve moderate to severe CD in several randomized control studies. There is a marked improvement in the CDAI and in the endoscopic/histologic appearance in the colitis.[27] This treatment also seems to be effective in patients who have abdominal or perianal fistulas, with 55% of patients having complete closure of the fistula, compared to 13% in the placebo group.[28] In vitro and in vivo, infliximab seems to bind to activated lymphocytes and induce apoptosis resulting in a decrease of pathogenic T cells.[29] Other treatments used in IBD may also act through this mechanism. Sulfasalazine, azathioprine, and thalidomide also induce T cell apoptosis. Thalidomide may reduce chronic inflammation by modifying the intestinal immune response in human IBD. The TNFα ΔARE model of murine colitis has been important in dissecting the pathophysiology of CD and in developing novel therapies.

TCRα KNOCKOUT MICE

Upon deletion of the alpha subunit of the T cell receptor, colitis develops in these mice at 16 weeks. TCRα knockout mice develop hypertrophy and inflammation of the colon from the rectum to cecum, with sparing of the small intestine. The histology of the large intestine demonstrates crypt abscesses with goblet cell depletion and infiltration of plasma cells, lymphocytes, and neutrophils. Interestingly, the mice develop autoantibodies due to polyclonal B cell activation.[30] As colitis is worse in double knockout mice deficient in TCRα and B cells (Igμ-/-), these autoantibodies are presumed to prevent inflammation and promote healing. The inflammation in this model is driven by Th2 immune response due to predominance of IL-4 and IL-5.[31] The pathologic lesions, autoantibodies, and Th2 immune response reflect a UC model. Recent studies suggest that anti-IL-4 antibody inhibits the activation of colitis in TCRα knockout mice, suggesting a possible novel agent for human ulcerative colitis.

TREFOIL FACTOR–DEFICIENT MICE

Intestinal trefoil factors (ITFs) are peptides secreted by mucus cells of the colon and small intestine after inflammation occurs. Mice deficient in ITF develop impaired wound healing and decreased epithelial regeneration. After induction of colitis by addition of DSS, ITF-deficient mice develop severe colitis and die. Addition of ITF has been shown to improve mucosal repair in chemical models of colitis.[32]

LIMITATIONS

Collectively, gene knockout models of murine colitis have helped identify the key components of immune regulation and oral tolerance in the gut. It is unlikely, however, that a single genetic mutation in key cytokines represents the underlying defect in IBD. No single gene defect in key molecules has been observed in the pathogenesis of human IBD. In fact, the most compelling evidence that genetic factors play a key role in the development of IBD comes from the identification of the NOD2 gene, which codes for a protein involved in the recognition of bacteria.[33] Data from two separate studies suggest that NOD2 mutations occur exclusively in patients with CD and not in patients with ulcerative colitis. Patients with heterozygous and homozygous NOD2 gene mutations have an increased relative risk for the development of CD (3-fold vs 38-fold).[34] Mutations in the NOD2 gene do not account for all cases of CD, however, suggesting the complex interplay of genetic predisposition and the mucosal microenvironment in the pathogenesis of IBD. In fact, studies have shown that normal individuals occasionally have NOD2 mutations on both chromosomes in the absence of disease. Also, none of the known mutations have been seen in 483 Japanese patients with CD.[35] These findings support the notion that single-gene knockout models are important but do not represent the causative factors in the development of human IBD.

TRANSGENIC MODELS OF COLITIS

Like knockout models, transgenic murine models result in colitis after genetic manipulation leads to either overexpression of proteins or loss of proteins in specific tissues. These models stress the importance of the loss of homeostasis in the mucosal immune system for the development of colitis. Three models will be discussed in detail, including IL-7 transgenic mice, HLA-B27 transgenic rats, and mice with myeloid-specific STAT 3 deficiency.

IL-7 TRANSGENIC MICE

IL-7 is derived from epithelial cells in the colon (along with thymic stromal cells and bone marrow cells) and plays a critical role in the regulation and proliferation of intraepithelial lymphocytes, intramucosal lymphocytes, and epithelial cells.[36] Studies with transgenic IL-7 mice, which overexpress IL-7, demonstrate increased incidence of acute colitis at 1 to 3 weeks of age. The mucosa of the large intestine has high levels of IL-7 with predominance of neutrophils, CD4+ T cells, and γδT cells. At 8 to 12 weeks of age, proctoptosis with anal bleeding and formation of crypt abscesses with monocyte infiltration occurs, resembling ulcerative colitis. Interestingly, IL-7 levels decrease at this stage, due to a decrease in goblet cells that are rich in IL-7.[37] UC patients have also been noted to have high serum levels of IL-7 during times of an acute flare. These findings demonstrate that IL-7 and IL-7 receptor–dependent signaling is important in the development of chronic colitis, suggesting a possible therapeutic target in human IBD.

HLA-B27 TRANSGENIC RATS

The class I MHC allele HLA-B27 is highly associated with the human spondyloarthropathies, but the basis for this is poorly understood. Rats transgenic for human HLA-B27 and β2-microglobulin genes spontaneously develop colitis, gastritis, arthritis, dermatitis, alopecia, and nail changes. The disease susceptibility correlates with HLA-B27 expression in the bone marrow–derived cells and is influenced by the genetic background. The mechanism of colitis in this model is still not completely understood. The entire colon is affected with crypt hyperplasia, mononuclear infiltration, and increased number of activated Th1 cells.[38] There is evidence that normal luminal bacteria play an essential role in initiating and perpetuating chronic colitis and gastritis in this system. Transgenic rats raised under germ-free conditions do not develop gastrointestinal disease, whereas littermates exposed to specific pathogen-free bacteria (*Bacteroides* spp.) develop colitis and gastritis within 2 to 4 weeks.[39] Similar to human IBD, antibiotic therapy and recently probiotics have been shown to decrease recurrence of colitis in this model.

MYELOID SPECIFIC STAT-3–DEFICIENT MICE

The STAT family of transcription factors, consisting of 7 members, is critically involved in cytokine signaling. The knockout of each member of the STAT family in mice has resulted in impaired responses to corresponding cytokines. Unlike other STAT knockout models, the knockout of STAT-3 results in early death in embryogenesis. Therefore, STAT-3 has been deleted in a cell- or tissue-specific manner via the Cre-loxP recombination system in myeloid cells (macrophages, neutrophils, and dendritic cells). These mice develop chronic enterocolitis due to an impaired response in IL-10 signaling and have increased secretion of IL-12, IL-6, and TNFα. Macrophages from the STAT-3 mutant mice do not show any anti-inflammatory response to IL-10 and produce increased levels of inflammatory cytokines in response to bacterial LPS.[40] These findings suggest that abnormal activation of myeloid cells is involved in the pathogenesis of chronic colitis via stimulation of effector T cells and disruption of homeostatic balance. This scenario may also be seen in CD, which is associated with mutations in NOD2 protein—a protein that senses bacterial peptidoglycans. Absence of NOD2 activity in myeloid cells may result in activated macrophages, which induce a strong effector T cell response and a weak regulatory T cell response.

LIMITATIONS

The transgenic mouse models have helped reveal other important pathways in mucosal inflammation. The myeloid-specific STAT-3 mouse model has identified the importance of the innate immune response in IBD. However, like knockout models, they represent genetic manipulation with artificial increases in cytokines or loss of signaling in certain cells. These changes may represent a final common pathway of mucosal inflammation in human IBD but are not the instigating factors.

SPONTANEOUS MODELS OF COLITIS

Spontaneous colitis models offer an exciting way to study human IBD because inflammation in the intestines occurs without direct exogenous manipulation. There are 3 important models of spontaneous colitis that will be discussed: C3H/HejBir mice, cotton top tamarins, and Boxer dogs.

C3H/HEJBIR MICE

Colitis and perianal ulcers have been occasionally seen in the C3H/Hej strain of mice. Selective interbreeding of the C3H/Hej mice with colitis resulted in the substrain of C3H/HejBir mice. These mice develop colitis limited to the ileocecal region and the right side of the colon at 3 to 4 weeks of life. The colitis develops spontaneously and usually regresses after 10 to 12 weeks of life. Ulcers, crypt abscesses, and regeneration of epithelium are noted, but granulomas and mucosal hypertrophy are not seen. Increased levels of IFN-γ and IL-2 suggest a Th1-mediated immune response.[41] Similar to SCID mice and some knockout mice models, there seems to be a correlation between *Helicobacter* infection and the onset of colitis. These findings stress the importance of gut flora in the development of IBD. When mice are kept in a germ-free environment, colitis does not occur. Even though no specific microorganisms have been associated with murine colitis or human disease, it is clear that normal mucosal microflora is required to initiate or maintain the inflammatory process in genetically susceptible hosts.

COLITIS IN THE COTTON TOP TAMARIN (*SAGUINUS OEDIPUS*)

Colitis is an important health problem in cotton top tamarins (*Saguinus oedipus*) housed in biomedical research institutes.[42-44] A prospective study in one research colony documented colitis in 24% of animals at 4 months of age and 52% at 48 months of age.[45] Clinical signs include weight loss, diarrhea, and rectal bleeding. The colitis is diffuse and characterized histologically by an inflammatory cell infiltrate in the lamina propria, hyperplasia of the colonic epithelium, decreased numbers of goblet cells, and crypt abscesses. Increased amounts of TNFα have been detected in feces of tamarins with colitis.[45] Treatment with sulfasalazine[46,47] or anti-TNFα antibody ameliorates colitis in affected tamarins.[48]

Tamarins in their native habitat are free of the disease,[49] tamarins housed in isolation are less frequently affected than colony-housed animals (56% vs 93%)[46] and diversion of the fecal stream ameliorates inflammation.[50] Hence, environmental factors such as diet and infectious agents are suspected to play a major role in the etiopathogenesis of colitis in cotton top tamarins.

Prospective evaluation of diets showed no effect on acute colitis, but chronic mucosal changes were significantly higher in animals fed a standard diet than semipurified diets.[46] *Campylobacter, Helicobacter,* and *Escherichia coli* have been variously implicated as infectious agents involved in the development of colitis. *Campylobacter* infection was not associated with colitis or diarrhea in colony-housed animals,[46,51] but was related to colitis in tamarins housed in isolation.[46] A novel group of *Helicobacter* resembling *Flexispira rappini* and *H fenelliae* has been isolated from affected individuals,[53] and spiral bacteria resembling *Helicobacter* were observed to invade colonic mucosa after re-introduction of the fecal stream.[50] However, luminal bacteria on their own are not considered sufficient to induce colitis, and both an adverse environment and the fecal contents appear to be required for expression of the disease.[50] A role for *E coli* is suggested by the finding that tamarins with fecal cultures positive for enteropathogenic *E coli* containing intimin sequences have a higher frequency of active colitis (75.0% vs 27.2%; *P*<0.005) and higher histological scores of colonic inflammation (0.875 vs 0.455, respectively; *P*<0.05).[53]

Cotton top tamarins with colitis are prone to develop colonic carcinoma and sclerosing cholangitis.[42,43] Approximately 25% to 40% of tamarins with active colitis progress to colonic adenocarcinoma.[52] In a prospective study, 7 of 212 animals in the study groups developed adenocarcinoma of the colon at 4 or more years of age.[46] Colonic adenocarcinoma arises spontaneously (ie, is not preceded by dysplasia) in areas of colonic inflammation, is multifocal, and shares lectin staining with UeA-1.[54]

GRANULOMATOUS COLITIS OF BOXER DOGS

Granulomatous colitis (GC) (also known as histiocytic ulcerative colitis) is a severe inflammatory bowel that typically affects Boxer dogs under 4 years of age.[55-57] Other breeds such as Mastiff, Alaskan Malamute, Doberman Pinscher, and French Bulldogs are sporadically affected.

Dogs are usually presented for the investigation of frequent bloody mucoid stools and weight loss. Clinicopathological abnormalities are generally limited to anemia and hypoalbuminemia. Abdominal ultrasonography may show thickening of the colon and regional lymphadenopathy. Lymph node aspirates may contain histiocytes. Colonoscopy is frequently characterized by thickening and ulceration of the colon.

The dominant histological features of colonic biopsies are loss of colonic epithelium and goblet cells, and the accumulation of large numbers of PAS-positive macrophages. The PAS-positive material is thought to be derived from remnants of bacterial cell wall glycoprotein, and the accumulation of PAS-positive material in macrophages may be due to defective phagocytosis. Immunopathological studies describe an increase in IgG3 and IgG4 plasma cells, CD3-T cells, and L1 and MHCII positive cells.[56]

Several studies have described bacteria within the mucosa of affected dogs but known enteropathogens such as *Salmonella, Campylobacter yersinia,* and *Shigella* have not been isolated. Ultrastructural studies suggest active phagocytosis of bacteria that in some instances resemble *Chlamydia*.[55] An attempt to reproduce colitis in Boxer dogs with *Mycoplasma* isolated from the colon and regional lymph nodes of 4 affected dogs was unsuccessful. The predilection for Boxer dogs, with only sporadic cases of this type of colitis reported in non-Boxer dogs, and absence of a causal infectious agent has led to GC being considered a breed-specific, immune-mediated disease of unknown etiology.

In contrast to the widely accepted view that GC is an incurable immune-mediated disease, the original description by Van Kruiningen[55] describes a favorable outcome in 6 of 9 dogs treated with chloramphenicol. The results of recent studies provide clear evidence of clinical and histological remission in Boxer dogs and 1 English Bulldog treated with antibiotic regimens containing fluoroquinolones.[57-60] Treatment with enrofloxacin induces resolution of clinical signs within 2 weeks, and sustained remission has been reported in 6 of 7 dogs examined to date (median disease-free interval to date of 47 months, range 17–62). [60]

From a comparative perspective, it is clear that GC in dogs has features in common with spontaneous idiopathic inflammatory bowel diseases in people such as UC (macroscopic appearance, regional distribution, immunopathology), CD (granulomatous inflammation, bacteria within macrophages, response to fluoroquinolones), and Whipple's disease (PAS-positive macrophages, bacteria within macrophages), but it is not identical to any one of these diseases.

Evidence is mounting that inflammatory bowel disease in people is a consequence of an abnormal host response to the enteric bacteria that can be viewed as normal flora or opportunistic pathogens. With this thought in mind, 2 studies have recently explored the possibility that an uncharacterized infectious agent such as *Trophyrema whippelii* (the causative agent of Whipple's disease)[61] or an abnormal mucosa-associated flora are involved in the etiopathogenesis of GC in Boxer dogs. One of these studies used a combination of culture-independent molecular techniques (16SrDNA sequencing and fluorescence in situ hybridization) to examine the mucosa associated bacterial flora of colonic biopsies from healthy dogs, dogs with lymphoplasmacytic colitis, and Boxer dogs with GC.[59] Those investigators demonstrated selective intramucosal colonization of GC biopsies by *E coli*. Another study described the immunolocalization of *E coli*, *Lawsonia intracellularis*, *Campylobacter*, and *Salmonella* to macrophages in the colon of 10/10, 3/10, 2/10, and 1/10 Boxer dogs with granulomatous colitis, respectively (dogs without colitis or other forms of colitis were not examined).[62] These findings strongly suggest that GC is a consequence of mucosal invasion by a subset of resident *E coli* in a susceptible individual (ie, an undefined breed-specific abnormality in Boxer dogs).

Interestingly, the *E coli* strains isolated from the colonic mucosa of dogs with GC adhered to, invaded, and persisted in cultured epithelial cells to the same degree as *E coli* strains associated with CD.[63,64] Initial investigations of GC and Crohn's-associated *E coli* indicate they are more similar in phylogeny and virulence gene profiles to extraintestinal pathogenic *E coli* (eg, uropathogenic *E coli*) than diarrheogenic *E coli* and point to the association of *E coli* that resemble extraintestinal pathogenic strains in genotype with chronic intestinal inflammation.[64]

Taken as a whole, granulomatous colitis in Boxer dogs represents an inability to kill a subset of resident *E coli* that selectively exploit a genetically susceptible individual. Identification of the genetic basis of susceptibility in Boxer dogs and virulence determinants of opportunistic pathogenic adherent and invasive *E coli* could provide useful insights into IBD in people.

SPONTANEOUS MODELS OF ILEITIS

In SAMP1/Yit and the SAMP1/YitFc mouse models, the mice develop ileitis and colitis, skin lesions, and perianal disease with fistula (findings that mimic CD).

SAMP1/Yit Mice

The SAMP1/Yit model, which was generated by more than 20 generations of brother-sister mating of a senescence-accelerated mouse line, develops spontaneous ileitis at 20 weeks of age. The ileitis develops without genetic or immunologic manipulation with almost 100% penetrance. These mice have segmental inflammation of the terminal ileum with transmural involvement, presence of granulomas, architectural distortion of the mucosa, and muscular hypertrophy. This chronic ileitis resembles human CD.[65] The ileitis can also be adoptively transferred to immunodeficient mice via CD4+ T cells isolated from SAMP1/Yit mice, again mediated by a Th1-induced immune response.[66]

SAMP1/YitFc Mice

Recent studies using this SAMP1/Yit of mice after an additional 20 generations or more of brother-sister matings have revealed new phenotypic features. The SAMP1/YitFc substrain develops ileitis as early as 10 weeks of age. These mice also have high levels of intestinal INF-γ by 4 weeks of age, preceding the onset of ileitis. The mesenteric lymph node lymphocytes develop an activated phenotype coincident with the development of ileitis. Finally, approximately 5% of the mice develop perianal disease with ulceration and fistulas. The emergence of perianal disease is the first report of such an occurrence in an animal model of IBD.[67] The ileitis noted in this model is driven by Th1-mediated cytokines. Administration of anti-TNF-α and anti-IL-12 antibodies can improve the colitis by induction of apoptosis in lamina propria mononuclear cells.[68] In addition to the benefit of anti-TNF-α antibodies, the role of antibiotics has also been tested in the SAMP1/YitFc model. The use of ciprofloxacin and metronidazole antibiotic therapy has been shown to prevent and treat colitis by decreasing the number of activated gut lymphocytes. As a consequence, there is a decrease in the characteristic Th1 cytokine production.[69] Finally, this mouse model has also been used to investigate the role of adhesion molecules such as integrins (VCAM-1 and ICAM-1) in colitis. These adhesion molecules have been implicated in T-cell homing and neutrophil trafficking during an inflammatory response. Blockade of ICAM-1 and α₄ integrins or a combination of ICAM-1 and VCAM-1 leads to a 70% improvement in the severity of inflammation in SAMP1/YitFc colitis.[70] Similar studies in human Crohn's disease have been encouraging using an antibody to α₄ integrins. The recombinant antibody natalizumab, with specificity to α₄β₁ and α₄β₇ integrins, has been used in a small trial involving 30 patients with Crohn's disease. A single infusion of this drug resulted in a 39% remission rate in the treated group versus 8% in placebo. Taken together, studies using the SAMP1/YitFc mice have had significant therapeutic implications in the management of IBD.

LIMITATIONS

Spontaneous colitis models mimic CD in many pathogenic features. Apart from ileal inflammation, the SAMP1/YitFc model is the first animal model to develop fistulizing disease with perianal ulcers. This model has increased our knowledge of the pathogenesis and treatment of CD. It may also help identify other genes that may be involved in the development of CD. Unlike monogenic disorders, the identification of mutated genes in complex genetic disorders (like IBD) is quite difficult. Generally, the whole genome of affected families is probed using polymorphic microsatellite markers. The whole genome screens are based on the principle that a marker that is located close to a disease gene is less likely to be separated during meiosis and can be co-inherited with the disease gene. Using cohorts of Crohn's patients, the NOD2 gene was recently identified in this manner. This approach can also be used to study an inbred strain of rodents in a controlled environment. The SAMP1/YitFc model develops colitis with a 100% penetrance, without exogenous environmental influence. The genetic analysis of this animal model of colitis may help identify disease susceptibility genes that are orthologues of human disease.

CONCLUSION

Animal models of colitis have increased our knowledge in understanding the pathogenesis and treatment of IBD. Immune therapies (anti-TNFα therapy) derived from colitis models have become the mainstay of disease management. It has become clear that CD results from a Th1-mediated immune response. New therapies that target the resultant cytokines may further add to the current arsenal (including anti-IL-12 and anti-IL-6). Because UC is influenced by a Th2-mediated immune response, antibody therapy that reduces this response may be useful in the treatment of UC (including anti-IL-13). In addition to limiting effector T cell response, augmenting the T regulatory response in human disease will serve as another avenue of novel treatments (TGF-β). Recognizing that results from 4-legged animals (ie, mice) do not always predict results in 2-legged animals (ie, humans), identification of disease susceptibility genes using murine colitis models holds great promise for the future.

REFERENCES

1. Croft M. Activation of naive, memory and effector T cells. *Curr Opin Immunol*. 1994;6:431-437.

2. Shevach EM, McHugh RS, Piccirillo CA, Thornton AM. Control of T-cell activation by CD4+ CD25+ suppressor T cells. *Immunol Rev*. 2001;182:58-67.

3. McHugh R S, Shevach EM. Cutting edge: depletion of CD4+CD25+ regulatory T cells is necessary, but not sufficient, for induction of organ-specific autoimmune disease. *J Immunol*. 2002;168;5979-5983.

4. Neurath MF, Fuss I, Kelsall BL, et al. Antibodies to interleukin 12 abrogate established experimental colitis in mice. *J Exp Med*. 1995;182:1281-1290.

5. Elson CO, Cong Y, Weaver CT, et al. Monoclonal anti-interleukin 23 reverses active colitis in a T cell-mediated model in mice. *Gastroenterology*. 2007;132:2359-2370.

6. Duerr RH, Taylor KD, Brant SR, et al. A genome-wide association study identifies IL23R as an inflammatory bowel disease gene. *Science*. 2006;314:1461-1463.

7. Sandborn WJ, Feagan BG, Fedorak RN, et al. A randomized trial of ustekinumab, a human interleukin-12/23 monoclonal antibody, in patients with moderate-to-severe Crohn's disease. *Gastroenterology*. 2008;135:1130-1141.

8. Boirivant M, Fuss IJ, Chu A, et al. Oxazolone colitis: a murine model of T helper cell type 2 colitis treatable by antibodies to interleukin-4. *J Exp Med*. 1998;188:1929-1939.

9. Heller F, Fuss IJ, Nieuwenhuis EE. Oxazolone colitis, a Th2 colitis model resembling ulcerative colitis, is mediated by IL-13 producing NK-T cells. *Immunity*. 2002;17:629-638.

10. Bouma G, Strober W, Bouma G, et al. The immunological and genetic basis of inflammatory bowel disease. *Nat Rev Immunol*. 2003;3:521-533.

11. Okayasu I, Hatakeyama S, Yamada M, et al. A novel method in the induction of reliable experimental acute and chronic ulcerative colitis in mice. *Gastroenterology*. 1990;98:694-702.

12. Dieleman LA, Palmen MJ, Akol H, et al. Chronic experimental colitis induced by dextran sulphate sodium (DSS) is characterized by Th1 and Th2 cytokines. *Clin Exp Immunol*. 1998;114:385-391.

13. Soriano A, Salas A, Salas A, et al. VCAM-1, but no ICAM-1 or Mad-CAM-1 immunoblockade ameliorated DSS induced colitis in mice. *Lab Invest*. 2000;80:1541-1551.

14. Powrie F, Correa-Oliveira R, Mauze S, Coffman RL. Regulatory interactions between C D45RBhigh and CD45RBlow CD4+ T cells are important for the balance between protective and pathogenic cell-mediated immunity. *J Exp Med*. 1994;179:589-600.

15. Neurath MF, Weigmann B, Finotto S, et al. The transcription factor T-beta regulates mucosal T cell activation in experimental colitis and Crohn's disease. *J Exp Med*. 2002;195:1129-1143.

16. Powrie F. T cells in inflammatory bowel disease: protective and pathogenic roles. *Immunity*. 1995;3(2):171-174.

17. Asseman C, Powrie F. Interleukin 10 is a growth factor for a population of regulatory T cells. *Gut*. 1998;42;157-158.

18. Mottet C, Uhlig HH, Powrie F. Cutting edge: cure of colitis by CD4+CD25+ regulatory T cells. *J Immunol*. 2003;170:3939-3943.

19. Fuss IJ, Boirivant M, Lacy B, Strober W. The interrelated roles of TGF-beta and IL-10 in the regulation of experimental colitis. *J Immunol*. 2002;168:900-908.

20. Sadlack B, Merz H, Schorle H, Schimpl A, Feller AC, Horak I. Ulcerative colitis-like disease in mice with a disrupted IL-2 gene. *Cell*. 1993;75:253-261.

21. Boone DL, Dassopoulos T, Lodolce JP, et al. Interleukin deficient mice develop colitis in the absence of CD28 costimulation. *Inflamm Bowel Dis*. 2002;8:35-42.

22. Kühn R, Löhler J, Rennick D, Rajewsky K, Müller W. Interleukin-10 deficient mice develop chronic enterocolitis. *Cell*. 1993;75:263-274.

23. Gratz R, Becker S, Sokolowski N, et al. Murine monoclonal anti-TNF antibody administration has a beneficial effect on IBD that develops in IL-10 knockout mice. *Dig Dis Sci*. 2002;47:1723-1727.

24. Schreiber S, Fedorak RN, Nielsen OH. Safety and efficacy of recombinant human IL-10 in chronic active Crohn's disease. Crohn's disease IL-10 cooperative study group. *Gastroenterology*. 2000;119:1461-1472.

25. Kontoyiannis D, Pasparakis M, Pizarro TT, Cominelli F, Kollias G. Impaired on/off regulation of TNF biosynthesis in mice lacking TNF AU-rich elements—implications for joint and gut-associated immunopathologies. *Immunity*. 1999;10:387-398.

26. Kontoyiannis D, Boulougouris G, Manoloukos M, et al. Genetics of dissection of the cellular pathways and signaling mechanisms in modeled TNF tumor necrosis factor-induced Crohn's-like IBD. *J Exp Med*. 2002;196:1563-1574.

27. Targan SR, Hanauer SB, van Deventer SJ. A short-term study of chimeric monoclonal antibody cA2 to TNF alpha for Crohn's disease. Crohn's Disease cA2 study group. *N Engl J Med*. 1997;337:1029-1035.

28. Present DH, Rutgeerts P, Targan S, et al. Infliximab for the treatment of fistulas in patient with Crohn's disease. *N Engl J Med*. 1999;340:1398-1405.

29. Di Sabatino A, Ciccocioppo R, Cinque B, et al. Defective mucosal T cell death is reverted by infliximab in Crohn's disease. *Gut*. 2004;53:70-77.

30. Mombaerts P, Mizoguchi E, Grusby MJ, Glimcher LH, Bhan AK, Tonegawa S. Spontaneous development of IBD in T cell receptor mutant mice. *Cell*. 1993;75:1-20.

31. Bhan AK, Mizoguchi E, Smith RN, Mizoguchi A. Colitis in transgenic and knockout animals as models of human IBD. *Immunol Rev*. 1999;169:195-207.

32. Mashimo H, Wu DC, Podolsky DK, Fishman MC. Impaired defense of intestinal mucosa in mice lacking intestinal trefoil factor. *Science*. 1996;272:262-265.

33. Ogura Y, Bonen DK, Inohara N, et al. A frameshift mutation in NOD2 associated with susceptibility to Crohn's disease. *Nature*. 2001;411:603-606.

34. Hugot JP, Chamaillard M, Zouali H, et al. Association of NOD2 leucine-rich repeat variants with susceptibility to Crohn's disease. *Nature*. 2001;411:599-603.

35. Yamazaki K, Takazoe M, Tanaka T, Kazumori T, Nakamura Y. Absence of mutation in the NOD2.Card15 gene among 483 Japanese patients with Crohn's disease. *J Hum Genet*. 2002;47:469-472.

36. Watanabe M, Watanabe N, Iwao Y, et al. The serum factor from patients with ulcerative colitis induces T cell proliferation in the mouse thymus is IL-7. *J Clin Immunol*. 1997;17:282-292.

37. Watanabe M, Yamazaki M, Kanai T. Mucosal T cells as a target for treatment of IBD. *J Gastroenterol*. 2003;38:48-50.

38. Rath HC, Ikeda JS, Linde HJ, Schölmerich J, Wilson KH, Sartor RB. Varying cecal bacterial loads influences colitis and gastritis in HLA-B27 transgenic rats. *Gastroenterology*. 1999;116:310-319.

39. Rath HC. Role of commensal bacteria in chronic experimental colitis: lessons from the HLA-B27 transgenic rat. *Pathobiology*. 2003;70:130-138.

40. Takeda K, Clausen BE, Kaisho T, et al. Enhanced Th1 activity and development of chronic enterocolitis in mice devoid of Stat3 in macrophages and neutrophils. *Immunity*. 1999;10:39-49.

41. Cong Y, Brandwein SL, McCabe RP, et al. CD4+ T cells reactive to enteric bacterial antigens in spontaneously colitic C3H/HejBir mice: increased T helper cell type 1 response and ability to transfer disease. *J Exp Med*. 1998;187:855-864.

42. Kirkwood JK, Pearson GR, Epstein MA. Adenocarcinoma of the large bowel and colitis in cottontop tamarins. *J Comp Pathol*. 1986;96:507-515.

43. Warren BF, Henke M, Clapp N. Extra-intestinal manifestations of cottontop tamarin colitis. In: Clapp N, ed. *A Primate Model for the Study of Colitis and Colonic Carcinoma*. Boca Raton, FL: CRC Press; 1993:127-132.

44. Leong KM, Terrell SP, Savage A. Causes of mortality in captive cotton-top tamarins (*Saguinus oedipus*). *Zoo Biol*. 2004;23:127-137.

45. Watkins PE, Foulkes R, Ward P, Stephens S, Warren BF. Faecal tumour necrosis factor alpha in cotton-top tamarin colitis [abstract]. *J Pathol*. 1993;170:364A.

46. Johnson LD, Ausman LM, Sehgal PK, King NW. A prospective study of the epidemiology of colitis and colon cancer in cotton-top tamarins (*Saguinus oedipus*). *Gastroenterology*. 1996;110:102-115.

47. Madara JL, Podolsky DK, King NW, Sehgal PK, Moore R, Winter HS. Characterization of spontaneous colitis in cotton-top tamarins (*Saguinus oedipus*) and its response to sulfasalazine. *Gastroenterology*. 1985;88(1 Pt 1):13-19.

48. Watkins PE, Warren BF, Stephens S, Ward P, Foulkes R. Treatment of ulcerative colitis in the cottontop tamarin using antibody to tumour necrosis factor alpha. *Gut*. 1997;40:628-633.

49. Wood JD, Peck OC, Tefend KS, et al. Colitis and colon cancer in cotton-top tamarins (*Saguinus oedipus oedipus*) living wild in their natural habitat. *Dig Dis Sci*. 1998;43:1443-1453.

50. Wood JD, Peck OC, Tefend KS, et al. Evidence that colitis is initiated by environmental stress and sustained by fecal factors in the cotton-top tamarin (*Saguinus oedipus*). *Dig Dis Sci*. 2000;45:385-393.

51. Johnson LD, Ausman LM, Rolland RM, Chalifoux LV, Russell RG. *Campylobacter*-induced enteritis and diarrhea in captive cotton-top tamarins (*Saguinus oedipus*) during the first year of life. *Comp Med*. 2001;51:257-261.

52. Saunders KE, Shen Z, Dewhirst FE, Paster BJ, Dangler CA, Fox JG. Novel intestinal Helicobacter species isolated from cotton-top tamarins (*Saguinus oedipus*) with chronic colitis. *J Clin Microbiol*. 1999;37:146-151.

53. Mansfield KG, Lin KC, Xia D, et al. Enteropathogenic *E. coli* and ulcerative colitis in cotton-top tamarins (*Saguinus oedipus*). *J Infect Dis*. 2001;184:803-807.

54. Moore R, King N, Alroy J. Differences in cellular glycoconjugates of quiescent, inflamed, and neoplastic colonic epithelium in colitis and cancer-prone tamarins. *Am J Pathol*. 1988;131(3):484-489.

55. Van Kruiningen HJ, Montali RJ, Strandberg JD, Kirk RW. A granulomatous colitis of dogs with histologic resemblance to Whipple's disease. *Pathol Vet*. 1965;2:521-544.

56. German AJ, Hall EJ, Kelly DF, Watson AD, Day MJ. An immunohistochemical study of histiocytic ulcerative colitis in boxer dogs. *J Comp Pathol*. 2000;122(2-3):163-175.

57. Hostutler RA, Luria BJ, Johnson SE, et al. Antibiotic-responsive histiocytic ulcerative colitis in 9 dogs. *J Vet Intern Med*. 2004;18:499-504.

58. Davies DR, O'Hara AJ, Irwin PJ, Guilford WG. Successful management of histiocytic ulcerative colitis with enrofloxacin in two Boxer dogs. *Aust Vet J*. 2004;82:58-61.

59. Simpson, KW, Dogan B, Rishniw M, et al. Adherent and invasive *Escherichia coli* is associated with granulomatous colitis in boxer dogs. *Infect Immun*. 2006;74:4778-4792.

60. Mansfield CS, James FE, Craven M, et al. Remission of histiocytic ulcerative colitis in Boxer dogs correlates with eradication of invasive intramucosal *Escherichia coli*. *J Vet Intern Med*. 2009;23(5):964-969.

61. Relman DA, Schmidt TM, MacDermott RP, Falkow S. Identification of the uncultured bacillus of Whipple's disease. *N Engl J Med*. 1992;327:293-301.

62. Van Kruiningen HJ, Civco IC, Cartun RW. The comparative importance of *E. coli* antigen in granulomatous colitis of Boxer dogs. *APMIS*. 2005;113:420-425.

63. Darfeuille-Michaud A, Boudeau J, Bulois P, et al. High prevalence of adherent-invasive *Escherichia coli* associated with ileal mucosa in Crohn's disease. *Gastroenterology*. 2004;127:412-421.

64. Baumgart M, Dogan B, Rishniw M, et al. Culture independent analysis of ileal mucosa reveals a selective increase in invasive *Escherichia coli* of novel phylogeny relative to depletion of Clostridiales in Crohn's disease involving the ileum. *ISME J*. 2007;1(5):403-418.

65. Matsumoto S, Okabe Y, Setoyama H, et al. Inflammatory bowel disease-like enteritis and caecitis in a senescence accelerated mouse P1/Yit strain. *Gut.* 1998;43:71-78.

66. Kosiewicz MM, Nast CC, Krishnan A, et al. Th1 type responses mediate spontaneous ileitis in a novel murine model of Crohn's disease. *J Clin Invest.* 2001;107:695-702.

67. Rivera-Nieves J, Bamias G, Vidrich A, et al. Emergence of perianal fistualizing disease in the SAMP1/YitFc mouse, a spontaneous model of chronic ileitis. *Gastroenterology.* 2003;124:972-982.

68. Marini M, Bamias G, Rivera-Nieves J, et al. TNF-a neutralization ameliorated the severity of murine Crohn's like ileitis by abrogation of intestinal cell apoptosis. *Proc Natl Acad Sci U S A.* 2003;100:8366-8371.

69. Bamias G, Marini M, Moskaluk CA, et al. Down regulation of intestinal lymphocyte activation and Th1 cytokine production by antibiotic therapy in a murine model of Crohn's disease. *J Immunol.* 2002;169:5308-5314.

70. Burns RC, Rivera-Nieves J, Moskaluk CA, Matsumoto S, Cominelli F, Ley K. Antibody blockade of ICAM-1 and VCAM-1 ameliorates inflammation in the SAMP-1/Yit adoptive transfer model of Crohn's disease in mice. *Gastroenterology.* 2001;121: 1428-1436.

PEDIATRIC CONSIDERATIONS IN MEDICAL THERAPY IN PATIENTS WITH INFLAMMATORY BOWEL DISEASE

Louis R. Ghanem, MD, PhD and Robert N. Baldassano, MD

Once considered rare in pediatric practice, chronic inflammatory bowel disease (IBD) is now being recognized with increasing frequency in children of all ages. In fact, 25% to 30% of all patients with Crohn's disease (CD) and 20% of those with ulcerative colitis (UC) present before the age of 20 years.[1] Four percent of pediatric IBD occurs before the age of 5 years, with a peak age of onset in the late adolescent years. With the increasing recognition of IBD among pediatric patients, it has become one of the most significant chronic diseases afflicting children and adolescents.[2]

Although the similarities between adult and pediatric patients diagnosed with IBD are numerous, several important differences should be emphasized. In addition to the usual gastrointestinal symptoms of diarrhea, abdominal pain, and rectal bleeding, children may exhibit prominent extraintestinal manifestations, such as growth failure, weight loss, anemia, delayed puberty, and joint symptoms. Other problems unique to pediatrics include the lack of appropriate numbers of controlled clinical trials and the psychological issues that occur in children and adolescents with IBD. These unique problems encountered in the pediatric population necessitate a different medical approach than is used for adult-onset IBD. This chapter reviews aspects in the management of pediatric inflammatory bowel disease that merit special consideration.

EPIDEMIOLOGY

Since the 1930s, the incidence of IBD has greatly increased. In the 1950s, ulcerative colitis was twice as prevalent as Crohn's disease, but recent studies in the United States show that CD has been steadily increasing.[3] IBD is now recognized as one of the most significant chronic diseases to affect children and adolescents.[4] Pediatric IBD population-based epidemiological studies are sparse. They are difficult to perform because of the large number of patients needed, high cost, and potential for surveillance error, and they are difficult to compare due to different criteria and designs.[5,6] Analysis of time trends indicates a rapid rise in incidence of Crohn's from the 1960s to 1980s with subsequent stabilization,[7] although some studies indicate a continuing rise in recent years.[5,8,9] The incidence of UC showed a more stable pattern, although again with a tendency for an increase over the years.[8,9] The incidence rates range for pediatric IBD from 0.2 to 8.5 per 100,000 for CD and 0.5 to 4.3 per 100,000 for UC.

The gender distribution of IBD among children indicates slightly increased preponderance of CD in boys,[2] whereas UC affects both genders equally. At the author's institution, there is a 2:1 male to female ratio for CD. A recent hypothesis regarding the etiology of IBD supports the multifactorial theory encompassing genetic predisposition, internal and external environmental influences, and immune system disorder.[10] Genetic factors are well recognized, with a high rate of concordance between monozygotic twins (44.4%) compared to dizygotic twins (3.8%).[11] Though there is no simple Mendelian genetic mechanism at work in the transmission of IBD, multiple familial occurrences are well documented in 30% of patients diagnosed with CD under 20 years of age compared to only 13% in patients diagnosed later. Familial IBD is particularly common with early onset IBD; in our institution, the incidence of IBD in first-degree relatives among the patients who present before 5 years of age is 56%. It is imperative that large, prospective

TABLE 5-1

FREQUENCY OF COMMON PRESENTING SYMPTOMS*

Symptom	Crohn's Disease (%)	Ulcerative Colitis (%)
Abdominal pain	62 to 95	54 to 76
Diarrhea	52 to 78	67 to 93
Hematochezia	14 to 60	52 to 97
Weight loss	43 to 92	22 to 55
Fever	11 to 48	4 to 34

*Courtesy of Mamula P, Markowitz J, Baldassano RN. Clinical features and natural history of pediatric inflammatory bowel disease. In: Sartor RB, Sandborn WJ, eds. *Kirsner's Inflammatory Bowel Diseases.* 6th ed. Philadelphia, PA: Saunders Company; 2004:301-315.

genetic studies as well as studies of environmental exposures to infections and living conditions are performed in children. The pediatric population is ideal for this type of research for various reasons. Environmental factors potentially leading to IBD may occur early in life; modification of early environment may be attempted. Patients with early onset disease tend to show more aggressive disease with a stronger genetic influence. Access to patients' relatives is easier than in adult populations when diagnosis is made in childhood.[4,10] Recent genomic-wide association studies have identified multiple genes that are associated with pediatric-onset IBD.

CLINICAL FEATURES

CROHN'S DISEASE

Unlike the findings in UC, the intestinal involvement in CD may occur in any portion of the gastrointestinal tract. The presentation is determined primarily by the location and extent of disease involvement. The majority of children have disease involving the terminal ileum (50%-70%), with more than half of these patients also having inflammation in variable segments of the colon, usually the ascending colon.[12-14] Ten percent to 20% of children have isolated colonic disease, and 10% to 15% have diffuse small bowel disease of the more proximal ileum or jejunum. Isolated gastroduodenal disease is uncommon (fewer than 5% of patients), but there may be endoscopic and histologic evidence of gastroduodenal inflammation in up to 30% to 40% of children with CD.[15] CD involving the small intestine usually presents with evidence of malabsorption including diarrhea, abdominal pain, growth deceleration, weight loss, and anorexia. Initially, these symptoms may be quite subtle, and any one may predominate the clinical picture. The onset of growth failure is usually insidious, and any child or adolescent with persistent alterations in growth should have an appropriate diagnostic evaluation for IBD. Growth failure may precede the onset of intestinal symptoms by years.[16] There are multiple causes of growth failure in patients with CD, but inadequate nutrient intake is usually present. Anorexia, reduced intake, malabsorption, increased losses, and increased metabolic demands all contribute to poor growth. Small bowel mucosal disease may result in malabsorption of iron, zinc, folate, or vitamin B_{12} deficiency. CD involving the colon may be clinically indistinguishable from UC, with symptoms of bloody mucopurulent diarrhea, crampy abdominal pain, and urgency to defecate. Table 5-1 summarizes common presenting symptoms in patients with CD and UC. Symptoms of painful defecation, bright red rectal bleeding, and perirectal pain may signal perianal disease, which may occur without symptomatic involvement in any other area of the intestinal tract. Perianal involvement includes simple skin tags, fissures, abscesses, and fistulae. The perineum should be inspected in all patients presenting with signs and symptoms of CD because abnormalities detectable in this region will substantially increase the clinical suspicion of IBD.

Delay in diagnosis of IBD in the pediatric population continues to be a concern, even with increasing incidence and heightened awareness of IBD. Mean delay in diagnosis for CD in children is reported to be between 7 and 11 months, in UC between 5 and 8 months, and in indeterminate colitis 14 months.[17-19] At the same time, the delay in the adult population is even longer and is measured in years.[20] The time lag between onset of symptoms and correct diagnosis of CD appears to be prolonged if the disease affects more proximal bowel, and if presenting symptoms do not include diarrhea. The diagnosis is particularly difficult when the presenting symptoms are uncharacteristic and consist mainly of extraintestinal manifestations.

ULCERATIVE COLITIS

UC is a diffuse mucosal inflammation limited to the colon; it invariably affects the rectum and may extend proximally in a symmetrical uninterrupted pattern to involve parts or all of the large intestine. Because UC is a mucosal disease limited to the colon, the most common presenting symptoms are rectal bleeding, diarrhea, and abdominal pain. Langholz et al reported that, at diagnosis, children with UC had more extensive disease than did adults.[12] Abdominal pain was also more common. The cumulative colectomy probability was 6% after 1 year and 29% after 20 years, not different from that of adults. They also reported that when a child presents with a proctitis at diagnosis there is a 65% chance of further spread of the disease to other parts of the large intestine during the course of the disease. This compares to a 39% chance of progression among adult-onset patients (not significant).[12] There are multiple patterns of presentation of UC in the pediatric age group, and 50% to 60% have mild disease. The diarrhea is insidious in onset and later associated with hematochezia. There are no systemic signs of fever, weight loss, or hypoalbuminemia. The disease is usually confined to the distal colon and responds well to therapy. Thirty percent of pediatric patients present with moderate disease characterized by bloody diarrhea, cramps, urgency to defecate, and abdominal tenderness according to population-based data. These patients have associated systemic signs, such as anorexia, weight loss, low-grade fever, and mild anemia. Severe colitis occurs in approximately 10% of patients. This presentation is characterized by more than 6 bloody stools per day, abdominal tenderness, fever, anemia, leukocytosis, and hypoalbuminemia. Severe hemorrhage, toxic megacolon, and perforation are serious complications in this group of patients.[21-23] Occasionally, children with UC may have a presentation dominated by extraintestinal manifestations, such as growth failure, arthropathy, skin manifestations, or liver disease. This is uncommon in adults and accounts for less than 5% of the pediatric disease.[13] Delay in diagnosis in UC is between 5 and 8 months.

COMPLICATIONS

CD and UC are both associated with significant gastrointestinal complications. The major intestinal complications of UC are massive bleeding, toxic megacolon, and carcinoma.

GASTROINTESTINAL COMPLICATIONS

CD is associated with significant gastrointestinal complications. The major intestinal complications of CD are due to the transmural nature of the disease. This leads to the formation of abscesses, fistulae, strictures, and adhesions, which may also contribute to the development of obstruction or bacterial overgrowth.

Colonic malignancy is a significant complication in both UC and CD in patients with pancolitis beginning in childhood.[24] Duration of disease and pancolitis are well recognized as risk factors for the development of malignancy, with the risk of cancer increasing over that of the general population after 10 years of disease.[25] Other less well-characterized risk factors include concomitant sclerosing cholangitis; an excluded, defunctionalized, or bypassed segment; and depressed red blood cell folate levels. Although the risk of malignancy in CD is not as high as in UC, the risk of adenocarcinoma of the colon for Crohn's colitis is 4 to 20 times that of the general population.[26] Patients with small intestinal disease are 50 to 100 times more likely to develop small intestinal carcinoma. Because small intestinal carcinoma is a rare event in the general population, it is also uncommon in CD.

Perforation is one of the more serious complications of IBD and is less common in CD than UC. Colonic perforation in UC usually occurs in association with toxic megacolon or severe fulminant disease. Perforation in CD usually occurs in the ileum and is not correlated with disease activity.[27] The presenting features of perforation are those of classic peritonitis, although these features may be masked by high-dose corticosteroid therapy.

Fistula and abscess formation is common in CD due to transmural bowel inflammation. Perianal and perirectal fistulization is the most common, with the most common enteroenteric fistula being between the ileum and sigmoid colon. Perianal disease occurs in 15% of pediatric patients with CD.[28] Perianal disease may precede the appearance of the intestinal manifestations of CD by several years and is seen most commonly in patients with colitis. Perianal disease may not respond to medical therapy, and surgical management would be necessary.

EXTRAINTESTINAL MANIFESTATIONS

Up to 35% of pediatric IBD patients in some series have at least one extraintestinal manifestation as a presenting sign.[29,30] Common symptoms in a series of pediatric IBD patients from Israel included anorexia, joint complaints, and anemia.[31] Table 5-2 lists extraintestinal manifestations commonly seen in children with IBD. These manifestations may also be noted concurrently with, or after, the diagnosis of IBD is made.[29]

Skin manifestations include erythema nodosum and pyoderma gangrenosum. Erythema nodosum is more common in CD and affects 3% of pediatric patients with CD.[32] It is estimated that 75% of the patients with erythema nodosum ultimately develop arthritis.[33]

TABLE 5-2

EXTRAINTESTINAL MANIFESTATIONS OF IBD*†

SKIN
Erythema nodosum
Pyoderma gangrenosum
Perianal disease
Metastatic Crohn's disease

MOUTH
Cheilitis
Stomatitis
Aphthae

LIVER
Primary sclerosing cholangitis
Hepatitis
Cholelithiasis

PANCREAS
Pancreatitis

KIDNEY
Nephrolithiasis
Obstructive hydronephrosis
Enterovesical fistula
Urinary tract infection
Amyloidosis

GROWTH
Delayed growth
Delayed puberty

BONE
Osteoporosis
Osteopenia

EYE
Uveitis
Episcleritis
Conjunctivitis

LUNGS
Pulmonary vasculitis
Fibrosing alveolitis

VASCULAR
Vasculitis
Thrombosis (pulmonary, limb, cerebrovascular)

JOINTS
Arthralgia
Arthritis
Ankylosing spondylitis

BLOOD
Iron deficiency anemia
Anemia of chronic disease
Thrombocytosis
Autoimmune hemolytic anemia
Vitamin B_{12} deficiency

GENERAL
Fever
Fatigue
Weight loss
Anorexia

*IBD indicates inflammatory bowel disease

†Courtesy of Mamula P, Markowitz J, Baldassano RN. Clinical features and natural history of pediatric inflammatory bowel disease. In: Sartor RB, Sandborn WJ, eds. *Kirsner's Inflammatory Bowel Diseases.* 6th ed. Philadelphia, PA: Saunders Company; 2004:301-315.

Mouth ulceration is the most common oral manifestation of IBD. It is more common in CD, frequently associated with skin and joint lesions, and together with skin and eye manifestations often parallels the activity of disease.[34]

Ophthalmologic manifestations occur in about 4% of the adult population with IBD but less frequently in children and adolescents with UC and CD.[35] The most common ocular findings are episcleritis and anterior uveitis.

Arthritis is the most common extraintestinal manifestation in children and adolescents, occurring in 7% to 25% of pediatric IBD patients.[36] The arthritis is usually transient, nondeforming synovitis, asymmetric in distribution, and involves the large joints of the lower extremities. In adults, the arthritis occurs when the disease is active, but in children the arthritis may occur years before any gastrointestinal symptoms develop.[37] Ankylosing spondylitis occurs in 2% to 6% of patients and is more common in males. It is associated with HLA-B27. Though not truly an arthritis, clubbing is common in children with CD involving the small intestine.[34]

Hepatobiliary manifestations in children may precede the onset of IBD, accompany active disease, or develop after surgical resection of all diseased bowel.[38] Hepatic manifestations include elevation of aminotransferases, chronic active hepatitis, granulomatous hepatitis, amyloidosis, fatty liver, and sclerosing cholangitis. Abnormal serum aminotransferases are commonly transient and appear to relate to medications or disease activity. If elevation persists, patients should be evaluated for the etiology of viral hepatitis. Chronic active hepatitis develops in less than 1% of children with IBD.[39] Colitis at the time may be relatively asymptomatic, although the hepatitis may proceed to cirrhosis. Sclerosing cholangitis develops in 3.5% of pediatric patients with UC, usually extensive disease, and less than 1% of pediatric patients with CD.[39] It is not related to disease activity and may appear years before any gastrointestinal disease develops or even years after a colectomy for UC. In a series of 36 pediatric patients with IBD who developed sclerosing cholangitis, only 4 had CD and 32 had UC.[40] The authors suggested heightened endoscopic surveillance once the diagnosis of IBD is made in the setting of sclerosing cholangitis because the time to dysplasia may be accelerated, as noted in 3 pediatric patients who underwent proctocolectomy due to dysplasia. Endoscopic retrograde cholangiopancreatography and magnetic resonance cholangiopancreatography have significantly improved the ability to diagnose this disease in the pediatric population. Cholelithiasis has been described in both UC and CD but more frequently in CD, especially after ileal resection.

The common urologic manifestations of IBD include nephrolithiasis, hydronephrosis, and enterovesicular fistulae. Nephrolithiasis is a common renal complication in pediatrics and occurs in approximately 5% of the children with IBD.[4] It usually is the result of fat malabsorption that occurs with small bowel CD. Dietary calcium binds to malabsorbed fatty acids in the colonic lumen, and free oxalate is absorbed. This results in hyperoxaluria and oxalate stones.[41] In patients with an ileostomy, increased fluid and electrolyte losses may lead to a concentrated, acidic urine and the formation of uric acid stones. External compression of the ureter by an inflammatory mass or abscess may lead to hydronephrosis. Enterovesical fistulae, which are more common in males, may present with recurrent urinary tract infections or pneumaturia.

Thromboembolic disease is a rare but severe complication of IBD. Both UC and CD are thought to be associated with a prothrombotic state with enhanced parameters of coagulation.[42] Several different coagulation abnormalities have been reported in patients with IBD, imparting an increased risk of thrombotic vascular disease over the general population: increased fibrinogen, thrombocytosis and abnormal platelet activation, accelerated thromboplastin generation, elevation of factors V and VIII, decreased antithrombin III, protein S and C deficiency, elevated anti-cardiolipin antibodies, high plasma factor VII coagulant activity, resistance to activated protein C, and prothrombin gene mutation (G20210).[43-45] Thromboembolic complications are reported in 1.3% to 6.4% of pediatric patients with IBD.[42,44] In the adult population, pulmonary, abdominal, and peripheral veins and arteries are more commonly involved than cerebral or retinal vessels. In pediatric IBD patients, cerebral and retinal vessels seem to be affected more frequently than other sites; thrombosis in these sites carries a better prognosis than in adults.[44,46] The majority of patients have active disease at the time of the thromboembolic event, more so in children than in the adult population.

Other extraintestinal manifestations may develop due to side effects of treatment. Those include pancreatitis, pericarditis, alopecia, osteoporosis, cataracts, acne, hepatitis, anemia, neutropenia, fibrosing alveolitis, interstitial pneumonitis, and peripheral neuropathy. For example, pancreatitis may result from therapy with 5-aminosalicylic acid, 6-mercaptopurine (6-MP), corticosteroids, and methotrexate; peripheral neuropathy may occur with metronidazole therapy; and corticosteroid therapy is associated with acne, cataracts, and osteoporosis.

GROWTH AND NUTRITION

Growth failure is a common problem in pediatric and adolescent patients with IBD. Abnormal nutritional status in IBD is now universally acknowledged. Poor growth in IBD is often attributed to chronic malnutrition related to decreased intake, as well as increased intestinal losses and metabolic demands, which if present concurrently produce a situation almost impossible to compensate for by oral intake alone.[47-49]

Growth failure may be the earliest sign of IBD in children and adolescents. Up to 85% of children with CD, and as many as 65% of those with UC, will demonstrate growth failure at the time of diagnosis.[50] A decreased rate of height accrual (growth velocity) may also precede diagnosis. In a review of 50 children and prepubescent adolescents with CD, 88% showed a decrease in height velocity before diagnosis.[51] Perhaps more importantly, 46% revealed evidence of decreased height velocity prior to the development of symptoms attributable to CD. Surprisingly, 34 of the 44 patients with decreased linear growth were still above the

5th percentile for height based on age. This fact may have contributed to further delay in diagnosis, as the duration between onset of growth failure and diagnosis was more than twice as long in the group with heights above the 5th percentile. Accordingly, growth velocity (rather than height for age percentile) has been incorporated into the scoring system of the Pediatric Crohn's Disease Activity Index (PCDAI). This index was developed and validated by a group of senior pediatric gastroenterologists in 1991[52] and correlates well with the original Crohn's Disease Activity Index (CDAI) developed for adult patients.[53]

Because decreasing height velocity is evident in the majority of CD patients several months or years before they develop symptoms attributable to the disease, there is a high likelihood they already demonstrate signs of chronic malnutrition at the time of diagnosis. Therefore, management of these patients should incorporate a plan for nutritional rehabilitation.

Poor intake is commonly felt to be the most important etiology of malnutrition in IBD.[4,54,55] Several studies have documented that dietary intake is chronically deficient in the majority of growth-retarded children with CD.[49,56,57] The causes of decreased food intake are multifactorial. Children and adolescents with IBD may limit their diet because eating exacerbates abdominal symptoms, including pain, nausea and bloating from partial obstruction, or diarrhea. Additionally, they may suffer from anorexia related to depression or increased inflammatory mediators such as tumor necrosis factor alpha (TNFα) and interleukin-1 (IL-1).[58] These repeated symptoms after eating lead to behavioral conditioning.[59] The impact of nutritional status is perhaps most significant during adolescence as the pubertal growth spurt accounts for about 16% of the adult height. Also, delays in skeletal maturation, onset of menarche, and epiphyseal fusion in long bones occur with undernutrition.

Several studies of patients with IBD demonstrate significant weight gain when calories are supplemented by a variety of means. Intravenous nutrition administered during acute exacerbations has been demonstrated to maintain fluid and electrolyte status and to arrest some of the early catabolism of protein stores.[58,60] Therapy for children with growth failure and IBD must initially be directed towards achieving remission and maximizing nutritional support. Kirschner et al demonstrated in a small series of children with CD that growth retardation responded to enterally administered calories, as measured by height velocity and height percentile.[61] To achieve these results, caloric intake was increased from 56% to 91% of the recommended goal for a period of 12 months. Improved linear growth rates and growth percentiles were seen in all patients. This study was among the first that was able to show that nutritional therapy was a useful adjunct to medical therapy of CD and suggested that enteral nutrition should be employed before more invasive therapies such as surgery or parenteral nutri-tion. The ability of enteral feeding to reverse malnutrition was also demonstrated by Motil et al.[56] In a series of 6 adolescents with active CD, caloric intake was increased by more than 40% (from 67 to 96 kcal/kg/day), with protein intake increasing from 2.3 to 3.2 g/kg/day for a period of 3 weeks. Patients gained an average of 3.3 kg over the study period, with a resultant increase in newly synthesized body protein stores as measured by radiolabeled leucine metabolism. The authors concluded that significant weight gain is achievable with short-term enteral nutritional supplementation and that the weight gain resulted largely from lean body mass accretion.

Despite the ability to induce both weight and height acquisition through calorie and nutrient supplementation, it is also clear that some effects of malnutrition are irreversible. When adjusting height for genetic potential based on parental height, many patients with CD never achieve expected levels, as demonstrated by measuring body composition in 132 subjects with CD and 66 controls aged 5 to 25 years.[55] In this population, adjusted height Z scores (which compare a pediatric patient in standard deviations from the mean for that age) were significantly lower than predicted heights. These findings were most pronounced in male patients, in whom the average adjusted height Z score was a full standard deviation below expected.

ASSESSMENT OF GROWTH AND NUTRITION

Accurately assessing growth and nutritional status is the first step in successfully addressing these issues in IBD. Growth irregularities in children with IBD have been measured in various ways, including weight for age, height for age, height and weight adjusted Z score, height velocity, and various anthropometric measures such as head circumference, midarm circumference, and triceps skinfold thickness.[50,62] When assessing a patient with IBD for growth failure, one must first use accurate measurements. Weight measurement should be performed on the same scale, with the patient wearing similar amounts of clothing each time. Height measurement should be obtained using a stadiometer, and the patient should be measured without shoes.

Accurate assessment of nutritional status, however, relies on more than just height and weight at a given time. Genetic height potential, determined by mid-parental height, should be calculated.[63] Previous height and weight points should be considered, with calculation of growth velocity. Height and weight deficit calculations expressed as a ratio of the actual height or weight divided by the expected value based on the 50th percentile for age can give insight into the duration of malnutrition. In cases of short-term deficiencies, one can expect weight deficit (wasting), whereas long-term malnutrition often results in height deficit (stunting).[62]

Stage of sexual maturation is an important reflection of nutritional status, with significant implications for the patient. Adolescents with CD often have delay in the onset of pubertal development, and active disease could potentially delay the onset of puberty indefinitely with a deleterious effect on growth.[64] Duration of puberty can also be affected in children with IBD, as active or relapsing disease during the years after puberty may slow down or even arrest the progression of puberty.

Patients who are in remission by the time they reach puberty may experience good catch-up growth with improved height velocity.[65] However, the persistence of growth deficits after the development of secondary sexual characteristics may signify irreversible loss of growth potential. Therefore, accurate staging of sexual development, using the parameters described by Tanner,[66] should be a routine component of the ongoing evaluation and care of any young patient with IBD.

Nutritional assessment should also include evaluation for macro- and micronutrient deficiencies. Overall caloric intake should be assessed using diet diaries, recorded for at least 3 consecutive days. This type of assessment allows accurate calculation of not just overall calories but the breakdown of fat, protein, and carbohydrate intake, as well as the amount of various micronutrients in the diet.

Iron intake is important in the diet of all children and adolescents, especially so in IBD, with more than 70% of patients manifesting iron deficiency.[67] Small bowel disease, a history of small bowel resection, and increased intestinal transit time may result in poor absorption of iron. Iron supplementation may cause frequent adverse side effects including indigestion and diarrhea, resulting in poor patient compliance.[68] Diet diaries may suggest that one is at risk of iron deficiency, with confirmation from objective measures such as hemoglobin, mean corpuscular volume, reticulocyte count, and levels of iron, ferritin, and transferrin saturation. Absorption of other micronutrients, in particular vitamin B_{12}, folic acid, vitamin D, and calcium, may also be impaired under various conditions in IBD. For example, extensive ileal disease or resection may result in B_{12} deficiency, whereas sulfasalazine administration can interfere with folate metabolism, resulting in megaloblastic anemia. Of all the micronutrients, calcium and vitamin D have received the greatest attention because of their role in bone disease.

BONE DISEASE AND OSTEOPOROSIS

Calcium homeostasis and bone growth is one of the most important aspects of malnutrition in pediatric IBD. Bone disease suffered by patients with IBD can be a combination of *osteomalacia*, defined as abnormal bone mineralization, and *osteoporosis*, defined as reduced bone mass.[69]

Osteopenia is the general term used for any abnormality of bone density and may occur in the context of either osteomalacia or osteoporosis.

Osteoporosis can be reliably detected by measurement of bone mineral density, of which dual energy x-ray absorptiometry (DEXA) is the favored approach.[70] When measured by DEXA, bone mineral density is expressed as the number of standard deviations above or below the mean for age-matched controls (Z score). One must be careful in interpreting bone density under circumstances of abnormal growth, however. For example, a patient with significant stunting may exhibit an abnormal Z score for age but may in turn have a normal Z score for height. Under these circumstances, the bone density changes over time have more clinical significance than any individual Z score. One should also be aware of the use of T scores in the expression of bone density. These scores express bone density as compared to other young adults and have little interpretive value for pediatric patients with IBD.

It is now believed that osteoporosis in the elderly has its roots in childhood. Adult levels of bone mineralization are predominantly achieved during childhood and adolescence,[71] and there remains no definitive treatment for significant osteoporosis. Therefore, derangements in calcium intake and bone growth early in life, such as those that occur with early onset IBD, may have profound permanent results on bone density. One of the serious consequences of osteoporosis is bone fracture, with vertebral compression fracture representing a frequent complication.[72] The health-care costs of disability from osteoporosis-related fractures are considerable.[73] As a result, childhood prevention of adult bone disease takes on a high level of significance. Effective prevention of osteoporosis and its consequences must occur during childhood, and identifying those patients at risk of abnormal bones is the cornerstone of successful prevention.

Rates of bone turnover are higher in children and adolescents than in adults. In a study of bone mass and biochemical markers of bone turnover in children at various stages of sexual development, bone formation markers were found to be highest at mid-puberty with reduction in late puberty.[74] Measures of bone formation correlated most highly with bone density, emphasizing the importance of this period of development on final bone composition.

The skeletal complications of IBD are in large part related to poor nutrition. Vitamin D deficiency is common among patients with IBD, and CD in particular, with more than 50% of patients demonstrating abnormal levels.[75] This deficiency could relate to decreased intake of dairy products, which may exacerbate abdominal symptoms in patients with lactose intolerance. Alternatively, patients with a history of ileal resection or active ileal disease may undergo treatment with cholestyramine, which binds vitamin D in addition to binding bile acids. Other disordered mechanisms of vitamin D homeostasis may be present in IBD patients

TABLE 5-3

PHARMACOLOGIC THERAPY FOR
INFLAMMATORY BOWEL DISEASE IN PEDIATRICS*†

	ULCERATIVE COLITIS	CROHN'S DISEASE
MILD DISEASE AND REMISSION	Sulfasalazine (Azulfidine) 50-75 mg/kg/day divided bid to qid (max. 5 g/day)	
	Mesalamine (Asacol, Pentasa) 50 to 75 mg/kg/day divided tid to qid (max. Asacol 4.8 g/day, Pentasa 4.0 g/day)	
	Mesalamine enema (Rowasa) 4 g qhs	
	Mesalamine suppository (Canasa) 500 mg qhs or bid	
	Hydrocortisone enema (Cortenema) qd to bid	
	Budesonide enema (Entocort enema 2 g/100 mL qd)	
MODERATE DISEASE		Metronidazole (Flagyl) 15 mg/kg/d divided tid (max. 1 g/day)
		Nutritional therapy
	Continue the above therapies with the addition of prednisone, to be tapered to every other day schedule over a 4- to 6-week period, depending on clinical remission. 1 to 2 mg/kg/daily qid (maximum oral dose of 40 mg/day)	
	Budesonide (Entocort) (controlled ileal release) 9 mg qd, may replace prednisone for acute flare	
REFRACTORY DISEASE	Azathioprine (Imuran) 2.0 to 2.5 mg/kg/day qd	
	6-Mercaptopurine (Purinethol) 1.0 to 1.5 mg/kg/day qd	
	Cyclosporin A (Sandimmune IV or PO) 4 to 6 mg/kg continuous infusion or bid	
	Infliximab (Remicade) 5-10 mg/kg/dose IV	

*bid indicates twice a day; qid, 4 times a day; tid, 3 times a day; qhs, every hour of sleep; qd, every day; IV, intravenously; PO, orally.

†Adapted from Baldassano RN, Piccoli DA. Inflammatory bowel disease in pediatric and adolescent patients. *Gastroenterol Clin North Am.* 1999;28:445-458.

such as changes in the metabolic clearance of vitamin D related to calcium deficiency[76,77] and could explain why ultraviolet light is not adequate to overcome dietary deficiencies. This would be of particular importance in IBD, as once established, a derangement in vitamin D or calcium homeostasis could become a self-perpetuating problem.[69]

Calcium homeostasis is another important factor in bone mineralization and density in IBD patients. As with vitamin D, decreased intake coupled with avoidance of dairy products may lead to inadequate dietary calcium. In contrast to vitamin D, however, calcium cannot be synthesized de novo. Furthermore, calcium deficiency may be exacerbated by fat malabsorption, present in patients with CD-related small bowel disease. The most important effects on calcium homeostasis may be secondary to the use of corticosteroids, as long-term corticosteroid therapy has been shown to inhibit intestinal calcium absorption and tubular resorption of calcium in the kidney.[78,79]

Beyond calcium malabsorption, corticosteroids may have a negative impact on bone remodeling in IBD patients. This includes the inhibition of osteoblastic activity, which limits bone formation, while osteoblastic activity continues unabated.[80,81] Corticosteroids also depress calcitonin levels, resulting in further bone resorption.[82] The clinician treating IBD is often faced with a double-edged sword when considering treatment with corticosteroids. Disease activity may be improved by treatment with corticosteroids, resulting in improved intake and absorption of vital nutrients. The use of corticosteroids may also undermine the development of adequate linear growth and bone density, however. It is unclear which situation is less desirable, but neither one is optimal. It is still debated whether the short-term benefits that corticosteroids offer for control of symptoms offset the long-term effects on bones. This dilemma may be resolved by rapidly metabolized corticosteroids such as budesonide or avoidance of corticosteroids by using alternatives such as anti-TNFα agents.

Various inflammatory cytokines also impact calcium homeostasis. IBD patients who have increased secretion of the proinflammatory cytokine IL-1β on a genetic basis are at increased risk of developing osteopenia.[83] In a study of 83 patients with IBD, it was shown that noncarriage of the allele for normal IL-1ra expression was independently associated with the development of increased bone loss.[84] In this same study, carrying an allele for increased expression of IL-6 was correlated with bone loss. Bone loss in this study was not, however, related to disease severity or use of corticosteroids. Based on these results, it was felt that genetic variation in the genes responsible for cytokine expression has a significant role in whether patients with IBD develop metabolic bone disease.

DELAYED PUBERTY

Children with Crohn's disease often have delay in the onset of pubertal development, and careful evaluation of pubertal staging should be part of their routine evaluation. Active disease uncontrolled by medical therapy could potentially delay the onset of puberty indefinitely with a deleterious effect on pubertal growth.[85] The duration of puberty could also be affected in children with CD. Active or relapsing disease during the years following the onset of puberty may slow down or even arrest the progression of puberty. Arrest of pubertal development in children with CD may be an early indication of disease relapse, and in the same way delay in pubertal onset may indicate persistent occult disease. Inducing disease remission before the onset of puberty and maintaining it during the pubertal years is crucial in order to avoid losing valuable height as a consequence of a missed pubertal growth spurt. Patients who are in remission by the time they go into puberty can experience good catch-up growth with peak height velocities greater than 12 cm/year.[65] The potential for catch-up growth may be severely compromised in those children who suffered relapse or whose disease activity is not controlled in the peripubertal years. Differing from healthy children, delayed puberty in CD may not allow future prolonged and/or greater linear growth.[55]

Factors affecting pubertal development in children with CD include nutritional deprivation, the inflammatory process, hormonal disturbances, and the effects of therapy. Severe protein-calorie malnutrition and weight loss can be associated with prepubertal levels of sex steroids, despite previous evidence of pubertal progression. Secondary amenorrhea is also observed following severe weight loss in these patients, similar to patients with anorexia nervosa where there is suppression of gonadotrophin secretion.[86]

Delayed puberty in patients with CD may affect the normal bone mineral accumulation peak that follows the pubertal growth spurt[87-89] and is another factor contributing to osteoporosis. Estrogen and testosterone are important for normal bone mineralization, as shown by the osteopenia found in estrogen-[90] and androgen-resistant[91] syndromes.

THERAPEUTIC OPTIONS

The physician or nurse practitioner caring for the pediatric patient with IBD faces many difficult challenges when considering the approach to treatment. Issues including growth, bone development, and sexual maturation should be considered when selecting therapies. General goals for optimizing outcome should achieve the best clinical and laboratory control of disease with the fewest side effects, promote growth through adequate nutrition, and permit the patient to function as normally as possible with consideration for school attendance and participation in activities. Table 5-3 summarizes current treatment options available. Because few randomized controlled drug trials have been performed in children, the gastroenterologist caring for a pediatric patient with IBD is often forced to use adult data or extrapolate success from anecdotal experiences. This section will provide treatment options that currently exist with a focus on the available pediatric literature.

Nutritional Therapies

Nutritional therapy in IBD is still underused, although it is gaining wider acceptance. One of the most appealing aspects of nutritional therapy is that it addresses the well-known effects of malnutrition, while providing a therapeutic option as well. Although parental nutrition is traditionally reserved for the sickest pediatric patients, enteral nutrition provides needed calories and eliminates dietary antigens that may trigger the immune system.

Perhaps the most basic form of nutritional therapy in IBD is the use of bowel rest and parenteral nutrition. In 1977, it was suggested that home total parenteral nutrition (TPN) be employed for the treatment of severe small bowel CD in children.[60] This study demonstrated that home TPN was safe and effective at promoting growth, while allowing the slow reintroduction of oral alimentation. Subsequently, trials of TPN and bowel rest have resulted in clinical remission of CD in adolescents and adults. Response rates as high as 90% have been reported with the use of exclusive TPN, even in steroid-refractory disease.[92] A study comparing TPN with a specified liquid diet and combined oral and parenteral nutrition showed that 71% of patients solely receiving TPN achieved remission after 21 days.[93] The other forms of nutritional support resulted in remission rates of 58% and 60% respectively, with 1-year remission rates decreasing to 42% in the TPN group and 55% in the other groups. A subsequent study similarly demonstrated superior response rates in a group receiving TPN, when compared to elemental diet and polymeric diet.[94]

Despite the reported success with TPN, enteral nutrition represents a more physiologic and safer delivery system and therefore would be preferable if similar results could be achieved. In 1995, Griffiths et al[95] reviewed 37 pediatric and adult trials of enteral nutrition as primary therapy for active CD. Thirteen trials met the inclusion criteria for meta-analysis, with 8 trials comprising 413 patients comparing liquid diet and corticosteroids. In this analysis, the pooled odds ratio for the likelihood of clinical remission with liquid diet therapy versus corticosteroids was 0.35, demonstrating that diet therapy alone was inferior to corticosteroid therapy for the induction of remission. Various sensitivity analyses did not significantly change the results. Approximately 20% of patients randomized to receive nutritional therapy failed to complete the trials due to intolerance to the formulas. The likelihood of intolerance was lower (8%) when the formula was administered strictly via nasogastric tube. The remaining 5 studies in the meta-analysis compared efficacy between polymeric and elemental diets. Out of 134 patients, tolerance for the liquid diets was quite high, with 94% completing the trials. In this analysis, there was no demonstrable difference in efficacy between the 2 types of diets. A subsequent meta-analysis demonstrated similar findings.[96] When including 10 studies comparing elemental diet with polymeric diet, no significant difference was found in efficacy of inducing remission. It should be noted that both TPN and enteral feeding are more effective for CD than for UC, where these interventions should be reserved for repletion of malnutrition rather than treatment of active disease.

AMINOSALICYLATES

The aminosalicylates, including sulfasalazine and the newer 5-aminosalicylic acid (5-ASA) compounds mesalamine and mesalazine, are first-line drugs with limited anti-inflammatory properties. They are felt to act locally with limited systemic absorption. The primary mechanism of action appears to be the drug's inhibition of the lipoxygenase pathway of arachidonic acid metabolism.[97]

There are limited pediatric data that evaluate the use of aminosalicylates in pediatric patients with IBD. Though there have been many studies evaluating the efficacy of these agents in adults with IBD, only a few randomized trials have been carried out in children. Based on findings from a large clinical trial, balsalazide is now 1 of 2 FDA-approved agents for treatment of UC in pediatric patients.[98] In a double-blind, placebo-controlled trial carried out by Griffiths et al, a small clinical and dose-related benefit was seen among the 6 patients treated with slow-release 5-ASA who completed the 20-week trial. A high drop-out rate among the placebo group and low recruitment rate led to termination of the study prior to its completion.[99] A novel high-strength formulation of 5-ASA—the Multimatrix mesalamine—is now available as 2.4 g and 4.8 g once daily (2 to 4 tablets at 1.2 g each tablet).[100,101] Although this formulation is not approved for children, because of the lower pill volume, it is an attractive option for use in the pediatric population.

Mesalamine (in Europe mesalazine) appears to be better tolerated than sulfasalazine among children.[102] Nausea and vomiting were more common with sulfasalazine. Other side effects including pancreatitis, hepatotoxicity, interstitial nephritis, and pericarditis have been described with the use of mesalamine. Rash and fever secondary to hypersensitivity can occur and are often linked to the sulfa moiety in sulfasalazine.[97]

Because of the limited number of controlled trials among children, dosing guidelines have not clearly been established for the use of the aminosalicylates. There is a trend towards using mesalamine in doses between 50 and 75 mg/kg/d, and doses as high as 100 mg/kg/d have been used. Limited availability of liquid preparations (azulfidine) of this class of drugs complicates its use among young patients who have difficulties swallowing pills or capsules, although patients are sometimes instructed to open Pentasa or Colazal capsules and place the microbeads or capsule contents in pudding, applesauce, or yogurt.

CORTICOSTEROIDS

Corticosteroids continue to be a mainstay of therapy for acute exacerbations of pediatric inflammatory bowel disease. Despite the known long list of side effects, no drug to date has shown a better ability to provide symptomatic relief. Previous studies have shown a 20% to 36% dependence rate among Crohn's patients and 20% of patients are steroid resistant.[97] There have been no controlled trials using corticosteroids versus placebo among pediatric patients. Previous studies have, however, evaluated enteral nutrition and corticosteroids. A recent meta-analysis found similar remission rates, close to 85%, among patients using corticosteroids and those treated with enteral nutrition.[103]

Budesonide, a newer steroid formulation with extensive first-pass hepatic metabolism, has been reported to reduce the unwanted side effects of corticosteroids. Although no placebo-controlled trials have been carried out using this drug in pediatrics, several studies comparing budesonide and prednisolone have been conducted recently. Levine et al performed an age-matched retrospective study using budesonide and prednisone in pediatric CD patients with mild to moderate disease.[104] Remission was achieved in 48% of patients in the budesonide group versus 77% of patients who received prednisone. They also demonstrated that budesonide was more effective than mesalamine and antibiotics at inducing remission. The authors concluded that budesonide should be considered a first-line agent in mild-to-moderate CD to induce remission. In 2004, Escher and the European Collaborative Research Group on Budesonide in Pediatric IBD conducted a prospective, double-blind trial comparing budesonide and prednisolone in active pediatric CD involving the ileum and/or the ascending colon. The study showed that both medications achieved some remission (55% among budesonide users versus 71% among prednisolone users). Though prednisolone showed a trend towards being more effective at inducing remission, budesonide demonstrated a better side effect profile with less adrenal suppression measured by mean cortisol levels and less cosmetic side effects.[105]

A prospective study of 128 children with severe UC identified several predictors of steroid unresponsiveness. Pediatric UC Activity Index (PUCAI) measures at days 3 and 5 after initiation of IV corticosteroid therapy were found to be strong predictors of treatment failure and an indication for salvage therapy.[106]

Although corticosteroids offer an effective short-term remediation of symptoms for active CD and UC, the side effect profiles prohibit long-term use. Side effects including fluid retention, fat redistribution, hypertension, hyperglycemia, cataracts, and weight gain are well known and appear to be related to dose and duration of therapy.[97] As discussed previously, bone demineralization and linear growth retardation that also occur with corticosteroid use are more damaging and often more difficult to correct. In the MATRIX study, budesonide was associated with a significantly smaller reduction in bone mass compared with prednisolone in corticosteroid-naïve patients with active ileocecal CD.[107]

IMMUNOMODULATORS

6-Mercaptopurine and Azathioprine

Used for more than 50 years in oncology patients, 6-MP and its predrug azathioprine (AZA) are being used with increasing frequency in pediatric patients with IBD. Markowitz et al conducted a survey among 718 pediatric gastroenterologists in North America that compared attitudes towards the use of immunomodulatory therapy in 1990 and 2000. His group found significant increases in physicians' willingness to prescribe these agents and an expansion in physicians' indications for prescribing this drug. Among the immunomodulators mentioned in this study, AZA and 6-MP were prescribed by the greatest number of responders.[108]

Among pediatric IBD patients, clinical evidence supporting the use of AZA and 6-MP was limited to retrospective studies until the past few years. In 1990, Verhave et al showed partial or complete clinical remission in 75% of patients with CD or UC who took AZA. Additionally, most of the patients who responded to the medication were able to discontinue corticosteroids within 6 months of starting AZA.[97,109] Markowitz et al also demonstrated a significant reduction in steroid use for patients who received 6-MP.

They reported that 57% were able to discontinue corticosteroids within 6 months and 80% within 1 year of the initiation of 6-MP.[110]

In 2000, Markowitz et al published the first randomized, placebo-controlled trial evaluating the early use of 6-MP in newly diagnosed pediatric patients with moderate to severe Crohn's. His group found a significantly shorter duration of steroid use and lower cumulative steroid dose at 6, 12, and 18 months among patients who received 6-MP versus placebo. And though remission was initially induced in 89% of both groups, only 9% of patients that were maintained on 6-MP relapsed versus 47% of controls. Long-term remission at 18 months was 89% in the 6-MP group versus 39% in the placebo group.[111]

Given the known side effects of the use of this class of medications including both allergic (pancreatitis, arthralgias, rash, and fever) and nonallergic reactions (leukopenia, thrombocytopenia, infection, hepatitis, and malignancy), safety remains a concern when prescribing this drug to pediatric patients. Kirschner reported that 28% of 95 pediatric patients who received 6-MP or AZA had some side effects (most commonly elevated aminotransferase levels) and that cessation of the drug occurred in 18% of patients because of drug hypersensitivity or infection.[112] Other retrospective studies showed mild side effects including leukopenia and elevated aminotransferases in almost 40% of pediatric patients.[97] Immunomodulators are generally well tolerated, although the potential for long-term exposure and the possibility of malignancy are a concern.[113] The risks of immunomodulators are contrasted with the benefits of steroids-sparing in vulnerable pediatric patients.[114]

Though the Markowitz study recommended the early use of 6-MP or AZA for all newly diagnosed pediatric patients with moderate to severe CD, clearer guidelines for selected use have not been reported. A study conducted at our institution found that patients with lower serum albumin at diagnosis (3.1 g/dL versus 3.75 g/dL) and higher PCDAI at diagnosis (40 versus 24) were significantly more likely to be started on immunomodulators. In addition, all patients with serum albumin 2.8 g/dL or less were placed on immunomodulators within 6 months of diagnosis versus only 45% of patients with serum albumin of 2.9 g/dL or greater.[115]

No studies to date have been performed with regards to appropriate pediatric dosing. Accepted practice among clinicians is to start with doses of 1 to 1.5 mg/kg when using 6-MP and 2.0 to 2.5 mg/kg when using AZA.

Methotrexate

Limited studies exist evaluating the use of methotrexate in pediatric IBD. In the only published full study to date assessing clinical outcomes with subcutaneous methotrexate, Mack et al established clinical efficacy with this medication. In a study of 14 patients with steroid-dependent

CD who failed or did not tolerate 6-MP, 9 (64%) showed improvement within 4 weeks of initiation of therapy.[116]

Side effects including gastrointestinal problems (nausea, anorexia, and diarrhea), headaches, dizziness, fatigue, and mood changes have been reported. Additionally, leukopenia, thrombocytopenia, pulmonary toxicity, and opportunistic infections are also possible. Hepatotoxicity, although still a concern, is less common than once thought.[97] Recent data in pediatrics suggest that oral methotrexate may be better tolerated and has similar bioavailability to the subcutaneous form.[117]

CYCLOSPORINE

Cyclosporine, developed initially for the prevention of organ rejection, has some role in the treatment of patients with IBD and in particular those patients with refractory, severe UC.[118-121] To date, no controlled trials have been conducted using cyclosporine in refractory UC in a pediatric population.

ANTIBIOTICS

Although bacteria flora has been given a central role in the development of IBD, the role of antibiotics in the treatment of pediatric IBD has only been studied on a limited basis. No randomized trials using antibiotics have been published in a pediatric population to date. In one pediatric reference, Hildebrand et al showed clinical efficacy of metronidazole among 20 children with CD with perianal involvement. Of the 20 patients, more than half showed some clinical improvement during 6 months of treatment. After discontinuation of therapy in 9 patients, 5 had a relapse within 1 month of discontinuation.[122]

Side effects with the use of metronidazole have been reported in children. Duffy et al documented peripheral neuropathies in 11 of 13 patients treated with metronidazole.[123] Other antibiotics including the fluoroquinolones, which have demonstrated some efficacy among adult patients with perianal and fistulous CD,[124] have been linked to cartilage damage in laboratory animals. Safety data for this class of drug have been published after studies in children in Great Britain and Japan; however, no safety data exist for pediatric IBD patients.[97] Fluoroquinolones and cephalosporins are strongly associated with the increasing incidence of *Clostridium difficile*-associated diarrhea (CDAD), which parallels the incidence of CDAD in patients with IBD.[125] Nitazoxanide 500 mg twice daily for 7 to 10 days is effective against *C difficile*. A recent study demonstrated the noninferiority of nitazoxanide compared with metronidazole in treating *C difficile* colitis.[126]

INFLIXIMAB

Infliximab, a humanized, chimeric, monoclonal anti-TNFα antibody, is approved by the Food and Drug Administration (FDA) for use in children with CD and represents the first biologic agent approved for use in children. In fact, the agent was first used in a 13-year-old girl with refractory Crohn's colitis. The first published controlled trial in children was carried out in a joint European–American trial. In this study, patients with severe refractory CD were randomized to receive either 1, 5, or 10 mg/kg of infliximab. The medication demonstrated clinical efficacy in the 5 and 10 mg/kg groups at 4, 12, and 20 weeks with better outcome at 20 weeks among the 5 mg/kg group versus the 10 mg/kg (50% versus 33%) group in achieving clinical remission.[127] A retrospective study conducted by Stephens et al reviewed the experience with infliximab at a large pediatric institution. A total of 432 infusions were given to 82 patients with severe refractory Crohn's disease. Of 33 patients who were using corticosteroids at the initiation of infliximab, almost 60% were able to discontinue their use. The study also showed significant decreases between steroid doses at 0 and 4 weeks and 0 and 8 weeks.[128] Several other open-label trials using infliximab have demonstrated clinical efficacy.[97] The REACH study evaluated the safety and efficacy of infliximab in children with moderately to severely active CD. After 1 year of treatment, 63.5% and 55.8% of patients who received infliximab every 8 weeks achieved clinical response and were in clinical remission, respectively, and did not require dose adjustment. Most importantly, at the end of 1 year, almost 50% of children receiving infliximab every 8 weeks were in remission and no longer required steroids, compared with only 17% of children receiving infliximab every 12 weeks.[129] Rare postmarketing cases of hepatosplenic T cell lymphoma have been reported; all of the cases occurred in patients on concomitant treatment with 6-MP or AZA. The role of early top-down infliximab or immunomodulators in steroid-naïve children with CD[130] or infliximab monotherapy in children with CD exposed to steroids[131] needs to be evaluated in light of the recent adult trials showing treatment efficacy and a reduced need for steroids in patients taking these agents.

Infliximab has also been used with some success in pediatric patients with UC.[132,133] Mamula et al demonstrated clinical efficacy with this medication among 9 patients consecutively treated with doses of infliximab at 0 and 2 weeks. Seven of 9 patients had a decrease of disease activity based on lowering of the Physician Global Assessment, and corticosteroids were discontinued in 6 of the 11 patients who received infliximab.[120] While this study showed some success in the short term, questions remain for the role of infliximab in the long-term management of pediatric UC.

Side effects of the medication, including opportunistic

infections, tuberculosis and herpes zoster, systemic lupus erythematosus drug-induced reaction serum sickness, and malignancies, although rare, have been reported. More common side effects from the medication are infusion reactions. Thought to occur in about 6% of patients who receive infliximab, reactions including diaphoresis, shortness of breath, blood pressure changes, and tachycardia are well documented.[97,127] Recent studies in pediatrics have focused on the role that human anti-chimeric antibodies (HACA, otherwise known as antibodies to infliximab or ATI) play in infusion reactions and efficacy of the medication. Miele et al evaluated the role that HACA plays in infusion reactions and found that they occurred in higher proportions in patients who were HACA-positive than in those who were HACA-negative. In addition, they found that patients with HACA levels above 8.0 μg/mL were more likely to have infusion reactions, and concomitant immunomodulator use was associated with a lower risk of developing HACA.[134]

TRANSITION OF THE PATIENT WITH INFLAMMATORY BOWEL DISEASE FROM PEDIATRIC TO ADULT CARE

Children with IBD should be cared for by a physician trained to manage issues unique to pediatric patients.[135] Pediatric gastroenterologists have the expertise to address a multitude of important problems that uniquely occur during childhood, particularly growth and development. Internist gastroenterologists have a different set of skills that are necessary to provide optimal care to adult patients with IBD.

The passage from adolescence to adulthood is a time of internal turmoil and intense examination of personal goals and wishes. Being ill during this time of growing and changing may cause frustration about the present and anxiety about the future. The growing adolescent must be able to progressively shed the sheltered environment of childhood and achieve self-reliance and independent living as a decision maker. Under normal circumstances, this process is painful for the healthiest of individuals. For the chronically ill adolescent, this period of transition can be stressful not only for the patient but for his or her family and health-care providers.[136-140]

During the transition to an internist-gastroenterologist, patients, parents, and other family members may feel threatened by changes in the pattern of care and resentful of the effort required to adjust to a new setting and different staff. They have weathered many crises and made vital decisions with the support of the pediatric team and frequently regard this strong source of advocacy as a permanent arrangement. In contrast, they may perceive the internist who expects to care for an independent individual as less involved or less sensitive to the developmental and social aspects of his or her medical condition.

Health-care providers may also feel ambivalent during this period of change. The pediatrician may view the maturation of the child as a professional and personal achievement and find difficulty in relinquishing the patient to others whose style of practice he or she may not know well.

The process of transition should begin when a patient enters early to middle adolescence. The pediatric gastroenterologist should begin seeing adolescent patients without their parents in order to build a relationship that promotes independence and self-reliance. It is important to discuss with the patient and the family that in the future they will need to transition to a gastroenterologist who is also trained in internal medicine with expertise in dealing with medical problems that occur during adulthood, including pregnancy, fertility, and cancer surveillance.

Once the decision to pursue a transition program has been made, the next step is to identify a skilled gastroenterologist who cares for young adults. This individual must realize that a young adult with childhood-onset IBD may have a different set of expectations than the young adult with a recent onset of IBD. These young adults also have a heightened risk for the development of cancer and will require an increased need for cancer surveillance. The pediatrician needs to provide all of the necessary medical records and medical summaries so that all providers are working together to deliver excellent care.

Timing for transition will require some flexibility, because many patients have special circumstances. Any adolescent who has additional growth potential as a result of delayed puberty should be followed by a pediatric gastroenterologist. Also, children with neurologic delay should be transitioned to an adult gastroenterologist who has the expertise and the support necessary to provide comprehensive care.

CONCLUSION

Due to the complex nature of issues surrounding the care of a child or adolescent with IBD, it is necessary to adopt a multidisciplinary approach and devise an individual plan for therapy. Pediatric patients with IBD are not "little" adults, and the specific set of problems that they face including issues around growth, sexual development and puberty, and osteoporosis should be thought about when caring for these individuals. Though many of the same medications are available for pediatric patients that exist in the management of adult IBD, the judicious use of corticosteroids should be remembered as it has demonstrated such profound deleterious effects on bone density and final height outcomes. Adopting a team approach that includes physicians, nurses and nurse practitioners, nutritionists, social workers, and psychologists is necessary to ensure comprehensive care that will allow pediatric IBD patients to achieve appropriate levels of physical, mental, and social well-being.

REFERENCES

1. Mendelhoff AI, Calkins BM. The epidemiology of idiopathic inflammatory bowel disease. In: Kirsner JB, Shorter RG, eds. *Inflammatory Bowel Disease.* Philadelphia, PA: Lea & Febiger; 1988:3-34.

2. Farmer RG, Michener WM. Prognosis of Crohn's disease with onset in childhood or adolescence. *Dig Dis Sci.* 1979;24:752-757.

3. Garland CF, Lilienfield AM, Mendelhoff AI, et al. Incidence rates of ulcerative colitis and Crohn's disease in 15 areas of the United States. *Gastroenterology.* 1981;81:1115.

4. Baldassano RN, Piccoli DA. Inflammatory bowel disease in pediatric and adolescent patients. *Gastroenterol Clin North Am.* 1999;28:445-458.

5. Fonager K, Sorensen HT, Olsen J. Change in incidence of Crohn's disease and ulcerative colitis in Denmark. A study based on the National Registry of Patients, 1981-1992. *Int J Epidemiol.* 1997; 26:1003-1008.

6. Lindberg E, Lindquist B, Holmquist L, et al. Inflammatory bowel disease in children and adolescents in Sweden, 1984-1995. *J Pediatr Gastroenterol Nutr.* 2000;30:259-264.

7. Russel MG, Stockbrugger RW. Epidemiology of inflammatory bowel disease: an update. *Scand J Gastroenterol.* 1996;31:417-427.

8. Logan RF. Inflammatory bowel disease incidence: Up, down or unchanged? *Gut.* 1998;42:309-311.

9. Bjornsson S, Johannsson JH, Oddsson E. Inflammatory bowel disease in Iceland, 1980-89. A retrospective nationwide epidemiologic study. *Scand J Gastroenterol.* 1998;33:71-77.

10. Oliva-Hemker M, Fiocchi C. Etiopathogenesis of inflammatory bowel disease: the importance of the pediatric perspective. *Inflamm Bowel Dis.* 2002;8:112-128.

11. Tysk C, Lindberg E, Jarnerot G, et al. Ulcerative colitis and Crohn's disease in an unselected population of monozygotic and dizygotic twins. A study of heritability and the influence of smoking. *Gut.* 1988;29:990-996.

12. Langholz E, Munkholm P, Krasilnikoff PA. Inflammatory bowel disease with onset in childhood. *Scand J Gastroenterol.* 1997;32: 139-147.

13. Grand RJ Homer DR. Inflammatory bowel disease in childhood and adolescence. *Pediatr Clin North Am.* 1975;22:835.

14. Griffiths AM. Crohn's disease. *Rec Adv Pediatr.* 1992;10:145.

15. Lenaerts C, Roy CC, Vaillancourt M, et al. High incidence of upper gastrointestinal tract involvement in children with Crohn's disease. *Pediatrics.* 1989;83:777.

16. Hildebrand H, Karlberg J, Kristiansson B. Longitudinal growth in children and adolescents with inflammatory bowel disease. *J Pediatr Gastroenterol Nutr.* 1994;18:165-173.

17. Tourtelier Y, Dabadie A, Tron I, et al. Incidence of inflammatory bowel disease in children in Brittany (1994-1997). Breton Association of Study and Research on Digestive System Diseases (Abermad). *Arch Pediatr.* 2000;7:377-384.

18. Heikenen JB, Werlin SL, Brown CW, et al. Presenting symptoms and diagnostic lag in children with inflammatory bowel disease. *Inflamm Bowel Dis.* 1999;5:158-160.

19. Spray C, Debelle GD, Murphy MS. Current diagnosis, management and morbidity in paediatric inflammatory bowel disease. *Acta Paediatr.* 2001;90:400-405.

20. Wagtmans MJ, Verspaget HW, Lamers CB, et al. Crohn's disease in the elderly: a comparison with young adults. *J Clin Gastroenterol.* 1998;27:129-133.

21. Fazio VW. Toxic megacolon in ulcerative colitis and Crohn's colitis. *Clin Gastroenterol.* 1980;9:271.

22. Huizenga KA, Schroeder KW. *Gastrointestinal Complications of Ulcerative Colitis and Crohn's Disease.* 3rd ed. Philadelphia, PA: Lea and Febiger; 1988.

23. Binder SC, Patterson JF, Glotzer DJ. Toxic megacolon in ulcerative colitis. *Gastroenterology.* 1974;66:1088.

24. Devroede GJ, Taylor WF, Sauer J, et al. Cancer risk and life expectancy of children with ulcerative colitis. *N Engl J Med.* 1973; 289:491.

25. Ekbom A, Melmick C, Zack M, et al. Ulcerative colitis and colorectal cancer: a population based study. *N Engl J Med.* 1990;323:1228-1233.

26. Griffiths AM, Sherman PM. Colonscopic surveillance for cancer in ulcerative colitis: a critical review. *J Pediatr Gastoenterol Nutr.* 1997;24:202-210.

27. Hoffley PM, Piccoli DA. Inflammatory bowel disease in children. *Med Clin North Am.* 1994;78:1281-1302.

28. Markowitz J, Daum F Algar M, et al. Perianal disease in children and adolescents with Crohn's disease. *Gastroenterology.* 1984; 86:829.

29. Danzi JT. Extraintestinal manifestations of idiopathic inflammatory bowel disease. *Arch Intern Med.* 1988;148:297-302.

30. Hyams JS. Crohn's disease in children. *Pediatr Clin North Am.* 1996;43:255-277.

31. Menachem Y, Weizman Z, Locker C, et al. Clinical characteristics of Crohn's disease in children and adults. *Harefuah.* 1998;134:173-175, 247.

32. Gryboski JD, Spiro HM. Prognosis in children with Crohn's disease. *Gastroenterology.* 1978;74:807-817.

33. Winesett M. Inflammatory bowel disease in children and adolescents. *Pediatr Ann.* 1997;26:227-234.

34. Hyams JS. Extraintestinal manifestations of inflammatory bowel disease in children. *J Pediatr Gastroenterol Nutr.* 1994;19:7-21.

35. Hofley P, Roarty J, McGinnity G, et al. Asymptomatic uveitis in children with chronic inflammatory bowel diseases. *J Pediatr Gastroenterol Nutr.* 1993;17:397-400.

36. Burbige EJ, Huang SH, Bayless TM. Clinical manifestations of Crohn's disease in children and adolescents. *Pediatrics.* 1975; 55:866-871.

37. Lindsley C, Schaller JG. Arthritis associated with inflammatory bowel disease in children. *J Pediatr.* 1974;86:76.

38. Kane W, Miller K, Sharp HL. Inflammatory bowel disease presenting as liver disease during childhood. *J Pediatr.* 1980;97:775-778.

39. Hyams J, Markowitz J, Treem W, et al. Characterization of hepatic abnormalities in children with inflammatory bowel disease. *Inflamm Bowel Dis.* 1995;1:27-33.

40. Faubion WA Jr, Loftus EV, Sandborn WJ, et al. Pediatric "PSC-IBD": a descriptive report of associated inflammatory bowel disease among pediatric patients with psc. *J Pediatr Gastroenterol Nutr.* 2001;33:296-300.

41. McLeod RS, Churchill DN. Urolithiasis complicating inflammatory bowel disease. *J Urol.* 1992;148:974-978.

42. Lloyd-Still JD, Tomasi L. Neurovascular and thromboembolic complications of inflammatory bowel disease in childhood. *J Pediatr Gastroenterol Nutr.* 1989;9:461-466.

43. Hudson M, Chitolie A, Hutton RA, et al. Thrombotic vascular risk factors in inflammatory bowel disease. *Gut.* 1996;38:733-737.

44. Markowitz RL, Ment LR, Gryboski JD. Cerebral thromboembolic disease in pediatric and adult inflammatory bowel disease: case report and review of the literature. *J Pediatr Gastroenterol Nutr.* 1989;8:413-420.

45. Reuner KH, Ruf A, Grau A, et al. Prothrombin gene G20210—a transition is a risk factor for cerebral venous thrombosis. *Stroke.* 1998;29:1765-1769.

46. Harper PH, Fazio VW, Lavery IC, et al. The long-term outcome in Crohn's disease. *Dis Colon Rectum.* 1987;30:174-179.

47. Motil KJ, Grand RJ, Maletskos CJ, et al. The effect of disease, drug, and diet on whole body protein metabolism in adolescents with Crohn disease and growth failure. *J Pediatr.* 1982;101:345-351.

48. Grill BB, Hillemeier AC, Gryboski JD. Fecal alpha 1-antitrypsin clearance in patients with inflammatory bowel disease. *J Pediatr Gastroenterol Nutr.* 1984;3:56-61.

49. Kelts D, Grand R, Shen G, et al. Nutritional basis of growth failure in children and adolescents with Crohn's disease. *Gastroenterology.* 1979;76:720-727.

50. Seidman E, LeLeiko N, Ament M, et al. Nutritional issues in pediatric inflammatory bowel disease. *J Pediatr Gastroenterol Nutr.* 1991;12:424-438.

51. Kanof ME, Lake AM, Bayless TM. Decreased height velocity in children and adolescents before the diagnosis of Crohn's disease. *Gastroenterology.* 1988;95:1523-1527.

52. Hyams JS, Ferry GD, Mandel FS, et al. Development and validation of pediatric Crohn's Disease Activity Index. *J Pediatr Gastroenterol Nutr.* 1991;12:439-447.

53. Otley A, Loonen H, Parekh N, et al. Assessing activity of pediatric Crohn's disease: which index to use? *Gastroenterology.* 1999;116:527-531.

54. Rigaud D, Cosnes J, Le Quintrec Y, et al. Controlled trial comparing two types of enteral nutrition in treatment of active Crohn's disease: elemental versus. polymeric diet. *Gut.* 1991;32:1492-1497.

55. Sentongo T, Semeao E, Piccoli D, et al. Growth, body composition, and nutritional status in children and adolescents with Crohn's disease. *J Pediatr Gastroenterol Nutr.* 2000;31:33-40.

56. Motil K, Grand R, Matthews D, et al. Whole body leucine metabolism in adolescents with Crohn's disease and growth failure during nutritional supplementation. *Gastroenterology.* 1982;82:1361-1368.

57. Layden T, Rosenberg F, Nemchausky G, et al. Reversal of growth arrest in adolescents with Crohn's disease after parenteral alimentation. *Gastroenterology.* 1976;70:1017-1021.

58. Christie P, Hill G. Effect of intravenous nutrition on nutrition and function in acute attacks of inflammatory bowel disease. *Gastroenterology.* 1990;99:730-736.

59. Ferguson A, Glen M, Ghosh S. Crohn's disease: nutrition and nutritional therapy. *Bailliere's Clin Gastroenterol.* 1998;12:93-114.

60. Byrne W, Halpin T, Asch M, et al. Home total parenteral nutrition: an alternative approach to the management of children with severe chronic small bowel disease. *J Ped Surg.* 1977;12:359-366.

61. Kirschner B, Klich J, Kalman S, et al. Reversal of growth retardation in Crohn's disease with therapy emphasizing oral nutritional restitution. *Gastroenterology.* 1980;80:10-15.

62. Motil K. Aggressive nutritional therapy in growth retardation. *Clin Nutr.* 1985;4:75-84.

63. Himes JH, Roche AF, Thissen D, et al. Parent-specific adjustments for evaluation of recumbent length and stature of children. *Pediatrics.* 1985;75:304-313.

64. Rosen DS. Pubertal growth and sexual maturation for adolescents with chronic illness or disability. *Pediatrician.* 1991;18:105-120.

65. Brain CE, Savage MO. Growth and puberty in chronic inflammatory bowel disease. *Bailliere's Clin Gastroenterol.* 1994;8:83-100.

66. Tanner JM. *Growth at Adolescence.* Oxford: Blackwell Scientific; 1972.

67. de Vizia B, Poggi V, Conenna R, et al. Iron absorption and iron deficiency in infants and children with gastrointestinal diseases. *J Pediatr Gastroenterol Nutr.* 1992;14:21-26.

68. Galloway R, McGuire J. Determinants of compliance with iron supplementation: supplies, side effects, or psychology? *Soc Sci Med.* 1994;39:381-390.

69. Mailloux R, Sitrin M. The skeletal complications of inflammatory bowel disease and their treatment. *Progr Inflamm Bowel Dis.* 1994;15:1-21.

70. Scott EM, Gaywood I, Scott BB. Guidelines for osteoporosis in coeliac disease and inflammatory bowel disease. British Society of Gastroenterology. *Gut.* 2000;46(suppl 1):1-8.

71. Caulfield L, Himes J, Rivera J. Nutritional supplementation during early childhood and bone mineralization during adolescence. *J Nutr.* 1995;125:1104-1110.

72. Kanis JA, Pitt FA. Epidemiology of osteoporosis. *Bone.* 1992;13(suppl 1):S7-15.

73. Kanis JA, McCloskey EV. Epidemiology of vertebral osteoporosis. *Bone.* 1992;13(suppl 2):S1-S10.

74. Mora S, Pitukcheewanont P, Kaufman F, et al. Biochemical markers of bone turnover and the volume and the density of bone in children at different stages of sexual development. *J Bone Miner Res.* 1999;14:1664-1671.

75. Compston JE, Creamer B. Plasma levels and intestinal absorption of 25-hydroxyvitamin D in patients with small bowel resection. *Gut.* 1977;18:171-175.

76. Bell NH, Shaw S, Turner RT. Evidence that calcium modulates circulating 25-hydroxyvitamin D in man. *J Bone Miner Res.* 1987;2:211-214.

77. Clements MR, Johnson L, Fraser DR. A new mechanism for induced vitamin D deficiency in calcium deprivation. *Nature.* 1987;325:62-65.

78. Caniggia A, Nuti R, Lore F, et al. Pathophysiology of the adverse effects of glucoactive corticosteroids on calcium metabolism in man. *J Steroid Biochem.* 1981;15:153-161.

79. Suzuki Y, Ichikawa Y, Saito E, et al. Importance of increased urinary calcium excretion in the development of secondary hyperparathyroidism of patients under glucocorticoid therapy. *Metabolism.* 1983;32:151-156.

80. Lukert BP, Raisz LG. Glucocorticoid-induced osteoporosis: pathogenesis and management. *Ann Intern Med.* 1990;112:352-364.

81. Schoon EJ, Geerling BG, Van Dooren IM, et al. Abnormal bone turnover in long-standing Crohn's disease in remission. *Aliment Pharmacol Ther.* 2001;15:783-792.

82. LoCascio V, Adami S, Avioli LV, et al. Suppressive effect of chronic glucocorticoid treatment on circulating calcitonin in man. *Calcif Tissue Int.* 1982;34:309-310.

83. Nemetz A, Toth M, Garcia-Gonzalez MA, et al. Allelic variation at the interleukin 1 beta gene is associated with decreased bone mass in patients with inflammatory bowel diseases. *Gut.* 2001;49:644-649.

84. Schulte CM, Dignass AU, Goebell H, et al. Genetic factors determine extent of bone loss in inflammatory bowel disease. *Gastroenterology.* 2000;119:909-920.

85. Brain C, Savage M, Leonard J, et al. Characteristics of pubertal development in inflammatory bowel disease (IBD). *Pediatr Res.* 1993;33(suppl):S86.

86. Kirschner BS. Growth and development in chronic inflammatory bowel disease. *Acta Paediatr Scand Suppl.* 1990;366:98-104.

87. Molgaard C, Thomsen BL, Michaelsen KF. Influence of weight, age and puberty on bone size and bone mineral content in healthy children and adolescents. *Acta Paediatr.* 1998;87:494-499.

88. Bonjour JP, Theintz G, Buchs B, et al. Critical years and stages of puberty for spinal and femoral bone mass accumulation during adolescence. *J Clin Endocrinol Metab.* 1991;73:555-563.

89. Bailey DA, Martin AD, McKay HA, et al. Calcium accretion in girls and boys during puberty: a longitudinal analysis. *J Bone Miner Res.* 2000;15:2245-2250.

90. Smith EP, Boyd J, Frank GR, et al. Estrogen resistance caused by a mutation in the estrogen-receptor gene in a man. *N Engl J Med.* 1994;331:1056-1061.

91. Bertolloni S, Cappa M, Lala R, et al. Altered bone mineralization in complete androgen insensitivity syndrome [abstract]. *Horm Res.* 1997;48(suppl):811A.

92. Forbes A. Crohn's disease—the role of nutritional therapy. *Aliment Pharmacol Ther.* 2002;16(suppl 4):48-52.

93. Greenberg G, Fleming C, Jeejeebhoy K, et al. Controlled trial of bowel rest and nutritional support in the management of Crohn's disease. *Gut.* 1988;29:1309-1315.

94. Kobayashi K, Katsumata T, Yokoyama K, et al. A randomized controlled study of total parenteral nutrition and enteral nutrition by elemental and polymeric diet as primary therapy in active phase of Crohn's disease. *Nippon Shokakibyo Gakkai Zasshi.* 1998;95:1212-1221.

95. Griffiths AM, Ohlsson A, Sherman PM, et al. Meta-analysis of enteral nutrition as a primary treatment of active Crohn's disease. *Gastroenterology.* 1995;108:1056-1067.

96. Zachos M, Tondeur M, Griffiths AM. Enteral nutritional therapy for inducing remission of Crohn's disease. *Cochrane Database Syst Rev.* 2001:CD000542.

97. Escher JC, Taminiau JA, Nieuwenhuis EE, et al. Treatment of inflammatory bowel disease in childhood: best available evidence. *Inflamm Bowel Dis.* 2003;9:34-38.

98. Bosworth BP, Pruitt RE, Gordon GL, et al. Balsalazide tablets 3.3 g twice daily improves signs and symptoms of mild-to-moderate ulcerative colitis [abstract]. *Gastroenterology.* 2008;134:A-495.

99. Griffiths A, Koletzko S, Sylvester F, et al. Slow release 5-aminosalicylic acid therapy in children with small intestinal Crohn's disease. *J Pediatr Gastroenterol Nutr.* 1993;17:186-192.

100. Lichtenstein GR, Kamm MA, Boddu P, et al. Effect of once or twice-daily MMX mesalamine (SPD476) for the induction of remission of mild to moderately active ulcerative colitis. *Clin Gastroenterol Hepatol.* 2007;5:95-102.

101. Kamm MA, Sandborn WJ, Gassull M, et al. Once-daily, high concentration MMX mesalamine in active ulcerative colitis. *Gastroenterology.* 2007;132:66-73.

102. Ferry GD, Kirschner BS, Grand RJ, et al. Olsalazine versus sulfasalazine in mild to moderate childhood ulcerative colitis: results of the Pediatric Gastroenterology Collaborative Research Group Clinical Trial. *J Pediatr Gastroenterol Nutr.* 1993;17:32-38.

103. Heuschkel RB, Menache CC, Megerian JT, et al. Enteral nutrition and corticosteroids in the treatment of acute Crohn's disease in children. *J Pediatr Gastroenterol Nutr.* 2000;31:8-15.

104. Levine A, Broide E, Stein M, et al. Evaluation of oral budesonide for treatment of mild and moderate exacerbations of Crohn's disease in children. *J Pediatr.* 2002;140:75-80.

105. Escher JC and the European Collaborative Research Group on Budesonide in Pediatric IBD. Budesonide versus prednisolone for the treatment of active Crohn's disease in children: a randomized, double-blind, controlled, multi-centre trial. *Eur J Gastroenterol Hepatol.* 2004;16:47-54.

106. Turner D, Mack D, Leleiko N, et al. Severe pediatric ulcerative colitis: a prospective multicenter study of outcomes and predictors of response. *Gastroenterology.* In press.

107. Schoon EJ, Bollani S, Mills PR, et al. Bone mineral density in relation to efficacy and side effects of budesonide and prednisolone in Crohn's disease. *Clin Gastroenterol Hepatol.* 2005;3:113-121.

108. Markowitz J, Grancher K, Kohn N, et al. Immunomodulatory therapy for pediatric inflammatory bowel disease: changing patterns of use, 1990-2000. *Am J Gastroenterol.* 2002;97:928-932.

109. Verhave M, Winter HS, Grand RJ. Azathiprine in the treatment of children with inflammatory bowel disease. *J Pediatr.* 1990;117:809-814.

110. Markowitz J, Rosa J, Grancher K, et al. Long-term 6-mercaptopurine treatment in adolescents with Crohn's disease. *Gastroenterology.* 1990;99:1347-1351.

111. Markowitz J, Grancher K, Kohn N, et al. A multicenter trial of 6-mercaptopurine and prednisone in children with newly diagnosed Crohn's disease. *Gastroenterology.* 2000;119:895-902.

112. Kirschner BS. Safety of azathiprine and 6-mercaptopurine in pediatric patients with inflammatory bowel disease. *Gastroenterology.* 1998;115:813-821.

113. Beaugerie L, Carrat F, Bouvier AM, et al, for the CESAME Study Group. Excess risk of lymphoproliferative disorders (LPD) in inflammatory bowel diseases (IBD): interim results of the CESAME cohort [abstract]. *Gastroenterology.* 2008;134(4 suppl 1):A116.

114. Griffiths AM. Specificities of inflammatory bowel disease in childhood. *Best Pract Res Clin Gastroenterol.* 2004;18:509-523.

115. Jacobstein D, Mamula P, Markowitz JE, et al. Predictors of immunomodulator use as early therapy in pediatric Crohn's disease [abstract]. *J Pediatr Gastroenterol Nutr.* 2004;39(suppl1):A678.

116. Mack DR, Young R, Kaufman SS, et al. Methotrexate in patients with Crohn's disease after 6-mercaptopurine. *J Pediatr.* 1998;132:830-835.

117. Stephens MC, Baldassano RN, York A, et al. The oral bioavailability of methotrexate in pediatric patients with inflammatory bowel disease [abstract]. *J Pediatr Gastroenterol Nutr.* 2004;39(suppl1):A287.

118. Treem WR, Cohen J, Davis PM, et al. Cyclosporine for the treatment of fulminant ulcerative colitis in children. Immediate response, long-term results, and impact on surgery. *Dis Colon Rectum.* 1995;38:474-479.

119. Nicholls SW, Domizio P, Williams CB, et al. Cyclosporin as initial treatment of Crohn's disease. *Arch Dis Child.* 1994;71:243-247.

120. Turner D, Walsh CM, Benchimol EI, et al. Severe paediatric ulcerative colitis: incidence, outcomes and optimal timing for second-line therapy. *Gut.* 2008;57:331-338.

121. Sandborn WJ. A critical review of cyclosporine therapy in inflammatory bowel disease. *Inflamm Bowel Dis.* 1995;1:48-63.

122. Hildebrand H, Berg NO, Hoevels J, et al. Treatment of Crohn's disease with metronidazole in childhood and adolescence. Evaluation of a six months trial. *Gastroenterol Clin Biol.* 1980;4:19-25.

123. Duffy LF, Daum F, Fisher SE, et al. Peripheral neuropathy in Crohn's disease patients treated with metronidazole. *Gastroenterology.* 1985;88:681-684.

124. Turunen U, Farkkila V, Valtonen V, et al. Long-term outcome of ciprofloxacin treatment in sever perianal of fistulous Crohn's disease [abstract]. *Gastroenterology.* 1993;104:A793.

125. Issa M, Ananthakrishnan AN, Binion DG. *Clostridium difficile* and inflammatory bowel disease. *Inflamm Bowel Dis.* 2008;14:1432-1442.

126. Musher DM, Logan N, Hamill RJ, et al. Nitazoxanide for the treatment of *Clostridium difficile* colitis. *Clin Infect Dis.* 2006;43:421-427.

127. Baldassano RN, Braegger CP, Escher JC, et al. Infliximab (REMICADE) therapy in the treatment of pediatric Crohn's disease. *Am J Gastroenterol.* 2003;98:833-838.

128. Stephens MC, Shepanski MA, Mamula P, et al. Safety and steroid-sparing experience using infliximab for Crohn's disease at a pediatric inflammatory bowel disease center. *Am J Gastroenterol.* 2003;98:104-111.

129. Hyams J, Crandall W, Kugathasan S, et al. Induction and maintenance infliximab therapy for the treatment of moderate-to severe Crohn's disease in children. *Gastroenterology.* 2007;132:863-873.

130. D'Haens G, Baert F, van Assche G, et al, and the Belgian Inflammatory Bowel Disease Research Group and North-Holland Gut Club. Early combined immunosuppression or conventional management in patients with newly diagnosed Crohn's disease: An open randomised trial. *Lancet.* 2008;371:660-667.

131. Sandborn W, Rutgeerts P, Reinisch W, et al. SONIC: A randomized, double-blind, controlled trial comparing infliximab and infliximab and azathioprine to azathioprine in patients with Crohn's disease naïve to immunomodulators and biologic therapy. Paper presented at: the American College of Gastroenterology 2008 Annual Scientific Meeting; Orlando, FL; October 7, 2008.

132. Mamula P, Markowitz JE, Brown, KA, et al. Infliximab as a novel therapy for pediatric ulcerative colitis. *J Pediatr Gastroenterol Nutr.* 2002;34:307-311.

133. Cucchiara S, Romeo E, Viola F, et al. Infliximab for pediatric ulcerative colitis: a retrospective Italian multicenter study. *Dig Liver Dis.* 2008;40(suppl 2):S260-S264.

134. Miele E, Markowitz JE, Mamula P, et al. Human antichimeric antibody in children and young adults with inflammatory bowel disease receiving infliximab. *J Pediatr Gastroenterol Nutr.* 2004;38:502-508.

135. Baldassano R, Ferry G, Griffiths A, et al. Transition of the patient with inflammatory bowel disease from pediatric to adult care: recommendations of the North American Society for Pediatric Gastroenterology, Hepatology and Nutrition. *J Pediatr Gastroenterol Nutr.* 2002;34:245-248.

136. Betz CL. Facilitating the transition of adolescents with chronic conditions from pediatric to adult health care and community settings. *Issues Compr Pediatr Nurs.* 1998;21:97-115.

137. Blum RW, Garell D, Hodgman CH, et al. Transition from child-centered to adult health-care systems for adolescents with chronic conditions. A position paper of the Society for Adolescent Medicine. *J Adolesc Health.* 1993;14:570-576.

138. Rosen D. Between two worlds: bridging the cultures of child health and adult medicine. *J Adolesc Health.* 1995;17:10-16.

139. Sawyer SM, Blair S, Bowes G. Chronic illness in adolescents: transfer or transition to adult services? *J Pediatr Child Health.* 1997;33:88-90.

140. American Academy of Pediatrics Committee on Children With Disabilities and Committee on Adolescence. Transition of care provided for adolescents with special health care needs. *Pediatrics.* 1996;98:1203-1206.

THE LIMITATIONS OF APPLYING EVIDENCE-BASED MEDICINE TO INFLAMMATORY BOWEL DISEASE
WHAT WE DO NOT LEARN FROM CLINICAL TRIALS

Joshua R. Korzenik, MD and Corey A. Siegel, MD

The support and enthusiasm for evidence-based medicine emerged from the hope that utilizing data from the best-performed studies would minimize the biases and inaccuracies inherent in relying heavily on personal experience to guide patient care. Though invaluable, clinical practice can present a random set of occurrences that alter the approach to particular patient circumstances. Evidence-based medicine aims to minimize those biases by grounding decision making in the data generated by studies conducted according to the highest standards. Randomized controlled trials have evolved to be conducted according to a rigorous set of criteria to provide evidence to direct clinical care. However, these trials have their weaknesses as well. This chapter aims to examine the limitations of the evidence we rely on to guide our clinical practice.

APPLICABILITY

The protean nature of inflammatory bowel disease (IBD) complicates the process of determining the applicability of trial results to an individual patient. The peculiarities of a particular study often are not generalizable to broader situations. The specific question that a study is designed to answer may not be applicable to the immediate dilemma facing the clinician. The inclusion and exclusion criteria for a study referred to for guidance may have excluded the patient that the physician is assessing for treatment. For instance, the medications a patient is taking or his or her level of disease activity may have prevented the patient from enrolling in the study, limiting the applicability of the results to that individual.

Often, a study is reduced to its bottom-line result: Is the study drug effective or not effective in the disease?

However, a positive trial does not imply that this drug is appropriate for any patient with the diagnosis. The specifics of the trial must be reviewed: What was the severity of patients enrolled—mild, moderate, or severe? What concomitant medications were permitted? What was the distribution of disease in patients? What was the duration of the study? Was this a maintenance study or evaluation of short-term efficacy? Were there subgroups that responded or failed to respond?

A central issue is whether the population studied resembles the individual being considered for therapy. Patients enrolled in clinical trials often have a disproportionate recruitment from academic centers, which by their nature differ from a typical community practice. An academic center will have a group of patients referred due to refractory disease, having failed numerous other agents. In addition, patients enrolled in a study may have fewer options for care as they may not have health insurance and are turning to a study as an opportunity to obtain medications. This population may have socioeconomic characteristics different from a typical community practice, as well as other associated complications such as nutritional deficits. In addition, as IBD management has changed in recent years, a shifting population may be enrolled in current trials compared to even just several years ago. As a variety of centers and countries are being brought in to enhance recruitment in the competitive proliferation of trials, there may be a shift in the nature of patients enrolled, making the applicability of the findings to an individual patient more in question. Placebo remission rates have had a significant amount of variability,[1] ranging from 4%[2] to as high as 27%,[3] reflecting the heterogeneity of patients included in studies, which further complicates the interpretation of trial results.

TRIAL DESIGN

The conduct of trials has changed over the years. Comparisons across trials are always dubious at best given different entry criteria, patient populations, and endpoints. In addition, trial methodology in IBD has evolved considerably over the years. The current standard assessment for clinical improvement in Crohn's trials—the Crohn's Disease Activity Index (CDAI)—is an imperfect tool developed in 1976.[4] However, some landmark studies did not use this and may not be appropriately compared to other studies.[5] Even in recent studies in CD, the standard for assessment of improvement is shifting. A 50-point decrease was used as a minimal response in earlier studies.[6] A 70-point decrease in CDAI was then considered a minimal criteria for clinical response. Due to an increase in placebo response as well as other factors, a 100-point decrement is increasingly considered as the minimum decrease required to be categorized as a response to therapy, which will make comparisons across trials increasingly difficult. The common acceptance and use of standard evaluation tools in UC trials is even more recent.

The use of the CDAI as an evaluative tool presents its own problems. The index, utilizing a composite score of 8 different factors, is heavily weighted to reflect a subjective assessment of disease activity. As this may be in part appropriate, it also suggests that it is more susceptible to influence by factors other than an improvement in the inflammation responsible for disease activity. Furthermore, a recent publication suggests that even skilled clinicians interpret the CDAI differently.[7] Few, if any, use the CDAI as a clinical tool. When considering a specific treatment, the patient may have a CDAI above or below the entry criteria of the reference trial. The relevance of the study findings to that patient would be in question. Furthermore, the expectations of a patient and treating physician for a response to a particular therapy may be misled by CDAI endpoints. A remission in a trial, defined as a CDAI below 150 points, can still reflect considerable disease activity that patients would not consider a clinical remission.

PATIENT SUBGROUPS

The broad brush of diagnosis in IBD, dividing patients into 2 basic categories, UC and CD, likely subsumes a number of subtypes of disease that may have a different pathophysiology, clinical behavior, and response to medications. Many of these subcategories of disease have been suggested but are poorly defined and even less well assessed in association with study results. The clinical relevance of these subgroups remains unclear but it is worth considering some potential subgroups of patients and trying to assess applicability.

Subgroups can be considered in terms of demographic characteristics, clinical behavior, biologic markers, genetic associations, or a more detailed microarray fingerprint. The patient characteristics and clinical behaviors suggested in the Vienna classification include age at diagnosis above or below 40 years, disease location, and disease behavior (nonstricturing/nonpenetrating, stricturing, penetrating).[8] Genetic subtypes are being increasingly well identified, though the clinical relevance remains incompletely defined. At least in a broader category, however, familial versus sporadic Crohn's may be important in disease behavior. More specific genotypes, such as NOD2/CARD15 genotypes, may predict behavior and identify distinct subgroups.[9] Biomarkers such as pANCA, ASCA, OmpC, I2, and anti-flagellin likely identify subgroups of patients[10] and may be useful to predict disease aggressiveness.[11] A distinct subpopulation is characterized by those with an elevated C-reactive protein (CRP), though its clinical significance remains uncertain.

The relevance and appropriate use of these markers are undefined. We are perhaps emerging into an era where microarray profiles hold a promise to identify patients more distinctly and allow for the identification of distinct pathophysiologic subgroups that have a common biologic behavior and response to therapy. The increasing number of agents available makes selection of the appropriate medication more challenging. In the future, the ability to identify which subgroups have an increased likelihood of response to a drug will hopefully allow for more targeted therapy. The size of most studies limits the close assessment of disease subtypes. It is possible, if not likely, that useful therapeutic agents have been discarded as ineffective because of the failure to determine a subgroup for which that medication might be highly beneficial.

ADVERSE EVENTS

In assessing the results of a clinical study, an additional issue involves understanding the risks associated with the study medication. Common events are likely to be identified in a large clinical trial. Less common side effects, however, are poorly defined even in relatively large studies. Most individual studies provide inadequate information to make clinical decisions and to explain risk to patients. Two cases in point are the assessment of lymphoma in relation to infliximab and the identification of progressive multifocal leukoencephalopathy (PML) in studies of natalizumab (Tysabri).

The association of infliximab and adalimumab with lymphoma is likely a rare event but how uncommon remains in dispute. Though one of the better studies based on a primary care database suggests that lymphoma is not increased in the Crohn's population,[12] this issue remains controversial. Best evidence suggests that lymphoma may occur in 1 or 2 per 1000 individuals treated with infliximab, information that has emerged after several other randomized controlled trials and observational studies have been completed.[13-18] Initial individual randomized trials were too inadequate to provide these data. Further data, which have emerged since the completion of randomized controlled trials, suggest an associated mortality with infliximab as high as 1% to 2%.[13,15] Though such observational studies must be taken with appropriate weight, the relevance to a community practice is in question—as are the results of the randomized clinical trials for reasons detailed previously. Additionally, it is typical to normalize the mortality to patient years of follow-up. Thus, the generally accepted number of 1% mortality per patient year of follow-up is often quoted. This also needs to be looked at in the context question of does this augment baseline risk for lymphoma? The available published data suggest that similar rates of mortality in IBD population cohorts were observed prior to the introduction of infliximab to general use. Recently, a large retrospective analysis of more than 20,000 CD and UC patients recruited into a French registry confirmed an increased risk of non-Hodgkin's lymphoma and Epstein-Barr virus (EBV)-associated lymphoma in patients treated with azathioprine and 6-mercaptopurine (6-MP).[19] A meta-analysis of 26 studies of anti-TNFα therapy with infliximab, adalimumab, and certolizumab showed an elevated incidence rate ratio of non-Hodgkin's lymphoma compared to the general population.[20] Identification of subgroups experiencing significant morbidity and mortality is critical but not yet possible on the basis of available data. In addition, a broader issue that remains poorly defined is the natural history of IBD itself.

The dilemmas raised by natalizumab involve a different set of issues. The recent information presented in part in the media has described 6 cases of progressive PML in patients treated with natalizumab, 5 with multiple sclerosis (MS), and 1 with Crohn's disease.[21] Only 2 cases have been fatal—1 patient with MS and 1 patient with CD in the controlled trials—and both patients were on combined immunosuppression. Some uncommon side effects not seen in clinical trials may emerge after Food and Drug Administration (FDA) approval in postmarketing surveillance, as was the case for use of natalizumab in MS. The relevance of the findings in MS to Crohn's was uncertain when the first 2 cases of PML were identified in patients with MS. The concern was whether these cases resulted from the concomitant use of natalizumab with interferon or whether there was a unique or particular risk of PML in MS. Until the third case was identified (in a patient with Crohn's disease), the medication was speculated as possibly safe or at least potentially safer in Crohn's patients than MS—though such an assessment was made on inadequate data. The risks involved in the use of this medication remain uncertain, as further evaluations of patients who have received this drug are underway. How to apply this developing information to an individual will remain a challenge if this drug is reintroduced into the market.

CLINICAL APPLICATION OF STUDIES

Translating the results of clinical trials into practice requires a detailed knowledge of the clinical data. But even then, for reasons detailed previously, clinical trials have significant limitations in guiding the care of patients. Many of our decisions, even when informed by the best research available, are based on inferences and suppositions one step removed from the data because of the differences between the individual patient being treated and the study population. In addition, conflicting data may further complicate an already difficult clinical decision. As examples of the difficulty of applying research results to an individual patient, we discuss 2 publications in the following paragraphs, 1 that changed clinical practice and another that has led us to question a long-time standard of care.

ACCENT 1, published by Hanauer et al in the *Lancet* in 2002,[14] changed the clinical practice of treating patients with Crohn's disease. ACCENT 1 studied 573 patients with moderate to severely active luminal Crohn's disease. All patients received an initial intravenous infusion of 5 mg/kg of infliximab. Two weeks later, patients were assessed for a clinical response. Responders, based on a drop in CDAI of 70 points, were randomized to receive repeat infusions of either infliximab or placebo at weeks 2 and 6 and then every 8 weeks thereafter until week 46. The primary endpoint of the study was the time to loss of response (up to 1 year). The results show that among initial responders, patients who received repeated infliximab infusions had a significantly longer time to loss of response when compared to the placebo group (46 weeks compared with 19 weeks, $P < 0.0002$). Furthermore, about 3 times as many patients in the treatment groups had discontinued corticosteroids, and significantly more patients maintained a remission ($P < 0.007$) and/or response ($P < 0.0001$) at the end of 1 year. Serious adverse events were infrequent (4% had serious infections, 1 death was attributable to infliximab), and most patients (90%) were able to continue receiving infusions for the 1-year study period. Based on these results, the use of infliximab for induction and maintenance of moderate to severely active CD has become standard of care.

What doesn't this study show us? Figure 6-1 shows us that the median age was 35 years old, the median disease duration was 7.9 years, and 51% of patients had already had a segmental bowel resection. Although we do see these characteristics in many patients with Crohn's disease, there is a large cohort of patients routinely receiving infliximab who differ significantly from this population. For example, younger patients with early aggressive disease in whom we

	All patients (n=573)	Week-2 responders (n=335)	Week-2 non-responders (n=238)
Sex			
Male	239 (42%)	130 (39%)	109 (46%)
Female	334 (58%)	205 (61%)	129 (54%)
Race			
White	549 (96%)	315 (94%)	234 (98%)
Black	12 (2%)	10 (3%)	2 (1%)
Asian	5 (1%)	4 (1%)	1
Other	7 (1%)	6 (2%)	1
Age (years), median (IQR)	35 (28–46)	35 (27–46)	37 (30–46)
Disease duration (years), median (range)	7·9 (3·9–14·7)	7·5 (3·7–14·2)	9·3 (4·6–15·3)
Involved intestinal area			
Ileum	137/568 (24%)	74/331 (22%)	63/237 (27%)
Colon	109/568 (19%)	74/331 (22%)	35/237 (15%)
Ileum and colon	322/568 (57%)	183/331 (55%)	139/237 (59%)
Gastroduodenum	43/573 (8%)	24/335 (7%)	19/238 (7%)
Previous segmental resection(s)	291/573 (51%)	148/335 (44%)	143/238 (60%)
CDAI*, median (IQR)	297 (260–342)	299 (264–342)	291 (249–340)
IBDQ, median (IQR)	127 (110–147)	129 (114–147)	125 (106–145)
C-reactive protein concentration (mg/dL), median (IQR)	0·8 (0·4–2·3)	1·1 (0·4–2·8)	0·6 (0·4–1·5)
Patients with concomitant medication			
5-aminosalicylates	288 (50%)	159 (47%)	129 (54%)
6-mercaptopurine and azathioprine	144 (25%)	81 (24%)	63 (27%)
Methotrexate	23 (4%)	10 (3%)	13 (6%)
Patients with concomitant corticosteroids			
Any	293 (51%)	175 (52%)	118 (50%)
>20 mg per day	93 (16%)	61 (18%)	32 (13%)

IBDQ=inflammatory bowel disease questionnaire (values can range from 32 to 224). *On final clinical data review, 13 enrolled patients had baseline Crohn's disease activity index (CDAI) <220. For nine of these patients, CDAI as calculated by investigator was ≥220. Remaining four patients were protocol violators.

FIGURE 6-1. Baseline patient characteristics from ACCENT 1. (Reproduced with permission from Hanauer SB, Feagan BG, Lichtenstein GR, et al. Maintenance infliximab for Crohn's disease: the ACCENT I randomised trial. *Lancet.* 2002;359:1541-1549.)

are trying to prevent surgery may benefit most from infliximab, but we do not get an indication of how these patients responded in ACCENT 1 (or whether they were adequately represented). Furthermore, only 25% of all patients were on 6-MP or azathioprine. In general, unless there is a contraindication, our practice is to maintain all patients on concomitant immunomodulators. Now, a few years later, the question of the clinical utility of this tactic is still controversial. We also do not know how concomitant medications (ie, immunomodulators, 5-aminosalicylic acid (5-ASAs), steroids, antibiotics) influenced response. This becomes very important when our patients ask us whether they need to continue their cocktail of drugs, and, unfortunately, we are not armed with an evidence-based answer. Patients also ask us how long they need to continue infliximab once started. The answer "until you lose a benefit or have an adverse event" is far from optimal. Although ACCENT 1 shows us the course of patients over a 1-year period, we still lack good data for long-term efficacy, expanding the dosing interval, or withdrawal studies.

When discussing risks of infliximab with patients, good evidence-based data are also inadequate. ACCENT 1 had limited severe toxicity, but adverse event reporting included only 385 patients and also did not have a complete placebo group as a comparison for safety (as all patients received at least one dose of the medication). What if severe, life-threatening toxicity were 1/500, 1/1000, 1/10,000, or even less common? Unfortunately, this is a question that can never be answered in trials like ACCENT 1 but waits for postmarketing analysis and future trials, which may be reported years later.

The role of a study like ACCENT 1 is to define efficacy in a homogeneous population, not explore alternative indications, long-term results, and adverse effects, or to characterize subpopulations of patients most likely to benefit from therapy. A single study can answer a limited set of questions. Once a landmark study like ACCENT 1 is presented, we are required to evaluate data critically and to heed further publications and our own clinical experience to guide our day-to-day management of patients. To that end, the follow-up REACH study confirmed safety and efficacy of infliximab in children with moderate to severely active Crohn's disease and confirms that infliximab every 8 weeks is more effective in maintaining remission than infliximab every 12 weeks.[22] An open randomized trial evaluating patients with Crohn's disease of short duration was recently performed. This study compared early use of combination therapy with infliximab and azathioprine and compared this to conventional step-up therapy where steroids are used initially and then after 2 courses of steroids, azathioprine is initiated. The early use of combination therapy with infliximab and azathioprine demonstrated a steroid-avoiding effect and significant mucosal healing (more so than with the corti-costeroid step-up approach) after 2 years of early combined therapy.[23]

SONIC is a large definitive randomized double-blind controlled trial comparing early intervention with inflix-imab/azathioprine combination therapy, infliximab mono-therapy, and azathioprine monotherapy for 1 year in patients with moderate-to-severe Crohn's disease of short duration. Patients in the trial were steroid exposed but naïve to bio-logics or immunomodulators. SONIC showed that patients with evidence of inflammation (elevated CRP level and endoscopic lesions at baseline colonoscopy) achieved supe-rior steroid-free clinical remission (50%, 42%, and 23%, respectively) associated with mucosal healing from early infliximab combination therapy or monotherapy.[24] These infliximab treatments were superior to azathioprine alone with similar safety outcome in all 3 arms. Just as ACCENT 1 was a pivotal study in establishing the role of maintenance therapy in Crohn's disease, SONIC is a landmark study sup-porting the tectonic shift toward early intervention with anti-tumor necrosis factor alpha (TNFα) therapy and away from unlimited steroid and azathioprine therapy.

A review of studies of 5-ASAs in Crohn's disease makes a different point about using evidence-based medicine to guide our medical decision making. Over time, new data may emerge, and on some occasions, old data may mate-rialize that changes the way we interpret the literature. In 1993, Singleton et al published a manuscript on the use of slow-release mesalamine capsules (Pentasa, Ferring, Van Lowes, Denmark) for the treatment of active Crohn's disease.[6] This was a double-blind, randomized, placebo-controlled trial that included 310 patients with Crohn's disease. The primary endpoint was a change in the CDAI from baseline. Patients taking 4 g/day of mesalamine had a mean decrease of 72 points in the CDAI compared with 21 points in the placebo group ($P < 0.01$). At the end of 16 weeks, 43% of patients in the 4 g/day mesalamine group were in remission compared to 18% in the placebo group. There was no significant toxicity related to mesalamine. The authors concluded that controlled-release mesalamine at 4 g/day was safe and effective in the treatment of Crohn's disease of the ileum and colon. This study changed clinical practice and went unchallenged by further published pla-cebo-controlled trials. It is worth noting that, to date, none of the 5-ASA agents have been approved by the FDA for the treatment of Crohn's disease.

It was not until 2004 that additional data became avail-able that questioned standard clinical practice. Hanauer's meta-analysis of double-blind, placebo-controlled trials of Pentasa in the treatment of active Crohn's disease[25] added 2 previously unpublished studies to the Singleton data for this analysis.[26,27] Although the authors confirmed that there was a statistically significant improvement of CDAI in Pentasa-treated patients as compared to controls, the net difference was a clinically insignificant 18 points in the

CDAI. These results, as argued by some experts,[28] should change our clinical practice by abandoning the use of newer 5-ASA agents for Crohn's disease.

Should new data like these cause us to change clinical practice? Certainly such studies should motivate more critical thinking about the utility of these agents, but we do not want to make the same mistake twice and too quickly rely on a single publication. The studies of 5-ASA agents in Crohn's disease overall present relatively limited support for a benefit, but it may be inappropriate to jettison the use of these medications in all Crohn's patients. For instance, what was not addressed in this meta-analysis was an evaluation of subgroups of patients with different clinical behaviors of Crohn's disease. Certain subgroups of patients may benefit from mesalamine, and it would be beneficial to treat them with this safe medication. Furthermore, per-haps other formulations or alternative dosing would make a difference. Is there a clinical benefit of 5-ASAs when used in combination with other agents? Are 5-ASAs protective against colorectal cancer in Crohn's disease, as it appears to be in ulcerative colitis?

This scenario also exposes the impact of publication bias. Publication bias refers to the fact that positive studies are more likely to be published than those that are negative. The 2 sets of data added to the meta-analysis were both from internal industry sources and not previously released publicly. Recent awareness of the gravity of this problem had led to a call from the International Committee of Medical Journal Editors to register all clinical trials in a public trial registry.[29]

Evidence guiding clinical practice evolves over time. A single "landmark" publication may tempt a change in the standard of care, but skepticism is healthy. A single study represents a reference point, or a guide. However, as above, it may not be entirely applicable to the patient sitting in front of us in clinic and may be one report in a large body of potentially conflicting data. These examples point out the limitations of even the best data from well-done random-ized clinical trials.

COMMON CLINICAL DECISIONS

Numerous commonly faced clinical dilemmas under-score the fact that many of the decisions we make everyday in clinical practice are guided by minimal or weak data at best. It may be fair to say that more clinical scenarios are without guiding evidence or with conflicting evidence than with a clear-cut answer. What is the optimal dose of steroids for a flare? How should steroids be tapered? Who is the appropriate patient for 6-MP or infliximab? How should 6-MP be initiated and monitored? Can we stop 5-ASAs once on an effective dose of 6-MP or infliximab? Should we pre-medicate patients with steroids prior to infliximab infu-sions? How do concomitant medications or environmental

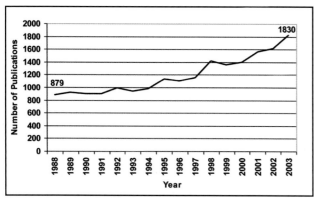

FIGURE 6-2. Number of publications per year on inflammatory bowel disease. Data compiled by a Medline search on the keywords "Crohn's disease," "ulcerative colitis," and "inflammatory bowel disease." (Reproduced with permission from Sands BE. How to read the inflammatory bowel disease literature. *Practical Gastroenterology.* 2005;March:30-43.)

exposures impact efficacy of drugs? Questions regarding practical and common circumstances are frequently without solid guiding evidence. In these cases, we must abandon dependence on evidence-based medicine, extrapolate from the literature, and rely on clinical experience.

CONCLUSION

The explosion of IBD publications (Figure 6-2) in recent years will require that we become even more astute in interpreting results and their applicability to our patients. The limitations of current clinical trials remain considerable and a variety of changes in the conduct of clinical trials could be hoped for to help enhance their utility. Over the next decade, an accepted set of biomarkers will hopefully be identified to assess biologic improvement in inflammation as well as to characterize distinct subsets of disease. It may be that trials have rejected a particular medication as being ineffective in a broad population of UC or Crohn's patients, while it may be highly useful in a particular subset of either disease. Though most authors identify biologic and environmental factors, such as the recent use of CRP and the characterization of disease location or smoking, those involved in the conduct of a trial should be encouraged to assess patients with other available markers such as pANCA, ASCA, as well as genetic markers and microarrays. This information will be critical to allow identification of subgroups of patients who may respond optimally to certain medications as well as others with a low likelihood of response. The blunt tools currently used for disease characterization cause a fundamental weakness in the data derived from clinical trials. As the knowledge of genetic and environmental factors in IBD develops further, it can be hoped that controlled trials will increase in sophistication to provide guidance in our clinical decision making and improve the care of patients with IBD.

REFERENCES

1. Su C, Lichtenstein GR, Krok K, Brensinger CM, Lewis JD. A meta-analysis of the placebo rates of remission and response in clinical trials of active Crohn's disease. *Gastroenterology.* 2004;126:1257-1269.

2. Targan SR, Hanauer SB, van Deventer SJ, et al. A short-term study of chimeric monoclonal antibody cA2 to tumor necrosis factor alpha for Crohn's disease. Crohn's Disease cA2 Study Group. *N Engl J Med.* 1997;337:1029-1035.

3. Ghosh S, Goldin E, Gordon FH, et al. Natalizumab for active Crohn's disease. *N Engl J Med.* 2003;348:24-32.

4. Best WR, Becktel JM, Singleton JW, Kern F Jr. Development of a Crohn's disease activity index. National Cooperative Crohn's Disease Study. *Gastroenterology.* 1976;70:439-444.

5. Present DH, Korelitz BI, Wisch N, Glass JL, Sachar DB, Pasternack BS. Treatment of Crohn's disease with 6-mercaptopurine. A long-term, randomized, double-blind study. *N Engl J Med.* 1980;302:981-987.

6. Singleton JW, Hanauer SB, Gitnick GL, et al. Mesalamine capsules for the treatment of active Crohn's disease: results of a 16-week trial. Pentasa Crohn's Disease Study Group. *Gastroenterology.* 1993;104:1293-1301.

7. Sands BE, Ooi CJ. A survey of methodological variation in the Crohn's disease activity index. *Inflamm Bowel Dis.* 2005;11:133-138.

8. Gasche C, Scholmerich J, Brynskov J, et al. A simple classification of Crohn's disease: report of the Working Party for the World Congresses of Gastroenterology, Vienna 1998. *Inflamm Bowel Dis.* 2000;6:8-15.

9. Abreu MT, Taylor KD, Lin YC, et al. Mutations in NOD2 are associated with fibrostenosing disease in patients with Crohn's disease. *Gastroenterology.* 2002;123:679-688.

10. Mow WS, Vasiliauskas EA, Lin YC, et al. Association of antibody responses to microbial antigens and complications of small bowel Crohn's disease. *Gastroenterology.* 2004;126:414-424.

11. Forcione DG, Rosen MJ, Kisiel JB, Sands BE. Anti-*Saccharomyces cerevisiae* antibody (ASCA) positivity is associated with increased risk for early surgery in Crohn's disease. *Gut.* 2004;53:1117-1122.

12. Lewis JD, Bilker WB, Brensinger C, et al. Inflammatory bowel disease is not associated with an increased risk of lymphoma. *Gastroenterology.* 2001;121:1080-1087.

13. Colombel JF, Loftus EV Jr, Tremaine WJ, et al. The safety profile of infliximab in patients with Crohn's disease: the Mayo clinic experience in 500 patients. *Gastroenterology.* 2004;126:19-31.

14. Hanauer SB, Feagan BG, Lichtenstein GR, et al. Maintenance infliximab for Crohn's disease: the ACCENT I randomised trial. *Lancet.* 2002;359:1541-1549.

15. Ljung T, Karlen P, Schmidt D, et al. Infliximab in inflammatory bowel disease: clinical outcome in a population based cohort from Stockholm County. *Gut.* 2004;53:849-853.

16. Rutgeerts P, D'Haens G, Targan S, et al. Efficacy and safety of retreatment with anti-tumor necrosis factor antibody (infliximab) to maintain remission in Crohn's disease. *Gastroenterology.* 1999;117:761-769.

17. Sands BE, Anderson FH, Bernstein CN, et al. Infliximab maintenance therapy for fistulizing Crohn's disease. *N Engl J Med.* 2004;350:876-885.

18. Seiderer J, Goke B, Ochsenkuhn T. Safety aspects of infliximab in inflammatory bowel disease patients. A retrospective cohort study in 100 patients of a German University Hospital. *Digestion.* 2004;70:3-9.

19. Beaugerie L, Carrat F, Bouvier A-M, et al. Excess risk of lymphopro-liferative disorders in inflammatory bowel disease: interim results of the Cesame cohort [abstract]. *Gastroenterology.* 2008;134(suppl 1):A116-A117.

20. Siegel C, Sadie M, Marden S, Persing SM, Larson RJ, Sands BE. Risk of lymphoma associated with anti-TNF agents for the treatment of Crohn's disease: a meta-analysis [abstract]. *Gastroenterology.* 2008;134(suppl 1):A144.

21. Van Assche G, Van Ranst M, Sciot R, et al. Progressive multifo-cal leukoencephalopathy after natalizumab therapy for Crohn's disease. *N Engl J Med.* 2005;353:362-368.

22. Hyams J, Crandall W, Kugathasan S, et al. Induction and mainte-nance infliximab therapy for the treatment of moderate-to-severe Crohn's disease in children. *Gastroenterology.* 2007;132:863-873.

23. D'Haens G, Baert F, van Assche G, et al. Early combined immuno-suppression or conventional management in patients with newly diagnosed Crohn's disease: an open randomised trial. *Lancet.* 2008;371:660-667.

24. Lichtenstein GR, Hanauer SB, Sandborn WJ, and the Practice Parameters Committee of American College of Gastroenterology. Management of Crohn's disease in adults. *Am J Gastroenterol.* 2009;104:465-483.

25. Hanauer SB, Stromberg U. Oral Pentasa in the treatment of active Crohn's disease: a meta-analysis of double-blind, placebo-con-trolled trials. *Clin Gastroenterol Hepatol.* 2004;2:379-388.

26. Nordic, Research Inc. Clinical research report: Efficacy and safety of oral Pentasa in the treatment of active Crohn's disease. October 23, 1991.

27. Hoechst, Marion Roussel Inc. Clinical study report: efficacy and safety of oral Pentasa in the treatment of active Crohn's disease. January 28, 1997.

28. Feagan BG. 5-ASA therapy for active Crohn's disease: old friends, old data, and a new conclusion. *Clin Gastroenterol Hepatol.* 2004;2:376-378.

29. DeAngelis CD, Drazen JM, Frizelle FA, et al. Clinical trial registra-tion: a statement from the International Committee of Medical Journal Editors. *JAMA.* 2004;292:1363-1364.

DISEASE MODIFIERS IN INFLAMMATORY BOWEL DISEASE

Jaime A. Oviedo, MD and Francis A. Farraye, MD, MSc, FACP, FACG

Although the individual susceptibility to develop inflammatory bowel disease (IBD) appears to be genetically determined, the actual occurrence of the disease is largely influenced by environmental factors. Though extraordinary advances have been made in our understanding of the genetics, pathogenesis, diagnosis, and medical management of patients with IBD, our emphasis on environmental modifiers, health maintenance, and lifestyle factors that can affect the course, complications, and severity of the disease has not been nearly as significant. Several modifying factors have been identified and are becoming increasingly relevant for physicians and patients alike. This chapter summarizes the available evidence surrounding the influence of disease modifiers on the natural history and course of IBD.

PERINATAL AND CHILDHOOD FACTORS

The first year of life is considered a crucial period for immune system maturation and development of tolerance. Exposure to specific antigens during early childhood is likely to lead to immune tolerance and might, at least in part, dictate the responses to antigens that are presumably involved in the pathogenesis of IBD.[1]

Based on these concepts, the influence of early life events such as mode of feeding, household hygiene, and perinatal infections on the development of IBD has been examined.

BREASTFEEDING

Evidence of a possible inverse association between breastfeeding and IBD remains controversial. Although several studies suggested a protective effect of breastfeeding against the development of IBD,[2-6] in some cases the association did not reach statistical significance and in others was not apparent at all.[7-10] In general, the association appears to be stronger for CD than for UC, but as mentioned the evidence is controversial at best, and no firm conclusions can be made.

Early weaning has also been implicated as a risk factor for both UC and CD.[9] Though the notion that early weaning has an impact on both immune system and bacterial colonization of the gut is appealing, a case-control study did not confirm an association between early formula feeding and IBD.[8] It is thus possible that in studies showing a positive association, early weaning may be a surrogate marker for higher socioeconomic status. In addition, long recall intervals and the potential for introduction of recall bias may also render studies on infant feeding unreliable.

SOCIOECONOMIC AND HYGIENIC FACTORS

Although in early reports, high socioeconomic status was postulated as a risk factor for both UC and CD,[11,12] subsequent studies have not confirmed this observation.[8,13] The contradicting results over time may be explained by the reduction or disappearance of differences in living conditions between socioeconomic groups following World War II.

Improvements in hygiene and living conditions during the 20th century have been associated with an increased risk of development of CD. Hygiene, especially early in life, appears to have an impact on the bacterial colonization of the gut and other infectious exposures that determine the development of the immune system.[14] In epidemiological studies, patients with CD were more likely to have running hot water, separate bathroom, less bed and bedroom sharing, and central heating compared to controls.[15,16]

Some authors advocate that the use of domestic refrigeration has contributed to the increasing incidence of CD during the 20th century. The hypothesis is based on the assumption that bacteria such as *Yersinia* spp. and *Listeria*, which can grow at cold temperatures, play a role in the pathogenesis of CD.[17]

Use of toothpaste in Western societies has also been implicated as a possible risk factor for IBD.[18] Dietary microparticles present in toothpaste are the theoretical culprit; however, no observational studies have corroborated this association.[14,19]

In an isolated report, exposure to soft toys during childhood was found to be protective against the development of IBD.[19] This finding has not been validated or reproduced in other studies.[14]

In summary, these reports suggest that strict attention to hygiene and environmental exposure during infancy might prevent the development of tolerance to many bacteria commonly found in the environment and perhaps predispose the individual to active immune-mediated events when the exposure occurs later in life. Although interesting from an epidemiological perspective, these findings are unlikely to lead to any specific recommendations to prevent IBD.

INFECTIONS AND IBD

In addition to the capacity to respond to sporadic challenges from pathogens, the mucosal immune system has the ability to recognize, tolerate, and avoid reacting against nonpathogenic intestinal bacteria. Available evidence from clinical observations and animal studies suggests that intestinal bacteria may play a role in triggering and perpetuating chronic bowel inflammation. IBD appears to result from the interaction of three essential cofactors: host susceptibility, enteric microflora, and mucosal immunity. In susceptible individuals, a breakdown in the regulatory constraints of the mucosal immune response to enteric bacteria may result in the development of IBD.[20]

Since the 1950s, infectious agents have been proposed to be causally related to the occurrence of IBD.[13] A wide range of different microorganisms including *Mycobacterium paratuberculosis* (MAP),[21] *Listeria*,[22] unspecified childhood gastroenteritis, and viral infections such as measles,[23]

TABLE 7-1

INFECTIOUS AGENTS POSSIBLY LINKED TO THE OCCURRENCE OF IBD*

BACTERIAL

Mycobacterium paratuberculosis[21]

Listeria[22]

Pharyngitis and otitis[49]

VIRAL

Unspecified childhood gastroenteritis

Measles and measles vaccination[23]

Mumps[38]

Influenza[24]

Varicella[24]

PARASITES

Helminthic parasites[20]

*IBD indicates inflammatory bowel disease.

---

influenza, and varicella[24] have been linked with either UC, CD, or both (Table 7-1).

MYCOBACTERIUM PARATUBERCULOSIS

MAP, a subspecies of *Mycobacterium avium*, known to cause Johne's disease (a granulomatous enterocolitis that resembles Crohn's disease in sheep and cattle), has been widely studied for its possible role in the development of CD. DNA from this organism has been detected by culture and molecular techniques in intestinal tissue of patients with CD.[1,25] In a recent study,[26] investigators detected viable MAP in peripheral blood in a higher proportion of patients with CD (13 out of 28) than in individuals without inflammatory bowel disease (0 out of 15). This evidence has, however, not been confirmed by other investigators as atypical mycobacteria have also been recovered from intestinal tissue of unaffected individuals.[27,28]

Recent microbiological studies have renewed the controversy by showing increased rates of detection of MAP in subepithelial Crohn's-related granulomas when compared to granulomas from other conditions such as foreign-body reaction or sarcoidosis.[28,29] In addition, several open-label studies that evaluated antibiotic regimens with antimycobacterial activity have shown clinical improvement in affected patients.[30-32] However, the results of randomized studies are not nearly as impressive, with a meta-analysis yielding conflicting results.[33] Furthermore, a recent study by Toracchio et al does not support MAP as a primary cause of Crohn's disease. The researchers examined ileal or colonic tissue from 29 patients with Crohn's disease and found MAP DNA in granuloma tissue from only 1 patient (5%); MAP DNA was not found in non-granuloma tissue samples.[34] Thus, although the hypothesis involving mycobacteria in the pathogenesis of CD is intriguing, the theory has not been unequivocally proven, and antimycobacterial therapy cannot be recommended in the management of affected patients.[35]

LISTERIA MONOCYTOGENES

Early reports suggested that *Listeria monocytogenes* may have the potential to cause IBD.[22,36] Recently, this theory has lost strength when studies utilizing tissue culture and polymerase chain reaction (PCR) have not found the bacteria in biopsy specimens from IBD patients.[37]

MEASLES INFECTION OR VACCINATION

A chronic granulomatous vasculitis of the mesenteric endothelium has been postulated as the mechanism to explain a possible association between exposure to measles and other viruses and the onset of IBD.[38] Although the possibility of this association was described as early as 1950, the supporting data have become increasingly controversial.

In a British cohort study,[39] mumps infection before age 2 was found to be a risk for UC (odds ratio [OR], 25.12, 95% confidence interval [CI], 6.35-99.36). Similarly, measles and mumps infections in the same year of life were significantly associated with UC and CD (OR 7.47, 95% CI 2.42-23.06 and OR 4.27, 95% CI 1.24-14.46, respectively). These relationships were reported to be independent of each other as well as of sex, social class at birth, household crowding in childhood, and family history of IBD. No significant relationship between measles infection or vaccination at a young age and subsequent IBD was found in this cohort. An increased incidence of IBD following concurrent epidemics of mumps and measles has also been reported in other parts of the world.[40] Similarly, the use of attenuated live measles vaccine was implicated as a possible cause of CD when the prevalence of the disease in a group of people who received the vaccine was 2 to 3 times higher than in the group that did not. However, the findings from population, as well as microbiological, studies do not support the relationship between viral infections or vaccinations and IBD.[41-44] A recent study showed no significant differences in the titers of serum anti-mumps immunoglobulin (Ig)G in IBD patients when compared to healthy controls.[45,46] Similarly, studies using amplification techniques found no evidence of mumps viral genome in intestinal mucosa or peripheral lymphocytes of patients with IBD.[47-49]

In general, the available evidence does not support the theory that measles infection or vaccination leads to IBD.

OTHER INFECTIONS

Childhood infections have also been postulated as a potential factor associated with the development of IBD. In a population study, patients with CD were more likely to report an increased frequency of childhood infections in general (OR 4.67, 95% CI 2.65-8.23), and pharyngitis specifically (OR 2.14, 95% CI 1.30-3.51), than healthy counterparts. Treatment with antibiotics for both otitis media (OR 2.07, 95% CI 1.03-4.14) and pharyngitis (OR 2.14, 95% CI 1.20-3.84) was also more common in the group with CD. Patients with UC also reported an excess of infections in general (OR 2.37, 95% CI 1.19-4.71) but not an excess of specific infections or treatments with antibiotics. Persons who reported an increased frequency of infections tended to have an earlier onset of CD ($P < 0.0001$) and ulcerative colitis ($P = 0.04$).[50]

Several studies have reported a higher frequency of gastroenteritis or diarrheal illness during infancy among future IBD patients.[3,9,13] As noted earlier, recall bias may affect the validity of the conclusions obtained from these studies.

An adhesive strain of *Escherichia coli* has been implicated in the pathogenesis of UC.[51] Adherent-invasive *E coli* (AIEC) strains have been described in patients with ileal CD.[52] A selective increase in a number of invasive *E coli* of novel phylogeny has been described in patients with ileal CD.[53] AIEC strains have been associated with Crohn's colitis and colonic cancer.[54] Many other agents including *Clostridium*, *Campylobacter*, *Pseudomonas*, *Mycoplasma*, *Cytomegalovirus*, herpes, and rotaviruses have been considered but not proven to have a role in IBD.[1]

Reduced immunologic exposure to helminthic parasites has also been proposed as a potential factor to explain the increased incidence of CD in industrialized societies when compared to developing countries.[20] Colonization with pathogenically attenuated helminths has been used to switch the mucosal cytokine profile in patients with CD. In a small open-label trial, the administration of porcine whipworm eggs was safe and resulted in improvement of CDAI scores for both CD and UC.[55]

In summary, although the bulk of evidence does not suggest that IBD is an infectious or a self-antigen-specific autoimmune disease, recent findings suggest that mucosal damage might be initiated and driven by common, ubiquitous microbial agents derived from the normal bacterial flora in the intestinal lumen.[56]

The role of the normal intestinal flora in the development and progression of IBD has thus generated considerable interest. Products of the commensal flora may promote inflammation in the presence of an impaired mucosal barrier or injury to the mucosa. There is also growing evidence suggesting that a change in the quantity or quality of bacterial luminal content may lead to induction or persistence of mucosal inflammation.[57] Conversely, the manipulation of the normal intestinal flora with antibiotics, or with other nonpathogenic organisms (probiotics), appears to be a promising method to modify mucosal cytokine balance and inflammatory response.

ANTIBIOTICS

Because the increasing exposure to antibiotics experienced after World War II coincided with an increase in the incidence of IBD, some investigators speculate that antibiotics may cause IBD.[58] However, the evidence supporting this hypothesis is limited, based on retrospective studies,[7,50] and likely influenced by indication bias (ie, patients receiving antibiotics for insidious symptoms not yet diagnosed as IBD) or by the increased susceptibility to other infections occasionally seen in patients with IBD. In addition, the prevalence of antibiotic use varies significantly between countries and does not appear to correlate well with the incidence of IBD.[14]

Antibiotics are widely used in patients with IBD and have been shown to be beneficial in the treatment of perianal and colonic CD and pouchitis.[20] Trials in both human IBD and experimental colitis have demonstrated that broad-spectrum antibiotics may influence the course of UC and CD. Antibiotics with narrow anaerobic coverage are effective for preventing relapse in CD after surgically induced remission.[59,60] The use of antibiotics in the management of IBD is reviewed in detail in chapters 15 and 41.

PROBIOTICS

Probiotics are live, nonpathogenic microbial food ingredients, usually of the genera *Bifidobacterium* or *Lactobacillus*, that alter the enteric flora and have been associated with beneficial effects on human health. Some noninvasive coliforms and nonbacterial organisms such as *Saccharomyces boulardii* are also categorized as probiotics.[20] Based on their ability to prevent the overgrowth of potentially pathogenic organisms and stimulate the intestinal immune defense system,[61] probiotics are being increasingly used as an adjuvant or alternative therapy for IBD. In 2 controlled studies,[62,63] a nonpathogenic strain of *E coli* was as effective as a 5-aminosalicylic acid (5-ASA) preparation maintaining remission in patients with UC. Probiotic combinations have also shown impressive results in the treatment of chronic pouchitis, reducing the relapse rate by up to 85% when compared to placebo.[64] VSL#3, a probiotic preparation with 450 billion live bacteria per packet, has been studied in 2 randomized, placebo-controlled trials evaluating 147 adults and 29 children with mild to moderate UC. Both studies suggested an induction

and maintenance response. Further studies evaluating VSL#3 in UC are warranted.[65,66] In CD, an open-label study of approximately 20 patients with mild to moderately active disease showed that probiotics reduced the need for corticosteroid therapy in more than 75% of the cases and were safe and well tolerated.[67] The use of probiotics in IBD is discussed in chapters 36 and 59.

APPENDECTOMY/APPENDICITIS

Appendectomy has been consistently found to be protective against the development of UC.[7,15,68,69] A meta-analysis of 17 case-control studies including more than 3600 cases and more than 4600 controls showed that appendectomy was associated with a 69% reduction in the subsequent risk of UC.[34,70] The results of cohort studies have been less consistent, with 2 large series producing conflicting results. A Swedish inpatient register of 212,963 patients with more than 5 million person-years of follow-up showed that patients who underwent appendectomy for appendicitis and mesenteric lymphadenitis had a 25% reduction of the risk of developing UC. The protective effect was only seen if the appendectomy was performed before the age of 20 years. Appendectomy for noninflammatory conditions such as nonspecific abdominal pain did not appear to confer protection against UC.[71] In another large cohort from Denmark, 154,000 patients who had undergone appendectomy were followed for more than 1 million person-years. Although the cohort was found to be 13% less likely to be diagnosed with UC than previously documented national averages, the difference was not statistically significant.[71] Despite these somewhat conflicting results, most evidence from case-control and cohort studies suggests that appendectomy is a protective factor against UC.[34]

The influence of appendicitis and appendectomy on UC is not limited to the onset of the disease. Appendectomy also appears to influence the clinical course of UC. When compared to patients with UC and an intact appendix, patients who have undergone appendectomy and develop UC are diagnosed at an older age,[72,73] develop less recurrent symptoms,[72] require colectomy less frequently,[69,74] and require less immunosuppressive therapy to control the disease.[69] The effect of appendectomy on the clinical course of patients with known UC is limited to case reports and small case series, and results are conflicting.[34]

The relationship between appendectomy and CD is less clear. Appendectomy has been associated with an increased risk of developing CD[75]; however, in many of the published studies, the results did not reach statistical significance. Appendicitis may mimic CD, and ileocolonic involvement by CD is frequently misdiagnosed as appendicitis, which may overestimate the strength of the association.[69,76]

The mechanism by which appendectomy protects against UC and increases the risk of CD is unknown. The appendix is part of the mucosa-associated lymphoid tissue system and is involved in B lymphocyte-mediated immune responses and extrathymic T lymphocytes. Because of its role as a reservoir for enteric bacteria, removal of the appendix may influence the mucosal immune system and the antigenic exposure in the bowel lumen.[1]

DIET

Various dietary exposures have been proposed as causative factors in IBD. Based on population and immigration studies, and considering the increase in the incidence of CD and UC in countries like Japan and South Korea during the 1990s, a Westernized diet has been implicated in the development of IBD.[14,77-79] Studies examining associations between diet and disease are difficult to perform because of recall bias and the possibility that the diet was modified before the formal diagnosis of IBD as a result of chronic gastrointestinal symptoms. Early dietary studies have been found to be poorly conducted and fraught with methodological deficiencies, making it impossible to draw any meaningful conclusion.[80]

The following dietary components are consistently cited in epidemiologic studies.

REFINED SUGAR

Consumption of refined sugar has been consistently found to be associated with CD in several retrospective case-control studies.[19,81,82] It is possible, however, that the increase in dietary sugar consumption may be driven by symptoms, as patients with CD tend to prefer easily digested foods.[14] Trials that have aimed to minimize difficulties with dietary recall bias by studying patients diagnosed within 1 year have shown contradictory results, with some[83-85] but not all studies showing an association.[82,86]

Because smoking is positively associated with sugar consumption, the interpretation of data derived from dietary studies is complicated. When analyzed separately, sugar intake and smoking have been shown to be independent risk factors; however, combined exposure did not result in a further increased risk.[87,88]

Although a positive association between consumption of refined sugar and the risk of UC has been proposed,[85] the studies are also affected by methodological problems and low statistical power.[14] The results of studies evaluating the effects of a low sugar diet on CD were disappointing.[89]

PROTEIN AND FAT

Although the results are inconsistent and the studies may also be affected by methodological problems, a posi-

tive association has been demonstrated for both protein and fat consumption with UC and CD.[71,85,90] In a recently published prospective study,[91] dietary factors such as a high intake of red and processed meat, protein, and alcohol were associated with an increased likelihood of relapse in patients with UC.

FRUIT AND VEGETABLES

High intake of dietary fiber, fruit, or vegetables may be protective against the development of IBD, but results vary among studies.[78,85,92] It is unclear whether this finding is the result of decreased fiber intake in response to symptoms of stricturing CD.[34]

FAST FOOD AND COLA DRINKS

Both fast food and cola drinks have been implicated as risk factors for UC and CD.[19,92] As mentioned earlier, the retrospective nature of the studies limits the validity of the association.

Many more foods have been implicated in the development or worsening of IBD, including margarine,[93] dairy products,[94] baker's yeast,[95,96] coffee,[92,97] alcohol,[97,98] cornflakes,[99,100] and curry,[101] among others. Lactase or other enzymatic deficiencies secondary to extensive mucosal involvement may be involved in specific food intolerance in patients with CD. In general, none of these associations has been irrefutably proven, and no firm clinical recommendations can be made in this regard.

The low incidence of IBD in populations with high consumption of curried and highly spiced food is intriguing. It has been postulated that curcumin, a major component of curry, has antioxidant and anti-inflammatory activity and acts as a protective factor against the development of IBD.[101]

Because dietary antigens may act as immunoregulators, it has been proposed that food allergies may play a role in the pathogenesis of IBD.[102,103] Small studies have shown that patients with CD feature a stronger response to food antigens than healthy individuals.[103] The success of treatment with elemental or exclusion diets would support food allergy as a biological pathway in patients with CD. Similarly, food additives present in modern urban diets may be involved in immune reactions both locally and systemically and have been proposed as an etiological factor in IBD, especially CD.[104,105] The role of elemental and exclusion diets and other dietary manipulations in IBD is discussed in chapters 37 and 38.

ORAL CONTRACEPTIVES

Since the 1970s, several case reports, as well as case-control and cohort studies, have described an increased risk of

IBD in women who use oral contraceptives (OCPs).[106-108] Although cohort studies compiling more than 80,000 women reported increases in IBD risk ranging from 40% to 3-fold, the results were not statistically significant, especially after adjusting for cigarette smoking.[34,107-109] In a meta-analysis of 2 cohort studies and 7 case-control studies, the pooled OR for CD among users of OCPs, after adjusting for smoking, was 1.4 (95% CI 1.1-1.9). OR for UC among OCP users was 1.29 but did not reach statistical significance (95% CI 0.9-1.8).[110] The association was thus found to be weak and not necessarily causal, as confounding factors could not be ruled out.[14]

Other case-control studies have also suggested an association between OCP use and IBD, and especially with CD.[111,112] The risk appears to be higher among longtime users[111,113,114] and among users of high-dose estrogen preparations.[111]

Although a single study reported an increased incidence of relapse among OCP users,[115] OCPs do not appear to increase the risk of relapse or modify the course of CD.[116]

In summary, available evidence supports a weak association between OCP use and IBD. The thrombogenic potential of OCPs, leading to multifocal gastrointestinal infarctions mediated by chronic mesenteric vasculitis, similar to those of smoking, are the proposed mechanism underlying the effect of OCPs on CD.[34,117]

ENVIRONMENTAL FACTORS

SMOKING

Smoking is the best characterized of the environmental factors that can affect the severity and natural history of IBD. Smoking cigarettes is associated with an increased prevalence of CD, and nonsmoking is associated with UC.[118] There is also strong evidence suggesting that smoking cigarettes has a negative effect on the course of CD and that smoking cigarettes may improve the disease severity or have a "protective" effect in some patients with UC.[119]

SMOKING AND UC

UC is predominately a disease of nonsmokers. Several meta-analyses as well as observational and case-control studies have confirmed that the relative risk of colitis is reduced in smokers when compared to people who have never smoked and to individuals who have quit smoking.[120,121] The incidence of UC in the Mormon community where smoking is discouraged is 5-fold higher than the general population.[122,123] Lifetime nonsmokers are almost 3 times more likely to have UC than current smokers.[124] Furthermore, approximately two thirds of former smokers with UC develop the disease after quitting smoking, with a particularly high incidence in the first few years.[125-127]

Smokers have also been noted to have a reduced incidence of conditions such as primary sclerosing cholangitis (PSC), with or without associated IBD[128-130] and pouchitis.[131] The protective effect against PSC suggests a systemic effect rather than a local effect on the colon.[34]

Smoking also appears to have an effect on the clinical course of UC. A significant proportion of patients report that their colitis improves while smoking ~20 cigarettes daily. Similarly, smokers with UC report fewer bowel complaints than their nonsmoking counterparts.[132] Most of the available evidence supports the contention that smoking is a significant disease modifier in UC. Several studies have reported lower hospitalization rates in smokers with UC, higher colectomy rates in ex-smokers who quit smoking before the onset of their colitis,[133] reduced rates of clinical relapse in patients who began smoking after diagnosis,[134] and reduced incidence of pouchitis in smokers following proctocolectomy.[131] Conversely, smoking cessation is usually followed by a statistically significant increase in disease severity, hospitalization rate, and a need for major medical therapy, when compared to continuing smoking.[135]

SMOKING AND CD

Smoking is a well-recognized risk factor for CD,[124] and patients with CD have higher rates of tobacco use than the general population.[124,136] Compared with non-smokers, patients with CD who smoke suffer more clinical relapses,[116,132,137] develop more complications,[138] require surgery more often,[119,139] and need more immunosuppressive therapy.[140,141]

There is also evidence suggesting that the detrimental effect of smoking on CD subsides after smoking cessation. Patients who quit smoking have a reduced risk of relapse[115,142] and postoperative recurrence when compared to current smokers.[139] On the basis of these associations, smoking cessation is a potential therapy for CD. However, many patients are unaware of the risk of worsening their CD by smoking and do not recall their physician ever informing them about these risks.[143]

Although it has been suggested that CD patients are poorly receptive to smoking cessation counseling,[144] which may explain why more efforts are not made to get these patients to quit, the percentages of people considering and attempting to quit are similar to those reported in other groups of smokers in the general population. Therefore, there is no evidence to conclude that patients with CD are any more refractory to smoking cessation than smokers in the general population.

Though remaining abstinent is as difficult for people with CD as it is for the smokers in the general population, the benefits of discontinuing smoking in patients with CD justify all the effort involved in achieving smoking cessation. Patients who successfully quit smoking for more than 1 year appear to significantly reduce their risk of

TABLE 7-2

EFFECTS OF SMOKING AND SMOKING CESSATION ON IBD*

	CROHN'S DISEASE	ULCERATIVE COLITIS
Smoking	Increased prevalence	Decreased prevalence
	Negative effect on course	"Protective" effect
	• More relapses	• Fewer flares
	• Increased complications	• Reduced hospitalizations
	• More surgeries	• Reduced colectomy rates
	• Increased need for use of immunomodulators	• Reduced incidence of pouchitis
Smoking cessation	Decreased risk of relapse and postoperative recurrence	Increased disease activity
	Decreased risk for steroids and immunomodulators	Increased need for hospitalization, steroids, and immunomodulators
		• Increased need for colectomy

*IBD indicates inflammatory bowel disease.

experiencing a flare, as well as reduce the need for the use of steroids or immunomodulators when compared to continuing smokers.[145]

Passive smoking has also been linked to increased IBD risk. In one study, passive smoking at birth was significantly associated with the development of either subtype of IBD.[146] The effect of passive smoking in childhood appears to be similar to that of active smoking in adults, as demonstrated by a study following children exposed to cigarette smoke at home who were found to be half as likely to develop UC.[147] In another study, exposure to cigarette smoke during childhood increased the risk of CD but not UC.[138]

Despite these well-described associations, the mechanism by which cigarette smoking affects UC and CD in opposite ways is not fully understood. In addition to nicotine, tobacco smoke contains hundreds of substances including free radicals and carbon monoxide (CO).[148] Several effects of nicotine are likely contributors to the role of smoking as a disease modifier in IBD. Nicotine modifies the thickness of mucus and abolishes the synthesis of inflammatory cytokines in the colonic mucosa in animal models.[58,112] In humans, nicotine is known to decrease the production of mucosal eicosanoids and some cytokines such as IL-2, IL-8, and tumor necrosis factor alpha (TNFα).[148-150] Nicotine also reduces smooth muscle tone and contractile activity as a result of nitric oxide release, changes in the microcirculation, and transient ischemia.[13,16] Cigarette smoke, in turn, increases lipid peroxidation and modifies the mucosal immune response.[151] Smoking increases CO concentration, which might amplify the impairment in vasodilation capacity in chronically inflamed microvessels, resulting in ischemia and perpetuating ulceration and fibrosis.[148,152]

Patient-related factors have also been found to play a role in the type and magnitude of the effects of smoking in IBD. The effects of nicotine on IBD appear to be dose related, with significant changes seen with 15 or more cigarettes per day. Women appear to be more susceptible than men to the harmful effect of smoking on CD, and as seen in patients with UC the protective effect of nicotine is more efficient in the distal intestine.[148] Table 7-2 summarizes the effects of smoking and smoking cessation on IBD.

Based on the known effects of cigarette smoking in the incidence and course of UC, nicotine has been studied as a potential therapeutic alternative. The role of nicotine therapy in the management of UC is discussed in chapter 34.

SMOKING AND IBD IN CLINICAL PRACTICE

Individuals with CD should be strongly encouraged to quit smoking. Like any other smokers, Crohn's patients will have low abstinence rates without additional support. Counseling, smoking cessation groups, and pharmacotherapy should be offered by providers treating these patients.

Although most evidence supports a beneficial effect of cigarette smoking on the course of UC, these patients should not be encouraged to smoke and should, as any other smoker, receive education about the health risks of nicotine use. Patients with UC should be educated about the relationship between smoking and their disease and should be allowed to make their own decisions based on the facts. Smokers with UC who plan to stop smoking should be informed of the potential risk of increase in disease activity, and, accordingly, therapy should be adjusted to prevent a flare of their colitis.

NONSTEROIDAL ANTI-INFLAMMATORY DRUGS

Nonsteroidal anti-inflammatory drugs (NSAIDs) are one of the most commonly used medications worldwide. In the United States alone, more than 70 million NSAID prescriptions and 30 billion over-the-counter preparations are sold every year.[153] Although NSAID use has typically been associated with the development of gastroduodenal injury, evidence implicating these agents in inducing and exacerbating damage in the distal gastrointestinal tract is also mounting. Colonic injury ranging from colitis resembling inflammatory bowel disease to colonic perforation and bleeding has been described.[154-156] NSAIDs have been associated with the onset of acute IBD lesions, as well as exacerbation of preexisting disease.[157] A relationship between NSAID use and the development of collagenous colitis has also been postulated.[158,159]

More than 80% of patients with IBD interviewed for one study reported use of NSAIDs within the previous month, and approximately one third of these patients thought that there was an association between their IBD symptoms and NSAID use. In contrast, only 2% of the IBS population used as control reported worsening symptoms following NSAID use.[160,161]

Although most of the available clinical evidence points toward an adverse influence of NSAIDs on the course of IBD, the exact mechanism by which NSAIDs can lead to exacerbations of the disease is not fully understood. Inhibition of colonic prostaglandin (PG) synthesis is likely a contributing factor.[162] The key enzyme in this pathway is cyclooxygenase (COX), which exists in 2 isoforms: COX-1, the constitutive enzyme involved in maintaining mucosal integrity in the gastrointestinal (GI) tract, and COX-2, an inducible enzyme that is expressed at sites of inflammation. COX-2 expression is significantly increased in the colonic mucosa of patients with active IBD when compared to inactive disease or healthy controls.[163] COX-2 appears to have a beneficial effect in healing experimental colitis and, in theory, COX-2 inhibition might impair colitis healing.[162]

Because of the evidence suggesting that COX-2-specific inhibitors are less toxic to the gastrointestinal tract than traditional NSAIDs, patients and physicians have assumed that coxibs would not increase the risk of exacerbation of IBD. However, cases of flares of IBD associated with use of COX-2 inhibitors have been reported in the literature.[164-166] In 2 case series of IBD patients who were prescribed COX-2 inhibitors, the risk of disease exacerbation was reported at 7%[167] and 13%,[168] respectively. In a recent series of 33 patients with IBD who were prescribed celecoxib or rofecoxib, 39% experienced exacerbation of their disease.[169] A recent randomized, placebo-controlled trial found no difference in relapse rate among 222 patients with ulcerative colitis in remission who were given oral celecoxib 200 mg or placebo twice daily for 14 days.[170] Until more information is available, however, the general expert consensus is that the use of COX-2-specific inhibitors in patients with IBD should be viewed with the same caution as the use of traditional NSAIDs.[171]

There is no simple solution for the small number of patients who require NSAIDs and have significant IBD activity. When patients are using NSAIDs to control the pain from IBD-related arthritis, the intestinal disease should be treated aggressively—in the hopes that the severity of the arthritis will decrease as the intestinal inflammatory activity resolves. Non-NSAID analgesics can be prescribed in the interim to control joint pain. In rheumatoid arthritis or other arthritides, this strategy may not be as successful because the course of the arthritis is independent of the activity of the intestinal disease.[172] Non-NSAID analgesics and local measures can be used for the treatment of trauma-related pain and inflammation in patients with IBD. If these fail, a short course of NSAIDs or COX-2-selective inhibitors may be prescribed with close monitoring of symptoms and side effects.

EXERCISE

Sedentary and physically less-demanding occupations have been associated with a higher incidence of IBD.[173-175] Regular exercise, in contrast, has been associated with significant improvements in quality of life and activity index scores, as well as with a reduction in the frequency of flares in patients with CD.[176]

Though GI symptoms such as nausea, heartburn, diarrhea, and occasionally GI bleeding are common during intense sports,[177-180] physical activity has also been associated with long-term benefits in the GI tract, especially a consistent reduction in colon cancer risk, which (although documented in non-IBD patients) is likely to also extend to individuals with IBD.[181,182]

Although the preventive effect of exercise remains inconclusive, it seems clear that physical activity is not harmful for patients with IBD. Another important reason to recommend regular physical activity is that IBD patients, especially those on chronic steroids, are at risk for osteoporosis and osteopenia.[182,183] A low-impact exercise program can potentially increase bone density in these patients.[184] Exercise may also alleviate stress and allow people to deal with stressful events more effectively, increasing the sense of general well-being and quality of life.[176] Physical activity should be recommended, keeping in mind that there are limited data regarding exactly how much exercise is appropriate[171] (Table 7-3).

TABLE 7-3

POSSIBLE EFFECTS OF EXERCISE IN IBD*

- Decreased incidence of CD and UC
- Possible reduction in incidence of colon cancer
- Increased bone density
- Improvement in quality of life in CD
- Reduction in flares and activity index in CD

*IBD indicates inflammatory bowel disease.

SEASONAL VARIATION

Whether the natural history of IBD follows a seasonal pattern remains controversial. Some patients report disease relapses at similar times during the year, and available evidence suggests that seasonal variation may occur, especially for UC. Study results are conflicting and difficult to reproduce, however. Though some studies demonstrated increased rates of UC flares in the spring,[185,186] others reported more flares in the fall and winter,[187,188] and a few others found no association at all.[189,190]

The results for CD are equally conflicting.[186,187,189,190] A seasonal increase in the incidence of upper respiratory infections has been implicated as a potential mechanism to explain flares that occur at similar times every year.[191,192] Most studies are limited by small sample size and difficulties determining exact temporal relationships between infections and IBD relapses, which makes any conclusions drawn from the data controversial at best. A recent retrospective study of more than 1500 patients with CD and more than 2700 patients with UC evaluated a population-based cohort of patients. The study reported a slight increase of UC exacerbations during the spring and no association between seasons and flares of CD.[193]

The potential variability of the natural history of IBD during different seasons of the year, although intriguing, is a factor that will be very difficult to completely elucidate and, if present, impossible to modify.

STRESS

Patients with IBD can experience considerable psychological stress. Factors such as potential disability caused by the symptoms of IBD and the uncertainty regarding disease outcomes can produce significant stress, anxiety, and depression.[194] Stress and emotional issues appear to play a significant role in increasing disease activity and frequency of relapses, as well as use of medical services

in patients with IBD.[194-198] Whether stress contributes to the onset or precipitates exacerbations of CD remains controversial. Although many patients and family members are convinced that stress is an essential factor in the onset and course of IBD, it has not been possible to correlate the development of disease with any psychological issues or disease exacerbations with stressful life events.[199] Though short-term stress does not appear to trigger disease flares in patients with UC in remission, perceived long-term stress has been associated with an increased risk of exacerbation.[200] A recent study found no evidence of an association between psychological stress, as measured by the death of a child, and the development of IBD.[201]

The possibility of concurrent IBS-related symptoms and their relation to stressful events should also be recognized to minimize the use of potent anti-inflammatory or disease-modifying therapies in the absence of a documented inflammatory component.

Strategies that improve social support, including local groups where individuals can share their experiences, can have a favorable impact on psychological distress and ultimately can improve health outcomes in patients with IBD.[198] Empathy, understanding, positive regard, and psychological support can improve the patient–physician relationship and lead to better quality of life for the patients.[202]

CONCLUSION

The role of certain environmental and lifestyle factors in the onset, severity, and course of IBD is significant. An approach that involves patients in the self-care of their condition includes open discussion, and (when possible) modifications of these factors should be part of the integral care provided to patients with IBD. Smoking is the best studied of the so-called disease-modifiers in IBD. Smoking cessation is of proven benefit for CD patients and is known to exert a negative impact on the course and severity of UC. Although achieving long-term smoking cessation is difficult, IBD patients, including those with UC, should be encouraged to quit smoking. The benefits of smoking cessation outweigh the risk of aggravating UC, and providers caring for these patients should be prepared to adjust the medical regimen to mitigate the adverse effects of nicotine discontinuation.

Though appendectomy appears to be protective against UC, the use of both traditional NSAIDs and selective COX-2 inhibitors appears to exert a negative effect on the onset and course of IBD. The influence of other factors such as diet, childhood infections, socioeconomic factors, psychological stress, and oral contraceptives is less clear, and specific recommendations cannot be generalized to all patients.

REFERENCES

1. Howlett M, Gibson P. Environmental influences on IBD. *IBD Monitor*. 2004;5:74-83.

2. Bergstrand O, Hellers G. Breast-feeding during infancy in patients who later develop Crohn's disease. *Scand J Gastroenterol*. 1983; 18:903-906.

3. Koletzko S, Sherman P, Corey M, Griffiths A, Smith C. Role of infant feeding practices in development of Crohn's disease in childhood. *BMJ*. 1989;298:1617-1618.

4. Rigas A, Rigas B, Glassman M, et al. Breast-feeding and maternal smoking in the etiology of Crohn's disease and ulcerative colitis in childhood. *Ann Epidemiol*. 1993;3:387-392.

5. Gruber M, Marshall JR, Zielezny M, Lance P. A case-control study to examine the influence of maternal perinatal behaviors on the incidence of Crohn's disease. *Gastroenterol Nurs*. 1996;19:53-59.

6. Thompson NP, Montgomery SM, Wadsworth ME, Pounder RE, Wakefield AJ. Early determinants of inflammatory bowel disease: use of two national longitudinal birth cohorts. *Eur J Gastroenterol Hepatol*. 2000;12:25-30.

7. Gilat T, Hacohen D, Lilos P, Langman MJ. Childhood factors in ulcerative colitis and Crohn's disease. An international cooperative study. *Scand J Gastroenterol*. 1987;22:1009-1024.

8. Ekbom A, Adami HO, Helmick CG, Jonzon A, Zack MM. Perinatal risk factors for inflammatory bowel disease: a case-control study. *Am J Epidemiol*. 1990;132:1111-1119.

9. Koletzko S, Griffiths A, Corey M, Smith C, Sherman P. Infant feeding practices and ulcerative colitis in childhood. *BMJ*. 1991;302:1580-1581.

10. Thompson NP, Pounder RE, Wakefield AJ. Perinatal and childhood risk factors for inflammatory bowel disease: a case-control study. *Eur J Gastroenterol Hepatol*. 1995;7:385-390.

11. Acheson ED, Nefzger MD. Ulcerative colitis in the United States Army in 1944. Epidemiology: comparisons between patients and controls. *Gastroenterology*. 1963;44:7-19.

12. Sonnenberg A. Disability from inflammatory bowel disease among employees in West Germany. *Gut*. 1989;30:367-370.

13. Whorwell PJ, Holdstock G, Whorwell GM, Wright R. Bottle feeding, early gastroenteritis, and inflammatory bowel disease. *Br Med J*. 1979;1:382.

14. Ekbom A, Montgomery SM. Environmental risk factors (excluding tobacco and microorganisms): critical analysis of old and new hypotheses. *Best Pract Res Clin Gastroenterol*. 2004;18:497-508.

15. Duggan AE, Usmani I, Neal KR, Logan RF. Appendicectomy, childhood hygiene, *Helicobacter pylori* status, and risk of inflammatory bowel disease: a case control study. *Gut*. 1998;43:494-498.

16. Gent AE, Hellier MD, Grace RH, Swarbrick ET, Coggon D. Inflammatory bowel disease and domestic hygiene in infancy. *Lancet*. 1994;343:766-767.

17. Hugot JP, Alberti C, Berrebi D, Bingen E, Cezard JP. Crohn's disease: the cold chain hypothesis. *Lancet*. 2003;362:2012-2015.

18. Sullivan SN. Hypothesis revisited: toothpaste and the cause of Crohn's disease. *Lancet*. 1990;336:1096-1097.

19. Russel MG, Engels LG, Muris JW, et al. Modern life in the epidemiology of inflammatory bowel disease: a case-control study with special emphasis on nutritional factors. *Eur J Gastroenterol Hepatol*. 1998;10:243-249.

20. Shanahan F. Inflammatory bowel disease: immunodiagnostics, immunotherapeutics, and ecotherapeutics. *Gastroenterology*. 2001; 120:622-635.

21. Morgan KL. Johne's and Crohn's. Chronic inflammatory bowel diseases of infectious aetiology? *Lancet*. 1987;1:1017-1019.

22. Van Kruiningen HJ, Colombel JF, Cartun RW, et al. An in-depth study of Crohn's disease in two French families. *Gastroenterology*. 1993;104:351-360.

23. Pardi DS, Tremaine WJ, Sandborn WJ, et al. Early measles virus infection is associated with the development of inflammatory bowel disease. *Am J Gastroenterol*. 2000;95:1480-1485.

24. Ekbom A, Adami HO, Helmick CG, Jonzon A, Zack MM. Perinatal risk factors for inflammatory bowel disease: a case-control study. *Am J Epidemiol*. 1990;132:1111-1119.

25. Greenstein RJ. Is Crohn's disease caused by a mycobacterium? Comparisons with leprosy, tuberculosis, and Johne's disease. *Lancet Infect Dis*. 2003;3:507-514.

26. Naser SA, Ghobrial G, Romero C, Valentine JF. Culture of *Mycobacterium avium* subspecies *paratuberculosis* from the blood of patients with Crohn's disease. *Lancet*. 2004;364:1039-1044.

27. Van Kruiningen HJ. Lack of support for a common etiology in Johne's disease of animals and Crohn's disease in humans. *Inflamm Bowel Dis*. 1999;5:183-191.

28. Ryan P, Kelly RG, Lee G, et al. Bacterial DNA within granulomas of patients with Crohn's disease-detection by laser capture microdissection and PCR. *Am J Gastroenterol*. 2004;99:1539-1543.

29. Ryan P, Bennett MW, Aarons S, et al. PCR detection of *Mycobacterium paratuberculosis* in Crohn's disease granulomas isolated by laser capture microdissection. *Gut*. 2002;51:665-670.

30. Gui GP, Thomas PR, Tizard ML, Lake J, Sanderson JD, Hermon-Taylor J. Two-year-outcomes analysis of Crohn's disease treated with rifabutin and macrolide antibiotics. *J Antimicrob Chemother*. 1997;39:393-400.

31. Shafran I, Kugler L, El-Zaatari FA, Naser SA, Sandoval J. Open clinical trial of rifabutin and clarithromycin therapy in Crohn's disease. *Dig Liver Dis*. 2002;34:22-28.

32. Borody TJ, Leis S, Warren EF, Surace R. Treatment of severe Crohn's disease using antimycobacterial triple therapy—approaching a cure? *Dig Liver Dis*. 2002;34:29-38.

33. Borgaonkar MR, MacIntosh DG, Fardy JM. A meta-analysis of antimycobacterial therapy for Crohn's disease. *Am J Gastroenterol*. 2000;95:725-729.

34. Toracchio S, El-Zimaity HM, Urmacher C, Katz S, Graham DY. *Mycobacterium avium* subspecies *paratuberculosis* and Crohn's disease granulomas. *Scand J Gastroenterol*. 2008;43:1108-1111.

35. Loftus EV Jr. Clinical epidemiology of inflammatory bowel disease: incidence, prevalence, and environmental influences. *Gastroenterology*. 2004;126:1504-1517.

36. Liu Y, van Kruiningen HJ, West AB, Cartun RW, Cortot A, Colombel JF. Immunocytochemical evidence of *Listeria, Escherichia coli*, and *Streptococcus* antigens in Crohn's disease. *Gastroenterology*. 1995;108:1396-1404.

37. Swidsinski A, Ladhoff A, Pernthaler A, et al. Mucosal flora in inflammatory bowel disease. *Gastroenterology*. 2002;122:44-54.

38. Wakefield AJ, Ekbom A, Dhillon AP, Pittilo RM, Pounder RE. Crohn's disease: pathogenesis and persistent measles virus infection. *Gastroenterology*. 1995;108:911-916.

39. Montgomery SM, Morris DL, Pounder RE, Wakefield AJ. Paramyxovirus infections in childhood and subsequent inflammatory bowel disease. *Gastroenterology*. 1999;116:796-803.

40. Montgomery SM, Bjornsson S, Johannsson JH, Thjodleifsson B, Pounder RE, Wakefield AJ. Concurrent measles and mumps epidemics in Iceland are a risk factor for later inflammatory bowel disease. *Gut*. 1998;42:A41.

41. Anonymous. Case control study finds no link between measles vaccine and inflammatory bowel disease. *Commun Dis Rep CDR Wkly*. 1997;7:339.

42. Feeney M, Ciegg A, Winwood P, Snook J. A case-control study of measles vaccination and inflammatory bowel disease. The East Dorset Gastroenterology Group. *Lancet*. 1997;350:764-766.

43. Morris DL, Montgomery SM, Thompson NP, Ebrahim S, Pounder RE, Wakefield AJ. Measles vaccination and inflammatory bowel disease: a national British Cohort Study. *Am J Gastroenterol*. 2000;95:3507-3512.

44. Davis RL, Kramarz P, Bohlke K, et al. Measles-mumps-rubella and other measles-containing vaccines do not increase the risk for inflammatory bowel disease: a case-control study from the Vaccine Safety Datalink project. *Arch Pediatr Adolesc Med*. 2001; 155:354-359.

45. Iizuka M, Saito H, Yukawa M, et al. No evidence of persistent mumps virus infection in inflammatory bowel disease. *Gut*. 2001; 48:637-641.

46. Peltola H, Patja A, Leinikki P, Valle M, Davidkin I, Paunio M. No evidence for measles, mumps, and rubella vaccine-associated inflammatory bowel disease or autism in a 14-year prospective study. *Lancet*. 1998;351:1327-1328.

47. Haga Y, Funakoshi O, Kuroe K, et al. Absence of measles viral genomic sequence in intestinal tissues from Crohn's disease by nested polymerase chain reaction. *Gut*. 1996;38:211-215.

48. Afzal MA, Armitage E, Begley J, et al. Absence of detectable measles virus genome sequence in inflammatory bowel disease tissues and peripheral blood lymphocytes. *J Med Virol*. 1998;55:243-249.

49. Folwaczny C, Jager G, Schnettler D, Wiebecke B, Loeschke K. Search for mumps virus genome in intestinal biopsy specimens of patients with IBD. *Gastroenterology*. 1999;117:1253-1255.

50. Wurzelmann JI, Lyles CM, Sandler RS. Childhood infections and the risk of inflammatory bowel disease. *Dig Dis Sci*. 1994;39:555-560.

51. Burke DA, Axon AT. Adhesive *Escherichia coli* in inflammatory bowel disease and infective diarrhoea. *BMJ*. 1988;297:102-104.

52. Darfeuille-Michaud A, Boudeau J, Bulois P, et al. High prevalence of adherent-invasive *Escherichia coli* associated with ileal mucosa in Crohn's disease. *Gastroenterology*. 2004;127:412-421.

53. Baumgart M, Dogan B, Rishniw M, et al. Culture independent analysis of ileal mucosa reveals a selective increase in invasive *Escherichia coli* of novel phylogeny relative to depletion of *Clostridiales* in Crohn's disease involving the ileum. *ISME J*. 2007;1:403-418.

54. Martin HM, Campbell BJ, Hart CA, et al. Enhanced *Escherichia coli* adherence and invasion in Crohn's disease and colon cancer. *Gastroenterology*. 2004;127:80-93.

55. Summers RW, Elliott DE, Qadir K, Urban JF Jr, Thompson R, Weinstock JV. *Trichuris suis* seems to be safe and possibly effective in the treatment of inflammatory bowel disease. *Am J Gastroenterol*. 2003;98:2034-2041.

56. Merger M, Croitoru K. Infections in the immunopathogenesis of chronic inflammatory bowel disease. *Semin Immunol*. 1998; 10:69-78.

57. Fiocchi C. Inflammatory bowel disease: etiology and pathogenesis. *Gastroenterology*. 1998;115:182-205.

58. Demling L. Is Crohn's disease caused by antibiotics? *Hepatogastroenterology*. 1994;41:549-551.

59. Schultz M, Scholmerich J, Rath HC. Rationale for probiotic and antibiotic treatment strategies in inflammatory bowel diseases. *Dig Dis*. 2003;21:105-128.

60. D'Haens GR, Vermeire S, Van Assche G, et al. Therapy of metronidazole with azathioprine to prevent postoperative recurrence of Crohn's disease: a controlled randomized trial. *Gastroenterology*. 2008;135:1123-1129.

61. Bengmark S. Colonic food: pre- and probiotics. *Am J Gastroenterol*. 2000;95(1 suppl):S5-S7.

62. Kruis W, Schulz T, Fric P, et al. Double blind comparison of an oral *Escherichia coli* preparation and mesalazine in maintaining remission of ulcerative colitis. *Aliment Pharmacol Ther*. 1997;11:853-858.

63. Rembacken BJ, Snelling AM, Hawkey PM, et al. Non-pathogenic *Escherichia coli* versus mesalazine for the treatment of ulcerative colitis: a randomized trial. *Lancet*. 1999;354:635-639.

64. Gionchetti P, Rizzello F, Venturi A, Campieri M. Probiotics in infective diarrhoea and inflammatory bowel diseases. *J Gastroenterol Hepatol*. 2000;15:489-493.

65. Makharia GK, Sood A, Midha V. A randomized, controlled trial of probiotic preperation VSL#3 for the treatment of mild to moderate ulcerative colitis [abstract]. *Gastroenterology*. 2008;134(suppl 1): A701.

66. Miele E, Baldessano R, Pascarella S. The effect of a probiotic preparation VSL#3 on induction and remission in mild UC [abstract]. *Gastoenterology*. 2008;134(suppl 1):1013.

67. Shanahan F. Probiotics: science or snake oil. *Clin Persp Gastroenterol*. 2001;4:47-50.

68. Rutgeerts P, D'Haens G, Hiele M, Geboes K, Vantrappen G. Appendectomy protects against ulcerative colitis. *Gastroenterology*. 1994;106:1251-1253.

69. Radford-Smith GL, Edwards JE, Purdie DM, et al. Protective role of appendectomy on onset and severity of ulcerative colitis and Crohn's disease. *Gut*. 2002;51:808-813.

70. Koutroubakis IE, Vlachonikolis IG, Kouroumalis EA. Role of appendicitis and appendectomy in the pathogenesis of ulcerative colitis: a critical review. *Inflamm Bowel Dis*. 2002;8:277-286.

71. Andersson RE, Olaison G, Tysk C, Ekbom A. Appendectomy and protection against ulcerative colitis. *N Engl J Med*. 2001;344:808-814.

72. Naganuma M, Iizuka B, Torii A, et al. Appendectomy protects against the development of ulcerative colitis and reduces its recurrence: results of a multicenter case-controlled study in Japan. *Am J Gastroenterol*. 2001;96:1123-1126.

73. Selby WS, Griffin S, Abraham N, Solomon MJ. Appendectomy protects against the development of ulcerative colitis but does not affect its course. *Am J Gastroenterol*. 2002;97:2834-2838.

74. Cosnes J, Carbonnel F, Beaugerie L, Blain A, Reijasse D, Gendre JP. Effects of appendectomy on the course of ulcerative colitis. *Gut*. 2002;51:803-807.

75. Andersson RE, Olaison G, Tysk C, Ekbom A. Appendectomy is followed by increased risk of Crohn's disease. *Gastroenterology*. 2003;124:40-46.

76. Kurina LM, Goldacre MJ, Yeates D, Seagroatt V. Appendectomy, tonsillectomy, and inflammatory bowel disease: a case-control record linkage study. *J Epidemiol Community Health*. 2002; 56:551-554.

77. Probert CS, Jayanthi V, Pinder D, Wicks AC, Mayberry JF. Epidemiological study of ulcerative proctocolitis in Indian migrants and the indigenous population of Leicestershire. *Gut*. 1992;33:687-693.

78. Shoda R, Matsueda K, Yamato S, Umeda N. Epidemiologic analysis of Crohn disease in Japan: increased dietary intake of n-6 polyunsaturated fatty acids and animal protein relates to the increased incidence of Crohn disease in Japan. *Am J Clin Nutr*. 1996;63:741-745.

79. Yang SK, Hong WS, Min YI, et al. Incidence and prevalence of ulcerative colitis in the Songpa-Kangdong District, Seoul, Korea, 1986-1997. *J Gastroenterol Hepatol*. 2000;15:1037-1042.

80. Persson PG, Ahlbom A, Hellers G. Crohn's disease and ulcerative colitis. A review of dietary studies with emphasis on methodologic aspects. *Scand J Gastroenterol*. 1987;22:385-389.

81. Mayberry JF, Rhodes J, Newcombe RG. Increased sugar consumption in Crohn's disease. *Digestion*. 1980;20:323-326.

82. Jarnerot G, Jarnmark I, Nilsson K. Consumption of refined sugar by patients with Crohn's disease, ulcerative colitis, or irritable bowel syndrome. *Scand J Gastroenterol.* 1983;18:999-1002.

83. Mayberry JF, Rhodes J, Allan R, et al. Diet in Crohn's disease two studies of current and previous habits in newly diagnosed patients. *Dig Dis Sci.* 1981;26:444-448.

84. Tragnone A, Valpiani D, Miglio F, et al. Dietary habits as risk factors for inflammatory bowel disease. *Eur J Gastroenterol Hepatol.* 1995;7:47-51.

85. Reif S, Klein I, Lubin F, Farbstein M, Hallak A, Gilat T. Pre-illness dietary factors in inflammatory bowel disease. *Gut.* 1997;40:754-760.

86. Brauer PM, Gee MI, Grace M, Thomson AB. Diet of women with Crohn's and other gastrointestinal diseases. *J Am Diet Assoc.* 1983;82:659-764.

87. Katschinski B, Logan RF, Edmond M, Langman MJ. Smoking and sugar intake are separate but interactive risk factors in Crohn's disease. *Gut.* 1988;29:1202-1206.

88. Thornton JR, Emmett PM, Heaton KW. Smoking, sugar, and inflammatory bowel disease. *Br Med J (Clin Res Ed).* 1985;290:1786-1787.

89. Riordan AM, Ruxton CH, Hunter JO. A review of associations between Crohn's disease and consumption of sugars. *Eur J Clin Nutr.* 1998;52:229-238.

90. Geerling BJ, Dagnelie PC, Badart-Smook A, Russel MG, Stockbrugger RW, Brummer RJ. Diet as a risk factor for the development of ulcerative colitis. *Am J Gastroenterol.* 2000;95:1008-1013.

91. Jowett SL, Seal CJ, Pearce MS, et al. Influence of dietary factors on the clinical course of ulcerative colitis: a prospective cohort study. *Gut.* 2004;53:1479-1484.

92. Persson PG, Ahlbom A, Hellers G. Diet and inflammatory bowel disease: a case-control study. *Epidemiology.* 1992;3:47-52.

93. Sonnenberg A. Geographic and temporal variations of sugar and margarine consumption in relation to Crohn's disease. *Digestion.* 1988;41:161-171.

94. Millar D, Ford J, Sanderson J, et al. IS900 PCR to detect *Mycobacterium paratuberculosis* in retail supplies of whole pasteurized cows' milk in England and Wales. *Appl Environ Microbiol.* 1996;62:3446-3452.

95. Main J, McKenzie H, Yeaman GR, et al. Antibody to *Saccharomyces cerevisiae* (bakers' yeast) in Crohn's disease. *BMJ.* 1988;297:1105-1106.

96. Barclay GR, McKenzie H, Pennington J, Parratt D, Pennington CR. The effect of dietary yeast on the activity of stable chronic Crohn's disease. *Scand J Gastroenterol.* 1992;27:196-200.

97. Boyko EJ, Perera DR, Koepsell TD, Keane EM, Inui TS. Coffee and alcohol use and the risk of ulcerative colitis. *Am J Gastroenterol.* 1989;84:530-534.

98. Hendriksen C, Binder V. Social prognosis in patients with ulcerative colitis. *Br Med J.* 1980;281:581-583.

99. James AH. Breakfast and Crohn's disease. *Br Med J.* 1977;1:943-945.

100. Mayberry JF, Rhodes J, Newcombe RG. Breakfast and dietary aspects of Crohn's disease. *Br Med J.* 1978;2:1401.

101. Ukil A, Maity S, Karmakar S, Datta N, Vedasiromoni JR, Das PK. Curcumin, the major component of food flavour turmeric, reduces mucosal injury in trinitrobenzene sulphonic acid-induced colitis. *Br J Pharmacol.* 2003;139:209-218.

102. Suchner U, Kuhn KS, Furst P. The scientific basis of immunonutrition. *Proc Nutr Soc.* 2000;59:553-563.

103. Van Den Bogaerde J, Cahill J, Emmanuel AV, et al. Gut mucosal response to food antigens in Crohn's disease. *Aliment Pharmacol Ther.* 2002;16:1903-1915.

104. Lomer MC, Thompson RP, Powell JJ. Fine and ultrafine particles of the diet: influence on the mucosal immune response and association with Crohn's disease. *Proc Nutr Soc.* 2002;61:123-130.

105. Lomer MC, Harvey RS, Evans SM, Thompson RP, Powell JJ. Efficacy and tolerability of a low microparticle diet in a double blind, randomized, pilot study in Crohn's disease. *Eur J Gastroenterol Hepatol.* 2001;13:101-106.

106. Rhodes JM, Cockel R, Allan RN, Hawker PC, Dawson J, Elias E. Colonic Crohn's disease and use of oral contraception. *Br Med J (Clin Res Ed).* 1984;288:595-596.

107. Ramcharan S, Pellegrin FA, Ray RM, Hsu JP. The Walnut Creek Contraceptive Drug Study. A prospective study of the side effects of oral contraceptives. Volume III, an interim report: a comparison of disease occurrence leading to hospitalization or death in users and nonusers of oral contraceptives. *J Reprod Med.* 1980;25(6 suppl):345-372.

108. Logan RF, Kay CR. Oral contraception, smoking and inflammatory bowel disease—findings in the Royal College of General Practitioners Oral Contraception Study. *Int J Epidemiol.* 1989;18:105-107.

109. Vessey M, Jewell D, Smith A, Yeates D, McPherson K. Chronic inflammatory bowel disease, cigarette smoking, and use of oral contraceptives: findings in a large cohort study of women of childbearing age. *Br Med J (Clin Res Ed).* 1986;292:1101-1103.

110. Godet PG, May GR, Sutherland LR. Meta-analysis of the role of oral contraceptive agents in inflammatory bowel disease. *Gut.* 1995;37:668-673.

111. Boyko EJ, Theis MK, Vaughan TL, Nicol-Blades B. Increased risk of inflammatory bowel disease associated with oral contraceptive use. *Am J Epidemiol.* 1994;140:268-278.

112. Corrao G, Tragnone A, Caprilli R, et al. Risk of inflammatory bowel disease attributable to smoking, oral contraception and breastfeeding in Italy: a nationwide case-control study. Cooperative Investigators of the Italian Group for the Study of the Colon and the Rectum (GISC). *Int J Epidemiol.* 1998;27:397-404.

113. Lesko SM, Kaufman DW, Rosenberg L, et al. Evidence for an increased risk of Crohn's disease in oral contraceptive users. *Gastroenterology.* 1985;89:1046-1049.

114. Katschinski B, Fingerle D, Scherbaum B, Goebell H. Oral contraceptive use and cigarette smoking in Crohn's disease. *Dig Dis Sci.* 1993;38:1596-1600.

115. Timmer A, Sutherland LR, Martin F. Oral contraceptive use and smoking are risk factors for relapse in Crohn's disease. The Canadian Mesalamine for Remission of Crohn's Disease Study Group. *Gastroenterology.* 1998;114:1143-1150.

116. Cosnes J, Carbonnel F, Carrat F, Beaugerie L, Gendre JP. Oral contraceptive use and the clinical course of Crohn's disease: a prospective cohort study. *Gut.* 1999;45:218-222.

117. Wakefield AJ, Sawyer AM, Hudson M, Dhillon AP, Pounder RE. Smoking, the oral contraceptive pill, and Crohn's disease. *Dig Dis Sci.* 1991;36:1147-1150.

118. Harries AD, Baird A, Rhodes J. Non-smoking: a feature of ulcerative colitis. *Br Med J.* 1982;284:706.

119. Sutherland LR, Ramcharan S, Bryant H, Fick G. Effect of cigarette smoking on recurrence of Crohn's disease. *Gastroenterology.* 1990;98:1123-1128.

120. Gareth AO, Thomas BS, Rhodes J, Green JT. Inflammatory bowel disease and smoking—a review. *Am J Gastroenterol.* 1998;93:144-149.

121. Reif S, Lavy A, Keter D, et al. Lack of association between smoking and Crohn's disease but the usual association with ulcerative colitis in Jewish patients in Israel: a multicenter study. *Am J Gastroenterol.* 2000;95:474-478.

122. Penny WJ, Penny E, Mayberry JF, Rhodes J. Mormons, smoking and ulcerative colitis. *Lancet.* 1983;2:1315.

123. Penny WJ, Penny E, Mayberry JF, et al. Prevalence of inflammatory bowel disease amongst Mormons in Britain and Ireland. *Soc Sci Med*. 1985;21:287-290.

124. Calkins BM. A meta-analysis of the role of smoking in inflammatory bowel disease. *Dig Dis Sci*. 1989;34:1841-1854.

125. Motley RJ, Rhodes J, Ford GA, et al. Time relationship between cessation of smoking and onset of ulcerative colitis. *Digestion*. 1987;37:125-127.

126. Doyko EJ, Koepsell TD, Perera DR, et al. Risk of ulcerative colitis among former and current cigarette smokers. *N Engl J Med*. 1987;316:707-710.

127. Lindberg E, Tysk C, Anderson K, et al. Smoking and inflammatory bowel disease. A case-control study. *Gut*. 1988;29:352-357.

128. Loftus EV Jr, Sandborn WJ, Tremaine WJ, et al. Primary sclerosing cholangitis is associated with nonsmoking: a case-control study. *Gastroenterology*. 1996;110:1496-1502.

129. van Erpecum KJ, Smits SJ, van de Meeberg PC, et al. Risk of primary sclerosing cholangitis is associated with nonsmoking behavior. *Gastroenterology*. 1996;110:1503-1506.

130. Mitchell SA, Thyssen M, Orchard TR, Jewell DP, Fleming KA, Chapman RW. Cigarette smoking, appendectomy, and tonsillectomy as risk factors for the development of primary sclerosing cholangitis: a case-control study. *Gut*. 2002;51:567-573.

131. Merrett MN, Mortensen N, Kettlewell M, Jewell DO. Smoking may prevent pouchitis in patients with restorative proctocolectomy for ulcerative colitis. *Gut*. 1996;38:362-364.

132. Russel MG, Nieman FH, Bergers JM, Stockbrugger RW. Cigarette smoking and quality of life in patients with inflammatory bowel disease. South Limburg IBD Study Group. *Eur J Gastroenterol Hepatol*. 1996;8:1075-1081.

133. Boyko EJ, Perera DR, Koepsell TD, et al. Effects of cigarette smoking on the clinical course of ulcerative colitis. *Scand J Gastroenterol*. 1988;23:1147-1152.

134. Fraga XF, Vergara M, Medina C, Casellas F, Bermejo B, Malagelada JR. Effects of smoking on the presentation and clinical course of inflammatory bowel disease. *Eur J Gastroenterol Hepatol*. 1997; 9:683-687.

135. Beaugerie L, Massot N, Carbonnel F, et al. Impact of cessation of smoking on the course of ulcerative colitis. *Am J Gastroenterol*. 2001;96:2113-2116.

136. Hilsden RJ, Hodgins D, Czechowsky D, Verhoef MJ, Sutherland LR. Attitudes toward smoking and smoking behaviors of patients with Crohn's disease. *Am J Gastroenterol*. 2001;96:1849-1853.

137. Breuer-Katschinski BD, Hollander N, Goebell H. Effect of cigarette smoking on the course of Crohn's disease. *Eur J Gastroenterol Hepatol*. 1996;8:225-228.

138. Lindberg E, Jarnerot G, Huitfeldt B. Smoking in Crohn's disease: effect on localization and clinical course. *Gut*. 1992;33:779-782.

139. Cottone M, Rosselli M, Orlando A, et al. Smoking habits and recurrence in Crohn's disease. *Gastroenterology*. 1994;106:643-648.

140. Cosnes J, Carbonnel F, Beaugerie L, Le Quintrec Y, Gendre JP. Effects of cigarette smoking on the long-term course of Crohn's disease. *Gastroenterology*. 1996;110:424-431.

141. Russel MG, Volovics A, Schoon EJ, et al. Inflammatory bowel disease: is there any relation between smoking status and disease presentation? European Collaborative IBD Study Group. *Inflamm Bowel Dis*. 1998;4:182-186.

142. Cosnes J, Carbonnel F, Carrat F, Beaugerie L, Cattan S, Gendre J. Effects of current and former cigarette smoking on the clinical course of Crohn's disease. *Aliment Pharmacol Ther*. 1999;13:1403-1411.

143. Shields PL, Low-Beer TS. Patients' awareness of adverse relation between Crohn's disease and their smoking: questionnaire survey. *BMJ*. 1996;313:265-266.

144. Cosnes J, Beaugerie L, Carbonnel F, Gendre JP. Decreased severity of Crohn's disease after smoking cessation, preliminary results of a prospective intervention study. *Gastroenterology*. 2000;118:A870.

145. Cosnes J, Beaugerie L, Carbonnel F, Gendre JP. Smoking cessation and the course of Crohn's disease: an intervention study. *Gastroenterology*. 2001;120:1093-1099.

146. Lashner BA, Shaheen NJ, Hanauer SB, et al. Passive smoking is associated with an increased risk of developing inflammatory bowel disease in children. *Am J Gastroenterol*. 1993;88:356-359.

147. Sandler RS, Sandler DP, McDonnell CW, Wurzelmann JI. Childhood exposure to environmental tobacco smoke and the risk of ulcerative colitis. *Am J Epidemiol*. 1992;135:603-608.

148. Cosnes J. Tobacco and IBD: relevance in the understanding of disease mechanisms and clinical practice. *Best Pract Res Clin Gastroenterol*. 2004;18:481-496.

149. Motley RJ, Rhodes J, Williams G, et al. Smoking, eicosanoids and ulcerative colitis. *J Pharm Pharmacol*. 1990;42:288-289.

150. Madretsma S, Wolters LM, van Dijk JP, et al. In-vivo effect of nicotine on cytokine production by human non-adherent mononuclear cells. *Eur J Gastroenterol Hepatol*. 1996;8:1017-1020.

151. Euler DE, Dave SJ, Guo H. Effect of cigarette smoking on pentane excretion in alveolar breath. *Clin Chem*. 1996;42:303-308.

152. Hatoum OA, Binion DG, Otterson MF, Gutterman DD. Acquired microvascular dysfunction in inflammatory bowel disease: loss of nitric oxide-mediated vasodilation. *Gastroenterology*. 2003; 125:58-69.

153. Wolfe MM, Lichtenstein DR, Singh G. Gastrointestinal toxicity of nonsteroidal antiinflamatory drugs. *N Engl J Med*. 1999;340: 1888-1899.

154. Katsinelos P, Christodoulou K, Pilpilidis I, et al. Colopathy associated with the systemic use of nonsteroidal antiinflammatory medications. An underestimated entity. *Hepatogastroenterology*. 2002;49:345-348.

155. Oren R, Ligumsky M. Indomethacin-induced colonic ulceration and bleeding. *Ann Pharmacother*. 1994;28:883-885.

156. Gibson GR, Whitacre EB, Ricotti CA. Colitis induced by nonsteroidal anti-inflammatory drugs. Report of four cases and review of the literature. *Arch Intern Med*. 1992;152:625-632.

157. O'Brien J. Nonsteroidal anti-inflammatory drugs in patients with inflammatory bowel disease. *Am J Gastroenterol*. 2000;95:1859-1861.

158. Kakar S, Pardi DS, Burgart LJ. Colonic ulcers accompanying collagenous colitis: implication of nonsteroidal anti-inflammatory drugs. *Am J Gastroenterol*. 2003;98:1834-1837.

159. Al-Ghamdi MY, Malatjalian DA, Veldhuyzen van Zanten S. Causation: recurrent collagenous colitis following repeated use of NSAIDs. *Can J Gastroenterol*. 2002;16:861-862.

160. Felder JB, Korelitz BI, Rajapakse R, Schwarz S, Horatagis AP, Gleim G. Effects of nonsteroidal antiinflammatory drugs on inflammatory bowel disease: a case-control study. *Am J Gastroenterol*. 2000;95:1949-1954.

161. Bonner GF, Walczak M, Kitchen L, Bayona M. Tolerance of nonsteroidal antiinflammatory drugs in patients with inflammatory bowel disease. *Am J Gastroenterol*. 2000;95:1946-1948.

162. Wallace JL. Nonsteroidal anti-inflammatory drugs and gastroenteropathy: the second hundred years. *Gastroenterology*. 1997; 112:1000-1016.

163. Hendel J, Nielsen OH. Expression of cyclooxygenase-2 mRNA in active inflammatory bowel disease. *Am J Gastroenterol*. 1997; 92:1170-1173.

164. Bonner GF. Exacerbation of inflammatory bowel disease associated with use of celecoxib. *Am J Gastroenterol*. 2001;96:1306-1308.

165. Goh J, Wight D, Parkes M, Middleton SJ, Hunter JO. Rofecoxib and cytomegalovirus in acute flare-up of ulcerative colitis: coprecipitants or coincidence? *Am J Gastroenterol.* 2002;97:1061-1062.

166. Gornet JM, Hassani Z, Modiglian R, Lemann M. Exacerbation of Crohn's colitis with severe colonic hemorrhage in a patient on rofecoxib. *Am J Gastroenterol.* 2002;97:3209-3210.

167. Mahadevan U, Loftus EV Jr, Tremaine WJ, Sandborn WJ. Safety of selective cyclooxygenase-2 inhibitors in inflammatory bowel disease. *Am J Gastroenterol.* 2002;97:910-914.

168. Reinisch W, Miehsler W, Dejaco C, et al. An open-label trial of the selective cyclo-oxygenase-2 inhibitor, rofecoxib, in inflammatory bowel disease-associated peripheral arthritis and arthralgia. *Aliment Pharmacol Ther.* 2003;17:1371-1380.

169. Matuk R, Crawford J, Abreu M, Targan S, Vasiliauskas E, Papadakis K. The spectrum of gastrointestinal toxicity and effect on disease activity of selective COX-2 inhibitors in patients with inflammatory bowel disease. *Inflamm Bowel Dis.* 2004;10:352-356.

170. Sandborn WJ, Stenson WF, Brynskov J, et al. Safety of celecoxib in patients with ulcerative colitis in remission: a randomized, placebo-controlled, pilot study. *Clin Gastroenterol Hepatol.* 2006;4:203-211.

171. Oviedo J, Farraye FA. Self-care for the inflammatory bowel disease patient: what can the professional recommend? *Semin Gastrointest Dis.* 2001;12:223-236.

172. Smale S, Bjarnason I. Nonsteroidal anti-inflammatory drugs, enterocolonic ulceration and inflammatory bowel disease. In: Bayless-Hanauer, ed. *Advance Therapy of Inflammatory Bowel Disease.* London: B.C Decker; 2001:625-627.

173. Sonnenberg A. Occupational distribution of inflammatory bowel disease among German employees. *Gut.* 1990;31:1037-1040.

174. Persson PG, Leijonmarck CE, Bernell O, Hellers G, Ahlbom A. Risk indicators for inflammatory bowel disease. *Int J Epidemiol.* 1993;22:268-272.

175. Klein I, Reif S, Farbstein H, Halak A, Gilat T. Preillness nondietary factors and habits in inflammatory bowel disease. *Ital J Gastroenterol Hepatol.* 1998;30:247-251.

176. Loudon CP, Corroll V, Butcher J, Rawsthorne P, Bernstein CN. The effects of physical exercise on patients with Crohn's disease. *Am J Gastroenterol.* 1999;94:697-703.

177. Oktedalen O, Lunde OC, Opstad PK, et al. Changes in the gastrointestinal mucosa after long-distance running. *Scand J Gastroenterol.* 1992;27:270-274.

178. Peters HP, Bos M, Seebregts L, et al. Gastrointestinal symptoms in long-distance runners, cyclists and triathletes: prevalence, medication, and etiology. *Am J Gastroenterol.* 1999;94:1570-1581.

179. Peters HP, Zweers M, Backx FJ, et al. Gastrointestinal symptoms during long-distance walking. *Med Sci Sports Exerc.* 1999;31:767-773.

180. Lucas W, Schroy PC. Reversible ischemic colitis in a high endurance athlete. *Am J Gastroenterol.* 1998;93:2231-2234.

181. Oliveria SA, Christos PJ. The epidemiology of physical activity and cancer. *Ann N Y Acad Sci.* 1997;833:79-90.

182. Peters HP, De Vries WR, Vanberge-Henegouwen GP, Akkermans LM. Potential benefits and hazards of physical activity and exercise on the gastrointestinal tract. *Gut.* 2001;48:435-439.

183. Robinson RJ, al-Azzawi F, Iqbal SJ, et al. Osteoporosis and determinants of bone density in patients with Crohn's disease. *Dig Dis Sci.* 1998;43:2500-2506.

184. Robinson RJ, Krzywicki T, Almond L, et al. Effect of a low-impact exercise program on bone mineral density in Crohn's disease: a randomized controlled trial. *Gastroenterology.* 1998;115:36-41.

185. Tysk C, Jarnerot G. Seasonal variation in exacerbations of ulcerative colitis. *Scand J Gastroenterol.* 1993;28:95-96.

186. Kangro HO, Chong SK, Hardiman A, Heath RB, Walker-Smith JA. A prospective study of viral and mycoplasma infections in chronic inflammatory bowel disease. *Gastroenterology.* 1990;98(3):549-553.

187. Myszor M, Calam J. Seasonality of ulcerative colitis. *Lancet.* 1984;2:522-523.

188. Sellu DP. Seasonal variation in onset of exacerbations of ulcerative proctocolitis. *J R Coll Surg Edinb.* 1986;31:158-160.

189. Don BA, Goldacre MJ. Absence of seasonality in emergency hospital admissions for inflammatory bowel disease. *Lancet.* 1984; 2:1156-1157.

190. Sonnenberg A, Jacobsen SJ, Wasserman IH. Periodicity of hospital admissions for inflammatory bowel disease. *Am J Gastroenterol.* 1994;89:847-851.

191. Dowell SF. Seasonal variation in host susceptibility and cycles of certain infectious diseases. *Emerg Infect Dis.* 2001;7:369-374.

192. Noah ND. Cyclical patterns and predictability in infection. *Epidemiol Infect.* 1989;102:175-190.

193. Lewis JD, Aberra FN, Lichtenstein GR, Bilker WB, Brensinger C, Strom BL. Seasonal variation in flares of inflammatory bowel disease. *Gastroenterology.* 2004;126:665-673.

194. Drossman DA, Leserman J, Mitchell M, et al. Health status and healthcare use in persons with inflammatory bowel disease. A national sample. *Dig Dis Sci.* 1991;36:1746-1755.

195. Porcelli P, Zaka S, Centonze S, Sisto G. Psychological distress and levels of disease activity in inflammatory bowel disease. *Ital J Gastroenterol.* 1994;26:111-115.

196. Porcelli P, Leoci C, Guerra V. A prospective study of the relationship between disease activity and psychologic distress in patients with inflammatory bowel disease. *Scand J Gastroenterol.* 1996;31:792-796.

197. North CS, Alpers DH, Helzer JE, et al. Do life events or depression exacerbate inflammatory bowel disease? A prospective study. *Ann Intern Med.* 1991;114:381-386.

198. Sewitch MJ, Abrahamowicz M, Bitton A, et al. Psychological distress, social support, and disease activity in patients with inflammatory bowel disease. *Am J Gastroenterol.* 2001;96:1470-1479.

199. Hanauer SB, Sandborn WJ; Practice Parameters Committee of the American College of Gastroenterology. Management of Crohn's disease in adults. *Am J Gastroenterol.* 2001;96:635-643.

200. Levenstein S, Prantera C, Varvo V, et al. Stress and exacerbation in ulcerative colitis: a prospective study of patients enrolled in remission. *Am J Gastroenterol.* 2000;95:1213-1220.

201. Li J, Norgard B, Precht DH, Olsen J. Psychological stress and inflammatory bowel disease: a follow-up study in parents who lost a child in Denmark. *Am J Gastroenterol.* 2004;99:1129-1133.

202. Moser G, Drossman DA. Managing patients' concerns. In: Bayless-Hanauer, ed. *Advanced Therapy of Inflammatory Bowel Disease.* London: BC Decker Inc; 2001:527-529.

FERTILITY AND PREGNANCY IN INFLAMMATORY BOWEL DISEASE

Jeffry A. Katz, MD and Vinita Elizabeth Jacob, MD

The incidence of inflammatory bowel disease (IBD) appears to be increasing worldwide, even in areas not previously described as having an increased prevalence of the disease. Given the bimodal age distribution of the onset of symptoms, the issue of inflammatory bowel disease during peak reproductive years is an important one to deal with. In this chapter, we discuss several relevant topics including fertility, the natural impact of pregnancy on the course of IBD, obstetric complications from IBD, and the effect of IBD medications on pregnancy outcomes.

IBD often presents before or during childbearing years, and young women with IBD are likely to become pregnant at some point. Patients with IBD naturally are concerned about the potential effects of their chronic illness on sexuality, fertility, pregnancy, and the fetus. Most evidence suggests that women with IBD can expect a normal pregnancy and delivery, provided their disease is inactive. Although Crohn's disease appears to be associated with an increased risk of premature delivery and low birth weight (LBW), children born to women with IBD are typically healthy. Neither ulcerative colitis nor Crohn's disease causes an increase in congenital abnormalities, and most of the usual medical therapies for IBD appear to be safe and well tolerated during pregnancy. Major concerns of the gastroenterologist and obstetrician should be the optimal timing of the pregnancy, the potential for symptomatic recurrence of IBD during pregnancy and after delivery, and the safety of and need for medical or surgical treatment during pregnancy. A clear understanding of the issues surrounding fertility and pregnancy in IBD help the physician better care for these patients. Although at times challenging, guiding a young person with IBD through conception and pregnancy to the delivery of a healthy child can be a tremendously rewarding experience for the treating physician.

FERTILITY

Little information exists exploring the factors that influence an IBD patient's decision to have children,[1] but difficulties with intimacy, body image, disease activity, surgery, chronic pain, fear of pregnancy, and inaccurate medical advice may all affect this decision. Older studies suggest that patients with IBD have fewer children than expected for the population.[2] Women with IBD whose first pregnancy occurred after disease onset have been reported to have fewer pregnancies than controls, whereas women whose first pregnancies occurred before the disease onset had the same average number of pregnancies as controls.[3] This decrease may, however, represent voluntary childlessness rather than a disease-related decrease in fertility. Newer data show normal female fecundity among 343 women with ulcerative colitis before and after their diagnosis.[4]

Fertility in women with Crohn's disease may be decreased compared to the normal population, though some of this is perceived to be voluntary.[5] A study by Khosla showed a 12% rate of infertility among women with Crohn's disease who were younger than age 45 years, a rate that is similar to that found among women without inflammatory bowel disease.[5] A study by Baird et al showed that measures of childlessness, infertility, and fecundability were mainly a consequence of the patient's choice rather than a disease-mediated process.[3] In an often-quoted study by Hudson et al, women with both ulcerative colitis and Crohn's disease

Lichtenstein GR, ed.
Crohn's Disease: The Complete Guide to Medical Management (pp 91-106).
© 2011 SLACK Incorporated

had normal fertility (~14%), a percentage similar to the general population of northeast Scotland.[6] In regards to ulcerative colitis, the Baird and Hudson studies showed that women with ulcerative colitis all had normal fertility when compared to the general population as well.

The study by Hudson et al suggested that infertility issues were more frequent in women who had undergone surgery for inflammatory bowel disease when compared to IBD pregnant women who had not, leading many to speculate that significant pelvic inflammation may scar and block fallopian tubes.[6] In addition, the inflammation that is present in patients with Crohn's disease occasionally affects the ovaries and the fallopian tubes, especially on the right side because of proximity to the terminal ileum, explaining some reduced fertility.[7] Additionally, Crohn's disease patients with perianal disease may have secondary dyspareunia and decreased libido contributing to lower fertility rates.[7] Fever, pain, diarrhea, and malnutrition have also been implicated in causing decreased fertility.[5,8] In large part, fertility is reduced in Crohn's disease in proportion to the disease activity, and IBD patients in general are less likely to conceive successfully while their disease is active.[6,9] Normal fertility can be restored when drug therapy achieves disease remission.[8] Patients with inactive Crohn's disease have normal fertility.

Although most data suggest that inactive IBD is associated with normal fecundity, it is becoming increasingly evident that surgical intervention is associated with decreased fertility, particularly in ulcerative colitis when a total proctocolectomy with an ileal pouch anal anastomosis is created.[4,6] A recent historical case-control study of 343 Scandinavian women with ulcerative colitis found an 80% reduction in fecundity after proctocolectomy and ileal pouch-anal anastomosis (IPAA) but not before diagnosis or before surgery. This observation persisted when examined by the length of time after surgery, as well as when analyzed only for women desiring conception. A second recent study of 153 Canadian women reported a 98% reduction in fertility after IPAA.[10] No difference in fertility rates was found before or after the diagnosis of ulcerative colitis. Pelvic adhesions are believed to play a role in decreased fertility after IPAA. Women with ulcerative colitis who wish to conceive should attempt to delay surgery until after having children. When this is not possible, early referral for in vitro fertilization should be considered.[4] Alternatively, the creation of an ileostomy with a Hartman's pouch or the creation of an ileorectal anastomosis has also been demonstrated to decrease the probability of infertility.

Infertility in male patients with IBD caused by sulfasalazine has been well documented.[11,12] Within 2 months of starting therapy, the density of the patient's semen decreases, abnormal forms of spermatozoa increase, and sperm motility is reduced.[11,13,14] These events are dose related and do not respond to supplemental folate.[13] Two to 3 months after withdrawal of the sulfasalazine, semen

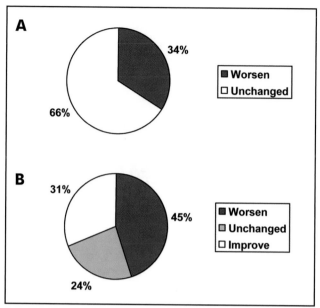

FIGURE 8-1. Effect of pregnancy on the activity of ulcerative colitis. (A) Ulcerative colitis inactive at time of conception. (B) Ulcerative colitis active at time of conception.

quality returns to normal.[15] A male patient who is trying to conceive should be switched to another oral mesalamine preparation. The overall reproductive capacity of men with IBD is not markedly diminished,[16] although male patients with Crohn's disease have been noted to have small families.[2,17]

PREGNANCY AND DISEASE ACTIVITY

Active IBD makes conception more difficult and a healthy pregnancy less certain. In pregnancy, the course of ulcerative colitis correlates with disease activity at the time of conception (Figure 8-1). A review of more than 500 pregnancies occurring in patients with inactive ulcerative colitis showed that approximately 34% relapsed during gestation, similar to the relapse rate in the nonpregnant ulcerative colitis patients.[18] Most relapses occur during the first trimester,[9,19] which may be partially related to patients stopping maintenance medications. Approximately two thirds of pregnant ulcerative colitis patients will have quiescent disease throughout the pregnancy.[18,19] Without drug therapy, active ulcerative colitis at conception is at risk of worsening during pregnancy.[20] In women with active ulcerative colitis at the time of conception, the disease activity worsens in 45%, remains unchanged in 24%, and decreases in 27%.[18] Nearly one third of the time, however, pregnancy will induce an improvement in disease activity or clinical remission, usually during the first trimester.[9] In about 5% of patients, the first presentation of ulcerative colitis

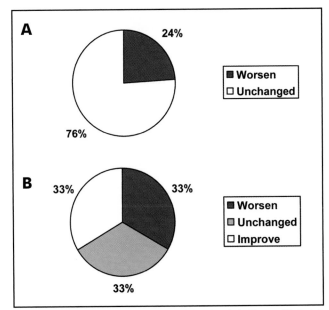

FIGURE 8-2. Effect of pregnancy on the activity of Crohn's disease. (A) Crohn's disease inactive at time of conception. (B) Crohn's disease active at time of conception.

will coincide with pregnancy. Additionally, some patients will have symptomatic disease only when pregnant, with quiescence between pregnancies and exacerbations during subsequent pregnancies.[9]

The course of Crohn's disease during pregnancy is similar to that of ulcerative colitis (Figure 8-2). Patients with quiescent disease at conception will typically remain in remission. In a study of 186 women with Crohn's disease, 27% of those with inactive disease at conception experienced a relapse.[18] Patients with active Crohn's disease during conception had an approximately 33% chance of worsened activity, continued activity, or decreased activity.[18] Khosla et al reported that 85% (44/52) of women with inactive Crohn's disease at conception remained well during the pregnancy, with almost all relapses occurring during the first trimester.[5] By contrast, active disease at conception is likely to remain active. Women who have active disease at conception remain active one third of the time and worsen one third of the time.[5] Additionally, patients with active Crohn's disease during pregnancy are at greater risk for spontaneous abortions[5,21] and preterm delivery.[22] A study by Beaulieu et al reviewed 51 pregnancies in 37 women (81% had Crohn's disease and 19% had ulcerative colitis).[23] The IBD flares mainly occurred in the first trimester (63.6%) and 1 month postpartum (13.7%) and were seen in 12.2% of patients. In the first-trimester and postpartum flares, 43% and 28.6% of patients discontinued their maintenance medications, respectively. No data exist on the optimal duration of remission before conception that will insure a good outcome for both mother and fetus; however, in general the longer the remission, the better the outcome.

The clinical course or outcome of previous pregnancies can predict neither the clinical course of IBD nor the outcome of pregnancy. The activity of IBD remains the primary predictor of the course of pregnancy. Interestingly, there has been one report suggesting that patients with distal ileal and colonic Crohn's disease who had been pregnant in the past subsequently need fewer surgical resections.[24] The authors hypothesized that pregnancy could influence the natural history of Crohn's disease by decreasing immune responsiveness or retarding fibrous stricture formation.

PREGNANCY OUTCOME

Retrospective studies have suggested no significant impact of ulcerative colitis on pregnancy outcome, including miscarriage, stillbirth, or fetal demise, when compared to non-IBD controls.[7,25] Rates of healthy offspring between 76% and 97%, spontaneous abortions of 5% to 13%, stillbirths of 1% to 3%, and congenital abnormalities of 1% to 3% do not differ significantly from those expected in the normal population.[7,25] Several large, controlled, population-based studies showed an increased risk of preterm delivery (before 37 weeks gestation) and LBW infants (less than 2500 g) in women with ulcerative colitis,[26-29] although not all population-based studies have confirmed LBW among the offspring of mothers with ulcerative colitis (Table 8-1).[28] The risk of preterm birth appears particularly increased when the first hospitalization for ulcerative colitis occurred during pregnancy.[28] Kornfeld et al evaluated the effect of IBD on birth outcomes in Sweden from 1991 to 1992.[27] The study involved 756 women with IBD and 239,000 controls. The adverse outcomes that carried higher risks for women with IBD were LBW infants, preterm births, and infants who were small for gestational age. The authors also found that the likelihood of delivery by cesarean section was higher for women with IBD than controls. These risks were overall low and not alarming to the newborn offspring of women with IBD. Kornfeld's findings were corroborated by Fonager et al[26] and Nørgård et al[28] in later studies in 1998 and 2000.

Most data support the position that Crohn's disease has a generally greater impact on fetal outcome than ulcerative colitis. Retrospective studies suggest that the rates of prematurity, fetal loss, and congenital anomalies in Crohn's disease approximate the incidence of these findings in the normal population.[25] Among IBD patients who experience stillbirths, spontaneous abortions, or children with birth defects, however, the majority of these women have Crohn's disease.[7] Recent population-based cohort studies have found children born to mothers with Crohn's disease to have LBW and be small for gestational age (see Table 8-1).[26,27,30] Patients who have ileal disease or have undergone previous surgery may be particularly at risk for these events.[31]

TABLE 8-1

OUTCOME OF PREGNANCY IN IBD: SUMMARY OF POPULATION-BASED STUDIES*

REFERENCE	YEAR	STUDY POPULATION	LBW (ODDS RATIO; 95% CI)	SGA (ODDS RATIO; 95% CI)	PRETERM BIRTH ODDS RATIO; (95% CI)	COMMENTS
Crohn's Disease						
Fonager et al[26]	1998	Denmark	2.4 (1.6-3.7)	NR	1.6 (1.1-2.3)	510 Crohn's births
Dominitz et al[30]	2002	Washington	3.6 (2.2-5.9)	2.3 (1.3-3.9)	2.3 (1.4-3.8)	155 mothers with Crohn's disease
Ludvigsson and Ludvigsson[29]	2002	Southeast Sweden	ND	NR	ND	13 mothers with Crohn's disease
Ulcerative Colitis						
Nørgård et al[28]	2000	Denmark	ND	NR	1.4 (1.1-1.9)	1531 ulcerative colitis births
Dominitz et al[30]	2002	Washington	ND	ND	ND	107 ulcerative colitis births
Ludvigsson and Ludvigsson[29]	2002	Southeast Sweden	Adjusted diff −330 g (−509 to −150 g)	NR	ND	26 ulcerative colitis births
IBD						
Kornfeld et al[27]	1997	Sweden	2.15 (1.11-4.15)	1.4 (0.97-2.02)	1.81 (1.06-3.07)	756 IBD births

*IBD indicates inflammatory bowel disease; CI, confidence interval; LBW, low birth weight; SGA, small for gestational age; ND, no difference; NR, not reported.

Reddy D, Murphy SJ, Kane SV, Present DH, Kornbluth AA. Relapses of inflammatory bowel disease during pregnancy: In-hospital management and birth outcomes. *Am J Gastroenterology.* 2008;103:1203-1209.

Understanding the cause of LBW in IBD is important, because LBW predisposes to future diseases, like diabetes.[29] The etiology of LBW infants in IBD remains unknown but may be related to the underlying disease itself, disease activity, or medication use. Unfortunately, none of the available analyses directly assesses the suspected critical impact of disease activity and medication history on fetal outcome.

Although several studies have shown no increase in congenital malformations among infants born to women with IBD,[8,9,19,32] a recent large population-based cohort study by Dominitz et al reported a 4-fold increased risk of fetal malformations in ulcerative colitis, but not Crohn's disease, as compared to the control population. In all, there

were 8 malformations in 107 exposed ulcerative colitis pregnancies, although no malformation occurred more than once and no clear pattern of malformation was evident.[30] The pregnancy outcome of greatest concern was the rate of congenital malformations of 7.9% in the ulcerative colitis group versus 1.7% in the general population. Other listed malformations, such as hip dislocation, are common, mild, and probably clinically unimportant. It is difficult to put these data into perspective for several reasons: the number of congenital malformations was small and it was difficult to identify any patterns, several of the malformations were of minor importance such as pilonidal cysts and congenital subluxation of the hip, and the medical histories of the mothers were not known (eg, nutritional status, disease activity, IBD medications, and possible effects of treatment). A second case-control population study by Nørgård et al has reported no significantly increased overall risk of congenital abnormalities in 22,000 children born to women with ulcerative colitis compared with 38,000 children born to controls.[33] The large size of this study allowed independent analysis of the risk for selected individual congenital abnormalities, and an increased risk of some selected congenital abnormalities was detected, including limb deficiencies, obstructive urinary complications, and multiple simultaneous congenital abnormalities.[33] Although both the studies by Dominitz et al[30] and Nørgård et al[33] seem to show a small increased risk of congenital abnormalities in ulcerative colitis, it remains unclear whether this risk is directly associated with the disease, its treatment, or some other bias. Certainly, the available data suggest that the risk of a woman with ulcerative colitis giving birth to a child with a congenital abnormality appears to be low. Women with ulcerative colitis who wish to have children should be encouraged to do so, ideally conceiving when their disease is quiescent and they are receiving appropriately attentive prenatal care.

A community-based study by Mahadevan et al in 2007 examined pregnancy outcomes in 461 pregnant women with a prebirth diagnosis of IBD (300 UC patients, 154 Crohn's patients, 7 indeterminate colitis) matched to 493 controls.[34] Adverse neonatal outcomes and congenital anomalies were not significantly increased in infants born to women with inflammatory bowel disease. Disease activity was not associated with any adverse outcomes; however, it is important to point out that the majority of both UC and CD patients had inactive or mild disease throughout the pregnancy.

Recently, Nørgård et al found an increased relative risk of 18.5% for preterm births in patients exposed to 6-mercaptopurine (6-MP) and azathioprine during pregnancy.[35] These findings were based on combined national data registries and national prescription databases. Most of the small number of patients on 6-MP and azathioprine were hospitalized, suggesting that disease activity rates rather than 6-MP/azathioprine were likely to be associated with adverse pregnancy outcomes. The effect of disease activity and immunomodulators or biologics on birth outcomes in pregnant IBD patients will best be assessed by a prospective pregnancy registry.

Retrospective analyses of pregnancy outcome in IBD have documented a higher rate of cesarean section for patients with Crohn's disease and ulcerative colitis versus controls (26% versus 13%, $P < 0.0001$).[9,30,36] In 2007, Cornish et al published a meta-analysis on the influence of IBD on pregnancy including at least 12 different studies.[37] The results suggest that women with IBD are more likely to experience adverse pregnancy outcomes than the general population. A greater risk of LBW babies and cesarean section birth was significant only in Crohn's disease patients; the rationale behind this increased mode of delivery was not discussed in the studies. IBD has also been associated with an increased risk for labor induction and chorioamnionitis.[22] Population studies have confirmed these findings.[27] The explanation for this finding is uncertain, though it may relate to concerns over the potential risk of perineal trauma causing postpartum complications. In a survey of Crohn's disease patients, the overall rate of developing perineal involvement after vaginal delivery, with or without episiotomy, in patients with no preexisting perineal involvement was 17.9%.[38] Others, however, have not reproduced these results.[39] Among 54 patients, 27 of 39 Crohn's disease patients without a history of perianal disease had an episiotomy at delivery. Of these, only 1 patient developed perianal disease after delivery, and this 1 patient had a third-degree laceration and an episiotomy. Ten of 15 Crohn's disease patients with inactive perianal disease had an episiotomy at delivery, and none of these patients progressed to develop recurrent perineal disease during a 2-year follow-up period.[39] Thus, women with Crohn's disease and either no perianal disease or inactive perianal disease at term do not require a cesarean section solely because of a concern about the integrity of the perineum. If an episiotomy is needed, a mediolateral episiotomy should be done to avoid trauma to the rectal sphincter.

EVALUATING INFLAMMATORY BOWEL DISEASE ACTIVITY DURING PREGNANCY

An accurate assessment of disease activity in the pregnant patient may be challenging. Many pregnant women will have intermittent abdominal discomfort related to changes in bowel habits or increased gastroesophageal reflux. In addition, abdominal pain in the pregnant IBD patient need not be due to ulcerative colitis or Crohn's disease but rather may be related to pregnancy-related disorders such as cholelithiasis, pancreatitis, toxemia, or a problem with the pregnancy itself. Despite these challenges, these acute processes can usually be distinguished from an IBD flare with a careful history, examination, and appropriate laboratory and diagnostic studies.

During pregnancy, a number of physiologically normal changes occur in routine laboratory parameters that should not be attributed to worsening IBD activity. These include a normal 1 g/dL fall in the hemoglobin due to dilution from an increased blood volume and reduced iron stores, a 2- to 3-fold increase in the erythrocyte sedimentation rate, a 1 g/dL fall in the serum albumin, and a 1.5-fold rise in the serum alkaline phosphatase.

When necessary in the evaluation of the pregnant patient with possible new-onset IBD or the IBD patient with worsening symptoms, flexible sigmoidoscopy can be safely used.[40,41] Although colonoscopy has been reported to be safe in pregnancy,[42] its use should probably be restricted to those patients where the information gained is critical to patient care. Colonoscopy is safest during the second trimester, and close fetal monitoring is indicated for the procedure.

Both ultrasound and magnetic resonance imaging can be safely used in pregnancy.[43] Clearly, it is best to avoid exposure of the fetus to radiation from abdominal x-rays, especially early in the pregnancy. The absolute risk to the fetus of abdominal radiography is minimal, however, and clinical necessity should guide the decision making.[44]

MEDICAL THERAPY

Two significant questions frame the issue of medical therapy for IBD in the pregnant patient: First, does the outcome of the pregnancy differ among pregnant IBD patients on drug therapy when compared to those not on treatment? And second, are medications used to treat the pregnant IBD patient safe and effective? Although some studies suggest an increase in the frequency of prematurity, spontaneous abortion, and fetal malformations among mothers with IBD undergoing medical treatment,[7,45] most investigations show that medical therapy, when analyzed as an independent variable, has no effect on pregnancy outcome.[5,9,21,37,46-48] As discussed previously, it is quite evident that disease activity, not medication, most strongly affects pregnancy outcome. In fact, although Baiocco and Korelitz[8] reported that their patients who received drug therapy during pregnancy had an increased complication rate compared to the general population, 50% of patients who had complications also had active disease. In addition, 50% of complications in untreated Crohn's disease patients occurred in the setting of active disease. Thus, there is at present little evidence that drug therapy increases the risk of pregnancy-related complications in the IBD patient.

The decision to stop or continue drug therapy during pregnancy needs to be carefully addressed with each individual couple prior to any decision to conceive. Most pregnant women are concerned about the risks of drugs to the fetus. Decisions surrounding continued medical therapy during pregnancy may be particularly difficult for the woman with IBD, who must balance concerns for the developing fetus against fears of increased disease activity. Counseling should stress the importance of controlling disease activity prior to an attempt at conception. Discussions with patients and their partners need to take into account the specific natural history of the individual patient's disease. Thus, patients with difficult-to-control disease may require continuation of multi-drug therapy during

pregnancy and consequently have potentially greater risk, whereas patients with stable quiescent disease may be able to discontinue maintenance therapy before or shortly after conception. An open dialogue between patient and physician facilitates the formulation of a prepregnancy management plan incorporating both the available data and the patient's wishes. Fortunately, much information exists on the safety of medical therapy for IBD during pregnancy, allowing for thorough and thoughtful counseling of the patient (Table 8-2).

5-AMINOSALICYLATES

SULFASALAZINE

Both sulfasalazine and sulfapyridine cross the placenta, with fetal serum levels equivalent to maternal levels.[49] Although sulfasalazine and sulfapyridine are excreted in breast milk, the levels are lower than in serum, and sulfasalazine is only occasionally detected in the serum of breast-fed infants whose mothers were taking the drug.[49] Because sulfa drugs can displace bilirubin bound to albumin, there has been concern that circulating fetal sulfasalazine and sulfapyridine could put newborns at risk for jaundice and kernicterus. The fetal levels of these drugs are low, however, and have minimal effect on displacing bilirubin from albumin.[49] Multiple studies have shown that there is no increased incidence of neonatal jaundice or kernicterus in the term infant associated with the use of sulfasalazine by pregnant women.[5,7,19,37,50]

Sulfasalazine has been used safely in many pregnant IBD patients. Although there are occasional case reports of congenital abnormalities associated with its use during pregnancy,[51-53] larger case series have proved sulfasalazine to be safe.[5,9,19,21,38] A recent population-based case-control study showed no increase in congenital abnormalities among Hungarian women taking sulfasalazine while pregnant, although the total number of women exposed was small.[53] Although a survey study of 1400 patients from the United Kingdom did report a statistically significant association between congenital abnormalities and sulfasalazine, the rate of congenital abnormalities was nearly identical to that in the general population.[54]

Sulfasalazine interferes with normal folate metabolism, and folate is critical to normal fetal development. Pregnant women are recommended to take 0.4 mg of supplemental folate daily; pregnant IBD patients on sulfasalazine should receive 2 mg of supplemental folate daily.[40]

MESALAMINE

Mesalamine remains a category B medication for pregnancy. 5-Aminosalicylic acid (5-ASA) and its metabolite acetyl-5-aminosalicylic acid (Ac-5-ASA) are found in both maternal and fetal plasma in women taking mesalamine, and the concentrations are comparable to those

TABLE 8-2

SAFETY OF DRUGS IN PREGNANCY

SAFE	PROBABLY SAFE	NOT SAFE
Loperamide	Azathioprine	Diphenoxylate
Sulfasalazine	6-Mercaptopurine	Methotrexate
Mesalamine	Ciprofloxacin	Thalidomide
Corticosteroids	Metronidazole	
Total parenteral nutrition	Cyclosporine	
	Infliximab	

found in women taking equivalent doses of sulfasalazine.[55] Mesalamine and its metabolites are also present at low levels in the breast milk of lactating women. Although these drugs have only been in clinical use for a little over a decade, information on their safety during pregnancy is gradually increasing.[56-58]

Diav-Citrin and colleagues conducted a prospective controlled cohort study of 165 women exposed to mesalamine during pregnancy; 146 women had first trimester exposure.[59] Pregnancy outcome was compared to a matched control group counseled for nonteratogenic medication exposure. The mean daily mesalamine dose was 2 g, with 20% of women taking between 2.4 g and 3.2 g and another 20% taking 3.2 g or more per day. No increase in major malformations or significant difference in the rates of live births, miscarriages, pregnancy termination, delivery method, or fetal distress was detected between the mesalamine-treated women compared to controls.[59] However, a statistically significant increase in preterm deliveries (13% versus 5%), a decrease in mean maternal weight gain (13 kg versus 15 kg), and a decrease in mean birth weight (3253 g versus 3461 g) occurred. Women with IBD who had active disease during pregnancy had babies with significantly LBW compared to women with inactive disease, and women who were treated with polytherapy had babies with significantly LBW and lower gestational ages compared to those women on monotherapy, suggesting a significant effect of disease activity on pregnancy outcome.

A new large epidemiological cohort study provides further evidence supporting the overall safety of 5-ASA during pregnancy.[60] Analyzing registry data over 10 years, the authors were able to identify all prescriptions for 5-ASA provided in either the 3 months prior to conception or throughout the pregnancy ($n = 148$) and a control group of women not prescribed medications during pregnancy ($n = 19,418$), including untreated pregnant women with IBD. No significant increase of congenital malformations or LBW infants was found. Although an increased risk of stillbirth and preterm birth was noted, this increased risk was restricted to women with UC. This risk remained ele-vated even when pregnant women with IBD using no medication were included as the control group. Interestingly, the odds ratio of stillbirth was highest in women using both 5-ASA and steroids, and the risk of preterm birth was highest in women treated with 5-ASA alone. Unfortunately, the authors were unable to adequately assess the precise relationship of disease activity, 5-ASA use, and birth outcome. Taken together, the smaller case series[56-58] and the larger studies[59,60] suggest that mesalamine is safe during pregnancy.

ANTIBIOTICS

For the treatment of IBD, metronidazole and ciprofloxacin are the most widely used antibiotics. Animal studies have not shown evidence of teratogenicity or increased fetal loss with metronidazole.[61] Although there have been reports of fetal malformation, particularly cleft lip, with use of metronidazole early in pregnancy,[62,63] 2 meta-analyses have found no relationship between metronidazole exposure during pregnancy and birth defects.[64,65]

In animal studies, no teratogenicity has been observed with ciprofloxacin, although arthropathy has been identified in immature animals.[66] This has led to restricted use of ciprofloxacin during pregnancy. A report of 35 women who received short-term ciprofloxacin during the first trimester for treatment of infections showed no association with fetal malformations or musculoskeletal problems,[67] however. A larger prospective controlled trial confirmed these preliminary results.[68] However, a higher rate of therapeutic abortions was observed in the quinolone-exposed women when compared to their controls (women treated with non-embryotoxic antimicrobials for similar indications).[68] The explanation for this observation remains uncertain.

Review of the non-IBD literature suggests that it is safe to use short courses of both metronidazole and ciprofloxacin during pregnancy. These agents are more commonly used for longer duration in IBD, however, and there currently exist no direct safety data on prolonged therapeutic use of these agents during pregnancy.

TABLE 8-3

FDA CLASSIFICATION OF DRUGS IN PREGNANCY*

CATEGORY A

Controlled studies in women fail to demonstrate a risk to the fetus, and the possibility of fetal harm appears remote.

CATEGORY B

Either animal reproduction studies have not demonstrated fetal risk but there are no controlled studies in pregnant women or animal reproduction studies have shown an adverse effect that was not confirmed in controlled studies in women.

CATEGORY C

Either studies in animals have revealed adverse effects on the fetus and there are no controlled studies in women or studies in women and animals are not available. Drugs should be given only if the potential benefits justify the potential risk to the fetus.

CATEGORY D

There is positive evidence of human fetal risk, but the benefits from use in pregnant women may be acceptable despite the risk.

CATEGORY X

Studies in animals or human beings have demonstrated fetal abnormalities. The risk of use of the drug in pregnant women clearly outweighs any possible benefit. The drug is contraindicated in women who are or may become pregnant.

CORTICOSTEROIDS

Corticosteroids have been used to treat a variety of illnesses during pregnancy. Case series examining corticosteroid therapy in asthma,[69] systemic lupus erythematosus,[70] and rheumatoid arthritis[71] have not revealed an increased risk of fetal malformation. Older animal studies in pregnant mice have shown an increase in cleft palate,[72] however, and similar concerns have been raised for the human fetus.[73,74] A recent case-control study reviewing data on 1184 live births with nonsyndromic oral clefts showed a relationship between first trimester exposure to corticosteroids and an increase in cleft lip among newborns (odds ratio [OR] = 6.55; 95% confidence interval [CI] + 1.44-29.76; $P = 0.015$).[73] Corticosteroids cross the placenta and are transferred into breast milk, but the ratio of maternal to fetal serum concentration depends upon the choice of corticosteroid used. Prednisolone is more efficiently metabolized compared to dexamethasone, and fetal levels are only approximately 10% of maternal levels.[75] Although there is a concern regarding possible adrenal suppression among the neonates of mothers taking corticosteroids, in practice this has rarely occurred.[74] If steroids must be used during pregnancy, it makes sense to use one more extensively metabolized by the placenta, such as prednisone or prednisolone.

Among patients with IBD, corticosteroid therapy has not been found to be harmful to the fetus.[19,50] In a study of 531 pregnant women, 168 received corticosteroids for an extended period of time, mostly during the second and third trimester.[50] No increased incidence of prematurity, spontaneous abortion, stillbirth, or developmental defects was noted. When necessary, corticosteroids can be safely used to control active disease during pregnancy. They are considered category C in pregnancy, given an association with cleft lip and cleft palate; however, the impact of the deformity they are associated with is usually more a cosmetic issue.

IMMUNOMODULATORS

AZATHIOPRINE/6-MERCAPTOPURINE

Azathioprine/6-mercaptopurine (AZA/6-MP) has been shown to be teratogenic in mice and rabbits but not in rats.[76] Given these known teratogenic effects, AZA/6-MP have been labeled as a class D medication during pregnancy. This rating means that there is positive evidence of human fetal risk but that the benefits from use in pregnant women may be acceptable despite the risk (Table 8-3). These differences among species suggest that variable metabolism may play a role in potential drug toxicity and make extrapolation of animal data to pregnant humans difficult. In addition, allelic variance for AZA/6-MP metabolism may make some people more susceptible than others to adverse drug effects.[77] AZA crosses the placenta, but the fetal liver lacks the enzyme inosinate pyrophosphorylase, which converts

AZA to its active metabolite, and, as expected, only trace amounts of its metabolites are detected in fetal serum.[78] Both AZA and 6-MP are excreted in low amounts in breast milk and rarely have immunosuppressant effects on the fetus.

The majority of the available published literature for IBD suggests that AZA/6-MP is safe and well tolerated during pregnancy. A retrospective analysis of 16 pregnancies among 14 women with IBD being treated with AZA found no increased in spontaneous abortion, fetal abnormalities, prematurity, or LBW.[76] Seven women continued AZA throughout the pregnancy, 5 stopped before week 16, and 2 had elective termination of pregnancy. One mother did contract hepatitis B infection during pregnancy. All pregnancies went to term, except for the voluntary termination and an elective cesarean section at 32 weeks gestation. No congenital anomalies or subsequent health problems occurred among 15 children. All neonates weighed 2.5 kg or greater. The authors recommended continuing AZA therapy throughout pregnancy if the drug is considered to play an important part in the control of the disease.

In contrast, small retrospective studies of the use of 6-MP during pregnancy have found an increased incidence of fetal demise[79] and an increase in fetal complications when fathers used 6-MP within 3 months of conception.[80] These studies were not carefully controlled, however, bringing into question their generalizability. The recent publication of a large retrospective analysis of the use of 6-MP during pregnancy provides much-needed additional safety information. Francella et al[81] evaluated drug treatment and pregnancy outcome among 155 IBD patients exposed to 6-MP. Compared to IBD patients not exposed to 6-MP, patients treated with 6-MP—prior to conception (40 women/44 men), at the time of conception (24 women/37 men), or throughout pregnancy (15 women)—showed no increased incidence of spontaneous abortion, major congenital abnormalities, neoplasia, or fetal infections.[81] It is important to keep in mind that most of these patients had quiescent disease. These results were further confirmed by a 2007 study by Mahadevan et al showing that "disease activity and medical treatment did not predict adverse outcomes in a large, nonreferral population."[34]

Data obtained from analysis of a Danish population database in 2003 contradict these findings, with Nørgård et al reporting increased risk of congenital malformations (OR 6.7, 95% CI 1.4-32.4), perinatal mortality (OR 20, 95% CI 2.5-161.4), and preterm birth (OR 3.8, 95% CI 0.4-33.3) in women exposed to AZA or 6-MP. Although the control group for this study included more than 19,000 pregnancies, only 11 women had exposure to AZA/6-MP, of whom only 6 had IBD.[82] The authors were unable to separate the effects of disease activity from drug effects and could not determine whether the observed associations are causal or occur through confounding. As already discussed, 2007 data from the Nørgård group showed an increased relative risk of 18.5% for preterm birth and 9.7% for congenital anomalies in patients exposed to these drugs during pregnancy.[35] This study impressively combined national data registries with a national prescription database. It is difficult to interpret these results, however, as disease activity was not measured by a review of the outpatient charts but was determined by hospitalizations.

In 2008, Jharap et al looked at the effect of thiopurine metabolites during pregnancy on mother and child.[83] This study was a prospective study of 10 IBD patients who were on azathioprine for at least 8 weeks before getting pregnant. 6-Methylmercaptopurine (6-MMP) and 6-thioguanine (6-TG) levels were drawn from the mothers before, during, and after pregnancy. These measurements were drawn in the infants from the umbilical cord directly after birth to test for intrauterine exposure. The metabolite levels varied highly during pregnancy in the mothers: 8 of 10 had decreased 6-TG levels, 3 of 8 had increased 6-MMP levels compared to prepregnancy baseline (one with elevated aspartate aminotransferase [AST]/alanine aminotransferase [ALT] that normalized after delivery), and 1 of 10 with increased 6-TG level and mild leukopenia that normalized after delivery. In the infants, the median 6-TG levels were significantly lower compared to the mothers at time of delivery. No 6-MMP was detected in the infants. There were no premature babies or congenital anomalies. The placenta appears to form a relative barrier to AZA. Where, then, are we with regard to AZA/6-MP use during pregnancy? The effects of disease activity and medication use on birth outcomes in pregnant inflammatory bowel disease patients will be best assessed by a prospective pregnancy registry. For now, given the years of experience in IBD, transplantation, and other autoimmune diseases (eg, rheumatoid arthritis), there has been no direct and clear association with immunomodulator therapy and congenital malformations. What needs to be assessed by the clinician is the risk of the medications versus the risk of uncontrolled symptomatic disease. The days of recommending voluntary termination following any fetal exposure to AZA/6-MP have passed. Because a flare of ulcerative colitis or Crohn's disease can result in significant fetal risk, patients taking AZA/6-MP should not unilaterally discontinue these medications when trying to conceive. All IBD couples considering conception should be carefully counseled regarding the limits of our knowledge regarding the safety of immunomodulator therapy during pregnancy but also reassured that most data support their safe use. Remembering that active disease represents the greatest difficulty to conception and pregnancy for the IBD patient, if AZA/6-MP is critical to maintain the health of the mother, then therapy with these drugs should be continued. For a couple who feels strongly that they do not wish to conceive while continuing AZA/6-MP, the drug should be stopped for at least 3 months before proceeding with attempts at conception. It must be emphasized to this group that should the disease flare during pregnancy, corticosteroid therapy would likely be recommended.

METHOTREXATE

Methotrexate (MTX) is increasingly used for the therapy of resistant Crohn's disease.[84] In a variety of animals, including chicks, rats, and mice, embryonic exposure to MTX has been associated with fetal loss and congenital anomalies, including neural tube and craniofacial defects.[78] In humans, high-dose MTX is an abortifacient.[85] Spontaneous abortions as high as 40% have been reported after MTX exposure, as have frequent neural tube defects, such as spina bifida.[86] Among 10 patients exposed to methotrexate during the first trimester, 30% had malformed fetuses.[87] It is not surprising, therefore, that MTX is contraindicated before conception and during pregnancy. With increasing use among IBD patients, however, inadvertent pregnancies are bound to occur. What advice should be given to a couple in this situation? Clearly, the risks of fetal loss and congenital malformation are high. Although some congenital abnormalities, such as spina bifida, can be screened for with blood tests and ultrasound, others are undetectable. Weighing against this increased risk is the fact not all infants will be adversely affected by MTX exposure. Although 5 of 10 pregnancies in women receiving low-dose MTX for rheumatoid arthritis resulted in abortion (2 elective, 3 spontaneous), the other 5 women delivered healthy, full-term infants.[88] In this difficult situation, it is probably best to carefully discuss the issue of pregnancy termination with each couple individually. It is certainly preferable, however, to avoid this situation through careful counseling and effective contraception prior to initiation of MTX therapy.

CYCLOSPORINE

Cyclosporine (CyA) is useful for the treatment of refractory ulcerative colitis unresponsive to high-dose intravenous corticosteroid therapy.[89,90] In this role, its safety is of particular interest given the occasional presentation of fulminant ulcerative colitis during pregnancy, where delaying surgery for even just a few weeks may profoundly affect fetal viability. At 10 mg/kg/day, CyA showed no fetal toxicity in rats; however, at higher doses, renal tubular damage was noted, as is seen in adult humans.[78] It is likely that this effect relates directly to the general nephrotoxicity of CyA, rather than any specific effects on the fetus. CyA crosses the placenta, but the concentration of the drug in the newborn falls rapidly within days.[78]

The National Transplant Registry was established to study outcomes in all solid-organ transplant recipients. The majority of the experience has been derived from female renal transplant recipients. Outcomes have shown no specific congenital abnormalities or birth defects associated with CyA use. There is a fairly high incidence of prematurity (56%) and LBW (49.5%), however.

In IBD, the literature is sparse and relegated to several case reports and 1 small study in *American Journal of Gastroenterology* in 2008 looking at 18 women with IBD out of which 5 patients required intravenous cyclosporine after high-dose intravenous steroids failed to achieve symptom control.[91] This study and the other case reports have shown no increase in the risk of congenital anomalies. These patients received CyA in the second or third trimesters.

In 2008, the first established case report describing the use of CyA in the first trimester was reported.[92] The case involved a young woman with ulcerative colitis who failed high-dose steroids and was given CyA at the end of her first trimester. The patient delivered a healthy baby who weighed 6 lbs 4 oz with normal Apgar scores. The baby was delivered at 37 weeks gestation via cesarean. In another case report, a pregnant patient was treated for steroid-resistant severe colitis in the 29th week. The disease flare was controlled with the addition of CyA, and a healthy baby was delivered at 36 weeks.[93] Marion and colleagues reported on 5 patients (4 ulcerative colitis and 1 Crohn's disease) with severe colitis treated initially with intravenous and then oral CyA.[94] Four of the 5 patients had live births; 1 patient whose colitis had responded to CyA had a spontaneous abortion at 8 weeks. No congenital abnormalities were observed, and no renal toxicity was noted in the neonates. Two of 4 infants were premature (<37 weeks) and weighed less than 2500 g. Two mothers needed a colectomy after delivery. These results were deemed favorable when compared to the results of surgery in the pregnant patient with severe colitis. In pregnancy, properly used and monitored CyA is probably as safe as AZA/6-MP. Use of CyA should be considered in cases of severe colitis as a means of avoiding urgent surgery and reaching a gestational age when the fetus can be safely delivered.

INFLIXIMAB

Infliximab (IFX) has dramatically improved the lives of many patients with Crohn's disease.[95] Given the peak incidence of IBD, it is not surprising that some women with Crohn's disease will inadvertently be exposed to infliximab either before conception or during pregnancy. Infliximab is currently FDA category B for pregnancy, which is surprising as it is a biologic; however, the limited studies thus far have shown relative safety in neonatal outcomes. The chimeric portion of the infliximab molecule contains human immunoglobulin (Ig)G1 constant region, which limits placental transfer during the first trimester. Maternal IgG concentrations in fetal blood increase from early in the second trimester through term, however, with most antibodies being acquired during the third trimester via placental transfer. This anti-tumor necrosis factor alpha (TNFα) agent is the medication in this class with the most safety literature thus far for pregnant IBD patients.

A single case report exists describing multiple congenital abnormalities and fetal death in a fetus exposed to infliximab; however, this mother had active luminal and fistulizing Crohn's disease and was also taking metronidazole, AZA, and 5-ASA.[96] Other case reports document the successful treatment of active Crohn's disease during pregnancy with infliximab.[97,98] A recent large study of postmarketing safety data by Katz et al suggested that inadvertent infliximab exposure either before conception or during pregnancy is safe and does not require termination of the pregnancy.[99] Among 82 pregnant Crohn's disease patients directly exposed to infliximab, live births occurred in 67%, miscarriages in 13%, and therapeutic termination in 20%, results not different from those expected for the general pregnant United States population or a population of pregnant women with CD not exposed to infliximab.[99] These findings were corroborated by data from the TREAT registry, a prospective registry of patients with Crohn's disease. The registry showed no fetal malformations, and the rates of miscarriage and neonatal complications were not statistically significant between IFX-treated and IFX-naïve patients.[99] In addition, a small number of pregnant patients with active Crohn's disease have been intentionally treated with infliximab with good outcome.[100] Interestingly, increased tumor necrosis factor has been associated with infertility, and TNFα blockade is being investigated as a potential therapy this condition.[101,102]

In 2005, Mahadevan et al performed a retrospective report on 10 women who had intentional infliximab use during pregnancy for induction or maintenance of remission in Crohn's disease.[103] All pregnancies resulted in healthy live births. Eight women had prior infliximab use and were maintained throughout pregnancy (mean of 5 weeks from last infliximab to start of pregnancy, mean dose 5 mg/kg, mean interval between doses 6.4 weeks). Two patients began infliximab in the first and third trimester, respectively.

Thus far, infliximab appears relatively safe to use during pregnancy with no obvious neonatal adverse events or congenital anomalies. What we do not yet know is the effect of infliximab on in utero and perinatal immune development of the infant.

A prospective study by Mahadevan et al in 2008 investigated 8 infants born to women with IBD (7 with CD and 1 with UC).[104] Seven of the patients were on maintenance infliximab and 1 on induction therapy. All women received infliximab in the third trimester. All infants received standard 6-month cycle of vaccines; their blood was collected up to 6 months postdelivery. Quantitative immunoglobulins A, G, and M; tetanus antibody titers; *Haemophilus influenzae* titers; and infliximab levels were drawn. The infants exposed to infliximab in utero generally mounted an appropriate response to routine childhood vaccinations. No child showed any immune deficits. Though 4 infants had decreased levels of IgM, the significance of this finding remains of unclear significance.

Two other anti-TNFα compounds are now approved for use in patients with Crohn's disease: adalimumab and etanercept. These formulations are administered subcutaneously and are in class B for pregnancy. At best in the literature, there have been case reports on adalimumab use during pregnancy in IBD patients.[105,106] In all cases, no increased incidence of congenital anomalies has been found.[105,106] A recently published abstract looking at pregnancy outcomes in women with autoimmune disease (mainly rheumatoid arthritis) exposed to adalimumab (OTIS project) found that pregnancy outcomes in the adalimumab-exposed group are comparable to disease-matched women with rheumatoid arthritis not treated with adalimumab (ADA) during pregnancy and women without rheumatoid arthritis with no exposure to ADA. Based on preliminary data from this ongoing study, there is no increased rate of congenital defects.[107]

SYMPTOMATIC THERAPY

There exists little evidence-based data on the use of antidiarrheal and antispasmodic agents during pregnancy. Bulking agents are safe during pregnancy, as kaolin is a category B medication. Codeine has been used for many years during pregnancy without report of associated fetal abnormalities but is a category C medication. Drug dependence and withdrawal in the newborn can occur but are rare.[40] A recent cohort controlled study in 108 women taking loperamide during the first trimester found no association with fetal malformation, abortion, premature delivery, or birth weight.[108] By contrast, diphenoxylate with atropine, a category C medication in pregnancy, is teratogenic in animals, and fetal malformations have been observed in infants exposed to diphenoxylate during the first trimester.[108] Both loperamide and diphenoxylate are excreted in breast milk. Bismuth subsalicylate should also not be used during pregnancy because salicylate absorption can occur. Salicylates, in general, have been associated with prolonged labor, decreased birth weight, and increased perinatal mortality.[109] Anticholinergics and antispasmodics have been associated with non-life-threatening fetal malformations and are best avoided during pregnancy.[110]

SURGICAL THERAPY

Elective nonobstetric surgery in the pregnant patient without IBD performed in the second trimester does not increase perinatal mortality.[111] In the pregnant IBD patient, however, elective surgical intervention is uncommon. When the need for surgery is obvious, as in the patient with fulminant colitis, toxic megacolon, or perforation, decision-making is relatively easy. The more typical and difficult scenario is a patient with a flare of ulcerative colitis or Crohn's disease incompletely responsive to medical therapy. In this situation, the natural tendency is to push on with medical therapy in the hope that the patient may eventually respond. Unfortunately, this approach may only further increase the risk to both mother and fetus,[112] and little information exists to help guide the physician and patient in making the difficult decision to proceed to surgery. In the ill and pregnant IBD patient not responding to medical therapy, the greater risk to the fetus is continued maternal illness rather than surgical intervention.[113] Doing what is best for the mother generally ends up being what is best for the fetus.

Numerous case reports can be found documenting successful surgical intervention for treatment of severe colitis in the pregnant patient[113,114-116]; however, it is difficult to find even small case series.[117] Anderson and colleagues reported the outcomes in 4 pregnant women whose IBD flared between the 28th and 37th weeks of gestation. Three patients were treated medically and allowed to progress to labor. Two babies were stillborn, and 1 child was normal. All 3 mothers required colectomy in the weeks after delivery. The fourth patient relapsed at 28 weeks gestation, had surgery for toxic megacolon at 31 weeks, and delivered at 34 weeks.[117] In patients with Crohn's disease, Hill and coworkers described 3 pregnant patients with intraperitoneal sepsis requiring surgery. All women recovered and delivered healthy infants.[118] As in these small case series, most isolated case reports also suggest proceeding to surgery when indicated.[112,114,115,117]

What operation to perform in the pregnant IBD patient depends on the disease and the specific indication for surgery. A variety of procedures have been performed, including panproctocolectomy, subtotal colectomy with ileostomy, hemicolectomy or segmental colectomy with primary anastomosis or ileostomy, and combined subtotal colectomy and cesarean section.[113] Two general points bear noting: First, primary anastomosis carries a greater risk of postoperative complications, and a temporary ileostomy is generally preferred. Second, if the fetus is sufficiently mature, cesarean section along with bowel resection is indicated.

Total proctocolectomy followed by IPAA is the preferred surgical procedure for ulcerative colitis. Ulcerative colitis patients who have had an IPAA and subsequently become pregnant typically do well, with little pouch dysfunction, either during the pregnancy or after delivery.[119,120] There is debate about whether women who have had IPAA should be allowed to deliver vaginally or whether cesarean section should be planned. In a study of 43 pregnancies in women who have had an IPAA, pregnancy was well tolerated, with a complication rate lower than in women who had an ileostomy.[121] Although more cesarean sections were performed in women with IPAA, the authors felt that this was likely due to uncertainty about pouch function in this

setting. An extended follow-up of women with an IPAA who delivered vaginally showed no adverse long-term effect on pouch function.[121] During pregnancy, however, women with IPAA may note increases in stool frequency, incontinence, and pad usage; these symptoms improved to baseline after delivery. Similarly, directly comparing pregnancy and delivery before and after IPAA in the same women ($n = 37$) has shown no differences in birth weight, duration of labor, pregnancy or delivery complications, vaginal delivery rates, or unplanned cesarean section.[122] Successful pregnancy and vaginal delivery do occur commonly after IPAA, despite the decrease in overall fertility. The mode of delivery in patients with an IPAA should be dictated by obstetric considerations.[121,122]

CONCLUSION

The past few years have seen significant additions to our knowledge of IBD and its relation to conception and pregnancy. Women with Crohn's disease appear to be at risk for early delivery and LBW infants, a significant finding given the association between LBW and the subsequent development of other illnesses later in life. Women with ulcerative colitis may be at increased risk for delivering children with congenital abnormalities, although this could be due to an unmeasured bias, such as disease activity or drug treatment. Despite lingering concerns, the preponderance of data supports the overall safety of the 5-ASA drugs, corticosteroids, and AZA/6-MP during pregnancy, and preliminary data suggest that inadvertent infliximab exposure may also be safe. Active disease, not drug treatment, remains the greatest risk to the pregnant mother and fetus. Despite recent advances, much of the available data remain tainted by small numbers and the inability to carefully assess the impact of disease activity on pregnancy course and fetal outcome. Until prospective, unbiased information arrives, the best advice is to recognize the limitations of our knowledge and carefully counsel each individual couple about the potential risks of IBD and its therapies during pregnancy. Although these risks are low, both potential parents and physicians are best served when such discussion takes place in advance of attempts at conception. To paraphrase an earlier author in this field,[123] the secret of the care of the pregnant IBD patient lies in caring for the patient before she becomes pregnant.

REFERENCES

1.   Trachter AB, Rogers AI, Leiblum SR. Inflammatory bowel disease in women: impact on relationship and sexual health. *Inflamm Bowel Dis.* 2002;8:413-421.

2.   Mayberry JF, Weterman IT. European survey of fertility and pregnancy in women with Crohn's disease: a case control study by European collaborative group. *Gut.* 1986;27:821-825.

3. Baird DD, Narendranathan M, Sandler RS. Increased risk of preterm birth for women with inflammatory bowel disease. *Gastroenterology.* 1990;99:987-994.

4. Ording KO, Juul S, Berndtsson I, Oresland T, Laurberg S. Ulcerative colitis: female fecundity before diagnosis, during disease, and after surgery compared with a population sample. *Gastroenterology.* 2002;122:15-19.

5. Khosla R, Willoughby CP, Jewell DP. Crohn's disease and pregnancy. *Gut.* 1984;25:52-56.

6. Hudson M, Flett G, Sinclair TS, Brunt PW, Templeton A, Mowat NA. Fertility and pregnancy in inflammatory bowel disease. *Int J Gynaecol Obstet.* 1997;58:229-237.

7. Fielding JF, Cooke WT. Pregnancy and Crohn's disease. *Br Med J.* 1970;2:76-77.

8. Baiocco PJ, Korelitz BI. The influence of inflammatory bowel disease and its treatment on pregnancy and fetal outcome. *J Clin Gastroenterol.* 1984;6:211-216.

9. Nielsen OH, Andreasson B, Bondesen S, Jarnum S. Pregnancy in ulcerative colitis. *Scand J Gastroenterol.* 1983;18:735-742.

10. Johnson P, Richard C, Ravid A, et al. Female infertility after ileal pouch-anal anastomosis for ulcerative colitis. *Dis Colon Rectum.* 2004;47:1119-1126.

11. Levi AJ, Fisher AM, Hughes L, Hendry WF. Male infertility due to sulfasalazine. *Lancet.* 1979;2:276-278.

12. Birnie GG, McLeod TI, Watkinson G. Incidence of sulfasalazine-induced male infertility. *Gut.* 1981;22:452-455.

13. O'Morain C, Smethurst P, Dore CJ, Levi AJ. Reversible male infertility due to sulfasalazine: studies in man and rat. *Gut.* 1984; 25:1078-1084.

14. Toth A. Reversible effect of salicylazosulfapyridine on semen quality. *Fertil Steril.* 1979;1:538-540.

15. Toovey S, Hudson E, Hendry WF, Levi AJ. Sulfasalazine and male infertility: reversibility and possible mechanism. *Gut.* 1981;22:445-451.

16. Narendranathan M, Sandler RS, Suchindran CM, Savitz DA. Male infertility in inflammatory bowel disease. *J Clin Gastroenterol.* 1989;11:403-406.

17. Burnell D, Mayberry J, Calcraft BJ, Morris JS, Rhodes J. Male fertility in Crohn's disease. *Postgrad Med J.* 1986;62:269-272.

18. Miller JP. Inflammatory bowel disease in pregnancy: a review. *J R Soc Med.* 1986;79:221-225.

19. Willoughby CP, Truelove SC. Ulcerative colitis and pregnancy. *Gut.* 1980;21:469-474.

20. Mogadam M, Korelitz BI, Ahmed SW, Dobbins WOD, Baiocco PJ. The course of inflammatory bowel disease during pregnancy and postpartum. *Am J Gastroenterol.* 1981;75:265-269.

21. Wolfson K, Cohen Z, McLeod RS. Crohn's disease and pregnancy. *Dis Colon Rectum.* 1990;33:869-873.

22. Bush M, Patel S, Lapinski R, Stone J. Perinatal outcomes in inflammatory bowel disease. *J Matern Fetal Med.* 2004;15:237-241.

23. Beaulieu DB, Otterson MF, Newcomer J, et al. Pregnancy complications and outcomes in the era of immunomodulator and biologic therapy: a tertiary referral center experience. *Gastroenterology.* 2005;128:A316.

24. Nwokolo CU, Tan WC, Andrews HA, Allan RN. Surgical resection in parous patients with distal ileal and colonic Crohn's disease. *Gut.* 1994;35:220-223.

25. Hanan IM, Kirsner JB. Inflammatory bowel disease in the pregnant woman. *Clin Perinatol.* 1985;12:669-682.

26. Fonager K, Sorensen HT, Olsen J, Dahlerup JF, Rasmussen SN. Pregnancy outcome for women with Crohn's disease: a follow-up study based on linkage between national registries. *Am J Gastroenterol.* 1998;93:2426-2430.

27. Kornfeld D, Cnattingius S, Ekbom A. Pregnancy outcomes in women with inflammatory bowel disease—a population-based cohort study. *Am J Obstet Gynecol.* 1997;177:942-946.

28. Nørgård B, Fonager K, Sorensen HT, Olsen J. Birth outcomes of women with ulcerative colitis: a nationwide Danish cohort study. *Am J Gastroenterol.* 2000;95:3165-3170.

29. Ludvigsson JF, Ludvigsson J. Inflammatory bowel disease in mother or father and neonatal outcome. *Acta Pediatr.* 2002;9:145-151.

30. Dominitz JA, Young JCC, Boyko EJ. Outcomes of infants born to mothers with inflammatory bowel disease: a population-based cohort study. *Am J Gastroenterol.* 2002;97:641-648.

31. Moser MA, Okun NB, Mayes DC, Bailey RJ. Crohn's disease, pregnancy, and birth weight. *Am J Gastroenterol.* 2000;95:1021-1026.

32. Nielsen OH, Andreasson B, Bondesen S, Jacobsen O, Jarnum S. Pregnancy in Crohn's disease. *Scand J Gastroenterol.* 1984;19:724-732.

33. Nørgård B, Puho E, Pedersen L, Czeizel AE, Sorensen HT. Risk of congenital abnormalities in children born to women with ulcerative colitis: a population-based, case-control study. *Am J Gastroenterology.* 2003;98:2006-2010.

34. Mahadevan U, Sandborn WJ, Li DK, Hakimian S, Kane S, Corley DA. Pregnancy outcomes in women with inflammatory bowel disease: a large community-based study from Northern California. *Gastroenterology.* 2007;133(4):1106-1112.

35. Nørgård B, Hundborg HH, Jacobsen BA, Nielsen GL, Fonager K. Disease activity in pregnant women with Crohn's disease and birth outcomes: a regional Danish cohort study. *Am J Gastroenterol.* 2007;102:1947-1954.

36. Porter RJ, Stirrat GM. The effects of inflammatory bowel disease on pregnancy: a case-controlled retrospective analysis. *Br J Obstet Gynecol.* 1986;93:1124-1131.

37. Cornish J, Tan E, Teare J, et al. A meta-analysis on the influence of inflammatory bowel disease on pregnancy. *Gut.* 2007;56:830-837.

38. Brandt LJ, Estabrook SG, Reinus JF. Results of a survey to evaluate whether vaginal delivery and episiotomy lead to perineal involvement in women with Crohn's disease. *Am J Gastroenterol.* 1995; 90:1918-1922.

39. Ilnyckyji A, Blanchard JF, Rawsthorne P, Bernstein CN. Perianal Crohn's disease and pregnancy: role of the mode of delivery. *Am J Gastroenterol.* 1999;94:3274-3278.

40. Present DH. Pregnancy and inflammatory bowel disease. In: Bayless TM, Hanauer SB, eds. *Advanced Therapy of Inflammatory Bowel Disease.* Hamilton, British Columbia: Dekker Inc; 2001:613-618.

41. Cappell MS, Sidhom O. Multicenter, multiyear study of safety and efficacy of flexible sigmoidoscopy during pregnancy in 24 females with follow-up of fetal outcome. *Dig Dis Sci.* 1995;40:472-479.

42. Cappell MS, Colon VJ, Sidhom OA. A study at 10 medical centers of the safety and efficacy of 48 flexible sigmoidoscopies and 8 colonoscopies during pregnancy with follow-up of fetal outcome and with comparison to control groups. *Dig Dis Sci.* 1996;41:2353-2361.

43. Shoenut JP, Smelka RC, Silverman R, Yaffe CS, Micflikier AB. MRI in the diagnosis of Crohn's disease in two pregnant women. *J Clin Gastroenterol.* 1993;17:244-247.

44. Brent RL. The effects of embryonic and fetal exposure to x-ray, microwave, and ultrasound: counseling the pregnant and nonpregnant patient about the risks. *Semin Oncol.* 1989;16:347-368.

45. Warrell DW, Taylor R. Outcome for the foetus of mothers receiving prednisolone during pregnancy. *Lancet.* 1968;1:117-118.

46. Schade RR, Thiel DHV, Gavaler JS. Chronic idiopathic ulcerative colitis. Pregnancy and fetal outcome. *Dig Dis Sci.* 1984;29:614-619.

47. Fedorkow DM, Persaud D, Nimrod CA. Inflammatory bowel disease: a controlled study of late pregnancy outcome. *Am J Obstet Gynecol.* 1989;160:998-1001.

48. Moskovitz DN, Bodian C, Chapman ML, et al. The effect on the fetus of medications used to treat pregnant inflammatory bowel disease patients. *Am J Gastroenterol.* 2004;99:656-661.

49. Esbjörner E, Järnerot G, Wranne L. Sulfasalazine and sulfapyridine levels in children to mothers treated with sulfasalazine during pregnancy and lactation. *Acta Paediatr Scand*. 1987;76:137-142.

50. Mogadam M, Dobbins WO, Korelitz BI, Ahmed SW. Pregnancy in inflammatory bowel disease: effect of sulfasalazine and corticosteroids on fetal outcome. *Gastroenterology*. 1981;80:72-76.

51. Newman NM, Correy JF. Possible teratogenicity of sulfasalazine. *Med J Aust*. 1983;1:528-529.

52. Hoo JJ, Hadro TA. Possible teratogenicity of sulfasalazine [letter]. *N Engl J Med*. 1988;318:1128.

53. Nørgård B, Czeizel AE, Rockenbauer M, Olsen J, Sorensen HT. Population-based case control study of the safety of sulfasalazine use during pregnancy. *Aliment Pharmacol Ther*. 2001;15:483-486.

54. Moody GA, Probert C, Jayanthi V, Mayberry JF. The effects of chronic ill health and treatment with sulfasalazine on fertility amongst men and women with inflammatory bowel disease in Leicestershire. *Int J Colorectal Dis*. 1997;12:220-224.

55. Christensen LA, Rasmussen SN, Hansen SH. Disposition of 5-aminosalicylic acid an N-acetyl-5-aminosalicylic acid in fetal and maternal body fluids during treatment with different 5-aminosalicylic acid preparations. *Acta Obstet Gynecol Scand*. 1994;74:399-402.

56. Marteau P, Crand J, Devaux CB. Mesalazine in pregnancy: fetal outcome in 76 IBD patients treated with Pentasa. *Gastroenterology*. 1995;108:A871.

57. Habal FM, Hui G, Greenberg GR. Oral 5-aminosalicylic acid for inflammatory bowel disease in pregnancy: safety and clinical course. *Gastroenterology*. 1993;105:1057-1060.

58. Bell CM, Habal FM. Safety of topical 5-aminosalicylic acid in pregnancy. *Am J Gastroenterol*. 1997;92:2201-2202.

59. Diav-Citrin O, Park YH, Veerasuntharam G, et al. The safety of mesalamine in human pregnancy: a prospective controlled cohort study. *Gastroenterology*. 1998;114:23-28.

60. Nørgård B, Fonager K, Pedersen L, Jacobsen BA, Sprensen HT. Birth outcome in women exposed to 5-aminosalicylic acid during pregnancy: a Danish cohort study. *Gut*. 2003;52:243-247.

61. Roe FJ. Toxicologic evaluation of metronidazole with particular reference to carcinogenic, mutagenic, and teratogenic potential. *Surgery*. 1983;93:158-164.

62. Czeizel AE, Rockenbauer M. A population based case-control teratologic study of oral metronidazole treatment during pregnancy. *Br J Obstet Gynaecol*. 1998;105:322-327.

63. Greenberg F. Possible metronidazole teratogenicity and clefting [letter]. *Am J Med Genet*. 1985;22:825.

64. Burtin P, Taddio A, Ariburnu O, Einarson TR, Koren G. Safety of metronidazole in pregnancy: a meta-analysis. *Am J Obstet Gynecol*. 1995;172:525-529.

65. Caro-Paton T, Carvajal A, Diego I, Martin-Arias LH, Requejo AA, Pinilla ER. Is metronidazole teratogenic? A meta-analysis. *Br J Clin Pharmacol*. 1997;44:179-183.

66. Linseman DA, Hampton LA, Branstetter DG. Quinolone-induced arthropathy in the neonatal mouse. Morphological analysis of articular lesions produced by pipemidic acid and ciprofloxacin. *Fundam Appl Toxicol*. 1995;28:59-64.

67. Berkovitch M, Pastuszak A, Garzarian M, Lewis M, Koren G. Safety of the new quinolones in pregnancy. *Obstet Gynecol*. 1994;84:535-538.

68. Loebstein R, Addis A, Ho E, et al. Pregnancy outcome following gestational exposure to fluoroquinolones: a multicenter prospective controlled study. *Antimicrob Agents Chemother*. 1998;42:1336-1339.

69. Fitzsimons R, Greenberger PA, Patterson R. Outcome of pregnancy in women requiring corticosteroids for severe asthma. *J Allergy Clin Immunol*. 1986;78:349-353.

70. Bulmash JM. Systemic lupus erythematosus and pregnancy. *Obstet Gynecol Annu*. 1978;7:153-194.

71. Bulmash JM. Rheumatoid arthritis and pregnancy. *Obstet Gynecol Annu*. 1979;8:223-276.

72. Pinsky L, DiGeorge AM. Cleft palate in the mouse: a teratogenic index of glucocorticoid potency. *Science*. 1965;147:402-403.

73. Rodriguez-Pinella E, Martinez-Frias ML. Corticosteroids during pregnancy and oral clefts: a case control study. *Teratology*. 1998;58:2-5.

74. Fraser FC, Sajoo A. Teratogenic potential of corticosteroids in humans. *Teratology*. 1995;51:45-46.

75. Beitens IZ, Bayarrd F, Ances IG, Kowarski A, Migeon CJ. The transplacental passage of prednisone and prenisolone in pregnancy near term. *J Pediatr*. 1972;81:936-945.

76. Alstead EM, Ritchie JK, Lennard-Jones JE, Farthing MJ, Clark ML. Safety of azathioprine in pregnancy in inflammatory bowel disease. *Gastroenterology*. 1990;99:443-446.

77. Sandborn WJ. A review of immune modifier therapy for inflammatory bowel disease: azathioprine, 6-mercaptopurine, cyclosporine, and methotrexate. *Am J Gastroenterology*. 1996;91:423-433.

78. Ramsey-Goldman R, Schilling E. Immunosuppressive drug use during pregnancy. *Rheum Clin NA*. 1997;23:149-167.

79. Zlatanic J, Korelitz BI, Rajapakse R, et al. Complications of pregnancy and child development after cessation of treatment with 6-mercaptopurine for inflammatory bowel disease. *J Clin Gastroenterol*. 2003;36:303-309.

80. Rajapaske RO, Korelitz BI, Zlatanic J, Baiocco PJ, Gleim GW. Outcome of pregnancies when fathers are treated with 6-mercaptopurine for inflammatory bowel disease. *Am J Gastroenterol*. 2000; 95:684-688.

81. Francella A, Dayan A, Bodian C, Rubin P, Chapman M, Present D. The safety of 6-mercaptopurine for childbearing patients with inflammatory bowel disease: a retrospective cohort study. *Gastroenterology*. 2003;124:9-17.

82. Nørgård B, Pedersen L, Fonager K, Rasmussen SN, Sorensen HT. Azathioprine, mercaptopurine and birth outcome: a population-based cohort study. *Aliment Pharmacol Ther*. 2003;17:827-834.

83. Jharap B, de Boer N, van der Woude CJ, et al. Thiopurine metabolite measurements during pregnancy in mother and child. *Gastroenterology*. 2008;134:A-69.

84. Feagan BG, Fedorak RN, Irvine EJ, et al. A comparison of methotrexate with placebo for the maintenance of remission in Crohn's disease. *N Engl J Med*. 2000;342:1627-1632.

85. Goldenberg M, Bider D, Admon D, Mashiach S, Oelsner G. Methotrexate therapy of tubal pregnancy. *Human Reprod*. 1993; 8:660-666.

86. Donnenfield AE, Pastuszak A, Noah JS, Schick B, Rose NC, Koren G. Methotrexate exposure prior to and during pregnancy. *Teratology*. 1994;49:79-81.

87. Briggs GG, Freeman RK, Yaffe SJ. *Drugs in Pregnancy and Lactation: A Reference Guide to Fetal and Neonatal Risk*. Baltimore, MD: Williams & Wilkins; 1998.

88. Kozlowski RD, Steinbrunner JV, MacKenzie AH, Clough JD, Wilke WS, Segal AM. Outcome of first-trimester exposure to low-dose methotrexate in eight patients with rheumatic disease. *Am J Med*. 1990;88:589-592.

89. Lichtiger A, Present D, Kornbluth A, et al. Cyclosporine in severe ulcerative colitis refractory to steroid therapy. *N Engl J Med*. 1994;330:1841-1845.

90. Cohen RD, Stein R, Hanauer SB. Intravenous cyclosporin in ulcerative colitis: a five year experience. *Am J Gastrorenterol*. 1999; 94:1587-1592.

91. Reddy D, Murphy SJ, Kane SV, Present DH, Kornbluth AA. Relapses of inflammatory bowel disease during pregnancy: in-hospital management and birth outcomes. *Am J Gastroenterology*. 2008;103:1203-1209.

92. Bertschinger P, Himmelmann A, Risti B, Follath F. Cyclosporine treatment of severe ulcerative colitis during pregnancy. *Am J Gastroenterol*. 1995;90:330.

93. Balzora S, Jacob V, Scherl E, Bosworth B. Cyclosporine in steroid refractory ulcerative colitis in the first trimester of pregnancy. *Am J Gastroenterol*. 2008;103:A663.

94. Marion JF, Rubin PH, Lichtiger S, Chapman M, Hanauer S, Present DH. Cyclosporine is safe for severe colitis complicating pregnancy [abstract]. *Am J Gastroenterol*. 1996;91:1975.

95. Feagan BG, Yan S, Bao W, Lichtenstein GR. The effects of infliximab maintenance therapy on health-related quality of life. *Am J Gastroenterol*. 2003;98:2232-2238.

96. Srinivasan R. Infliximab treatment and pregnancy outcome in active Crohn's disease. *Am J Gastroenterol*. 2001;96:2274-2275.

97. Burt MJ, Frizelle FA, Barbezat GO. Pregnancy and exposure to infliximab (anti-tumor necrosis factor-alpha monoclonal antibody). *J Gastroenterol Hepatol*. 2003;18:465-466.

98. James RL, Pearson LL. Successful treatment of pregnancy-triggered Crohn's disease complicated by severe recurrent life-threatening gastrointestinal bleeding [abstract]. *Am J Gastroenterol*. 2001;296:S295.

99. Katz JA, Antoni C, Keenan GF, Smith DE, Jacobs SJ, Lichtenstein GR. Outcome of pregnancy in women receiving infliximab for the treatment of Crohn's disease and rheumatoid arthritis. *Am J Gastroenterol*. 2004;99:2385-2392.

100. Mahadevan U, Kane S, Sandborn WJ, et al. Intentional infliximab use for maintenance or acute Crohn's disease (CD) flare in pregnancy. *Gastroenterology*. 2004;126:A629.

101. Sills ES, Perloe M, Tucker MJ, Kaplan CR, Palermo GD. Successful ovulation induction, conception, and normal delivery after chronic therapy with etanercept: a recombinant fusion anti-cytokine treatment for rheumatoid arthritis. *Am J Reprod Immunol*. 2001;46:366-368.

102. Wallace DJ. The use of etanercept and other tumor necrosis factor-alpha blockers in infertility: it's time to get serious. *J Rheumatol*. 2003;30(9):1897-1899.

103. Mahadevan U, Kane S, Sandborn WJ, et al. Intentional infliximab use during pregnancy for induction or maintenance of remission in Crohn's disease. *Aliment Pharmacol Ther*. 2005;21:733-738.

104. Mahadevan U, Kane SV, Church JA, et al. The effect of maternal peripartum infliximab use on neonatal immune response. *Gastroenterology*. 2008;134:A499.

105. Mishkin DS, Van Deinse W, Becker JM, Farraye FA. Successful use of adalimumab (Humira) for Crohn's disease in pregnancy. *Inflamm Bowel Dis*. 2006;12:827-828.

106. Coburn LA, Wise PE, Schwartz DA. The successful use of adalimumab to treat active Crohn's disease of an ileoanal pouch during pregnancy. *Dig Dis Sci*. 2006;51:2045-2047.

107. Johnson D, Lyons Jones K, Chambers C. Pregnancy outcomes in women exposed to adalimumab: the OTIS autoimmune diseases in pregnancy project. *Am J Gastroenterol*. 2008;103(suppl 1):958.

108. Einarson A, Mastroiacovo P, Arnon J, et al. Prospective, controlled, multicentre study of loperamide in pregnancy. *Can J Gastroenterol*. 2000;14:185-187.

109. Collins E. Maternal and fetal effects of acetaminophen and salicylates in pregnancy. *Obstet Gynecol*. 1981;58:57S.

110. Bonapace ES, Fisher RS. Constipation and diarrhea in pregnancy. *Gastroenterol Clin NA*. 1998;27:197-211.

111. Levine W, Diamond B. Surgical procedures during pregnancy. *Am J Obstet Gynecol*. 1961;81:1046-1052.

112. Kelly MJ, Hunt TM, Wicks ACB, Mayne CJ. Fulminant ulcerative colitis and parturition: A need to alter current management? *Br J Obstet Gynecol*. 1994;101:166-167.

113. Subhani JM, Hamiliton MI. Review article: the management of inflammatory bowel disease during pregnancy. *Aliment Pharmacol Ther*. 1998;12:1039-1053.

114. Bohe MG, Ekelund GR, Genell SN, et al. Surgery for fulminating colitis during pregnancy. *Dis Colon Rectum*. 1983;26:119-122.

115. Boulton R, Hamilton M, Lewis A, Walker P, Pounder R. Fulminant ulcerative colitis in pregnancy. *Am J Gastroenterol*. 1994;89:931-933.

116. Greenfield C, Craft IL, Pounder RE, Lewis AAM. Severe ulcerative colitis during successful pregnancy. *Postgrad Med J*. 1983;59:459-461.

117. Anderson JB, Turner GM, Williamson RC. Fulminant ulcerative colitis in late pregnancy and the puerperium. *J R Soc Med*. 1987;80:492-494.

118. Hill J, Clark A, Scott NA. Surgical treatment of acute manifestations of Crohn's disease during pregnancy. *J R Soc Med*. 1997;90:64-66.

119. Wax JR, Pinette MG, Cartin A, Blackstone J. Female reproductive health after ileal pouch anal anastomosis for ulcerative colitis. *Obstet Gynecol Surv*. 2003;58:270-274.

120. Ravid A, Richard CS, Spencer LM, et al. Pregnancy, delivery, and pouch function after ileal pouch-anal anastomosis for ulcerative colitis. *Dis Colon Rectum*. 2002;45:1283-1288.

121. Juhasz ES, Fozard B, Dozois RR, Ilstrup DM, Nelson H. Ileal pouch-anal anastomosis function following childbirth. An extended evaluation. *Dis Colon Rectum*. 1995;38:159-165.

122. Hahnloser D, Pemberton JH, Larson BGW, Harrington J, Farouk R, Dozois RR. Pregnancy and delivery before and after ileal pouch-anal anastomosis for inflammatory bowel disease: immediate and long-term consequences and outcomes. *Dis Colon Rectum*. 2004; 47:1127-1135.

123. Donaldson RM Jr. Management of medical problems in pregnancy—inflammatory bowel disease. *N Engl J Med*. 1985;312:1616-1619.

MEDICATION ADHERENCE IN INFLAMMATORY BOWEL DISEASE

Sunanda Kane, MD, MSPH, FACG, FACP, AGAF

Though literature on other chronic diseases such as coronary artery disease, congestive heart failure, and diabetes has tried to address the issue of medication nonadherence and its effect on disease outcomes, the impact of medication adherence on specific inflammatory bowel disease (IBD) outcomes has not been fully explored. The published literature on the efficacy of IBD maintenance medications underestimates the extent of the problem, as patients often conceal their failure to take medications as directed once outside of controlled clinical trial environments. The remainder of this chapter will discuss the state of knowledge regarding the issues surrounding nonadherence in the management of IBD, with special attention to ulcerative colitis, as the literature in this area is more substantial than that for Crohn's disease.

CURRENT DATA ON NONADHERENCE

NONADHERENCE TO MEDICATIONS

Multiple studies have demonstrated the efficacy of aminosalicylates as first-line therapy to induce and maintain remission in ulcerative colitis.[1-5] These well-designed multicenter trials have used pill count and patient inquiry to assess adherence, with rates ranging from 70% to >95%. Based upon community-based follow-up studies in other chronic illnesses, the percentage of long-term adherence tends to be much lower, about 40% to 50%.[6] This wide variance across studies can be explained by 1) a study's

definition of adherence, 2) the degree to which the investigators were proactive in adherence measures, and 3) patient population. Particularly after remission has been established, patients may not believe (or understand) the importance of continuing on maintenance therapy. Many patients openly admit they do not take their medications as prescribed; medication-taking probably makes patients more uncomfortably aware of their chronic illness status, they have a fear of long-term side effects from medications, and they question the need for medication in the setting of quiescent disease.

Patient adherence is defined as the extent to which an individual's behavior coincides with medical or health advice.[7] The term *adherence* replaces *compliance*, the latter a term that conveys a paternalistic concept of medical care and patient obedience to the physician's authority. Despite research attempting to profile nonadherent patients, there are no characteristics consistently linked to nonadherence. This is not surprising, given that patient nonadherence varies between and within individuals as well as across time, recommended behaviors, and diseases.

The issue of adherence was first introduced several decades ago, in several published studies addressing long-term sulfasalazine use in UC. Das and colleagues defined its metabolism in patients with ulcerative colitis, during both the active and quiescent phases of the disease. They subsequently studied the relationship between clinical status and serum concentrations of sulfasalazine and its metabolites.[8] Levels of total sulfapyridine (SP) were demonstrated to be different in slow versus rapid acetylators, and a serum concentration of 20 to 50 µg/mL appeared to coincide with clinical improvement in the absence of side effects. One-year follow-up on 64 outpatients revealed that of the 43 patients with quiescent disease, 32 with total SP levels above 20 μg/mL remained in remission.[9] Ten of 21 with active disease had levels below 20 μg/mL and remained symptomatic. The correlation between "therapeutic" levels and disease activity suggested that adherence was associated with an improved outcome and that following metabolite levels may be a method to monitor patient adherence.

In a second study, Van Hees and Van Tongeren measured urine levels of acetylated sulfasalazine as a marker for adherence in 51 patients 1 to 6 months after hospital discharge and in 171 outpatients over several years.[10] The authors found that nonadherence, as defined by undetectable urine levels, in the months after hospital discharge approximated 40%. In the cohort of outpatients followed on maintenance doses of sulfasalazine, 12% had undetectable urine levels at 6-month follow-up.

In a study by a group of Italian psychiatrists treating IBD patients, Nigro et al examined the effect of psychiatric disorders on adherence with medications.[11] They found a correlation between duration of disease and adherence but an inverse relationship between disease severity and the presence of significant psychiatric disorders with regular medication consumption. Their recommendation was preventive liaison interventions for these patients to improve disease outcomes.

In an attempt to understand the possible effect of adherence on disease outcome, Riley and colleagues included adherence as a potential factor leading to disease relapse in patients with quiescent UC.[12] Medication adherence was determined by pill count and direct patient inquiry. After 48 weeks, there was no difference in adherence rates between the patients who relapsed versus those who remained in remission. However, the total adherence for both groups was >95% throughout the study, making the interpretation of these findings difficult.

Farup et al, in their trial of mesalazine (European term for mesalamine) versus hydrocortisone foam enemas, incorporated the issue of tolerability, ease, and adherence into the data collection.[13] In this 4-week trial, patients were asked to mark on a 100-mm visual analog scale an assessment of their medication regimen with regard to ease of administration and practicality. Adherence, as measured by the return of unused bottles, was >80% at 2 weeks in both groups, then dropped to 73% for the foam patients but remained >90% for the mesalazine group. The authors suggested that the better outcome in the mesalazine group was in part due to convenience and simplicity and thus better adherence to that treatment regimen.

Shale and Riley, in another more recent prospective study, evaluated 98 outpatients with IBD who were prescribed maintenance delayed-release mesalazine.[14] Adherence was studied by both direct inquiry and by analysis of urine samples for the presence of 5-aminosalicylic acid (5-ASA) and N-acetyl 5-ASA. Demographic variables, disease- and treatment-related factors, quality of life, psychiatric morbidity, and aspects of the doctor–patient relationship were all assessed as possible determinants of adherence. Self-reporting revealed nonadherence (ie, taking less than 80% of the prescribed dose) in 42 patients (43%). Logistic regression revealed 3 times daily dosing (odds ratio [OR] 3.1, 95% confidence ratio [CI] 1.8-8.4), full-time employment (OR 2.7, 95% CI 1.8-8.9), and depression (Hospital Anxiety and Depression rating scale >7) (OR 10.5, 95% CI 1.8-79) were the only independent predictors of nonadherence. Urinary drug measurements revealed 12 patients with no detectable 5-ASA or N-acetyl 5-ASA. Of interest, self-reporting correctly identified 66% of patients judged to be nonadherent on the basis of urinary drug measurements, but only 2 of the 12 patients with undetectable drug levels admitted to complete nonadherence.

In a recently published prevalence survey, Kane and colleagues found the overall adherence rate with a maintenance dose of Asacol to be only 40%.[15] Adherence was measured by pharmacy refill data rather than patient inquiry or pill count. The median amount of medication dispensed per patient was 71% (range 8% to 130%) of the prescribed regimen over a 6-month period. Noncompliant patients were more likely to be male (67% versus 52%, $P < 0.05$), single (68% versus 53%, $P = 0.04$), and to have disease limited to the left side of the colon versus pancolitis (83% versus 51%, $P < 0.01$). Sixty-eight percent of patients who took >4 prescription medications were found to be noncompliant versus only 40% of those patients taking fewer medications ($P = 0.05$). Age, occupation, a family history of IBD, length of remission, or quality-of-life score was not associated with nonadherence. Logistic regression identified that a history of >4 prescriptions (OR 2.5, 95% CI 1.4-5.7) and male gender (OR 2.06, 95% CI 1.17-4.88) increased the risk of nonadherence. Two statistically significant variables that were protective against nonadherence were endoscopy within the past 24 months (OR 0.96, 95% CI 0.93-0.99), and being married (OR 0.46, 95% CI 0.39-0.57).

The advent of biologic therapy and its intravenous administration potentially eases the burden of daily oral therapies. Regular infusions to some patients seem more attractive than pills or tablets frequently throughout the day. A study examining the adherence rate for scheduled infliximab appointments in a large tertiary IBD center found the no-show rate to be only 4%.[16]

NONADHERENCE WITH NON-MEDICATION-RELATED TREATMENT AND THERAPIES

Patient adherence rates with surveillance colonoscopy are not well documented. In the only study that directly addressed this issue, Woolrich et al reported on 7 patients of their cohort of 121 who were found to have cancer.[17] In

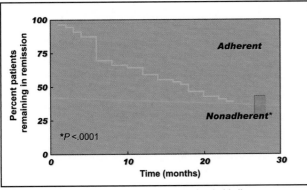

FIGURE 9-1. Nonadherence with medications is associated with disease recurrence.

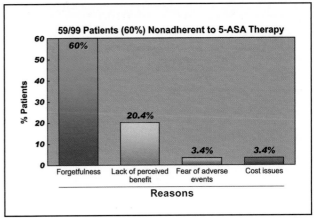

FIGURE 9-2. Reasons cited for patient nonadherence with maintenance medications. 5-ASA indicates 5-aminosalicylic acid.

2 of these patients, previous colonoscopy had found dysplasia in the setting of quiescent disease, and neither of these patients was adherent with recommendations for close follow-up colonoscopy or colectomy. It was the conclusion of the authors that quiescent disease was a risk factor for nonadherence with physician recommendations.

Long-term adherence rates with enteral feeding are dismal. In a dietary intervention trial by Levenstein et al, 24% (17/70) randomized to either a low residue or Mediterranean diet had dropped out prior to the end of the 24-month trial.[18] In another dietary intervention trial, adherence at 3 months for Ensure supplementation was only 39%.[19] In a postoperative recurrence study, patients were randomized to placebo, omega-3 fatty acid supplementation, or a low carbohydrate diet. At the end of 12 months, only 16% of patients were adherent to the diet.[20]

ADHERENCE AND OUTCOMES

What data do we have that would compel a patient to continue taking medication in the setting of well-being? A prospective 2-year follow-up on a cohort of patients with quiescent UC was done to help answer this question.[21] Patients in remission were enrolled and then stratified by adherence based on the previous 6-month pharmacy refill data. At 6 months, 12 patients (12%) had clinical recurrence of disease symptoms, all of whom were noncompliant with medication. At 12 months, 19 of 86 patients had recurrent disease, 13 (68%) of whom were noncompliant. A multiple Cox proportional hazards model revealed that patients not compliant with medication had more than 5-fold greater risk of recurrence than the compliant patients (hazard ratio 5.47, 95% [CI] 2.26-13.22, $P < 0.001$) (Figure 9-1). As part of the study, nonadherent patients were asked why they were not taking their medications.[22] The majority stated that they simply forgot one of their doses. Fewer than 10% of patients complained of side effects and cost (Figure 9-2).

The detrimental effects of tobacco smoking on Crohn's disease are well known. Cosnes et al prospectively followed 59 patients who quit smoking and were able to remain adherent to the smoking cessation program.[23] During a median follow-up of 29 months, the risk for need for steroids or immunosuppressive medications was similar to that in nonsmokers and lower than in current smokers.

There are now several studies that suggest that documented medication consumption is protective for colon cancer, which is an important concern for the long-term natural history of UC. Moody et al studied 168 patients with UC diagnosed between 1972 and 1981 and correlated sulfasalazine nonadherence with risk of colorectal cancer.[24] A patient was classified as noncompliant if there was clear evidence in the medical record of medications not taken or if upon the advice of a physician medication was discontinued. Their crude colectomy rate was 23% in 10 years, with a 3% rate in those patients on maintenance sulfasalazine and 31% in patients either noncompliant or off all medications. Because the authors found colectomy rate and cancer incidence similar to previously published series, they concluded that medications were beneficial in reducing cancer risk. In a second retrospective case-control study, Pinczowski et al found that a record of at least a 3-month history of therapy with sulfasalazine had a protective effect for colon cancer.[25] There was a 62% reduction in risk with any history of therapy in the 102 patients studied. It is difficult to interpret this finding, however, as documentation of dose and duration of therapy for each patient was not known. However, a recent meta-analysis by Velayos et al demonstrated a 50% reduction in development of either dysplasia or colorectal cancer with continued use of 5-ASAs.[26]

Eaden and colleagues found in a case-control study that mesalamine at a dose of 1.2 g/day or greater reduced colorectal cancer risk by 91% in patients with UC compared to no treatment.[27] There was also a protective effect of >2 visits to the physician per year, but the same was not

TABLE 9-1

METHODS TO ENHANCE PATIENT COMPLIANCE

- Communication regarding medication concerns
- Education about necessity of medications long-term
- Simplification of patient regimens as much as possible
- Provision of patient autonomy and self-management

found for the number of surveillance colonoscopies. More data on mesalamine come from investigators at Mount Sinai Medical Center in New York who followed patients whose colon biopsies were indeterminate for dysplasia.[28] Those patients on 2 g or more of 5-ASA per day did not progress to definite dysplasia, suggesting that any chemoprotective effect occurs early in the cancer progression pathway. Rubin and colleagues studied the University of Chicago experience with all forms of 5-ASA in ulcerative colitis patients.[29] The use of at least 1.2 g daily of a 5-ASA carried a 72% relative risk reduction for the development of colorectal cancer, when controlled for disease extent, duration, and folic acid use. In contrast, IBD patients on 5-ASA agents followed in Canada did not appear to have the same protective effect.[30]

METHODS TO OPTIMIZE ADHERENCE

Optimizing adherence is most effective when open lines of communication characterize the relationship between physician and patient (Table 9-1). Allowing the patient the time to voice his or her concerns and questions is the first step in effective education. Open-ended questions during a patient visit can be time consuming, but setting an appropriate tone so as not to overestimate the patient's level of education is paramount in establishing a good relationship. One study from the psychology literature featuring IBD patients revealed that, when asked, their greatest concern was the uncertain nature of their disease.[31] In addition, patients expressed a significant concern about the effect of medications on their disease.

It has been suggested that physicians may overestimate patient comprehension in regard to instructions and education. Martin and colleagues showed that of IBD patients polled, 62% of ulcerative colitis patients felt ill informed about their disease.[32] Though 86% of patients responding knew of the increased risk of cancer, only 44% knew that it was possible to screen for dysplasia and possible prevention of invasive cancer. Other literature also suggests that nonadherence is linked to patient noncomprehension.[33] A

recent study (yet to be published in full form) reported that in a GI outpatient clinic 15% of patients did not know how their medication worked; 22% felt dissatisfied with their medications, primarily from unexpected side effects; and 12% admitted that they do not tell their physician all the medications that they take.[34]

A new model of patient adherence has been proposed in which effective patient–physician dialog is central to promoting patient adherence.[35] This theoretical framework is in part supported by findings that higher patient–physician discordance has been associated with unfavorable health outcomes as well as with decreased patient satisfaction, a variable that is related to poorer adherence. In a study of 153 patients, the nonadherence rate for IBD medications within 2 weeks of a clinic visit was 41%.[36] Eighty-one percent of these patients were found to have "nonintentional" nonadherent behavior (ie, forgetfulness or carelessness in taking medication). Intentional nonadherence was found to be associated with patients who were considered "nondistressed" by psychosocial measurements but showed high discordance with their physician in terms of disease activity. The clinical implications of these findings suggest that the therapeutic relationship can influence adherence just as much as individual clinical and psychosocial characteristics.

Simplifying patient regimens is an effective way to increase adherence. A recent pilot feasibility trial assessed short-term outcomes in patients on once-daily mesalamine compared to a conventional (twice or 3 times daily) regimen for maintenance of ulcerative colitis.[37] Secondary aims included overall medication consumption rates and patient satisfaction. Twenty-two patients were randomized and followed for 6 months. The number of clinical relapses after 6 months was similar in the once-daily and conventional dosing groups. Though there was no statistically significant difference in 6-month adherence rates between the 2 groups, there was a numerical advantage for overall consumption with a once-daily regimen. Patients in the once-daily group were generally more satisfied with their regimen as compared to the conventional dosing patients. There is an emerging trend toward once- and twice-daily dosing.[38,39] A recent study confirms maintenance of remission with once-a-day 1.5-g granulated mesalamine.[40,41]

Patient autonomy is also a means to enhance adherence with medications. Realizing the potential difficulties for long-term adherence with sulfasalazine, Dickinson et al studied continuous versus "on demand" sulfasalazine in 28 patients with quiescent ulcerative colitis.[42] Of the 18 patients in the "on demand" group directed to take 3 g of sulfasalazine per day starting within 24 hours of symptom recurrence, 7 relapsed within the study period and 4 within the first 2 months of the trial. Three of the 10 patients randomized to the continuous group relapsed. Adherence was measured by serum sulfapyridine levels every 4 months for 1 year or until relapse and was reported as adequate

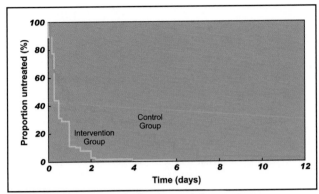

FIGURE 9-3. Self-management leads to improved disease outcomes.

for patients in either group. The authors concluded that because there was no difference in relapse rates between the 2 groups, and because by serologic testing sulfapyridine levels were therapeutic, an "on demand" regimen may be as efficacious as continuous therapy. These results were published as preliminary, and unfortunately no larger studies have been published to date that corroborate these results.

This patient-centered, self-management approach offers the opportunity to improve outcomes through patient education and empowerment. In a British study, 203 patients with UC were randomized to either routine treatment by a specialist or patient-centered self-management in the primary care setting.[43] Patient training included a written algorithm for treatment and a 15- to 30-minute training session. In the self-management group, relapses were treated significantly more rapidly than in the conventional group (14.8 versus 49.6 hours, $P < 0.01$), had fewer office visits (0.9 versus 2.9/year, $P < 0.01$), and the length of the flares that did occur was shorter (Figure 9-3).

CONCLUSION

Medication nonadherence is prevalent in chronic illnesses, and ulcerative colitis is no exception. The problem is still not well understood, because it is difficult to predict who and when nonadherence becomes a clinically important issue. As discussed previously, there are emerging data to show the long-term benefits of adherence, and the risks of nonadherence, with medications or other physician recommendations. Through physician and patient education, the clinical relevance of adherence can be emphasized, and outcomes will be improved in the long-term disease.

REFERENCES

1. An oral preparation of mesalamine as long-term maintenance therapy for ulcerative colitis: a randomized, placebo-controlled trial. The Mesalamine Study Group. *Ann Intern Med.* 1996;124:204-211.

2. Ardizzone S, Petrillo M, Molteni P, et al. Coated oral 5-aminosalicylic acid (Claversal) is equivalent to sulfasalazine for remission maintenance in ulcerative colitis. A double-blind study. *J Clin Gastroenterol.* 1995;21:287-289.

3. Fockens P, Mulder CJ, Tytgat GN, et al. Comparison of the efficacy and safety of 1.5 compared with 3.0 g oral slow-release mesalazine (Pentasa) in the maintenance treatment of ulcerative colitis. Dutch Pentasa Study Group. *Eur J Gastroenterol Hepatol.* 1995;7:1025-1030.

4. Green JR, Gibson JA, Kerr GD, et al. Maintenance of remission of ulcerative colitis: a comparison between balsalazide 3 g daily and mesalazine 1.2 g daily over 12 months. ABACUS Investigator group. *Aliment Pharmacol Ther.* 1998;12:1207-1216.

5. Miner P, Hanauer S, Robinson M, et al. Safety and efficacy of controlled-release mesalamine for maintenance of remission in ulcerative colitis. Pentasa UC Maintenance Study Group. *Dig Dis Sci.* 1995;40:296-304.

6. Miller NH. Compliance with treatment regimens in chronic asymptomatic diseases. *Am J Med.* 1997;102:43-49.

7. Haynes RB. Determinants of compliance: the disease and the mechanisms of treatment. In Haynes RB, Taynor, DW, Sackett DL, eds. *Compliance in Health Care.* Baltimore, MD: Johns Hopkins University Press; 1979:1-21.

8. Das K, Estwood MA, McManus JPA, et al. The metabolism of salicylazaosulphapyridine in ulcerative colitis. *Gut.* 1973;14:631-641.

9. Cowan GO, Das KM, Eastwood MA. Further studies of sulfasalazine metabolism in the treatment of ulcerative colitis. *Br Med J.* 1977;2:1057-1059.

10. van Hees PA, van Tongeren JH. Compliance to therapy in patients on a maintenance dose of sulfasalazine. *J Clin Gastroenterol.* 1982;4:333-336.

11. Nigro G, Angelini G, Grosso SB, et al. Psychiatric predictors of noncompliance in inflammatory bowel disease. Psychiatry and compliance. *J Clin Gastroenterol.* 2001;32:66-68.

12. Riley S, Mani V, Goddman MJ, et al. Why do patients with ulcerative colitis relapse? *Gut.* 1990;31:179-183.

13. Farup PG, Hovde O, Halvorsen FA, et al. Mesalazine suppositories versus hydrocortisone foam in patients with distal ulcerative colitis. A comparison of the efficacy and practicality of two topical treatment regimens. *Scand J Gastroenterol.* 1995;30:164-170.

14. Shale MJ, Riley SA. Studies of compliance with delayed-release mesalazine therapy in patients with inflammatory bowel disease. *Aliment Pharmacol Ther.* 2003;18:191-198.

15. Kane SV, Aikens J, Hanauer SB. Medication regimens are associated with nonadherence in quiescent ulcerative colitis. *Am J Gastroenterol.* 2002;97:S770.

16. Kane SV, Crivens L. Infliximab infusions are associated with high adherence rate. *Gastroenterol.* 2004;126:A476.

17. Woolrich AJ, DeSilva MD, Korelitz BI. Surveillance in the routine management of ulcerative colitis: the predictive value of low-grade dysplasia. *Gastroenterology.* 1992;103:431-438.

18. Levenstein L, Prantera C, Luzi C, D'Ubali A. Low residue or normal diet in Crohn's disease: a prospective controlled study in Italian patients. *Gut.* 1985;26:989-993.

19. Imes A, Pinchbeck B, Dinwoodie A, et al. Effect on Ensure, a defined formula diet, in patients with Crohn's disease. *Digestion.* 1986;35:158-169.

20. Lorenz-Mayer H, Bauer P, Nicolay C, et al. Omega-3 fatty acids and low carbohydrate diet for maintenance of remission in Crohn's disease: a randomized controlled multicenter trial. *Scand J Gastroenterol.* 1996;31:778-785.

21. Kane SV, Aikens J, Huo D, et al. Medication adherence is associated with improved outcomes in patients with quiescent ulcerative colitis. *Am J Med.* 2003;113:39-42.

22. Kane SV. Medication adherence and the physician-patient relationship. *Am J Gastroenterol.* 2002;97:1853.

23. Cosnes J, Beaugerie L, Carbonnel F, et al. Smoking cessation and the course of Crohn's disease: an intervention study. *Gastroenterology.* 2001;120:1093-1099.

24. Moody GA, Jayanthi V, Probert CS, et al. Long-term therapy with sulfasalazine protects against colorectal cancer in ulcerative colitis: a retrospective study of colorectal cancer risk and compliance with treatment in Leicestershire. *Eur J Gastroenterol Hepatol.* 1996;8:1179-1183.

25. Pinczowski D, Ekbom A, Baron J, et al. Risk factors for colorectal cancer in patients with ulcerative colitis: a case-control study. *Gastroenterology.* 1994;107:117-120.

26. Velayos FS, Terdiman JP, Walsh JM. Effect of 5-aminosalicylate use on colorectal cancer and dysplasia risk: a systematic review and metaanalysis of observational studies. *Am J Gastroenterol.* 2005;100:1345-1353.

27. Eaden J, Abrams K, Ekbom A, et al. Colorectal cancer prevention in ulcerative colitis: a case-control study. *Aliment Pharmacol Ther.* 2000;14:145-153.

28. Matula S, Croog V, Itzkowitz S, et al. Chemoprevention of colorectal neoplasia in ulcerative colitis: the effect of 6-mercaptopurine. *Clin Gastroenterol Hepatol.* 2005;3:1015-1021.

29. Rubin DT, LoSavio A, Yadron N, Huo D, Hanauer SB. Aminosalicylate therapy in the prevention of dysplasia and colorectal cancer in ulcerative colitis. *Clin Gastroenterol Hepatol.* 2006;4:1346-1350.

30. Bernstein CN, Blanchard JF, Metge C, et al. Does the use of 5-aminosalicylates in inflammatory bowel disease prevent the development of colorectal cancer? *Am J Gastroenterol.* 2003;98:2784-2788.

31. Drossman DA, Leserman K, Li Z, et al. The rating form of IBD patient concerns. A new measure of health status. *Psychosom Med.* 1991;53:701-712.

32. Martin A, Leone L, Fries W, et al. What do patients want to know about their inflammatory bowel disease. *Ital J Gastroenterol.* 1992;24:477-480.

33. Levy R, Feld AD. Increasing patient adherence to gastroenterology treatment and prevention regimens. *Am J Gastroenterol.* 1999;94:1733-1742.

34. Kane SV, Dang J. Medication taking behavior in a gastroenterology clinic: a disconnect between patient behavior and physician knowledge. *Gastroenterology.* 2004;126:A605.

35. Nobel LM. Doctor-patient communication and adherence to treatment. In: Myers LB, Midence K, eds. *Adherence to Treatment in Medical Conditions.* New York, NY: Harwood Academic Publishers; 1998:51-82.

36. Sewitch MJ, Abrahamowicz M, Barkun A, et al. Patient nonadherence to medication in inflammatory bowel disease. *Am J Gastroenterol.* 2003;98:1535-1544.

37. Kane SV, Huo D, Magnanti K. A pilot feasibility trial of once daily versus. conventional dosing of mesalamine for treatment of ulcerative colitis. *Clin Gastroenterol Hepatol.* 2003;1:170-173.

38. Rubin DT, Rosen AA, Sedghi S, et al. Twice-daily balsalazide tablets improve patient quality of life after 2 and 8 weeks of treatment: results of a phase 3, randomized, double-blind, placebo-controlled, multicenter study [abstract]. *Gastroenterology.* 2008;134(4 suppl 1): A494.

39. Bosworth BP, Pruitt RE, Gordon GL, et al. Balsalazide tablets 3.3 g twice daily improves signs and symptoms of mild to moderate ulcerative colitis [abstract]. *Gastroenterology.* 2008;134(4 suppl 1): A495.

40. Lichtenstein G, Merchant K, Shaw A, Yuan J, Bortey E, Forbes W. Once-daily 1.5-g granulated mesalamine effectively maintains remission in patients with ulcerative colitis who switch from different 5-ASA formulations [abstract 1100]. *Am J Gastroenterol.* 2008;13(suppl 1):s429-s430.

41. Kruis W, Kiudelis G, Racz I, et al. Once-daily versus three-times-daily mesalazine granules in active ulcerative colitis: A double-blind, double-dummy, randomised non-inferiority trial. *Gut.* 2009;58:233-240.

42. Dickinson RJ, King A, Wight DG, et al. Is continuous sulfasalazine necessary in the management of patients with ulcerative colitis? Results of a preliminary study. *Dis Colon Rectum.* 1985;28:929-930.

43. Robinson A, Thompson DG, Wilkin D, et al. Guided self-management and patient-directed follow-up of ulcerative colitis: A randomized trial. *Lancet.* 2001;358:976-981.

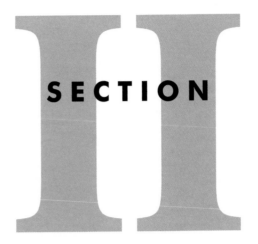

SECTION II

MEDICATIONS

MESALAMINE FOR MAINTENANCE THERAPY IN ULCERATIVE COLITIS

HOW MUCH, HOW LONG?

Miles P. Sparrow, MD, MBBS, FRACP; Wee-Chian Lim, MD, MBBS, MMed, MRCP; and Stephen B. Hanauer, MD

Crohn's disease and ulcerative colitis (UC), which together comprise the idiopathic inflammatory bowel diseases (IBDs), are chronic, relapsing, and remitting conditions that require biphasic pharmacologic therapy, first with induction agents and then with maintenance agents. Aminosalicylates or 5-aminosalicylic acid (5-ASA, mesalamine) remain the mainstay of therapy for both the induction and maintenance of remission in UC, and with these agents annual relapse rates can be reduced to 30% to 50%, as compared to 80% if no maintenance agent is added.[1]

Sulfasalazine, the prototype aminosalicylate that combines sulfapyridine (an antibiotic) with the anti-inflammatory 5-ASA, was found to be efficacious for UC in the 1940s. It was not until the 1970s that 5-ASA was recognized as the active moiety, with the sulfapyridine component acting as an inert carrier molecule that delivers the 5-ASA to the site of active mucosal inflammation in the colon only.[2] This discovery and the recognition that the "sulfa" component was responsible for most of the allergic and dose-dependent side effects of sulfasalazine led to the development of various sulfa-free mesalamine formulations that carry 5-ASA to the inflamed small bowel and colonic mucosa.

Broadly speaking, the newer 5-ASA formulations can be categorized as either sulfa-free azo-bonded prodrugs or sulfa-free coated 5-ASAs. Prodrugs (sulfasalazine, balsalazide, olsalazine) contain azo-bonds that conjugate different carrier molecules to the 5-ASA moiety, which is then released when the azo-bond is cleaved by colonic bacterial azo-reductases. In balsalazide, the inert carrier molecule is 4-aminobenzoyl-β alanine; olsalazine consists of two 5-ASA molecules joined by an azo-bond. The sulfa-free coated 5-ASA preparations include pH-dependent delayed-release (Asacol, Proctor & Gamble, Ohio) and time-dependent controlled-release (Pentasa) formulations. Delayed-release Asacol is a 5-ASA coated with Eudragit-S, an acrylic-based resin that dissolves at pH 7 or higher, beginning in the terminal ileum or cecum. Controlled-release Pentasa incorporates 5-ASA into microgranules of ethylcellulose, a semi-permeable membrane that dissolves when hydrated and releases mesalamine in a time-dependent fashion throughout the small bowel and colon. At the molecular level, aminosalicylates are known to possess a wide array of anti-inflammatory and immunomodulatory actions, but the exact mechanism of action of 5-ASAs in IBD is unknown; it is theorized that the 5-ASAs exert a topical effect on the intestinal mucosa rather than a systemic effect.[3] On the background of this brief introduction to aminosalicylate formulations and their delivery, the evidence regarding their use in UC, with emphasis on their role as maintenance agents, will now be reviewed.

MESALAMINE MAINTENANCE THERAPY OF ULCERATIVE COLITIS: HOW MUCH SHOULD BE GIVEN?

As an induction agent in mild to moderate UC, mesalamine induces remission in 40% to 74% of patients at doses of 1.5 to 4.8 g daily,[4] with a dose-response demonstrated for doses up to 3 g (olsalazine),[5] 4.8 g (Asacol),[6] and 6.75 g (balsalazide).[7] Despite this knowledge, the optimal 5-ASA dose for the treatment of active disease is yet to be

Lichtenstein GR, ed.
Crohn's Disease: The Complete Guide to Medical Management (pp 115-118).
© 2011 SLACK Incorporated

determined. Based on trials with Asacol, however, the current recommendation is for dose titration up to 4.8 g/day.[6]

Once complete remission of UC has been induced, maintenance therapy should be instituted, but again, the optimal dose of 5-ASA therapy needed to prevent relapse is unknown. Sulfasalazine maintains remission in 71% to 88% of patients when given at doses of 1 to 4 g/day, with a dose-response demonstrated up to 4 g/day. At these higher doses, adverse effects attributable to the sulfapyridine component become problematic in 30% to 40% of patients; maintenance doses of 2 g/day are more commonly employed.[8] In the only maintenance dose-ranging studies for mesalamine, there was no dose-response between 800 mg and 1.6 g daily of Asacol.[9] In another study comparing 1.5 g daily and 3 g daily Pentasa, there was a trend favoring the higher dose that nearly reached statistical significance ($P = 0.057$).[10] Neither of these trials looked at the dose-response in patients who required higher doses of mesalamine to achieve remission, however, and it is probable that a dose-response exists up to 4.8 g daily.[11]

A recent Cochrane systematic review showed that mesalamine at doses of 0.8 to 4 g daily was superior to placebo at maintaining remission in UC, with a pooled odds ratio (OR) for relapse of 0.47 (95% confidence interval [CI] 0.36-0.62) and a number needed to treat (NNT) of 6; however, a dose-dependent trend was not seen ($P = 0.489$). This same meta-analysis compared the efficacy of sulfasalazine and mesalamine formulations as maintenance agents, and the OR for maintenance of remission favored sulfasalazine over mesalamine (OR 1.20, 95% CI 1.05-1.57), unlike for induction therapy where the odds ratio favored mesalamine (OR 0.87, 95% CI 0.63-1.21).[12]

Lialda (Multimatrix [MMX] mesalamine) is a novel, once-daily high-strength (1.2 g tablet) formulation of mesalamine, utilizing MMX Multimatrix System technology designed to deliver the active drug throughout the colon. Two studies have shown MMX mesalamine, given either once or twice a day in 2.4 or 4.8 g/day doses, to be more effective than placebo.[13,14] This formulation is currently approved by the Food and Drug Administration (FDA) for treatment of active UC with a dose of 2.4 to 4.8 g daily. A granulated formulation of mesalamine called Apriso (that releases mesalamine at a Ph $\geq$ 6) and is administered once daily has recently been approved by the FDA at a dose of 1.5 g daily (in four 375-mg capsules).[15,16]

Previously, it was common to reduce the aminosalicylate dosage once remission had been attained; the current standard of care is to maintain the same dose of mesalamine for induction and maintenance therapy.[17] There is evidence to demonstrate the long-term safety of mesalamine at doses of up to 5 g daily.[18] Numerous gaps in the data remain, such as confirmation of the dose-response for maintenance therapy, and dose-ranging studies needed to clarify whether oral mesalamine can maintain corticosteroid-induced remissions.

With respect to choosing which formulation of mesalamine should be used for maintaining remission in UC, there is currently insufficient evidence to suggest that one formulation is superior to another, and a recent systematic review found no difference in the pharmacokinetic profile of the various oral 5-ASA formulations.[19] Hence, the selection of oral 5-ASA formulation or 5-ASA prodrug as a maintenance agent should be based on a combination of efficacy data, the potential for adverse effects, and practical issues such as compliance and cost.[20]

Patients with left-sided UC should be treated with topical (rectal) 5-ASA for both the induction and maintenance of remission. Given that 80% of incident cases of UC have endoscopic disease distal to the splenic flexure and 95% of incident cases are mild or moderate in severity, the majority of patients with UC could benefit from rectal 5-ASA therapy over the course of their disease. In practice, oral aminosalicylates are used more commonly in this setting due to patient preferences.[21] The delivery formulations available as topical 5-ASA therapy include suppositories, foams, and liquid enemas; the appropriate form for each patient depends on the proximal extent of mucosal disease. Suppositories reach the upper rectum, foams typically reach the proximal sigmoid, and enemas typically reach the splenic flexure. As induction agents in left-sided disease, meta-analyses have shown topical mesalamine to be superior to placebo, oral mesalamine, and topical corticosteroids, although a dose-response has not been demonstrated for doses greater than 1 g/day.[22,23] In patients not responding to either topical mesalamine or topical corticosteroid, the combination of the two is superior to using either agent alone,[24] and similarly, the combination of oral and topical mesalamine therapy is more efficacious than using either agent alone.[25]

As maintenance agents in left-sided UC, topical mesalamine in doses as low as 1 g/day have been shown to be as efficacious as oral mesalamine,[26] and efficacy can be maintained even if the dosing interval is reduced to every other day or every third day.[23] A combination of oral and topical mesalamine may prove to be the most effective way to maintain remission. In a 1-year double-blind study of 72 patients who had experienced 2 or more relapses in the previous year but were currently in remission, relapse occurred in 64% of patients taking oral therapy alone but in only 36% of patients receiving the combination of oral mesalamine 1.6 g/day and twice weekly mesalamine enemas 4 g/100 mL.[27] In patients with proctitis, suppositories of 5-ASA are effective in maintaining remission. In a double-blind study comparing 5-ASA suppositories 500 mg twice daily with placebo, cumulative 1-year relapse rates were 47% in the placebo group versus 10% in the treatment group.[28]

MESALAMINE FOR MAINTENANCE THERAPY IN UC: HOW LONG SHOULD IT BE USED?

Although aminosalicylates are effective maintenance agents in quiescent UC,[12] the duration of therapy remains controversial. It is not clear whether all patients should be treated indefinitely or whether there exists a subgroup of patients whose treatment can be discontinued. Foundational 5-ASA maintenance trials had follow-up durations of less than 2 years, and "longer-term" maintenance efficacy rates compared with placebo remain unexplored. Although a recent prospective cohort study revealed that all patients with newly diagnosed UC relapsed within 10 years despite long-term 5-ASA maintenance therapy—in particular those with extensive disease with the majority of patients doing so in the first 2 to 3 years—the oral maintenance dose of 1.6 g daily may not have been optimal.[29] Several randomized trials that have attempted to answer these questions also produced conflicting results. An early withdrawal trial did not find a difference in relapse rates at 6 months in patients who had been in remission for at least 1 year with sulfasalazine after randomization to either continuing maintenance treatment with sulfasalazine or placebo, suggesting that perhaps maintenance treatment may be discontinued in this group of patients.[30] This finding was disputed by a subsequent study that recommended indefinite maintenance therapy. Sixty-four patients with prolonged clinical, endoscopic, and histological remission while taking sulfasalazine were randomized to continue treatment or placebo in a double-blind, double-dummy trial; at 6 months, placebo-treated patients had more than 4 times the relapse rate of those receiving sulfasalazine.[31] These early studies do suffer from methodological flaws and failed to clearly define the baseline characteristics of enrolled patients (duration and extent of disease, length of remission, previous treatment received). Therefore, these studies did not allow identification of patient subgroups with higher relapse risks who would benefit from continuing therapy.

In the latest placebo-controlled trial with a longer duration of follow-up (12 months), mesalamine maintenance therapy significantly reduced the relapse rates in UC patients who had been in clinical, endoscopic, and histological remission for 1 to 2 years with aminosalicylates therapy; this was true in a subset of older patients who had been in remission for more than 2 years and had a longer duration of disease and a lower mean risk of relapse per year.[32] The statistical power of this study was compromised, however, due to insufficient recruitment and should be interpreted with caution. Until more convincing data emerge, aminosalicylates maintenance therapy should be continued on a long-term basis to prevent disease relapse.

The recent flurry of data demonstrating the potential for aminosalicylates to reduce cancer risk provides yet another compelling reason to continue long-term maintenance therapy. Although one study did not find a significant difference in 5-ASA use between colorectal cancer cases and controls, the duration of 5-ASA therapy was less than 2 years.[33] In contrast, data from retrospective case control and cohort studies support a protective effect for sulfasalazine in adherent patients[34] who had taken doses of >2 g/day[35] for at least 3 months.[36] Similarly, regular mesalamine (in patients on it for less than 1 year, and without medications in a 5- to 10-year period) conferred a protective effect, decreasing the risk of cancer by 81% at doses of >1.2 g/day.[35] These findings were corroborated in a similar study that demonstrated a 76% cancer risk reduction for patients taking >1.2 g/day of mesalamine.[37]

Finally, patient adherence is crucial to the success of long-term pharmacological maintenance therapy. Single men, multiple concomitant medications,[38] and frequent dosing[39] are associated with nonadherence and increasing the risk of relapse among patients with quiescent ulcerative colitis.[40] Patient education, self-directed management strategies,[41] and single dosing schedules[42] will help improve patient compliance and eventual outcome.

REFERENCES

1. Klotz U. The role of aminosalicylates at the beginning of the new millennium in the treatment of chronic inflammatory bowel disease. *Eur J Clin Pharmacol.* 2000;56:353-362.

2. Azad Khan AK, Piris J, Truelove SC. An experiment to determine the active therapeutic moiety of sulfasalazine. *Lancet.* 1977;2:892-895.

3. MacDermott RP. Progress in understanding the mechanisms of action of 5-aminosalicylic acid. *Am J Gastroenterol.* 2000;95:3343-3345.

4. Sutherland L, MacDonald JK. Oral 5-aminosalicylic acid for induction of remission in ulcerative colitis. *Cochrane Database Syst Rev.* 2003(3):CD000543.

5. Meyers S, Sachar DB, Present DH, et al. Olsalazine sodium in the treatment of ulcerative colitis among patients intolerant of sulfasalazine. A prospective, randomized, placebo-controlled, double-blind, dose-ranging clinical trial. *Gastroenterology.* 1987;93:1255-1262.

6. Schroeder KW, Tremaine WJ, Ilstrup DM. Coated oral 5-aminosalicylic acid therapy for mildly to moderately active ulcerative colitis. A randomized study. *N Engl J Med.* 1987;317:1625-1629.

7. Levine DS, Riff DS, Pruitt R, et al. A randomized, double blind, dose-response comparison of balsalazide (6.75 g), balsalazide (2.25 g), and mesalamine (2.4 g) in the treatment of active, mild-to-moderate ulcerative colitis. *Am J Gastroenterol.* 2002;97:1398-1407.

8. Azad Khan AK, Howes DT, Piris J, Truelove SC. Optimum dose of sulfasalazine for maintenance treatment in ulcerative colitis. *Gut.* 1980;21:232-240.

9. Hanauer SB, Sninsky CA, Robinson M, et al. An oral preparation of mesalamine as long-term maintenance therapy for ulcerative colitis. A randomized, placebo-controlled trial. The Mesalamine Study Group. *Ann Intern Med.* 1996;124:204-211.

10. Fockens P, Mulder CJ, Tytgat GN, et al. Comparison of the efficacy and safety of 1.5 compared with 3.0 g oral slow-release mesalazine (Pentasa) in the maintenance treatment of ulcerative colitis. Dutch Pentasa Study Group. *Eur J Gastroenterol Hepatol.* 1995;7:1025-1030.

11. Kornbluth A, Sachar DB. Ulcerative colitis practice guidelines in adults. American College of Gastroenterology, Practice Parameters Committee. *Am J Gastroenterol.* 1997;92:204-211.

12. Sutherland L, Roth D, Beck P, et al. Oral 5-aminosalicylic acid for maintenance of remission in ulcerative colitis. *Cochrane Database Syst Rev.* 2002;(4):CD000544.

13. Lichtenstein GR, Kamm MA, Boddu P, et al. Effect of once or twice-daily MMX mesalamine (SPD476) for the induction of remission of mild to moderately active ulcerative colitis. *Clin Gastroenterol Hepatol.* 2007;5:95-102.

14. Kamm MA, Sandborn WJ, Gassull M, et al. Once-daily, high concentration MMX mesalamine in active ulcerative colitis. *Gastroenterology.* 2007;132:66-73.

15. Lichtenstein G, Merchant K, Shaw A, Yuan J, Bortey E, Forbes W. Once-daily 1.5-g granulated mesalamine effectively maintains remission in patients with ulcerative colitis who switch from different 5-ASA formulations [abstract]. *Am J Gastroenterol.* 2008;13(suppl 1):s429-s430.

16. Kruis W, Kiudelis G, Racz I, et al. Once-daily versus three-times-daily mesalazine granules in active ulcerative colitis: a double-blind, double-dummy, randomised non-inferiority trial. *Gut.* 2008;8:233-240.

17. Hanauer SB, Present DH. The state of the art in the management of inflammatory bowel disease. *Rev Gastroenterol Disord.* 2003;3:81-92.

18. Cunliffe RN, Scott BB. Review article: monitoring for drug side-effects in inflammatory bowel disease. *Aliment Pharmacol Ther.* 2002;16:647-662.

19. Sandborn WJ, Hanauer SB. Systematic review: The pharmacokinetic profiles of oral mesalazine formulations and mesalazine pro-drugs used in the management of ulcerative colitis. *Aliment Pharmacol Ther.* 2003;17:29-42.

20. Sandborn WJ. Rational selection of oral 5-aminosalicylate formulations and prodrugs for the treatment of ulcerative colitis. *Am J Gastroenterol.* 2002;97:2939-2941.

21. Marshall JK, Irvine EJ. Putting rectal 5-aminosalicylic acid in its place: the role in distal ulcerative colitis. *Am J Gastroenterol.* 2000;95:1628-1636.

22. Marshall JK, Irvine EJ. Rectal aminosalicylate therapy for distal ulcerative colitis: a meta-analysis. *Aliment Pharmacol Ther.* 1995;9:293-300.

23. Cohen RD, Woseth DM, Thisted RA, Hanauer SB. A meta-analysis and overview of the literature on treatment options for left-sided ulcerative colitis and ulcerative proctitis. *Am J Gastroenterol.* 2000;95:1263-1276.

24. Mulder CJ, Fockens P, Meijer JW, et al. Beclamethasone dipropionate (3 mg) versus 5-aminosalicylic acid (2 g) versus the combination of both (3 mg/2 g) as retention enemas in active ulcerative proctitis. *Eur J Gastroenterol Hepatol.* 1996;8:549-553.

25. Safdi M, DeMicco M, Sninsky C, et al. A double-blind comparison of oral versus rectal mesalamine versus combination therapy in the treatment of distal ulcerative colitis. *Am J Gastroenterol.* 1997;92:1867-1871.

26. Trallori G, Messori A, Scuffi C, et al. 5-Aminosalicylic acid enemas to maintain remission in left-sided ulcerative colitis: a meta- and economic analysis. *J Clin Gastroenterol.* 1995;20:257-259.

27. d'Albasio G, Pacini F, Camarri E, et al. Combined therapy with 5-aminosalicylic acid tablets and enemas for maintaining remission in ulcerative colitis: a randomized double-blind study. *Am J Gastroenterol.* 1997;92:1143-1147.

28. d'Albasio G, Paoluzi P, Campieri M, et al. Maintenance treatment of ulcerative proctitis with mesalazine suppositories: a double-blind placebo-controlled trial. The Italian IBD Study Group. *Am J Gastroenterol.* 1998;93:799-803.

29. Bresci G, Parisi G, Bertoni M, et al. Long-term maintenance treatment in ulcerative colitis: a 10-year follow-up. *Dig Liver Dis.* 2002;34:419-423.

30. Riis P, Anthonisen P, Wulff HR, et al. The prophylactic effect of salazosulfapyridine in ulcerative colitis during long-term treatment. A double-blind trial on patients asymptomatic for one year. *Scand J Gastroenterol.* 1973;8:71-74.

31. Dissanayake AS, Truelove SC. A controlled therapeutic trial of long-term maintenance treatment of ulcerative colitis with sulfasalazine (Salazopyrin). *Gut.* 1973;14:923-926.

32. Ardizzone S, Petrillo M, Imbessi V, et al. Is maintenance therapy always necessary for patients with ulcerative colitis in remission? *Aliment Pharmacol Ther.* 1999;13:373-379.

33. Bernstein CN, Blanchard JF, Metge C, et al. Does the use of 5-aminosalicylates in inflammatory bowel disease prevent the development of colorectal cancer? *Am J Gastroenterol.* 2003;98:2784-2788.

34. Moody GA, Jayanthi V, Probert CS, et al. Long-term therapy with sulfasalazine protects against colorectal cancer in ulcerative colitis: a retrospective study of colorectal cancer risk and compliance with treatment in Leicestershire. *Eur J Gastroenterol Hepatol.* 1996;8:1179-1183.

35. Eaden J, Abrams K, Ekbom A, et al. Colorectal cancer prevention in ulcerative colitis: a case-control study. *Aliment Pharmacol Ther.* 2000;14:145-153.

36. Pinczowski D, Ekbom A, Baron J, et al. Risk factors for colorectal cancer in patients with ulcerative colitis: a case-control study. *Gastroenterology.* 1994;107:117-120.

37. Rubin D. Use of 5-ASA is associated with decreased risk of dysplasia and colon cancer in ulcerative colitis. *Gastroenterology.* 2003;124:A279.

38. Kane SV, Cohen RD, Aikens JE, et al. Prevalence of nonadherence with maintenance mesalamine in quiescent ulcerative colitis. *Am J Gastroenterol.* 2001;96:2929-2933.

39. Shale MJ, Riley SA. Studies of compliance with delayed-release mesalazine therapy in patients with inflammatory bowel disease. *Aliment Pharmacol Ther.* 2003;18:191-198.

40. Kane S, Huo D, Aikens J, et al. Medication nonadherence and the outcomes of patients with quiescent ulcerative colitis. *Am J Med.* 2003;114:39-43.

41. Robinson A, Thompson DG, Wilkin D, et al. Guided self-management and patient-directed follow-up of ulcerative colitis: a randomised trial. *Lancet.* 2001;358:976-981.

42. Kane S, Huo D, Magnanti K. A pilot feasibility study of once daily versus conventional dosing mesalamine for maintenance of ulcerative colitis. *Clin Gastroenterol Hepatol.* 2003;1:170-173.

ANTIBIOTIC USE IN THE TREATMENT OF CROHN'S DISEASE

Manuel Mendizabal, MD; Wojciech Blonski, MD, PhD; David Kotlyar, MD;
and Gary R. Lichtenstein, MD, FACP, FACG, AGAF

Antibiotics have been extensively used for treating infectious complications of patients with inflammatory bowel disease (IBD), such as sepsis, wound infections, and pelvic abscess; however, their ability to serve as primary therapy for treating patients with IBD has not been well established by clinical trials. The rationale for using antibiotics in IBD, particularly Crohn's disease, is based upon an increasing amount of evidence showing that intestinal bacteria are implicated in the pathogenesis of the disease.[1] In those patients affected by IBD, a dysregulation of the normal immune system directed against enteric flora or their biologically active products has been described.[2,3] Many transgenic and knockout mutant murine models do not develop IBD when they are raised in a sterile (germ-free) environment,[4,5] and T lymphocyte–mediated intestinal inflammation occurs after commensal bacteria is introduced in the intestines.[5] Furthermore, patients with CD consistently improved after diversion of the fecal stream, with rapid recurrence of inflammation once intestinal continuity is restored or luminal content is infused into the bypassed ileum.[6,7] Moreover, an alteration in the function and composition of the microbiota has been reported.[7-9] Many studies demonstrate decreased microbial diversity in active IBD; increased numbers of *Enterobacteriaceae*, including mucosa-adherent *Escherichia coli*; and decreased firmicutes, with selectively decreased *Clostridium* species.[8-11] Mycobacteria has also been identified as a possible etiologic agent, usually only isolated by sensitive DNA detection.[12,13] On the other hand, it is not clear whether the number of protective bifidobacteria and lactobacilli are decreased or not.[7,11,14,15] Active CD preferentially occurs in the distal ileum and colon; fluorescent in situ hybridization

studies have demonstrated dramatically increased mucosally associated bacteria.[11] Consequently, bacteria invade mucosal ulcers and fistulae; and bacterial DNA, especially *E coli*, is present within granulomas.[16-18]

Bacterial pathogens have evolved several strategies to escape phagocytic killing by macrophages, including avoidance of phagocytosis[19-21] and escape from autophagic recognition.[22] Recently, Mpofu et al[23] described mannan-induced inhibition of bacterial killing as an additional mechanism by which phagocytosed bacteria may survive and replicate within macrophages. These represent plausible mechanisms wherein bacteria and lipopolysaccharide (LPS) are translocated to the portal vein with the consequent finding of circulating antibodies against bacterial flagellar antigens.[24]

These and other studies support the hypothesis that CD may result from defective mucosal defense against the gut microbiota. The epithelial mucosal barrier extends along the gastrointestinal tract, preventing infectious pathogens from interacting with lamina propia-immune cells and acting as innate immune sensors of microbial pathogens and commensal bacteria.[25] Although still inconclusive, alterations in this barrier have been associated with IBD.[25] Further support comes from identification of NOD2/CARD15 as a gene that is mutated in a significant minority of patients.[26,27] The gene is expressed in intestinal epithelial cells (mostly Paneth cells) and mononuclear cells and encodes a protein that regulates macrophage activation in response to bacterial LPS.[28] The NOD2 mutations associated with patients with CD result in reduced macrophage activation of nuclear factor (NF)-κB in response to LPS.[29] In addition, decreased production of antibacterial defensins by Paneth cells has also been described in patients with NOD2 variants.[30] Homozygous persons for NOD2 variants may have a 20-fold or more increase in susceptibility to CD, particularly of the ileal region, and those who are heterozygous are also at an increased risk.[31-33] Less than 20% of patients with CD are homozygous for NOD2 variants, however.[31-33]

So far, the compelling evidence suggests that CD origin is multifactorial. Host genetic polymorphisms most likely interact with functional luminal flora to stimulate an aberrant immune response that led to chronic intestinal mucosa injury.[33] Other possibilities include increased exposure to normal luminal bacteria caused by altered mucosal barrier function or continuous infection with a specific pathogen.[1] All of these observations suggest that CD may be treated via manipulation of the intestinal microflora; consequently, increasing evidence supports a therapeutic role of antimicrobials in the management of CD.[34-36]

ANTIBIOTICS

Treatment with antibiotics has the potential to influence the course of CD by several mechanisms. Some of these drugs may also act as immunomodulators and thereby exert their benefit by mechanisms other than their antimicrobial effects.[37,38] The use of antimicrobials as the primary therapy in CD is poorly documented, and large controlled trials are needed to define the optimal antibiotic regimen. The most frequently used maintenance antibiotics in management of CD are metronidazole and ciprofloxacin. Based on several observations suggesting a link between CD and mycobacteria,[12] clarithromycin has been commonly used. Recently, rifaximin has been evaluated in the treatment-naïve patients with encouraging results.[39]

Metronidazole is a prodrug and a member of the nitroimidazole group. After bacterial enzymes activate the drug, its primary target is bacterial DNA, which is fragmented by the drug. It is one of the mainstay drugs for the treatment of facultative anaerobic bacteria. An unpleasant taste and disulfiram-like reaction in response to drinking alcohol may occur, as well as occasional transient darkening of the urine.[40] Peripheral neuropathy is a common side effect with extensive prolonged use, particularly among those receiving high doses of the drug, and it may be irreversible if therapy is not stopped on time.[41] Seizures and reversible neutropenia have also been reported, although these events are rare.[42,43]

Ciprofloxacin is a fluoroquinolone, the only class of antimicrobial agents in clinical use that are direct inhibitors of bacterial DNA synthesis. It possesses potent activity against aerobic Gram-negative bacilli, particularly *Enterobacteriaceae*, and less potency against Gram-positive organisms. Although it is generally well tolerated, the most frequent category of adverse effect involves the gastrointestinal tract with anorexia, nausea, vomiting, and abdominal

discomfort (which are mild when they occur).[44-46] Less commonly, mild headache and dizziness can occur.[44-46] Phototoxicity reactions also occur in some patients after exposure to type A UV light; therefore, the use of sunblock is recommended.[44-46] Tendinitis and tendon rupture have been reported uncommonly in adults given fluoroquinolones, with highest risk among elderly patients receiving glucocorticoids.[44-46]

Clarithromycin is a macrolide that inhibits bacterial protein synthesis by binding to the 50S subunit of bacterial ribosomes.[47] It presents activity against Gram-positive and Gram-negative bacteria. Side effects are uncommon, and they include nausea, diarrhea, and abdominal pain. Clarithromycin has also been associated with QT interval prolongation.[48]

Promising results in the treatment of IBD have also been recently shown with rifaximin.[39] It has excellent coverage against most Gram-negatives, Gram-positives (including aerobes and anaerobes), and *Mycobacterium* isolates by inhibiting bacterial RNA synthesis.[49] Less than 0.4% of the drug is absorbed; thus, the majority of the drug when ingested is excreted unchanged in feces. It has very good tolerability and an excellent safety profile; infrequently, it presents side effects including headache, abdominal cramps, flatulence, and urticarial rash.[49]

ACTIVE LUMINAL CROHN'S DISEASE

Clinical experience with antibiotics in the treatment of CD has far outpaced published scientific evidence. Most studies were small, short-term, used different inclusion criteria, and focused on different endpoints, thus limiting direct comparisons between studies (Table 11-1). Therefore, the published literature has not clearly established a role for antibiotics in the treatment for primary or adjunctive therapy of active mild to moderate CD. Metronidazole alone or in combination with ciprofloxacin suggested a modest benefit for colonic CD but not for isolated small intestine disease. Other antibiotics, such as clarithromycin and rifaximin, alone or in combination regimens, appear to be effective, although there is somewhat less experience. Strategies to reduce side effects should be applied and, because of antibiotics' potential to alter the composition of luminal microflora, particular attention should be taken to the emergence of resistant strains.

METRONIDAZOLE AND CIPROFLOXACIN

Ursing and Kamme[50] first reported the use of metronidazole in CD in 1975. They described 5 patients with CD who were treated with metronidazole 400 to 600 mg/day for 1 to 7 months. In 3 patients, metronidazole was discontinued after 4 to 6 months of treatment, and 2 had no signs or symptoms of relapse after 3 and 6 months.[50] In 1978, Blichfeldt et al,[51] in a placebo-controlled, double-blind, crossover trial, gave placebo or metronidazole 250 mg qid to 22 patients with active CD for 2 months. After 1 to 4 weeks of rest, they were crossed over to the other drug for an additional 2 months. There was no significant improvement in the metronidazole group, but a positive trend in favor of metronidazole was observed in the 6 patients with colonic involvement.[51]

In the National Cooperative Swedish study,[52] metronidazole (400 mg twice daily) was compared to sulfasalazine (1.5 g twice daily) for the treatment of active CD using a double-blind, crossover design. A total of 78 patients were randomly assigned and followed up for two 4-month periods. Both treatments were comparable in the first treatment period, metronidazole being slightly more efficacious.[52] Patients who initially were treated with sulfasalazine and then switched over to metronidazole showed a significant improvement in the CD activity index (CDAI), whereas initial treatment with metronidazole followed by sulfasalazine gave no changes.[52] In addition, a subgroup analysis suggested that treatment was more effective in patients with colitis or ileocolitis compared with patients with only ileitis. It was concluded that metronidazole was slightly more effective than sulfasalazine in the treatment of CD.[52]

Sutherland et al[53] performed a double-blind, placebo-controlled study to compare the efficacy of 2 doses of metronidazole (10 mg/kg/day and 20 mg/kg/day) versus placebo. Only 56 of the 105 patients completed the 16 weeks of treatment.[53] Results indicated significant improvement, as measured by both CDAI and serum orosomucoid, in the metronidazole groups as compared with placebo.[53] No difference was found in the rates of remission in patients receiving metronidazole, however.[53] Patients receiving higher doses of metronidazole did not experience significant differences when compared to those treated with lower doses.[53] Preliminary analysis suggested that metronidazole was more effective in patients with disease confined to the large intestine or affecting both small and large bowel than in those with small bowel disease only.[53]

Several studies evaluated the use of ciprofloxacin alone or in combination with other drugs to treat active CD (Table 11-1). Arnold et al[54] assessed the efficacy of ciprofloxacin 1 g/day as adjunctive therapy in patients with moderately active but resistant cases of CD. Forty-seven patients with moderately active CD were randomly assigned treatment with ciprofloxacin versus placebo for 6 months in addition to their conventional therapy.[54] Patients treated with antibiotics had a statistically significant decrease in CDAI from 187 to 112, and in the placebo group CDAI dropped from 230 to 205.[54] Of note, only 37 patients completed the trial, and there were twice as many patients in the treatment group as compared with the placebo.[54] The authors concluded that ciprofloxacin may be an effective agent when added to the treatment of moderately active, resistant CD.[54]

Colombel et al[55] carried out a randomized controlled study involving 40 patients with a mild to moderate flare of CD and investigated the efficacy of ciprofloxacin (1 g/day) versus mesalamine (4 g/day). The treatment trial was 6 weeks with endpoints based on improvement in the CDAI.[55] The study, however, was underpowered. Complete remission was achieved in 10 patients (56%) treated with ciprofloxacin and in 12 patients (55%) treated with mesalazine; partial remission was observed in 3 and 1 patients, respectively.[55] They concluded that ciprofloxacin 1 g/day is as effective as mesalazine 4 g/day in treating mild to moderate flares of CD.[55]

Some studies evaluated the efficacy of combined antibiotic treatment with ciprofloxacin and metronidazole against active CD. Greenbloom et al[56] performed an open study that examined the efficacy and safety of combination ciprofloxacin and metronidazole for patients with active CD of the ileum and/or colon. Seventy-two patients were treated with ciprofloxacin 1 g/day and metronidazole 750 mg/day for a mean of 10 weeks.[56] Clinical remission, defined as a Harvey-Bradshaw index of 3 points or less, was observed in 49 patients (68%); 55 patients (76%) showed a clinical response.[56] A clinical remission was noted in 29 of 43 patients (67%) who were not taking concurrent prednisone treatment and in 26 of 29 patients (90%) receiving prednisone (mean dose of 15 mg/day).[56] A clinical response also occurred in a greater proportion of patients with colonic disease (84%) compared with patients with isolated ileal disease (64%).[56] Therapy was generally well tolerated. After a mean follow-up of 9 months, clinical remission was maintained in 26 patients off treatment and in 12 patients who continued antibiotic therapy.[56] The authors concluded that ciprofloxacin in combination with metronidazole appears to play a beneficial role in achieving clinical remission for patients with active CD, particularly when there is colonic involvement.[56]

Prantera et al[57] performed a prospective, randomized controlled study in which metronidazole (250 mg 4 times daily) plus ciprofloxacin (500 mg twice daily) was compared to methylprednisolone (0.7 to 1 mg/kg/day followed by tapering 4 mg weekly) for 3 months in 41 patients with active CD. There were no significant differences in responses between the 2 groups, with a 63% remission rate (12 out of 19 patients) in the methylprednisolone group and 45.5% remission rate (10 out of 22 patients) in the antibiotic-treated group.[57] Treatment failure was reported in 22.7% of the patients on the antibiotic-treated group and in 26.3% of the patients on steroids.[57] The authors concluded that metronidazole and ciprofloxacin could be an alternative to steroids in treating the acute phase of CD.[57]

The same Italian group reviewed the records of 233 patients with active CD treated with metronidazole (1 g/day) and/or ciprofloxacin (1 g/day).[58] Achievement of a complete or partial remission was 70.6%, 72.8%, and 69% with combination therapy, metronidazole, and ciprofloxacin, respectively.[58] Discontinuation of therapy due to side

TABLE 11-1

ANTIBIOTICS IN CROHN'S DISEASE: REPRESENTATIVE STUDIES*

Author	Year	Patients	Study Design	Antibiotic Scheme	Length	Outcome
Ursing and Kamme[50]	1975	5	Case study	Metronidazole 400 to 600 mg/day	1 to 7 months	Clinical response in 2 patients
Blichfeldt et al[51]	1978	22	Double-blind crossover study	Metronidazole 250 mg qid	8 weeks	Symptomatic improvement in 6 patients with colonic involvement
Ursing et al[52]	1982	78	Double-blind crossover study	Metronidazole 400 mg bid	16 weeks	Slightly more effective than sulfasalazine
Sutherland et al[53]	1991	105	Double-blind RCT	Metronidazole 10 or 20 mg/kg/day	16 weeks	Reduction CDAI in patients with colonic disease\nNo difference in remission rates
Prantera et al[57]	1996	41	Double-blind RCT	Ciprofloxacin 500 mg bid and Metronidazole 250 mg qid	12 weeks	Equally effective as methylprednisolone
Greenbloom et al[56]	1998	72	Uncontrolled study	Ciprofloxacin 500 mg bid and Metronidazole 250 mg tid	10 weeks	Clinical remission in 68% of patients\nMore likely in colonic involvement
Prantera et al[58]	1998	233	Retrospective study	Ciprofloxacin 1 g/day and/or Metronidazole 1 g/day		No benefit of combination therapy over either antibiotic alone
Colombel et al[55]	1999	40	Double-blind RCT	Ciprofloxacin 1 g/day	6 weeks	Equally effective as mesalamine
Arnold et al[54]	2002	47	Non-blind RCT	Ciprofloxacin 500 mg bid	6 months	Superior to placebo reducing CDAI
Steinhart et al[59]	2002	134	Double-blind RCT	Ciprofloxacin 500 mg bid and Metronidazole 250 mg tid	8 weeks	Antibiotic combination may be beneficial in colonic disease
Leiper et al[63]	2000	25	Open-label	Clarithromycin 250 mg bid	4 weeks	48% remission rate, 64% response
Inoue et al[62]	2007	14	Open-label	Clarithromycin 200 mg bid	4 weeks	36% remission rate, 57% response
Leiper et al[63]	2008	41	Double-blind RCT	Clarithromycin 1 g/day	12 weeks	Ineffective, some benefit at 1 month
Shafran et al[66]	2005	29	Open-label	Rifaximin 200 mg tid	16 weeks	59% remission rate, 78% response
Prantera et al[67]	2006	83	Double-blind RCT	Rifaximin 800 mg/day or 800 mg bid	12 weeks	High-dose rifaximin is superior to placebo in inducing clinical remission
Shafran et al[39]	2008	5	Open-label	Rifaximin 400 mg bid	16 weeks	3 patients had endoscopic and clinical improvement

*Bid indicates 2 times a day; tid, 3 times a day; qid, 4 times a day; RCT, randomized controlled trial; CDAI, Crohn's Disease Activity Index.

effects was reported in about 20% of the patients.[58] They concluded that metronidazole and ciprofloxacin seem to be useful in treating active phases of Crohn's disease, supporting the important role of fecal flora in causing CD symptoms.[58]

Steinhart el al[59] conducted a multicenter, placebo-controlled trial including 134 patients with ileal CD, with or without colonic involvement. Patients were randomly assigned to metronidazole and ciprofloxacin (both at 1 g/day) or placebo for 8 weeks.[59] All patients received budesonide (9 mg/day).[59] At the end of treatment, 33% (21 of 64 patients) in the antibiotic-treated group and 38% (25 of 66 patients) in the placebo group achieved remission ($P = 0.55$).[59] Discontinuation of therapy because of adverse events occurred in 20% of patients treated with antibiotics, compared with 0% in the group who received placebo ($P < 0.001$).[59] Again, there was a significant difference when results by site of disease were analyzed. Patients with colonic involvement treated with antibiotics presented a 53% (9 of 17) remission rate compared with only 25% (4 of 16) of the patients who received placebo.[59] The authors concluded that in patients with ileal active CD, the addition of ciprofloxacin and metronidazole to budesonide was ineffective, but this antibiotic combination may be beneficial when there is involvement of the colon.[59]

CLARITHROMYCIN

Clarithromycin is a macrolide antibiotic that accumulates in extremely high levels within macrophages, enhancing their efficacy against intracellular organisms. Also, immunomodulatory properties have been described, such as macrophage proliferation, phagocytosis, and cytocidal activity.[60] Clarithromycin suppresses NF-κB and reduces the production of proinflammatory cytokines (IL-1, IL-6, IL-8, and tumor necrosis factor alpha [TNFα]).[60,61] Different studies assessed its therapeutic efficacy for the treatment of patients with active CD.[62-64] Leiper et al[64] performed an open-label study that included 25 patients with active CD treated with clarithromycin 500 mg/day for 4 weeks; treatment was then continued to up to 12 weeks in those who responded. All patients receiving corticosteroids or azathioprine had been on unchanged treatment for at least 12 weeks. Remission was achieved in 12 patients (48%), and 16 patients (64%) presented with clinical response.[64] Treatment was continued in 11 patients for a median of 28 weeks, during which 8 patients (73%) remained in clinical remission.[64] The authors suggested that patients with active CD who are resistant to other therapy may benefit by adding clarithromycin.[64] Subsequently, the same group of investigators performed a placebo-controlled trial in which patients were randomly assigned to clarithromycin (1 g/day) or placebo.[63] After 41 patients were recruited, the trial was stopped because no benefit was shown at 3 months; however, a post hoc analysis observed a possible benefit in the clarithromycin group at 1 month.[63]

A Japanese uncontrolled study trial evaluated the effect of clarithromycin therapy (200 mg twice daily) in 14 patients for 4 weeks.[62] Treatment was continued up to 24 weeks in those who showed clinical response.[62] After 4 weeks, 57.1% of the patients showed clinical improvement, and 36% of the patients achieved remission.[62] Eight patients continued clarithromycin therapy after 4 weeks, and 4 (28.6%) remained in remission after 24 weeks.[62] No severe side effects were observed during the study period.[62] The authors suggested that Japanese patients with active CD may benefit from clarithromycin therapy.[62] In summary, open-label studies assessing clarithromycin monotherapy for treating active CD have shown positive results[62,64]; however, the only randomized clinical trial performed so far was not able to reproduce those findings.[63] Further controlled trials are needed to assess the effect of clarithromycin, combined or alone, in the treatment active CD.

RIFAXIMIN

Rifaximin is approved by the FDA for the treatment of traveler's diarrhea.[65] It has been suggested by some to consider the use of rifaximin for the treatment of patients with active CD subsequent to its antimicrobial activity against *Bacteroides* and *E coli*, 2 bacteria frequently found in the intestinal mucosa of CD patients.[11] It has been suggested in 2 open-label studies that rifaximin may be an effective and well-tolerated treatment of CD.[39,66] Shafran and Johnson[66] conducted an open-label study assessing rifaximin (200 mg 3 times a day) in 29 patients with active CD for 16 weeks duration. Clinical improvement and remission, assessed by the CDAI, was reported in 59% and 41% of the patients at 1 month, and at 4 months it was 78% and 59%, respectively.[66] The same group recently reported another open-label study, where 5 patients newly diagnosed with mild CD were treated with rifaximin 800 mg/day as the first-line therapy for a minimum of 3 months.[39] Three patients presented a substantial clinical and endoscopic improvement, and no side effects were reported.[39] The authors suggested that rifaximin may be useful for active CD.[39]

Prantera et al[67] conducted a controlled trial including 83 patients with mild-to-moderate CD who were randomly assigned to rifaximin 1600 mg/day, rifaximin 800 mg/day, and placebo. Clinical response was achieved in 67% (18 of 29) of the high-dose rifaximin group, 48% (12 of 25) of the low-dose rifaximin group, and 41% (11 of 27) of the placebo group (P = ns).[67] However, treatment failure was significantly less likely in the high- and low-dose rifaximin treated group when compared to placebo, 4%, 12%, and 33%, respectively.[67] They concluded that rifaximin 1600 mg/day was superior to placebo in inducing clinical remission of active Crohn's disease, and the number of the failures in the placebo group was significantly higher than those who received rifaximin 1600 mg/day.[67] At this point, it seems probable that rifaximin will benefit patients with active CD; however, there is not yet prospective randomized, placebo-controlled data from large clinical trials that have proven its efficacy in patients with active CD. Further randomized, placebo-controlled trials are warranted to investigate the role and the dose of rifaximin in the management and treatment of CD.

TABLE 11-2

ANTIMYCOBACTERIAL IN CROHN'S DISEASE: REPRESENTATIVE STUDIES*

Author	Year	Patients	Study Design	Antibiotic Scheme	Length	Outcome
Shafran et al[76]	2002	36	Open-label	Clarithromycin 250 mg bid and Rifabutin 150 mg bid	4 to 17 months	58% response rate in patients with MAP infection
Goodgame et al[83]	2001	31	Double-blind RCT	Clarithromycin 500 mg bid and ethambutol 15 mg/day	12 weeks	No benefit
Borody et al[84]	2002	52	Open-label	Clarithromycin 1 g/day, rifabutin 600 mg/day, and clofazimine 100 mg/day	6 months to 9 years	56% endoscopic and 39% histological improvement
Selby et al[85]	2007	213	Double-blind RCT	Clarithromycin 750 mg/day, rifabutin 450 mg/day, and clofazimine 50 mg/day	16 weeks	No long-term benefit

*Bid indicates 2 times a day; MAP, *Mycobacterium avium paratuberculosis*; RCI, randomized controlled trial.

ANTIMYCOBACTERIAL THERAPY IN CROHN'S DISEASE

It was Sir T. Kennedy Dalziel in the early 1900s who first described pathologic similarities between CD and tuberculous gastroenteritis,[68] but it was not until 1984 when *M. avium* subspecies *paratuberculosis* (MAP) was cultured from resected CD tissues.[69] It was then isolated from the bloodstream of CD patients[70] and its specific DNA insertion sequence IS900 was recovered in a significant number of patients with CD but not in controls.[71] Interestingly, MAP causes Johne's disease, an infectious enteritis in animals that resembles CD clinically and histologically.[72] There is no current evidence, however, that suggests a causal association of MAP and CD.[13,73]

MAP is an obligate intracellular organism that appears to exist as a cell wall–deficient form, making conventional anti tuberculous drugs ineffective as treatment. Macrolide compounds, such as clarithromycin and azithromycin, are considered to be the most effective antibiotics against MAP. In this context, several studies assessed the efficacy of antimycobacterial therapy in CD (Table 11-2). Four open-label studies assessed the efficacy of clarithromycin, alone or in combination with other drugs, in patients with active CD.[64,74-76] One of these open-label studies was conducted by Shafran et al[76] and included 36 patients with active CD who tested positive against p35 and p36 antigens, recombinant proteins of MAP, who were treated with clarithromycin 500 mg/day and rifabutin 300 mg/day accompanied with a probiotic. Seven patients withdrew from the study due to side effects, and of the 29 patients

who remained on the study, 21 (58.3%) reached a sustained improvement assessed by CDAI without needing other Crohn's medication.[76] The authors concluded that those patients with active CD and evidence of MAP could benefit from rifabutin and macrolide antibiotic therapy.[76]

Multiple randomized, controlled studies have tried to evaluate the efficacy of various combinations of antimycobacterial agents in patients with CD,[77-81] with no clear benefit. In the year 2000, a meta-analysis included a total of 8 randomized, placebo-controlled trials, of which 2 were published as abstracts.[82] The studies administered a wide range of antibiotic combinations and for different periods of time. The authors concluded that antimycobacterial therapy may be effective in maintaining remission in patients with CD after a course of corticosteroids combined with antimycobacterial therapy to induce remission; however, because of the heterogeneity of the trials, no definitive recommendations could be drawn.[82]

Later, Goodgame et al[83] assessed the efficacy of clarithromycin (1 g/day) and ethambutol (15 mg/kg/day) in patients with CD and a lactulose-mannitol permeability test of >0.03. Patients were randomly assigned to receive the antibiotic combination (n = 15) or placebo (n = 16) for 3 months in addition to their regular therapy with no difference between the drug or placebo groups regarding active disease (33% vs 44%) and mean lactulose-mannitol test (0.06 vs 0.10).[83] After a 12-month follow-up period, there were no statistically significant differences in the mean Harvey-Bradshaw index or lactulose-mannitol test between the 2 groups.[83]

A retrospective study that included 39 patients with severe CD evaluated histologic response to antibiotic

TABLE 11-3

ANTIBIOTICS IN PERIANAL FISTULOUS DISEASE: REPRESENTATIVE STUDIES*

Author	Year	Patients	Study Design	Antibiotic Scheme	Length	Outcome
Bernstein et al [88]	1980	21	Open-label	Metronidazole	–	All the patients presented clinical improvement
Brandt et al [89]	1982	26	Open-label	Metronidazole	12 to 36 months	Exacerbation after dose reduction 50% of paresthesias
Dejaco et al [90]	2003	52	Open-label	Ciprofloxacin 500 to 1000 mg/day and/or metronidazole 1000 to 1500 mg/day	8 weeks	Combination with azathioprine may be effective for fistula improvement
West et al [92]	2004	24	Double-blind RCT	Ciprofloxacin 500 mg bid	12 weeks	Combination with infliximab is more effective than infliximab alone
Thia et al [91]	2009	25	Double-blind RCT	Ciprofloxacin 500 mg bid or Metronidazole 500 mg bid	10 weeks	Ciprofloxacin presented higher remission and response rate

*Bid indicates 2 times a day; RCT, randomized controlled trial.

therapy.[84] Patients received rifabutin (up to 600 mg/day), clofazimine (up to 100 mg/day), and clarithromycin (up to 1 g/day) for 6 months to 9 years.[84] Twenty-two patients (56.4%) presented with mucosal healing. Histologically, a marked reduction in inflammation occurred in 15 of 39 patients (38.5%).[84] They concluded that anti-MAP therapy can be more effective than standard anti-inflammatory and immunosuppressant drugs in patients with active CD.[84]

Recently, Selby et al[85] conducted the largest prospective, double-blind, randomized, placebo-controlled antibiotic trial in patients with active CD. Two hundred and thirteen patients were randomized to clarithromycin (750 mg/day), rifabutin (450 mg/day), and clofazimine (50 mg/day) or placebo, in addition to a 16-week tapering course of corticosteroids.[85] After 16 weeks, 122 patients achieved remission and continued maintenance therapy with trial medication for 2 years.[85] After 2 years, trial medications were discontinued, and patients on remission were followed for 1 more year. At week 16, there were significantly more subjects in remission in the antibiotic arm (66%) than the placebo arm (50%; $P = 0.02$).[85] The rate of relapse was not significantly different in the 3 following years. After 1 year in the maintenance phase, 39% of the patients in the antibiotics arm relapsed, compared with 56% taking placebo ($P = 0.054$); 26% and 43% relapsed after 2 years ($P = 0.14$); and during the following year, 59% of the antibiotic group and 50% of the placebo group relapsed ($P = 0.54$).[85] The authors concluded that combination

antibiotic therapy does not support a significant role for MAP in the pathogenesis of CD; furthermore, the short-term improvement seen in antibiotic combination added to corticosteroids might be secondary to nonspecific antibacterial effects.[85] In conclusion, we do not have enough evidence to assert any true connection between CD and MAP. Further trials assessing histological progress and serologic responses to MAP before and after treatment together with higher antimycobacterial doses are currently warranted. Thus, antimycobacterial therapy is not recommended for the treatment of active CD.

PERIANAL FISTULOUS DISEASE

Perianal fistulae affect approximately 20% to 40% of the patients with CD over their lifetime,[86] and it can develop either as a result of an anal gland abscess or secondary to a penetrating ulcer in the rectum or anus.[87] Several uncontrolled trials evaluated the efficacy of antibiotics for perianal disease.[88-92] Despite the relative paucity of evidence, antibiotics are routinely used for this complication (Table 11-3). Bernstein et al[88] studied the efficacy of metronidazole in 21 patients suffering perianal CD. All patients presented clinical improvement, and complete healing was obtained in 10 of 18 patients maintained on therapy.[88] A follow-up article in those patients evaluated drug safety and effectiveness.[89] Dose reduction was associated with exacerbation of the disease (6 of 6 patients), but they responded to reinstitution of the drug, and metronidazole was successfully discontinued in only 28% of the patients.[89] Of note, paresthesias occurred in 50% of the patients after a mean treatment duration of 6.5 months.[89] Dejaco et al[90] performed another open-label study, including 52 patients with CD and perianal fistulas. Patients started with an 8-week regimen of ciprofloxacin (500 to 1000 mg/day) and/or metronidazole (1 to 1.5 g/day); azathioprine was added at enrollment or after 8 weeks of antibiotic treatment in 17 and 14 patients, respectively.[90] After completing 8 weeks, 26 patients (50%) responded to antibiotic treatment, with complete healing in 25% of patients.[90] Forty-nine patients were treated for 20 weeks; response was noted in 17 of the 49 patients (35%), with complete healing in 9 patients (18%).[90] Patients who received azathioprine were more likely to achieve a response (48%) than those without immunosuppression (15%) ($P = 0.03$).[90] The authors concluded that there is a role for antibiotics in the short-term treatment of perianal disease and azathioprine may be essential for the maintenance of fistula improvement.[90]

West et al[92] conducted a placebo-controlled study to evaluate whether the concomitant use of ciprofloxacin enhanced the efficacy of infliximab in patients with perianal fistulas in CD. Twenty-four patients were randomly assigned to receive 1 g/day of ciprofloxacin or a placebo for 12 weeks; in addition, they received 5 mg/kg infliximab at weeks 6, 8, and 12 and were then followed for 18 weeks.[92] Clinical response was 73% (8 of 11) in the ciprofloxacin group and 39% (5 of 13) in the placebo group, but it was not statistically significant.[92] However, logistic regression analysis showed that there was a tendency towards better clinical response with ciprofloxacin than with a placebo (odds ratio [OR] = 2.37, 95% confidence interval [CI] 0.94-5.98, $P = 0.07$).[92] The authors suggested that a combination of ciprofloxacin and infliximab tended to be more effective than infliximab alone.[92]

Recently, Thia et al[91] performed the first placebo-controlled pilot trial assessing the efficacy and safety of ciprofloxacin and metronidazole in patients with perianal CD. Patients were randomly assigned to ciprofloxacin ($n = 10$) or metronidazole ($n = 7$), both 1 g/day, or placebo ($n = 8$).[91] After 10 weeks, remission and response rates were 30% and 40% in the ciprofloxacin group, 0% and 14% in the metronidazole group, and 12.5% and 12.5% in those who received placebo, respectively.[91] Adverse events were reported in 7 of 10 patients in the ciprofloxacin group and in all 7 patients who received metronidazole, with 3 of them discontinuing treatment.[91] Although the authors recognized that an important limitation of their study was the small number of patients evaluated, they concluded that those patients treated with ciprofloxacin had a higher chance of remission and response.[91]

An interesting study exploring the association between NOD2/CARD15 variants and clinical response of perianal fistulae in patients using antibiotic therapy was recently conducted by Angelberger et al.[93] Of note, 13 of 39 patients with NOD2/CARD15 wild-type (33%) presented with complete response after receiving treatment with ciprofloxacin or metronidazole for 7 weeks.[93] On the other hand, none of the patients carrying NOD2/CARD15 variants developed any improvement after treatment ($P = 0.02$).[93] This study raises the question of whether patients with fistulizing CD might benefit from individualized antibiotic therapy regarding their NOD2/CARD15 variant carrier status. Further studies are needed to corroborate these findings.

On the basis of these small randomized controlled trials and open-label studies, antibiotics are routinely used for treating perianal CD. Ciprofloxacin 500 mg twice daily and metronidazole 10 to 20 mg/kg/day, alone or in combination, are used as first-line therapy of uncomplicated perianal fistulae, following drainage of associated abscesses. Antibiotics are continued for 8 to 12 weeks with careful observations of potential side effects, specifically peripheral neuropathy in metronidazole-treated patients. Addition of immunosuppressive therapy with azathioprine, 6-mercaptopurine, and infliximab is usually reserved for more complex or refractory cases.

POSTOPERATIVE RECURRENCE

Patients with CD have a 50% to 70% chance of requiring surgery during the course of their disease, with resection of the terminal ileum and cecum the most common intervention.[94] Approximately 73% of the patients will eventually develop recurrence 1 year after resection and 85% after 3 years.[95,96] During the early stages after endoscopic recurrence, patients may remain asymptomatic with only 20% and 34% of the patients developing symptoms after 1 and 3 years, respectively.[96] After 10 years, 26% to 65% of the patients who underwent ileocolonic resection will require further surgery.[97] Luminal bacteria may be involved in the pathogenesis of recurrent lesions. Patients with an ileocolonic anastomosis and temporary proximal loop ileostomy do not develop recurrent disease; however, infusion of intestinal contents through a proximal loop ileostomy triggers recurrent inflammation.[6,7] The theoretical role of luminal bacteria as inducers of recurrent disease led to studies of antibiotics as prophylactic therapy in this setting (Table 11-4).[98-100]

A double-blind, placebo-controlled trial conducted by Rutgeerts et al[99] explored the effect of starting metronidazole 20 mg/kg/day within 1 week from surgery for 3 months. Patients who underwent a curative resection of the terminal ileum and partial colectomy with a new ileocolonic anastomosis were eligible for the study.[99] At 12 weeks, 21 of 28 patients (75%) in the controlled group and 12 of 23 patients (52%) in the metronidazole arm had recurrent lesions in the neoterminal ileum ($P = 0.09$).[99] The incidence of severe endoscopic recurrence was significantly

TABLE 11-4

ANTIBIOTICS IN POSTOPERATIVE RECURRENCE: REPRESENTATIVE STUDIES*

AUTHOR	YEAR	PATIENTS	STUDY DESIGN	ANTIBIOTIC SCHEME	LENGTH	OUTCOME
Rutgeerts et al[99]	1995	60	Double-blind RCT	Metronidazole 20 mg/kg/day	12 weeks	Decreases severity of early recurrence
Rutgeerts et al[100]	2005	80	Double-blind RCT	Ornidazole 1 g/day	12 months	Reduces clinical and endoscopic recurrence
D'Haens et al[98]	2008	81	RCT	Metronidazole 750 mg/day	12 weeks	Combination with azathioprine is more effective than metronidazole alone

*RCT indicates randomized controlled trial.

reduced in the metronidazole-treated group (3 of 23, 13%) compared with the placebo group (12 of 28, 43%).[99] In addition, after 1 year, the clinical symptomatic recurrence rate was reduced to 4% in the metronidazole group and 25% in the placebo group ($P < 0.05$); however, reductions at 2 years (26% vs 43%) and 3 years (30% vs 50%) were not significant.[99] Adverse events were more frequent in the metronidazole group. The authors concluded that metronidazole therapy for 3 months decreases the severity of early recurrence of CD in the neoterminal ileum after resection and seems to delay symptomatic recurrence.[99]

The same group investigated the safety and efficacy of another nitroimidazole antibiotic, ornidazole, for the prevention of postoperative clinical recurrence of CD.[100] Eighty patients were randomized to receive ornidazole 1 g/day or placebo for 1 year starting 1 week after ileal or ileocolonic resection.[100] The endoscopic recurrence rate at 12 months was significantly lower in the antibiotic group (54%, 15 of 28) compared with the placebo group (79%, 26 of 33).[100] The clinical recurrence rate at 1 year was 8% (3 of 38 patients) in the ornidazole group and 37.5% (15 of 40) in the placebo group ($P = 0.002$). Endoscopic recurrence at 3 and 12 months predicted clinical recurrence.[100] Significantly more patients in the ornidazole group dropped out from the study because of side effects. The authors concluded that ornidazole is effective for the prevention of recurrence of CD after ileocolonic resection.[100]

Recently, D'Haens et al[98] examined whether metronidazole with azathioprine is superior to metronidazole alone to reduce CD postoperative recurrence. Patients who underwent curative ileal or ileocolonic resection with ileocolonic anastomosis were randomized to receive either azathioprine or placebo for 12 months, in addition to metronidazole 750 mg/day during 3 months, and therapy was started within 2 weeks after surgery.[98] The study assessed significant endoscopic recurrence after 3 and 12 months defined as an endoscopic index ≥ 2 according to the Rutgeerts endoscopic score,[96] and only patients considered

"high risk" for postoperative recurrence were included. Significant endoscopic recurrence in the azathioprine group was 44% (14 of 32) and 69% (20 of 29) in the placebo group at 12 months postsurgery ($P = 0.048$).[98] The intention-to-treat analysis revealed endoscopic recurrence in 22 of 40 (55%) in the azathioprine group and 32 of 41 (78%) in the placebo group at month 12 ($P = 0.035$).[98] Absence of inflammatory lesions at 1 year was seen in 7 of 32 patients and 1 of 29 patients in the azathioprine and placebo group, respectively.[98] The authors concluded that concomitant use of metronidazole and azathioprine resulted in lower endoscopic recurrence rates and less severe recurrences 12 months postsurgery.[98]

Prevention of postoperative recurrence of CD remains a challenge to physicians and patients. The use of nitroimidazole antibiotics has been shown to have benefit in reducing clinical and endoscopic CD recurrence during the first year after resection surgery.[99] The addition of an immunomodulator, such as azathioprine, might enhance the antibiotic effectiveness in controlling postsurgery recurrence with better tolerability.[98] However, it remains unclear what the optimal antibiotic dose is, in order to balance efficacy with toxicity, as well as the exact timing for initiation of therapy after surgery and for how long prophylactic therapy should be maintained. Nonetheless, antibiotics, with or without immunomodulators, are routinely used after ileal or ileocolonic resection for active CD.

PROBIOTICS

Probiotics have been defined as "living micro-organisms, which upon ingestion in certain numbers, exert health benefits beyond inherent basic nutrition."[101] Microbial species used as probiotics include *Lactobacilli*, *Bifidobacteria*, Gram-positive cocci, *E coli*, *Saccharomyces cerevisiae*, *Saccharomyces boulardii*, and fungi (*Aspergillus oryzae*) or VSL #3, a combination of 8 probiotic bacterial species (4 lactobacilli, 3 bifidobacteria, and *Streptococcus salivarius spp. thermophilus*).[102,103]

TABLE 11-5

CLINICAL EVIDENCE FOR BACTERIA IN THE PATHOGENESIS OF INFLAMMATORY BOWEL DISEASE*

EVIDENCE	CROHN'S DISEASE	ULCERATIVE COLITIS	POUCHITIS
Disease in area of ↑ bacterial concentration	Terminal ileum, colon	Colon	Ileal pouch
↑ Mucosal adherence	Yes	Yes	?
↑ Mucosal invasion	Yes	Yes	?
↓ Inflammation with bypass, bowel rest	Yes	No	Yes
Response to antibiotics	Colon only	No	Yes
Protection by probiotics	?	Yes	Yes
Pathogenetic immune response to bacteria	Yes	Yes	?
Exacerbation by pathogens	Yes	Yes	?

*↑ indicates increased; ↓, decreased; ?, not studied.

Reprinted with permission from Sartor RB. Therapeutic manipulation of the enteric microflora in inflammatory bowel diseases: antibiotics, probiotics, and prebiotics. *Gastroenterology.* 2004;126:1620-1633. Copyright 2004 Elsevier.

The possibility of using probiotics to alter enteric bacterial microflora has been explored (Table 11-5).[103] Proposed mechanisms of action of probiotics in diminishing the inflammatory response are listed in Table 11-6. Several trials studied the use of various probiotics in inducing and maintaining remission of Crohn's disease.

INDUCTION OF REMISSION IN CROHN'S DISEASE

A recent Cochrane review by Butterworth et al[104] identified only one small randomized, placebo-controlled study that evaluated the efficacy of orally administered probiotics (*Lactobacillus* GG at the dose of 2×10^9 colony forming units [CFU]/day) for 6 months in active Crohn's disease.[105] Eleven patients were randomized after a preceding 7-day treatment with antibiotics (ciprofloxacin 1000 mg daily and metronidazole 750 mg daily) and corticosteroids (60 mg with subsequent tapering).[105] The rates of remission (CDAI < 150) were comparable between patients treated with probiotics and placebo after 12 weeks of treatment (80% vs 83%, OR 0.80, 95% CI 0.04-17.20).[104,105]

Currently, there is no evidence to suggest that there is efficacy for using probiotics in induction of remission in patients with Crohn's disease, given the lack of well-designed randomized controlled trials.[104]

MAINTENANCE OF REMISSION IN CROHN'S DISEASE

Several studies evaluated the efficacy of probiotics in maintaining clinical remission in Crohn's disease (Table 11-7). A Cochrane review analyzed 6[105-110] small randomized controlled trials that compared maintenance

TABLE 11-6

MECHANISMS OF ACTION OF PROBIOTICS

INHIBIT PATHOGENIC ENTERIC BACTERIA

- Decrease luminal pH
- Secrete bactericidal proteins
- Colonization resistance (occupy ecologic niche)
- Block epithelial binding—induction of MUC 2

INHIBIT EPITHELIAL INVASION—RHO-DEPENDENT AND -INDEPENDENT PATHWAYS

- Improve epithelial and mucosal barrier function
- Produce short-chain fatty acids, including butyrate
- Enhance mucus production
- Increase barrier integrity

ALTER IMMUNOREGULATION

- Induce IL-10, transforming growth factor β expression and secretion
- Stimulate secretory immunoglobulin A production
- Decrease tumor necrosis factor expression

Reprinted with permission from Sartor RB. Therapeutic manipulation of the enteric microflora in inflammatory bowel diseases: antibiotics, probiotics, and prebiotics. *Gastroenterology.* 2004;126:1620-1633. Copyright 2004 Elsevier.

therapy with probiotics alone or with other concomitant treatment to placebo or aminosalicylates in adult patients

TABLE 11-7

RANDOMIZED CONTROLLED TRIALS COMPARING THE EFFICACY OF VARIETY OF PROBIOTICS TO PLACEBO OR OTHER TREATMENT IN MAINTAINING REMISSION IN PATIENTS WITH QUIESCENT CROHN'S DISEASE*

Study	Probiotic Name	Daily Probiotic Dose	Duration of Treatment	Number of Patients in Clinical Remission at Study Entry		Clinical Relapse Rate at the End of the Study		P Value	Risk Ratio (95% CI)
				Probiotic	Control	Probiotic	Control		
Malchow et al[106]	Escherichia coli strain Nissle, 1917	2 capsules (2.5 x 1010 viable bacteria per capsule)	12 months	10	10 (placebo)	3 (30%)	7 (70%)	0.11	0.43 (0.15-1.20)
Prantera et al[107]	Lactobacillus GG	12 x 109 CFU	12 months	18	19 (placebo)	3 (16.7%)	2 (10.5%)	0.59	1.58 (0.30-8.40)
Schultz et al[105]	Lactobacillus GG	2 x 109 CFU	6 months	4	5 (placebo)	2 (50%)	3 (60%)	0.77	0.83 (0.25-2.80)
Zocco et al[108]	Lactobacillus GG	18 x 109 CFU	12 months	12	12 (mesalazine)	2 (16.7%)	3 (25%)	0.62	0.67 (0.13-3.30)
Guslandi et al[110]	Saccharomyces boulardii yeast + mesalazine 2 g daily	1 g	6 months	16	16 (mesalazine)	1 (6.25%)	6 (37.5%)	0.079	0.17 (0.02-1.23)
Bousvaros et al[111] (pediatric trial)	Lactobacillus GG + aminosalicylates, low-dose corticosteroids, 6-MP/azathioprine	20 x 109 CFU	11 months	39	36 (placebo + aminosalicylates, low-dose corticosteroids, 6-MP/azathioprine)	12 (31%)	6 (16.7%)	0.17	1.85 (0.77-4.40)
Van Gossum et al[113]	Lactobacillus johnsonii, LA1	1010 CFU	12 weeks	27	22 (placebo)	4 (14.7%)	3 (13.6%)	0.91	1.1 (0.163-8.449)

*CI indicates confidence interval; CFU, colony forming unit; 6-MP, 6-mercaptopurine.

with medically or surgically induced remission, with one pediatric placebo-controlled trial[111] with patients receiving conventional maintenance therapy in conjunction with either probiotics or placebo.[112] Treatment with probiotics was not found to be superior to other treatments in reducing the risk of recurrence of the disease.[112] Data from eligible trials were not pooled together due to differences in probiotics evaluated, methodology, and medication regimen.[112] Pooled data from placebo-controlled studies demonstrated similar clinical relapse rates at the end of the study period between probiotics and placebo in patients who had remission induced either medically or surgically (25% vs 35%, $P = 0.39$, relative risk [RR] = 0.68, 95% CI

0.34-1.39).[105-107,112] In addition, one placebo-controlled trial did not show any advantage of Lactobacillus GG with respect to reducing endoscopic recurrence of CD at the end of the study.[107,112] Instead, 50% relapse rate was observed in patients treated with probiotics and a 31.5% relapse rate was observed among placebo recipients ($P = 0.26$, RR = 1.58, 95% CI 0.71-3.55).[107,112]

Campieri et al compared the rates of endoscopic recurrence among 40 patients with Crohn's disease, whose remission was induced surgically and who were randomly assigned to receive either rifaximin at a daily dose of 1.8 g for 3 months followed by 6 g of a VSL #3 probiotic cocktail including 300 billion bacteria per gram for 9 months or mesalamine at daily dose of 4 g for 12 months.[109] That study, published only in the abstract form, yielded 20% and 40% (P = 0.19) endoscopic recurrence rates among probiotics and mesalamine recipients, respectively (RR = 0.50, 95% CI 0.18-1.40).[109,112] A small study of 32 patients randomized to maintenance treatment with mesalazine 2 g/day in conjunction with yeast (*Saccharomyces boulardii*) or mesalazine at 3 g/day alone did not find a significant difference in clinical relapse rates between treatment arms (6.25% vs 37.5%, P = 0.079) with an insignificant relative risk of 0.17 (95% CI 0.02-1.23).[110] One pediatric randomized and multicenter trial of 75 children with Crohn's disease in remission compared maintenance therapy with *Lactobacillus* GG to placebo.[111] All patients were also receiving maintenance treatment of aminosalicylates, 6-mercaptopurine/azathioprine, and low-dose corticosteroids.[111] The addition of probiotics did not prolong the disease-free time, with 31% and 17% of patients relapsing in the probiotics and placebo group, respectively (P = 0.17, RR = 1.85; 95% CI 0.77-4.40).[111] Data from the aforementioned trials were not pooled together due to differences in the probiotics evaluated, methodology, and medication regimen.[112]

Recently, Rahimi et al published results of a meta-analysis of 8 randomized placebo-controlled trials[105-108,110,111,113,114] assessing the efficacy of probiotics in maintaining remission of CD.[115] That meta-analysis did not find that probiotics were superior to placebo in preventing clinical (7 trials[105-108,110,111,113]: pooled OR = 0.92, 95% CI 0.52-1.62, P = 0.9) or endoscopic recurrence (3 trials[107,113,114]: pooled OR = 0.97, 95% CI 0.54-1.78, P = 0.9) of CD.[115]

CONCLUSION

Strong evidence has shown that enteric commensal bacteria are involved in the pathogenesis of CD, and several studies have evaluated whether suppression of intestinal flora with antibiotics is beneficial in these patients. Thus far, few controlled trials support the use of antibiotics in perianal CD and postoperative recurrence; however, they are routinely used in this setting. On the other hand, the efficacy of metronidazole, ciprofloxacin, or their combination as first-line treatment for mild to moderately active CD remains unclear, although they appear to be more beneficial in ileocolonic or colonic involvement when compared to ileal disease alone. Of note, long-term use of metronidazole is associated with peripheral neuropathy that does resolve for most patients once the drug is discontinued. Rifaximin has emerged as an alternative to metronidazole and ciprofloxacin with fewer side effects and better tolerability; however, its role and dosing in the treatment of active CD remain to be conclusively elucidated.

Many questions still need to be answered regarding the utilization of antibiotics in patients with active CD.

Ciprofloxacin and metronidazole are the most frequently used antibiotics, but some authors have questioned whether this selection is the best option.[116] Individualization of antibiotic therapy depending on the clinical phenotype also requires further evaluation. The optimal antibiotic regimen with concomitant use of immunomodulating agents remains unclear.

Rigorous multicenter, randomized controlled trials are needed to define the role of antibiotics in CD and better assess their risks and benefits.

REFERENCES

1. Sartor RB. Microbial influences in inflammatory bowel diseases. *Gastroenterology.* 2008;134:577-594.
2. Duchmann R, Kaiser I, Hermann E, Mayet W, Ewe K, Meyer zum Buschenfelde KH. Tolerance exists towards resident intestinal flora but is broken in active inflammatory bowel disease (IBD). *Clin Exp Immunol.* 1995;102:448-455.
3. Macpherson A, Khoo UY, Forgacs I, Philpott-Howard J, Bjarnason I. Mucosal antibodies in inflammatory bowel disease are directed against intestinal bacteria. *Gut.* 1996;38:365-375.
4. Rath HC, Herfarth HH, Ikeda JS, et al. Normal luminal bacteria, especially *Bacteroides* species, mediate chronic colitis, gastritis, and arthritis in HLA-B27/human beta2 microglobulin transgenic rats. *J Clin Invest.* 1996;98:945-953.
5. Sellon RK, Tonkonogy S, Schultz M, et al. Resident enteric bacteria are necessary for development of spontaneous colitis and immune system activation in interleukin-10-deficient mice. *Infect Immun.* 1998;66:5224-5231.
6. D'Haens GR, Geboes K, Peeters M, Baert F, Penninckx F, Rutgeerts P. Early lesions of recurrent Crohn's disease caused by infusion of intestinal contents in excluded ileum. *Gastroenterology.* 1998;114:262-267.
7. Neut C, Bulois P, Desreumaux P, et al. Changes in the bacterial flora of the neoterminal ileum after ileocolonic resection for Crohn's disease. *Am J Gastroenterol.* 2002;97:939-946.
8. Bibiloni R, Mangold M, Madsen KL, Fedorak RN, Tannock GW. The bacteriology of biopsies differs between newly diagnosed, untreated, Crohn's disease and ulcerative colitis patients. *J Med Microbiol.* 2006;55:1141-1149.
9. Frank DN, St Amand AL, Feldman RA, Boedeker EC, Harpaz N, Pace NR. Molecular-phylogenetic characterization of microbial community imbalances in human inflammatory bowel diseases. *Proc Natl Acad Sci USA.* 2007;104:13780-13785.
10. Martin HM, Campbell BJ, Hart CA, et al. Enhanced *Escherichia coli* adherence and invasion in Crohn's disease and colon cancer. *Gastroenterology.* 2004;127:80-93.
11. Swidsinski A, Ladhoff A, Pernthaler A, et al. Mucosal flora in inflammatory bowel disease. *Gastroenterology.* 2002;122:44-54.
12. Ryan P, Bennett MW, Aarons S, et al. PCR detection of *Mycobacterium paratuberculosis* in Crohn's disease granulomas isolated by laser capture microdissection. *Gut.* 2002;51:665-670.
13. Shanahan F, O'Mahony J. The mycobacteria story in Crohn's disease. *Am J Gastroenterol.* 2005;100:1537-1538.
14. Scanlan PD, Shanahan F, O'Mahony C, Marchesi JR. Culture-independent analyses of temporal variation of the dominant fecal microbiota and targeted bacterial subgroups in Crohn's disease. *J Clin Microbiol.* 2006;44:3980-3988.
15. Tamboli CP, Neut C, Desreumaux P, Colombel JF. Dysbiosis in inflammatory bowel disease. *Gut.* 2004;53:1-4.

16. Cartun RW, Van Kruiningen HJ, Pedersen CA, Berman MM. An immunocytochemical search for infectious agents in Crohn's disease. *Mod Pathol.* 1993;6:212-219.

17. Liu Y, van Kruiningen HJ, West AB, Cartun RW, Cortot A, Colombel JF. Immunocytochemical evidence of *Listeria, Escherichia coli,* and *Streptococcus* antigens in Crohn's disease. *Gastroenterology.* 1995;108:1396-1404.

18. Ryan P, Kelly RG, Lee G, et al. Bacterial DNA within granulomas of patients with Crohn's disease—detection by laser capture microdissection and PCR. *Am J Gastroenterol.* 2004;99:1539-1543.

19. Ernst JD. Bacterial inhibition of phagocytosis. *Cell Microbiol.* 2000; 2:379-386.

20. Finlay BB, Cossart P. Exploitation of mammalian host cell functions by bacterial pathogens. *Science.* 1997;276:718-725.

21. Subramanian S, Roberts CL, Hart CA, et al. Replication of colonic Crohn's disease mucosal *Escherichia coli* isolates within macrophages and their susceptibility to antibiotics. *Antimicrob Agents Chemother.* 2008;52:427-434.

22. Ogawa M, Sasakawa C. Intracellular survival of *Shigella. Cell Microbiol.* 2006;8:177-184.

23. Mpofu CM, Campbell BJ, Subramanian S, et al. Microbial mannan inhibits bacterial killing by macrophages: a possible pathogenic mechanism for Crohn's disease. *Gastroenterology.* 2007;133:1487-1498.

24. Lodes MJ, Cong Y, Elson CO, et al. Bacterial flagellin is a dominant antigen in Crohn disease. *J Clin Invest.* 2004;113:1296-1306.

25. Wyatt J, Vogelsang H, Hubl W, Waldhoer T, Lochs H. Intestinal permeability and the prediction of relapse in Crohn's disease. *Lancet.* 1993;341:1437-1439.

26. Hugot JP, Chamaillard M, Zouali H, et al. Association of NOD2 leucine-rich repeat variants with susceptibility to Crohn's disease. *Nature.* 2001;411:599-603.

27. Ogura Y, Bonen DK, Inohara N, et al. A frameshift mutation in NOD2 associated with susceptibility to Crohn's disease. *Nature.* 2001;411:603-606.

28. Lala S, Ogura Y, Osborne C, et al. Crohn's disease and the NOD2 gene: a role for paneth cells. *Gastroenterology.* 2003;125:47-57.

29. Barnich N, Aguirre JE, Reinecker HC, Xavier R, Podolsky DK. Membrane recruitment of NOD2 in intestinal epithelial cells is essential for nuclear factor-{kappa}B activation in muramyl dipeptide recognition. *J Cell Biol.* 2005;170:21-26.

30. Wehkamp J, Harder J, Weichenthal M, et al. NOD2 (CARD15) mutations in Crohn's disease are associated with diminished mucosal alpha-defensin expression. *Gut.* 2004;53:1658-1664.

31. Ahmad T, Armuzzi A, Bunce M, et al. The molecular classification of the clinical manifestations of Crohn's disease. *Gastroenterology.* 2002;122:854-866.

32. Cuthbert AP, Fisher SA, Mirza MM, et al. The contribution of NOD2 gene mutations to the risk and site of disease in inflammatory bowel disease. *Gastroenterology.* 2002;122:867-874.

33. Podolsky DK. Inflammatory bowel disease. *N Engl J Med.* 2002; 347:417-429.

34. Perencevich M, Burakoff R. Use of antibiotics in the treatment of inflammatory bowel disease. *Inflamm Bowel Dis.* 2006;12:651-664.

35. Sartor RB. Therapeutic manipulation of the enteric microflora in inflammatory bowel diseases: antibiotics, probiotics, and prebiotics. *Gastroenterology.* 2004;126:1620-1633.

36. Isaacs KL, Sartor RB. Treatment of inflammatory bowel disease with antibiotics. *Gastroenterol Clin North Am.* 2004;33:335-345, x.

37. Morikawa K, Watabe H, Araake M, Morikawa S. Modulatory effect of antibiotics on cytokine production by human monocytes in vitro. *Antimicrob Agents Chemother.* 1996;40:1366-1370.

38. Williams AC, Galley HF, Watt AM, Webster NR. Differential effects of three antibiotics on T helper cell cytokine expression. *J Antimicrob Chemother.* 2005;56:502-506.

39. Shafran I, Burgunder P. Rifaximin for the treatment of newly diagnosed Crohn's disease: a case series. *Am J Gastroenterol.* 2008; 103:2158-2160.

40. Navarro F, Hanauer SB. Treatment of inflammatory bowel disease: safety and tolerability issues. *Am J Gastroenterol.* 2003;98:S18-S23.

41. Frytak S, Moertel CH, Childs DS. Neurologic toxicity associated with high-dose metronidazole therapy. *Ann Intern Med.* 1978; 88:361-362.

42. Halloran TJ. Convulsions associated with high cumulative doses of metronidazole. *Drug Intell Clin Pharm.* 1982;16:409.

43. Smith JA. Neutropenia associated with metronidazole therapy. *Can Med Assoc J.* 1980;123:202.

44. van der Linden PD, Sturkenboom MC, Herings RM, Leufkens HG, Stricker BH. Fluoroquinolones and risk of Achilles tendon disorders: case-control study. *BMJ.* 2002;324:1306-1307.

45. van der Linden PD, Sturkenboom MC, Herings RM, Leufkens HM, Rowlands S, Stricker BH. Increased risk of achilles tendon rupture with quinolone antibacterial use, especially in elderly patients taking oral corticosteroids. *Arch Intern Med.* 2003;163:1801-1807.

46. Owens RC Jr, Ambrose PG. Antimicrobial safety: focus on fluoroquinolones. *Clin Infect Dis.* 2005;41(suppl 2):S144-S157.

47. Sturgill MG, Rapp RP. Clarithromycin: review of a new macrolide antibiotic with improved microbiologic spectrum and favorable pharmacokinetic and adverse effect profiles. *Ann Pharmacother.* 1992;26:1099-1108.

48. Volberg WA, Koci BJ, Su W, Lin J, Zhou J. Blockade of human cardiac potassium channel human ether-a-go-go-related gene (HERG) by macrolide antibiotics. *J Pharmacol Exp Ther.* 2002;302:320-327.

49. Scarpignato C, Pelosini I. Rifaximin, a poorly absorbed antibiotic: pharmacology and clinical potential. *Chemotherapy.* 2005;51 (suppl 1):36-66.

50. Ursing B, Kamme C. Metronidazole for Crohn's disease. *Lancet.* 1975;1:775-777.

51. Blichfeldt P, Blomhoff JP, Myhre E, Gjone E. Metronidazole in Crohn's disease: a double blind cross-over clinical trial. *Scand J Gastroenterol.* 1978;13:123-127.

52. Ursing B, Alm T, Barany F, et al. A comparative study of metronidazole and sulfasalazine for active Crohn's disease: the Cooperative Crohn's Disease Study in Sweden. II. Result. *Gastroenterology.* 1982;83:550-562.

53. Sutherland L, Singleton J, Sessions J, et al. Double blind, placebo controlled trial of metronidazole in Crohn's disease. *Gut.* 1991;32:1071-1075.

54. Arnold GL, Beaves MR, Pryjdun VO, Mook WJ. Preliminary study of ciprofloxacin in active Crohn's disease. *Inflamm Bowel Dis.* 2002;8:10-15.

55. Colombel JF, Lemann M, Cassagnou M, et al. A controlled trial comparing ciprofloxacin with mesalazine for the treatment of active Crohn's disease. Groupe d'Etudes Therapeutiques des Affections Inflammatoires Digestives (GETAID). *Am J Gastroenterol.* 1999;94:674-678.

56. Greenbloom SL, Steinhart AH, Greenberg GR. Combination ciprofloxacin and metronidazole for active Crohn's disease. *Can J Gastroenterol.* 1998;12:53-56.

57. Prantera C, Zannoni F, Scribano ML, et al. An antibiotic regimen for the treatment of active Crohn's disease: a randomized, controlled clinical trial of metronidazole plus ciprofloxacin. *Am J Gastroenterol.* 1996;91:328-332.

58. Prantera C, Berto E, Scribano ML, Falasco G. Use of antibiotics in the treatment of active Crohn's disease: experience with metronidazole and ciprofloxacin. *Ital J Gastroenterol Hepatol.* 1998; 30:602-606.

59. Steinhart AH, Feagan BG, Wong CJ, et al. Combined budesonide and antibiotic therapy for active Crohn's disease: a randomized controlled trial. *Gastroenterology*. 2002;123:33-40.

60. Xu G, Fujita J, Negayama K, et al. Effect of macrolide antibiotics on macrophage functions. *Microbiol Immunol*. 1996;40:473-479.

61. Desaki M, Takizawa H, Ohtoshi T, et al. Erythromycin suppresses nuclear factor-kappaB and activator protein-1 activation in human bronchial epithelial cells. *Biochem Biophys Res Commun*. 2000;267:124-128.

62. Inoue S, Nakase H, Matsuura M, et al. Open label trial of clarithromycin therapy in Japanese patients with Crohn's disease. *J Gastroenterol Hepatol*. 2007;22:984-988.

63. Leiper K, Martin K, Ellis A, Watson AJ, Morris AI, Rhodes JM. Clinical trial: randomized study of clarithromycin versus placebo in active Crohn's disease. *Aliment Pharmacol Ther*. 2008;27:1233-1239.

64. Leiper K, Morris AI, Rhodes JM. Open label trial of oral clarithromycin in active Crohn's disease. *Aliment Pharmacol Ther*. 2000;14:801-806.

65. Robins GW, Wellington K. Rifaximin: a review of its use in the management of traveller's diarrhoea. *Drugs*. 2005;65:1697-1713.

66. Shafran I, Johnson LK. An open-label evaluation of rifaximin in the treatment of active Crohn's disease. *Curr Med Res Opin*. 2005; 21:1165-1169.

67. Prantera C, Lochs H, Campieri M, et al. Antibiotic treatment of Crohn's disease: results of a multicentre, double blind, randomized, placebo-controlled trial with rifaximin. *Aliment Pharmacol Ther*. 2006;23:1117-1125.

68. Dalziel T. Chronic intestinal enteritis. *BMJ*. 1913;2:1068-1070.

69. Chiodini RJ, Van Kruiningen HJ, Thayer WR, Merkal RS, Coutu JA. Possible role of mycobacteria in inflammatory bowel disease. I. An unclassified *Mycobacterium* species isolated from patients with Crohn's disease. *Dig Dis Sci*. 1984;29:1073-1079.

70. Naser SA, Ghobrial G, Romero C, Valentine JF. Culture of *Mycobacterium avium* subspecies *paratuberculosis* from the blood of patients with Crohn's disease. *Lancet*. 2004;364:1039-1044.

71. Autschbach F, Eisold S, Hinz U, et al. High prevalence of *Mycobacterium avium* subspecies *paratuberculosis* IS900 DNA in gut tissues from individuals with Crohn's disease. *Gut*. 2005;54:944-949.

72. Morgan KL. Johne's and Crohn's. Chronic inflammatory bowel diseases of infectious aetiology? *Lancet*. 1987;1:1017-1019.

73. Sartor RB. Does *Mycobacterium avium* subspecies *paratuberculosis* cause Crohn's disease? *Gut*. 2005;54:896-898.

74. Borody TJ, Leis S, Warren EF, Surace R. Treatment of severe Crohn's disease using antimycobacterial triple therapy—approaching a cure? *Dig Liver Dis*. 2002;34:29-38.

75. Gui GP, Thomas PR, Tizard ML, Lake J, Sanderson JD, Hermon-Taylor J. Two-year-outcomes analysis of Crohn's disease treated with rifabutin and macrolide antibiotics. *J Antimicrob Chemother*. 1997;39:393-400.

76. Shafran I, Kugler L, El-Zaatari FA, Naser SA, Sandoval J. Open clinical trial of rifabutin and clarithromycin therapy in Crohn's disease. *Dig Liver Dis*. 2002;34:22-28.

77. Afdhal NH, Long A, Lennon J, Crowe J, O'Donoghue DP. Controlled trial of antimycobacterial therapy in Crohn's disease. Clofazimine versus placebo. *Dig Dis Sci*. 1991;36:449-453.

78. Elliott PR, Burnham WR, Berghouse LM, Lennard-Jones JE, Langman MJ. Sulphadoxine-pyrimethamine therapy in Crohn's disease. *Digestion*. 1982;23:132-134.

79. Prantera C, Kohn A, Mangiarotti R, Andreoli A, Luzi C. Antimycobacterial therapy in Crohn's disease: results of a controlled, double-blind trial with a multiple antibiotic regimen. *Am J Gastroenterol*. 1994;89:513-518.

80. Shaffer JL, Hughes S, Linaker BD, Baker RD, Turnberg LA. Controlled trial of rifampicin and ethambutol in Crohn's disease. *Gut*. 1984;25:203-205.

81. Swift GL, Srivastava ED, Stone R, et al. Controlled trial of anti-tuberculous chemotherapy for two years in Crohn's disease. *Gut*. 1994;35:363-368.

82. Borgaonkar MR, MacIntosh DG, Fardy JM. A meta-analysis of antimycobacterial therapy for Crohn's disease. *Am J Gastroenterol*. 2000;95:725-729.

83. Goodgame RW, Kimball K, Akram S, et al. Randomized controlled trial of clarithromycin and ethambutol in the treatment of Crohn's disease. *Aliment Pharmacol Ther*. 2001;15:1861-1866.

84. Borody TJ, Bilkey S, Wettstein AR, Leis S, Pang G, Tye S. Antimycobacterial therapy in Crohn's disease heals mucosa with longitudinal scars. *Dig Liver Dis*. 2007;39:438-444.

85. Selby W, Pavli P, Crotty B, et al. Two-year combination antibiotic therapy with clarithromycin, rifabutin, and clofazimine for Crohn's disease. *Gastroenterology*. 2007;132:2313-2319.

86. Schwartz DA, Loftus EV Jr, Tremaine WJ, et al. The natural history of fistulizing Crohn's disease in Olmsted County, Minnesota. *Gastroenterology*. 2002;122:875-880.

87. Present DH. Crohn's fistula: current concepts in management. *Gastroenterology*. 2003;124:1629-1635.

88. Bernstein LH, Frank MS, Brandt LJ, Boley SJ. Healing of perineal Crohn's disease with metronidazole. *Gastroenterology*. 1980;79:357-365.

89. Brandt LJ, Bernstein LH, Boley SJ, Frank MS. Metronidazole therapy for perineal Crohn's disease: a follow-up study. *Gastroenterology*. 1982;83:383-387.

90. Dejaco C, Harrer M, Waldhoer T, Miehsler W, Vogelsang H, Reinisch W. Antibiotics and azathioprine for the treatment of perianal fistulas in Crohn's disease. *Aliment Pharmacol Ther*. 2003; 18:1113-1120.

91. Thia KT, Mahadevan U, Feagan BG, et al. Ciprofloxacin or metronidazole for the treatment of perianal fistulas in patients with Crohn's disease: a randomized, double-blind, placebo-controlled pilot study. *Inflamm Bowel Dis*. 2009;15:17-24.

92. West RL, van der Woude CJ, Hansen BE, et al. Clinical and endosonographic effect of ciprofloxacin on the treatment of perianal fistulae in Crohn's disease with infliximab: a double-blind placebo-controlled study. *Aliment Pharmacol Ther*. 2004;20:1329-1336.

93. Angelberger S, Reinisch W, Dejaco C, et al. NOD2/CARD15 gene variants are linked to failure of antibiotic treatment in perianal fistulating Crohn's disease. *Am J Gastroenterol*. 2008;103:1197-1202.

94. Sachar DB. The problem of postoperative recurrence of Crohn's disease. *Med Clin North Am*. 1990;74:183-188.

95. Olaison G, Smedh K, Sjodahl R. Natural course of Crohn's disease after ileocolic resection: endoscopically visualised ileal ulcers preceding symptoms. *Gut*. 1992;33:331-335.

96. Rutgeerts P, Geboes K, Vantrappen G, Beyls J, Kerremans R, Hiele M. Predictability of the postoperative course of Crohn's disease. *Gastroenterology*. 1990;99:956-963.

97. Chardavoyne R, Flint GW, Pollack S, Wise L. Factors affecting recurrence following resection for Crohn's disease. *Dis Colon Rectum*. 1986;29:495-502.

98. D'Haens GR, Vermeire S, Van Assche G, et al. Therapy of metronidazole with azathioprine to prevent postoperative recurrence of Crohn's disease: a controlled randomized trial. *Gastroenterology*. 2008;135:1123-1129.

99. Rutgeerts P, Hiele M, Geboes K, et al. Controlled trial of metronidazole treatment for prevention of Crohn's recurrence after ileal resection. *Gastroenterology*. 1995;108:1617-1621.

100. Rutgeerts P, Van Assche G, Vermeire S, et al. Ornidazole for prophylaxis of postoperative Crohn's disease recurrence: a randomized, double-blind, placebo-controlled trial. *Gastroenterology.* 2005;128:856-861.

101. Guarner F, Schaafsma GJ. Probiotics. *Int J Food Microbiol.* 1998; 39:237-238.

102. Fooks LJ, Gibson GR. Probiotics as modulators of the gut flora. *Br J Nutr.* 2002;88(suppl 1):S39-S49.

103. Sartor RB. Probiotic therapy of intestinal inflammation and infections. *Curr Opin Gastroenterol.* 2005;21:44-50.

104. Butterworth AD, Thomas AG, Akobeng AK. Probiotics for induction of remission in Crohn's disease. *Cochrane Database Syst Rev.* 2008:CD006634.

105. Schultz M, Timmer A, Herfarth HH, Sartor RB, Vanderhoof JA, Rath HC. *Lactobacillus* GG in inducing and maintaining remission of Crohn's disease. *BMC Gastroenterol.* 2004;4:5.

106. Malchow HA. Crohn's disease and *Escherichia coli.* A new approach in therapy to maintain remission of colonic Crohn's disease? *J Clin Gastroenterol.* 1997;25:653-658.

107. Prantera C, Scribano ML, Falasco G, Andreoli A, Luzi C. Ineffectiveness of probiotics in preventing recurrence after curative resection for Crohn's disease: a randomised controlled trial with *Lactobacillus* GG. *Gut.* 2002;51:405-409.

108. Zocco M, Zileri Dal Verme L, Armuzzi A, et al. Comparison of *Lactobacillus* GG and mesalazine in maintaining remission of ulcerative colitis and Crohn's disease. *Gastroenterology.* 2003;124: A201.

109. Campieri M, Rizzello F, Venturi A, et al. Combination of antibiotic and probiotic treatment is efficacious in prophylaxis of post-operative recurrence of Crohn's disease: a randomized controlled study vs. mesalamine. *Gastroenterology.* 2000;4:A781.

110. Guslandi M, Mezzi G, Sorghi M, Testoni PA. *Saccharomyces boulardii* in maintenance treatment of Crohn's disease. *Dig Dis Sci.* 2000;45:1462-1464.

111. Bousvaros A, Guandalini S, Baldassano RN, et al. A randomized, double-blind trial of *Lactobacillus* GG versus placebo in addition to standard maintenance therapy for children with Crohn's disease. *Inflamm Bowel Dis.* 2005;11:833-839.

112. Rolfe VE, Fortun PJ, Hawkey CJ, Bath-Hextall F. Probiotics for maintenance of remission in Crohn's disease. *Cochrane Database Syst Rev.* 2006:CD004826.

113. Van Gossum A, Dewit O, Louis E, et al. Multicenter randomized-controlled clinical trial of probiotics (*Lactobacillus johnsonii*, LA1) on early endoscopic recurrence of Crohn's disease after Ileo-caecal resection. *Inflamm Bowel Dis.* 2007;13:135-142.

114. Marteau P, Lemann M, Seksik P, et al. Ineffectiveness of *Lactobacillus johnsonii* LA1 for prophylaxis of postoperative recurrence in Crohn's disease: a randomised, double blind, placebo controlled GETAID trial. *Gut.* 2006;55:842-847.

115. Rahimi R, Nikfar S, Rahimi F, et al. A meta-analysis on the efficacy of probiotics for maintenance of remission and prevention of clinical and endoscopic relapse in Crohn's disease. *Dig Dis Sci.* 2008;53:2524-2531.

116. West RL, Van der Woude CJ, Endtz HP, et al. Perianal fistulas in Crohn's disease are predominantly colonized by skin flora: implications for antibiotic treatment? *Dig Dis Sci.* 2005;50:1260-1263.

CORTICOSTEROIDS IN CROHN'S DISEASE

Lene Riis, MD and Pia Munkholm, MD, DMSCi

Corticosteroids are a mainstay in the treatment of inflammatory bowel diseases (IBDs). Administered topically, orally, or intravenously, corticosteroids rapidly and consistently improve moderate to severe active Crohn's disease, although they are ineffective in maintaining remission and endoscopic healing. The beneficial effects of corticosteroid therapies are counterbalanced by their many side effects.

HISTORY

The potent anti-inflammatories were first described in rheumatoid arthritis patients in 1949, which led to clinical trials in numerous other chronic inflammatory disorders, including IBD.[1]

Since the beginning of the 1950s, we have learned from Weedon and colleagues' data[2] that corticosteroids have had a great impact on survival. Identical data were obtained when surgery was introduced in this decade.[3] Cumulative survival rates declined 20% over the following 20 years after the introduction of corticosteroids in Crohn's disease (Figure 12-1).

The first controlled trials documenting the beneficial effects of corticosteroids and adrenocorticotropic hormones (ACTH)[4] in the treatment of UC and CD appeared more than 50 years ago in the United States and in Europe.[1,5,6] In 1979, the National Cooperative Crohn's Disease Study[7] (NCCDS) was the first randomized, double-blind, placebo-controlled trial consisting of 569 patients showing remission rates of 60% compared with the placebo-treated patients of 30%. A dose of 0.25 to 0.75 mg/kg/day was applied in accordance with the patients' Crohn's disease activity index (CDAI) score. Using a slightly higher dose of methylprednisolone of 48 mg initially and tapered by 8 mg weekly, the European Cooperative Crohn's Disease Study[8] (ECCDS) reported even better results; with 80% of the patients achieving remission at week 18 compared with 40% of placebo-treated patients.[8] No prevention of relapse by steroids in quiescent CD could be found.[7,8]

The slow mucosal endoscopic healing after corticosteroid treatment was surprisingly elucidated by the GETAID group in France[9] in the 1990s. One hundred forty-two patients with active colonic or ileocolonic CD were included in a multicenter prospective study. Seven weeks after initializing corticosteroid, a high dose of oral prednisolone at 1 mg/kg bodyweight, 92% went into clinical remission; however, only 29% responded with endoscopic healing of the mucosa.[9] At initial colonoscopy, mucosal lesions were (by decreasing order of frequency) superficial ulcerations, deep ulcerations, mucosal edema, erythema, pseudopolyps, aphthoid ulcers, ulcerated stenosis, and nonulcerated stenosis. No correlation was found between the clinical activity index and any of the endoscopical data (lesion frequency and surface, endoscopic severity index). Corticosteroids obviously were not the drugs of choice when targeting endoscopic remission.[9] To obtain endoscopic healing, discontinuing corticosteroids should be considered along with alternative therapies, such as azathioprine, 6-mercaptopurine, methotrexate, or infliximab.

Lichtenstein GR, ed.
Crohn's Disease: The Complete Guide to Medical Management (pp 135-142).
© 2011 SLACK Incorporated

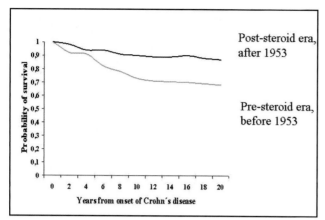

FIGURE 12-1. Cumulative probability of survival before and after introduction of corticosteroids in 1953. A significant increase in survival of 20% was found after corticosteroid treatment was introduced.[2]

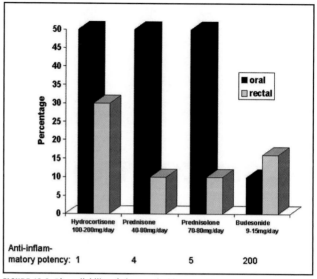

FIGURE 12-2. Bioavailability of glucocorticoid preparations.

PHARMACOKINETICS

MECHANISMS OF ACTION

Corticosteroids are lipophilic hormones; dissociated molecules diffuse across cell membranes and bind to the cytoplasmatic glucocorticosteroid receptors (GR), complexed to heat-shock protein 90 (hsp90).[10] The corticosteroid complex translocates to the nucleus, where the dimer binds to a glucocorticosteroid-response element (GRE) on the promoter region of steroid responsive genes, resulting in increased or decreased transcription of m-RNA and production of proteins. Effects of corticosteroids include inhibition of the production of proinflammatory proteins, such as tumor necrosis factor alpha (TNFα), IL-1, and chemokines, such as IL-8; repression of the transcription of the genes for certain enzymes, such as inducible nitric oxide synthase, phospholipase A_2, and cyclooxygenase II; and blockade of adhesion molecules expression.[11-15] These molecular actions of corticosteroids lead to reduced leucocyte migration and function and inhibition of numerous mediators of inflammation.

Recent studies have also shown that interaction between activated corticosteroid receptors and nuclear factor κB (NF-κB) plays a role in the anti-inflammatory action of corticosteroids. The action of NF-κB is inhibited by activated corticosteroid receptors via a direct protein–protein interaction and stimulation of the NF-κB inhibitor I-κB.[16] NF-κB is known to play a key role in the inflammatory process.

Resistance to corticoid therapy in patients with IBD is often caused by an increased expression of the multidrug resistance-1 gene (MDR1) resulting in increased expression of membrane-based drug efflux pump, which pumps corticosteroids out of cells, lowering the intracellular concentration.[17]

FORMULATION

Prednisone and prednisolone are the most widely used corticosteroids in the treatment of CD. Both drugs are easily absorbed from the gut, with a bioavailability of 70% after oral administration (Figure 12-2). Prednisone is converted to the active metabolite prednisolone in the liver. The maximum plasma concentration is reached after 1 to 3 hours, and plasma half-life is 3 to 4 hours. Prednisolone and prednisone can be administered orally or intravenously. When given orally, absorption may be decreased in patients with CD of the small bowel and in severe UC.[18-20] Oral administration of prednisolone resulted in a lower peak plasma concentration than in healthy volunteers.[20] In this study, continuous infusion resulted in a greater mean serum concentration over time compared to bolus injection. Thus, intravenous administration with prednisolone, prednisone, and corticotropin is preferable in these cases.

Formulation designed to administer topical corticosteroids at the site of the disease as rectal enema/suppository or orally via an ileal or colonic slow release formulation (see Chapter 13) have been developed to reduce the toxicity of corticosteroids. However, a certain amount of adrenal suppression of the steroid production cannot be avoided. Systemic absorption of hydrocortisone from enemas is less than from oral administration, because rectal bioavailability is ranging from 15% to 30%.[21,22] Furthermore, results from bone turnover indicate that a significant systemic corticosteroid activity is present when patients with distal UC are treated.[23,24]

REGIMEN AND TAPERING

In the NCCDS study, dose adjustment in accordance with disease activity was demonstrated and a daily initial dose recommended: moderate to severe disease 0.75 mg/kg, mild to moderate disease 0.5 mg/kg, and mild inflammation 0.25 mg/kg.[7] In the European study, 48 mg/day of 6-methylprednisolone was sufficient to obtain the same remission rates of 60% to 80%.[8] Tapering steroids down is generally done differently in Europe compared to North America. Crohn's disease patients admitted to the ward are started with 1 mg/kg prednisolone orally and subsequently tapered down during 3 months. In North America, the typical initial dose is 40 mg/kg in 14 to 30 days, tapered by 5 mg/kg per week to 20 mg/day, then a slower tapering by 2.5 mg per week until cessation of the drug. One trial has shown that there is no difference in the outcome in CD patients whether you taper over 2 or 4 months.[25]

ADVERSE EVENTS

Numerous toxicities after 17 weeks with corticosteroids were found in the NCCDS study[7]: moon face 47%, acne 30%, infection 27%, ecchymosis 17%, hypertension 15%, hirsutism 7%, striae 6%, and petechial subcutaneous bleeding 6%.

A summary of the most common and serious adverse events is given in Table 12-1.

METABOLIC EFFECTS

The metabolic effects of steroid therapy include hyperglycemia and an unmasking of a genetic predisposition to diabetes mellitus and hyperlipidemia. Alteration of fat distribution with development of a Cushingoid appearance and hepatic steatosis might be irreversible.

OCULAR EFFECT

Glaucoma has been described in both children and adults and correlates with the intensity and duration of treatment.[26] Likewise, a dose-response relationship has been found between the length of steroid therapy and the development of subcapsular cataract.[27]

NEUROPSYCHIATRIC

Milder and more common reactions to steroids are insomnia, irritability, excessive talkativeness, and anger. Severe neuropsychiatric complications including psychosis, depression, mania, and delirium occur in 25%, of which 6% are severe.[28] Thus, at high doses, it is essential to observe the patients' reactions, as hallucinations have been reported.[29]

TABLE 12-1

ADVERSE EFFECTS ASSOCIATED WITH SYSTEMIC CORTICOSTEROID THERAPY

METABOLIC
Hyperglycemia
Diabetes mellitus
Hyperlipidemia
Hypertension
Hypokalemia

NEUROPSYCHIATRIC
Neuropathy
Insomnia
Psychosis
Depression
Pseudotumor cerebri

GASTROINTESTINAL
Nausea
Vomiting
Dyspepsia
Esophagitis
Pancreatitis
Intestinal perforation

IMMUNOLOGIC
Increased risk of infection
Lymphocytosis
Leukocytosis
Immunosuppression

OCULAR
Cataracts
Glaucoma

GYNECOLOGIC/OBSTETRICAL
Amenorrhea
Gestational diabetes
Adrenal suppression of the child

MUSCULOSKELETAL
Osteoporosis
Aseptic necrosis of bone
Myopathy
Growth retardation

DERMATOLOGIC
Acne
Telangiectasia
Striae
Alopecia

ENDOCRINE
Moon face
Hypothalamic-pituitary-adrenal axis suppression
Hirsutism
Buffalo hump
Weight gain

GASTROINTESTINAL

The use of corticosteroids alone may not increase the risk of peptic ulcer, but studies indicated that the risk of upper gastrointestinal bleeding is increased in patients taking nonsteroidal antiinflammatory drugs (NSAIDs) concomitantly with corticosteroids.[30,31] Important considerations in patients with CD include promoting intestinal perforation with the use of corticosteroids.

IMMUNOLOGIC

Patients treated with high doses of steroids for prolonged periods of time are at an increased risk of infectious complications.[32]

GYNECOLOGIC/OBSTETRICAL

Corticosteroids cross the placenta and are transferred into breast milk, but the ratio of maternal to fetal serum concentration depends on the corticosteroid used. Prednisolone is more efficiently metabolized compared with dexamethasone, and fetal levels are only approximately 10% of maternal levels.[33] These concentrations are not thought to present a clinically significant risk to the fetus, and no adverse events have been reported. Corticosteroids are safe for the breast-feeding infant; thus, women on steroid therapy should be encouraged to continue breast-feeding. In 531 pregnant women,[34] 30% received corticosteroids for an extended period of time, mostly during the second and third trimesters, with no increased incidence of prematurity, spontaneous abortion, stillbirth, or developmental defects noted.

MUSCULOSKELETAL

Osteopenia and osteoporosis are common complications of IBD, which is also seen in nonsteroid-treated patients. In recent years, it has been shown that patients with CD have an increased risk of fractures,[35,36] and several population-based studies have shown decreased bone mineral density in a substantial part of patients with CD[37]; only one population-based study from the Mayo Clinic came to the opposite conclusion.[38] Risk factors are high cumulative dose of corticosteroids, low body weight, malabsorption of calcium and lipid-soluble vitamins, and the inflammatory process. Corticosteroids affect both bone resorption and formation, ultimately resulting in decreased bone density and fractures.[39] In IBD, the higher total lifetime steroid dose, the lower the bone density.[40] All patients with CD should have an x-ray absorptiometry scanning at diagnosis and after treatment with oral steroids for more than 3 months/year. At each steroid course and at osteopenia (T-score between –1.5 and –2.5), each patient should be treated with calcium and vitamin D supplementation. Patients with osteoporosis (T-score less than or equal to –2.5) should further have bisphosphonate compound, such as alendronate or risedronate.[39,41]

DERMATOLOGIC

Steroid-induced subcutaneous tissue atrophy causes striae and predisposes to purpura and telangiectasia. The latter changes can be removed by laser techniques, but for striae the only option is surgical intervention.

ENDOCRINE

Adrenal insufficiency and Addisonian crisis after discontinuation of steroid treatment can occur due to suppression of the hypothalamic-pituitary-adrenal axis. It is difficult to predict the risk of developing adrenal suppression.[42] After longer courses of steroid, adrenal function may be suppressed for up to 1 year after treatment cessation. A simple Synacthen test should be done immediately. Patients on long-term steroids should have a supplemental "stress" dose before any surgery.

CLINICAL TRIALS FOCUSING ON CORTICOSTEROID USE IN CROHN'S DISEASE

MILD TO MODERATELY ACTIVE CROHN'S DISEASE

The algorithm of mild to moderately active CD and first-line therapy has changed recently due to the evidence provided from the budesonide trials in ileum and/or right-sided colonic CD (Figure 12-3).[43,44] Sulfasalazine 3 to 6 g/day are used as first-line therapy induction for 16 weeks. The less toxic mesalamines should be considered for cancer chemoprevention in CD patients as maintenance treatment.[45] Two small placebo-controlled comparative studies demonstrated a trend towards greater efficacy of prednisolone 30 mg/day versus ciprofloxacin 1 g/day combined with metronidazole.[46]

When treatment fails with budesonide and sulfasalazine, oral prednisolone should be offered 40 mg/day to 60 mg/day initially. The tapering regimen has never been tested with regard to long-term efficacy. In Europe, we tend to start with 1 mg/kg/day body weight administered as a single dose. There is no evidence that prolonged tapering over 4 to 6 months improves the long-term outcome, and such an approach leads to a greater steroid exposure. There have never been any adjunctive benefits for sulfasalazine and steroids shown.[8,47]

SEVERE CROHN'S DISEASE

Severe CD includes severely active, toxic enteritis; colitis and complications of megacolon; small bowel obstruction; and abdominal abscess. Severely active disease presents variably as severe abdominal pain and/or diarrhea, fever, tachycardia, dehydration, and severe anemia. Toxic megacolon is demonstrated by abdominal x-ray and defined by colonic distension of 5 to 6 cm or more, decreased or absent bowel sounds, and sometimes absent or decreased bowel movements. Abdominal computed tomography (CT) scan

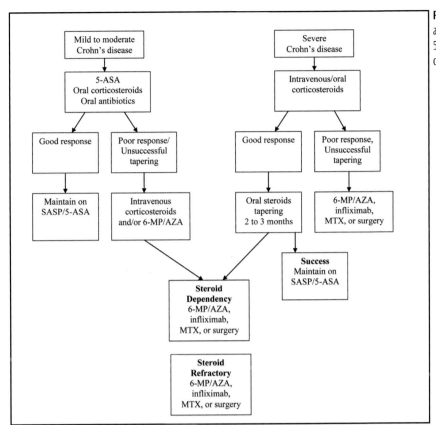

FIGURE 12-3. Management algorithm for mild to moderate and severely active Crohn's disease. 5-ASA indicates 5-aminosalicylates; SASP, salazopyrine; 6-MP, 6-mercaptopurine; AZA, azathioprine; MTX, methotrexate.

or ultrasound should be performed to exclude abscesses and fistulae. In the acute stage,[48] it is important to treat the patient with intravenous fluids, electrolyte supplements, bowel rest, transfusion if indicated, intravenous antibiotics, and intravenous corticosteroids, although published data are lacking. Factors that have been implicated in the development of toxic megacolon should be avoided in patients with severe Crohn's colitis, such as barium enema, narcotic antidiarrheal agents (loperamide, tincture opium, codeine, and diphenoxylate), anticholinergic agents, antidepressants, and electrolyte imbalance.

Intravenous corticoid therapy should be initiated with hydrocortisone 300 to 400 mg/day or methylprednisolone 40 to 60 mg/day. A pharmacokinetic study has shown that patients can benefit from continuous infusion regimen rather than intermittent bolus therapy. Patients failing to respond to intravenous corticosteroid therapy after 7 to 10 days and who are nonresponders to the addition of infliximab after approximately 5 days should undergo surgical resection (see Figure 12-3).

It is recognized that clinically many patients who initially respond to corticosteroid therapy and who relapse with tapering can be maintained in an asymptomatic state by long-term therapy with prednisone 10 to 30 mg/day or its equivalent. Such patients are termed *steroid-dependent*.[49,50] The short- and long-term response to steroid treatment in CD has been analyzed in 2 studies by Munkholm et al[49] and

Faubion et al[50] (Figures 12-4 and 12-5), with very concordant results. A flare-up of CD responding to medical treatment with corticosteroids within 1 month causes complete remission in 48% to 58% of patients and causes improvement in an additional 26% to 32% of patients. No response at all was found in 16% to 20%. Furthermore, close to 30% of the patients became steroid dependent, with immediate flare-up after treatment cessation. The definition of steroid dependency in the Copenhagen inception cohort was that patients who initially obtained a fair response either by complete response or partial response after cessation of corticosteroids, who either relapsed within 30 days or at tapering, had to continue corticosteroids for more than 1 year to maintain the response.

SONIC is a large definitive randomized double-blind controlled trial comparing early intervention with infliximab/azathioprine combination therapy, infliximab monotherapy, and azathioprine monotherapy for 1 year in patients with moderate-to-severe Crohn's disease of short duration. Patients in the trial were steroid exposed but naïve to biologics or immunomodulators. SONIC showed that patients with evidence of inflammation (elevated C-reactive protein level and endoscopic lesions at baseline colonoscopy) achieved superior steroid-free clinical remission (50%, 42%, and 23%, respectively) associated with mucosal healing from early infliximab combination therapy or monotherapy.[51] These infliximab treatments

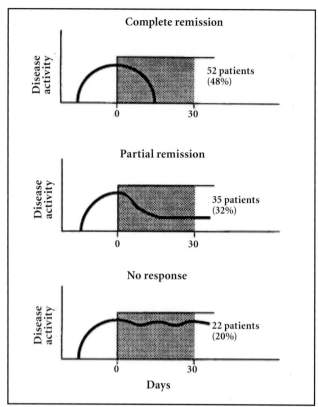

FIGURE 12-4. Initial outcome of the first steroid treatment course after 1 month of prednisolone (1 mg/kg) administration in 109 patients with Crohn's disease.[49] Reprinted with permission from Munkholm P, Langholz E, Davidsen M, Binder V. Frequency of glucocorticoid resistance and dependency in Crohn's disease. *Gut.* 1994;35:360-362.

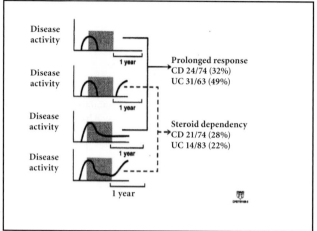

FIGURE 12-5. One-year outcomes for Crohn's disease were prolonged response in 24 (32%), corticosteroid dependence in 21 (28%), operation in 28 (38%), and lost to follow-up in 1. One-year outcomes for ulcerative colitis were prolonged response in 31 (49%), corticosteroid dependence in 14 (22%), and operation in 18 (29%).[50] Reprinted with permission from Faubion WA Jr, Loftus EV Jr, Harmsen WS, Zinsmeister AR, Sandborn WJ. The natural history of corticosteroid therapy for inflammatory bowel disease: a population-based study. *Gastroenterology.* 2001;121:255-260.

were superior to azathioprine alone with similar safety outcome in all 3 arms. Just as ACCENT 1 was a pivotal study in establishing the role of maintenance therapy in Crohn's disease, SONIC is a landmark study supporting the tectonic shift toward early intervention with anti-TNFα therapy and away from unlimited steroid and azathioprine therapy. There is no role for systemic oral steroids as maintenance treatment. However, it has been shown that maintenance treatment with 6-methylprednisolone 0.25 mg/kg/day in asymptomatic patients with elevated inflammation markers has the benefit of suppressing subclinical inflammation.[52] Newer corticosteroids, such as budesonide (see Chapter 13), have shown in an initial study that the time to relapse was prolonged; however, sustained benefit is not observed after 1 year.

FUTURE DIRECTIVES

The therapeutic indications of corticosteroids in CD are induction of remission for moderate to severely active disease. Intravenous therapy should be considered for more severe disease. Corticosteroid should be tapered and cessation obtained within 2 to 3 months. Since the late 1980s, the algorithm in the case of steroid dependency and resistance has been to supplement with azathioprine/6-mercaptopurine and thus should be applied to wean off the steroid faster. The "top-down" model in future studies in case of acute severe CD will elucidate the efficacy of infliximab and other biological modifiers in patients not responding to steroids.

REFERENCES

1.   Truelove SC, Witts LJ. Cortisone in ulcerative colitis; final report on a therapeutic trial. *Br Med J.* 1955:1041-1048.

2.   Weedon DD, Shorter RG, Ilstrup DM, Huizenga KA, Taylor WF. Crohn's disease and cancer. *N Engl J Med.* 1973;289:1099-1103.

3.   Devroede GJ, Taylor WF, Sauer WG, Jackman RJ, Stickler GB. Cancer risk and life expectancy of children with ulcerative colitis. *N Engl J Med.* 1971;285:17-21.

4.   Standley MM, Rosenberg IN, Cleroux AP. The use of corticotropin (ACTH) in the treatment of chronic regional enteritis. *Med Clin N Am.* 1951;35:1255-1265.

5.   Dearing WH, Brown PJ. Experiences with cortisone and ACTH in chronic ulcerative colitis. *Proc Mayo Clin.* 1950;25:486.

6.   Elliott JM, Kiefer ED, Hurxthal LM. The treatment of chronic ulcerative colitis with pituitary adrenocorticotropic hormone (ACTH). A clinical study of 28 cases. *N Engl J Med.* 1951;245:288-292.

7.   Summers RW, Switz DM, Sessions JT Jr, et al. National Cooperative Crohn's Disease Study: results of drug treatment. *Gastroenterology.* 1979;77:847-869.

8.   Malchow H, Ewe K, Brandes JW, et al. European Cooperative Crohn's Disease Study (ECCDS): results of drug treatment. *Gastroenterology.* 1984;86:249-266.

9. Modigliani R, Mary JY, Simon JF, et al. Clinical, biological, and endoscopic picture of attacks of Crohn's disease. Evolution on prednisolone. Groupe d'Etude Therapeutique des Affections Inflammatoires Digestives. *Gastroenterology.* 1990;98:811-818.

10. Hollenberg SM, Weinberger C, Ong ES, et al. Primary structure and expression of a functional human glucocorticoid receptor cDNA. *Nature.* 1985;318:635-641.

11. Brostjan C, Anrather J, Csizmadia V, Natarajan G, Winkler H. Glucocorticoids inhibit E-selectin expression by targeting NF-kappaB and not ATF/c-Jun. *J Immunol.* 1997;158:3836-3844.

12. Paliogianni F, Raptis A, Ahuja SS, Najjar SM, Boumpas DT. Negative transcriptional regulation of human interleukin 2 (IL-2) gene by glucocorticoids through interference with nuclear transcription factors AP-1 and NF-AT. *J Clin Invest.* 1993;91:1481-1489.

13. Colotta F, Re F, Muzio M, et al. Interleukin-1 type II receptor: a decoy target for IL-1 that is regulated by IL-4. *Science.* 1993;261:472-475.

14. Wissink S, van Heerde EC, vand der BB, van der Saag PT. A dual mechanism mediates repression of NF-kappaB activity by glucocorticoids. *Mol Endocrinol.* 1998;12:355-363.

15. Barnes PJ, Karin M. Nuclear factor-kappaB: a pivotal transcription factor in chronic inflammatory diseases. *N Engl J Med.* 1997;336:1066-1071.

16. Auphan N, Didonato JA, Rosette C, Helmberg A, Karin M. Immunosuppression by glucocorticoids: inhibition of NF-kappa B activity through induction of I kappa B synthesis. *Science.* 1995;270:286-290.

17. Farrell RJ, Murphy A, Long A, et al. High multidrug resistance (P-glycoprotein 170) expression in inflammatory bowel disease patients who fail medical therapy. *Gastroenterology.* 2000;118:279-288.

18. Shaffer JA, Williams SE, Turnberg LA, Houston JB, Rowland M. Absorption of prednisolone in patients with Crohn's disease. *Gut.* 1983;24:182-186.

19. Tanner AR, Halliday JW, Powell LW. Serum prednisolone levels in Crohn's disease and coeliac disease following oral prednisolone administration. *Digestion.* 1981;21:310-315.

20. Elliott PR, Powell-Tuck J, Gillespie PE, et al. Prednisolone absorption in acute colitis. *Gut.* 1980;21:49-51.

21. Petitjean O, Wendling JL, Tod M, et al. Pharmacokinetics and absolute rectal bioavailability of hydrocortisone acetate in distal colitis. *Aliment Pharmacol Ther.* 1992;6:351-357.

22. Cann PA, Holdsworth CD. Systemic absorption from hydrocortisone foam enema in ulcerative colitis. *Lancet.* 1987;1:922-923.

23. Robinson RJ, Iqbal SJ, Whitaker RP, Abrams K, Mayberry JF. Rectal steroids suppress bone formation in patients with colitis. *Aliment Pharmacol Ther.* 1997;11:201-204.

24. Luman W, Gray RS, Pendek R, Palmer KR. Prednisolone metasulphobenzoate foam retention enemas suppress the hypothalamo-pituitary-adrenal axis. *Aliment Pharmacol Ther.* 1994;8:255-258.

25. Brignola C, De SG, Belloli C, et al. Steroid treatment in active Crohn's disease: a comparison between two regimens of different duration. *Aliment Pharmacol Ther.* 1994;8:465-468.

26. Tripathi RC, Kirschner BS, Kipp M, et al. Corticosteroid treatment for inflammatory bowel disease in pediatric patients increases intraocular pressure. *Gastroenterology.* 1992;102:1957-1961.

27. Cumming RG, Mitchell P, Leeder SR. Use of inhaled corticosteroids and the risk of cataracts. *N Engl J Med.* 1997;337:8-14.

28. Ismail K, Wessely S. Psychiatric complications of corticosteroid therapy. *Br J Hosp Med.* 1995;53:495-499.

29. Jacob R, Walsh C, Hunter JO. Road traffic accident as an iatrogenic complication of steroid treatment in Crohn's disease. *Am J Gastroenterol.* 2002;97:2154-2155.

30. Keenan GF. Management of complications of glucocorticoid therapy. *Clin Chest Med.* 1997;18:507-520.

31. Carson JL, Strom BL, Schinnar R, Duff A, Sim E. The low risk of upper gastrointestinal bleeding in patients dispensed corticosteroids. *Am J Med.* 1991;91:223-228.

32. Stuck AE, Minder CE, Frey FJ. Risk of infectious complications in patients taking glucocorticosteroids. *Rev Infect Dis.* 1989;11:954-963.

33. Beitins IZ, Bayard F, Ances IG, Kowarski A, Migeon CJ. The transplacental passage of prednisone and prednisolone in pregnancy near term. *J Pediatr.* 1972;81:936-945.

34. Mogadam M, Dobbins WO III, Korelitz BI, Ahmed SW. Pregnancy in inflammatory bowel disease: effect of sulfasalazine and corticosteroids on fetal outcome. *Gastroenterology.* 1981;80:72-76.

35. Vestergaard P, Krogh K, Rejnmark L, Laurberg S, Mosekilde L. Fracture risk is increased in Crohn's disease, but not in ulcerative colitis. *Gut.* 2000;46:176-181.

36. Bernstein CN, Blanchard JF, Leslie W, Wajda A, Yu BN. The incidence of fracture among patients with inflammatory bowel disease. A population-based cohort study. *Ann Intern Med.* 2000;133:795-799.

37. Jahnsen J, Falch JA, Aadland E, Mowinckel P. Bone mineral density is reduced in patients with Crohn's disease but not in patients with ulcerative colitis: a population based study. *Gut.* 1997;40:313-319.

38. Loftus EV Jr, Crowson CS, Sandborn WJ, Tremaine WJ, O'Fallon WM, Melton LJ III. Long-term fracture risk in patients with Crohn's disease: a population-based study in Olmsted County, Minnesota. *Gastroenterology.* 2002;123:468-475.

39. Valentine JF, Sninsky CA. Prevention and treatment of osteoporosis in patients with inflammatory bowel disease. *Am J Gastroenterol.* 1999;94:878-883.

40. Silvennoinen JA, Karttunen TJ, Niemela SE, Manelius JJ, Lehtola JK. A controlled study of bone mineral density in patients with inflammatory bowel disease. *Gut.* 1995;37:71-76.

41. Scott EM, Gaywood I, Scott BB. Guidelines for osteoporosis in coeliac disease and inflammatory bowel disease. British Society of Gastroenterology. *Gut.* 2000;46(suppl 1):i1-i8.

42. Schlaghecke R, Kornely E, Santen RT, Ridderskamp P. The effect of long-term glucocorticoid therapy on pituitary-adrenal responses to exogenous corticotropin-releasing hormone. *N Engl J Med.* 1992;326:226-230.

43. Greenberg GR, Feagan BG, Martin F, et al. Oral budesonide for active Crohn's disease. Canadian Inflammatory Bowel Disease Study Group. *N Engl J Med.* 1994;331:836-841.

44. Tremaine WJ, Hanauer SB, Katz S, et al. Budesonide CIR capsules (once or twice daily divided-dose) in active Crohn's disease: a randomized placebo-controlled study in the United States. *Am J Gastroenterol.* 2002;97:1748-1754.

45. Riis L, Vind I, Jess T, Winther K, Munkholm P. Chemoprevention of colorectal cancer in chronic inflammatory bowel disease: which candidate drugs? *Acta Endoscopica.* 2004;34:199-213.

46. Prantera C, Zannoni F, Scribano ML, et al. An antibiotic regimen for the treatment of active Crohn's disease: a randomized, controlled clinical trial of metronidazole plus ciprofloxacin. *Am J Gastroenterol.* 1996;91:328-332.

47. Singleton JW, Summers RW, Kern F Jr, et al. A trial of sulfasalazine as adjunctive therapy in Crohn's disease. *Gastroenterology.* 1979;77:887-897.

48. Shepherd HA, Barr GD, Jewell DP. Use of an intravenous steroid regimen in the treatment of acute Crohn's disease. *J Clin Gastroenterol.* 1986;8:154-159.

49. Munkholm P, Langholz E, Davidsen M, Binder V. Frequency of glucocorticoid resistance and dependency in Crohn's disease. *Gut.* 1994;35:360-362.

50. Faubion WA Jr, Loftus EV Jr, Harmsen WS, Zinsmeister AR, Sandborn WJ. The natural history of corticosteroid therapy for inflammatory bowel disease: a population-based study. *Gastroenterology.* 2001;121:255-260.

51. Lichtenstein GR, Hanauer SB, Sandborn WJ. Practice Parameters Committee of American College of Gastroenterology. Management of Crohn's disease in adults. *Am J Gastroenterol.* 2009;104:465-483.

52. Brignola C, Campieri M, Farruggia P, et al. The possible utility of steroids in the prevention of relapses of Crohn's disease in remission. A preliminary study. *J Clin Gastroenterol.* 1988;10:631-634.

Oral Budesonide for Inflammatory Bowel Disease

Gordon R. Greenberg, MD, FRCP(C)

Although the therapeutic armamentarium for the management of patients with Crohn's disease has expanded considerably during the past decade, corticosteroids continue to be a cornerstone treatment for active Crohn's disease. After 10 weeks of treatment with prednisone, remission rates of 60% to 80% are reported.[1-3] This benefit is offset by a substantial risk of serious side effects that impact negatively on quality of life, however.[4] The frequent adverse event profile associated with corticosteroids prompted the development of a new group of steroid agents that provide distinct advantages over conventional steroids by achieving nearly equivalent efficacy with a lower adverse event profile. First developed for the treatment of asthma and allergic rhinitis, budesonide was formulated into an oral delayed-release preparation for the treatment of patients with Crohn's disease.

PHARMACOLOGY

Budesonide is a nonhalogenated glucocorticosteroid that provides a different structure-activity profile when compared to prednisone, primarily via alterations of the D-ring of the basic hydrocortisone molecule (Figure 13-1). Substitution of a lipophilic acetyl group at the 16α and 17α positions of budesonide facilitates higher affinity for the glucocorticoid receptor that is 195-fold greater than hydrocortisone and 15-fold greater than prednisolone (Table 13-1). Therefore, budesonide has a substantially enhanced topical antiinflammatory activity, which is about 1000-fold higher than hydrocortisone.[5] Budesonide is stable in extrahepatic tissues and, after oral administration and absorption, undergoes approximately a 90% first-pass hepatic metabolism to form 6β-hydroxy-budesonide and 16α-hydroxy-prednisolone, both of which have less than 1% corticosteroid activity of the parent drug. The metabolites are excreted primarily in urine and to a lesser extent in feces. The rapid hepatic breakdown of budesonide via cytochrome P450 CYP3A4 reduces systemic bioavailability and therefore decreases the potential for steroid-related side effects. Budesonide also has relatively high water solubility that allows for adequate intraluminal dissolution and high lipid solubility that facilitates efficient mucosal uptake and high local concentrations in intestinal tissues. In the intestinal mucosa and submucosa, approximately 30% to 50% of budesonide is converted to reversible fatty acid esters (which lack receptor affinity, causing the formation of an intracellular pool of inactive drug). As the intracellular concentration of free budesonide decreases, budesonide esters are gradually hydrolyzed back to the active state, causing a slow release of active budesonide. This unique property of budesonide increases its retention time, prolongs the duration of action, and contributes in part to the lower risk of systemic side effects.[6]

Two oral preparations of budesonide are available for the treatment of inflammatory bowel disease (IBD), and both agents are formulated for targeted delivery to the ileum and colon. A controlled ileal-release (CIR) preparation of budesonide (Entocort, AstraZeneca, Lund, Sweden) contains multiple acid-stable microgranules composed of an inner sugar core surrounded by a layer of budesonide in ethylcellulose and an outer coat of methacrylic acid copolymer (Eudragit L 100-55) that dissolves above pH 5.5. For patients with CD, the absorption of this preparation in

Lichtenstein GR, ed.
Crohn's Disease: The Complete Guide to Medical Management (pp 143-156).
© 2011 SLACK Incorporated

TABLE 13-1

PHARMACOLOGIC PROPERTIES OF PREDNISOLONE VS BUDESONIDE*

	PREDNISOLONE	BUDESONIDE
Relative affinity for glucocorticoid receptor	13	195
Relative topical anti-inflammatory activity	1	1000
Clearance (L/min)	0.23	1.20
Systemic availability (%)	80	9

*Adapted from Brattsand R. Overview of newer glucocorticoid preparations for inflammatory bowel disease. *Can J Gastroenterol.* 1990;4:407-414.

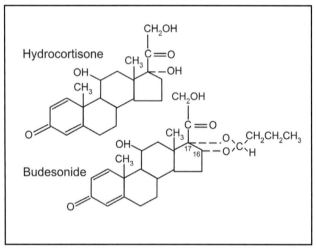

FIGURE 13-1. Chemical structure of hydrocortisone and budesonide.

the ileocecal region is 68.7% (95% confidence interval [CI] 53.8-83.6), and in the transverse and descending colon, it is 26.2% (6.6-45.8), with a mean absorption time of 6.4 hours (95% CI 5.1-7.8); these values are similar to absorption parameters observed for healthy volunteers.[7] The systemic bioavailability of oral budesonide 9 mg/day is 11 ± 7% in adults and 9 ± 5% in children,[8] compared with approximately 80% for prednisone. This low systemic availability accords with the extensive first-pass hepatic metabolism of budesonide. Food ingestion does not significantly affect the systemic availability or the mean time to maximum plasma concentrations.[9] In patients with an ileostomy, the mean budesonide concentration in the effluent is higher after administration of budesonide CIR capsules than after standard budesonide.

The second oral preparation is pH-modified-release budesonide (Budenofalk, Dr. Falk Pharma, Freiberg, Germany) formulated in capsules containing 400 pellets with a 1-mm diameter of budesonide coated with a Eudragit that dissolves above pH 6.0. Approximately 60%

to 80% of pH-modified-release budesonide is absorbed in the ileum and ascending colon, and 20% to 40% reaches more distal sites in the colon.[10]

The systemic oral availability of budesonide is increased by approximately 2.5-fold in patients with hepatic cirrhosis, and a reduction of dosage should be considered for patients with severe liver disease. In patients with renal sufficiency, budesonide treatment may cause higher concentrations of budesonide metabolites; however, the corticosteroid activity of the metabolites is minimal and should not be associated with a greater adverse event profile.

Because budesonide is metabolized via the cytochrome P450 CYP3A4 pathway, plasma contractions may increase when the drug is administered to patients receiving inhibitors of CYP3 A4. Thus, co-administration of budesonide with ketoconazole increases systemic budesonide concentrations by 8-fold; co-ingestion of grapefruit juice, an inhibitor of intestinal mucosal CYP3A, causes an approximately 2-fold increase of systemic budesonide concentrations. The estrogen portion of oral contraceptives is metabolized via the CYP3A4 pathway, but women receiving oral contraceptives do not show significantly altered plasma concentrations of budesonide. Although formulated for dissolution above pH 5.5, the absorption and pharmacokinetics of budesonide are not influenced by co-administration of omeprazole.

CLINICAL OUTCOMES

Oral budesonide has been evaluated with randomized, double-blind clinical trials for the treatment of patients with Crohn's disease, including induction of remission for active Crohn's disease, maintenance therapy for quiescent Crohn's disease after medically induced remission, prevention of postoperative recurrence after ileocecal resection, and as replacement therapy for steroid-dependent patients. Oral budesonide has also been evaluated for the treatment of active ulcerative colitis and collagenous colitis.

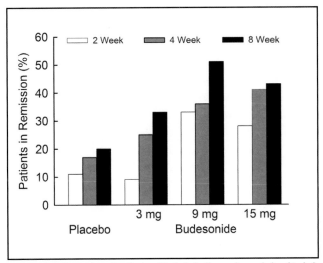

FIGURE 13-2. Proportion of patients with Crohn's disease in remission (Crohn's disease activity index (CDAI) < 150) after treatment with placebo or budesonide. (Adapted from Greenberg GR, Feagan BG, Martin F, et al. Oral budesonide for active Crohn's disease. *N Engl J Med*. 1994;331:836-841.)

ACTIVE CROHN'S DISEASE

The major indication for oral budesonide is induction of remission for patients with mild to moderately active CD of the ileum and right colon. For this indication, the clinical efficacy of oral budesonide has been evaluated with randomized, double-blind clinical trials comparing budesonide to placebo; to mesalamine; and to the conventional corticosteroids, prednisolone and prednisone.

BUDESONIDE VS PLACEBO

Two short-term trials[11,12] compared budesonide with placebo for the treatment of active mild to moderate Crohn's disease of the ileum and ascending colon. The primary outcome measure in both trials was clinical remission defined by a Crohn's disease activity index (CDAI) of 150 or less. In a dose-finding study,[11] 258 patients were randomly assigned to placebo or 1 of 3 doses of budesonide—3, 9, or 15 mg daily. After 8 weeks of treatment, the remission observed with 9 and 15 mg/day was similar (51% vs 43%; *P* = 0.70), and both doses were more effective than the placebo response of 20% (*P* < 0.001 and *P* = 0.009, respectively) (Figure 13-2). The rate of remission for the 3 mg/day group of 33% was not different from placebo (*P* = 0.13). Health-related quality of life also rapidly improved by 2 weeks in both the 9-mg and 15-mg budesonide groups to a greater extent than placebo.[13] The findings established 9 mg/day of budesonide as the optimal dose required to achieve induction of remission for patients with mild to moderately active Crohn's disease.

A second trial[12] compared budesonide 9 mg/day given as a single dose or as a split dose of 4.5 mg twice daily against placebo. The 2 budesonide dose regimens achieved similar rates of remission (48% vs 53%) but, because of

a higher than usual placebo response of 33%, the differences between active treatment and placebo did not reach statistical significance. However, a meta-analysis[14] of the 2 trials found that budesonide induced remission of active Crohn's disease more often than placebo with a relative risk (RR) = 1.85 (95% CI 1.31-2.61). Further, the effectiveness of budesonide compared with placebo was shown not only for patients with lower disease activity (entry CDAI 200-300); (RR = 1.54, 95% CI 1.01-2.35) but also for patients with high disease activity (entry CDAI > 300) (RR = 4.25, 95% CI 1.39-12.15).

No clinical trials have been undertaken to evaluate a comparison of the efficacy of the pH-modified-release formulation of budesonide with placebo for the treatment of active Crohn's disease. However, in a randomized, double-blind, dose-ranging study[15] of pH-modified budesonide 6, 9, and 18 mg /day, at 6 weeks, remission rates were 36%, 55%, and 66%, respectively (18 mg vs 6 mg budesonide; *P* = 0.017). A subgroup analysis indicated that budesonide at 18 mg/day compared with 6 mg/day was more effective for induction of remission for patients with an entry CDAI > 300 (75% vs 0%; *P* = 0.028) and for patients with disease distal to the transverse colon (73% vs 31%; *P* = 0.042). For patients with ileal and/or right colon involvement and for patients with an entry CDAI < 300, which comprised 75% of total entry population, remission rates were similar after treatment with budesonide 9 or 18 mg daily.

Together, the results from these studies provide controlled evidence that oral budesonide is effective therapy for patients with mild to moderately active Crohn's disease of the ileum and right colon. For most patients, the optimal therapeutic dose of budesonide is 9 mg given once daily. The 2 oral formulations of budesonide cause similar efficacy when disease involvement is limited to the ileum and right colon. The pH-modified formulation of budesonide may also provide clinical benefit for patients with active Crohn's disease extending beyond the hepatic flexure.

BUDESONIDE VS MESALAMINE

Only 1 trial[16] has been undertaken comparing budesonide 9 mg once daily and mesalamine (Pentasa) 2 g twice daily. The rates of remission (CDAI < 150) after 8, 12, and 16 weeks of treatment were significantly higher at all time points in the budesonide group than in the mesalamine group (Figure 13-3). At 16 weeks of treatment, the respective rates of remission for budesonide and mesalamine groups were 62% and 36% (*P* < 0.001), producing a relative risk of 1.73 (95% CI 1.26-2.39). Thus, a patient with flare-up CD of the ileum and right colon who receives budesonide is 73% more likely to achieve remission compared to a similar patient who receives mesalamine. In a subgroup analysis of patients with involvement of the right colon, budesonide was more effective than mesalamine (56% vs 23%; *P* < 0.001). Among patients who presented

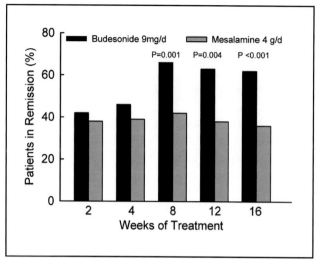

FIGURE 13-3. Proportion of patients with Crohn's disease in remission (Crohn's disease activity index [CDAI] < 150) after treatment with budesonide or mesalamine. (Adapted from Thomsen OØ, Cortot A, Jewell D, et al. A comparison of budesonide and mesalamine for active Crohn's disease. *N Engl J Med.* 1998;339:370-374.)

with low disease activity (entry CDAI 200-300), budesonide induced the remission of Crohn's disease more frequently than mesalamine (73% vs 49%; *P* < 0.01) (RR = 1.49, 95% CI 1.10-2.03).[14] Similarly, for patients who present with high disease activity (initial CDAI > 300), budesonide induced remission more frequently than mesalamine (41% vs 11%; *P* = 0.001) (RR = 3.80, 95% CI 1.19-12.2). The absolute benefit increase was 30%, and the number needed to treat (NNT) was 3. For patients with mild to moderately active CD, health-related quality of life also was improved to a greater extent after budesonide 9 mg/day than mesalamine 2 g twice daily.[17]

The composite findings provide evidence that budesonide is a more effective treatment option than mesalamine for patients with active CD of the ileum and right colon. Coupled with conclusions from a meta-analysis indicating the low therapeutic utility of mesalamine (Pentasa) for active Crohn's disease,[18] the results also provide support for recommendations[19,20] that budesonide and not mesalamine should be considered first-line therapy for the treatment of mild to moderately active Crohn's disease of the ileum and right colon.

BUDESONIDE VS PREDNISOLONE IN ADULTS

For patients with active Crohn's disease, the efficacy of budesonide 9 mg/day has been compared with prednisolone in 4 clinical trials of 8 to 12 weeks' duration (Table 13-2). Two studies[21,22] evaluated budesonide CIR and included patients with Crohn's disease restricted to the ileum or ileocecal region. In 2 other studies,[23,24] pH-modified budesonide was evaluated without restriction on disease location. Notwithstanding these differences in drug for-

mulation and disease location, the remission rates observed in the 4 trials were remarkably similar (see Table 13-2).

In a study by Rutgeerts et al,[21] remission rates at 8 weeks of 52% with budesonide CIR 9 mg/day and 65% with prednisolone 40 mg once daily for 2 weeks (tapered to 5 mg daily by the last week) were not statistically different (*P* = 0.12). However, the mean CDAI score was decreased to a greater extent in the prednisolone group (270 to 136) compared with the budesonide group (275 to 175) (*P* = 0.001). A randomized, 3-arm trial by Campieri et al[22] found after 8 weeks' treatment equivalent remission rates of 60% in patients receiving budesonide CIR 9 mg once daily or prednisolone 40 mg (tapered to 5 mg daily by the last week). Patients treated with budesonide CIR 4.5 mg twice daily had a lower remission rate of 42%, although the overall differences between groups were not statistically significant (*P* = 0.062). Together, the results from the 2 studies indicate that single-dose administration of budesonide CIR 9 mg daily is nearly as effective as prednisolone for the treatment of patients with ileal and/or right colon Crohn's disease.

Two clinical trials evaluated the efficacy of pH-modified budesonide compared with conventional corticosteroids (Table 13-2). Bar-Meier et al[23] compared budesonide 9 mg once daily with prednisone 40 mg/day (tapered after 2 weeks) and after 8 weeks' treatment found similar rates of remission of 51.0% and 52.5%, respectively (*P* = 0.8). For patients with disease localized only in the terminal ileum and/or right colon, budesonide was as effective as prednisone (55.6% vs 50%); however, budesonide seemed less effective than prednisone when the disease extended beyond the hepatic flexure (47% vs 62.5%). In the second study,[24] a higher dose of 6-methylprednisolone 48 mg/day (tapered after 2 weeks) appeared more effective than pH-modified budesonide 9 mg once daily with remission rates of 73% versus 56%, respectively, but the difference between groups was not statistically significant (see Table 13-2).

Two meta-analyses[14,25] have been undertaken to assess the effectiveness of oral budesonide compared with conventional corticosteroids for the treatment of active Crohn's disease. Papi et al[25] evaluated 4 studies[21-24] and found at 8 weeks 177 of the 341 patients (52%) receiving budesonide entered remission compared to 169 of 280 patients (60%) treated with conventional corticosteroids (Figure 13-4). The pooled rate difference for response to budesonide versus conventional corticosteroids was −8.5% (95% CI −1.64 to −0.7%; *P* = 0.02) and the NNT was 12. The results of the meta-analysis suggested that budesonide was slightly but significantly less effective than conventional corticosteroids for induction of remission in patients with active Crohn's disease of the ileum and right colon.

A more recent meta-analysis by Kane et al[14] evaluated the same 4 clinical trials[21-24] as Papi et al,[25] and also included a small trial[26] of budesonide 9 mg/day versus short-term methylprednisolone, although the latter study

TABLE 13-2

BUDESONIDE FOR INDUCTION OF REMISSION IN ACTIVE CROHN'S DISEASE*†

REFERENCE	TREATMENT REGIMEN (MG/DAY)	TREATMENT DURATION (WEEKS)	PATIENTS EVALUATED (N)	REMISSION (CDAI < 150) AT 8 WEEKS	RD (%) (95% CI)
COMPARISON WITH PLACEBO					BUDESONIDE VS PLACEBO
Greenberg et al[11]	Bud CIR 7.5 mg bid	8	258	28/64 43%	22.5 (10.6-34.3)
	Bud CIR 4.5 mg bid			31/61 51%	
	Bud CIR 3 mg od			22/67 33%	
	Placebo			13/66 20%	
Tremaine et al[12]	Bud CIR 9 mg od	8	197	37/79 48%	17.2 (−0.13 to 34.5)
	Bud CIR 4.5 mg bid			41/78 53%	
	Placebo			13/40 33%	
COMPARISON WITH PREDNISOLONE/ PREDNISONE					BUDESONIDE VS PREDNISOLONE/ PREDNISONE
Rutgeerts et al[21]	Bud CIR 9 mg od	10	176	46/88 52%	−12.5 (−26.9 to 1.9)
	Prednisolone 40 mg			57/88 65%	
Campieri et al[22]	Bud CIR 9 mg od	12	177	46/58 60%	−9.0 (−24.5 to 6.3)
	Bud CIR 4.5 mg bid			57/61 42%	
	Prednisolone 40 mg			57/58 60%	
Bar-Meier et al[23]	Bud pH mod 9 mg od	8	201	51/100 51%	−1.4 (−15.2 to 12.3)
	Prednisone 40 mg			53/101 52%	
Gross et al[24]	Bud pH mod 9 mg od	8	67	19/34 56%	−16.8 (−39.4 to 5.7)
	6-methylprednisolone 48 mg			24/33 73%	

*CDAI indicates Crohn's disease activity index; RD, rate difference; CI, confidence interval; CIR, controlled ileal response; bid, 2 times a day; od, 1 time a day.
†Adapted from Papi C, Luchetti R, Gili L, et al. Budesonide in the treatment of Crohn's disease: a meta-analysis. *Aliment Pharmacol Ther.* 2000;14:1419-1428.

was not designed to evaluate efficacy. The overall conclusions by Kane et al[14] were similar to the study by Papi et al[25] in that conventional corticosteroids induced the remission of CD more frequently than budesonide (RR = 0.87, 95% CI 0.76-0.995). A subgroup analysis of entry disease activity found that for patients with lower disease activity (entry CDAI 200-300), budesonide and conventional corticosteroids induced remission of active Crohn's disease at similar rates (RR = 0.91, 95% CI 0.77-1.07).

Thus, the composite data evaluating oral budesonide compared with conventional corticosteroids allow the following conclusions. For the treatment of patients with active Crohn's disease of the ileum and right colon, conventional corticosteroids such as prednisone and methylprednisolone are more effective than oral budesonide, although the absolute differences are small. Clinical outcomes are similar after treatment with either formulation of budesonide. For the subgroup of patients with mild to moderately active CD (entry CDAI < 300), budesonide is as effective as the conventional corticosteroids for induction of remission. For patients who present with more severe disease activity (entry CDAI > 300) or with involvement of disease beyond the right colon, however, conventional corticosteroids are likely to be a more effective treatment.

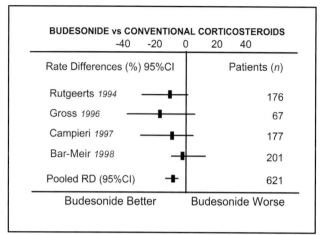

FIGURE 13-4. Rate differences (RD) of response in randomized controlled studies of budesonide versus conventional corticosteroids for inducing remission in active Crohn's disease. Remission was defined as a Crohn's Disease Activity Index score of 150 or less after 8 weeks of treatment. The pooled RD for response of budesonide versus conventional corticosteroids is –8.5% (95% CI –16.4 to –0.7%; *P* = 0.02). The number needed to treat is 12. (Reproduced with permission from Papi C, Luchetti R, Gili L, et al. Budesonide in the treatment of Crohn's disease: a meta-analysis. *Aliment Pharmacol Ther.* 2000;14:1419-1428.)

BUDESONIDE VS PREDNISONE IN CHILDREN

Oral budesonide has been evaluated in children with active Crohn's disease in 2 randomized, controlled trials. A study by Levine et al[27] of 33 children (mean age: 14.3 years) compared pH-modified budesonide 9 mg/day with prednisone 40 mg (tapered after 2 weeks) and at 12 weeks found similar remission rates of 47% and 50%, respectively. In a second trial[28] of 48 children (ages 6 to 16 years), budesonide CIR 9 mg/day was compared with prednisolone (1 mg/kg/day tapered after 4 weeks). After 8 weeks of treatment, the rate of remission in the budesonide group appeared lower than the prednisolone group (55% vs 71%), although the difference did not reach statistical significance (difference –16%; 95% CI –45 to 13; *P* = 0.25). The mean CDAI values at 8 weeks in the budesonide group did, however, remain higher compared with prednisolone (149 vs 97; *P* = 0.047). Therefore, as in adults, either of the 2 formulations of budesonide administered to children with mild to moderately active Crohn's disease of the ileum and right colon are nearly as effective as prednisolone for induction of remission.

BUDESONIDE VS BUDESONIDE PLUS ANTIBIOTICS

Recent experimental evidence suggests that an altered immune system to commensal enteric flora in a genetically susceptible host contributes to the development of intestinal inflammation in CD. The hypothesis that broad-spectrum antibiotics might enhance the efficacy of budesonide was evaluated in a double-blind study of patients with active CD of the ileum, right colon, or both.[29] Patients were randomized to receive oral ciprofloxacin and metro-

nidazole, both 500 mg twice daily, or placebo for 8 weeks, and all patients received budesonide 9 mg once daily. At 8 weeks, remission rates in the antibiotic group of 33% and in the placebo group of 38% were similar (absolute difference –5%, 95% CI –21% to 11%; *P* = 0.55). However, an interaction between treatment allocation and disease location was identified, as 53% of patients with Crohn's disease of the colon achieved remission with the addition of antibiotics compared with 25% of those who received placebo (*P* = 0.025). Therefore, the addition of metronidazole and ciprofloxacin to budesonide is ineffective therapy for patients with uncomplicated active CD restricted to the ileum, but this antibiotic-budesonide combination may improve outcome in patients who also have disease involvement of the colon. For the treatment of patients with ileocecal Crohn's disease complicated by an inflammatory mass, the addition of antibiotics, such as metronidazole and ciprofloxacin, warrants consideration to accelerate remission and avoid the potential for septic complications.

BUDESONIDE FOR MAINTENANCE TREATMENT OF CROHN'S DISEASE

The efficacy of oral budesonide as maintenance therapy for quiescent Crohn's disease has been evaluated with randomized, double-blind clinical trials comparing budesonide to placebo for maintenance of medically induced remission, for prevention of postoperative recurrence after ileocecal resection, and as replacement therapy of prednisolone for steroid-dependent patients.

MAINTENANCE OF MEDICALLY INDUCED REMISSION

The role of oral budesonide as maintenance treatment for patients with medically induced remission of Crohn's disease has been assessed with 4 clinical trials. Three of the trials compared budesonide CIR 3 or 6 mg once daily with placebo[30-32] and 1 trial[33] compared pH-modified budesonide 3 mg/day with placebo. After 1 year of treatment, the 4 trials showed similar results; budesonide, at the doses evaluated, was an ineffective intervention for maintenance of medically induced remission (Table 13-3). Although a life table analysis based on time to relapse or discontinuation of pooled data from 2 trials[30,31] indicated that budesonide CIR 6 mg/day increased the duration of remission compared with placebo, the response was not sustained at 1-year follow-up (Figure 13-5).

A meta-analysis[25] of the 4 trials[30-33] further supports the lack of benefit provided by budesonide administered as maintenance therapy after medically induced remission. Comprising a total of 449 patients, the meta-analysis showed relapse rates at 1 year of 57.7% for the 90 patients receiving budesonide 6 mg/day compared with 65.5% for 174 patients treated with budesonide 3 mg/day and 64.3% for 185 patients treated with placebo. The estimated common odds ratio for response to budesonide was 0.96%

TABLE 13-3

BUDESONIDE VS PLACEBO FOR PREVENTION OF CLINICAL RELAPSE IN QUIESCENT CROHN'S DISEASE*†

Reference	Treatment Regimen (mg/day)	Treatment Duration (months)	Patients Evaluated (N)	Relapse (CDAI > 150)	RD (%) (95% CI) Budesonide vs Placebo
Greenberg et al[30]	Bud CIR 3 mg	12	105	23/33 70%	-1.4 (-20.5 to 17.6)
	Bud CIR 6 mg			22/36 61%	
	Placebo			24/36 67%	
Lofberg et al[31]	Bud CIR 3 mg	12	90	23/31 74%	3.7 (-17.9 to 25.3)
	Bud CIR 6 mg			19/32 59%	
	Placebo			17/27 63%	
Ferguson et al[32]	Bud CIR 3 mg	12	75	12/26 46%	-11.3 (-34.6 to 11.9)
	Bud CIR 6 mg			11/22 48%	
	Placebo			16/27 60%	
Gross et al[33]	Bud pH mod 3 mg	12	179	56/84 67%	1.4 (-12.5 to 15.3)
	Placebo			62/95 65%	
				Pooled rate difference (95% CI)	-0.8 (-9.9 to 8.3)

*CDAI indicates Crohn's disease activity index; RD, rate difference; CI, confidence interval; CIR, controlled ileal release.
†Adapted from Papi C, Luchetti R, Gili L, et al. Budesonide in the treatment of Crohn's disease: a meta-analysis. *Aliment Pharmacol Ther.* 2000;14:1419-1428.

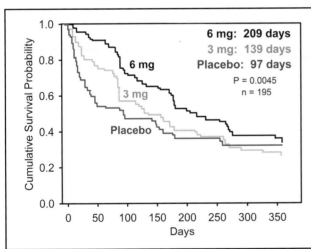

FIGURE 13-5. Life table analysis based on time to relapse or discontinuation for patients receiving budesonide or placebo as maintenance treatment for Crohn's disease. Results are pooled data from 2 separate trials undertaken in Canada (*n* = 105) and Europe (*n* = 95). (Data from Greenberg GR, Feagan BR, Martin F, et al. Oral budesonide as maintenance treatment for Crohn's disease: a placebo-controlled dose-ranging study. *Gastroenterology.* 1996;110:45-51; and Lofberg R, Rutgeerts P, Malchow H, et al. Budesonide prolongs time to relapse in ileal and ileocecal Crohn's disease. A placebo-controlled one year study. *Gut.* 1996;39:82-86.)

(95% CI 0.69-1.93), and the pooled rate difference for response to budesonide was −0.8% (95% CI −9.9 to 8.3%; *P* = 0.42).

The efficacy of budesonide CIR 6 mg/day has also been compared with a slow-release formulation of mesalamine (Pentasa) for maintenance of medically induced remission of Crohn's disease. Mantzaris et al[34] evaluated 57 patients with Crohn's disease who were eligible for maintenance therapy with azathioprine but were either intolerant to the drug (*n* = 36) or refused the treatment. At 1 year, the rate of relapse was significantly lower in the budesonide group than in the mesalamine group (55% vs 82%) (95% CI 12.4%-41%; *P* = 0.045). Budesonide also prolonged the period of remission compared with mesalamine (241 ± 114 days vs 147 ± 117 days) (95% CI 32.7-155.3; *P* = 0.003). Although the findings suggested that budesonide is more effective than mesalamine for maintenance of remission in patients with CD, it is noteworthy that the relapse rate at 1 year in the budesonide group of 55% was similar to the mean relapse rate of 57.7% observed for other budesonide maintenance trials,[25] and the values in turn are not different from the mean relapse rate of 64.3% observed for patients receiving placebo.

Because budesonide at a single daily dose of 6 mg is not beneficial for maintenance of medically induced remission, a multicenter, 1-year trial[35] was undertaken to address the question of whether a flexible dose regimen of 3, 6, or 9 mg once daily—adjusted according to the severity of Crohn's disease symptoms assessed at 13-week interval clinic visits—would be a more effective treatment strategy compared with a fixed budesonide dose at 6 mg once daily. At the 1-year follow-up, there was no difference between the 2 groups with a similar proportion of patients discontinued due to uncontrolled CD (flexible group: 38% versus fixed group: 37%; $P = 0.9$). Further, the average consumed dose of budesonide was comparable (flexible group: 5.8 mg versus fixed group: 6.0 mg). Therefore, a flexible dose schedule of budesonide to accommodate patients with intermittent increments of disease activity does not appear to provide any additional clinical benefit over a fixed-dose regimen for maintenance of remission up to 1 year.

Together, the results show budesonide at a dosage up to 6 mg/day is ineffective therapy for the prevention of relapse after medically induced remission in patients with Crohn's disease. The findings are similar to previous large, randomized clinical trials,[1,2] indicating the lack of benefit provided by low-dose treatment with prednisone or methylprednisolone for maintenance of remission. Whether long-term therapy with budesonide 9 mg/day, the minimum effective dose for active disease, prolongs remission without adverse effects has not been studied and requires prospective evaluation.

MAINTENANCE OF SURGICALLY INDUCED REMISSION

Two randomized, double-blind clinical trials[36,37] have been undertaken to evaluate whether oral budesonide is effective therapy for prevention of postoperative recurrence after ileal or ileocecal resection. Assessment of outcome included endoscopic recurrence, defined as a score of ≥ 2 according to an endoscopic scoring system,[38] and clinical recurrence, defined as an increase in CDAI score > 200. One trial[36] compared budesonide CIR 6 mg/day with placebo and found no difference in the frequency of endoscopic recurrence at 3 months (31% vs 35%) or at 12 months (52% vs 58%). However, at 12 months, the endoscopic recurrence rate for patients undergoing resection for disease activity was lower in the budesonide group compared with placebo (32% vs 65%; $P = 0.047$); the same difference was not observed for patients who required resection for fibrostenotic disease. The rates of clinical recurrence at 12 months were very similar in the budesonide and placebo groups (32% vs 31%), independent of the indication for surgery. A second trial[37] evaluated pH-modified budesonide 3 mg/day compared with placebo and also showed no differences at 1 year between the groups in the rates of endoscopic (47% vs 48%) or clinical (19% vs 28%) recurrence.

A meta-analysis[25] of the 2 trials found the pooled rate difference for response to budesonide versus placebo was −3.5% (95% CI −16.9 to 9.8%; $P = 0.3$) for prevention of endoscopic recurrence and −3.0% (95% CI −15.0% to 8.8%; $P = 0.33$) for prevention of clinical recurrence.

Thus, budesonide administered for 1 year at a daily dose of up to 6 mg is not effective for prevention of clinical recurrence of CD after ileocecal resection. The reduction of endoscopic recurrence found after budesonide treatment for patients undergoing resection for disease activity[36] is unlikely to impact long-term rates of clinical recurrence. The observation does suggest, however, that stratification by surgical indication may be a relevant requirement for future studies investigating other therapies for prevention of postoperative recurrence in Crohn's disease.

REPLACEMENT OF PREDNISOLONE WITH BUDESONIDE

Treatment with conventional corticosteroids is associated with a substantial spectrum of clinically relevant side effects.[4] Two studies[39,40] therefore examined the utility of replacement of prednisolone with oral budesonide in steroid-dependent patients with assessments of clinical outcome and rate of glucocorticosteroid-related side effects. In 1 double-blind trial,[39] patients receiving treatment with prednisolone (mean dose: 16.5 mg/day, range: 10 to 30 mg) were randomly assigned to budesonide CIR 6 mg/day or placebo for 12 weeks; the prednisolone was tapered to zero over the first 4 to 10 weeks. At 13 weeks, the rate of clinical relapse (CDAI > 200) was 32% in the budesonide group and 65% in the placebo group ($P < 0.001$). The median time to relapse was significantly longer for budesonide at > 160 days than for placebo at 75 days ($P < 0.001$). The initial dose of prednisolone and the use of azathioprine did not influence relapse rates. At 13 weeks, the number of glucocorticoid-related symptoms was similar in both groups and was reduced by 50% after prednisolone discontinuation.

In a second prospective, open-design trial,[40] patients receiving prednisolone (range: 5 to 30 mg daily) were treated with pH-modified budesonide 9 mg/day for 9 weeks and the prednisolone was tapered over the first 3 weeks. At 9 weeks, the remission rate for patients entered with active CD while receiving prednisolone was 38.6%; for patients entered with clinical remission on prednisolone, 78% maintained the remission after replacement with budesonide. The total number of glucocorticoid side effects related to prednisolone treatment was decreased by 67% after replacement with budesonide.

Thus, the results of the 2 studies[39,40] indicate that a substantial proportion of patients with ileocecal Crohn's disease who are conventional corticosteroid dependent may be switched to budesonide without loss of clinical response and with an important reduction in the incidence of glucocorticosteroid-related side effects. This therapeutic strategy may be of particular benefit to steroid-dependent patients for whom immunomodulators are ineffective or are not tolerated.

BUDESONIDE FOR EXTRA-INTESTINAL MANIFESTATIONS

The effect of budesonide on joint pain, a frequent extra-intestinal manifestation of active Crohn's disease, was evaluated in a retrospective analysis[41] of all patients reporting symptoms of arthralgia or arthritis (291 of 611 patients) at entry into 3 budesonide CIR trials.[11,21,22] The results showed a nearly 2-fold higher clinical remission of joint pain in the budesonide-treated group compared with placebo (74% vs 41%), and the rate was similar to the 72% remission observed for prednisolone-treated patients. Because the actions of budesonide on intestinal inflammation are predominantly local and not systemic, the findings regarding the benefit of budesonide for joint pain lend support to the notion that normalization of intestinal immune functions plays an important role in the management of extra-intestinal manifestations of Crohn's disease.

Ulceration of the oral buccal mucosa is another of the extra-intestinal manifestations that may be successfully managed with budesonide. The approach is to dissolve one budesonide 2.3-mg tablet into 100 cc of diluent (both provided in the rectal budesonide preparation; Entocort enema, AstraZeneca, Lund, Sweden); the mixture is taken orally, using a swish-and-swallow technique, once or twice daily for 7 to 14 days.

Active CD is known to negatively impact on linear growth in children. The mechanisms are not entirely elucidated, but disease activity, poor nutritional status, and administration of conventional corticosteroids are among the factors likely contributing to the growth retardation associated with Crohn's disease. A prospective, longitudinal study[42] therefore evaluated growth in 32 children treated with budesonide CIR 9 mg/day for 8 weeks followed by 6 mg/day for 6 to 13 months. Although a clinical response occurred in 59% of patients, the mean height velocity was only 2.3 ±1.0 cm/year, and none grew at a rate of more than 4 cm/year. Thus, notwithstanding the clinical benefit of budesonide for children with CD, subnormal growth persists. The mechanisms underlying these findings are unclear. The most likely explanation is less than optimal control of disease activity, as budesonide at 6 mg/day is an ineffective dose for maintenance of remission. An unrecognized secondary corticosteroid effect on growth associated with budesonide administration remains plausible but seems less likely.

Conventional corticosteroids increase water absorption and electrolyte transport in the intestinal mucosa, independent from any antiinflammatory effects. To evaluate whether budesonide causes similar effects, intestinal outputs were studied in quiescent CD patients with an ileostomy where the majority (31 of 34 patients) had no evidence of macroscopic disease.[43] After 8 days of treatment with pH-modified budesonide 3 mg 3 times daily, reduction of intestinal output was substantially greater than occurred with placebo (30.2% vs 0.3%), suggesting that budesonide improves absorptive capacity of the intestinal mucosa, independent of an antiinflammatory effect. Therefore, oral budesonide may provide an additional treatment option for patients who develop high intestinal outputs after intestinal resection. The results also point to a plausible mechanism distinct from an antiinflammatory action whereby budesonide improves bowel function in symptomatic Crohn's disease patients with an intact intestinal tract.

BUDESONIDE FOR ACTIVE ULCERATIVE COLITIS

Budesonide as an enema formulation has been extensively evaluated and shown to be efficacious for the treatment of distal ulcerative colitis involving the rectum and/or sigmoid colon. However, clinical trials examining the role of oral budesonide for the treatment of more extensive ulcerative colitis are limited. A study by Lofberg et al[44] randomized 72 patients with left-sided or more extensive UC to treatment with budesonide 10 mg/day formulated for delivery to the colon or prednisolone 40 mg/day (tapered after 2 weeks). After 9 weeks, a mean decrease in the overall endoscopic score was similar in budesonide and prednisolone groups (1.20 vs 1.36; P = 0.12). However, analysis of endoscopic colonic segments showed significantly greater improvement in the descending and sigmoid colon with the prednisolone group than the budesonide group (P = 0.04). Although budesonide was associated with treatment benefit, the results suggested the budesonide formulation employed in the study did not provide sufficient delivery of the active drug to the distal colon. The investigators proposed the requirement for a revised formulation with improved distribution to the left colon, but the product has not been developed for clinical investigation.

A smaller study[45] of 14 conventional steroid-dependent ulcerative colitis patients evaluated the efficacy of pH-modified budesonide 3 mg administered 3 times daily as a steroid-sparing agent. At 3 months, the results showed that 11 patients had the conventional steroids discontinued and clinical remission was maintained to 6 months with daily administration of budesonide.

Thus, oral budesonide appears to provide treatment benefit for patients with panulcerative colitis, but the controlled evidence is inadequate to draw firm conclusions regarding indications, dosage, or efficacy. Further clinical trials are required with new formulations of oral budesonide that achieve adequate distribution of the active drug to the entire colon. Areas of particular interest for study include ulcerative colitis patients who are intolerant or unresponsive to oral 5-aminosalicylic acid (5-ASA) preparations, develop major adverse effects to conventional corticosteroids, or are conventional corticosteroid dependent and intolerant or unresponsive to immunomodulators.

TABLE 13-4

BUDESONIDE VS PLACEBO FOR TREATMENT OF COLLAGENOUS COLITIS*

Reference	Treatment Regimen (mg/day)	Treatment Duration (weeks)	Patients Evaluated (N)	Clinical Remission (≤3 stools /d) (N)	P	Histologic Improvement (N)	P
Baert et al[47]	Bud pH mod 9 mg Placebo	8	28	8/14 57% 3/14 21%	0.05	14/14 100% 4/12 33%	0.05
Miehlke et al[48]	Bud CIR 9 mg Placebo	6	45	20/23 87% 3/22 14%	<0.001	14/23 61% 1/22 5%	<0.001
Bonderup et al[49]	Bud CIR 9 mg Placebo	8	20	10/10 100% 2/10 20%	<0.001	Inflammation grade score 2.3 to 1.0 1.9 to 1.5	<0.01 NS

*CIR indicates controlled ileal release; NS, not significant.

BUDESONIDE FOR COLLAGENOUS COLITIS

Collagenous colitis is a distinct form of colitis characterized by chronic watery diarrhea, normal endoscopy of the colon, and typical histologic features of diffuse thickening of the subepithelial collagen layer between the basement membrane with a lymphoplasmacytic infiltrate of the lamina propria.[46] Several treatment options have been advocated for collagenous colitis including mesalamine, antibiotics, prednisone, and bismuth subsalicylate but with only moderate degrees of success and with high relapse rates after discontinuation of therapy.[46] The efficacy of oral budesonide for patients with collagenous colitis has been evaluated with 3 clinical trials[47-49] comparing budesonide 9 mg/day with placebo. After 6 to 8 weeks, the studies found closely similar results—oral budesonide was highly effective for the treatment of collagenous colitis (Table 13-4). Together, the 3 trials comprising a total of 93 patients showed a rate of clinical remission (stool frequency ≤ 3 stools/day) for the budesonide group of 80.9% compared with 15.2% for the placebo group (95% CI 0.43-0.84; $P < 0.001$). A decrease of the lamina propria inflammatory infiltrate[47] and reduction of the thickness of the collagen band[49] were also higher in the budesonide groups than in patients receiving placebo. Long-term follow-up data are limited, but preliminary experience from pilot studies[50,51] suggests that the clinical remission may last up to 1 year in some patients or can be maintained with a rather low dose of budesonide at 3 mg/day. Placebo-controlled trials[47,49] reporting short-term follow-up indicate relapse rates of 63% to 80% at 8 weeks after discontinuation of budesonide.

Therefore, oral budesonide is highly effective therapy for patients with collagenous colitis, but the risk of relapse after cessation of therapy appears high, and long-term administration of budesonide may be a requirement for the majority of patients. How oral budesonide, particularly the budesonide CIR formulation, causes improvement is unclear because involvement of the entire colon is usual with collagenous colitis. Reduced net Na^+ and Cl^- absorption, accompanied by active chloride secretion, is a major mechanism contributing to the diarrhea in collagenous colitis,[52] and, notably, oral budesonide causes direct and reversible improvement of water and electrolyte transport capacity in the intestinal mucosa.[43] Thus, in addition to the anti-inflammatory actions of budesonide, effects on water and electrolyte transport may account for the clinical improvement observed in patients with collagenous colitis.

ADVERSE EVENT PROFILE

The tolerability of budesonide has been evaluated in clinical trials by assessment of general adverse events, effects on metabolic functions, clinical corticosteroid-related symptoms and signs, and effects on bone loss.

GENERAL ADVERSE EVENTS

Controlled trials evaluating clinical outcomes after budesonide treatment (see Tables 13-2 and 13-4) provide supporting evidence to indicate whether the drug is generally well tolerated. The incidence of general adverse events is similar to placebo and to treatment with mesalamine. Importantly, as discussed in further detail later, corticosteroid-related clinical effects associated with budesonide are significantly lower than those that occur with prednisone treatment and are similar to patients receiving placebo. Further, a multinational, multicenter, uncontrolled, open-label study[53] evaluated 4092 patients who received oral budesonide for up to 5 years at daily doses of 2 to 21 mg, with 9 mg the most commonly used dose. Serious adverse events were found in only 3% of patients, most of which were gastrointestinal, and < 0.24% were considered treatment related.

EFFECTS ON METABOLIC FUNCTIONS AND CORTICOSTEROID-RELATED CLINICAL EVENTS

In controlled trials, changes in basal and adrenocorticotropic hormone (ACTH)-stimulated plasma cortisol levels were evaluated as a measure of systemic corticosteroid activity and for the assessment of the potential for causing adverse effects. Budesonide administered for up to 10 weeks at doses of 9 and 15 mg/day caused a mean plasma reduction of cortisol levels greater than placebo[11] but significantly less than occurred after treatment with prednisolone.[21,22] The proportion of patients with a mean plasma cortisol below 150 nmol/L was also significantly higher in patients receiving prednisolone than in those receiving budesonide.[21,22] Oral budesonide 9 mg/day impairs the response to ACTH greater than placebo (50% vs 19%; $P = 0.006$) but causes less suppression when compared with prednisolone (42% vs 84%; $P = 0.013$).[11,21,22]

Clinical trials show that the overall incidence of glucocorticosteroid-related adverse events is not different between budesonide 9 mg/day and placebo-treated patients after 8 weeks' administration.[11,12] In only 1 study,[11] moon face was more common in patients treated with budesonide at 3, 9, or 15 mg/day than placebo (17% vs 2%; $P = 0.001$). The incidence of glucocorticosteroid-related adverse events was not different between budesonide 9 mg/day and mesalamine-treated patients after 16 weeks' administration.[16] In contrast, after 10 weeks' treatment, glucocorticosteroid-related adverse events observed in patients receiving prednisolone were significantly more frequent than for patients receiving budesonide 9 mg daily. A meta-analysis[25] of 341 patients treated for active Crohn's disease found at least 1 corticosteroid-related adverse event in 41% of patients receiving budesonide compared with 62% of patients treated with conventional corticosteroids (odds ratio [OR]= 0.42, 95% CI 0.30-0.58). The rate difference of glucocorticosteroid-related adverse effects in the budesonide-treated patients was −22.4% (95% CI −32 to −12.8%; $P < 0.01$), and the NNT was 5. In longer-term maintenance trials, of 370 patients receiving budesonide 3 to 6 mg/day, the occurrence of at least 1 corticosteroid-related adverse effect was similar in budesonide and placebo-treated patients (23% vs 19%; rate difference [RD] 5.3%, 95% CI −3.9% to 14.5%; $P = 0.30$) after 1 year of treatment.[25]

Hematological and biochemical parameters assessed in clinical trials did not differ between patients receiving budesonide 3 to 15 mg/day and those receiving placebo. One case of severe hypokalemia has been reported in an 18-year-old patient with Crohn's disease after treatment with budesonide 9 mg/day.[54] Symptoms resolved, and serum potassium normalized with cessation of budesonide and potassium supplementation.

Benign intracranial hypertension, rarely associated with conventional corticosteroid therapy, has been reported in 3 adolescents with CD and poor nutritional status who received treatment with budesonide.[55] Symptoms of headache resolved upon withdrawal of budesonide and did not recur with subsequent use of prednisone. Conversely, severe neuropsychiatric symptoms occurring in patients with CD receiving prednisone are abrogated by cessation of prednisone and replacement with budesonide 9 mg/day, with control of the disease activity.[56,57]

Thus, the incidence of clinically relevant glucocorticosteroid-related adverse events is not different between patients receiving budesonide and placebo, but biochemical adrenal function is impaired in approximately 50% of budesonide-treated patients. Clinical practice guidelines employed for conventional corticosteroid therapy should, therefore, also be followed for treatment with budesonide. To avoid possible effects of adrenal suppression, before discontinuation of therapy, tapering of the dosage of budesonide to 6 mg/day for 1 week followed by 3 mg/day for 1 week may be considered. For budesonide-treated patients who encounter surgical emergencies, short-term supplementation with conventional corticosteroids is required. Budesonide, as a replacement therapy for prednisone, generally should be initiated only after the prednisone dose has been tapered to ≤ 15 mg/day. Additional clinical monitoring is warranted for budesonide-treated patients with hypertension, diabetes mellitus, and/or cataracts.

EFFECTS ON BONE DENSITY

Reduction of bone mineral density is a recognized complication of Crohn's disease.[58] The mechanisms contributing to bone loss are unclear, but factors implicated include a direct effect of proinflammatory cytokines and administration of corticosteroids. Conventional systemic steroid therapy causes preferential loss of trabecular bone relative to cortical bone, and this effect occurs predominantly in the first 12 months of therapy.[59] Four studies[23,26,60,61] have evaluated parameters related to bone loss in CD patients receiving treatment with budesonide. After 8 weeks' treatment, serum osteocalcin (a marker of osteoblast activity) did not change with budesonide CIR[26] or pH-modified budesonide[23] at 9 mg/day, but in 1 study,[26] serum osteocalcin was significantly suppressed after treatment with methylprednisolone. Budesonide or methylprednisolone did not change urinary pyridinolines and deoxypyridinolines, markers of bone degradation.[26] Therefore, in contrast to short-term treatment with methylprednisolone, budesonide does not impair osteoblast activity in patients with CD.

A 2-year prospective annual evaluation of bone mineral density in patients with quiescent CD was undertaken to examine a comparison of patients treated with mean daily doses of 8.5 mg budesonide CIR, 10.5 mg prednisone, or nonsteroid drugs.[60] Between baseline and 1 year, a mean decrease of 2.36% occurred at the lumbar spine in the budesonide group compared with 0.61% in the prednisone group and 0.09% in the nonsteroid group. The difference between budesonide and nonsteroid groups was significant ($P = 0.003$). At the femoral neck, no differences occurred between the 3 groups at the 2-year follow-up. However, the proportion of patients with bone loss of > 2% per annum at the lumbar spine and at the femoral neck was higher in the budesonide group than in the nonsteroid group ($P < 0.01$) and the prednisone group ($P < 0.05$). A second 2-year prospective study[61] indicated that steroid-naïve active Crohn's disease patients showed less bone loss after treatment with budesonide CIR than with prednisolone; no differences occurred between budesonide-treated patients and previously steroid-treated or steroid-dependent patients.

Together, the results suggest that short-term budesonide treatment does not impact on bone metabolism. Patients with Crohn's disease receiving long-term treatment with oral budesonide may incur bone loss, however, particularly at the lumber spine, in the first year of treatment. Therefore, with long-term budesonide therapy, evaluation of annual bone density and administration of calcium and vitamin D supplementation warrants consideration.

CONCLUSION

Oral budesonide is an effective drug for the treatment of adults and children with mild to moderately active Crohn's disease involving the ileum and/or right colon. The optimal dose of budesonide required to achieve induction of remission is 9 mg, administered once daily for 8 weeks. For patients who derive clinical improvement, but not complete remission, a further 8 weeks of therapy may be considered. In the absence of a clinical response, there is no benefit in continuing therapy beyond 2 months. Because biochemical adrenal suppression may occur after budesonide treatment, a 2-week dose-tapering schedule before discontinuation of therapy may be considered. Patients who encounter surgical emergencies require short-term supplementation with conventional corticosteroids.

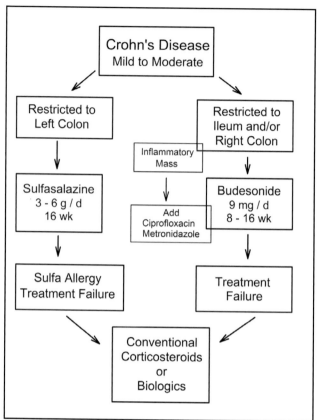

FIGURE 13-6. Algorithm for induction of remission in patients with mild to moderately active Crohn's disease.

Compared with mesalamine (Pentasa), budesonide causes a rate of remission that is more rapid and more effective, and the adverse event profiles are similar. Mesalamine is often employed as the initial treatment for active Crohn's disease, but the marginal efficacy casts doubt on the utility of this strategy. Rather, evidence-based analysis leads to the conclusion that budesonide should now be considered as the first-line treatment for induction of remission of mild to moderately active Crohn's disease in patients with involvement of the ileum and/or right colon (Figure 13-6).

Budesonide is only marginally less effective than the standard conventional corticosteroids: prednisone, prednisolone, and 6-methylprednisolone. Further, when compared to conventional corticosteroids, budesonide is associated with a significantly lower frequency of glucocorticosteroid-associated adverse events that is not different from the frequency observed in patients treated with placebo. The improved efficacy/adverse event ratio of budesonide compared with conventional corticosteroids implies that prednisone should be considered only after failure of treatment with budesonide (see Figure 13-6). Budesonide can also replace prednisone and thus be of benefit to patients unable to taper off of conventional corticosteroid therapy.

Budesonide at a dose of 6 mg daily is an ineffective intervention for maintenance of medically induced remission and for prevention of postoperative recurrence after ileocecal resection. Whether a higher maintenance dose of 9 mg/day prolongs the time to clinical relapse in these settings has not been evaluated but warrants study. Assessment of clinical efficacy and evaluation of adverse events, notably effects on bone loss, are both areas of interest.

For the treatment of panulcerative colitis, controlled evidence in support of a role for oral budesonide is limited. For this indication, the one oral formulation available in North America, budesonide CIR (Entocort), has not been evaluated but is unlikely to be helpful given its pharmacoscintographic characteristics. The pH-modified formulation of budesonide, Budenofalk (available only in Europe), may provide benefit for selected patients with panulcerative colitis but requires further controlled evaluation. Conclusions regarding indications, dosage, and efficacy for patients with panulcerative colitis await additional controlled clinical trials with new formulations of oral budesonide that achieve adequate distribution of the active drug to the entire colon.

For the treatment of collagenous colitis, budesonide is highly effective, and the drug should now be considered first-line therapy for this condition. Relapse rates appear high after discontinuation of treatment, however, necessitating clinical follow-up and the possible requirement for long-term budesonide therapy.

REFERENCES

1. Summers RW, Switz DM, Sessions JT, et al. National Cooperative Crohn's Disease Study: results of drug treatment. *Gastroenterology.* 1979;77:847-869.

2. Malchow H, Ewe K, Brandes JW, et al. European Cooperative Crohn's Disease Study (ECDDS): results of drug treatment. *Gastroenterology.* 1984;86:249-266.

3. Modigliani R, Mary JY, Simon JF, et al. Clinical, biological and endoscopic picture of attacks of Crohn's disease. Evolution on prednisolone. *Gastroenterology.* 1990;98:811-818.

4. Rutgeerts PJ. The limitations of cortocosteroid therapy in Crohn's disease. *Aliment Pharmacol Ther.* 2001;15:1515-1525.

5. Brattsand R. Overview of newer glucocorticoid preparations for inflammatory bowel disease. *Can J Gastroenterol.* 1990;4:407-414.

6. Miller-Larsson A, Gustafsson, B, Jerre A, et al. Topical anti-inflammatory activity of budesonide (Entocort®) in intestinal tissue may be prolonged due to budesonide reversible esterification [abstract]. *Gut.* 2002;51(suppl 3):A 305.

7. Edsbächer S, Bengtsson B, Larsson P, et al. A pharmacoscintographic evaluation of oral budesonide given as controlled-release (Entocort) capsules. *Aliment Pharmacol Ther.* 2003;17:525-536.

8. Lundin PDP, Edsbächer S, Bergstend M, et al. Pharmacokinetics of budesonide controlled release capsules in children and adults with active Crohn's disease. *Aliment Pharmacol Ther.* 2003;17:85-92.

9. Lundin P, Naber T, Nilsson M, Edsbächer S, et al. Effect of food on the pharmacokinetics of budesonide controlled ileal release capsules in patients with active Crohn's disease. *Aliment Pharmacol Ther.* 2001;15:45-51.

10. Möllmann HW, Hochhaus G, Tromm A, et al. Pharmacokinetics and evaluation of systemic side effects after oral administration of modified release capsules in healthy volunteers, ileostoma patients and patients with Crohn's disease [abstract]. *Gastroenterology.* 1996;110:A972.

11. Greenberg GR, Feagan BG, Martin F, et al. Oral budesonide for active Crohn's disease. *N Engl J Med.* 1994;331:836-841.

12. Tremaine W, Hanauer S, Katz S, et al. Budesonide CIR capsules (once or twice daily divided-dose) in active Crohn's disease. A randomized placebo-controlled study in the United States. *Am J Gastroenterol.* 2002;97:1748-1754.

13. Irvine EJ, Greenberg GR, Fegan BG, et al. Quality of life improves with budesonide therapy for active Crohn's disease. Canadian Inflammatory Bowel Disease Study Group. *Inflamm Bowel Dis.* 2000;6:181-187.

14. Kane SV, Schoenfeld P, Sandborn WJ, et al. The effectiveness of budesonide therapy for Crohn's disease. *Aliment Pharmacol Ther.* 2002;16:1509-1517.

15. Herfarth H, Gross V, Andus T, et al. Analysis of the therapeutic efficacy of budesonide in patients with active Crohn's ileocolitis depending on disease activity and localization. *Int J Colorectal Dis.* 2004;19:147-152.

16. Thomsen OØ, Cortot A, Jewell D, et al. A comparison of budesonide and mesalamine for active Crohn's disease. *N Engl J Med.* 1998;339:370-374.

17. Thomsen OØ, Cortot A, Jewell D, et al. Budesonide and mesalamine in active Crohn's disease. A comparison of the effects on quality of life. *Am. J Gastroenterol.* 2002;97:649-653.

18. Hanauer SB, Strömberg U. Oral Pentasa in the treatment of active Crohn's disease: a meta-analysis of double-blind, placebo-controlled trials. *Clin Gastroenterol Hepatol.* 2004;2:379-388.

19. Feagan BG. 5-ASA therapy for active Crohn's disease: old friends, old data and a new conclusion. *Clin Gastroenterol Hepatol.* 2004; 2:376-378.

20. Sandborn WJ, Feagan BG. Mild to moderate Crohn's disease: Defining the basis for a new treatment algorithm. *Aliment Pharmacol Ther.* 2003;18:263-277.

21. Rutgeerts P, Lofberg R, Malchow H, et al. A comparison of budesonide with prednisolone for active Crohn's disease. *N Engl J Med.* 1994;331:842-845.

22. Campieri M, Ferguson A, Doe W, et al. Oral budesonide is as effective as oral prednisolone in active Crohn's disease. *Gut.* 1997; 41:209-214.

23. Bar-Meir S, Chowers Y, Lavy A, et al. Budesonide versus prednisone in the treatment of active Crohn's disease. *Gastroenterology.* 1998;115:835-840.

24. Gross V, Andus T, Caesar I, et al. Oral pH modified release budesonide versus 6-methylprednisolone in active Crohn's disease. *Eur J Gastroenterol Hepatol.* 1996;8:905-910.

25. Papi C, Luchetti R, Gili L, et al. Budesonide in the treatment of Crohn's disease: A meta-analysis. *Aliment Pharmacol Ther.* 2000; 14:1419-1428.

26. D'Haens G, Verstraete A, Cheyns K, et al. Bone turnover during short-term therapy with methylprednisolone or budesonide in Crohn's disease. *Aliment Pharmacol Ther.* 1998;12:419-424.

27. Levine A, Weizman Z, Broide E, et al. A comparison of budesonide and prednisone for the treatment of active pediatric Crohn's disease. *J Pediatr Gastroenterol Nutr.* 2003;36:248-252.

28. Escher JC and the European Collaborative Research Group on Budesonide in Paediatric IBD. Budesonide versus prednisolone for the treatment of active Crohn's disease in children: a randomized, double-blind, controlled, multicentre trial. *Eur J Gastroenterol Hepatol.* 2004;16:47-54.

29. Steinhart AH, Feagan BG, Wong CJ, et al. Combined budesonide and antibiotic therapy for active Crohn's disease: A randomized controlled trial. *Gastroenterology.* 2002;123:33-40.

30. Greenberg GR, Feagan BR, Martin F, et al. Oral budesonide as maintenance treatment for Crohn's disease: a placebo-controlled dose-ranging study. *Gastroenterology.* 1996;110:45-51.

31. Lofberg R, Rutgeerts P, Malchow H, et al. Budesonide prolongs time to relapse in ileal and ileocecal Crohn's disease. a placebo-controlled one year study. *Gut.* 1996;39:82-86.

32. Ferguson A, Campieri M, Doe W, et al. Oral budesonide as maintenance therapy in Crohn's disease: results of a 12 month study. *Aliment Pharmacol Ther.* 1998;12:175-183.

33. Gross V, Andus T, Ecker KW, et al. Low dose oral pH modified release budesonide for maintenance of steroid induced remission in Crohn's disease. *Gut.* 1998;42:493-496.

34. Mantzaris GJ, Petraki K, Sfakianakis M, et al. Budesonide versus mesalamine for maintaining remission in patients refusing other modulators for steroid-dependent Crohn's disease. *J Clin Gastroenterol Hepatol.* 2003;1:122-128.

35. Green JRB, Lobo AJ, Giaffer M, et al. Maintenance of Crohn's disease over 12 months: fixed versus flexible dosing regimen using budesonide controlled release capsules. *Aliment Pharmacol Ther.* 2001;15:1331-1341.

36. Hellers G, Cortot A, Jewell D, et al. Oral budesonide for prevention of post-surgical recurrence in Crohn's disease. *Gastroenterology.* 1999;116:294-300.

37. Ewe K, Bottger T, Buhr HJ, et al. Low dose budesonide treatment for prevention of postoperative recurrence of Crohn's disease: a multicentre randomized placebo-controlled trial. *Eur J Gastroenterol Hepatol.* 1999;11:277-282.

38. Rutgeerts P, Geboes K, Vantrappen G, et al. Predictability of the postoperative course of Crohn's disease. *Gastroenterology.* 1990;99:956-963.

39. Cortot A, Colombel FJ, Rutgeerts P, et al. Switch from systemic steroids to budesonide in steroid-dependent patients with inactive Crohn's disease. *Gut.* 2001;48:86-90.

40. Andus T, Gross V, Caesar I, et al. Replacement of conventional glucocorticoids by oral pH-modified release budesonide in active and inactive Crohn's disease. Results of an open, prospective, multicenter trial. *Dig Dis Sci.* 2003;48:373-378.

41. Florin TH, Graffner H, Nilsson LG, et al. Treatment of joint pain in Crohn's patients with budesonide controlled ileal release. *Clin Exp Pharmacol Physiol.* 2000;27:295-298.

42. Kundhal P, Zachos M, Holmes JL, et al. Controlled ileal release budesonide in pediatric Crohn's disease: efficacy and effect on growth. *J Pediatr Gastroenterol Nutr.* 2001;33:75-80.

43. Ecker KW, Stallmach A, Seitz G, et al. Oral budesonide significantly improves water absorption in patients with ileostomy for Crohn's disease. *Scand J Gastroenterol.* 2003;288:293-298.

44. Lofberg R, Danielsson A, Suhr O, et al. Oral budesonide versus prednisolone in patients with active extensive and left-sided ulcerative colitis. *Gastroenterology.* 1996;110:1713-1718.

45. Keller R, Stoll R, Foerser EC, et al. Oral budesonide therapy for steroid-dependent ulcerative colitis: a pilot trial. *Aliment Pharmacol Ther.* 1997;11:1047-1052.

46. Zins BJ, Sandborn WJ, Tremaine WJ. Collagenous and lymphocytic colitis: subject review and therapeutic alternatives. *Am J Gastroenterol.* 1995;90:1394-1400.

47. Baert F, Schmidt A, D'Haens G, et al. Budesonide in collagenous colitis: a double-blind placebo-controlled trial with histologic follow-up. *Gastroenterology.* 2002;122:20-25.

48. Miehlke S, Heymer P, Bethke B, et al. Budesonide treatment for collagenous colitis: a randomized double-blind, placebo-controlled, multicenter trial. *Gastroenterology.* 2002;123:978-984.

49. Bonderup OK, Hansen JB, Birket-Smith L, et al. Budesonide treatment of collagenous colitis: a randomized, double-blind, placebo controlled trial with morphometric analysis. *Gut.* 2003;52:248-251.

50. Tromm A, Griga T, Möllman HW, et al. Budesonide for the treatment of collagenous colitis: first results of a pilot trial. *Am J Gastroenterol.* 1999;94:1871-1875.

51. Bohr J, Olesen M, Tysk C, et al. Budesonide and bismuth in microscopic colitis. *Int J Colorectal Dis.* 1999;14;58-61.

52. Bürgel N, Bojarski C, Mankertz J, et al. Mechanisms of diarrhea in collagenous colitis. *Gastroenterology.* 2002;123:433-443.

53. Lyckegaard E, Hakansson K, Bengtsson B. Compassionate use of budesonide capsules (Entocort® EC) in patients with Crohn's disease [abstract]. *Gastroenterology.* 2002;122(T-1665):A-500.

54. Rosenbach Y, Zahavi I, Rachmal A, et al. Severe hypokalemia after budesonide treatment for Crohn's disease. *J Pediatr Gastroenterol Nutr.* 1997;24:352-355.

55. Levine A, Watenberg N, Hager H. Benign intracranial hypertension associated with budesonide treatment in children with Crohn's disease. *J Chil Neurol.* 2001;16:458-461.

56. Nahon S, Pisante L, Delas N. A successful switch from prednisone to budesonide for neuropsychiatric adverse effects in a patient with ileal Crohn's disease. *Am J Gastroenterol.* 2001;96:1953-1954.

57. Sandborn W, Bengtsson B. Budesonide capsules (Entocort® EC) decrease the frequency of psychiatric adverse events compared with prednisolone in Crohn's disease patients [abstract]. *Gastroenterology.* 2002;122(T-1664):A-500.

58. Lichenstein GR. Evaluation of bone mineral density in inflammatory bowel disease: current safety focus. *Am J Gastroenterol.* 2003;98(suppl):S24-S30.

59. Laan RFJM, van Riel PLCM, van de Putte, et al. Low dose prednisone induces rapid reversible axial bone loss in patients with rheumatoid arthritis. *Ann Intern Med.* 1993;119:963-968.

60. Cino M, Greenberg GR. Bone mineral density in Crohn's disease: a longitudinal study of budesonide, prednisone and non-steroid therapy. *Am J Gastroenterol.* 2002;97:915-920.

61. Schoon EJ, Bollani S, Mills PR, et al. Bone mineral density in relation to efficacy and side effects of budesonide and prednisolone in Crohn's disease. *Clin Gastroenterol Hepatol.* 2005;3(2):113-121.

6-MERCAPTOPURINE AND AZATHIOPRINE IN CROHN'S DISEASE

Mark T. Osterman, MD and Gary R. Lichtenstein, MD, FACP, FACG, AGAF

Since its initial use for treatment of patients with CD in an uncontrolled study by Brooke et al in 1969,[1] 6-mercaptopurine (6-MP) and its derivative azathioprine (AZA) have gained popular acceptance and are now standard therapy for many patients with inflammatory bowel disease (IBD), particularly those with CD. As thiopurine analogues, 6-MP and AZA are potent immunomodulators used to control the dysregulated immune response in IBD. These medications are not only efficacious in inducing and maintaining clinical remission but they appear to aid in the sparing or cessation of corticosteroids; in the postoperative setting to maintain remission; in the healing and closure of fistulae; in minimizing antibody formation against infliximab, adalimumab, certolizumab, and other biologic therapies; and in mucosal healing. Although 6-MP and AZA are widely used by many physicians throughout the world to treat IBD, there is a great deal of heterogeneity in the clinical administration of these medications. This variation can most likely be attributed to the limited data on dosing and duration of use of these agents. In addition, specific guidelines regarding monitoring of 6-MP and AZA metabolite levels are lacking, although a number of retrospective studies addressing this issue have been published.

In this chapter, the clinical efficacy of 6-MP and AZA in CD will be discussed at length first. Specifically, clinical trial data regarding their use in the induction of remission, maintenance of remission (including postoperative), treatment of fistulizing disease, corticosteroid sparing, and minimization of immunogenicity to infliximab will be addressed. The other main section of the chapter will be devoted to the pharmacology of 6-MP and AZA. The metabolism, mechanism of action, pharmacokinetics, monitoring of metabolite levels, dosing and duration

of therapy, adverse effects, safety in pregnancy, and drug interactions with these agents will be reviewed.

CLINICAL EFFICACY

The clinical efficacy of 6-MP and AZA has been fairly well studied in IBD, particularly in CD (for which many of the clinical trials have been performed). These medications are currently indicated in CD in the following settings: induction of remission for moderate to severe active disease, maintenance of remission (including in the postoperative setting), treatment of fistulizing CD, sparing of corticosteroids, and minimization of immunogenicity to infliximab adalimumab and other biologics.

INDUCTION OF REMISSION

A number of studies, both uncontrolled and controlled, have been performed with respect to induction of remission with 6-MP or AZA in patients with active CD. To date, 8 randomized controlled trials focusing on the treatment of active CD have been published (Table 14-1).[2-9] Taken individually, these studies report a wide range of clinical efficacies with 6-MP and AZA for induction of remission in patients with moderate to severe active CD. An improvement with 6-MP or AZA compared to placebo was observed in 5 of the studies,[2,5-8] 2 of which demonstrated statistical significance[6,7] and another of which also would likely have shown statistical significance had a statistical test been performed.[2] However, one must be cognizant of the fact that these studies are rather heterogeneous with respect to study design; specifically, the number of patients included,

Lichtenstein GR, ed.
Crohn's Disease: The Complete Guide to Medical Management (pp 157-176).
© 2011 SLACK Incorporated

TABLE 14-1

RANDOMIZED CONTROLLED TRIALS FOR INDUCTION OF REMISSION WITH 6-MP OR AZA IN ACTIVE CROHN'S DISEASE*

Author (Year)	N	Drug Dose	Length of Rx	Response 6-MP/AZA	Response Placebo	P value	Co-therapy 5-ASA/ Steroids
Willoughby (1971)	12	AZA 2 mg/kg/day	24 weeks	6/6 (100%)	1/6 (17%)	NR	Steroids in all
Rhodes (1971)	16	AZA 2 mg/kg/day	2 months	0/9 (0%)	0/7 (0%)	NR	5-ASA in 3 Steroids in 3
Klein (1974)	26	AZA 3 mg/kg/day	4 months	6/13 (46%)	6/13 (46%)	NR	Steroids in 17
Summers (1979) (Part I, Phase 1)	136	AZA 2.5 mg/kg/day	17 weeks	21/59 (36%)	20/77 (26%)	0.25	No
Present (1980)	72	6-MP 1.5 mg/kg/day	1 year	26/36 (72%)	5/36 (14%)	<0.001	5-ASA in 43 Steroids in 60
Ewe (1993)	42	AZA 2.5 mg/kg/day	4 months	16/21 (76%)	8/21 (38%)	0.03	Steroids in all
Candy (1995)	63	AZA 2.5 mg/kg/day	12 weeks	24/33 (73%)	19/30 (63%)	0.6	Steroids in all
Oren (1997)	58	6-MP 50 mg/day	9 months	13/32 (41%)	12/26 (46%)	NS	5-ASA in 39 Steroids in 45

*6-MP indicates 6-mercaptopurine; AZA, azathioprine; 5-ASA, 5-aminosalicylic acid; NR, not reported; NS, not significant.

disease extent and location (small versus large bowel), presence of fistulizing disease, prior abdominal surgery, choice of 6-MP or AZA, dosage of medication, duration of therapy, concomitant or prior treatment with 5-amino-salicylic acid (5-ASA) or corticosteroids, and definition of treatment response and clinical remission (various clinical, laboratory, radiographic, and endoscopic markers and disease activity indices were used in these studies). For this reason, it is not very surprising that different results were obtained and different conclusions were drawn.

When looking at the data collectively, however, it is clear that 6-MP and AZA have efficacy in the treatment of active CD. A meta-analysis evaluated the first 7 of these randomized controlled trials and found that 6-MP and AZA were more efficacious than placebo in achieving clinical remission.[10] The authors reported an overall response rate (defined as clinical improvement or remission) of 56% in patients taking 6-MP or AZA compared to 32% in patients taking placebo. The corresponding pooled odds ratio for response was 3.09 (95% confidence interval [CI] 2.45-3.91) with 6-MP or AZA compared to placebo. In addition, the meta-analysis reported a statistically significant increase in response with increasing duration of therapy. Studies

of longer duration also tended to cite higher response rates with 6-MP or AZA ($P = 0.03$). The authors felt that 17 weeks of treatment appeared to be the minimum period of time for an adequate trial of 6-MP or AZA. A more recent meta-analysis, which included all 8 randomized controlled trials, reported a slightly lower pooled odds ratio of 2.36 (95% CI 1.57-3.53) with a corresponding number needed to treat of only 5 patients.[11] Thus, the current available data indicate that 6-MP and AZA have clinical efficacy in inducing remission for patients with moderate to severe active CD.

Another important factor to consider is that in 6 of the 8 randomized controlled trials, the majority of patients were concomitantly taking 5-ASA compounds, corticosteroids, or both. The National Cooperative Crohn's Disease Study was the only one of these trials to compare monotherapy with AZA to placebo.[5] In this study, although the response rate was higher in patients taking AZA, the difference did not attain statistical significance. Hence, it is likely that 6-MP and AZA have their greatest clinical utility and most appropriate applicability in the setting of cotherapy with other medications used to treat CD.

TABLE 14-2

RANDOMIZED CONTROLLED TRIALS FOR MAINTENANCE OF REMISSION WITH 6-MP OR AZA IN CROHN'S DISEASE*

AUTHOR (YEAR)	N	DRUG DOSE	LENGTH OF RX	RESPONSE 6-MP/AZA	RESPONSE PLACEBO	P VALUE	REMISSION INDUCED BY
Willoughby (1971)	10	AZA 2 mg/kg/day	24 weeks	4/5 (80%)	2/5 (40%)	NR	Steroids ± AZA
Rosenberg (1975)	20	AZA 2 mg/kg/day	26 weeks	8/10 (80%)	5/10 (50%)	NR	Steroids
O'Donoghue (1978)	51	AZA 2 mg/kg/day	1 year	13/24 (54%)	8/27 (30%)	<0.01	AZA ± steroids/5-ASA
Summers (1979) (Part I, Phase 2)	39	AZA 2.5 mg/kg/day	35 weeks	16/19 (84%)	15/20 (75%)	NS	AZA or placebo
Summers (1979) (Part II)	155	AZA 1 mg/kg/day	1 year	37/54 (69%)	65/101 (64%)	0.53	Any drug or surgery
Candy (1995)	43	AZA 2.5 mg/kg/day	12 months	14/24 (58%)	2/19 (11%)	0.001	Steroids ± AZA/placebo

*6-MP indicates 6-mercaptopurine; AZA, azathioprine; 5-ASA, 5-aminosalicylic acid; NR, not reported; NS, not significant.

MAINTENANCE OF REMISSION

AZA has also been studied with regard to maintenance of remission in CD. To date in adults, 6 randomized controlled trials have been published to address this issue (Table 14-2).[2,5,8,12,13] All 6 studies observed that AZA maintained remission at higher rates than placebo, although the results were quite variable among the studies. Statistical significance was achieved in 2 trials[8,13] and likely would have been achieved in 2 others[2,12] had statistical testing been conducted. Similar to the studies on induction of remission, these trials on maintenance also displayed great variation with respect to study design, specifically in the number of patients included, disease location and extent (small versus large bowel), presence of fistulizing disease, use of surgery, medications used to induce remission, dose of AZA, duration of treatment, and definition of remission and clinical activity indices used.

A meta-analysis of these trials found that AZA is more efficacious than placebo at maintaining remission in CD.[10] In this study, remission maintenance rates were 67% for patients taking AZA compared to 52% in patients taking placebo, with a corresponding odds ratio of 2.27 (95% CI 1.76-2.93). In addition, a dose-response effect was observed, with a statistically significant benefit at 2 mg/kg/day and an even greater benefit at 2.5 mg/kg/day.

SONIC is a large, definitive, randomized double-blind controlled trial comparing early intervention with infliximab/azathioprine combination therapy, infliximab monotherapy, and azathioprine monotherapy for 1 year in patients with moderate-to-severe CD of short duration. Patients in the trial were steroid exposed but naïve to biologics or immunomodulators. SONIC showed that patients with evidence of inflammation (elevated C-reactive protein [CRP] level and endoscopic lesions at baseline colonoscopy) achieved superior steroid-free clinical remission (50%, 42%, and 23%, respectively) associated with mucosal healing from early infliximab combination therapy or monotherapy.[14] These infliximab treatments were superior to azathioprine alone with similar safety outcomes in all 3 arms. Just as ACCENT 1 was a pivotal study in establishing the role of maintenance therapy in CD, SONIC is a landmark study supporting the tectonic shift toward early intervention with anti-tumor necrosis factor alpha (TNFα) therapy and away from unlimited steroid and azathioprine therapy. There have been no randomized controlled trial studies on 6-MP for maintenance of remission in adults with CD. One randomized controlled study in 55 pediatric patients showed that 6-MP was superior to placebo in maintaining remission in CD.[15] In this trial, 6-MP at a dose of 1.5 mg/kg/d maintained remission in 91% of patients compared to 53% in the placebo group (P = 0.007). Given these data, and knowing that AZA is actually a precursor of 6-MP, it seems reasonable to assume that the benefits incurred with AZA would be translatable to 6-MP.

TABLE 14-3

RANDOMIZED CONTROLLED TRIALS FOR TREATMENT OF FISTULIZING CROHN'S DISEASE WITH 6-MP OR AZA*

Author (Year)	N	Drug Dose	Length of Rx	Response 6-MP/AZA	Response Placebo	P value
Willoughby (1971)	3	AZA 2 mg/kg/day	24 weeks	0/2 (0%)	0/1 (0%)	NR
Rhodes (1971)	6	AZA 2 mg/kg/day	2 months	2/4 (50%)	0/2 (0%)	NR
Klein (1974)	10	AZA 3 mg/kg/day	4 months	4/5 (80%)	2/5 (40%)	NR
Rosenberg (1975)	5	AZA 2 mg/kg/day	26 weeks	0/4 (0%)	1/1 (100%)	NR
Present (1980)	46	6-MP 1.5 mg/kg/day	1 year	16/29 (55%)	4/17 (24%)	NR

*6-MP indicates 6-mercaptopurine; AZA, azathioprine; NR, not reported.

6-MP and AZA have also been used to maintain remission postoperatively in patients who required surgical intervention in order to induce remission. Although the data in this setting are limited, 2 studies have been published. The first, an uncontrolled study in 10 patients who were started on 6-MP after surgical resection-induced remission, revealed that 9 patients (90%) were still in remission after a mean follow-up period of 41 months.[16] The other trial, which is the only randomized controlled study on this topic to date, examined 131 postoperative CD patients from 5 centers who were treated with 6-MP (at 50 mg/day), Pentasa (at 3 g/day), or placebo for 24 months.[17] Clinical, endoscopic, and radiographic endpoints were investigated. The authors found that 6-MP was superior to placebo or Pentasa in preventing clinical, endoscopic, and radiographic postoperative relapse in CD. Clinical, radiographic, and endoscopic recurrence rates were 50%, 43%, and 33%, respectively, for 6-MP; 58%, 63%, and 46%, respectively, for Pentasa; and 77%, 64%, and 49%, respectively, for placebo. The differences reached statistical significance for 6-MP compared to placebo over 2 years when clinical and endoscopic indices were used (P < 0.05).

TREATMENT OF FISTULIZING DISEASE

6-MP and AZA also have proven to be efficacious in the healing of fistulae, thereby allowing patients to delay or avoid surgical intervention. In the very first publication documenting use of AZA in CD, Brooke et al reported that all 6 patients with fistulizing disease who had received AZA demonstrated marked clinical improvement in their fistulae.[1] Since then, 5 randomized controlled trials that investigated healing of fistulae as a secondary endpoint have been published (Table 14-3).[2-4,6,12] There have been no studies to date that have evaluated the efficacy of AZA/6-MP for fistulae healing as a primary endpoint in patients with CD. The studies used improvement or complete healing of fistulae as the outcome measure. With the exception of the trial by Present et al,[6] the studies had very few patients with fistulizing disease. The studies were quite heterogeneous with respect to duration of therapy; there was also some variability in medication used and dosage. Three of the 5 trials observed higher rates of fistula improvement with 6-MP or AZA.[3,4,6] Of note, the study by Present et al observed a 31% rate (9/29) of complete closure of the fistulae in the group receiving 6-MP vs 6% (1/17) for the placebo group.[6] A subsequent series published by the same group showed that fistulae remained closed for 1 to 5 years in 54% (7/13) of patients who remained on 6-MP and that relapses tended to occur within 2 weeks to 9 months after discontinuation of 6-MP.[18] The authors also noted that although all types of fistulae responded to 6-MP, abdominal wall and enteroenteric fistulae responded particularly well.

A meta-analysis of these 5 trials reported an overall response rate (defined as improvement or complete healing) in 54% of patients treated with 6-MP or AZA, compared to 21% in patients treated with placebo.[10] The corresponding pooled odds ratio for fistula healing with 6-MP or AZA was 4.44 (95% CI 1.50-13.20). When interpreting the results of this meta-analysis, it is important to keep in mind that the majority of the fistulous cases (46/70

= 66%) were derived from a single study conducted at a single center.[6] Thus, the results of the meta-analysis were driven largely by that 1 study.

CORTICOSTEROID-SPARING EFFECTS

Another highly beneficial effect of 6-MP and AZA is their corticosteroid-sparing capability, which is important clinically because of the vast array of damaging side effects incurred during prolonged use of corticosteroids. Corticosteroid sparing with 6-MP and AZA has been investigated with respect to both induction of remission and maintenance of remission in CD.

Six randomized controlled trials have examined the corticosteroid-sparing effects of 6-MP or AZA during induction of remission.[2-4,6-8] Each of the studies suggested that corticosteroid dose and/or duration could be lessened with 6-MP or AZA compared to placebo. A meta-analysis analyzed 5 of these studies[2,3,6-8] and defined reduction in corticosteroid use as successful completion of a corticosteroid-tapering regimen or reduction in dose of prednisone or prednisolone to ≤ 10 mg/day with control of symptoms. This study found that corticosteroid use was reduced in 65% (76 of 117) of patients receiving 6-MP or AZA versus 36% (39 of 109) of those receiving placebo.[10] The corresponding pooled odds ratio favoring reduction in corticosteroids with 6-MP or AZA was 3.69 (95% CI 2.12-6.42).

Three randomized controlled trials have addressed the same question in the context of maintenance of remission.[2,12,15] All 3 studies observed a protective effect of 6-MP or AZA compared to placebo. Two of the studies[2,12] were further analyzed in the same meta-analysis as mentioned previously.[10] Using the same definition of reduction in corticosteroid use as in the induction-of-remission case, the authors reported that 87% (13 of 15) of patients taking AZA reduced their corticosteroid consumption compared to 53% (8 of 15) of those taking placebo. The corresponding pooled odds ratio favoring the use of AZA was 4.64 (95% CI 1.00-21.54). The third randomized controlled trial differed in 2 important ways, for it looked at children who were taking 6-MP.[15] Corticosteroid sparing is especially important in pediatric populations, given the growth impairment caused by this class of medications. In this study of 55 pediatric patients, those who were taking 6-MP at 1.5 mg/kg/day required fewer days and lower cumulative doses of corticosteroid therapy and were able to remain off prednisone for significantly longer than patients taking placebo. Only 1 patient in the 6-MP arm required a further course of corticosteroids within 540 days compared with 31% of control subjects at 90 days and 57% of controls at 1 year ($P < 0.0001$).

In a randomized, placebo-controlled trial involving patients shortly after diagnosis of disease with CD with C-reactive protein levels of more than 8.0 and endoscopic lesions, 28%, 56.9%, and 68.8% of patients were in remission and off steroids following 26 weeks of treatment with azathioprine, infliximab alone, and infliximab plus azathioprine, respectively.[14]

MINIMIZATION OF IMMUNOGENICITY TO INFLIXIMAB

Recently, infliximab, a chimeric monoclonal immunoglobulin (Ig)G1 antibody against tumor necrosis factor, has been approved for the treatment of moderate to severe CD in patients who have inadequate response to conventional therapy. Unfortunately, infliximab therapy can result in the formation of antibodies to infliximab (ATI), which can predispose patients to infusion reactions and also lead to loss of response to infliximab. There are several strategies that can be implemented to decrease immunogenicity to infliximab (to be discussed in detail in a later chapter), one of which is the use of concomitant immunosuppression with 6-MP and AZA. In addition to infliximab, adalumimab (and certolizumab) acts in a similar fashion and the use of immunomodulators can be associated with a reduction in the formation of antibodies against adalimumab. Several studies published in the past 2 years have examined the effect of 6-MP and AZA in this capacity.[19-22] Baert et al demonstrated that patients who were taking immunomodulators (6-MP, AZA, or methotrexate) had a lower incidence of ATI formation, 43% versus 75% ($P < 0.01$), as well as lower concentrations of ATIs ($P < 0.001$) compared to those not taking these drugs.[19] In this study of 125 consecutive patients who received infliximab only during flares of disease activity, the relative risk of a clinically significant antibody titer (> 8.0 µg/mL) favoring treatment with immunomodulators was 2.40 (95% CI 1.56-3.65, $P < 0.001$) in the group without fistulae and 2.85 (95% CI 1.54-5.25, $P < 0.001$) in the group with fistulae. A few months later, Farrell et al published a study of 53 patients taking infliximab in an episodic fashion and also found a significantly lower incidence of ATI formation in patients on concurrent immunosuppression (6-MP, AZA, methotrexate, or prednisone for ≥ 3 months duration), 24% versus 63% ($P = 0.007$), compared to subjects not taking these medications.[20] In multivariable logistic regression, concurrent administration of 6-MP, AZA, or methotrexate for ≥ 3 months' duration was a significant independent protective factor against the development of ATIs with an odds ratio of 0.16 (95% CI 0.04-0.7, $P = 0.007$), which exceeded the protective effect of concomitant prednisone therapy.

The ACCENT I trial (A Crohn's disease Clinical trial Evaluating infliximab in a New long-term Treatment regimen) was a large multicenter study designed to assess the safety and efficacy of repeated infliximab infusions, specifically episodic versus scheduled repeated infusions at doses of 5 mg/kg versus 10 mg/kg.[23] In a posthoc analysis by Hanauer et al, concomitant therapy with immunomodulators (6-MP, AZA, or methotrexate) decreased

FIGURE 14-1. Metabolism of 6-MP and AZA. 6-MP indicates 6-mercaptopurine; AZA, azathioprine; XO, xanthine oxidase; 6-TU, 6-thiouric acid; TPMT, thiopurine methyltransferase; 6-MMP, 6-methylmercaptopurine; 6-MMPR, 6-methylmercaptopurine ribonucleotides; HPRT, hypoxanthine phosphoribosyltransferase; 6-TIMP, 6-thioinosine 5'-monophosphate; IMPDH, inosine monophosphate dehydrogenase; 6-TXMP, 6-thioxanthosine 5'-monophosphate; GMPS, guanosine monophosphate synthetase; 6-TGN, 6-thioguanine nucleotides.

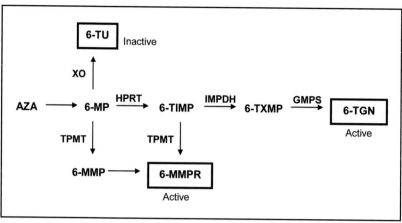

the incidence of ATIs in patients receiving scheduled infliximab at 5 mg/kg and 10 mg/kg, although these differences did not attain statistical significance.[21] Because only about 29% of patients in the ACCENT I trial were receiving concomitant therapy with immunomodulators, however, this post hoc analysis may have been underpowered to detect a significant difference. In the ACCENT II trial, which was designed to evaluate the efficacy of infliximab maintenance therapy in patients with fistulizing CD, the authors also reported a protective effect of immunomodulators (and corticosteroids) against formation of ATIs.[22] In this study, the incidence of ATI formation was 24% in patients with no concomitant immunosuppression, 13% with corticosteroids alone, 11% with immunomodulators alone, and 4% with both corticosteroids and immunomodulators. With the emerging concern about the combination of anti-TNFα therapy and immunosuppression associated with hepatosplenic T-cell lymphoma, there is a trend toward infliximab or immunomodulator monotherapy. Interestingly, in the SONIC trial, rates of adverse events were similar in patients who received infliximab plus azathioprine compared with those who received infliximab or azathioprine monotherapy in patients with early onset disease (average duration of disease < 2.5 years).[14] Therefore, it may prove over time that combination therapy is associated with fewer adverse events if initiated earlier in the disease course as compared with late introduction, where we know from the TREAT registries and other studies that there is an increased risk of infectious complications.[24] Over time, there is likely a higher risk of lymphoma as well.

PHARMACOLOGY

In this section, the metabolism, mechanism of action, and pharmacokinetics will first be discussed. Next, attention will be given to the use of laboratory testing, specifically for thiopurine methyltransferase (TPMT) genotype and enzyme activity, 6-thioguanine nucleotides (6-TGN) levels, and 6-methylmercaptopurine (6-MMP) levels, in the management of IBD patients receiving 6-MP and AZA.

The dosing of these drugs and duration of therapy will then be addressed. Finally, this section will conclude with a discussion of the adverse effects of these agents, their safety in pregnancy, and important interactions they have with other drugs.

METABOLISM

6-MP and its nitroimidazole derivative, AZA, are members of the thiopurine class of medications and, as such, have potent immunomodulatory effects. They are both inactive prodrugs that require extensive chemical alteration by a number of different enzymes in order to achieve their active forms (Figure 14-1). Upon oral administration, AZA is absorbed into the plasma and cleaved rapidly to 6-MP and glutathionyl imidazole by a nonenzymatic reaction occurring within erythrocytes. Three major pathways then ensue to convert 6-MP into its various metabolites.[25] The 3 critical enzymes corresponding to these pathways are xanthine oxidase, TPMT, and hypoxanthine phosphoribosyltransferase (HPRT). Xanthine oxidase, which is present in high concentrations within enterocytes and hepatocytes, rapidly and extensively metabolizes 6-MP into the inactive compound 6-thiouric acid (6-TU). As a result, the absolute oral bioavailability of 6-MP is only 5% to 37%.[26] The anabolic conversion of 6-MP into its active metabolites occurs along 2 competing pathways via the enzymes TPMT and HPRT. TPMT actually participates in 2 reactions, the first of which directly transforms 6-MP into 6-MMP, and the second of which leads to the formation of 6-MMP ribonucleotides by way of an intermediate in the HPRT pathway. These metabolites are thought to be responsible for some of the toxic effects (particularly hepatotoxicity) of 6-MP and AZA. HPRT begins the process of converting 6-MP into its therapeutically active metabolites, 6-TGN, which help quell the inflammatory response in IBD but may lead to the untoward effect of myelosuppression, which can affect all 3 bone marrow cell lines.

The TPMT gene, located on chromosome 6, is inherited as an autosomal codominant trait. An apparent genetic polymorphism has been observed in TPMT activity, resulting in a trimodal distribution. Approximately 0.3% of the general population exhibits low to absent activity due to inheritance of 2 mutant copies of the TPMT gene (TPMT^L/TPMT^L). Roughly 11% of the population is heterozygous for the mutation (TMPT^H/TPMT^L) and therefore has intermediate enzyme activity. The vast majority of the population (89%) is homozygous for the wild-type of TPMT (TPMT^H/TPMT^H) with normal to high enzyme activity.[27] A number of ethnic variations in the mutant TPMT alleles have also been identified.[28-33] To date, at least 11 allelic variants for the TPMT gene have been found. Overall, the most common allele is the wild-type allele, TPMT*1. The most common mutant allele, which is also the most common mutation in whites, is TPMT*3A. The most common mutant allele in African Americans and Asians is TPMT*3C. Each mutant allele corresponds to different degrees of reduction in TPMT activity; for example, TPMT*3A mutations are associated with complete loss of activity. It is believed that inherited differences in TPMT account for the majority of the observed variability in response to 6-MP or AZA among different people.

MECHANISM OF ACTION

The precise molecular mechanism of the immunomodulatory action of 6-MP and AZA are unknown. However, several putative mechanisms likely coexist to produce the composite effect of these drugs. At the molecular level, the 6-TGNs, which are the active metabolites of the HPRT pathway, are known purine antagonists that have the ability to interfere with both DNA and RNA synthesis.[25] AZA and 6-MP are also believed to work at the cellular level in a variety of ways. These medications have been shown to inhibit the proliferation of both T and B lymphocytes, to decrease suppressor T lymphocyte function and cellular immunity, to induce apoptosis of T lymphocytes, and to interfere with the cytotoxic ability of natural killer cells.[25,34,35]

PHARMACOKINETICS

As mentioned previously, the oral bioavailability of AZA and 6-MP is only 5% to 37% due to the rapid and extensive metabolism of 6-MP to 6-TU by the enzyme xanthine oxidase. Another limitation of these drugs is their slow onset of action. One randomized controlled study observed a mean time to response of 3.1 months in subjects with active CD.[6] A meta-analysis of 7 randomized controlled trials involving patients with active CD found that the odds ratio of response to 6-MP or AZA increased from 1.25 (95% CI 0.51-3.05) with less than 17 weeks of treatment to 1.95 (95% CI 1.10-3.46) at 17 weeks of treatment, to 19.2 (95% CI 6.27-58.8) with greater than 17 weeks of treatment, with a corresponding significant trend toward increased response with longer duration of therapy ($P = 0.03$).[10] The authors thus concluded that 17 weeks was likely the minimum amount of time necessary for a trial of 6-MP or AZA to be considered adequate.

The reason underlying their slow onset of action is not entirely clear but most likely involves the pharmacokinetics of the 6-TGN compounds. 6-MP and AZA themselves have a short plasma half-life of approximately 1 to 2 hours, but their active metabolites, the 6-TGNs, have a much longer half-life in the erythrocyte, ranging from 3 to 13 days.[25,26,36,37] In addition, data from pharmacological studies indicate that a steady-state level of the 6-TGNs may be reached in as little as 4 days or as long as 3 years.[38-43] Thus, the biology of AZA and 6-MP is not only highly variable among patients but also may take a very long time to reach equilibrium. One randomized controlled trial aimed at shortening this time course via intravenous loading of AZA, but no difference was observed between the treatment group and control group.[44] However, the authors also noticed that equilibrium of 6-TGN level was reached much earlier than expected, at 2 weeks. In addition, they reported that most of the responders attained clinical remission within 8 weeks of treatment. Thus, although 6-MP and AZA have a relatively slow onset of action, this time course may actually be shorter than originally thought.

MEASUREMENT OF TPMT GENOTYPE AND ACTIVITY, 6-TGN LEVELS, AND 6-MMP LEVELS

In order to understand the interplay between enzymes, metabolites, clinical efficacy, and toxicity, the metabolism of 6-MP and AZA will be reviewed (Figure 14-2). In this simplified diagram, the TPMT enzyme catalyzes the transformation of 6-MP to the hepatotoxic metabolite 6-MMP, which at levels of at least 5700 pmol/8 x 10^8 red blood cells (RBCs) may predispose one to this adverse effect. It should be noted that this specific level of 6-MMP has not been assessed in prospective randomized fashion to assess its positive and negative predictive value. The other major competing pathway in the metabolism of 6-MP leads to the formation of the clinically active metabolite 6-TGN. 6-TGN levels of 230 to 260 pmol/8 x 10^8 RBCs have been reported to be associated with clinical response, whereas levels of at least 450 pmol/8 x 10^8 RBCs have been linked to bone marrow suppression. The use of measuring TPMT genotype and/or enzyme activity, 6-TGN levels, and 6-MMP levels has been investigated in the context of clinical remission and toxicity in IBD patients. Most patients in these studies were CD patients receiving AZA.

TPMT GENOTYPE AND ENZYME ACTIVITY

As discussed previously, over 11% of the population exhibits reduced activity of TPMT due to inheritance of mutant alleles, with 0.3% of individuals having low or absent activity (homozygous recessive). Lennard et al first suggested that mutations in the TPMT gene may be associated with an increased risk of leukopenia, as the metabolism of 6-MP is shunted preferentially to the HPRT

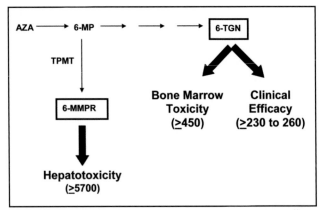

FIGURE 14-2. Metabolism of 6-MP and AZA in relationship to clinical efficacy and toxicities (all metabolite units are in pmol/8 x 10[8] RBCs.). 6-MP indicates 6-mercaptopurine; AZA, azathioprine; 6-TGN, 6-thioguanine nucleotides; TPMT, thiopurine methyltransferase; 6-MMPR, 6-methylmercaptopurine ribonucleotides.

pathway leading to the production of 6-TGNs, which are thought to be responsible for the bone marrow–suppressive effects of 6-MP and AZA.[45] A more recent study confirmed this mechanism by showing that 6-TGN levels were higher in patients heterozygous for TPMT than in those who were homozygous for the wild-type.[46] In addition, Colombel et al observed that the time to development of leukopenia was shorter in subjects with TPMT mutations than in wild-type individuals.[47]

The important question that arises from these data is whether or not measurement of TPMT genotype and/or phenotype (ie, enzyme activity) predicts therapy-limiting leukopenia in patients treated with 6-MP or AZA. Five studies addressing this issue have been published.[46-50] Only 1 of these (and possibly a second), however, has shown that measurement of TPMT enzyme activity (phenotype) predicts therapy-limiting leukopenia in patients treated with 6-MP or AZA. In this study of 67 consecutive rheumatologic patients (mostly with rheumatoid arthritis and systemic lupus erythematosus) taking AZA, 5 of the 6 patients heterozygous for TMPT genotype developed leukopenia—necessitating drug discontinuation within the first month of therapy.[48] In comparison, the 61 patients with wild-type TPMT genotype remained on AZA for a median duration of 39 weeks ($P = 0.018$). Another study of 30 consecutive patients on AZA status postcardiac transplantation also reported a positive result, but this result must be interpreted with caution.[49] The authors of this study found that therapy-ending leukopenia occurred in all 4 patients heterozygous for TPMT genotype, compared to none of the 26 patients with wild-type genotype. However, 9 of these 26 patients (35%) required cessation of AZA for reasons other than leukopenia and therefore may have developed drug-limiting leukopenia had they not developed other adverse effects of AZA.

Three other studies, all in IBD patients on 6-MP or AZA, showed that TPMT genotype and/or activity was not

associated with an increased risk of leukopenia.[46,47,50] In addition, in 2 of these studies, only 27% and 8% (respectively) of patients with leukopenia had a mutation in the TPMT gene.[46,47] Thus, relying solely on TPMT genotype and/or phenotype to monitor leukopenia is insufficient. Many patients who have decreased TPMT enzyme activity do not develop leukopenia when administered 6-MP or AZA, and leukopenia develops in many patients with normal TPMT enzyme activity when taking these medications. This underscores the importance of measuring complete blood counts (CBC) on a regular basis.

The other potential use of measuring TPMT genotype and/or phenotype is to predict clinical response. To date, there have been no studies published that examined clinical efficacy in relation to TPMT status. Only 4 published studies have investigated the association between TPMT genotype and/or enzyme activity and 6-TGN levels.[46,50-52] Three of these reported significantly higher 6-TGN levels among patients with intermediate TPMT enzyme activity compared to those with normal TPMT enzyme activity.[46,50,51] One study by Dubinsky et al reported a dissenting result, for TPMT enzyme activity did not correlate with 6-TGN levels.[52]

Taken collectively, the previous studies do not present compelling evidence that measurement of baseline TPMT genotype and/or enzyme activity levels predict either development of leukopenia or clinical response, especially in heterozygotes and even more so in homozygous wild-type subjects. Still, many authors advocate measurement of TPMT genotype and/or phenotype in all patients prior to initiation of therapy with 6-MP or AZA. The one group of individuals who may benefit from TPMT genotype and/or enzyme activity measurement is the homozygous mutants. In this small subpopulation of patients (representing roughly 1 in every 300 individuals), bone marrow suppression with 6-MP or AZA is nearly guaranteed and may result in severe leukopenia and sepsis, which have been associated with a high mortality rate.[53] Thus, in this subgroup of people, 6-MP and AZA should be avoided, and alternate treatment should be sought. Even though the cost to identify such patients is high (knowing that 299 tests will be negative for every 1 positive test), the consequences of not finding these individuals could be catastrophic. For this reason, we advocate the practice of testing every patient who is contemplating treatment with 6-MP or AZA.[54] Furthermore, such testing of all patients has recently been shown to be cost effective in the IBD population.[55,56]

6-TGN LEVELS

The association between 6-TGN levels and clinical response in IBD has been investigated by a number of studies. We have just completed a meta-analysis of the 12 studies[46,50-52,57-64] that contained data sufficient for inclusion.[65,66] These studies varied widely in sample size, in the proportion of patients who were in remission, and in

TABLE 14-4

STUDIES REPORTING AN ASSOCIATION BETWEEN 6-TGN THRESHOLD VALUES AND CLINICAL REMISSION*†‡

AUTHOR (YEAR)	N	6-TGN THRESHOLD (PMOL/8 x 10^8 RBC)	PROPORTION ABOVE THRESHOLD IN REMISSION	PROPORTION BELOW THRESHOLD IN REMISSION	ODDS RATIO (95% CI) FOR REMISSION
Achkar (2004)	60	235	0.51	0.22	3.80 (1.17, 12.39)
Goldenberg (2004)	74	235	0.24	0.18	1.47 (0.47, 4.62)
Belaiche (2001)	28	230	0.75	0.65	1.62 (0.26, 10.23)
Cuffari (2001)	82	250	0.86	0.35	11.63 (3.78, 35.72)
Gupta (2001)	101	235	0.56	0.43	1.65 (0.73, 3.75)
Dubinsky (2000)	92	235	0.78	0.40	5.07 (2.62, 9.93)
Pooled results			0.62 (0.43, 0.80)	0.36 (0.25, 0.48)	3.27 (1.71, 6.27) $P < 0.001$

*Random effects results shown only.

†6-TGN indicates 6-thioguanine nucleotides; RBC, red blood cell; CI, confidence interval.

‡Adapted from Kundu R, Osterman MT, Lichtenstein GR, Lewis JD. Association of 6-thioguanine nucleotide levels and inflammatory bowel disease (IBD) activity—a meta-analysis. *Gastroenterology.* 2005;128:A309-A310.

the activity indices used. Each study also included patients who varied considerably with respect to duration of disease and duration of 6-MP or AZA use. The studies appeared less heterogeneous in other respects, as the majority of patients in each study were adults with CD who had been using 6-MP or AZA for at least 10 weeks. In addition, the vast majority of the studies were retrospective. Moreover, assays for 6-TGN levels were performed in a uniform fashion in most studies via a modification of the high-performance liquid chromatography (HPLC) assay developed initially by Lennard and Singleton.[67]

Eight studies reported differences in mean (with standard deviations) or median (with ranges) 6-TGN levels between patients with active and inactive disease, thus allowing calculation of a pooled difference with 95% CI.[46,50-52,57-59,61] Mean/median 6-TGN levels were significantly higher among patients in remission than in those with active disease with a pooled difference of 66 pmol/8 x 10^8 RBC (95% CI 18-113, $P = 0.006$).[65] Six studies reported sufficient data on threshold values of 6-TGN level to allow calculation of odds ratios of remission based on each threshold value, as well as calculation of the proportion of patients above and below the threshold values who were in remission (Table 14-4).[46,57,58,61-63] Threshold values ranged from 230 to 260 pmol/8 x 10^8 RBC. Pooled analysis showed that 62% of patients above the threshold value were in remission, compared to 36% of patients below the threshold value who were in remission. Patients in remission were more likely to have 6-TGN levels above

the threshold value in all studies based on calculated odds ratios; statistical significance was reached in 3 of the 6 studies when considered individually. Pooled analysis demonstrated that patients in remission were significantly more likely to have 6-TGN levels above the threshold value, with a pooled odds ratio of 3.27 (95% CI 1.71-6.27, $P < 0.001$).[65] Thus, measurement of 6-TGN levels may be of benefit in optimizing clinical response in IBD patients treated with 6-MP or AZA. A large prospective trial designed to address this issue is currently underway.

Another potential value of measuring 6-TGN levels with respect to clinical remission concerns the nonresponders to 6-MP and AZA. Dubinsky et al proposed that clinical nonresponders to 6-MP and AZA fall into 3 categories.[52] The first group consists of patients with low 6-TGN levels and low 6-MMP levels. This scenario may occur with true underdosing of the drugs, medical nonadherence with therapy, or malabsorption of the agents. These patients may respond to increased doses of 6-MP and AZA (or to their regular dose, in the case of nonadherence). The second category is comprised of individuals manifesting relatively low 6-TGN levels but relatively high 6-MMP levels. These subjects are refractory to therapy because their metabolism of 6-MP is preferentially shunted toward forming 6-MMP via the TPMT enzyme and away from the HPRT enzyme that forms the 6-TGNs. This shunting is therefore one possible mechanism that can lead to resistance to 6-MP and AZA. These patients will likely not benefit from increased doses of medication. The third group contains patients who exhibit relatively high levels of 6-TGN but low levels of 6-MMP, hence preferentially shunting toward the HPRT/6-TGN pathway. These individuals are truly refractory to treatment and should seek alternate therapies. Thus, measurement of 6-TGN and 6-MMP levels may be helpful in identifying a subpopulation of patients who are nonadherent, underdosed, or malabsorbing their medications, conditions that are potentially reversible with dose increase. Identification of refractory patients is also useful in that toxicities of 6-MP and AZA may be spared as an alternate treatment is sought.

The use of measuring 6-TGN levels has also been investigated in relation to development of leukopenia. It has been suggested that 6-TGN levels above 450 pmol/8 x 10^8 RBCs can increase the risk of leukopenia.[68] To date, at least 9 studies have been published that examined the correlation between 6-TGN levels and leukopenia.[46,50-52,58,61,63,64,69] Seven of these have found no correlation between these 2 entities.[50-52,58,61,64,69] Two other studies did report that 6-TGN levels were higher in patients with leukopenia.[46,63] The study by Dubinsky et al revealed that the median 6-TGN level was 286 pmol/8 x 10^8 RBCs in patients with leukopenia, compared to 232 pmol/8 x 10^8 RBCs in those without leukopenia, a result that nearly attained statistical significance ($P = 0.06$).[46] Similarly, Gupta et al found corresponding median 6-TGN levels of 286 pmol/8 x 10^8 RBCs in leukopenic subjects versus 178 pmol/8 x 10^8 RBCs in those with normal leukocyte count, which reached statistical significance ($P = 0.03$).[63] Of note, in all 9 of these studies, leukopenia was seen at low or normal 6-TGN levels in many cases, and many patients who had high 6-TGN levels ($\geq$ 450 pmol/8 x 10^8 RBCs) did not develop leukopenia. Thus, measurement of 6-TGN levels should not supplant regular monitoring of CBC and appears to be of limited value in reducing bone marrow suppression in IBD patients receiving 6-MP and AZA (see Adverse Effects section for discussion of measuring CBC in these patients).

One other point that deserves mention is that intentional induction of leukopenia with the goal of achieving clinical remission with 6-MP and AZA is to be discouraged.[54] In pediatric patients receiving 6-MP for acute lymphoblastic leukemia, 6-TGN levels appear to correlate inversely with the risk of relapse and with absolute neutrophil count.[38,45,70-72] One early study by Colonna et al in CD patients treated with 6-MP reported that significantly more patients with leukopenia achieved remission than those whose leukocyte counts remained normal.[73] Since then, 4 published studies have refuted this finding.[44,48,64,69] The majority of patients in these studies attained remission without developing leukopenia. Furthermore, 2 additional studies have documented significant harm, specifically severe leukopenia, infection, and death, associated with such a management strategy.[74,75]

Overall, although not yet part of standard practice, measurement of 6-TGN levels may have a role in optimizing clinical response in IBD patients treated with 6-MP and AZA. 6-TGN levels may also be of use in identifying individuals who are nonadherent or underdosed, as well as those who are truly resistant to the medication and need alternate therapy. With respect to reduction of leukopenia, however, there is no compelling evidence that measurement of 6-TGN levels is helpful.

6-MMP LEVELS

As indicated previously, measurement of 6-MMP levels in conjunction with 6-TGN levels may have a role in identifying individuals who are either nonadherent or underdosed or those who are truly refractory to medical treatment with 6-MP and AZA. 6-MMP levels by themselves, however, do not have any significant association with clinical response, as demonstrated by at least 9 studies.[46,50-52,57-59,61,64]

Measurement of 6-MMP levels has also been postulated to be potentially helpful in predicting hepatotoxicity. At least 9 studies have examined this issue to some degree.[46,51,52,58-61,63,64] Two studies by the same group of investigators have shown that subjects with hepatotoxicity were more likely to have higher levels of 6-MMP, especially above 5700 pmol/8 x 10^8 RBCs.[46,52] Two other studies reported the opposite, ie, that 6-MMP levels were no different in patients with and without hepatotoxicity.[59,63] The other 5 studies had a very limited number of patients with hepatotoxicity and consequently reported no associations.[51,58,60,62,64] Overall, the majority of these 9 studies (even the 2 positive studies) have observed that hepatotoxicity can occur at low levels of 6-MMP and, conversely, that many patients with very elevated 6-MMP levels do not develop hepatotoxicity. Given the lack of convincing data supporting the routine measurement of 6-MMP levels in the assessment of hepatotoxicity, there is no current role for this laboratory test in this setting. Instead, periodic monitoring of liver-associated laboratory chemistries is the preferred modality of testing for hepatotoxicity (to be discussed in more detail in Adverse Effects section).

DRUG DOSAGE AND DURATION OF THERAPY

The dosing of 6-MP and AZA in IBD is one of the unresolved matters in this disease. The first question to ask is whether or not dosage of these agents correlates with clinical response or with potential surrogates of clinical response, namely 6-TGN and 6-MMP levels. With respect to 6-TGN levels, at least 6 studies have found that dosage of 6-MP and AZA does not correlate with 6-TGN levels.[46,51,57-59,63] Only 1 study by Dubinsky et al found a positive correlation but only in patients who responded to 6-MP or AZA with $r = 0.59$ (among nonresponders, $r = 0.12$).[52] When considering

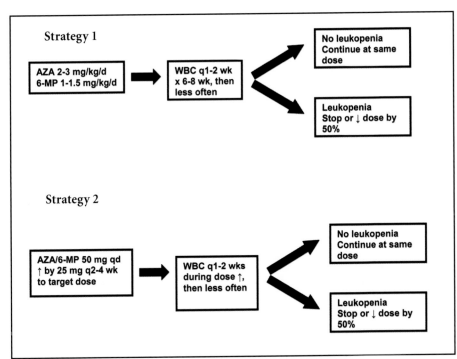

FIGURE 14-3. Recommended treatment strategies for initiation of 6-MP and AZA in IBD patients. 6-MP indicates 6-mercaptopurine; AZA, azathioprine; IBD, inflammatory bowel disease; WBC, white blood cell.

the correlation between drug dose and 6-MMP levels, on the other hand, all 5 studies that measured this association found positive correlations, albeit weak in most cases (range $r = 0.32\text{-}0.52$).[46,51,52,57,58] One of these studies also noted a positive correlation between drug dosage and the ratio of 6-MMP to 6-TGN level.[51] As discussed previously, some patients may preferentially shunt their metabolism of 6-MP to the TPMT/6-MMP pathway and therefore will not benefit from higher doses of medication.

The association between dose of 6-MP or AZA and clinical response has also been addressed in a number of studies. At least 6 studies have shown that the 6-MP or AZA dose was no different in patients with active versus inactive disease.[46,51,52,59,61,63] Only one study, by Achkar et al, reported that doses of 6-MP and AZA were significantly higher in patients who were complete or partial responders than in those who were nonresponders ($P = 0.002$).[57] Hence, it appears that drug dosage beyond a certain point does not play a large role in determining who will respond to treatment (in all studies on dosing, most patients were on substantial doses of 6-MP and AZA).

Unfortunately, the optimal dosages of 6-MP and AZA for treating IBD are unknown. Clinical trials have achieved clinical efficacy with 6-MP at 1 to 1.5 mg/kg/day and with AZA at 2 to 3 mg/kg/day. There is a multiplicative conversion factor of 2.07 to 2.08 when adjusting 6-MP doses to the equivalent doses of AZA.[44,76] In general, 2 dosing strategies for 6-MP and AZA in IBD patients are well accepted,[54] as shown in Figure 14-3. Prior to initiation of therapy, however, TPMT genotype and/or enzyme activity should be established in all patients. Only patients who are not homozygous mutant (ie, having low or absent TPMT activity) should be offered therapy with these agents. At this point, the treating physician has 2 options: begin at target dose (strategy 1) or begin at low dose and slowly uptitrate the dose over several months until the target dose is reached (strategy 2). Both strategies involve diligent and regular monitoring of the CBC, especially the white blood cell count (WBC) portion. Strategy 2 seems appealing from a toxicity standpoint, as the dose can be decreased or the drug can be stopped altogether at lower doses in the event that leukopenia occurs. Its major disadvantage is that it delays the achievement of the target dose, thereby likely delaying attainment of clinical response. In patients who have intermediate TMPT enzyme activity (heterozygotes), however, this strategy is very reasonable; alternatively, these patients can be started at 50% of target dose. Overall, we prefer strategy 1, largely because time to response is more rapid and many clinical trials have provided evidence that this pathway is well tolerated.[54]

The last aspect of drug therapy with 6-MP and AZA concerns the duration of treatment after achievement of clinical remission. Currently, it is not known how long patients should remain on treatment to maintain remission and, thus, when it is acceptable to stop therapy. The randomized controlled trials on maintenance of remission (see Table 14-2) treated patients with 6-MP and AZA for at most 1 year. The earliest study that addressed this specific question was a retrospective study of 157 CD patients in remission who were taking 6-MP or AZA for a median of 60 months.[77] The 1- and 5-year relapse rates in these patients were 11% and 32%, respectively. Among the 42 patients within this group who discontinued therapy, the 1- and 5-year relapse rates were higher at 38% and 75%, respectively. In addition, the authors found that duration of remission less than 4 years was associated with a higher risk of relapse. A retrospective study published a few years later also reported that discontinuation of 6-MP led to higher relapse rates in CD patients who were maintained in remission for at least 6 months.[78] In this study, relapse rates at 1, 2, 3, and 5 years were 29%, 45%, 55%, and 61%, respectively, for the 84 patients maintained on 6-MP compared to 36%, 71%, 85%, and 85%, respectively, for the 36 patients who discontinued 6-MP. The corresponding median lengths of remission were 32 months for the group that continued therapy and 16 months for the subjects who stopped treatment ($P < 0.004$). More recently, Fraser et al published a 30-year review of AZA use in IBD and observed that remission was maintained in 95%, 90%, 69%, 63%, and 62% at 1, 2, 3, 4, and 5 years, respectively, among the 324 patients who had achieved remission.[79] Two hundred twenty-two of these patients discontinued therapy at some point during the study period and had lower remission rates of 63%, 44%, 34%, 28%, and 25% at 1, 2, 3, 4, and 5 years, respectively. In contrast to the study by Bouhnik et al, they found that duration of treatment was not associated with risk of relapse following drug withdrawal.[77]

A randomized controlled trial by Lémann et al examined CD patients on AZA who maintained remission for at least 42 months.[80] They observed that relapse rates at 18 months were significantly lower in patients who remained on therapy (7.9%) versus those who stopped the drug (21%). Long-term follow-up of patients given the bridging strategy of infliximab plus AZA showed a probability of relapse at 4 years of 85% and 88% in the infliximab plus AZA group and placebo groups, respectively. Most of the relapses (80%) occurred despite maintenance treatment with AZA.[81] Using a Markov model, Lewis et al showed that the benefits of maintenance 6-MP and AZA outweighed the risks for up to 10 years in patients under the age of 65.[82] The benefit-to-risk ratios increased with younger age and interestingly with longer duration of therapy (10 years versus 4 years). Thus, though it is still unclear how long patients should remain on 6-MP or AZA before discontinuing therapy, it seems reasonable to continue treatment as long as patients can tolerate it with the goal of maintaining remission, particularly in the younger population. Of course, all treatment decisions need to be individualized upon discussion between patient and physician.

ADVERSE EFFECTS

Adverse events are common with 6-MP and AZA. The most frequently reported adverse effects include allergic reactions, leukopenia, pancreatitis, and other gastrointestinal side effects. Less common but clinically important side effects include infection, hepatotoxicity, and malignancy. A meta-analysis of 9 randomized controlled trials[2-8,12,13]

of CD patients receiving 6-MP or AZA found that adverse effects severe enough to cause withdrawal from a trial occurred in 8.9% of patients taking 6-MP or AZA versus 1.7% of those receiving placebo.[10] The corresponding pooled odds ratio was 5.26 (95% CI 2.20-12.60). In this study, the most common adverse events necessitating discontinuation of medication were allergic reactions in 2.0%, leukopenia in 1.7%, pancreatitis in 1.3%, and nausea in 1.3%. Of note, no malignancies were reported, but 1 death occurred in a patient on long-standing AZA who developed persistent leukopenia and subsequently died of infectious complications. In this meta-analysis, the authors noted a trend toward higher incidence of adverse events with greater cumulative dosage of 6-MP or AZA.

ALLERGIC REACTIONS

Allergic reactions caused by 6-MP and AZA are idiosyncratic and therefore dose independent. Allergic reactions typically consist of fever and/or rash or arthritis and generally resolve following cessation of therapy and may recur with rechallenge.[10,68] However, some patients who develop an allergic reaction to 6-MP may be able to tolerate AZA.[83]

PANCREATITIS

Pancreatitis associated with 6-MP and AZA therapy also represents an idiosyncratic response. Pancreatitis most commonly occurs during the first month of therapy and is also reversible after withdrawal of the drug. To date, no cases of chronic pancreatitis attributed to 6-MP or AZA have been reported. Routine measurement of pancreatic enzyme levels is not recommended unless clinical suspicion of pancreatitis arises.[68]

OTHER GASTROINTESTINAL ADVERSE EFFECTS

Other gastrointestinal toxicities may occur with 6-MP or AZA irrespective of pancreatitis. These include nausea, vomiting, and abdominal pain and are likely dose related. These events usually occur early in the course of treatment, are mild in severity, and often improve with time.[68]

BONE MARROW SUPPRESSION

Bone marrow suppression is a relatively common and clinically important adverse event caused by 6-MP and AZA, occurring in 2% to 5% of individuals.[84,85] Although all 3 cell lines may be affected, the white cell line is by far the most common, resulting in leukopenia. Unlike allergic reactions and pancreatitis, 6-MP– and AZA-induced leukopenia is dose dependent. For this reason, management of this condition consists primarily of dose reduction and, when necessary, drug cessation. Not surprisingly, routine monitoring of the CBC, especially the WBC count, is indicated in IBD patients receiving these medications. In addition to obtaining baseline values prior to commencement of treatment with 6-MP or AZA, it is reasonable to collect weekly CBCs for the first 4 weeks of therapy, followed by biweekly CBCs for the next 4 weeks, followed by monthly or bimonthly CBCs thereafter.[68] Leukopenia has been reported as long as 11 years after starting these medications[85] and, hence, continued monitoring of the CBC for the duration of treatment with 6-MP or AZA is warranted. The potential use of measuring TPMT genotype and/or enzyme activity prior to initiation of therapy and monitoring 6-TGN levels with respect to leukopenia have already been discussed in previous sections.

INFECTIOUS COMPLICATIONS

Even in the absence of leukopenia, 6-MP and AZA are potent immunosuppressive agents and thus place individuals at a higher risk of infectious complications. Serious infections that have been reported in association with these agents include both viral and bacterial causes.[79,84,86-88] Viral infections include cytomegalovirus with colitis, hepatitis and disseminated infection, varicella zoster virus, viral hepatitis, and genital warts. Reported bacterial infections include listeria cerebritis, Q fever, liver abscess, pneumonia, and septic phlebitis with arthritis. In reference to the risk of postoperative infectious complications associated with 6-MP or AZA in IBD patients undergoing elective surgery, a recent retrospective cohort study found no increased risk in patients treated with these agents alone or in combination with corticosteroids.[89]

HEPATOTOXICITY

Hepatotoxicity is another potential adverse effect of therapy with 6-MP and AZA and appears to occur in a dose-dependent fashion. The entity of hepatotoxicity in this case encompasses a spectrum of uncommon adverse occurrences, including elevation of liver-associated chemistries, cholestasis with inflammation, nodular regenerative hyperplasia, and peliosis hepatis.[77,84] Abnormal liver-associated chemistries (mostly alanine aminotransferase, aspartate aminotransferase, and alkaline phosphatase) may be seen in up to 2% of patients receiving 6-MP or AZA but typically normalize upon withdrawal of the drug.[77] Because liver biopsy is rarely performed in these instances, the exact pattern of injury is not known. However, drug-induced hepatitis with cholestasis has been reported.[84] Nodular regenerative hyperplasia and peliosis hepatis have been reported but appear to occur less rarely.[77] Monitoring of liver-associated chemistries is reasonable when treating with 6-MP or AZA. It is advisable to obtain baseline liver-associated chemistries prior to initiation of therapy, followed by repeated samples every 3 to 4 months for the first year and then every 4 to 6 months thereafter.[68] The use of measuring 6-MMP levels with regard to hepatotoxicity has already been addressed in a prior section.

MALIGNANCY

Finally, possibly the most alarming adverse event induced by 6-MP and AZA is the development of malignancy, which can occur in up to 3% to 4% of IBD patients treated with these agents.[84,90] Overall, this risk does not appear to exceed that of the population not receiving these medications.[90] However, treatment with 6-MP and AZA may increase the risk of lymphoma. Several studies have suggested an increased risk of non-Hodgkin's lymphoma in patients with rheumatoid arthritis and patient status after solid organ transplantation who are treated with 6-MP or AZA.[91-96] A number of case reports in IBD patients treated with these agents triggered similar concerns.[77,84,97-99] Five studies examining this issue in IBD patients have been published, 3 of which found no statistically significant increased risk of lymphoma with 6-MP or AZA (Table 14-5).[90,100-103]

One of these studies, which reported no increased risk, was the only population-based study conducted on this topic to date.[101] It was a retrospective cohort study using the General Practice Research Database in the United Kingdom, which included nearly 17,000 IBD patients, 1465 of whom were taking 6-MP or AZA. The study found that the risk of lymphoma in this subgroup of IBD patients treated with 6-MP or AZA was not significantly higher than that of the remaining IBD patients not taking these medications (risk ratio [RR] = 1.27, 95% CI 0.03-8.20).

Two studies, however, suggested that these agents may be associated with an increased risk of lymphoma.[100,103] One study by Farrell et al included patients taking AZA or methotrexate with or without cyclosporine A.[100] This study reported 2 cases of non-Hodgkin's lymphoma among patients treated with AZA and 2 other cases in patients treated with methotrexate with or without cyclosporine A. Methotrexate and cyclosporine A may themselves be associated with an increased risk of lymphoma that may differ from that of 6-MP and AZA. In addition, this study (like the study by Connell et al[90]) used indirect standardization to calculate standardized incidence ratios and P values, rather than using a dedicated control group. Only the studies by Lewis et al,[101] Fraser et al,[102] and Dayharsh et al[103] used true control groups (ie, IBD patients not taking 6-MP or AZA but derived from the same population) and 2 of these showed no increased risk of lymphoma with these drugs. The other study observing an increased risk, by Dayharsh et al, suggested that the lymphomas developing in IBD patients treated with 6-MP or AZA may be caused by Epstein-Barr virus (EBV).[103]

Recently, a large retrospective analysis of more than 20,000 Crohn's and ulcerative colitis patients recruited into a French registry confirmed an increased risk of non-Hodgkins lymphoma and EBV-associated lymphoma in patients treated with azathioprine and 6-MP.[104]

Hence, the data on 6-MP and AZA being risk factors for the development of lymphoma in IBD patients are far from conclusive. The general consensus opinion regarding lymphoma in IBD patients treated with 6-MP and AZA is that if an association truly exists, it is likely to be of small magnitude and unlikely to outweigh the potential benefit

TABLE 14-5

STUDIES ON RISK OF LYMPHOMA IN INFLAMMATORY BOWEL DISEASE WITH 6-MP AND AZA*

Author (Year)	N (Treatment) N (Controls)	Drug	Average Follow-Up	Lymphoma Treatment	Lymphoma Controls	P Value
Connell (1994)	755 Gen pop. rates	AZA	9 years	0/755 (0%)	0.52 Expected	0.69
Farrell (2000)	238 Gen pop. rates	AZA MTX CyA	8 years	4/238 (1.7%)	0.13 Expected	0.0001
Lewis (2001)	1465 15531	AZA 6-MP	3.8 years	1/1465 (0.07%)	14/15,531 (0.09%)	0.98
Fraser (2002)	626 1578	AZA	6.9 years	3/626 (0.5%)	5/1578 (0.3%)	0.5
Dayharsh (2002)	1200 8898	AZA 6-MP	NR	6/1200 (0.5%)	6/8898 (0.07%)	NR

*6-MP indicates 6-mercaptopurine; AZA, azathioprine; Gen pop., general population; MTX, methotrexate; CyA, cyclosporine A; NR, not reported.

of therapy, at least during the first decade and especially among younger patients.[68]

SAFETY IN PREGNANCY

It is currently believed that 6-MP and AZA can be used safely in pregnant patients with IBD. Animal data suggest that these medications may be teratogenic, causing hydrops fetalis, skeletal anomalies, cleft palate, decreased thymic size, and bone marrow suppression.[105,106] In addition, several studies have demonstrated chromosomal abnormalities in the spermatocytes of male mice exposed to 6-MP.[106-110] Human data have shown that AZA readily crosses the placenta, primarily in its inactive form as the metabolite 6-thiouric acid.[111] A few studies have documented fetal chromosomal anomalies and hematopoietic suppression in cultured cells of the progeny of mothers taking AZA during pregnancy.[112-115] Nonetheless, studies in patients receiving immunosuppressive therapy for renal transplants and systemic lupus erythematosus have shown these agents to be generally safe in pregnancy.[116-120]

In IBD, prospective controlled data regarding the safety of 6-MP and AZA during pregnancy are lacking. However, 3 retrospective studies have been published.[121-123] The first study, a descriptive analysis of 16 pregnancies among 14 women receiving AZA during pregnancy, found no congenital anomalies or other health problems in the offspring,

except for 1 case of hepatitis B infection.[121] A larger more recent retrospective cohort study of 325 pregnancies in 155 women with IBD found that exposure to 6-MP before conception, at conception, or during pregnancy was not associated with a significant increase in the rates of prematurity, spontaneous abortion, congenital defects, infections (neonatal and childhood), or neoplasia.[122] The third study (also a retrospective cohort study), however, did report an increase in adverse events with 6-MP used prior to conception.[123] The authors noted that 16 (22%) spontaneous abortions and 2 abnormal amniocenteses (resulting in therapeutic abortions) occurred in women who conceived at least 6 months (median 6 years) after discontinuation of 6-MP, compared to 18 spontaneous abortions (13%) and no abnormal amniocenteses in those without prior exposure to 6-MP. Among offspring in each group, long-term follow-up did not suggest an increased risk of developmental abnormalities with 6-MP use prior to conception.

Recently, Nørgård et al suggested that there was an increased relative risk of 18.5% for preterm births in women exposed to 6-MP and azathioprine during pregnancy.[124] These findings were based on combined national data registries and national prescription databases. Most of the small number of patients on 6-MP and azathioprine were hospitalized, suggesting that disease activity rates rather than 6-MP/azathioprine were likely to be associated with adverse pregnancy outcomes. The effect of disease activity and immunomodulators or biologics on birth outcomes in pregnant IBD patients will best be assessed by a prospective pregnancy registry.

With respect to paternal use of 6-MP and AZA and risk to the neonate or child, organ transplant data have shown these agents to be generally safe.[120,124-126] In IBD, 2 studies have been published that address the paternal use of these drugs, one of which raises concern regarding the safety of these medications.[127,128] In the first study, a retrospective cohort study of 50 pregnancies in which the father previously or currently received 6-MP, the authors found that 2 spontaneous abortions and 2 congenital anomalies occurred among 13 pregnancies fathered by male patients receiving 6-MP within 3 months of conception.[127] In comparison, only 2 complications were observed in 90 pregnancies fathered by male patients without prior 6-MP exposure ($P < 0.002$), and 1 complication was seen in 37 pregnancies fathered by men who had stopped taking 6-MP more than 3 months prior to conception ($P < 0.0013$). The other study in IBD patients concluded that paternal use of AZA was safe.[128] This study was primarily concerned with semen quality in 23 patients taking AZA and found that AZA did not adversely affect sperm density, morphology, motility, total sperm count, or ejaculate volume. In addition, the authors noted that no fetal abnormalities were observed among the 7 children fathered by 6 men receiving AZA and that all 7 children displayed normal growth and development after 3 years of follow-up.

Thus, overall, 6-MP and AZA appear to be generally safe in pregnancy, based on a number of studies in the solid organ transplant literature and a small number of studies in IBD patients. The use of these medications may be associated with a slightly increased risk of spontaneous abortions and an even smaller risk of chromosomal abnormalities or congenital anomalies among pregnancies in which either the mother or father are receiving these agents. However, this risk must be balanced against the benefit of inducing or maintaining remission, as flare of disease during pregnancy is the most important predictor of poor outcome.[68] Currently, 6-MP and AZA are Food and Drug Administration (FDA) pregnancy category D. Thus, termination of pregnancy is not mandatory for women who conceive while receiving these agents. The use of 6-MP and AZA in female and male patients planning to conceive should be individualized based on informed discussions between patients and physicians, weighing the benefits of therapy against the potential risks.

DRUG INTERACTIONS

A number of medications, when taken concomitantly with 6-MP or AZA, may influence their metabolism and clinical efficacy. The 2 most important drug interactions with 6-MP and AZA occur with the 5-ASA compounds and allopurinol.[68]

The 5-ASA compounds mesalamine, sulfasalazine, olsalazine, and balsalazide have been shown in in vitro studies to be potent inhibitors of TPMT enzyme activity.[129-131] In vivo data, which are limited, have reached conflicting conclusions. Two studies in CD patients observed that cotherapy with mesalamine had no effect on TPMT enzyme activity or metabolite levels.[46,52] Another study found that concomitant mesalamine or sulfasalazine, but not balsalazide, increased erythrocyte 6-TGN levels.[132] There is currently 1 case report that did find an important drug interaction in a CD patient taking olsalazine concurrently with 6-MP.[130] This patient developed 2 episodes of bone marrow suppression while on both drugs, thus necessitating discontinuation of each.

Allopurinol is an inhibitor of the enzyme xanthine oxidase and therefore may theoretically decrease the rapid and extensive metabolism of 6-MP into 6-thiouric acid, thereby increasing the oral bioavailability of 6-MP.[68] In this fashion, with more 6-MP available to the enzyme HPRT, the levels of 6-TGNs may be increased, which could lead to higher levels of bone marrow suppression. The clinical settings in which allopurinol is most commonly used, ie, gout and tumor lysis in cancer patients, are not typically encountered with great frequency in CD patients.

Other medications that may potentially interact with 6-MP and AZA are aspirin and furosemide.[133,134] However, the clinical significance of these interactions has not been clearly elucidated.

CONCLUSION

Since their introduction into the world of IBD in the 1960s,[1,135] 6-MP and AZA have become some of the most commonly prescribed medications for this disease, particularly in CD. A number of randomized controlled trials and meta-analyses have shown these agents to be efficacious in CD patients for induction of remission and maintenance of remission. In addition, these agents have proven benefit in treating fistulizing disease, in corticosteroid sparing, and more recently in minimizing immunogenicity to infliximab. 6-MP and AZA have a complex metabolism with several competing pathways, which combined with population heterogeneity in the TMPT enzyme results in wide variation in bioavailability and active metabolite levels. For this reason, dosing of these agents is not straightforward. The use of measuring metabolite levels and enzyme activity will likely be explored in more detail in the near future. Even though 6-MP and AZA have a slow onset of action of no less than 1 to 2 months, their safety profile is quite good, especially if care is taken to monitor CBC and liver-associated enzymes. These agents also appear to be safe in pregnancy. Thus, when considering their efficacy and broad applications in patients with CD, the benefits of these agents appear to exceed the risks, especially over the long run.

REFERENCES

1. Brooke BN, Hoffman DC, Swarbrick ET. Azathioprine for Crohn's disease. *Lancet.* 1969;2:612-614.

2. Willoughby JM, Beckett J, Kumar PJ, et al. Controlled trial of azathioprine in Crohn's disease. *Lancet.* 1971;2:944-947.

3. Rhodes J, Bainton D, Beck P, et al. Controlled trial of azathioprine in Crohn's disease. *Lancet.* 1971;2:1273-1276.

4. Klein M, Binder HJ, Mitchell M, et al. Treatment of Crohn's disease with azathioprine: a controlled evaluation. *Gastroenterology.* 1974;66:916-922.

5. Summers RW, Switz DM, Sessions JT Jr, et al. National Cooperative Crohn's Disease Study: results of drug treatment. *Gastroenterology.* 1979;77:847-869.

6. Present DH, Korelitz BI, Wisch N, et al. Treatment of Crohn's disease with 6-mercaptopurine: a long-term, randomized, double-blind study. *N Engl J Med.* 1980;302:981-987.

7. Ewe K, Press AG, Singe CC, et al. Azathioprine combined with prednisolone or monotherapy with prednisolone in active Crohn's disease. *Gastroenterology.* 1993;105:367-372.

8. Candy S, Wright J, Gerber M, et al. A controlled double blind study of azathioprine in the management of Crohn's disease. *Gut.* 1995;37:674-678.

9. Oren R, Moshkowitz M, Odes S, et al. Methotrexate in chronic active Crohn's disease: a double-blind, randomized, Israeli multicenter trial. *Am J Gastroenterol.* 1997;92:2203-2209.

10. Pearson DC, May GR, Fick GH, et al. Azathioprine and 6-mercaptopurine in Crohn's disease: a meta-analysis. *Ann Intern Med.* 1995;123:132-142.

11. Sandborn WJ, Sutherland L, Pearson DC, et al. Azathioprine or 6-mercaptopurine for inducing remission of Crohn's disease. *Cochrane Database Syst Rev.* 2000;2:CD000545.

12. Rosenberg JL, Levin B, Wall AJ, et al. A controlled trial of azathioprine in Crohn's disease. *Am J Dig Dis.* 1975;20:2203-2209.

13. O'Donoghue DP, Dawson AM, Powell-Tuck J, et al. Double-blind withdrawal trial of azathioprine as maintenance treatment for Crohn's disease. *Lancet.* 1978;2:955-957.

14. Lichtenstein GR, Hanauer SB, Sandborn WJ, and the Practice Parameters Committee of American College of Gastroenterology. Management of Crohn's disease in adults. *Am J Gastroenterol.* 2009;104:465-483.

15. Markowitz J, Grancher K, Kohn N, et al. A multicenter trial of 6-mercaptopurine and prednisone in children with newly diagnosed Crohn's disease. *Gastroenterology.* 2000;119:895-902.

16. Korelitz BI, Adler DJ, Mendelsohn RA, et al. Long-term experience with 6-mercaptopurine in the treatment of Crohn's disease. *Am J Gastroenterol.* 1993;88:1198-1205.

17. Hanauer SB, Korelitz BI, Rutgeerts P, et al. Postoperative maintenance of Crohn's disease remission with 6-mercaptopurine, mesalamine, or placebo: a 2-year trial. *Gastroenterology.* 2004;127:723-729.

18. Korelitz BI, Present DH. Favorable effect of 6-mercaptopurine on fistulae of Crohn's disease. *Dig Dis Sci.* 1985;30:58-64.

19. Baert F, Noman M, Vermeire S, et al. Influence of immunogenicity on the long-term efficacy of infliximab in Crohn's disease. *N Engl J Med.* 2003;348:601-608.

20. Farrell RJ, Alsahli M, Jeen Y-T, et al. Intravenous hydrocortisone premedication reduces antibodies to infliximab in Crohn's disease: a randomized controlled trial. *Gastroenterology.* 2003;124:917-924.

21. Hanauer SB, Wagner CL, Bala M, et al. Incidence and importance of antibody responses to infliximab after maintenance or episodic treatment in Crohn's disease. *Clin Gastroenterol Hepatol.* 2004;2:542-553.

22. Sands BE, Anderson FH, Bernstein CN, et al. Infliximab maintenance therapy for fistulizing Crohn's disease. *N Engl J Med.* 2004;350:876-885.

23. Rutgeerts P, Feagan BG, Lichtenstein GR, et al. Comparison of scheduled and episodic treatment strategies of infliximab in Crohn's disease. *Gastroenterology.* 2004;126:402-413.

24. Lichtenstein GR, Feagan BG, Cohen RD, et al. Serious infections and mortality in association with therapies for Crohn's disease: TREAT registry. *Clin Gastroenterol Hepatol.* 2006;4:621-630.

25. Lennard L. The clinical pharmacology of 6-mercaptopurine. *Eur J Clin Pharmacol.* 1992;43:329-339.

26. Zimm S, Collins JM, Riccardi R, et al. Variable bioavailability of oral mercaptopurine: is maintenance chemotherapy in acute lymphoblastic leukemia being optimally delivered? *N Engl J Med.* 1983;308:1005-1009.

27. Weinshilboum RM, Sladek SL. Mercaptopurine pharmacogenetics: monogenic inheritance of erythrocyte thiopurine methyltransferase activity. *Am J Hum Genet.* 1980;32:651-662.

28. Yates CR, Krynetski EY, Loennechen T, et al. Molecular diagnosis of thiopurine S-methyltransferase deficiency: genetic basis for azathioprine and mercaptopurine intolerance. *Ann Intern Med.* 1997; 126:608-614.

29. Otterness D, Szumlanski C, Lennard L, et al. Human thiopurine methyltransferase pharmacogenetics: gene sequence polymorphisms. *Clin Pharmacol Ther.* 1997;62:60-73.

30. Ameyaw MM, Collie-Duguid ES, Powrie RH, et al. Thiopurine methyltransferase alleles in British and Ghanaian populations. *Hum Mol Genet.* 1999;8:367-370.

31. Hon YY, Fessing MY, Pui CH, et al. Polymorphisms of the thiopurine S-methyltransferase gene in African Americans. *Hum Mol Genet.* 1999;8:371-376.

32. Krynetski EY, Evans WE. Genetic polymorphism of thiopurine S-methyltransferase: molecular mechanisms and clinical importance. *Pharmacology.* 2000;61:136-146.

33. Weinshilboum RM. Thiopurine pharmacogenetics: clinical and molecular studies of thiopurine methyltransferase. *Drug Metab Dispos.* 2001;29:601-605.

34. Brogan M, Hiserodt J, Oliver M, et al. The effect of 6-mercaptopurine on natural killer-cell activities in Crohn's disease. *J Clin Immunol.* 1985;5:204-211.

35. Tiede I, Fritz G, Strand S, et al. CD28-dependent Rac1 activation is the molecular target of azathioprine in primary human CD4+ T lymphocytes. *J Clin Invest.* 2003;111:1133-1145.

36. Lennard L, Keen D, Lilleyman JS. Oral 6-mercaptopurine in childhood leukemia: parent drug pharmacokinetics and active metabolite concentrations. *Clin Pharmacol Ther.* 1986;40:287-292.

37. Van Os EC, Zins BJ, Sandborn WJ, et al. Azathioprine pharmacokinetics after intravenous, oral, delayed release oral and rectal foam administration. *Gut.* 1996;39:63-68.

38. Lennard L, Rees CA, Lilleyman JS, et al. Childhood leukaemia: a relationship between intracellular 6-mercaptopurine metabolites and neutropenia. *Br J Clin Pharmacol.* 1983;16:359-363.

39. Lennard L, Brown CB, Fox M, et al. Azathioprine metabolism in kidney transplant recipients. *Br J Clin Pharmacol.* 1984;18:693-700.

40. Zimm S, Ettinger LJ, Holcenberg JS, et al. Phase I and clinical pharmacological study of mercaptopurine administered as a prolonged intravenous infusion. *Cancer Res.* 1985;45:1869-1873.

41. Lennard L, Harrington CI, Wood M, et al. Metabolism of azathioprine to 6-thioguanine nucleotides in patients with pemphigus vulgaris. *Br J Clin Pharmacol.* 1987;23:229-233.

42. Lennard L, Lilleyman JS. Variable mercaptopurine metabolism and treatment outcome in childhood lymphoblastic leukemia. *J Clin Oncol.* 1989;7:1816-1823.

43. Chan GL, Erdmann GR, Gruber SA, et al. Azathioprine metabolism: pharmacokinetics of 6-mercaptopurine, 6-thiouric acid and 6-thioguanine nucleotides in renal transplant patients. *J Clin Pharmacol.* 1990;30:358-363.

44. Sandborn WJ, Tremaine WJ, Wolf DC, et al. Lack of effect of intravenous administration on time to respond to azathioprine for steroid-treated Crohn's disease. *Gastroenterology.* 1999;117:527-535.

45. Lennard L, Van Loon JA, Weinshilboum RM. Pharmacogenetics of acute azathioprine toxicity: relationship to thiopurine methyltransferase genetic polymorphism. *Clin Pharmacol Ther.* 1989; 46:149-154.

46. Dubinsky MC, Lamothe S, Yang HY, et al. Pharmacogenomics and metabolite measurement for 6-mercaptopurine therapy in inflammatory bowel disease. *Gastroenterology.* 2000;118:705-713.

47. Colombel JF, Ferrari N, Debuysere H, et al. Genotypic analysis of thiopurine S-methyltransferase in patients with Crohn's disease and severe myelosuppression during azathioprine therapy. *Gastroenterology.* 2000;118:1025-1030.

48. Black AJ, McLeod HL, Capell HA, et al. Thiopurine methyltransferase genotype predicts therapy-limiting severe toxicity from azathioprine. *Ann Intern Med.* 1998;129:716-718.

49. Sebbag L, Boucher P, Davelu P, et al. Thiopurine S-methyltransferase gene polymorphism is predictive of azathioprine-induced myelosuppression in heart transplant recipients. *Transplantation.* 2000;69:1524-1527.

50. Lowry PW, Franklin CL, Weaver AL, et al. Measurement of thiopurine methyltransferase activity and azathioprine metabolites in patients with inflammatory bowel disease. *Gut.* 2001;49:665-670.

51. Hindorf U, Lyrenas E, Nilsson A, et al. Monitoring of long-term thiopurine therapy among adults with inflammatory bowel disease. *Scand J Gastroenterol.* 2004;39:1105-1112.

52. Dubinsky MC, Yang HY, Hassard PV, et al. 6-MP metabolite profiles provide a biochemical explanation for 6-MP resistance in patients with inflammatory bowel disease. *Gastroenterology.* 2002;122:904-915.

53. Ansley A, Lennard L, Mayou SC, et al. Pancytopenia related to azathioprine—an enzyme deficiency caused by a common genetic polymorphism: a review. *J R Soc Med.* 1992;85:752-756.

54. Lichtenstein GR. Use of laboratory testing to guide 6-mercaptopurine/azathioprine therapy. *Gastroenterology.* 2004;127:1558-1564.

55. Winter J, Walker A, Shapiro D, et al. Cost-effectiveness of thiopurine methyltransferase genotype screening in patients about to commence azathioprine therapy for treatment of inflammatory bowel disease. *Aliment Pharmacol Ther.* 2004;20:593-599.

56. Dubinsky MC, Reyes E, Ofman J, Chiou CF, Wade S, Sandborn WJ. A cost-effectiveness analysis of alternative disease management strategies in patients with Crohn's disease treated with azathioprine or 6-mercaptopurine. *Am J Gastroenterol.* 2005;100:2239-2247.

57. Achkar JP, Stevens T, Easley K, et al. Indicators of clinical response to treatment with six-mercaptopurine or azathioprine in patients with inflammatory bowel disease. *Inflamm Bowel Dis.* 2004;10:339-345.

58. Goldenberg BA, Rawsthorne P, Bernstein CN. The utility of 6-thioguanine metabolite levels in managing patients with inflammatory bowel disease. *Am J Gastroenterol.* 2004;99:1744-1748.

59. Wright S, Sanders DS, Lobo AJ, et al. Clinical significance of azathioprine active metabolite concentrations in inflammatory bowel disease. *Gut.* 2004;53:1123-1128.

60. Mardini HE, Arnold GL. Utility of measuring 6-methylmercaptopurine and 6-thioguanine nucleotide levels in managing inflammatory bowel disease patients treated with 6-mercaptopurine in a clinical setting. *J Clin Gastroenterol.* 2003;36:390-395.

61. Belaiche J, Desager JP, Horsmans Y, et al. Therapeutic drug monitoring of azathioprine and 6-mercaptopurine metabolites in Crohn's disease. *Scand J Gastroenterol.* 2001;36:71-76.

62. Cuffari C, Hunt S, Bayless T. Utilisation of erythrocyte 6-thioguanine metabolite levels to optimise therapy in patients with inflammatory bowel disease. *Gut.* 2001;48:642-646.

63. Gupta P, Gokhale R, Kirschner B. 6-mercaptopurine metabolite levels in children with inflammatory bowel disease. *J Pediatr Gastroenterol Nutr.* 2001;33:450-454.

64. Cuffari C, Theoret Y, Latour S, et al. 6-Mercaptopurine metabolism in Crohn's disease: correlation with efficacy and toxicity. *Gut.* 1996;39:401-406.

65. Kundu R, Osterman MT, Lichtenstein GL, Lewis JD. Association of 6-thioguanine nucleotide levels and inflammatory bowel disease (IBD) activity–A meta-analysis. *Gastroenterology.* 2005;128: A309-A310.

66. Osterman MT, Kundu R, Lichtenstein GR, Lewis JD. Association of 6-thioguanine nucleotide levels and inflammatory bowel disease activity: a meta-analysis. *Gastroenterology.* 2006;130:1047-1053.

67. Lennard L, Singleton HJ. High-performance liquid chromatographic assay of human red blood cell thiopurine methyltransferase activity. *J Chrom Biomed Appl.* 1994;661:25-33.

68. Su C, Lichtenstein GL. Treatment of inflammatory bowel disease with azathioprine and 6-mercaptopurine. *Gastroenterol Clin N Am.* 2004;33:209-234.

69. Sandborn WJ, Van Os EC, Zins BJ, et al. An intravenous loading dose of azathioprine decreases the time to response in patients with Crohn's disease. *Gastroenterology.* 1995;109:1808-1817.

70. Lennard L, Van Loon JA, Lilleyman JS, et al. Thiopurine pharmacogenetics in leukemia: correlation of erythrocyte thiopurine methyltransferase activity and 6-thioguanine nucleotide concentrations. *Clin Pharmacol Ther.* 1987;41:18-25.

71. Lennard L, Lilleyman JS, Van Loon JA, et al. Genetic variation in response to 6-mercaptopurine for childhood acute lymphoblastic leukaemia. *Lancet.* 1990;336:225-229.

72. Lilleyman JS, Lennard L. Mercaptopurine metabolism and risk of relapse in childhood lymphoblastic leukaemia. *Lancet.* 1994;343:1188-1190.

73. Colonna T, Korelitz BI. The role of leucopenia in the 6-mercaptopurine-induced remission of refractory Crohn's disease. *Am J Gastroenterol.* 1994;89:362-366.

74. Campbell S, Ghosh S. Is neutropenia required for effective maintenance of remission during azathioprine therapy in inflammatory bowel disease? *Eur J Gastroenterol Hepatol.* 2001;13:1073-1076.

75. Wallace TM, Veldhuyzen van Zanten SJ. Frequency of use and standards of care for the use of azathioprine and 6-mercaptopurine in the treatment of inflammatory bowel disease: a systematic review of the literature and survey of Canadian gastroenterologists. *Can J Gastroenterol.* 2001;15:21-28.

76. Sandborn WJ. A review of immune modifier therapy for inflammatory bowel disease: azathioprine, 6-mercaptopurine, cyclosporine and methotrexate. *Am J Gastroenterol.* 1996;91:423-433.

77. Bouhnik Y, Lemann M, Scemama G, et al. Long-term follow-up of patients with Crohn's disease treated with azathioprine or 6-mercaptopurine. *Lancet.* 1996;347:215-219.

78. Kim PS, Zlatanic J, Korelitz BI, et al. Optimum duration of treatment with 6-mercaptopurine for Crohn's disease. *Am J Gastroenterol.* 1999;94:3254-3257.

79. Fraser AG, Orchard TR, Jewell DP. The efficacy of azathioprine for the treatment of inflammatory bowel disease: a 30 year review. *Gut.* 2002;50:485-489.

80. Lémann M, Mary JY, Colombel JF, et al. A randomized, double-blind, controlled withdrawal trial in Crohn's disease patients in long-term remission on azathioprine. *Gastroenterology.* 2005;128:1812-1818.

81. Costes L, Colombel J-F, Mary J-Y, et al. Long term follow-up of a cohort of steroid-dependent Crohn's disease patients included in a randomized trial evaluating short term infliximab combined with azathioprine [abstract]. *Gastroenterology.* 2008;134;A-134.

82. Lewis JD, Schwartz JS, Lichtenstein GR. Azathioprine for maintenance of remission in Crohn's disease: benefits outweigh the risks of lymphoma. *Gastroenterology.* 2000;118:1018-1024.

83. Cheng BK, Lichtenstein GR. Are individuals with Crohn's disease who are intolerant to 6-mercaptopurine able to tolerate azathioprine? *Gastroenterology.* 2000;118:A1336.

84. Present DH, Meltzer SJ, Krumholz MP, et al. 6-mercaptopurine in the management of inflammatory bowel disease: short- and long-term toxicity. *Ann Intern Med.* 1989;111:641-649.

85. Connell WR, Kamm MA, Ritchie JK, et al. Bone marrow toxicity caused by azathioprine in inflammatory bowel disease: 27 years of experience. *Gut.* 1993;34:1081-1085.

86. George J, Present DH, Pou R, et al. The long-term outcome of ulcerative colitis treated with 6-mercaptopurine. *Am J Gastroenterol.* 1996;91:1711-1714.

87. Korelitz BI, Fuller SR, Warman JI, et al. Shingles during the course of treatment with 6-mercaptopurine for inflammatory bowel disease. *Am J Gastroenterol.* 1999;94:424-426.

88. Pfau P, Kochman ML, Furth EE, et al. Cytomegalovirus colitis complicating ulcerative colitis in the steroid-naïve patient. *Am J Gastroenterol.* 2001;96:895-899.

89. Aberra FN, Lewis JD, Hass H, et al. Corticosteroids and immunomodulators: postoperative infectious complication risk in inflammatory bowel disease patients. *Gastroenterology.* 2003;125:320-327.

90. Connell WR, Kamm MA, Dickson M, et al. Long-term neoplasia risk after azathioprine treatment in inflammatory bowel disease. *Lancet.* 1994;343:1249-1252.

91. Penn I. Chemical immunosuppression and human cancer. *Cancer.* 1974;34(suppl 4):80.

92. Kinlen LJ. Incidence of cancer in rheumatoid arthritis and other disorders after immunosuppressive treatment. *Am J Med.* 1985;78:44-49.

93. Silman AJ, Petrie J, Hazleman B, et al. Lymphoproliferative cancer and other malignancy in patients with rheumatoid arthritis treated with azathioprine: a 20 year follow-up study. *Ann Rheum Dis.* 1988;47:988-992.

94. Wilkinson AH, Smith JL, Robinson EM, et al. Increased frequency of posttransplant lymphomas in patients treated with cyclosporine, azathioprine, and prednisone. *Transplantation.* 1989;47:293-296.

95. Opelz G, Henderson R. Incidence of non-Hodgkin lymphoma in kidney and heart transplant recipients. *Lancet.* 1993;342:1514-1516.

96. Asten P, Barrett J, Symmons D. Risk of developing certain malignancies is related to duration of immunosuppressive drug exposure in patients with rheumatic diseases. *J Rheumatol.* 1999;26:1705-1714.

97. Gelb A, Zalusky R. The use of azathioprine and 6-mercaptopurine (6-MP) as immunosuppressive therapy in inflammatory bowel disease and its role in the etiology of lymphocytic lymphoma. *Am J Gastroenterol.* 1983;78:316.

98. Larvol L, Soule JC, Le Tourneau A. Reversible lymphoma in the setting of azathioprine therapy for Crohn's disease. *N Engl J Med.* 1994;331:883-884.

99. Bickston SJ, Lichtenstein GR, Arseneau KO, et al. The relationship between infliximab treatment and lymphoma in Crohn's disease. *Gastroenterology.* 1999;117:1433-1437.

100. Farrell RJ, Ang Y, Kileen P, et al. Increased incidence of non-Hodgkin's lymphoma in inflammatory bowel disease patients on immunosuppressive therapy but overall risk is low. *Gut.* 2000;47:514-519.

101. Lewis JD, Bilker WB, Bresinger C, et al. Inflammatory bowel disease is not associated with an increased risk of lymphoma. *Gastroenterology.* 2001;121:1080-1087.

102. Fraser AG, Orchard TR, Robinson EM, et al. Long-term risk of malignancy after treatment of inflammatory bowel disease with azathioprine. *Aliment Pharmacol Ther.* 2002;16:1225-1232.

103. Dayharsh GA, Loftus EV Jr, Sandborn WJ, et al. Epstein-Barr virus-positive lymphoma in patients with inflammatory bowel disease treated with azathioprine or 6-mercaptopurine. *Gastroenterology.* 2002;122:72-77.

104. Beaugerie L, Carrat F, Bouvier A-M, et al. Excess risk of lymphoproliferative disorders in inflammatory bowel disease: interim results of the Cesame cohort [abstract]. *Gastroenterology.* 2008;134(suppl 1):A116-A117.

105. Rosenkrantz JG, Githens JH, Cox SM, et al. Azathioprine (imuran) and pregnancy. *Am J Obstet Gynecol.* 1967;97:387-394.

106. Polifka JE, Friedman JM. Teratogen update: azathioprine and 6-mercaptopurine. *Teratology.* 2002;65:240-261.

107. Generoso WM, Preston RJ, Brewen JG, et al. 6-Mercaptopurine, an inducer of cytogenetic and dominant-lethal effects in premeiotic and early meiotic germ cells of male mice. *Mutat Res.* 1975;28:437-447.

108. Oakberg EF, Crosthwait CD, Raymer GD. Spermatogenic stage sensitivity to 6-mercaptopurine in the mouse. *Mutat Res.* 1982;94:165-178.

109. Meistrich ML, Finch M, da Cunha MF, et al. Damaging effects of fourteen chemotherapeutic drugs on mouse testis cells. *Cancer Res.* 1982;42:122-131.

110. Mosesso P, Palitti F. The genetic toxicology of 6-mercaptopurine. *Mutat Res.* 1993;296:279-294.

111. Saarikoski S, Seppala M. Immunosuppression during pregnancy: transmission of azathioprine and its metabolites from the mother to the fetus. *Am J Obstet Gynecol.* 1973;115:1100-1106.

112. Price HV, Salaman JR, Laurence KM, et al. Immunosuppressive drugs and the foetus. *Transplantation.* 1976;21:294-298.

113. McGeown MG, Nevin NC. Cytogenetic analysis on children born of parents treated with immunosuppressive drugs. *Proc Eur Dial Transplant Assoc.* 1978;15:384-390.

114. DeWitte DB, Buick MK, Cyran SE, et al. Neonatal pancytopenia and severe combined immunodeficiency associated with antenatal administration of azathioprine and prednisone. *J Pediatr.* 1984;105:625-628.

115. Davison JM, Dellagrammatikas H, Parkin JM. Maternal azathioprine therapy and depressed haemopoiesis in the babies of renal allograft patients. *Br J Obstet Gynecol.* 1985;93:233-239.

116. Erkman J, Blythe JG. Azathioprine therapy complicated by pregnancy. *Obstet Gynecol.* 1972;40:708-710.

117. Farber M, Kennison RD, Jackson HT, et al. Successful pregnancy renal transplantation. *Obstet Gynecol.* 1976;48(suppl 1):2S-4S.

118. Meehan RT, Dorsey JK. Pregnancy among patients with systemic lupus erythematosus receiving immunosuppressive therapy. *J Rheumatol.* 1987;14:252-258.

119. Hou S. Pregnancy in organ transplant recipients. *Med Clin N Am.* 1989;73:667-683.

120. Huynh LA, Min DI. Outcomes of pregnancy and the management of immunosuppressive agents to minimize fetal risks in organ transplant patients. *Ann Pharmacother.* 1994;28:1355-1357.

121. Alstead EM, Ritchie JK, Lennard-Jones JE, et al. Safety of azathioprine in pregnancy in inflammatory bowel disease. *Gastroenterology.* 1990;99:443-446.

122. Francella A, Dyan A, Bodian C, et al. The safety of 6-mercaptopurine for childbearing patients with inflammatory bowel disease: a retrospective cohort study. *Gastroenterology.* 2003;124:9-17.

123. Zlatanic J, Korelitz BI, Rajapakse RO, et al. Complications of pregnancy and child development after cessation of treatment with 6-mercaptopurine for inflammatory bowel disease. *J Clin Gastroenterol.* 2003;36:303-309.

124. Nørgård B, Hundborg HH, Jacobsen BA, Nielsen GL, Fonager K. Disease activity in pregnant women with Crohn's disease and birth outcomes: a regional Danish cohort study. *Am J Gastroenterol.* 2007;102:1947-1954.

125. Golby M. Fertility after renal transplantation. *Transplantation.* 1970;10:201-207.

126. Penn I, Makowski E, Droegemueller W, et al. Parenthood in renal homograft recipients. *JAMA.* 1971;216:1755-1761.

127. Lingardh G, Andersson L, Osterman B. Fertility in men after renal transplantation. *Acta Chir Scand.* 1974;140:494-497.

128. Rajapakse RO, Korelitz BI, Zlatanic J, et al. Outcome of pregnancies when fathers are treated with 6-mercaptopurine for inflammatory bowel disease. *Am J Gastroenterol.* 2000;95:684-688.

129. Dejaco C, Mittermaier C, Reinisch W, et al. Azathioprine treatment and male fertility in inflammatory bowel disease. *Gastroenterology.* 2001;121:1048-1053.

130. Szumlanski CL, Weinshilboum RM. Sulphasalazine inhibition of thiopurine methyltransferase: possible mechanism for interaction with 6-mercaptopurine and azathioprine. *Br J Pharmacol.* 1995; 39:456-459.

131. Lewis LD, Benin A, Szumlanski CL, et al. Olsalazine and 6-mercaptopurine-related bone marrow suppression: a possible drug-drug interaction. *Clin Pharmacol Ther.* 1997;62:464-475.

132. Lowry PW, Szumlanski CL, Weinshilboum RM, et al. Balsalazide and azathioprine or 6-mercaptopurine: evidence for a potentially serious drug interaction. *Gastroenterology.* 1999;116:1505-1506.

133. Lowry PW, Franklin CL, Weaver AL, et al. Leukopenia resulting from a drug interaction between azathioprine or 6-mercaptopurine and mesalamine, sulphasalazine, or balsalazide. *Gut.* 2001;49:656-664.

134. Woodson LC, Ames MM, Selassie CD, et al. Thiopurine methyltransferase: aromatic thiol substrates and inhibition by benzoic acid derivatives. *Mol Pharmacol.* 1983;24:471-478.

135. Lysaa RA, Giverhaug T, Wold HL, et al. Inhibition of human thiopurine methyltransferase by furosemide, bendroflumethiazide and trichlormethiazide. *Eur J Clin Pharmacol.* 1996;49:393-396.

METHOTREXATE IN THE TREATMENT OF CROHN'S DISEASE

15

Ellen J. Scherl, MD, FACP, AGAF; Arun Swaminath, MD;
Ryan Urquhart Warren, MD; and Harrison Lakehomer, BA

Methotrexate, a folate antagonist and potent anti-inflammatory agent, is an analog of dihydrofolic acid that inhibits dihydrofolate reductase and folate-dependent enzymes that are pivotal in the synthesis of purines and pyrimidines.[1-3] It is an effective therapy in rheumatoid arthritis, Crohn's disease, and psoriasis.[4-9] The efficacy of methotrexate in the treatment of ulcerative colitis (UC) is not yet established.

Although steroids have been a mainstay of therapy for moderate-to-severe Crohn's disease, recently, there has been a tectonic shift toward earlier use of biologic or immunomodulator therapy aimed at steroid-free remission.[10-13] It has been long recognized that while steroids are effective in inducing remission, they are ineffective in maintaining remission in Crohn's disease[14,15] with approximately two thirds of patients being either steroid dependent or refractory.[16,17] Furthermore, cost benefit analyses confirm that steroid use of more than 3 months is associated with increased cost to society in terms of time out of work and hospitalization.[18]

In the context of limiting steroids, there is an increasing role for immunomodulator therapy for moderate-to-severe Crohn's disease. The thiopurines 6-mercaptopurine (6-MP) and azathioprine are associated with nonresponse in approximately 30% of patients, intolerance in 20% of patients,[19,20] and an excess risk for lymphoproliferative disorders.[21,22] The onset of action of 6-MP and azathioprine may also limit their use as it may be as long as 3 to 6 months[23] and nearly two thirds of steroid-exposed Crohn's disease patients receiving azathioprine maintenance therapy have relapsed after 1 year of therapy.[24]

This chapter will discuss the role of methotrexate in thioprine-naïve and thioprine-experienced patients with Crohn's disease.

MECHANISM OF ACTION

Methotrexate is an analog of dihydrofolic acid with a substitution of a hydroxyl group by an amino acid and an insertion of a methyl group allowing methotrexate to enter the cell by active transport or facilitated diffusion. It inhibits dihydrofolate reductase and inhibits the synthesis of purines and pyrimidines. These molecular mechanisms explain its antiproliferative effect although the antiinflammatory effects remain to be elucidated. It is felt that, in part, the antiinflammatory effects of methotrexate are related to binding adenosine on target cells, which may lead to inhibition of tumor necrosis factor alpha (TNFα) and other proinflammatory cytokines.[25-27]

TOXICITY

The most common adverse events associated with low-dose methotrexate use in UC are nausea, vomiting, occasional diarrhea, abdominal pain, and increased liver transaminase levels. Rare central nervous system effects such as insomnia and paresthesias have been described, and infectious events have also been noted along with bone marrow suppression, but these effects are transient. Methotrexate-induced pneumonitis may be severe or life threatening. Hepatic fibrosis and cirrhosis is a concern with long-term maintenance therapy, but data suggest that even with cumulative doses of greater than 1.5 g, there is no significant toxicity.[1,3,28]

Neurotoxicity is rare with low-dose methotrexate and is mostly related to higher doses.[29,30] While the mechanism is not clear, high-dose methotrexate has been shown to decrease 5-methyltetrahydrofolate in the cerebrospinal fluid of some patients not given folate rescue, which underscores the importance of folate supplementation in methotrexate low- or high-dose treatment.[30]

Methotrexate is contraindicated in pregnancy because of its teratogenicity and must be discontinued 6 months prior to conception. Folic acid plays a significant role in hematopoiesis and the growth and development of the central nervous system.[31] During pregnancy, methotrexate may pose a risk to normal fetal development, as folic acid deficiency can lead to fetal abnormalities.[31] Neural tube defects leading to conditions such as spina bifida and anencephaly in the fetus can result from administration of methotrexate during pregnancy.[32] High-dose methotrexate has been shown to induce spontaneous abortion in the third trimester.[32] Whether low-dose methotrexate with folic acid supplementation will have the same effect is not clear. Pending further trials, the authors speculate that perhaps the category X should be reevaluated in low-dose methotrexate with folate replacement. Nonetheless, methotrexate is also contraindicated in breast feeding. Folic acid supplementation at a dose of 1 to 5 mg per day is common when prescribing methotrexate.[33] In addition, the risk of lymphoproliferative disorders observed in thiopurines is not associated with methotrexate in the treatment of rheumatoid arthritis, psoriasis, and Crohn's disease.[34-36]

Hypersensitivity pneumonitis, although rare, is a recognized complication of methotrexate use. A baseline chest x-ray as well as follow-up monitoring of complete blood counts and liver chemistries is advocated.[37-39] The risk of methotrexate-associated hepatotoxicity is low in patients who do not have one of the following risk factors: obesity, diabetes mellitus, history of excessive or long-term ethanol use, elevated baseline hepatocellular laboratory chemistries, a cumulative dose of methotrexate exceeding 1.5 g total drug dose, and daily dosing of methotrexate.[3,37]

INDUCTION AND MAINTENANCE TRIALS

The first 2 randomized controlled trials showed the efficacy of low-dose methotrexate in induction and maintenance of remission in thiopurine-naïve Crohn's disease[7,8] used 25 mg/week intramuscularly for inducing remission and 15 mg/week intramuscularly for maintaining remission. One hundred and forty-one steroid-dependent patients with chronic active Crohn's disease received either intramuscular methotrexate 25 mg/week or placebo. After 4 months of therapy, 40% of the methotrexate-treated patients achieved steroid-free remission compared with only 20% in the placebo group. The greatest efficacy was found in patients who required greater than 20 mg prednisone.[8] Methotrexate 25 mg intramuscularly or subcutaneously is effective in the treatment of steroid-dependent or steroid-refractory Crohn's disease with a number needed to treat of 5.[40] Subcutaneous methotrexate at doses of 15 to 25 mg/week achieved therapeutic serum and mucosal concentrations as well as clinical response.[41] Patients who failed to respond or maintain remission at 15 mg/week may respond to methotrexate dose escalation to 25 mg/week.[7,41] Ultra-low-dose oral dosing with 12.5 mg/week was not more effective than placebo or 50 mg of 6-MP when administered to patients with chronic active Crohn's disease.[42] In 84 patients who received steroid and 5-aminosalicylic acid in addition to ultra-low dose placebo, methotrexate (12.5 mg), or low-dose 6-MP (50 mg), methotrexate was moderately better but not significantly better than 6-MP or placebo.

Another randomized, double-blind controlled trial evaluating oral methotrexate 15 mg/week up to 22.5 mg/week and placebo in patients with steroid-dependent Crohn's disease who were refractory to 6-MP for up to 1 year or until treatment failure showed that only 46% of methotrexate-treated patients flared compared with 80% of placebo-treated patients. Laboratory indices of inflammation were similar in the 2 groups.[43]

Methotrexate was first reported to be effective in the treatment of Crohn's disease (15 patients) and ulcerative colitis (7 patients) in an uncontrolled study using an induction dose of intramuscular methotrexate 25 mg/week and a maintenance dose of methotrexate 15 mg/week per os.[44] Two thirds of patients had symptom improvements with steroid-sparing effects, and one third of Crohn's disease patients showed histologic improvements. Nonrandomized studies confirm the efficacy of low-dose methotrexate in moderate chronic active steroid-dependent Crohn's disease with significant steroid sparing and low toxicity.[45-48]

A large prospective randomized controlled trial confirmed the efficacy of low-dose intramuscular methotrexate (15 mg/week) for maintenance therapy[7] over 40 weeks in chronic active thiopurine-naïve, steroid-dependent Crohn's disease who were successfully induced into remission with 25 mg/week intramuscular methotrexate over 6 months.[8] At the end of 40 weeks, almost two thirds (65%) of patients maintained remission compared with only 40% in the placebo group. The methotrexate-treated patients were less likely to require steroids (approximately one quarter compared to two thirds in the placebo group). More than one half of patients who relapsed were successfully reinduced with intramuscular methotrexate 25 mg/week and were in steroid-free remission. No serious adverse events were noted.

In contrast, thiopurine-experienced Crohn's disease patients (patients who are intolerant or unresponsive to 6-MP/azathioprine) may be candidates for methotrexate therapy prior to considering anti-TNFα therapy.[46,49,50] A recent retrospective study evaluating 99 patients with CD showed that 29% had no response to weight-based 6-MP or azathioprine and 71% were intolerant to treatment.[51] Intolerance was due to leukopenia (23%) and nonspecific symptoms, which included arthralgias, alopecia, rash, and flu-like symptoms. The initial induction doses were 25 mg/week with a range of 7.5 to 25 mg/week, followed by a maintenance dose of 15 to 25 mg/week for an average duration of 72 weeks (7-208 weeks) in thiopurine-refractory patients and 15 mg/week for 96 weeks (12-378 weeks) in thiopurine-intolerant patients. All patients received folic acid supplements of 5 mg/day for 5 days or 5 mg/day weekly 48 hours after taking the methotrexate dose. Clinical response at 6 months was approximately 60% in both thiopurine-refractory and thiopurine-intolerant groups. Complete steroid withdrawal occurred in all thiopurine nonresponders (6 out of 6 patients). Fifteen out of the 99 patients were receiving concomitant infliximab. This retrospective study confirms that methotrexate is effective, provides steroid-sparing effect, and is well tolerated.

These results are consistent with another recent retrospective study where remission was achieved in 71% of 39 patients at 16 weeks.[52] A pediatric study of 61 thiopurine-experienced Crohn's disease patients also reported more than two-thirds clinical response to methotrexate at 6 months, where the majority of patients were thiopurine refractory.[53,54] Methotrexate 25 mg/week achieved response in 40% of thiopurine-refractory patients, of whom more than half also received infliximab.

Only one third of steroid-exposed Crohn's disease patients achieve mucosal healing.[55] Steroid-sparing with thiopurine 6-MP/azathioprine or methotrexate achieves clinical efficacy but mucosal healing is generally achieved in only approximately one third of patients.[28,56] However, 2 small series reported higher rates of mucosal healing associated with methotrexate.[57,58]

In steroid-dependent Crohn's disease patients, there was no difference between methotrexate in combination with infliximab or infliximab alone during a forced steroid taper over 14 weeks, suggesting that with regularly scheduled infliximab there is no need for immunosuppression.[59] Low-dose orally administered methotrexate (7.5 to 20 mg/week) has been combined not only with infliximab but also with sulfasalazine,[60] hydroxychloroquine,[61] cyclosporine,[62] azathioprine,[63] and infliximab.[64-66] Infliximab and methotrexate were effective in severe fistulizing Crohn's disease, with complete closure found in nearly three quarters of patients.[67] There appears to be an expanding role for methotrexate in the treatment of Crohn's disease in both thiopurine-naïve and thiopurine-experienced refractory and intolerant patients. Larger prospective head-to-head randomized controlled trials evaluating steroid-free remission and mucosal healing with early intervention using low-dose methotrexate alone and in combination with anti-TNFα therapy in thiopurine-naïve and thiopurine-experienced patients are warranted.

REFERENCES

1. Schröder O, Stein J. Low dose methotrexate in inflammatory bowel disease: current status and future directions. *Am J Gastroenterol.* 2003;98:530-537.

2. El-Matary W, Vandermeer B, Griffiths AM. Methotrexate for maintenance of remission in ulcerative colitis. *Cochrane Database Syst Rev.* 2009;CD007560.

3. Te HS, Schiano TD, Kuan SF, Hanauer SB, Conjeevaram HS, Baker AL. Hepatic effects of long-term methotrexate use in the treatment of inflammatory bowel disease. *Am J Gastroenterol.* 2000;95:3150-3156.

4. Schnabel A, Gross WL. Low-dose methotrexate in rheumatic diseases—efficacy, side effects, and risk factors for side effects. *Semin Arthritis Rheum.* 1994;23:310-327.

5. Klippel JH, Decker JL. Methotrexate in rheumatoid arthritis. *N Engl J Med.* 1985;312:853-854.

6. Weinblatt ME, Coblyn JS, Fox DA, et al. Efficacy of low-dose methotrexate in rheumatoid arthritis. *N Engl J Med.* 1985;312:818-822.

7. Feagan BG, Fedorak RN, Irvine EJ, et al. A comparison of methotrexate with placebo for the maintenance of remission in Crohn's disease. North American Crohn's Study Group Investigators. *N Engl J Med.* 2000;342:1627-1632.

8. Feagan BG, Rochon J, Fedorak RN, et al. Methotrexate for the treatment of Crohn's disease. The North American Crohn's Study Group Investigators. *N Engl J Med.* 1995;332:292-297.

9. Feagan BG, McDonald JWD, Panaccione R, et al. A randomized trial of methotrexate (MTX) in combination with infliximab (IFX) for the treatment of Crohn's disease (CD). *Gastroenterology.* 2008;134(4 suppl 1):682c.

10. D'Haens G, Baert F, van Assche G, et al. Early combined immunosuppression or conventional management in patients with newly diagnosed Crohn's disease: an open randomised trial. *Lancet.* 2008;371:660-667.

11. Sandborn WJ, Rutgeerts PJ, Reinisch W, et al. One year data from the SONIC Study: a randomized, double-blind trial comparing infliximab and infliximab plus azathioprine to azathioprine in patients with Crohn's disease naive to immunomodulators and biologic therapy [abstract]. Presented at: Digestive Diseases Week 2009; June 2, 2009; Chicago, IL.

12. Colombel JF, Sandborn WJ, Rutgeerts P, et al. Adalimumab for maintenance of clinical response and remission in patients with Crohn's disease: the CHARM trial. *Gastroenterology.* 2007;132:52-65.

13. Schreiber S, Khaliq-Kareemi M, Lawrance IC, et al, and the PRECiSE 2 Study Investigators. Maintenance therapy with certolizumab pegol for Crohn's disease. *N Engl J Med.* 2007;357:239-250.

14. Lennard-Jones JE, Misiewicz JJ, Connell AM, Baron JH, Jones FA. Prednisone as maintenance treatment for ulcerative colitis in remission. *Lancet.* 1965;1:188-189.

15. Truelove SC, Witts LJ. Cortisone in ulcerative colitis; final report on a therapeutic trial. *Br Med J.* 1955;2:1041-1048.

16. Munkholm P, Langholz E, Davidsen M, Binder V. Frequency of glucocorticoid resistance and dependency in Crohn's disease. *Gut.* 1994;35:360-362.

17. Faubion WA Jr, Loftus EV Jr, Harmsen WS, Zinsmeister AR, Sandborn WJ. The natural history of corticosteroid therapy for inflammatory bowel disease: a population-based study. *Gastroenterology.* 2001;121:255-260.

18. Feagan BG, Loftus EV, Kamm MA, et al. Impact of steroid discontinuation on healthcare resource utilization in Crohn's disease. *Am J Gastroenterol.* 2007;102(suppl 2):S445-S446.

19. Ansari A, Arenas M, Greenfield SM, et al. Prospective evaluation of the pharmacogenetics of azathioprine in the treatment of inflammatory bowel disease. *Aliment Pharmacol Ther.* 2008;28:973-983.

20. Dubinsky MC, Lamothe S, Yang HY, et al. Pharmacogenomics and metabolite measurement for 6-mercaptopurine therapy in inflammatory bowel disease. *Gastroenterology.* 2000;118:705-713.

21. Beaugerie L, Carrat F, Bouvier AM, et al, for the CESAME Study Group. Excess risk of lymphoproliferative disorders (LPD) in inflammatory bowel diseases (IBD): interim results of the CESAME cohort [abstract]. *Gastroenterology.* 2008;134(4 suppl 1):A116.

22. Dayharsh GA, Loftus EV Jr, Sandborn WJ, et al. Epstein-Barr virus-positive lymphoma in patients with inflammatory bowel disease treated with azathioprine or 6-mercaptopurine. *Gastroenterology.* 2002;122:72-77.

23. Present DH, Meltzer SJ, Krumholz MP, Wolke A, Korelitz BI. 6-mercaptopurine in the management of inflammatory bowel disease: short- and long-term toxicity. *Ann Intern Med.* 1989;111:641-649.

24. Candy S, Wright J, Gerber M, Adams G, Gerig M, Goodman R. A controlled double blind study of azathioprine in the management of Crohn's disease. *Gut.* 1995;37:674-678.

25. Cronstein BN, Naime D, Ostad E. The antiinflammatory mechanism of methotrexate. Increased adenosine release at inflamed sites diminishes leukocyte accumulation in an in vivo model of inflammation. *J Clin Invest.* 1993;92:2675-2682.

26. Krump E, Lemay G, Borgeat P. Adenosine A2 receptor-induced inhibition of leukotriene B4 synthesis in whole blood ex vivo. *Br J Pharmacol.* 1996;117:1639-1644.

27. Schröder O, Stein J. Low dose methotrexate in inflammatory bowel disease: current status and future directions. *Am J Gastroenterol.* 2003;98:530-537.

28. Kozarek RA, Bredfeldt JE, Rosoff LE, et al. Does chronic methotrexate (MTX) cause liver toxicity when used for refractory inflammatory bowel disease? *Gastroenterology.* 1991;100:A223.

29. Raghavendra S, Nair MD, Chemmanam T, Krishnamoorthy T, Radhakrishnan VV, Kuruvilla A. Disseminated necrotizing leukoencephalopathy following low-dose oral methotrexate. *Eur J Neurol.* 2007;14:309-314.

30. Vezmar S, Schüsseler P, Becker A, Bode U, Jaehde U. Methotrexate-associated alterations of the folate and methyl-transfer pathway in the CSF of ALL patients with and without symptoms of neurotoxicity. *Pediatr Blood Cancer.* 2009;52:26-32.

31. Lloyd ME, Carr M, McElhatton P, Hall GM, Hughes RA. The effects of methotrexate on pregnancy, fertility and lactation. *QJM.* 1999;92:551-563.

32. Hausknecht RU. Methotrexate and misoprostol to terminate early pregnancy. *N Engl J Med.* 1995;333:537-540.

33. van Ede AE, Laan RF, Blom HJ, De Abreu RA, van de Putte LB. Methotrexate in rheumatoid arthritis: an update with focus on mechanisms involved in toxicity. *Semin Arthritis Rheum.* 1998;27:277-292.

34. Kandiel A, Fraser AG, Korelitz BI, Brensinger C, Lewis JD. Increased risk of lymphoma among inflammatory bowel disease patients treated with azathioprine and 6-mercaptopurine. *Gut.* 2005;54:1121-1125.

35. Rosh JR, Gross T, Mamula P, Griffiths A, Hyams J. Hepatosplenic T-cell lymphoma in adolescents and young adults with Crohn's disease: a cautionary tale? *Inflamm Bowel Dis.* 2007;13:1024-1030.

36. Beaugerie L, Seksik P, Carrat F. Thiopurine therapy is associated with a three-fold decrease in the incidence of advanced colorectal neoplasia in IBD patients with longstanding extensive colitis: results from the CESAME cohort [abstract]. Presented at: Digestive Disease Week; June 1, 2009; Chicago, IL. Abstract 281.

37. Lichtenstein GR, Hanauer SB, Sandborn WJ, and the Practice Parameters Committee of American College of Gastroenterology. Management of Crohn's disease in adults. *Am J Gastroenterol.* 2009;104:465-483.

38. Travis SP, Stange EF, Lémann M, et al. European evidence based consensus on the diagnosis and management of Crohn's disease: current management. *Gut.* 2006;(55 suppl 1):i16-i35.

39. Lichtenstein GR, Abreu MT, Cohen R, Tremaine W, and the American Gastroenterological Association. American Gastroenterological Association Institute medical position statement on corticosteroids, immunomodulators, and infliximab in inflammatory bowel disease. *Gastroenterology.* 2006;130:935-939.

40. Alfadhli AA, McDonald JW, Feagan BG. Methotrexate for induction of remission in refractory Crohn's disease. *Cochrane Database Syst Rev.* 2005;CD003459.

41. Egan LJ, Sandborn WJ, Tremaine WJ, et al. A randomized dose-response and pharmacokinetic study of methotrexate for refractory inflammatory Crohn's disease and ulcerative colitis. *Aliment Pharmacol Ther.* 1999;13:1597-1604.

42. Oren R, Moshkowitz M, Odes S, et al. Methotrexate in chronic active Crohn's disease: a double-blind, randomized, Israeli multicenter trial. *Am J Gastroenterol.* 1997;92:2203-2209.

43. Arora S, Katkov W, Cooley J, et al. Methotrexate in Crohn's disease: results of a randomized, double-blind, placebo-controlled trial. *Hepatogastroenterology.* 1999;46:1724-1729.

44. Kozarek RA, Patterson DJ, Gelfand MD, et al. Methotrexate induces clinical and histologic remission in patients with refractory inflammatory bowel disease. *Ann Intern Med.* 1989;110:353-356.

45. Vandeputte L, D'Haens G, Baert F, Rutgeerts P. Methotrexate in refractory Crohn's disease. *Inflamm Bowel Dis.* 1999;5:11-15.

46. Lémann M, Zenjari T, Bouhnik Y, et al. Methotrexate in Crohn's disease: long-term efficacy and toxicity. *Am J Gastroenterol.* 2000;95:1730-1734.

47. Chong RY, Hanauer SB, Cohen RD. Efficacy of parenteral methotrexate in refractory Crohn's disease. *Aliment Pharmacol Ther.* 2001;15:35-44.

48. Fraser AG, Morton D, McGovern D, Travis S, Jewell DP. The efficacy of methotrexate for maintaining remission in inflammatory bowel disease. *Aliment Pharmacol Ther.* 2002;16:693-697.

49. Soon SY, Ansari A, Yaneza M, Raoof S, Hirst J, Sanderson JD. Experience with the use of low-dose methotrexate for inflammatory bowel disease. *Eur J Gastroenterol Hepatol.* 2004;16:921-926.

50. Mack DR, Young R, Kaufman SS, Ramey L, Vanderhoof JA. Methotrexate in patients with Crohn's disease after 6-mercaptopurine. *J Pediatr.* 1998;132:830-835.

51. Wahed M, Louis-Auguste JR, Baxter LM, et al. Efficacy of methotrexate in Crohn's disease and ulcerative colitis patients unresponsive or intolerant to azathioprine/mercaptopurine. *Aliment Pharmacol Ther.* 2009;30:614-620.

52. Din S, Dahele A, Fennel J, et al. Use of methotrexate in refractory Crohn's disease: the Edinburgh experience. *Inflamm Bowel Dis.* 2008;14:756-762.

53. Uhlen S, Belbouab R, Narebski K, et al. Efficacy of methotrexate in pediatric Crohn's disease: a French multicenter study. *Inflamm Bowel Dis.* 2006;12:1053-1057.

54. Garg M, Wilson J, De Crus PP, et al. Methotrexate in thiopurine refractory Crohn's Disease—a retrospective cohort study. Presented at: Digestive Disease Week; June 3, 2009; Chicago, IL.

55. Olaison G, Sjödahl R, Tagesson C. Glucocorticoid treatment in ileal Crohn's disease: relief of symptoms but not of endoscopically viewed inflammation. *Gut*. 1990;31:325-328.

56. D'Haens G, Geboes K, Rutgeerts P. Endoscopic and histologic healing of Crohn's (ileo-) colitis with azathioprine. *Gastrointest Endosc*. 1999;50:667-671.

57. Panaccione R. The use of methotrexate is associated with mucosal healing in Crohn's disease. *Gastroenterology*. 2005;128(suppl):A49.

58. Mañosa M, Naves JE, Leal C, et al. Does methotrexate induce mucosal healing in Crohn's disease? *Inflamm Bowel Dis*. 2010;16:377-378.

59. Feagan BG, McDonald J, Ponich T, et al. A randomized trial of methotrexate (MTX) in combination with infliximab (IFX) for the treatment of Crohn's disease (CD) [late-breaking abstract]. *Gastroenterology*. 2008;134:682c.

60. Haagsma CJ, van Riel PL, de Jong AJ, van de Putte LB. Combination of sulphasalazine and methotrexate versus the single components in early rheumatoid arthritis: a randomized, controlled, double-blind, 52 week clinical trial. *Br J Rheumatol*. 1997;36:1082-1088.

61. O'Dell JR, Haire CE, Erikson N, et al. Treatment of rheumatoid arthritis with methotrexate alone, sulfasalazine and hydroxychloroquine, or a combination of all three medications. *N Engl J Med*. 1996;334:1287-1291.

62. Tugwell P, Pincus T, Yocum D, et al. Combination therapy with cyclosporine and methotrexate in severe rheumatoid arthritis. The Methotrexate-Cyclosporine Combination Study Group. *N Engl J Med*. 1995;333:137-141.

63. Willkens RF, Urowitz MB, Stablein DM, et al. Comparison of azathioprine, methotrexate, and the combination of both in the treatment of rheumatoid arthritis. A controlled clinical trial. *Arthritis Rheum*. 1992;35:849-856.

64. Maini R, St Clair EW, Breedveld F, et al. Infliximab (chimeric anti-tumour necrosis factor alpha monoclonal antibody) versus placebo in rheumatoid arthritis patients receiving concomitant methotrexate: a randomised phase III trial. ATTRACT Study Group. *Lancet*. 1999;354:1932-1939.

65. Lipsky PE, van der Heijde DM, St Clair EW, et al. Infliximab and methotrexate in the treatment of rheumatoid arthritis. Anti-Tumor Necrosis Factor Trial in Rheumatoid Arthritis with Concomitant Therapy Study Group. *N Engl J Med*. 2000;343:1594-1602.

66. St Clair EW, van der Heijde DM, Smolen JS, et al. Combination of infliximab and methotrexate therapy for early rheumatoid arthritis: a randomized, controlled trial. *Arthritis Rheum*. 2004; 50:3432-3443.

67. Roumeguere P, Bouchard D, Pigot F, et al. Combined approach with infliximab, surgery, and methotrexate in severe fistulizing anoperineal Crohn's disease: results from a prospective study. *Inflamm Bowel Dis*. 2010;Jul 8. [Epub ahead of print].

CALCINEURIN INHIBITORS (CYCLOSPORINE A, TACROLIMUS, AND SIROLIMUS) AND MYCOPHENOLATE MOFETIL IN CROHN'S DISEASE

Gerassimos J. Mantzaris, MD, PhD, AGAF

Patients with active steroid-refractory or steroid-dependent CD in whom the use of conventional immune modulators such as azathioprine (AZA), 6-mercaptopurine (6-MP), or methotrexate is precluded by slow onset of action, lack of response, or intolerance, are currently treated with rapidly acting anti-tumor necrosis factor alpha (TNFα) agents such as infliximab. Patients who fail to respond to all these therapies may benefit from the use of calcineurin inhibitors or mycophenolate mofetil either as rescue or adjunctive immunosuppressive therapy. Calcineurin inhibitors (cyclosporine or CyA, tacrolimus, and sirolimus) are natural products derived from fungi.[1] They exert potent but noncytotoxic effects on the immune system. This is due to inhibition of calcineurin, the rate-limiting cytoplasmic phosphatase enzyme for the T cell receptor, signaling transduction pathway leading onto synthesis of IL-2.[2-4] The use of calcineurin inhibitors in organ transplantation, autoimmune diseases, and inflammatory bowel disease (IBD) was based on the premise that these conditions are T cell dependent. CyA and tacrolimus have been approved for the treatment of CD.

CYCLOSPORINE (SANDIMMUNE, NEORAL, GENGRAF)

BACKGROUND

CyA, first described in 1983, revolutionized treatment in organ transplantation by preventing allograft rejection, despite quick tapering of steroids in the posttransplant period. In the field of autoimmune diseases, it emerged as an alternative therapy to slow-acting, nonspecific, and often cytotoxic anti-rheumatoid drugs. CyA was welcome as a promising drug for steroid-refractory IBD, but a decade later the advent of anti-TNFα biologics has dramatically changed the therapy of refractory CD.

PHARMACOKINETICS

CyA is a neutral, lipophilic cyclic endecapeptide (mol. wt. 1202 daltons) extracted from the soil fungus *Tolypocladium inflatum gams.*[2] CyA inhibits calcineurin and calcineurin complexed with calmodulin (Figure 16-1).[2] Under normal circumstances, the activated calcineurin dephosphorylates the cytoplasmic component of the nuclear factor of activated T cells (NF-AT). The latter then crosses into the nucleus and joins with its nuclear counterpart, facilitating the assembly of a transcription factor for IL-2 and its receptor. CyA binds to a 17-kDa receptor, cyclophilin, but tacrolimus binds to a 12-kDa receptor, the FK506 binding protein. These dimeric complexes inhibit the enzymatic activity of calcineurin.[4-6] As a result, the NF-AT is not activated and shuts off the transcription of genes crucial for the activation of T helper cells and T cell–dependent activation of B cells, such as IL-2 and IL-2 receptor, IL-3, IL-4, interferon-γ, and TNFα. CyA may also shift the immune response towards a Th2 direction. It is not known which of these mechanisms mediates the effect of CyA in IBD. CyA is commercially available as an intravenous (IV) concentrate (Sandimmune, 50 mg/mL), oral liquid preparation (Sandimmune, 100 mg/mL), oral gelatin capsules (Sandimmune, 25, 50, and 100 mg), and oral microemulsion formulation (Neoral, Gengraf).

Lichtenstein GR, ed.
Crohn's Disease: The Complete Guide to Medical Management (pp 183-196).
© 2011 SLACK Incorporated

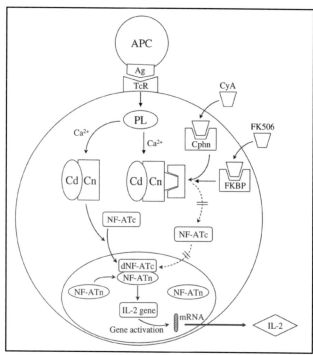

FIGURE 16-1. Simplified model showing the mechanism of action of cyclosporine and tacrolimus. APC, antigen presenting cell; Ag, antigen; TcR, T-cell receptor; PL, phospholipase; Cn, calcineurin; Cd, calmodulin; NF-ATc, cytoplasmic component of the Nuclear Factor of Activated T-cells; dNF-ATc, dephosphorylated NF-AT; NF-ATn, nuclear component of NF-AT; CyA, cyclosporine; Cphn, cyclophilin; FKBP, FK 506 binding protein (Adapted from Prograf [product monograph]. UK; Fujisawa Ltd: 1999.)

Oral absorption of CyA is dependent on patient population and formulations. Absorption from Sandimmune formulations is very unpredictable because it is dose independent and influenced by small intestinal motility, mucosal integrity, presence of bile, and first-pass metabolism in the gut.[6-11] Thus, partial gastrectomy, short bowel syndrome, graft-versus-host disease, radiation enteritis, bile diversion, intrahepatic cholestasis, and CD of the small bowel may lead to malabsorption of CyA. Vitamin E, ursodeoxycholic acid, and metoclopramide may improve the bioavailability of Sandimmune.[12] Peak blood concentration after a single oral dose of Sandimmune occurs at approximately 4 hours (interindividual range 1 to 8 hours) and bioavailability ranges from 12% to 35%.[9,13-15] Neoral has a less variable absorption profile and higher bioavailability because in contact with water it forms a decreased CyA-oil-water emulsion droplet size relative to Sandimmune.[6] As a result, absorption of CyA from Neoral is rapid, dose dependent, and less dependent on mixing with food, bile solubilization, or small bowel disease.[16,17] Pharmacokinetics of Neoral in patients with CD is broadly similar to that in healthy subjects or other patient groups except for patients with long intestinal resections or intestinal bypass.[17] All studies in CD have been performed using Sandimmune formulations, however. CyA administered orally or as an

enema is poorly absorbed from the colon; in contrast, IV administration results in high intracolonic concentrations of CyA.[7,8,18]

In the circulation, the distribution of CyA between blood and plasma, binding to lipoproteins, and uptake by erythrocytes is a function of temperature.[19] Because this induces variability during handling of samples for plasma determinations, trough concentrations of CyA should be measured preferably in whole blood using high-performance liquid chromatography (HPLC), monoclonal radioimmunoassay (mRIA), or fluorescence polarization immunoassays, which are specific for native CyA.[20,21] CyA is metabolized by the hepatic cytochrome P450-3A isoenzyme to at least 25 inactive metabolites. Erythromycin, doxycycline, diltiazem, ketoconazole, and oral contraceptives increase but rifampicin, carbamazepine, phenobarbital, phenytoin, octreotide, co-trimoxazole, and omeprazole reduce the blood concentrations of CyA.[22] High-dose corticosteroids may interfere with the metabolism of CyA. Elimination half-life of CyA from Neoral is ~8 hours. CyA is primarily eliminated through the bile.

ADVERSE EVENTS

CyA therapy for CD is associated with many, usually dose-dependent, adverse events. Doses of oral CyA ≤ 5 mg/kg/day do not cause major toxicity. The frequency of serious adverse events in 3 controlled trials of low-dose oral CyA was 0.13% (42 of 312 patients).[23-25] However, doses of oral CyA > 5 mg/kg/day or IV therapy (4 mg/kg/day) may cause life-threatening complications.[26] In a review of CyA treatment, 321 adverse events were reported in 343 IBD patients (0.94 events per patient), the most common being paresthesias, hypertrichosis, and hypertension.[13] The majority of these events were reversible after CyA withdrawal or on dose reduction.

The foremost concern in CyA therapy is nephrotoxicity, manifested as acute transient or severe renal failure or chronic nephropathy. Acute renal dysfunction is characterized by a decreased glomerular filtration rate occurring in the first days of treatment. This is due to a dose-dependent vasoconstriction of the afferent arteriole resulting in reduced renal blood flow and is thought to reverse soon after CyA is withdrawn.[14,27] Calcium blockers may oppose the acute renal toxic effect of CyA. However, data from the Kidney Biopsy Registry of Cyclosporin in Autoimmune Diseases Study revealed that 1 of 5 patients receiving long-term oral CyA in doses > 5 mg/kg/day develops chronic nephropathy despite having normal serum creatinine levels. This is manifested histologically as striped interstitial fibrosis and tubular atrophy and less often as arteriolar alterations, or both.[28] Risk factors include mean oral CyA doses greater than 8 mg/mL/day, greater maximum increase in serum creatinine and advancing age, but not hypertension or duration of therapy. Thus, nephropathy results from repeated, brief insults of toxic blood CyA levels rather than from a cumulative toxic drug effect. It has, therefore, been recommended that patients with rheumatoid arthritis or psoriasis be treated with ≤ 5 mg/mL/day oral CyA with dose adjustments when serum creatinine exceeds pretreatment levels by more than 30%.[28] If this holds true, it is reasonable to assume that nearly 20% of patients with CD on high-dose oral or IV CyA therapy are expected to have clinically silent, permanent nephropathy.

Neurotoxicity is manifested mainly as burning or tingling paresthesias, tremor of the hands, headache, malaise, and (less often) seizures or peripheral neuropathy.[13,29] Patients on CyA therapy may develop grand mal seizures de novo or in the setting of specific risk factors such as hypocholesterolemia, hypomagnesemia, hypertension, underlying seizure disorder, or cotreatment with high-dose methylprednisolone.[29] CyA-induced optic neuropathy, external ophthalmoplegia and nystagmus,[30] reversible cortical atrophy,[31] and cerebral vasculopathy[32] have also been reported.

Serious infections were noted in 4 controlled trials of oral CyA.[23-25,33] However, life-threatening infections and fatalities have been reported in CD patients who were treated concomitantly with steroids, high-dose oral or IV CyA, and immune modulators and had a pretreatment deteriorating health condition: 1 case of carotid mycotic aneurysm; 2 cases of cytomegalovirus infection; and 3 fatalities of *Pneumocystis carinii* pneumonia (PCP), invasive aspergillosis, and sepsis were reported.[34-37] Co-trimoxazole prophylaxis against PCP should be considered in selected patients.

Only 1 case of cholestatic hepatitis has been reported in CD.[38] Hepatotoxicity is usually manifested as biochemical cholestasis, which is due to inhibition of the adenosine triphosphate (ATP)-dependent excretion of bile salts by CyA metabolites.[39] If a primary cholestatic liver disease preexists, accumulation of CyA metabolites may initiate a vicious circle of worsening cholestasis. Total parenteral nutrition may also aggravate cholestasis during CyA therapy. Cholestasis usually resolves upon dose reduction or cessation of treatment. There is no evidence that CyA increases the risk for colon cancer or lymphomas in CD.[24,40] Because CyA does not inhibit the activity of hemopoietic stem cell, hematological toxicity is also not expected. Two uncomplicated pregnancies have been reported during CyA therapy for CD.[24] CyA is not teratogenic but is associated with prematurity and growth retardation. If initiation of treatment during pregnancy is inevitable, patients should be closely monitored because they may develop hypertension and/or seizures.

Before starting CyA therapy, a history of seizures and cancer and a pregnancy test should be obtained. Full blood counts, serum electrolytes, creatinine, total cholesterol, and liver function tests should be checked before starting, and every 1 to 2 days during therapy. Hypomagnesemia should be corrected before starting therapy. Therapy should not be initiated if total serum cholesterol levels are below 120 mg/dL. Whole blood CyA concentrations must be measured daily. Blood pressure should be measured several times daily. Patients must be closely monitored for early detection of nephrotoxicity, infections, and hepatotoxicity. When IV therapy is switched to oral therapy, tight measures may be relaxed slightly, bearing always in mind that patients treated concurrently with oral CyA and azathioprine/6-MP are still at risk for severe toxicity.

CLINICAL TRIALS

In the first controlled trial, 71 patients with active CD resistant or intolerant of corticosteroids received oral CyA (mean final dose 7.6 mg/kg/day) or placebo for 3 months (Table 16-1).[33] At the end of the trial, two thirds of the patients showed substantial or moderate improvement in clinical and laboratory indices of disease activity. The therapeutic effect of CyA was apparent after 2 weeks, was greater in patients receiving corticosteroids, and was independent of the site of disease. A similar number of patients were withdrawn from the 2 arms of the study. During a 3-month CyA tapering off period, 14 (38%) of 37 CyA-treated patients but only 5 (15%) of 34 placebo-treated patients maintained improvement (*P* = 0.034). However, the therapeutic effect of CyA waned off during a 6-month post-treatment follow-up.[41]

In contrast, 3 large controlled trials confirmed that low-dose (5 mg/kg/day) oral CyA is ineffective for both induction of remission and remission maintenance of chronically active CD (see Table 16-1).[23-25] The Great Britain and Ireland Cyclosporine Trial[23] included patients who required prednisolone and/or azathioprine to control symptoms but relapsed soon after 1 of these treatments was discontinued. Patients were randomized to oral CyA or placebo for 3 months. Prednisolone (20 mg/day) was co-administered for 4 weeks, with tapering to less than 10 mg in the next 2 to 4 weeks. Clinical response was defined as resolution/improvement of symptoms on withdrawal or reduction of prednisolone. At the end of the trial, more patients on placebo achieved clinical remission compared with CyA. The outcome of therapy did not change in 55 patients who continued treatment off-protocol for a further 12 weeks (24 CyA, 31 placebo) because 64% of placebo-treated but only 46% of CyA-treated patients remained in remission. No serious adverse events were noted. In the Canadian Trial,[24] patients with chronic active CD activity index (CDAI) > 150 (*n* = 112) or quiescent disease (CDAI ≤ 150) were treated with oral CyA (final mean dose 4.8 mg/kg/day) or placebo for 18 months. Patients were stratified according to center and score of disease activity. The primary endpoint was as a 100-point increase in the CDAI over each patient's baseline value. Again, more patients worsened with CyA than with placebo. Deterioration of

TABLE 16-1

RANDOMIZED, PLACEBO-CONTROLLED TRIALS OF ORAL CYCLOSPORINE FOR ACTIVE CROHN'S DISEASE*†

Author	Year	No. of Patients	Site of Disease	Initial Dose of CyA (mg/kg/day)	Steroids (% of Patients)	Duration of Treatment (Months)	No. of Patients on CyA	Clinical Response (%) CyA, Placebo, P	Therapeutic Advantage % (95% CI)
Brynskov et al[33]	1989	71	SB, IC, C, PA	5-7.5	34	3	37	59, 32, 0.03	27 (5 to 49)
Jewell et al[23]	1994	146	SB, IC, C	5	100	3	72	36, 43, NS	−7 (−23 to 9)
Feagan et al[24]	1994	305	SB, IC, C	5	61	18	151	40, 48, NS	−8 (−19 to 3)
Stagne et al[25]	1995	182	SB, IC, C, AR	5	77	12	89	20, 20, NS	0 (−12 to 12)

*CyA indicates cyclosporine; CI, confidence interval; SB, small bowel; IC, ileocolonic; C, colonic; PA, perianal; AR; anorectal; NS, nonsignificant.

†Adapted from Sandborn WJ. A critical review of cyclosporine therapy in inflammatory bowel disease. *Inflamm Bowel Dis.* 1995;1:48-63; Loftus CG, Egan LJ, Sandborn WJ. Cyclosporine, tacrolimus, and mycophenolate mofetil in the treatment of inflammatory bowel disease. *Gastroenterol Clin N Am.* 2004;33:141-169.

disease occurred earlier in CyA-treated than in placebo-treated patients (mean time 338 days vs 492 days, respectively). Finally, in the European Trial,[25] 182 patients were randomized to oral CyA or placebo for 12 months. Patients were stratified at entry to a low or high disease activity stratum according to baseline score of CDAI (≤ 200 and > 200, respectively). Patients in the former stratum received the pretrial dose of steroids; those in the latter stratum received 1 mg/kg/day prednisone. Steroids were tapered within 4 months to 5 mg/day prednisone. Efficacy was measured by changes in CDAI scores. Primary outcome was remission rates at 12 months. After 4 months (steroid-tapering period), no significant differences were seen in remission rates between patients treated with CyA or placebo (35% vs 27%). At 12 months, only 20% of patients had sustained clinical remission.

In the past 20 years, numerous uncontrolled trials of high-dose CyA therapy for active CD have been published.[26,42-63] Most centers have used 4 mg/kg/day CyA as continuous IV infusion (range 1 to 5 mg/kg/day). Centers that preferred the oral route have used an overall mean dose of 10 mg/kg/day CyA (range 5 to 15 mg/kg/day). Treatment was given for a period of 2 to 156 weeks. These trials have been reviewed recently in detail by Loftus et al.[15] Although a formal meta-analysis is impossible due to differences in patient characteristics, lack of control population, doses and duration of CyA therapy, primary outcome measures, etc, the results of these trials are strikingly similar to those in the controlled trial of high-dose oral CyA.[33] In summary, the overall short-term mean clinical response of 227 patients treated in 26 uncontrolled trials was 64%, ranging from 0% to 100%[15] compared with 59% in the Brynskov et al study.[33] Clinical improvement was very rapid and inde-

pendent from the site of disease; however, two thirds of the responders deteriorated soon after stopping therapy.[15] In contrast, long-term clinical improvement was substantially better when CyA was offered as "bridge" therapy to slower-acting immune modulators.[35,57,59-61]

Some uncontrolled trials were performed on or included patients with fistulizing CD (Table 16-2).[64-66] To summarize data, a 7- to 14-day continuous IV infusion of 4 mg/kg/day CyA was effective in healing active fistulae that were nonresponsive to treatment with antibiotics, corticosteroids, and immune modulators. Overall, short-term fistulae improvement or closure was achieved in 75 of 93 patients (81%, range 0% to 100%) within 3 to 10 days and was independent of the number and the anatomical site of the fistulae. Sustained fistula closure was reported in 34 (39%) patients but the majority of these were on maintenance treatment with oral CyA and/or immune modulators.

Uncontrolled trials have reported successful healing with CyA of pyoderma gangrenosum complicating CD, which was refractory to antibiotics, corticosteroids, dapsone, and/or azathioprine/6-MP in more than 90% of patients.[68-70] Clinicians have used CyA in doses 3 to 10 mg/kg/day orally or 4 mg/kg/day IV for 7 to 22 days. Responding patients received 4 to 8 mg/kg/day oral CyA and azathioprine/6-MP to maintain healing. Improvement was usually seen within days, but complete healing took longer.[70] Intralesional administration may also be effective. Refractory ocular manifestations of CD were treated with CyA and corticosteroids.[71]

Can whole blood CyA concentrations predict the outcome of treatment? In the transplantation setting, the therapeutic window using HPLC is 150 to 300 ng/mL.[14] In

TABLE 16-2

INITIAL AND SUSTAINED FISTULA RESPONSE IN UNCONTROLLED TRIALS OF CYCLOSPORINE FOR PATIENTS WITH ACTIVE FISTULIZING CROHN'S DISEASE*†

Author	No. of Study Patients	No. of Fistula Patients	Site of Disease	Site of Fistula	Initial Daily Dose (mg/kg)	Duration of Trial (Weeks)	Concomitant Treatments, No. of Patients	Fistula Response Initial	Fistula Response Sustained
Fukushima[47]	7	2	IC, C	EC (1), ns (1)	8, oral	16	None	1	1
Peltekian[44]	7	4	IC, C, PA	EE, EC, PA	10, oral	16	CS, 10	2	0
Stagne[50]	11	4	SB, IC, C, PA	PA, EV	Variable, oral	2-150	CS, 11	4	1
Ardizzone[51]	8	3	SB, IC, C	EC, ns (2)	10, oral	6-36	CS, 3	1	0
Hanauer[35]	5	5	SB, IC, C, PA	EV, EC, PA	4, IV	8-56	CS, 2	5	2‡
Present[66]	16	16	SB, IC, C, PA	PA, EC, EV	4, IV	4-37	CS, 8	14	9‡
Markowitz[54]	1	1	PA	PA	4, IV	14	None	0	1
Abreu-Martin[37]	2	2	SB, C	ns	2.5, IV	variable	CS, 2; AZA, 1	2	1
O'Neil[62]	8	8	SB, IC, C, PA	PA, RV, EC, EV, EE	4, IV	6-34	CS, 8; AZA, 8	7	0
Hinterleitner[65]	9	9	SB, IC, C, PA	PA, EC, EV	5, IV	12	CS, 9; AZA, 9	9	4‡
Egan[58]	18	9	SB, C, PA, PG, IP	PA, EC, EV	4, IV	5-24	CS, 2; AZA, 8	7	2‡
Gurudu[60]	6	3	SB, C	EE, EC, RV	4, IV	5-124	CS, 6	2	1
Haslam[26]	6	4	SB, C, PA	PA (1), ns (3)	ns, oral	variable		3	2
Bararino[64]	4	3	IC, C, PA	PA	ns, IV/oral	1-93	CS, 3; AZA, 2	2	1
Cat[67]	20	20	PA	PA	4, IV	13-30		16	9‡
Total	141	93						75 (81%)	34 (39%)

*IC indicates ileocolonic; C, colonic; SB, small bowel; PA, perianal; PG, proximal gut; EE, enteroenteric; EC, enterocutaneous; EV, enterovesicular; IV, intravenous; IP, ileal pouch; RV, rectovaginal; IP, ileal pouch; AZA, azathioprine; CS, corticosteroids; 6-MP, 6-mercaptopurine; MTX, methotrexate; ns, not stated.

† Adapted from Sandborn WJ. A critical review of cyclosporine therapy in inflammatory bowel disease. *Inflamm Bowel Dis.* 1995;1:48-63; Hanauer SB, Smith MB. Rapid closure of Crohn's disease fistulas with continuous intravenous cyclosporine A. *Am J Gastroenterol.* 1993;88:646-649; Ngo MD, Hagege H, Rosa I, et al. Acute hepatitis in the course of cyclosporine therapy of Crohn's disease. *Presse Med.* 1999;28:1873-1875.

‡Patients were also on CyA and/or immune modulators.

FIGURE 16-2. Patients with steroid-refractory Crohn's disease who fail treatment with conventional immune modulators and anti-TNFα biologics should be treated with a non anti-TNFα biologic agent; if unavailable or failed, patients may be treated with cyclosporine A or tacrolimus (dotted line indicates 2nd option). If remission is achieved, patients may receive maintenance therapy but due to limited efficacy of these agents to maintain remission and considering long-term toxicity, surgical options should be discussed with the patient. Anti-TNFα, anti-tumor necrosis factor alpha.

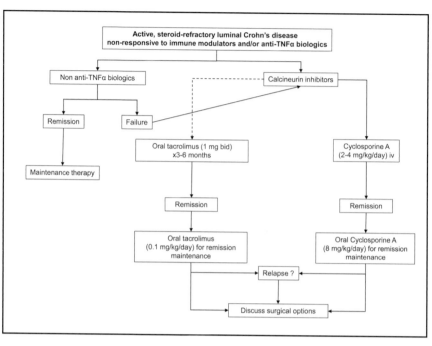

rheumatoid arthritis, the range of whole blood CyA levels (HPLC, mRIA) is 150 to 250 ng/mL for low-dose (≤ 5 mg/mL) and 251 to 400 ng/mL for high-dose (> 5 mg/mL) oral CyA therapy.[15] In 3 controlled trials of low-dose oral CyA, the mean whole blood CyA levels fell within the intended therapeutic range (100 to 250 ng/mL), but there were no differences between responders and nonresponders.[23-25] Using oral CyA in doses adjusted to whole blood CyA levels of 200 to 300 ng/mL (HPLC), a strong correlation was seen between clinical response and endoscopic healing but not mean CyA levels in blood or intestinal tissues.[72] This indicates that the minimum whole blood CyA concentrations that are essential for a clinical response of an individual patient with CD are not quite clear. However, responding patients to CyA doses 8 to 10 mg/kg/day orally or 4 mg/kg/day IV are more likely to have whole blood CyA levels > 400 ng/mL.[15,33] This extremely narrow window between therapeutic levels and toxic concentrations of CyA in CD stresses the need for close monitoring.

FUTURE DIRECTIVES

Based on available data, the use of CyA in CD should be limited to the occasional patient with highly active luminal disease who is confronted with limited surgical options and is refractory to treatment with corticosteroids, anti-TNFα agents and newer non anti-TNFα biologics (Figure 16-2). In this setting, CyA should be offered as rescue continuous IV infusion therapy (2 to 4 mg/kg/day) for approximately 10 days. Because predictable recurrence of disease occurs following cessation of treatment, whereas adverse events preclude its long-term use, responders to IV therapy should be given cautiously oral CyA (8 to 10 mg/kg/day) as a

short-term (3 to 6 months) bridge therapy to slower-acting immune modulators, if the patient is naïve to their use, or to elective surgery.[13,15] A similar approach has been advocated for refractory fistulizing CD,[35,66] but this approach is purely empiric. Controlled trials are needed in CD to compare the efficacy of low- versus high-dose IV as well as oral versus IV CyA therapy, but these trials are unlikely to perform in the era of anti-TNFα therapy.

TACROLIMUS (FK 506, PROGRAF)

BACKGROUND

Tacrolimus was isolated from the culture broth of the soil fungus *Streptomyces tsukubaensis* in 1984.[73] Tacrolimus was a major therapeutic advantage for liver and kidney allograft recipients because it reduced the incidence of acute steroid-resistant rejection and chronic rejection. It was introduced in the treatment of IBD in the 1990s.

PHARMACOKINETICS

Tacrolimus is a water-insoluble macrolide lactone antibiotic that shares similar immunomodulatory properties with CyA (see Figure 16-1).[3] The oral bioavailability is relatively low (mean 20%; range 6% to 43%) because tacrolimus is hydrophobic, is partially metabolized by intestinal P450-3A, and as a macrolide lactone may exert prokinetic effects on the small intestine.[3,73] Absorption is affected by food, and the drug should be taken on an empty stomach. Because absorption does not depend on bile or mucosal integrity, however, tacrolimus has more reliable bioavailability and is a more advantageous immune modifier for the treatment of complicated small bowel CD than CyA.[3,6] A solid dispersible formulation in hydroxypropyl methylcellulose has developed to allow rapid and more consistent oral absorption.[3]

After oral or IV dosing, tacrolimus binds strongly to erythrocytes. The distribution in the blood depends on blood concentration of the drug, the levels of plasma proteins, and hematocrit. Tacrolimus is metabolized by the hepatic P450-3A4 isoenzyme to produce at least 8 metabolites.[3] Drug interactions with tacrolimus are very similar to that with CyA.[3,22] The elimination half-life is approximately 40 hours. Caution is needed when tacrolimus is coadministered with nephrotoxic or neurotoxic drugs or drugs competing for binding to plasma proteins. Tacrolimus is commercially available in formulations for oral (capsules 0.5, 1, and 5 mg) and IV use (5 mg/mL concentrate). An ointment for topical use can be compounded from capsules or IV solution.

Whole blood tacrolimus concentration measurements using sensitive enzyme immunoassays is the preferred method for routine therapeutic monitoring.[21] Results are available within 1 hour. Tacrolimus has a 10- to 100-fold greater immunosuppressive activity in vitro than CyA, and whole blood tacrolimus concentration should be ~20-fold lower than corresponding CyA concentrations.[21] In CD, the recommended dose is 0.1 to 0.2 mg/kg/day orally and 0.01 to 0.02 mg/kg IV. Higher oral doses (0.2 mg/kg/day) should be adjusted to whole blood tacrolimus levels of 10 to 20 ng/mL and for nephrotoxicity (ie, avoiding increases in serum creatinine levels greater than 30% over pretreatment levels).[15] However, these doses are near toxic for kidney/liver allograft recipients in whom a concentration range of 5 to 15 ng/mL tacrolimus has been shown to minimize toxicity without compromising efficacy.[20] Recent uncontrolled data suggest that oral tacrolimus in doses 0.05 to 0.10 mg/kg/day targeting for whole blood concentrations of 5 to 10 ng/mL is also effective in CD.[74,75]

ADVERSE EVENTS

Adverse events have been reported from many organ systems during tacrolimus treatment. Some may be idiosyncratic, but the majority are dose related and reversible on dose reduction or discontinuation of treatment. The most serious adverse events in a controlled trial of oral tacrolimus for fistulizing CD were neurotoxicity and nephrotoxicity.[76] Common adverse events are also nausea, vomiting, paresthesias, tremor, arthralgias, insomnia, pruritus, hypertension, opportunistic infections, hyperkalemia, hyperglycemia, hyperlipidemia, diabetes mellitus, and alopecia.[74-82] Lymphomas are unlikely to develop in CD due to the short duration of treatment. The outcome of pregnancy in tacrolimus-treated women before conception is similar to that with CyA. Tacrolimus crosses the human placenta and is detectable in breast milk.[3] In view of insufficient data, it is contraindicated in pregnancy. The safety protocol includes weekly measurements of blood pressure, serum electrolytes, whole blood tacrolimus levels, and renal function tests during the first month, biweekly during the second month, and monthly thereafter. The dose of the drug must be adjusted to avoid increases in serum creatinine >30% above pretreatment levels.

CLINICAL TRIALS

One controlled trial has been reported in fistulizing CD.[76] Forty-six of 54 screened patients were randomized to oral tacrolimus (0.2 mg/kg/day) or placebo for 10 weeks (Table 16-3). Fistulae had not healed on antibiotics. Infliximab was also unsuccessful in some patients. The rate of fistula remission was similar in the 2 groups but fistula improvement was significantly better in tacrolimus-treated patients. Enterocutaneous fistulae in placebo-treated patients did not improve. During the trial, 19 (90%) of 21 patients required at least 1 dose reduction to maintain the levels of tacrolimus within the target range of 10 to 20 ng/mL or serum creatinine to levels ≤ 1.5 mg/dL. Yet, the mean whole blood tacrolimus levels were similar in patients with or without fistula improvement. Adverse events were more common with tacrolimus, but only 2 patients were withdrawn. Thus, tacrolimus improved draining of perianal fistula at an acceptable safety profile but did not lead to sustained fistula closure.

In contrast, a number of uncontrolled trials and case series reported favorable results of tacrolimus in the treatment of luminal and/or fistulizing CD.[74,75,77-82] Sandborn was the first to report successful use of tacrolimus as a bridge to maintenance treatment with methotrexate or 6-MP in 3 patients with complicated proximal small bowel and/or fistulizing disease.[77] In a more recent report from the Mayo Clinic, 11 patients with refractory single or multiple perianal fistulae received 0.15 to 0.31 mg/kg/day oral tacrolimus for 5 to 47 (mean 22) weeks.[78] Seven patients were already receiving azathioprine/6-MP, and 4 started treatment concomitantly with tacrolimus. Partial fistula healing was seen in 4 and complete fistula closure in 7 patients after a mean period of 2.4 and 12.2 weeks, respectively. Fistula closure was maintained long-term with azathioprine/6-MP in 6 patients but 9 patients underwent surgery in the perianal region during the study period.

In another series,[80] 6 patients with CD and 2 with indeterminate colitis refractory to corticosteroids and/or azathioprine received IV tacrolimus (0.01 to 0.02 mg/kg/day) for 7 days, followed by oral tacrolimus (0.1 to 0.2 mg/kg/day) for a mean period of 8 months (range 0.25 to 16). Mesalamine and azathioprine were given when indicated. Six (75%) of 8 patients improved, and 4 (50%) achieved remission. Fistula draining was decreased in 2 patients with fistulizing disease. However, 4 of 6 responders relapsed, and 3 underwent surgery soon after cessation of treatment.

TABLE 16-3

RESULTS OF A RANDOMIZED, PLACEBO-CONTROLLED TRIAL OF ORAL TACROLIMUS FOR FISTULIZING CROHN'S DISEASE*†

Treatment	No. of Patients	Fistula Location (No. of Patients)			CDAI Mean (SD)	Previous IFX (No. of Patients)	Initial Dose (mg/kg/day)	Concomitant Treatments (No. of Patients)				Trial Duration (Weeks)	Outcome Measures	
		PA	EC	PA/EC				5-ASA	Abx	CS	AZA/6-MP		Primary‡ No. of Patients (%)	Secondary§
Tacrolimus	21	20	0	1	195 (93)	15	20	9	13	5	13	10	9 (43%)	2 (10%)
Placebo	25	22	3	0	196 (108)	14		10	19	4	14	10	2 (8%)	2 (8%)
P value													0.01	1

*PA indicates perianal; EC, enterocutaneous; SD, standard deviation; CDAI, Crohn's Disease Activity Index; IFX, infliximab; 5-ASA, 5-aminosalicylic acid; Abx, antibiotics; CS, corticosteroids; AZA/6-MP, azathioprine/6-mercaptopurine.

†Adapted from Sandborn WJ, Present DH, Isaacs KL, et al. Tacrolimus for the treatment of fistulas in patients with Crohn's disease: a randomized, placebo-controlled trial. *Gastroenterology.* 2003;125:380-388; Loftus CG, Egan LJ, Sandborn WJ. Cyclosporine, tacrolimus, and mycophenolate mofetil in the treatment of inflammatory bowel disease. *Gastroenterol Clin N Am.* 2004;33:141-169.

‡ Fistula improvement: Closure of ≥ 50% of fistulas that were draining at baseline; maintenance of closure for ≥ 4 weeks.

§ Fistula remission: Closure of all fistulas; maintenance of closure for ≥ 4 weeks.

In the prospective, open-label study of Ierardi et al,[81] 13 patients with active, steroid-refractory Crohn's ileocolitis (6), colitis (6), or duodenitis and distal colitis (1) who had developed side effects to CyA received an initial dose of 0.1 to 0.2 mg/kg/day tacrolimus for 2 to 93 months (median 27.3). Mesalamine was allowed but steroids were tapered off. Only 1 patient achieved full remission, but significant reduction in CDAI scores was achieved in 11 (85%) of 13 patients at 6 months and was maintained in 9 (69%) for 12 months and in 2 (15%) for 7 years. Five patients required low-dose steroids for clinical relapse of disease. Three of 6 patients with fistulizing disease had complete closure of perianal, enterocutaneous, and enterocolic fistulae, and 1 had decreased fistula draining. One patient dropped out due to severe tremor. In an open-label, multicenter pediatric IBD trial, Bousvaros et al[82] included 4 children with CD and 2 with indeterminate colitis. Patients received oral tacrolimus (0.1 mg/kg bid aiming for whole blood levels of 10 to 15 ng/mL) for 3 to 4 months as a bridge therapy to azathioprine/6-MP. Clinical improvement was rapid, and 3 children maintained remission for 1 year.

Two trials have reported effective treatment with low-dose oral tacrolimus (0.1 mg/kg/day) of luminal[75] and fistulizing[76] CD. In the first retrospective trial, 3 of 6 patients with disease refractory to steroids and CyA improved, and 1 achieved remission.[75] In the second trial, 15 patients with perianal, enterocutaneous, and rectovaginal fistulae nonresponsive to infliximab were treated concomitantly with tacrolimus and azathioprine/6-MP for 6 to 18 months.[76] Rapid improvement of fistulae was observed in 9 patients but most fistulae needed 6 to 8 months of treatment to close. Fistula closure was maintained with 6-MP. Nephrotoxicity was not reported.

Tacrolimus ointment has been effectively used in the treatment of recalcitrant parastomal pyoderma gangrenosum,[83] oral, and perineal lesions of CD.[84]

FUTURE PERSPECTIVES

Evidence from controlled and uncontrolled clinical trials indicates that tacrolimus is rapidly effective in patients with active fistulizing CD who have failed treatment with antibiotics, conventional immune modulators, and infliximab. In the absence of controlled data for CyA, tacrolimus should be preferred over CyA for fistulizing CD (see Figure 16-2). Despite encouraging preliminary data in uncontrolled clinical trials and case reports, controlled trials are needed to evaluate the efficacy, dosing, and safety of tacrolimus for the induction and maintenance of remission of active luminal disease that is refractory to treatment with steroids and anti-TNFα agents before recommending its general use.

SIROLIMUS (RAPAMYCIN, RAPAMUNE)

Sirolimus is a natural fermentation product of the actinomycete *Streptomyces hygroscopicus* isolated from soil samples from Rapa Nui, in the Easter Islands, in 1975.[2] Sirolimus is a macrocyclic lactone.[5] At a molecular level, sirolimus binds to FKBP12. The complex directly inhibits the TOR1 and TOR2 (targets of rapamycin) enzymes arresting the transition of the G1 to S phase of the T cell cycle and prevents the proliferation of T helper cells. Sirolimus is used in vitro to upregulate autophagy in cell cultures but has not been tested in randomized controlled trials in CD. However, sporadic case reports claim sustained benefit in patients with luminal and/or fistulizing CD unresponsive to immune modulators and anti-TNFα biologics. Everolimus, an immunosuppressive agent similar to sirolimus, was tested recently in active CD but after an interim analysis, this trial was stopped prematurely due to lack of differences in efficacy between everolimus and its comparators, azathioprine and placebo.[85]

MYCOPHENOLATE MOFETIL (CELLCEPT)

BACKGROUND

Mycophenolate mofetil (MMF) was isolated from cultures containing *Penicillium* spp. It was initially used for the treatment of psoriasis and subsequently as an adjunct immunosuppressive for the prevention of rejection in organ transplantation.[86]

PHARMACOKINETICS

Human lymphocytes, unlike other rapidly dividing cells such as macrophages, are almost totally dependent on the de novo pathway for purine biosynthesis.[80] MMF is a morpholino ester prodrug of mycophenolic acid, the active metabolite that exerts immunosuppressive activity. This is due to a selective, noncompetitive, reversible inhibition of type 2 inosine monophosphate dehydrogenase, the rate-limiting enzyme in the de novo synthesis of guanosine nucleotides, which prevents the de novo purine synthesis and arrests T and B cell division and the formation of antibodies.[87] Deficiency of guanosine nucleotides affects the glycosylation of leukocyte adhesion molecules, inhibiting leukocyte and monocyte trafficking to sites of inflammation.[87] This effect may be crucial for downregulating inflammation in IBD. MMF may also prevent the formation of intestinal strictures in CD by inhibiting fibronectin synthesis and smooth muscle growth.

Studies in several animal species have shown that oral bioavailability of MMF is better than mycophenolic acid.[86] MMF either alone or as adjunct immunosuppressive prevents the rejection of various allografts and reverses acute rejection of kidney or heart allografts.[86] These effects are coupled with a low toxicity and a good safety profile. Studies in healthy volunteers and allograft recipients have demonstrated that absorption of MMF after oral administration is rapid and almost complete. MMF undergoes extensive de-esterification resulting in complete systemic delivery of mycophenolic acid.[88] Because >98% of mycophenolic acid in the circulation is bound to albumin, patients with CD and hypoalbuminemia may have more active drug available for pharmacological action and may be prone to adverse events. Mycophenolic acid is metabolized to phenolic acid glucuronide, which is excreted through the kidneys.[88] Commercially available formulations of MMF include an oral capsule (250 mg), an oral tablet (500 mg), powder for solution (200 mg/mL), and suspension (200 mg/mL). A new enteric-coated mycophenolate sodium formulation that delivers mycophenolic acid has been developed to improve tolerability. It has a similar efficacy and safety to MMF in renal transplant patients.

Adverse Events

Allograft recipients who receive long-term 2 to 3 g/day of MMF are prone to serious adverse events, especially myelosuppression, infections, and lymphoproliferative disorders. Serious adverse events are not as common in CD, probably because of smaller doses (2 g/day) and shorter duration of treatment. Overall, 34 (22%) of 157 patients in 11 clinical trials of CD discontinued therapy for MMF-related adverse events (0.37 events per patient).[89-99] These include nausea and/or vomiting (15%), skin rashes (15%), diarrhea (12%), malaise (12%), headache and/or migraine (9%), arthralgias (6%), pancreatitis (6%), behavioral changes (6%), and (less often) medullary aplasia, constipation, depression, parotitis, and elevated liver enzymes. In the controlled trial of Neurath et al,[89] only 2 MMF-treated patients compared with 7 azathioprine-treated patients developed serious side effects. Cases of serious drug-induced colitis or lymphoproliferative disorders have not been reported in CD. MMF is contraindicated in pregnancy. The safety protocol should include full blood counts every week during the first month of treatment and monthly thereafter.

Clinical Trials

Motivation to use MMF in the transplantation setting was the efficacy of the drug in psoriasis. In patients receiving CyA and corticosteroids, 2 oral doses of MMF (1 g and 1.5 g bid) were superior to placebo or azathioprine (100 to 150 mg/day) for the prevention of treatment failure or biopsy-proven acute rejection in the first 6 months after transplantation.[100] During the annual follow-up, the number of patients with a first episode of acute rejection or biopsy-proven rejection was significantly lower with MMF treatment. MMF has also been used in the treatment of rheumatoid arthritis, lupus nephritis, and pemphigus vulgaris. In allograft recipients, the efficacy and safety of MMF was better with the 2 g/day dose. In CD, most physicians use 2 g/day.

A randomized clinical trial and a number of case series have suggested a possible role of MMF for active, steroid-refractory CD. In the open, randomized, single-center, 6-month trial, 70 patients with moderately active (CDAI 150 to 300) or highly active (CDAI > 300) steroid-dependent CD received oral MMF (15 mg/kg/day) or azathioprine (2.5 mg/kg/day) in a 1:1 ratio.[89] All patients received 50 mg prednisolone with tapering to a maintenance dose of 5 mg within 7 weeks. The results showed that although differences in remission rates with MMF or azathioprine were not significant at the end of the trial, the decrease in laboratory indices of disease activity was significantly higher for MMF than azathioprine after 1 month of treatment, indicating an earlier response to MMF. However, this study has several limitations: because neither patients nor physicians were blinded to treatment, a decrease in CDAI scores was not a primary endpoint, patients received initially a high-dose pulse prednisolone therapy, and intention-to-treat analysis was not performed.

A number of case series evaluating the efficacy of MMF (mean dose 2 g/day; range 0.75 to 3 g/day) in refractory CD have reported both positive and negative results.[90-99,101] These trials should be interpreted with caution because of high variability regarding criteria for efficacy, disease activity, concomitant treatments, doses, and potential loss of MMF efficacy with prolonged treatment. Pooled data show an initial response rate to MMF of 44.2% (61 of 138 patients) but only 39 (28.3%) patients were in remission 6 months later despite tolerance of treatment. Eight trials reported initial closure of 1 or more active perianal fistulae in 10 (31%) and decreased draining in 10 (31%) of 32 patients.[90-92,95-97,99,101] Four trials reported sustained fistula closure in 9 (47%) of 19 patients on chronic MMF treatment.[91,95,97,99] Patients with arthritis or pyoderma-gangrenosum improved during MMF treatment.[95]

Future Directives

MMF is superior to azathioprine/6-MP in inducing a rapid clinical response of steroid-dependent/refractory CD, regardless of disease location. However, few of the initial responders maintain long-term remission. Drug toxicity, especially hemorrhagic colitis, may be another limitation in IBD. Further controlled trials are needed to clarify a role for MMF in the treatment of CD. Because this target seems unrealistic, the use of MMF should be limited to patients who are intolerant or have failed treatment with first-line immune modulators and anti-TNFα agents.

REFERENCES

1. Sigal NH, Dumont FJ. Cyclosporin A, FK-506, and rapamycin: pharmacologic probes of lymphocyte signal transaction. *Ann Rev Immunol.* 1992;10:519-560.

2. Schreiber SL. Chemistry and biology of the immunophilins and their immunosuppressive ligands. *Science.* 1991;251:283-287.

3. Prograf [product monograph]. London, UK: Fujisawa Ltd; 1999.

4. Reed JC, Prystowsky MB, Nowell PC. Regulation of gene expression in lectin-stimulated or lymphokine-stimulated lymphocytes. *Transplantation.* 1988;46(2 suppl):858-898.

5. Morris RE. Mechanisms of action of new immunosuppressive drugs. *Ther Drug Monit.* 1995;17:564-569.

6. Choc MG. Cyclosporine: pharmacology. In: Yocum DE, ed. *Cyclosporine: Clinical Application in Autoimmune Diseases.* Philadelphia, PA: Mosby-Wolfe Medical Communications; 2000: 15-30.

7. Drewe J, Berlinger C, Kissel T. The absorption site of cyclosporin in the human gastrointestinal tract. *Br J Clin Pharmacol.* 1992; 33:39-43.

8. Brynskov J, Freund L, Campanini MC, Kampmann JP. Cyclosporin pharmacokinetics after intravenous and oral administration in patients with Crohn's disease. *Scand J Gastroenterol.* 1992;27:961-967.

9. Fahr A. Cyclosporin clinical pharmacokinetics. *Clin Pharmacokinet.* 1993;24:472-495.

10. Roberts R, Sketris IS, Abraham I, Givner ML, MacDonald AS. Cyclosporin absorption in two patients with short-bowel syndrome. *Drug Intell Clin Pharm.* 1988;22:570-572.

11. Kolars JC, Awni WM, Merion RM, Watkins PB. First-pass metabolism of cyclosporin by the gut. *Lancet.* 1991;338:1488-1490.

12. Gutzler F, Zimmermann R, Ring GH, Sauer P, Stiehl A. Ursodeoxycholic acid enhances the absorption of cyclosporine in a heart transplant patient with short bowel syndrome. *Transplant Proc.* 1992;24:2620-2621.

13. Sandborn WJ. A critical review of cyclosporine therapy in inflammatory bowel disease. *Inflamm Bowel Dis.* 1995;1:48-63.

14. Kahan BD. Cyclosporine. *N Engl J Med.* 1989;321:1725-1738.

15. Loftus CG, Egan LJ, Sandborn WJ. Cyclosporine, tacrolimus, and mycophenolate mofetil in the treatment of inflammatory bowel disease. *Gastroenterol Clin N Am.* 2004;33:141-169.

16. Kahan BD, Dunn J, Fitts C, et al. Reduced inter- and intra-subject variability in cyclosporine pharmacokinetics in renal transplant recipients treated with a microemulsion formulation in conjunction with fasting, low-fat meals, or high-fat meals. *Transplantation.* 1995;59:505-511.

17. Latteri M, Angeloni G, Silveri NG, Manna R, Gasbarrini G, Navarra P. Pharmacokinetics of cyclosporin microemulsion in patients with inflammatory bowel disease. *Clin Pharmacokinet.* 2001;40:473-483.

18. Sandborn WJ, Strong RM, Forland SC, Chase RE, Cutler RE. The pharmacokinetics and colonic tissue concentrations of cyclosporine after IV, oral, and enema administration. *J Clin Pharmacol.* 1991;31:76-80.

19. Wenk M, Follath F, Abisch E. Temperature dependency of apparent cyclosporine A concentrations in plasma. *Clin Chem.* 1983; 29:1865.

20. Oellerich M, Armstrong VW, Schutz E, Shaw LM. Therapeutic drug monitoring of cyclosporine and tacrolimus. Update on Lake Louise Consensus Conference on Cyclosporine and Tacrolimus. *Clin Biochem.* 1998;31:309-316.

21. Armstrong VW, Oellerich M. New developments in the immunosuppressive drug monitoring of cyclosporine, tacrolimus, and azathioprine. *Clin Biochem.* 2001;34:9-16.

22. Castelao AM, Sabate I, Grino JM, et al. Cyclosporine-drug interactions. *Transplant Proc.* 1988;20(5 suppl 6):66-69.

23. Jewell DP, Lennard-Jones JE. Oral cyclosporin for chronic active Crohn's disease: a multicentre controlled trial. *Eur J Gastroenterol Hepatol.* 1994;6:499-505.

24. Feagan BG, McDonald JW, Pochon J, et al. Low-dose cyclosporine for the treatment of Crohn's disease. The Canadian Crohn's Relapse Prevention Trial Investigators. *N Engl J Med.* 1994;330: 1846-1851.

25. Stange EF, Modigliani A, Pena AS, Wood AJ, Feutren G, Smith PR. European trial of cyclosporine in chronic active Crohn's disease: a 12-month study. The European Study Group. *Gastroenterology.* 1995;109:774-782.

26. Haslam N, Hearing SD, Prombert CSJ. Audit of cyclosporine use in inflammatory bowel disease: limited benefits, numerous side-effects. *Eur J Gastroenterol Hepatol.* 2000;12:657-660.

27. Gunliffe RN, Scott BB. Review article: monitoring for the drug side-effects in inflammatory bowel disease. *Aliment Pharmacol Ther.* 2002;16:647-662.

28. Feutren G, Mihatsch MJ, for the International Kidney Biopsy Registry of Cyclosporine in Autoimmune Diseases. Risk factors for cyclosporine-induced nephropathy in patients with autoimmune diseases. *N Engl J Med.* 1992;326:1654-1660.

29. Rosencrantz R, Moon A, Raynes H, Spivac W. Cyclosporine-induced neurotoxicity during treatment of Crohn's disease: lack of correlation with previously reported risk factors. *Am J Gastroenterol.* 2001;96:2778-2781.

30. Porges Y, Blumen S, Fireman Z, Sternberg A, Zamir D. Cyclosporine-induced optic neuropathy, ophthalmoplegia and nystagmus in a patient with Crohn's disease. *Am J Ophthalmol.* 1998;126:607-609.

31. Barabino A, Castellano A, Gandullia P, Biscaldi F. A girl with severe fistulizing Crohn's disease. *Dig Liv Dis.* 2000;32:792-794.

32. Shbarou RM, Chao NJ, Morgenlander JC. Cyclosporin-related cerebral vasculopathy. *Bone Marrow Transplant.* 2000;26:801-804.

33. Brynskov J, Freund L, Rasmussen SN, et al. A placebo-controlled, double-blind, randomized trial of cyclosporine therapy in active chronic Crohn's disease. *N Engl J Med.* 1989;321:845-850.

34. Vega P, Bertràn X, Menacho M, et al. Cytomegalovirus infection in patients with inflammatory bowel disease. *Am J Gastroenterol.* 1999;94:1053-1056.

35. Hanauer SB, Smith MB. Rapid closure of Crohn's disease fistulas with continuous intravenous cyclosporine A. *Am J Gastroenterol.* 1993;88:646-649.

36. Scalzini A, Barni C, Stellrini R, Sueri L. Fatal invasive aspergillosis during cyclosporine and steroids treatment for Crohn's disease. *Dig Dis Sci.* 1995;40:528-540.

37. Abreu-Martin MT, Vasiliauskas EA, Gaiennie J, Voigt B, Targan SR. Continuous infusion cyclosporine ineffective for severe acute Crohn's disease ... But for how long [abstract]. *Gastroenterology.* 1996;110:A851.

38. Ngo MD, Hagege H, Rosa I, et al. Acute hepatitis in the course of cyclosporine therapy of Crohn's disease. *Presse Med.* 1999;28:1873-1875.

39. Bluhm RE, Rodgers WH, Black DL, Wilkinson GR, Branch R. Cholestasis in transplant patients—what is the role of cyclosporine? *Aliment Pharmacol Ther.* 1992;6:207-219.

40. Bebb JR, Logan RP. Does the use of immunosuppressive therapy in inflammatory bowel disease increase the risk of developing lymphoma? *Aliment Pharmacol Ther.* 2001;15:1843-1849.

41. Brynskov J, Freund L, Norby Rasmussen S, et al. Final report on a placebo-controlled, double-blind, randomized, multicentre trial of cyclosporin treatment in active Crohn's disease. *Scand J Gastroenterol.* 1991;26:689-695.

42. Allison MC, Pounder RE. Cyclosporin for Crohn's disease. *Aliment Pharmacol Ther.* 1987;1:39-43.

43. Parrott NR, Taylor RM, Venables CW, Record CO. Treatment of Crohn's disease in relapse with cyclosporine A. *Br J Surg.* 1988; 75:1185-1188.

44. Peltekian KM, Williams CN, MacDonald AS, Roy PD, Czolpinska E. Open trial of cyclosporine in patients with severe active Crohn's disease refractory to conventional therapy. *Can J Gastroenterol.* 1988;2:5-11.

45. Brynskov J, Binder V, Riis P, et al. Low-dose cyclosporin for Crohn's disease: implications for clinical trials. *Aliment Pharmacol Ther.* 1989;3:135-142.

46. Baker K, Jewell DP. Cyclosporin for the treatment of severe inflammatory bowel disease [erratum appears in *Aliment Pharmacol Ther.* 1989;3:414]. *Aliment Pharmacol Ther.* 1989;3:143-149.

47. Fukushima T, Sugita A, Masuzawa S, Yamazaki Y, Tsuchiya S. Effects of cyclosporin A on active Crohn's disease. *Gastroenterol Jpn.* 1989;24:12-15.

48. Lofberg R, Angelin B, Einarsson K, Gabrielsson N, Ost L. Unsatisfactory effect of cyclosporine A treatment in Crohn's disease: a report of five cases. *J Intern Med.* 1989;226:157-161.

49. Ranzi T, Campanini MC, Quarto Di Palo F, Velio P, Bianchi PA. Cyclosporin A in Crohn's disease. *Curr Ther Res.* 1989;45:245-252.

50. Stagne EF, Fleig WE, Rehklau E, Ditschuneit H. Cyclosporin A treatment in inflammatory bowel disease. *Dig Dis Sci.* 1989;34:1387-1392.

51. Ardizzone S, Fasoli R, Sangaletti O, Petrillo M, Bianchi-Porro G. The treatment of chronically active Crohn's disease with cyclosporine A. *Curr Ther Res.* 1990;48:1-4.

52. Lichtiger S. Cyclosporine therapy in inflammatory bowel disease: open-label experience. *Mt Sinai J Med.* 1990;57:315-319.

53. Lobo AJ, July LD, Rothwell J, Poole TW, Axon AT. Long-term treatment of Crohn's disease with cyclosporine: the effect of a very low dose on maintenance of remission. *J Clin Gastroenterol.* 1991;13:42-45.

54. Markowitz J, Grancher K, Rosa J, Simpser E, Aiges H, Daum F. Highly destructive perianal disease in children with Crohn's disease. *J Pediatr Gastroenterol Nutr.* 1995;21:149-153.

55. Santos JV, Baudet JA, Casellas FJ, Guarner LA, Vilaseca JM, Malagelada JR. Intravenous cyclosporine for steroid-refractory attacks of Crohn's disease: short- and long-term results. *J Clin Gastroenterol.* 1995;20:207-210.

56. Mahdi G, Israel DM, Hasall E. Cyclosporine and 6-mercaptopurine for active, refractory Crohn's disease in children. *Am J Gastroenterol.* 1996;91:1355-1359.

57. Ramakrishna J, Langhans N, Calenda K, Grand RJ, Verhave M. Combined use of cyclosporine and azathioprine or 6-mercaptopurine in pediatric inflammatory bowel disease. *J Pediatr Gastroenterol Nutr.* 1996;22:296-302.

58. Egan LJ, Sandborn WJ, Tremaine WJ. Clinical outcome following treatment of refractory inflammatory and fistulizing Crohn's disease with intravenous cyclosporine. *Am J Gastroenterol.* 1998;93:442-448.

59. Taylor AC, Connell WR, Elliott R, d'Apice AJF. Oral cyclosporine in inflammatory bowel disease. *Austr NZ J Med.* 1998;28:179-183.

60. Gurudu SR, Griffel LH, Gialanella RJ, Das KM. Cyclosporine therapy in inflammatory bowel disease: Short-term and long-term results. *J Clin Gastroenterol.* 1999;29:151-154.

61. Lavy A. Long-term cyclosporine for resistant Crohn's disease. *J Clin Gastroenterol.* 1999;28:254-255.

62. O'Neil J, Pathmakanthan S, Coh J. Cyclosporine A induces remission of Crohn's disease but relapse occurs upon cessation of treatment [abstract]. *Gastroenterology.* 1997;112:A1056.

63. Hermida-Rodriguez C, Cantero Perona J, Garcia-Valriberas R, Pajares Garcia JM, Mate-Jimenez J. High-dose intravenous cyclosporine in steroid refractory attacks of IBD. *Hepatogastoenterology.* 1999;46:2265-2268.

64. Bararino A, Torrente F, Castellano E, et al. The use of ciclosporin in pediatric inflammatory bowel disease: an Italian experience. *Aliment Pharmacol Ther.* 2002;16:1503-1507.

65. Hinterleitner TA, Petritsch W, Aichbicher B, Fickert P, Ranner G, Krejs GJ. Combination of cyclosporine, azathioprine and prednisolone for perianal Crohn's disease. *Z Gastroenterol.* 1997;35:603-608.

66. Present DH, Lichtiger S. Efficacy of cyclosporine in treatment of fistula in Crohn's disease. *Dig Dis Sci.* 1994;39:374-380.

67. Cat H, Sophani I, Lemann M, Modigliani R, Solue JC. Cyclosporin treatment of anal and perianal lesions associated with Crohn's disease. *Turk J Gastroenterol.* 2003;14:121-127.

68. Tjandra JJ, Hughes LE. Parastomal pyoderma gangrenosum in inflammatory bowel disease. *Dis Colon Rectum.* 1994; 37:938-942.

69. Carp JM, Onuma E, Das K, Gottlieb AB. Intravenous cyclosporine therapy in the treatment of pyoderma gangrenosum secondary to Crohn's disease. *Cutis.* 1997;60:135-138.

70. Friedman S, Marion JF, Scherl E, Rubin PH, Present DH. Intravenous cyclosporine in refractory pyoderma gangrenosum complicating inflammatory bowel disease. *Inflamm Bowel Dis.* 2001;7:1-7.

71. Nussenblatt RB, Palestine AG, Chan CC, Stevens G Jr, Mellow SD, Green SB. Randomized, double-masked study of cyclosporine compared to prednisolone in the treatment of endogenous uveitis. *Am J Ophthalmol.* 1991;112:138-146.

72. Sandborn WJ, Tremaine WJ, Lawson GM. Clinical response does not correlate with intestinal or blood cyclosporine concentrations in patients with Crohn's disease treated with high-dose oral cyclosporine. *Am J Gastroenterol.* 1996;91:37-43.

73. Kino T, Hatanaka H, Hashimoto M, et al. FK-506, a novel immunosuppressant isolated from a *Streptomyces*. I. Fermentation, isolation and physico-chemical and biological characteristics. *J Antibiot.* 1987;40:1249-1255.

74. Baumgart DC, Wiedenmann B, Dignass AU. Rescue therapy with tacrolimus is effective in patients with severe and refractory inflammatory bowel disease. *Aliment Pharmacol Ther.* 2003;17:1273-1281.

75. Gonzalez Lama Y, Abreu LE, Vera MI, de la Revilla J, Fernandez-Puga N, Escartin P. Long-term oral tacrolimus in refractory to infliximab fistulizing Crohn's disease: comments from the Spanish experience [erratum appears in *Gastroenterology.* 2004;126:1500]. *Gastroenterology.* 2004;126:942-943.

76. Sandborn WJ, Present DH, Isaacs KL, et al. Tacrolimus for the treatment of fistulas in patients with Crohn's disease: a randomized, placebo-controlled trial. *Gastroenterology.* 2003;125:380-388.

77. Sandborn WJ. Preliminary report on the use of oral tacrolimus (FK506) in the treatment of complicated proximal small bowel and fistulizing Crohn's disease. *Gastroenterology.* 1997;92:876-879.

78. Lowry PW, Weaver AL, Teamaine WJ, Sandborn WJ. Combination therapy with oral tacrolimus (FK506) and azathioprine or 6-mercaptopurine for treatment-refractory Crohn's disease perianal fistulae. *Inflamm Bowel Dis.* 1999;5:239-245.

79. Ierardi E, Principi M, Bendina M, et al. Oral tacrolimus (FK 506) in Crohn's disease complicated by fistulae of the perineum. *J Clin Gastroenterol.* 2000;30:200-202.

80. Fellermann K, Ludwig D, Stahl M, David-Walek T, Stange EF. Steroid-unresponsive acute attacks of inflammatory bowel disease: immunomodulation by tacrolimus. *Am J Gastroenterol.* 1998; 93:1860-1866.

81. Ierardi E, Principi M, Francavilla R, et al. Oral tacrolimus long-term therapy in patients with Crohn's disease and steroid resistance. *Aliment Pharmacol Ther.* 2001;15:371-377.

82. Bousvaros A, Kirschner BS, Werlin SL, et al. Oral tacrolimus treatment for severe colitis in children. *J Pediatr.* 2000;137:794-799.

83. Khurrum Baig M, Marquez H, Nogueras JJ, Weiss EG, Wexner SD. Topical tacrolimus (FK506) in the treatment of recalcitrant parastomal pyoderma gangrenosum associated with Crohn's disease: report of two cases. *Colorectal Disease.* 2004;6:250-253.

84. Casson DH, Eltumi M, Tomlin S, Walker-Smith JA, Murch SH. Topical tacrolimus may be effective in the treatment of oral and perineal Crohn's disease. *Gut.* 2000;47:436-440.

85. Reinisch W, Panés J, Lémann M, et al. A multicenter, randomized, double-blind trial of everolimus versus azathioprine and placebo to maintain steroid-induced remission in patients with moderate-to-severe active Crohn's disease. *Am J Gastroenterol.* 2008;103:2284-2292.

86. Sollinger HW. Mycophenolates in transplantation. *Clin Transplant.* 2004;18:485-492.

87. Allison AC, Eugui EM. Purine metabolism and immunosuppressive effects of mycophenolate mofetil (MMF). *Clin Transplant.* 1996;10(1 pt 2):77-84.

88. Bullingham RE, Nicholls AJ, Kamm BR. Clinical pharmacokinetics of mycophenolate mofetil. *Clin Pharmacokinet.* 1998;34:429-455.

89. Neurath MF, Wanitschke R, Peters M, Krummenauer F, Meyer Zum Büschenfelde KH, Schlaak H. Randomized trial of mycophenolate mofetil versus azathioprine for treatment of chronic active Crohn's disease. *Gut.* 1999;44:625-628.

90. Horgan K. Initial experience with mycophenolate mofetil in the treatment of severe inflammatory bowel disease. *Gastroenterology.* 1997;112:A999.

91. Fickert P, Hinterleitner TA, Wenzl HH, Aichbichler BW, Petritsch W. Mycophenolate mofetil in patients with Crohn's disease. *Am J Gastroenterol.* 1998;93:2529-2532.

92. Radford-Smith GL, Taylor P, Florin THJ. Mycophenolate mofetil in IBD patients. *Lancet.* 1999;354:1386-1387.

93. Hassard P, Vasilauskas E, Kam L, Targan S, Abreu-Martin MT. Efficacy of mycophenolate mofetil in patients failing 6-mercaptopurine or azathioprine therapy for Crohn's disease. *Inflamm Bowel Dis.* 2000;6:16-20.

94. Fellermann K, Steffen M, Stein J, et al. Mycophenolate mofetil: lack of efficacy in chronic active inflammatory bowel disease. *Aliment Pharmacol Ther.* 2000;14:171-176.

95. Miehsler W, Reinisch W, Moser G, Gangl A, Vogeslang H. Is mycophenolate mofetil an affective alternative in azathioprine-intolerant patients with chronic active Crohn's disease. *Am J Gastroenterol.* 2001;96:782-787.

96. Skelly MM, Logan RFA, Jenkins D, Mahida YR, Hawkey CJ. Toxicity of mycophenolate mofetil in patients with inflammatory bowel disease. *Inflamm Bowel Dis.* 2002;8:93-97.

97. Hafraoui S, Dewit O, Marteau P, et al. Mycophenolate mofetil in refractory Crohn's disease after failure of treatments by azathioprine or methotrexate. *Gastroenterol Clin Biol.* 2002;26:17-22.

98. Ford AC, Towler RJ, Moayyedi P, Chalmers DM, Axon AT. Mycophenolate mofetil in refractory inflammatory bowel disease. *Aliment Pharmacol Ther.* 2003;17:1365-1369.

99. Wenzl HH, Hinterleitner TA, Aichbichler BW, Fickert P, Petritsch W. Mycophenolate mofetil for Crohn's disease: short-term efficacy and long-term outcome. *Aliment Pharmacol Ther.* 2004;19:427-434.

100. Halloran P, for the International Mycophenolate Mofetil Renal Transplant Study Groups. Mycophenolate mofetil in renal allograft recipients: a pooled efficacy analysis of three randomized, double-blind, clinical studies in prevention of rejection. *Transplantation.* 1997;63:39-47.

101. Nehme OS, Overley CA, O'Brien JJ. The role of mycophenolate mofetil in the management of refractory inflammatory bowel disease [abstract]. *Gastroenterology.* 1998;114:A1049.

INFLIXIMAB IN CROHN'S DISEASE

Lawrence W. Comerford, MD and Stephen J. Bickston, MD, AGAF

CD is a chronic inflammatory disorder of the gastrointestinal tract that results in significant morbidity and health-care expenditure. More than 400,000 individuals in the United States have been diagnosed with CD, and the prevalence continues to increase as a result of both increasing incidence and improved survival.[1] The chronic nature of CD results in frequent hospitalizations, with a majority of patients eventually requiring surgery as a result of complications such as strictures, abscesses, fistula, or refractory disease.

The etiology of CD is currently unknown, but the disease apparently occurs when the intestinal immune cascade is triggered by an antigen in genetically susceptible individuals.[2] Mucosal damage is caused by overactivation of the enteric immune and inflammatory pathways, resulting in the clinical signs and symptoms of CD. Various medications, including 5-aminosalicylates, antibiotics, corticosteroids, and immunomodulators such as purine antimetabolites and methotrexate, have traditionally been used to control this inflammatory response. None of these medications completely resolves the disease; however, with their use serving only to minimize the need for surgery and hopefully improve the patient's quality of life. Although immunomodulators are effective maintenance drugs, they have a slow onset of action with clinical remission rates of approximately 40%. Unfortunately, many patients require steroids to control their symptoms, which is far from optimal due to their wide range of dose-related adverse effects. The limitations of conventional agents therefore leave the clinician in need of a medication that is steroid sparing, has a rapid onset of action, and is capable of maintaining remission.[3]

Advances in genetic engineering techniques have allowed the production of endogenous proteins in sufficient quantities to be viable for therapeutic use. This recombinant technology involves the incorporation of mammalian DNA encoding a specific protein into bacteria or cells, which then produce the protein in large quantities that are relatively easy to purify. The monoclonal antibody is a useful class of protein that has evolved from recombinant technology[4]; these antibodies bind to a particular antigen with high affinity and specificity.[5] Monoclonal antibodies are currently used in the treatment of immune-mediated inflammatory diseases, transplant rejection, and malignancies.[6] Parallel advances in our understanding of the molecular biology of intestinal inflammation in animal models have allowed specific application to CD in humans.

Infliximab (Remicade/cA2; Centocor Inc, Malvern, PA) is a chimeric monoclonal antibody (75% human and 25% mouse) that targets tumor necrosis factor alpha (TNFα), a potent proinflammatory cytokine that plays a pivotal role in the initiation and promotion of intestinal inflammation. The international nonproprietary name (INN) infliximab derives from the nomenclature where *mab* denotes a monoclonal antibody, *xi* conveys its chimeric nature, and *infli* indicates that its target is the inflammatory cascade. This novel biological agent is now used extensively in the treatment of patients with moderate-to-severe luminal and fistulizing CD, as well as for the alleviation of symptoms of rheumatoid arthritis (RA). Since marketing approval in August 1998, more than 492,000 patients with more than 900,000 patient-years of exposure have received infliximab commercially worldwide. This includes approximately 277,000 RA patients and approximately 200,000

Lichtenstein GR, ed.
Crohn's Disease: The Complete Guide to Medical Management (pp 197-212).
© 2011 SLACK Incorporated

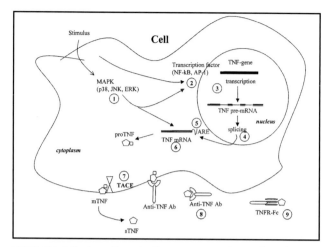

FIGURE 17-1. Activation pathways leading to tumor necrosis factor (TNFα) production. Anti-TNFα strategies using antibodies and TNFα receptors (TNFα-R) target membrane-bound and soluble TNFα. ARE indicates adenosine-uracil rich elements; ERK, extracellular regulated kinase; JNK, c-Jun N-terminal kinase; MAPK, mitogen-activated protein kinase; TACE, TNFα-converting enzyme. (Reprinted from Papadakis KA, Targan SR. Tumor necrosis factor: biology and therapeutic inhibitors. *Gastroenterology.* 2000;119:1148-1157.)

CD patients.[7] Thus far, this agent has proven to be safe and effective in patients afflicted with CD.

BACKGROUND

TNFα is an important proinflammatory cytokine that plays a key role in several disease states. Interest in the potential of TNFα as a therapeutic target was first raised 20 years ago, with the investigation of its role in endotoxin-induced sepsis.[4] Elevated TNFα concentrations have been found in inflamed tissues of patients with CD, RA, and multiple sclerosis (MS).[8] In addition, stool and mucosal concentrations of TNFα in CD patients correlate with the clinical activity of the disease.[9]

The TNFα precursor is a 157 amino acid protein produced by T cells, monocytes, and macrophages. Initially secreted in this inactive precursor form, the protein is rapidly proteolyzed to a 17 kD monomer that trimerizes to form the biologically active 51 kD mature cytokine. TNFα binds to either a 55 or 75 kD transmembrane TNFα receptor (TNFα-R) located on the surface of a number of different cell types (TNFα-R p55 and TNFα-R p75, respectively).[4,10] Binding of TNFα to one of these receptors triggers intracellular signaling events via the nuclear factor-κB (NF-κB) and c-Jun N-terminal kinase (JNK) pathways (Figure 17-1). These include the initiation of transcription of genes involved in the inflammatory response and induction of apoptosis via members of the caspase family of proteins.[4,8] In addition, the interaction causes upregulation of endothelial cell adhesion molecules, proliferation of fibroblasts, induction of metalloproteinases critical to

tissue destruction; induction of inflammatory mediators such as interferon-γ, platelet-activating factor, nitric oxide synthetase, and cyclooxygenase; activation of the coagulation cascade; and formation of granulomas. Another consequence is increased intestinal permeability.[10-15]

The demonstration of the important role that TNFα plays in the inflammatory cascade has led considerable research efforts to investigate the effects of blocking this cytokine with novel biological agents. Indeed, clinical and histological improvement has been demonstrated in animal models of colitis, arthritis, and myelin destruction in response to TNFα inhibitors.[4] Investigators therefore postulated that, because TNFα was involved in granuloma formation, a TNFα inhibitor may have potential for the treatment of granulomatous bowel diseases such as CD.[16] Recombinant technology subsequently enabled the development of monoclonal antibodies that inhibit TNFα. In preliminary open-label trials, mucosal healing and clinical improvement were observed in CD patients administered one of these monoclonal antibodies.[16]

Infliximab is a chimeric antibody that was configured by linking the constant regions of the human immunoglobulin G1k (IgG1k) to the variable antigen-binding regions of a murine anti-human TNFα antibody.[12,17] Infliximab neutralizes the biological activity of TNFα by binding to both the soluble and transmembrane forms of this cytokine, and thereby inhibiting binding of TNFα to its receptors.[17,18] Binding to transmembrane or cell-bound TNFα causes antibody-dependent cell-mediated cytotoxicity or complement fixation and lysis of cells bearing TNFα on their surface.[18] The IgG1 Fc portion of the antibody causes apoptosis of T lymphocytes.[19] Blockade of TNFα also decreases expression of interleukins-1 and -6, interferon-γ, and other proinflammatory cytokines. In addition, downregulation of acute phase proteins, adhesion molecules, and inducible nitric oxide synthetase occurs.[20,21]

THE CONTEXT OF ANTI-TNFα THERAPY

The scientific and commercial success of infliximab rekindled interest in thalidomide and led to efforts to develop other anti-TNFα biological agents. Thalidomide has some of the characteristics of a more ideal therapy, as it is an orally available agent with an easy dosing schedule. Its anti-TNFα activity in CD is supported by a small study of cytokine effects,[22] and clinical benefit has been seen in small trials.[23,24] Thalidomide may share some aspects of the apoptotic mechanism described for infliximab.[25] A subsequent open-label study reported beneficial effects of thalidomide (100 mg) in maintaining remission induced by infliximab in 15 patients. The authors reported remission rates with thalidomide of 92%, 83%, and 83% at 3, 6, and 12 months, respectively; after the last infliximab infusion, therapy was terminated in 4 patients (27%) because of perceived toxicity.[26] The tragic history of teratogenicity

TABLE 17-1

CHARACTERISTICS OF APPROVED ANTI-TNFα BIOLOGICAL AGENTS ETANERCEPT, INFLIXIMAB, ADALIMUMAB, AND CERTOLIZUMAB*†

	ETANERCEPT	INFLIXIMAB	ADALIMUMAB	CERTOLIZUMAB
Class	Soluble TNFα receptor	TNFα mAb	TNFα mAb	Pegylated anti-TNFα
Construct	Recombinant fusion protein	Chimeric mAb	Human mAb	Humanized Fab fragment
Neutralizes soluble TNFα	Yes	Yes	Yes	Yes
Neutralizes cell-bound TNFα	Yes	Yes	Yes	Yes
Neutralizes TNFα-ß lymphotoxin	Yes	No	No	No
Lyses TNFα-producing cells/T cell apoptosis	No	Yes	Yes	No
Develops anti-DNA antibodies	—	13%	12%	< 4%
Human origin	Entirely	Partially	Entirely	Humanized
Half-life in days	4.8	9.5	12 to 14	14
Incidence of anti-agent antibodies	< 5	13	< 12	< 8
Dosing schedule	Twice/week	q 4 to 8 weeks	q 2 weeks	q 4 weeks

*TNFα indicates tumor necrosis factor alpha.

†Adapted from Haraoui B. Is there a rationale for switching from one anti-tumor necrosis factor agent to another? *J Rheumatology.* 2004;31:6:1021-1022. Sources: Baert F, Noman M, Vermeire S, et al. Influence of immunogenicity on the long-term efficacy of infliximab in Crohn's disease. *N Engl J Med.* 2003;348:601-608; Colombel JF, Sandborn WJ, Rutgeerts P, et al. Adalimumab for maintenance of clinical response and remission in patients with Crohn's disease: the CHARM trial. *Gastroenterology.* 2007;132:52-65; Sandborn WJ, Feagan BG, Stoinov S, et al, and the PRECISE 1 Study Investigators. Certolizumab pegol for the treatment of Crohn's disease. *N Engl J Med.* 2007;357:228-238; Schreiber S, Khaliq-Kareemi M, Lawrance IC, et al, and the PRECISE 2 Study Investigators. Maintenance therapy with certolizumab pegol for Crohn's disease. *N Engl J Med.* 2007;357:239-250.

remains a problem, as do the drug's abilities to sedate and to cause neuropathy.

Adalimumab is a fully human IgG1 monoclonal antibody approved by the Food and Drug Administration (FDA) in December 2002 for RA. It blocks p55 and p75 cell surface TNFα receptors and lyses TNFα-expressing cells in the presence of complement proteins. A placebo-controlled trial of 299 patients randomized to loading doses of 40, 80, or 160 mg injections, followed by 20, 40, or 80 mg injections every other week, demonstrated a dose-response relationship. At the highest dose, 35% of patients achieved remission, and 49% of patients dropped their Crohn's disease activity index (CDAI) score by 100 points.[27] The commercial drug is formulated currently at a concentration of 40 mg/0.8 cc; a 160-mg dose requires a 3 cc subcutaneous injection. Because 1 cc is the typical volume of subcutaneously administered medications, and greater costs are associated with higher doses, it seems likely that a reformulation may be considered.[28]

Etanercept is a fully human-soluble TNFα receptor fusion protein. It binds reversibly to circulating TNFα and, while very effective in RA, fell short in trials for CD.[29] It does not induce apoptosis of activated lymphocytes, a mechanistic difference from infliximab that may provide a biological basis for the difference in efficacy of the 2 drugs.[30] Table 17-1 lists characteristics of the currently approved anti-TNFα biological agents.

Oxpentifylline is a methyl-xanthine-phosphodiesterase (PDE4) inhibitor, which has shown anti-TNFα effects in vitro.[31] It is commercially available, but strong supporting data on its use in CD are lacking.[32]

After demonstrating only mild benefit from CDP571, a humanized monoclonal antibody to TNFα, the developing company, Celltech, has shifted its focus to a pegylated humanized anti-TNFα fragment.[33] Certolizumab pegol (CDP870 currently Cimzia) was assessed in 292 adults with active CD in a randomized, double-blind, placebo-controlled trial. Subjects were randomized to receive subcutaneous 100, 200, or 400 mg or placebo at weeks 0, 4, and 8. The therapeutic effects of certolizumab pegol were evident by week 2. The greatest response was observed in the high-dose group at all time points, with maximal response at week 10. At that time, the high-dose certolizumab pegol response was 52.8% versus 30.1% with placebo ($P = 0.006$). However, benefit was lost at week 12. In a subgroup of 118 patients with elevated C-reactive protein (CRP) levels at baseline, a greater dose separation was observed. Remission rates were also the highest in the high-dose group (400 mg) at all time points and peaked at week 10 with a remission rate of 41.9% ($n = 31$) versus placebo 10.7% ($n = 28$) rate ($P = 0.009$). In patients with CRP levels of <10 mg/L at baseline ($n = 173$), no significant differences were observed.[34]

HISTORY AND PHARMACOLOGY

Initial support for the use of infliximab was obtained from uncontrolled studies and was subsequently supported by evidence from well-designed clinical trials. An early study by Derkx et al reported clinical improvement in a CD patient after administration of infliximab.[35] In a subsequent open-label pilot study, van Dullemen et al provided direct evidence that a single infusion of infliximab induced remission in 8 of 10 patients; the infusions significantly decreased the CDAI and improved colonoscopic and histopathologic findings within 4 weeks of infusion.[16] Sedimentation rates and CRP levels fell within days of treatment.

Positive results obtained in these initial studies led to a multicenter, randomized, placebo-controlled, double-blind trial of 108 patients with active CD.[36] Patients were administered a single infusion of infliximab (5, 10, or 20 mg/kg) or placebo. By 4 weeks, 22 of 27 patients (81%) administered 5 mg/kg had achieved the primary endpoint, a clinical response defined as a reduction of 70 or more points in the CDAI score. Of the patients administered 10 mg/kg, 14 of 28 (50%) achieved the desired clinical response, and 18 of 28 patients (64%) administered 20 mg/kg improved their CDAI by at least 70 points. Overall response in the infliximab group was 65%, whereas only 4 of 24 patients (17%) administered placebo responded at 4 weeks ($P < 0.001$). In addition, 33% of the patients who received an infusion of infliximab achieved complete remission (defined as a CDAI score of less than 150), including 48% of patients administered 5 mg/kg, compared with only 4% of patients administered placebo ($P = 0.005$). At 12 weeks, 34 of 83 patients in the infliximab group (41%) maintained their clinical response compared with 3 of 25 in the placebo group (12%; $P = 0.008$). The investigators concluded that a single infusion of infliximab was an effective short-term treatment in patients with moderate-to-severe CD. Although this was a landmark study in the clinical investigation of infliximab, constructive criticisms of the study included the observations that the placebo response rate was unusually low, the mean concentration of CRP at baseline was lower in the placebo group, and significantly more patients with ileal disease alone were included in the placebo group compared with the 3 treatment groups.

Approximately one third of CD patients develop fistulae, and therefore the efficacy of infliximab in closing these has been studied.[37] In a multicenter, randomized, placebo-controlled, double-blind trial, 94 adults with active draining perianal or abdominal fistulae were administered either placebo or infliximab (5 or 10 mg/kg, intravenously at 0, 2, and 6 weeks).[38] At 5 mg/kg infliximab, 55% of patients had closure of all fistulas, and at 10 mg/kg, 38% of patients had closure of all fistulas, compared with only 13% of patients who received placebo ($P = 0.001$ and $P = 0.04$, respectively). In addition, 68% of the patients administered 5 mg/kg and 56% of the patients administered 10 mg/kg achieved closure of at least half of their fistulae compared with 26% of the placebo group ($P = 0.002$ and 0.02, respectively). The median length of time the fistulas remained closed was 3 months.

Infliximab is administered intravenously, with the standard dose being 5 mg/kg over a period of at least 2 hours. Data collected from clinical trials using single infusions of infliximab (5, 10, and 20 mg/kg) reveal a linear and direct relationship between the dose administered, the maximum serum concentration (Cmax), and the area under the concentration-time curve. The volume of distribution at steady-state was determined to be independent of dose, indicating that infliximab was primarily distributed within the vascular compartment.[4,15] The terminal half-life of infliximab was determined to be 8 to 10 days after infusion of 3 and 5 mg/kg; after a single infusion, detectable levels of infliximab were present for 8 to 12 weeks. No systemic accumulation was observed in patients administered up to 4 infusions of infliximab (doses as high as 10 mg/kg) at 4- or 8-week intervals. The route(s) of drug metabolism and secretion are yet to be determined, and it is unknown whether gender and severe renal or hepatic dysfunction affect the clearance or volume of distribution of infliximab.[4,39]

APPROVED GASTROINTESTINAL INDICATIONS

INFLIXIMAB AS AN INDUCTION THERAPY

In accordance with the results of clinical trials published thus far, the FDA approved the use of infliximab as an induction therapy for the following CD-related indications: reduction in signs and symptoms and induction of clinical remission in patients with moderately to severely active inflammatory CD where there is an inadequate response to conventional therapy; and reduction in the number of draining enterocutaneous and rectovaginal fistulas in patients with CD.[40] Off-label but clinically accepted indications for induction therapy include avoidance of initiation of steroid therapy by using infliximab as a rapidly acting induction therapy, followed by maintenance treatment with azathioprine, 6-mercaptopurine, or methotrexate; and steroid-sparing in patients who are currently treated with steroids. Improvement of nutritional status in sick, malnourished patients with active disease may also be a reasonable indication.[40]

INFLIXIMAB AS A MAINTENANCE THERAPY

The clinical effect from a single infusion of infliximab wanes with time, and relapses are common.[41] This means that patients often require repeat administration of infliximab. Clinical trials investigating infliximab as a maintenance therapy were therefore conducted, resulting in FDA approval of the use of infliximab for maintenance of clinical improvement and remission in patients who previously had moderate to severe active inflammatory CD and had not adequately responded to conventional therapy but who responded to initial induction therapy with infliximab.[40] Infliximab is also indicated for maintaining fistula closure in patients with CD who responded to initial induction therapy with infliximab.

A study was conducted by Rutgeerts et al to determine whether response could be maintained with repeated infusions in patients who responded to an initial infusion.[42] Patients ($n = 73$) were randomized to receive 10 mg/kg of infliximab or placebo at 8-week intervals for 36 weeks, with follow-up until week 48. Maintenance of remission was achieved in 53% of the patients receiving infliximab through week 44 compared with 20% of placebo-treated patients. The majority of the patients administered infliximab eventually relapsed 8 to 12 weeks after the final dose (administered at week 36), suggesting that the duration of the beneficial effects with infliximab in patients is approximately 8 weeks.[19] Repeated administration of infliximab maintained median values for CDAI and inflammatory bowel disease (IBD) questionnaire (a quality of life measurement), and serum CRP concentrations were maintained at remission levels.

A phase III clinical trial was conducted to compare the long-term efficacy of maintenance infliximab therapy with no further treatment for CD patients who respond to a single dose of infliximab.[3] The ACCENT 1 (A Crohn's disease Clinical trial Evaluating infliximab in a New long-term Treatment regimen) study was a multicenter, randomized, placebo-controlled, double-blind trial that included 573 patients with active CD. All patients received an open-label dose of 5 mg/kg infliximab at week 0. Responders at week 2 (335 of 573, or 59%) were then randomized into 1 of 3 groups. The first group received infusions of placebo at weeks 2 and 6 and then every 8 weeks until week 46, and the second group received infusions of 5 mg/kg infliximab at the same time points. The final treatment group received infusions of 5 mg/kg infliximab at weeks 2 and 6, followed by 10 mg/kg every 8 weeks until week 46. Study endpoints were the proportion of patients who responded at week 2 and were in remission (CDAI < 150) at week 30 and the time to loss of response up to week 54. At week 30, 23 of 110 patients (21%) in the placebo group were in remission, compared with 44 of 113 (39%) patients ($P = 0.003$) from the second group, and 50 of 112 (45%) patients from the third ($P = 0.0002$). These results demonstrate that repeat administration of infliximab every 8 weeks in initial responders is more effective than placebo in maintaining remission. Analysis of a nested study at week 10 demonstrated that a 3-dose induction regimen with infliximab (at 0, 2, and 6 weeks) was more effective at inducing remission than a

single induction dose. After a 3-dose induction, 40% of the patients achieved remission compared with 28% remission after a single-dose induction.[19,43] Other regimens have also been advocated to improve response or decrease adverse events, with 1 study suggesting that a single second infusion within 8 weeks is beneficial.[44]

ACCENT II went on to evaluate the efficacy of infliximab as maintenance therapy for fistulizing disease over 54 weeks. This was a multicenter, randomized, placebo-controlled trial in which patients were infused with 5 mg/kg infliximab at 0, 2, and 6 weeks. Of the 282 patients who completed the 14-week lead-in period, 195 patients (69%) responded, with closure of at least 50% of draining fistulas sustained over 1 month. The responders were then randomized to receive either 5 mg/kg infliximab (96 patients) or placebo (99 patients) every 8 weeks. Sands et al reported significantly greater rates for fistula improvement (reduction in the number of draining fistulas) and fistula remission (no draining fistulas) in the group administered infliximab. Specifically, almost half (48%) of the infliximab-treated patients maintained fistula response at week 30 compared with 27% of the placebo group. At week 54, 36% of the infliximab-treated group maintained fistula response compared with 19% of the placebo group. The median time to loss of response was over 40 weeks in the infliximab-treated group compared with 14 weeks in the placebo group.[45]

Infliximab is approved for reducing signs and symptoms and inducing and maintaining clinical remission in pediatric patients with moderately to severely active CD who have had an inadequate response to conventional therapy. The REACH study showed that at week 54 of treatment, 63.5% and 55.8% of children who received infliximab every 8 weeks achieved clinical response and were in clinical remission, respectively, and did not require dose adjustment.[46] At the end of 1 year, almost 50% of children receiving infliximab every 8 weeks were in remission and off steroids, compared with only 17% of children receiving infliximab every 12 weeks. Rare postmarketing cases of hepatosplenic T cell lymphoma have been reported, all of which occurred in patients receiving concomitant treatment with azathioprine or 6-mercaptopurine.[46]

Adalimumab is now approved by the FDA for inducing and maintaining clinical remission in adult patients with moderate to severe CD who have had an inadequate response to conventional therapy and for inducing remission in these patients if they have also lost response to or are intolerant to infliximab. Adalimumab, a fully humanized anti-TNFα antibody, was demonstrated to be superior to placebo for the induction of remission in patients with moderate to severe CD who were naïve to anti-TNFα therapy[47] and to maintain clinical remission for up to 56 weeks in these patients.[48] Among patients who were intolerant or did not respond to infliximab therapy, adalimumab was shown to induce remission more frequently than placebo[49] among patients who initially responded to adalimumab. Colombel et al reported significantly higher rates of remission with adalimumab versus placebo at 1 year.[50] In patients with CD for less than 2 years, approximately 50% remained in remission more than 1 year after receiving 40 mg of adalimumab subcutaneously every other week or weekly, again arguing for earlier aggressive treatment.[51]

Certolizumab pegol is a pegylated Fab' fragment of a humanized monoclonal antibody that neutralizes TNFα. A phase III, randomized, double-blind, multicenter study that assessed the efficacy and tolerability of certolizumab in patients with moderate to severe CD showed a modest improvement in response rates, as compared with placebo, but no significant improvement in remission rates.[52] In addition, patients who had a response to induction therapy with certolizumab were more likely to have maintained response and remission at 26 weeks with continued monthly subcutaneous injection compared to those who switched to placebo.[53]

The results from the induction phase of the PRECiSE 2 trial compared favorably to other monoclonal anti-TNFα induction studies. The 6-week response rates of approximately two thirds of patients in the study and remission rates of 40% were unaffected by concomitant immunosuppressants or corticosteroids.[54] Long-term data of certolizumab (at 52 and 54 weeks) suggest that 400-mg subcutaneous injections given monthly are well tolerated with low anti-double-stranded DNA—3.2% in PRECiSE 3 and 2.7% in PRECiSE 4—possibly because of the low apoptosis rates associated with certolizumab. In more than 900 patients treated with certolizumab for 1 year, the incidence of infections and malignancy is similar to other anti-TNFα agents.[55] In the WELCOME study, nearly two thirds of patients who had lost response or were intolerant to infliximab responded to induction with certolizumab at 0, 2, and 4 weeks, with maintenance every 2 or 4 weeks. In addition, almost 40% of those patients achieved remission on certolizumab.[56]

SONIC is a large definitive randomized double-blind controlled trial comparing early intervention with infliximab/azathioprine combination therapy, infliximab monotherapy, and azathioprine monotherapy for 1 year in patients with moderate-to-severe Crohn's disease of short duration. Patients in the trial were steroid exposed but naïve to biologics or immunomodulators. SONIC showed that patients with evidence of inflammation (elevated CRP level and endoscopic lesions at baseline colonoscopy) achieved superior steroid-free clinical remission (50%, 42%, and 23%, respectively) associated with mucosal healing from early infliximab combination therapy or monotherapy.[57] These infliximab treatments were superior to azathioprine alone with similar safety outcome in all 3 arms. Just as ACCENT I was a pivotal study in establishing the role of maintenance therapy in Crohn's disease, SONIC is a landmark study supporting the tectonic shift toward early intervention with anti-TNFα therapy and away from unlimited steroid and azathioprine therapy.

MUCOSAL HEALING

Mucosal healing after infliximab treatment was evaluated in a multicenter, randomized, placebo-controlled trial. Patients ($n = 39$) underwent colonoscopy with terminal ileum intubation prior to administration of infliximab (5, 10, or 20 mg/kg) or placebo; an endoscopy was carried out 4 weeks later. Biopsy specimens were taken from 9 of 30 patients pre- and post treatment, and mucosal lesions were scored using a validated Crohn's Disease Endoscopic Index of Severity (CDEIS). CDEIS scores decreased significantly in the majority of patients administered infliximab, although no dose response was noted. In contrast, no endoscopic improvement was observed for patients administered placebo. The inflammatory infiltrate observed in the initial biopsies resolved after treatment with infliximab but not placebo.[58] Rutgeerts et al demonstrated that endoscopy documented mucosal healing correlated with improved outcomes; specifically, fewer individuals underwent hospitalization and surgery in the group where mucosal healing had occurred compared with the group with no mucosal healing. The findings of this small study are provocative but will require validation in larger trials.[59]

STEROID-SPARING

Infliximab is an option for patients who are intolerant of, resistant to, or dependent on steroids.[60] Of the first 100 patients administered infliximab at the Mayo Clinic, 29 of 40 patients (73%) were able to completely withdraw from steroids.[41] Cohen et al reported that corticosteroid tapering was achieved in more than 90% of patients with luminal disease, and complete withdrawal of steroids was possible for 54% of patients after the second infusion of infliximab.[61] This study included 81 patients with luminal disease and 48 patients with fistulizing disease, who received at least 1 infusion of infliximab. At study entry in the ACCENT I trial, more than half of the patients were taking corticosteroids; one third of the patients receiving maintenance infliximab discontinued steroids and maintained clinical benefit.[3]

OTHER MANIFESTATIONS OF CROHN'S DISEASE

Efficacy of infliximab for the treatment of other gastrointestinal-related conditions has also been reported. For example, the medical records of 7 patients with CD who underwent an ileal pouch anal anastomosis for an original diagnosis of presumed UC were reviewed at the Mayo Clinic. The patients received between 1 and 4 doses of infliximab (5 mg/kg) for active inflammatory or fistulizing disease after no improvement in their symptoms was achieved with conventional therapies. All patients improved clinically after administration of infliximab, with 6 of 7 achieving a complete response and 1 achieving a partial response. Six of the 7 patients received concurrent treatment with immunomodulators.[62]

Patients with CD frequently experience extraintestinal manifestations of their disease, which are often debilitating and difficult to manage. These include ankylosing spondylitis, peripheral arthritis, pyoderma gangrenosum, and erythema nodosum. There is evidence that infliximab likely has a role in treating these conditions.[63-66]

CD patients are at increased risk for low bone mineral density (BMD), with reports of prevalence of osteopenia and osteoporosis as high as 50% and 10%, respectively. Infliximab may improve BMD in CD patients, both directly through inhibition of TNFα and indirectly through steroid-sparing. The etiology for low BMD is multifactorial, with low body mass index through poor nutrition, corticosteroid use, decreased intake of calcium and vitamin D, and malabsorption of nutrients secondary to inflamed or resected bowel all implicated. The systemic inflammatory aspect of CD may also cause bone loss through the action of cytokines, including TNFα. Stimulation of osteoclast function by these cytokines affects bone resorption, as has been demonstrated in numerous in vitro and in vivo studies.[67,68] A prospective study was conducted by Abreu et al to evaluate the effect of infliximab on surrogate markers of bone turnover in 38 CD patients.[69] The data obtained demonstrated that bone synthesis markers were increased in the infliximab-treated patients. Longer-term studies are needed to clarify the effect of infliximab on BMD.

SAFETY

Safety data are available from a variety of sources. The clinical trials data discussed here are inclusive through the Integrated Safety Summary (ISS) submitted to the FDA on September 29, 2003. In addition to the data from clinical trials, data from the infliximab Postmarketing Surveillance (PMS) program are presented. This includes infliximab data from spontaneous reports, registries, phase IV and expanded access programs, and investigator-initiated studies. The data are inclusive through the 8th Periodic Safety Update Report (PSUR 8), submitted to European Health Authorities on October 17, 2003. The manufacturers have also collected data through the TREAT registry (Crohn's Therapy Resource Evaluation and Assessment Tool) on top of these sources.

Although efficacy of infliximab for the treatment of CD has clearly been demonstrated, serious side effects have been reported. In particular, these include acute infusion reactions, delayed hypersensitivity reactions, infections including reactivation of tuberculosis (TB), autoantibody formation, and a Lupus-like syndrome. Clinicians need to be aware of these potential outcomes to enable accurate diagnosis and appropriate management of these complications. In addition, it is important to counsel candidates for therapy about these toxicities prior to infusions.

ACUTE INFUSION REACTIONS

Acute infusion reactions are adverse events that occur during infusion or within 2 hours after completion of the infusion. They are common, occurring in approximately 22% of patients administered infliximab compared with 9% of patients administered placebo, according to the manufacturer's drug insert.[39] However, the Mayo Clinic reported a much lower incidence in their clinical experience; only 19 of 500 patients (3.8%) who received infusions experienced an acute infusion reaction.[70] The reactions are non-IgE-mediated anaphylactoid events that include, but are not limited to, headache, nausea, dyspnea, urticaria, and chest tightness. Generally, these reactions can be managed relatively easily by first slowing or temporarily stopping the infusion and then administering oral acetaminophen and serial doses of intravenous diphenhydramine (25 to 50 mg) if symptoms persist. It has also been demonstrated that intravenous famotidine can be helpful for the histamine component of the allergic response.[71] After the symptoms have resolved, the infusion can generally be recommenced at a slower rate and then titrated upwards as tolerated. The majority of patients are able to complete their infusion.

Patients with a history of infusion reactions should be considered for premedication with the clinician's choice of antihistamines, acetaminophen, or corticosteroids approximately 30 minutes prior to the infusion, but there is no evidence that routine premedication in patients without a history of infusion reaction is necessary.[40] In certain situations, premedication with prednisone may be necessary in patients who have infusion-associated symptoms that are not alleviated by diphenhydramine and acetaminophen or those who are at risk because of a long interval (greater than 4 months) since their last infusion.

DELAYED-HYPERSENSITIVITY REACTIONS

Delayed-hypersensitivity or serum sickness-like reactions can also occur several days after the infusion. Symptoms include severe pruritus, headaches, hand, facial or lip swelling, myalgias, rash, sore throat, and dysphagia. One study of 40 CD patients demonstrated a 25% incidence rate, with 6 patients requiring hospitalization.[72] These patients had initially received infusions of an investigational liquid formulation of the drug (development of which was subsequently discontinued), with a follow-up infusion 2 to 4 years later with the approved formulation (lyophilized powder). These events occur much less frequently in clinical practice when the intervals between infusions are up to 1 year; in ACCENT I, where patients received repeat infusions every 8 weeks, the frequency of delayed hypersensitivity reaction was 2%.[3] Of 500 patients investigated by researchers at the Mayo Clinic, only 14 (2.8%) had serum sickness related to infliximab.[70]

INFECTIONS

Infections requiring treatment have been associated with infliximab therapy during clinical trials. Specifically, these occurred in 36% of patients administered infliximab compared with 26% of patients receiving placebo,[39] although no statistically significant increases in serious infections or sepsis were observed in patients administered infliximab compared to placebo.[40] Mayo Clinic physicians reported different infection frequencies, with 41 of 500 patients (8.2%) developing an infection related to infliximab.[70] Of these, 28 patients had a serious infection: 2 cases of lethal sepsis; 8 pneumonias, of which 2 were lethal; 6 viral infections, including 3 varicella-zoster virus infections; 2 abdominal abscesses requiring surgery; 1 arm cellulitis; and 1 histoplasmosis. No cases of TB were observed.

In postmarketing experience, infections have been observed with pathogens, including viral, bacterial, fungal, and protozoal organisms. Although the majority of infections involved the respiratory (ie, pharyngitis, sinusitis, and bronchitis) and urinary tracts, serious and even fatal infections have been reported, including abscess, sepsis, pneumonia, cellulitis, TB, disseminated coccidioidomycoses, *Pneumocystis carinii* pneumonia, histoplasmosis, listeriosis, and aspergillosis.

Reactivation of latent TB after infusion with infliximab has occurred, mandating screening of patients for TB prior to infusion. This likely reflects the impact of infliximab on the TNFα-driven apoptosis of cells within granulomas. More than 70 cases were originally reported; 48 of the patients developed TB after 3 or fewer infusions.[73] The majority of cases occurred within the first 2 months after initiation of therapy with infliximab, suggesting activation of latent disease rather than new infection, although the majority of cases (64 of 70) were from countries with a low incidence of TB. Forty of 70 patients had extrapulmonary disease. Interestingly, the majority of cases involved patients being treated for RA; only 22% of these patients had CD.[40] Overall through August 2003, 441 reports of active TB have been received out of more than 492,000 patients worldwide. While the majority of patients have been treated in the United States, the majority of TB reports have originated from countries other than the United States.[7]

A purified protein derivative (PPD) should be administered to all patients being considered for treatment with infliximab, with the results interpreted according to the risk strata adapted from the American Thoracic Society (ATS).[39,74] Patients with negative readings and no risk factors for previous exposure from history and physical examination can receive infliximab therapy, whereas patients with a positive PPD should undergo a chest radiograph. If the radiograph is normal, patients should be treated for latent TB according to ATS guidelines prior to commencement of infliximab therapy (a 9-month course of isoniazid is currently the preferred treatment).[40,75] If the radiograph is abnormal, infliximab should not be administered until the active TB is adequately treated. Chronically ill patients taking corticosteroids and immune modulators may be anergic.[76] For these patients, a positive PPD is greater than or equal to 5 mm in duration, as is used in clinical practice for patients with human immunodeficiency virus (HIV). In addition, the importance of taking a thorough medical history to check for risk factors for TB cannot be overemphasized. A chest radiograph should be performed if warranted by the medical history, even if the PPD is negative. Having the pharmacy confirm clearance for TB before releasing vials of infliximab is a practical fail-safe mechanism.

PREGNANCY

The safety of infliximab in reproduction and pregnancy was not investigated in animal reproduction studies, as infliximab does not cross-react with TNFα from species other than humans and chimpanzees. However, a toxicity study in mice was conducted using an analogous antibody that selectively inhibits the functional activity of mouse TNFα, and no evidence of maternal toxicity, embryotoxicity, or teratogenicity was observed.[39] Data are now accumulating that demonstrate that patients are delivering healthy children after exposure to the drug, although infliximab is currently a pregnancy category B drug. (Case reports describe patients delivering healthy babies after being infused with infliximab during their pregnancy.) Katz et al recently surveyed data stored in the infliximab safety database maintained by the manufacturer (Centocor Inc, Malvern, PA) for pregnancy outcomes in 133 female patients and 14 male partners exposed to infliximab.[77] Pregnancy outcome data were available for approximately 50% (65 of 133) of these patients. Of the female patients, 56% (74 of 133) were exposed to infliximab within 3 months prior to conception, and 45% (33 of 74) received infliximab both prior to conception and during the first trimester. Live births occurred in 65% (42 of 65) of cases, miscarriages in 17% (11 of 65), and therapeutic terminations in 22% (14 of 65); these incidences did not differ from expected outcomes in the general pregnant US population. For the 14 male partners, there were 7 live births, 1 miscarriage, 3 ongoing pregnancies, and 3 unknown outcomes. The available data therefore suggest that inadvertent exposure does not harm the fetus. Nonetheless, infliximab should ideally only be administered to pregnant patients when a flare uncontrolled by other medications poses a greater health risk to the mother and unborn child than the risks associated with infliximab.

As with many other medications, immunoglobulins are secreted in breast milk; however, it is unknown whether infliximab is secreted in this way.[39] In addition, it is currently unknown whether infliximab is absorbed systematically after oral administration. Due to the theoretical risk for adverse reactions in nursing infants, patients should either discontinue infliximab therapy prior to breast-feeding or discontinue breast-feeding if therapy is required.

LYMPHOMA

Lymphoma has been reported in association with all 3 approved TNFα antagonists, causing considerable concern, although a causal relationship is debated.[78,79] One reason for the ambiguity is that the risk of lymphoma is also increased among patients with RA who have never received infliximab, particularly in severe cases.[80,81] Data from clinical trials for both CD and RA, representing 2421 patients with 4148 patient-years of follow-up, indicate that lymphoma was seen in 6 patients who were receiving active treatment but none of the control patients, supporting the possibility of a causal relationship.[82] The incidence of other cancers is not significantly altered, though researchers from the Mayo Clinic reported that 3 of 500 patients developed a malignancy (2 lung cancers and 1 non-Hodgkin's lymphoma) potentially related to infliximab.[70] A recent meta-analysis by Siegel et al has suggested an increased risk of lymphoma in patients receiving infliximab for Crohn's disease.[83]

DEMYELINATING SYNDROMES

There are reports of both the new appearance of MS and aggravation of existing disease in patients receiving anti-TNFα therapy.[84] Although a causal relationship has not been established, such reports suggest that anti-TNFα agents should be used with extreme caution if at all in patients with these neurological syndromes.[85]

CONGESTIVE HEART FAILURE

Initial reports on anti-TNFα therapy for heart failure were encouraging. However, subsequent studies of etanercept and infliximab in heart failure were terminated early because of lack of evidence of benefit and, in the case of infliximab, increased mortality. In a further study, 150 patients with stable New York Heart Association class III or IV heart failure and left ventricular ejection fraction ≤ 35% were randomly assigned to receive placebo ($n = 49$), infliximab 5 mg/kg ($n = 50$), or infliximab 10 mg/kg ($n = 51$). Patients were followed up prospectively for 28 weeks, and the combined risk of death from any cause or hospitalization for heart failure through 28 weeks was increased in the patients randomized to 10 mg/kg infliximab.[86] Infliximab does not appear to induce cardiac problems de novo. In clinical trials where congestive heart failure was an exclu-sion factor, no increased incidence of cardiac adverse events was reported with active therapy compared to placebo.[3,36]

SPECIAL CONSIDERATIONS

Infliximab contains exogenous proteins that can prompt the formation of antibodies-to-infliximab (ATIs), the clinical implications of which are currently being investigated. As part of the ACCENT I trial, patients were assessed for the presence of ATIs up to week 54.[3] Of the 442 patients assessed, 64 (14.5%) developed antibodies, whereas 173 (39%) did not. Results for the remaining patients (46%) were inconclusive due to the presence of infliximab in their serum, which can compete for the detection of antibodies to infliximab in the immunoassay. Patients administered a single dose of infliximab followed by either placebo or episodic infliximab retreatment had higher incidence of ATI formation than patients administered scheduled maintenance regimens of 5 or 10 mg/kg (28% compared with 9% and 6% of patients, respectively). Similar rates of clinical response were observed in patients independent of their antibody status: 64% of patients with ATIs responded clinically to infliximab (decrease in CDAI of >70 points from baseline and >25 points reduction in total CDAI score) compared to 62% who did not form ATIs. The rate of infusion reactions was slightly higher in the ATI-positive group, with 38% of these patients having 1 or more infusion reactions compared with 24% of patients without ATIs. However, only a small minority of infusions in the ATI group caused an infusion reaction: 16% of infusions in the ATI-positive group compared with 8% of infusions in the ATI-negative group. The majority of the infusion reactions were mild to moderate, and severe reactions and serum sickness-like reactions were rare and not increased in the ATI-positive group.

Baert et al conducted a study of 125 CD patients who received "on demand" (ie, episodic) infliximab therapy; patients with luminal disease were administered a single 5 mg/kg infusion, whereas patients with fistulizing disease were administered 3 infusions of 5 mg/kg infliximab at 0, 2, and 6 weeks.[87] Responders were re-treated as needed when symptoms recurred. In this trial, 61% of patients developed ATIs, much higher than the 14% detected in ACCENT I. Of these patients, only 37% had clinically significant levels of infliximab (> 8 μg/mL). A higher incidence of infusion reactions was observed in the ATI-positive group (relative risk 2.4), but more importantly, an association of high ATI levels with loss of response was also observed. Patients with high ATI levels had a substantially shorter duration of response (35 days) compared with patients who did not form antibodies (71 days).

The impact of ATIs on durability of response is reshaping treatment strategies. Three approaches have been examined thus far: premedication/concomitant steroids; concomitant antimetabolite therapy; and regular, rather than episodic, infusions. The incidence of development of ATIs has generally been lower in patients receiving concomitant immunosuppressants. For example, fewer RA patients administered methotrexate in addition to infliximab formed antibodies. In ACCENT I, only 4 of the 64 (6%) patients who were receiving corticosteroids plus immunomodulator therapy developed ATIs.[3] In comparison, 17% of patients receiving steroids alone, 10% of patients receiving immunomodulators, and 18% of patients receiving no additional immunomodulators formed ATIs. The lowest incidence of infusion reactions in the ACCENT I trial occurred in patients receiving both steroids and immunomodulators (8%) compared with patients receiving neither (32%). In the study by Baert et al, patients receiving concomitant immunomodulator therapy had a decreased incidence of antibody formation, higher concentrations of infliximab, reduced incidence of infusion reactions, and increased duration of response, prompting the authors to recommend their use.[87] In a randomized trial of 53 consecutive patients receiving 199 infusions, Farrell et al went on to demonstrate that loss of initial response and infusion reactions post-infliximab were strongly related to ATI formation and level.[44] Both administration of a second infusion within 8 weeks of the first and concurrent immunosuppressant therapy significantly reduced ATI formation.

Patients administered infliximab can also develop autoantibodies; in clinical trials, antinuclear antibodies (ANA) and anti-double-stranded DNA antibodies developed in 44% and 22% of patients, respectively.[39] The vast majority of these patients were asymptomatic and re-administration of infliximab is not contraindicated in these patients.[40] Three patients with CD developed signs of drug-induced lupus.[40] Again, the frequency of development of autoantibodies is lowered by concomitant immunosuppressive therapy.

COST

At a cost of more than US $2000 per infusion, infliximab is an expensive medication. This raises the consideration of whether or not it is a cost-effective therapy for CD patients, especially in the current health-care climate. To attempt to answer this question, it is first necessary to study the general costs of CD on society. Hay and Hay in 1990 provided landmark economic analysis of this disease.[88] They found that the lifetime direct medical cost of the illness per case was US $18,000 to $178,000. For comparison, the estimated cost of heart disease per case was US $10,000 to $60,000. Estimates of the annual average medical cost per patient are approximately US $9,500, with a total annual cost for CD in 1996 of US $1.4 to 1.7 billion.[88,89] Surgery and hospitalizations accounted for approximately 80% of the direct costs for CD, and the

remaining 20% was composed of medications, outpatient resources, complications, and diagnostic testing. Indirect costs were also significant, with 5% to 10% of patients out of work and receiving disability benefits annually; the average number of workdays missed per month due to CD among full-time workers was 3.3 days.[90] In the United States, the proportion of patients not working because of their disease was estimated to be 1 in 6.

In their study of insurance claims for more than 600 patients with CD over a 1-year period, Feagan et al obtained similar results to Hay and Hay.[91] Patients were stratified into 3 disease severity groups: group 1 required hospitalization, group 2 required chronic steroid or immunomodulator therapy, and group 3 included all remaining patients. Group 1 consumed the most health-care dollars at US $37,135 per patient-year, compared with US $10,033 and US $6277 for patients from groups 2 and 3, respectively. In this study, hospitalization accounted for 57% of all direct health-care costs in CD. A minority of patients was responsible for the majority of the costs, with approximately 25% of patients requiring 80% of the cost. These data indicate that new therapeutics could reduce overall costs if they reduce the need for hospitalization.

Cohen et al reviewed the computer database at the University of Chicago for all hospitalizations with a primary diagnosis of CD during a 1-year period.[92] The major charge during hospitalization was for surgery, accounting for nearly 40% of all hospital charges. The authors concluded that more effective medical therapies could result in an overall decrease in health-care costs, providing that they reduce the need for hospitalization and surgery. Finally, a study was conducted by Rubenstein et al to determine whether infliximab decreased the utilization of health-care services by CD patients.[93] The investigation involved an electronic and paper chart review up to 3 years prior to infusion and 1 year following the initial infusion. Patients served as their own controls, and utilization rates prior to and after infliximab infusion were compared. Several health-care resource utilizations decreased by a statistically significant percentage following infusion of infliximab, including gastrointestinal surgeries (–18%), emergency room visits (–66%), endoscopies (–43%), radiology exams (–12%), and all outpatient visits (–16%). Fewer hospitalizations occurred for patients treated for fistulas (–59%) and gastrointestinal surgeries (–59%).

These studies indicate that savings can be accrued by attempting to reduce hospitalizations and surgical procedures, possibly with infliximab. However, there is a need for further studies of cost-effectiveness that factor in medication costs of infliximab, with its direct and indirect cost savings, including improvement in quality of life aspects.

OPTIMIZING THERAPY WITH INFLIXIMAB

Defining the best strategy for using infliximab to optimize treatment results while limiting expense and exposure to possible side effects is under constant review. Current data allow the extrapolation of various practical recommendations that can be applied to the clinical use of infliximab.

INDUCTION OF REMISSION

For induction of remission in luminal disease, a single 5 mg/kg intravenous (IV) infusion is beneficial, although a 3-dose induction regimen of 5 mg/kg IV at 0, 2, and 6 weeks offers an addition margin of efficacy. Generally, if a patient has no clinical response after 2 doses, this should be considered a treatment failure. The 3-dose induction regimen at 0, 2, and 6 weeks is recommended for the treatment of fistulizing disease.

In several studies, concomitant use of immunomodulators, such as azathioprine (2 to 2.5 mg/kg/day), 6-mercaptopurine (1 to 1.5 mg/kg/day), or methotrexate (15 mg intramuscular [IM] per week), reduced the formation of ATIs and therefore the clinical consequences of immunogenicity of chimeric antibodies.[87,94] The formation of antibodies to infliximab is associated with the occurrence of infusion reactions and with a shortened duration of response.[44,87] Patients should therefore have fewer infusion reactions and decreased loss of response rates if treated simultaneously with immunomodulators, although prospective data are not currently available. Patients who receive infliximab episodically should generally be treated with concomitant immunomodulator therapy.

What is the best timing for commencement with immunomodulators? In the ACCENT trials, 3 months of stable dosing of immunomodulators was required for study inclusion, but a 3-month delay prior to the first infliximab infusion may not be tolerable for ill patients. As azathioprine steady-state pharmacokinetics are established at approximately 4 weeks, 1 month of immunomodulation prior to the first infusion may be reasonable.[95] For particularly ill patients, immunomodulation can be started simultaneously.

MAINTENANCE THERAPY

Patients with a positive clinical response to infliximab induction therapy should generally be continued on maintenance therapy. ACCENT I demonstrated that patients with luminal disease infused every 8 weeks had higher rates of response and remission at 54 weeks than those who received episodic treatment. In that series, the proportion of patients with ATIs was significantly lower in the maintenance infusion group (11%) compared with the episodic treatment group (38%). Baert et al[87] have demonstrated that duration of response is correlated to ATI levels, but the role of testing for ATI in clinical practice has not been established. It is likely that ATIs are to blame when patients suffer progressive shortening of the beneficial effects of infusion. In such patients, the interval between infusions can safely be shortened as needed, but increasing the dose to 10 mg/kg may allow less frequent infusions and decrease both direct and indirect costs. Crossover from 5 mg/kg to 10 mg/kg was successful in a substantial proportion of patients in the ACCENT trials. In these trials, patients who crossed over to 10 mg/kg were then maintained on the higher dose. Supporting data have not been published, but some clinicians advocate a single dose of 10 mg/kg to "mop up" ATI, followed by resumption of maintenance at lower dosing.

For patients with fistulizing CD who responded to the 3-dose induction regimen, systematic 8-week re-treatment with 5 mg/kg is advised based on the results of the ACCENT II trial. Fistula healing is often slow, and response may be lost, necessitating dose escalation or more frequent infusions. Surgical intervention may also be required, including the incision and drainage of abscesses, performance of fistulotomy or advancement flap-plasty, placement of setons, and sphincter repair. Infliximab should not be given until the abscesses are draining. Setons should probably be kept in place until after the induction infusions are administered and then removed once the patient is receiving maintenance therapy and is improving.[94]

MANAGEMENT AND PROPHYLAXIS FOR INFUSION REACTIONS

Prophylactic pretreatment with 650 mg of acetaminophen, H1 antagonists (diphenhydramine 25 to 50 mg PO or IV), or corticosteroids (methylprednisolone dose pack, hydrocortisone 200 mg IV, or prednisone) prior to infliximab infusions are generally not recommended, unless the patient has had a prior infusion reaction. If a patient has had an interval of generally more than 14 weeks without an infliximab infusion, then prophylaxis with these agents is recommended to avoid a potential infusion reaction. Cheifetz et al offer a practical guideline to the management of infusion reactions and premedication from Mt Sinai School of Medicine.[96]

The length of time for which patients can safely continue to receive infusions of infliximab is controversial, because there are no controlled data beyond 1 year. It is difficult to withhold a medication if the patient is enjoying substantial clinical response or, better yet, remission. However, expense and concern for long-term side effects may tempt clinicians and patients to stop the infusions once treatment goals such as fistula healing or discontinuation of steroids have been achieved. If it is elected to withdraw the infliximab until possible disease relapse, then immunomodulator therapy should be continued and infliximab therapy reinstated if the disease reflares. Hopefully, a placebo-controlled infliximab discontinuation study will better answer this important clinical question.

CONCLUSION

Infliximab has been administered to hundreds of thousands of patients since its approval in 1998. In both clinical trials and practice, it has been demonstrated to be safe, effective, and generally well tolerated. On its debut as the earliest effective biological agent for CD, infliximab was considered to be the first truly novel therapy for CD in half a century. It was the first anti-TNFα product to demonstrate complement activation and destruction of effector cells, which distinguishes it from humanized monoclonal antibodies such as CDP571 and other anti-TNFα agents investigated thus far.

The critical factors affecting patient response remain to be determined. Drug factors aside, what about patient characteristics? Parsi et al demonstrated that nonsmoking and concurrent use of immunomodulators were predictors of response to infliximab.[97] Another study demonstrated that various genetic factors and antibodies identified as playing a role in susceptibility to CD, such as NOD2/CARD15, ASCA, and ANCA, were not predictive of outcome with infliximab treatment for CD.[98,99] It is important to find and investigate other factors that could identify the patients who are more likely to accrue benefit from this drug. Other topics for future investigation include infliximab's role after surgical resection of disease to prevent recurrence; assessment of a possible synergy with immunomodulators; and finally, the potential of infliximab as a first-line drug in the treatment of CD. Because it is a relatively new medication, expensive, and novel in its mechanism of action, the strategy for employing infliximab needs further refinement at this stage.

The substantial concerns expressed in 1998 regarding the safety and cost of infliximab were very similar to the gastroenterology community's response to 6-mercaptopurine decades ago. The majority of clinicians are now comfortable with 6-mercaptopurine, and likely a similar time period will have the same effect for biological therapeutics. As acceptance of infliximab becomes more widespread, more than 70 new biological agents are progressing along the development pipeline. Although the speed of the development process from concept to biologic agent is far faster than in the days when antimetabolites were newcomers, it remains prudent to continue to examine infliximab closely for lessons in therapeutic success.

REFERENCES

1. Loftus EV, Sandborn WJ. Epidemiology of inflammatory bowel disease. *Gastroenterol Clin North Am.* 2002;31:1-20.
2. Ardizzone S, Porro GB. Inflammatory bowel disease: new insights into pathogenesis and treatment. *J Intern Med.* 2002;252:475-496.
3. Hanaeur SB, Feagan BG, Lichtenstein GR, et al. Maintenance infliximab for Crohn's disease: the ACCENT I randomized trial. *Lancet.* 2002;359:1541-1549.
4. Valle E, Gross M, Bickston SJ. Infliximab. *Expert Opin Pharmacother.* 2001;2:1015-1025.
5. Breedveld FC. Therapeutic monoclonal antibodies. *Lancet.* 2000; 355:735-740.
6. Gura T. Therapuetic antibodies: magic bullets hit the target. *Nature.* 2002;417:584-586.
7. Data on file, Centocor, Inc.
8. Ksontini R, MacKay SLD, Moldawer LL. Revisiting the role of tumor necrosis factor a and the response to surgical injury and inflammation. *Arch Surg.* 1998;133:558-567.
9. van Deventer SJ. Review article: targeting TNF alpha as a key cytokine in the inflammatory processes of Crohn's disease—the mechanisms of action of infliximab. *Aliment Pharmacol Ther.* 1999;13(suppl 4):3-8.
10. Beutler BA. The role of tumour necrosis factor in health and disease. *J Rheumatol.* 1999;26(suppl 57):16-21.
11. Yacyshyn BR. Novel manipulations of inflammatory mediator pathways. In: Bayless TM, Hanauer SB, eds. *Advanced Therapy of Inflammatory Bowel Disease.* Hamilton, London: B.C. Decker; 2001:165-169.
12. Sandborn WJ. Transcending conventional therapies: the role of biologic and other novel therapies. *Inflamm Bowel Dis.* 2001;1(suppl 7):s9-s16.
13. van Deventer SJ. Tumour necrosis factor and Crohn's disease. *Gut.* 1997;40:443-448.
14. Kalogeris T, Grisham MB. Mode of action of anti-inflammatory agents. In: Bayless TM, Hanauer SB, eds. *Advanced Therapy of Inflammatory Bowel Disease.* Hamilton, London: B.C. Decker; 2001:63-67.
15. Mouser JF, Hyams JS. Infliximab: a novel chimeric monoclonal antibody for the treatment of Crohn's disease. *Clin Ther.* 1999; 21:932-942.
16. van Dullemen HM, van Deventer SJ, Hommes DW, et al. Treatment of Crohn's disease with anti-tumor necrosis factor chimeric monoclonal antibody (cA2). *Gastroenterology.* 1995;109:129-135.
17. Knight DM, Trinh H, Le J, et al. Construction and initial characterization of a mouse-human chimeric anti-TNF antibody. *Mol Immunol.* 1993;30:1443-1453.
18. Scallon BJ, Moore MA, Trinh H, Knight DM, Ghrayeb J. Chimeric anti-TNF-alpha monoclonal antibody cA2 binds recombinant transmembrane TNF-alpha and activates immune effector functions. *Cytokine.* 1995;7:251-259.
19. Sandborn WJ, Targan SR. Biologic therapy of inflammatory bowel disease. *Gastroenterology.* 2002;122:1592-1608.
20. Eigler A, Sinha B, Hartmann G, Endres S. Taming TNF: strategies to restrain this proinflammatory cytokine. *Immunol Today.* 1997; 18:487-492.
21. Sands BE. Crohn's disease. In: Feldman M, Friedman LS, Sleisenger MH, eds. *Sleisenger & Fordtran's Gastrointestinal and Liver Disease.* 7th ed. Philadelphia, PA: Saunders; 2002:2028-2029.

22. Bauditz J, Wedel S, Lochs H. Thalidomide reduces tumour necrosis factor-α and interleukin 12 production in patients with chronic active Crohn's disease. *Gut.* 2002;50:196-200.

23. Ehrenpreis ED, Kane SV, Cohen LB, Cohen RD, Hanauer SB. Thalidomide therapy for patients with refractory Crohn's disease: an open-label trial. *Gastroenterolgy.* 1999;117:1271-1277.

24. Vasiliauskas EA, Kam LY, Abreu-Martin MT, et al. An open-label pilot study of low-dose thalidomide in chronically active, steroid-dependent Crohn's disease. *Gastroenterology.* 1999;117:1278-1287.

25. Gockel HR, Lugering A, Heidemann J, et al. Thalidomide induces apoptosis in human monocytes by using a cytochrome c-dependent pathway. *J Immunol.* 2004;172:5103-5109.

26. Sabate JM, Villarejo J, Lemann M, Bonnet J, Allez M, Modigliani R. An open-label study of thalidomide for maintenance therapy in responders to infliximab in chronically active and fistulizing refractory Crohn's disease. *Aliment Pharmacol Ther.* 2002;16:1117-1124.

27. Hanauer SB, Sandborn WJ, Rutgeerts P, et al. Human anti-tumor necrosis factor monoclonal antibody (adalimumab) in Crohn's disease: the CLASSIC-I trial. *Gastroenterology.* 2006;130:323-333.

28. Shargel L, Mutnick H, Souney P, Swanson L, Block L, eds. *Comprehensive Pharmacy Review.* 3rd ed. Baltimore, MD; Williams and Wilkins: 1997.

29. Sandborn WJ, Hanauer SB, Katz S, et al. Etanercept for active Crohn's disease: a randomized, double-blind, placebo-controlled trial. *Gastroenterology.* 2001;121:1088-1094.

30. Van den Brande JM, Braat H, van den Brink GR, et al. Infliximab but not etanercept induces apoptosis in lamina propria T-lymphocytes from patients with Crohn's disease. *Gastroenterology.* 2003;124:1774-1785.

31. Reimund JM, Dumont S, Muller CD, et al. In vitro effects of oxpentifylline on inflammatory cytokine release in patients with inflammatory bowel disease. *Gut.* 1997;40:475-480.

32. Bauditz J, Haemling J, Ortner M, et al. Treatment with tumour necrosis factor inhibitor oxpentifylline does not improve corticosteroid dependent chronic active Crohn's disease. *Gut.* 1997;40:470-474.

33. Sandborn WJ, Feagan BG, Hanauer SB, et al. CDP571 Crohn's Disease Study Group. An engineered human antibody to TNF (CDP571) for active Crohn's disease: a randomized double-blind placebo-controlled trial. *Gastroenterology.* 2001;120:1330-1338.

34. Schreiber S, Rutgeerts P, Fedorak R, et al. CDP870, a humanized anti-TNF fragment, induces clinical response with remission in patients with active Crohn's disease [abstract]. *Gastroenterology.* 2003;124:468.

35. Derkx B, Taminiau J, Radema S, et al. Tumour-necrosis-factor antibody treatment in Crohn's disease. *Lancet.* 1993;342:173-174.

36. Targan SR, Hanauer SB, van Deventer SJH, et al. A short-term study of chimeric monoclonal antibody cA2 to tumor necrosis factor a for Crohn's disease. *N Engl J Med.* 1997;337:1029-1035.

37. Williams DR, Collier JA, Corman ML, Nugent FW, Veidenheimer MC. Anal complications in Crohn's disease. *Dis Colon Rectum.* 1981;24:22-24.

38. Present DH, Rutgeerts P, Targan S, et al. Infliximab for the treatment of fistulas in patients with Crohn's disease. *N Engl J Med.* 1999;340:1398-1405.

39. Remicade (infliximab) for IV injection [package insert]. Malvern, PA: Centocor, Inc; 2002.

40. Sandborn WJ, Hanauer SB. Infliximab in the treatment of Crohn's disease: a user's guide for clinicians. *Am J Gastroenterol.* 2002;97:2962-2972.

41. Ricart E, Panaccione R, Loftus E, Tremaine W, Sandborn W. Infliximab for Crohn's disease in clinical practice at the Mayo Clinic: the first 100 patients. *Am J Gastroenterol.* 2001;96:722-729.

42. Rutgeerts P, D'Haens G, Targan S, et al. Efficacy and safety of retreatment with anti-tumor necrosis factor antibody (infliximab) to maintain remission in Crohn's disease. *Gastroenterology.* 1999;117:761-769.

43. Mayer L, Han C, Bala M, et al. Three dose induction regimen of infliximab (Remicade) is superior to a single dose in patients with Crohn's disease (CD). *Am J Gastroenterol.* 2001;96:S303.

44. Farrell RJ, Alsahli M, Jeen YT, Falchuk KR, Peppercorn MA, Michetti P. Intravenous hydrocortisone premedication reduces antibodies to infliximab in Crohn's disease: a randomized controlled trial. *Gastroenterology.* 2003;124:917-924.

45. Sands B, van Deventer S, Bernstein C, et al. Long-term treatment of fistulizing Crohn's disease: response to infliximab in the ACCENT II trial through 54 weeks. *Gastroenterology.* 2002;122:A81.

46. Hyams J, Crandall W, Kugathasan S, et al. Induction and maintenance infliximab therapy for the treatment of moderate-to-severe Crohn's disease in children. *Gastroenterology.* 2007;132:863-873.

47. Hanauer SB, Sandborn WJ, Rutgeerts P, et al. Human anti-tumor necrosis factor monoclonal antibody (adalimumab) in Crohn's disease: the CLASSIC-I trial. *Gastroenterology.* 2006;130:323-333.

48. Sandborn WJ, Hanauer SB, Rutgeerts P, et al. Adalimumab for maintenance treatment of Crohn's disease: results of the CLASSIC II trial. *Gut.* 2007;56:1232-1239.

49. Sandborn WJ, Rutgeerts P, Enns R, et al. Adalimumab induction therapy for Crohn disease previously treated with infliximab: a randomized trial. *Ann Intern Med.* 2007;146:829-838.

50. Colombel JF, Sandborn WJ, Rutgeerts P, et al. Adalimumab for maintenance of clinical response and remission in patients with Crohn's disease: the CHARM trial. *Gastroenterology.* 2007;132:52-65.

51. Schreiber S, Reinisch W, Colombel JF, et al. Early Crohn's disease shows high levels of remission to therapy with adalimumab: subanalysis of CHARM [abstract]. *Gastroenterology.* 2007;132(4 suppl 1):A147.

52. Sandborn WJ, Feagan BG, Stoinov S, et al, and the PRECiSE 1 Study Investigators. Certolizumab pegol for the treatment of Crohn's disease. *N Engl J Med.* 2007;357:228-238.

53. Schreiber S, Khaliq-Kareemi M, Lawrance IC, et al, and the PRECiSE 2 Study Investigators. Maintenance therapy with certolizumab pegol for Crohn's disease. *N Engl J Med.* 2007;357:239-250.

54. Thomsen OO, Schreiber S, Khaliq-Kareemi M, Hanauer SB, Bloomfield R, Sandborn WJ. Rapid onset of response and remission to subcutaneous certolizumab pegol and lack of influence of concomitant baseline medications in active Crohn's disease: results from the open-label induction phase of the PRECiSE 2 study [abstract]. *Gastroenterology.* 2007;132(4 suppl 1):A505.

55. Colombel JF, Schreiber S, Hanauer SB, Rutgeerts P, Sandborn WJ. Long-term tolerability of subcutaneous certolizumab pegol in active Crohn's disease: results from PRECiSE 3 and 4 [abstract]. *Gastroenterology.* 2007;132(4 suppl 1):A503.

56. Vermeire S, Abreu MT, D'Haens G, et al. Efficacy and safety of certolizumab pegol in patients with active Crohn's disease who previously lost response or were intolerant to infliximab: open-label induction preliminary results of the WELCOME study [abstract]. *Gastroenterology.* 2008;134(4 suppl 1):A67.

57. Lichtenstein GR, Hanauer SB, Sandborn WJ, and the Practice Parameters Committee of American College of Gastroenterology. Management of Crohn's disease in adults. *Am J Gastroenterol.* 2009;104:465-483.

58. D'Haens G, van Deventer S, van Hogezand R, et al. Endoscopic and histologic healing with infliximab anti-tumor necrosis factor antibodies in Crohn's disease: a European multicenter trial. *Gastroenterology.* 1999;116:1029-1034.

59. Rutgeerts P, Malchow H, Vatn MH, et al. Mucosal healing in Crohn's disease patients is associated with reduction in hospitalizations and surgeries. *Gastroenterology.* 2002;123:M2138.

60. Lichtenstein GR. Approach to corticosteroid-dependent and corticosteroid-refractory Crohn's disease. *Inflammatory Bowel Dis.* 2001;7:S23-S29.

61. Cohen RD, Tsang JF, Hanauer SB. Infliximab for Crohn's disease: first anniversary clinical experience. *Am J Gastroenterol.* 2000; 95:3469-3477.

62. Ricart E, Panaccione R, Loftus EV, Tremaine WJ, Sandborn WJ. Successful management of Crohn's disease of the ileoanal pouch with infliximab. *Gastroenterology.* 1999;117:429-432.

63. Braun J, Brandt J, Listing J, et al. Treatment of active ankylosing spondylitis with infliximab: a randomized controlled multicenter trial. *Lancet.* 2002;359:1187-1193.

64. Parsi MA, Achkar JP, Brzezinski A, Shen B, Lashner B. Extraintestinal manifestations of Crohn's disease respond to infliximab. *Am J Gastroenterol.* 2002;97:S265.

65. Tan MH, Gordon M, Lebwohl O, George J, Lebwohl MG. Improvement of *Pyoderma gangrenosum* and psoriasis associated with Crohn's disease with anti-tumor necrosis factor alpha monoclonal antibody. *Arch Dermatol.* 2001;137:930-933.

66. Su CG, Judge TA, Lichtenstein GR. Extraintestinal manifestations of inflammatory bowel disease. *Gastroenterol Clin North Am.* 2002;31:307-327.

67. Bertolini DR, Nedwin GE, Bringman TS, Smith DD, Mundy GR. Stimulation of bone resorption and inhibition of bone formation in vitro by human tumour necrosis factors. *Nature.* 1986;319:516-518.

68. Manolagas SC, Jilka RL. Bone marrow, cytokines, and bone remodeling—emerging insights into the pathophysiology of osteoporosis. *N Engl J Med.* 1995;332:305-311.

69. Abreu MT, Kam LY, Vasiliauskas EA, et al. Treatment with infliximab is associated with increased markers of bone synthesis in patients with Crohn's disease. *Am J Gastroenterol.* 2002;97:S269.

70. Colombel JF, Loftus EV, Tremaine WJ, et al. The safety profile of infliximab for Crohn's disease in clinical practice: the Mayo Clinic experience in 500 patients. *Gastroenterology.* 2003;124:A7.

71. Runge JW, Martinez JC, Caravati EM, et al. Histamine antagonists in the treatment of acute allergic reactions. *Ann Emerg Med.* 1992; 21:237-242.

72. Hanauer SB, Rutgeerts PJ, D'Haens G, et al. Delayed hypersensitivity to infliximab (Remicade) re-infusion after a 2-4 year interval without treatment. *Gastroenterology.* 1999;116:A731.

73. Keane J, Gershon S, Wise RP, et al. Tuberculosis associated with infliximab, a tumor necrosis factor alpha-neutralizing agent. *N Engl J Med.* 2001;345:1098-1104.

74. Diagnostic standards and classification of tuberculosis in adults and children. Official statement of the American Thoracic Society and the Centers for Disease Control and Prevention, adopted by the American Thoracic Society Board of Directors, July 1999. Endorsed by the Council of the Infectious Diseases Society of America, September 1999. *Am J Respir Crit Care Med.* 2000;161:1376-1395.

75. Targeted tuberculin testing and treatment of latent tuberculosis infection. Official statement of the American Thoracic Society, adopted by the American Thoracic Society Board of Directors, July 1999. Joint statement of the American Thoracic Society and the Centers for Disease Control and Prevention, endorsed by the Council of the Infectious Diseases Society of America, September 1999. *Am J Respir Crit Care Med.* 2000;161:S221-S247.

76. Mow WS, Abreu MT, Papadakis KA, Targan SR, Vasiliauskas EA. High incidence of anergy limits the usefulness of PPD screening for tuberculosis (TB) prior to Remicade in inflammatory bowel disease (IBD). *Gastroenterology.* 2002;122:A100.

77. Katz JA, Keenan GF, Snith DE, Lichtenstein GR. Outcome of pregnancy in patients receiving infliximab for the treatment of Crohn's disease and rheumatoid arthritis. *Gastroenterology.* 2003;124:A63.

78. Brown SL, Greene MH, Gershon SK, Edwards ET, Braun MM. Tumor necrosis factor antagonist therapy and lymphoma development: twenty-six cases reported to the Food and Drug Administration. *Arthritis Rheum.* 2002;46:3151-3158.

79. Bickston SJ, Lichtenstein GR, Arseneau KO, Cohen RB, Cominelli F. The relationship between infliximab treatment and lymphoma in Crohn's disease. *Gastroenterology.* 1999;117:1433-1437.

80. Ekstrom K, Hjalgrim H, Brandt L, et al. Risk of malignant lymphomas in patients with rheumatoid arthritis and in their first degree relatives. *Arthritis Rheum.* 2003;48:963-970.

81. Baecklund E, Ekbom A, Sparen P, Feltelius N, Klareskog L. Disease activity and risk of lymphoma in patients with rheumatoid arthritis: nested case-control study. *BMJ.* 1998;317:180-181.

82. Potential serious adverse events of the anti-TNF alpha drugs. US Food and Drug Administration, Center for Drug Evaluation and Research Web site. Available at http://www.fda.gov. Accessed.

83. Siegel CA, Hur C, Korzenik JR, Gazelle GS, Sands BE. Risks and benefits of infliximab for the treatment of Crohn's disease. *Clin Gastroenterol Hepatol.* 2006;4:1017-1024.

84. Mohan N, Edwards ET, Cupps TR, et al. Demyelination occurring during anti-tumor necrosis factor alpha therapy for inflammatory arthritides. *Arthritis Rheum.* 2001;44:2863-2869.

85. Lenercept Multiple Sclerosis Study Group and the University of British Columbia MS/MRI Analysis Group. TNF neutralization in MS: results of a randomized, placebo-controlled multicenter study. *Neurology.* 1999;53:457-465.

86. Chung ES, Packer M, Lo KH, Fasanmade AA, Willerson JT. Randomized, double-blind, placebo-controlled, pilot trial of infliximab, a chimeric monoclonal antibody to tumor necrosis factor-alpha, in patients with moderate-to-severe heart failure: results of the anti-TNF Therapy Against Congestive Heart Failure (ATTACH) trial. *Circulation.* 2003;107:3133-3140.

87. Baert F, Noman M, Vermeire S, et al. Influence of immunogenicity on the long-term efficacy of infliximab in Crohn's disease. *N Engl J Med.* 2003;348:601-608.

88. Hay JW, Hay AR. Inflammatory bowel disease: costs-of-illness. *J Clin Gastroenterol.* 1992;14:309-317.

89. Hanauer SB, Cohen RD, Becker RV, Larson LR, Vreeland MG. Advances in the management of Crohn's disease: economic and clinical potential of infliximab. *Clinical Therapeutics.* 1998;20:1009-1028.

90. Lichtenstein GR, Feagan BG, Cohen RD, et al. Serious infections and mortality in association with therapies for Crohn's disease: TREAT registry. *Clin Gastroenterol Hepatol.* 2006;4:621-630.

91. Feagan BG, Vreeland MG, Larson LR, Bala MV. Annual cost of care for Crohn's disease: a payor perspective. *Am J Gastroenterol.* 2000;95:1955-1960.

92. Cohen RD, Larson LR, Roth JM, Becker RV, Mummert LL. The cost of hospitalization in Crohn's disease. *Am J Gastroenterol.* 2000;95:524-530.

93. Rubenstein JH, Chong RY, Cohen RD. Infliximab decreases resource use among patients with Crohn's disease. *J Clin Gastroenterol.* 2002;35:151-156.

94. McNamara DA, Brophy S, Hyland JM. Perianal Crohn's disease and infliximab therapy. *Surgeon.* 2004;2:258-263.

95. Sandborn WJ. Azathioprine: state of the art in inflammatory bowel disease. *Scand J Gastroenterol.* 1998;225(suppl):92-99.

96. Cheifetz A, Smedley M, Martin S, et al. The incidence and management of infusion reactions to infliximab: a large center experience. *Am J Gastroenterol.* 2003;98:1315-1324.

97. Parsi MA, Achkar JP, Richardson S, et al. Predictors of response to infliximab in patients with Crohn's disease. *Gastroenterology.* 2002;123:707-713.

98. Vermeire S, Louis E, Rutgeerts P, et al. NOD2/CARD15 does not influence response to infliximab in Crohn's disease. *Gastroenterology.* 2002;123:106-111.

99. Esters N, Vermeire S, Joossens S, et al. Serological markers for prediction of response to anti-tumor necrosis factor treatment in Crohn's disease. *Am J Gastroenterol.* 2002;97:1458-1462.

ANTI-TNFα THERAPY FROM SYMPTOMS TO MOLECULES

IMPACT OF INDIVIDUAL VARIABILITY ON ANTI-TNFα OPTIMIZATION STRATEGIES

Ellen J. Scherl, MD, FACP, AGAF

"If it were not for the great variability among individuals, medicine might as well be a science and not an art."
—*Sir William Osler, 1892*

The greatest challenge for physicians treating Crohn's disease today is to move from generalized symptom-oriented step-up strategies to individualized prevention-oriented—early intervention/top-down—strategies involving personalized and proactive targeting of molecules. The recent advent of molecular-targeted therapies such as anti-tumor necrosis factor (anti-TNFα) agents has the potential to change the immunobiology of inflammation, clinical outcomes, and natural history of Crohn's disease in select patients. Whether biologic therapies should be introduced earlier in the disease course or whether they should be used as monotherapy or combination therapy differs for different patients, and these topics remain a source of lively debate.

This chapter will review the evolution of anti-TNFα agents and novel biologic therapies in the context of corticosteroids and immunomodulators, focusing on anti-TNFα agents as a steroid-sparing and steroid-avoiding strategy and focusing on the rationale for evaluating combination therapy versus monotherapy; intervening early; and personalizing medicine predicated on a constellation of symptoms, diagnostics (endoscopy, laboratory, and radiographic testing), and molecular signatures. Our goal is to reverse progression of disease and favorably affect the natural history of inflammatory bowel disease (IBD), while making existing therapies safer by stratifying therapeutic responses and identifying individuals who are likely to benefit from early aggressive biologic therapy either in combination or as monotherapy.

Prior to the introduction of anti-TNFα therapy, steroids were recognized to be ineffective in maintaining clinical remission in IBD,[1-3] with nearly one third of steroid-treated ulcerative colitis patients requiring colectomy and nearly 50% of steroid-treated patients with Crohn's disease being refractory to treatment and requiring surgical intervention.[4,5] Among the predictors of disabling course in Crohn's disease is a requirement for steroids during the first flare or a requirement of 2 or more courses of steroids.[6] More than one half of steroid-exposed Crohn's disease patients receiving thiopurine (6-mercaptopurine [6-MP] or azathioprine) maintenance therapy will relapse after 1 year,[7,8] and more than 3 months of steroid therapy is associated with increased cost to society in terms of time out of work and hospitalization.[9]

Approximately one third of steroid-treated, azathioprine-treated, or methotrexate-treated patients achieve mucosal healing.[10,11] In steroid-naïve patients treated with combination infliximab and azathioprine, up to three quarters achieve mucosal healing.[12] While there is a weak correlation between symptomatic improvement and mucosal healing, there is a stronger correlation between mucosal healing and decreased hospitalization and surgical rates.[13-17]

In contrast to steroids, anti-TNFα therapies have proven effective in both induction and maintenance of remission for Crohn's disease.[18-23]

Lichtenstein GR, ed.
Crohn's Disease: The Complete Guide to Medical Management (pp 213-224).
© 2011 SLACK Incorporated

IBD IMMUNOBIOLOGY: ANTI-TNFα MECHANISM OF ACTION

TNFα is a proinflammatory cytokine that is pivotal in the dysregulated immune response to luminal microbial antigens that characterizes chronic recurrent Crohn's disease.[24,25] An uncontrolled exaggerated immune response to luminal bacteria results in an increase in proinflammatory cytokines and a decrease in antiinflammatory cytokines, resulting in tissue damage. TNFα is secreted into intestinal mucosa by macrophages and monocytes and is bound to T lymphocytes and monocytes. Its biological activity is mediated by cell surface TNFα receptors binding to either membrane-bound or soluble TNFα.[26-28] TNFα may increase adhesion molecules, allowing for increased cell infiltration and enhanced metalloproteinase and collagenase production, which help form ulcers and fistulas.

Antibodies to TNFα (infliximab, adalimumab, certolizumab, and golimumab) bind to TNFα on cell surfaces as well as to soluble TNFα, and this may be responsible for its prolonged effect.[29] Infliximab is a chimeric immunoglobulin (Ig)G1 monoclonal antibody to TNFα composed of 25% murine variable fragment antigen binding (Fab) sections and 75% human constant region and is produced by a recombinant cell line. Adalimumab is humanized recombinant IgG1 monoclonal antibody to TNFα (95% human/5% murine). It is produced by recombinant DNA technology in a mammalian cell expression system. Certolizumab is a recombinant humanized Fab fragment with high affinity to TNFα attached to a polyethylene backbone in order to increase plasma stability, and this may also increase tissue bioavailability as well as confer diminished transfer to the placenta.[30] The Fab fragment of certolizumab is produced by *Escherichia coli*. Etanercept and onercept are Fc fusion proteins with less avidity for TNFα and only bind to circulating soluble TNFα, which may explain why they are not as effective in Crohn's disease.[31] Thalidomide binds to TNFα receptors, thereby blocking the production of proinflammatory mediators, but its effect is short lived and only lasts as long as thalidomide is perfusing the monocytes or target cells.[32,33] The real problem is that the gene responsible for TNFα production is still activated with all of these therapies, and until the gene is inhibited, permanent anti-TNFα response will not occur. Nonetheless, antibodies to TNFα provide the best and most durable antiinflammatory effect compared to other anti-TNFα treatments such as thalidomide or the Fc receptor proteins etanercept and onercept.[32,33]

TNFα is one of many proinflammatory cytokines, chemokines, and growth factors mediating intestinal inflammation. TNFα mediates recruitment of leukocytes from blood vessels into intestinal mucosa through circulating cells interacting with adhesion molecules on the vascular endothelium.[34,35]

In contrast, anti-integrins such as natalizumab (an alpha$_4$ anti-integrin) and vedolizumab (an alpha$_4$beta$_7$ anti-integrin) bind to receptors on the cell surface of leukocytes, which inhibit alpha$_4$-mediated adhesion of leukocytes to vascular endothelium, preventing transmigration of leukocytes across the vascular endothelium into inflamed intestinal mucosa, thereby reducing leukocyte delivery of proinflammatory cytokines.[23,36] Chemokine inhibitors block T lymphocyte trafficking and activation of CCR9 T lymphocytes into the intestinal lymphoid tissue, thereby diminishing inflammation.[37]

INFLIXIMAB COMBINATION TREATMENT IN MEDICALLY REFRACTORY CROHN'S DISEASE: INDUCTION TRIALS (1995 TO 1999)

The original open-label trial of infliximab for steroid and immunomodulator refractory Crohn's colitis demonstrated dramatic mucosal healing after only 4 weeks of treatment.[38] This pivotal study ushered in the first of many randomized controlled trials evaluating the role of anti-TNFα therapies in inducing remission in medically refractory (ie, both steroid and immunomodulator refractory) Crohn's disease.[39] The first infliximab induction trial for medically refractory Crohn's disease revealed that 81% of patients treated with a single dose of infliximab 5 mg/kg achieved clinical response by week 4, with many patients achieving response within 2 weeks and 48% of patients achieving clinical remission at 4 weeks compared to only 4% in the placebo group.[39] The trial also introduced the concept of anti-TNFα mucosal healing. The exceptionally low placebo rate underscores the importance of the study design, which included patients who had failed conventional therapies such as steroids and immunomodulators. This was the first large-scale study evaluating combination therapy in medically refractory Crohn's disease excluding internal fistulizing or stricturing disease. Those patients with perianal fistula noted improvement, but the study was not powered to address the impact of infliximab on perianal fistula.

The follow-up study to evaluate the role of infliximab in perianal fistula, which also excluded internal fistulizing and stricturing disease, was equally compelling and included a 3-dose infliximab induction.[40] The study showed that more than 50% of patients in the infliximab group had a complete closure of all fistulas compared with only 13% in the placebo group.

INFLIXIMAB COMBINATION TREATMENT IN MEDICALLY REFRACTORY CROHN'S DISEASE: MAINTENANCE TRIALS (1999 TO 2006)

Prior to establishing the role of infliximab in maintaining remission in Crohn's disease, large randomized controlled trials failed to demonstrate a role for steroids, sulfasalazine, or azathioprine maintenance therapy in Crohn's disease.[41,42] Therefore, patients who responded to infliximab in the induction trial[37] were cautiously enrolled in a retreatment trial to evaluate the potential role of infliximab in maintaining remission.[43] At week 12, patients were randomized to receive infliximab 5 mg/kg every 8 weeks or placebo. The peak remission rates were achieved by week 8. A proportion of patients, therefore, had lost response by the time of the 12-week randomization. Based on the every 8-week maintenance regimen in this trial and the robust maintenance of remission, maintenance randomized controlled trials were conducted. We now have adopted an every 8-week maintenance schedule based on the original retreatment trial and subsequent randomized controlled maintenance trials.

In the ACCENT I trial, which involved maintenance infliximab therapy given every 8 weeks, 39% and 45% of patients receiving 5 and 10 mg/kg of infliximab, respectively, were in clinical remission at week 30, compared with 21% of patients receiving placebo.[20] In another controlled trial, 5 mg/kg of infliximab, given in 3 doses, completely closed fistulas for a median of 3 months in 46% of patients and achieved a 50% reduction in fistula drainage in 62% of patients.[44]

Infliximab has been approved for induction and maintenance of remission in pediatric patients with moderate-to-severe active Crohn's disease who have had an inadequate response to conventional therapy. The REACH study evaluated the safety and efficacy of infliximab in children with moderate-to-severe active Crohn's disease and confirmed that infliximab 5 mg/kg every 8 weeks was more effective than every 12 weeks.[45]

IMMUNOGENICITY: INFLIXIMAB AND COMBINATION THERAPY (1999 TO PRESENT)

Once the role of infliximab for maintenance of remission in Crohn's disease was established, consideration of the optimal dosing schedule began. Those patients in the maintenance trials[20,44] who responded and were randomized into the placebo arm were treated episodically with infliximab when they required therapy for disease exacerbation. It was noted that the incidence of antibodies to infliximab was greater in the episodic treatment arm when compared to the regularly scheduled 5 mg/kg and 10 mg/kg every 8-week maintenance arms.[20,44] It was also noted that the percentage of patients forming antibodies to infliximab in both ACCENT I and ACCENT II maintenance studies was nearly twice the percentage of patients forming antibodies in the ATTRACT rheumatoid arthritis maintenance trial.[46,47] Unlike the rheumatoid arthritis trials where all patients received scheduled therapy and the majority received methotrexate in combination with infliximab, approximately one third of patients in the maintenance Crohn's disease trials received episodic treatment, and only one third received concomitant immunosuppression.

A study following the long-term outcome of the episodic treatment strategy confirmed that the majority of patients treated episodically (the patients who were initially treated in the Targan induction trial[39] who were enrolled into the retreatment study)[48] developed antibodies to infliximab.[49] These antibodies were associated with an increased risk of infusion reaction and a reduction in the median duration of response from 71 to 35 days only if the antibody titer was greater than 8.0 mcg/mL, which occurred in 37% of patients. In contrast, in the scheduled maintenance arm, approximately 10% of patients developed antibodies to infliximab.[50] Maintenance therapy dosed episodically is less effective than scheduled every 8-week dosing, which has been associated with prolonged mucosal healing and improved pharmacoeconomic and quality-of-life outcomes.[13] Scheduled maintenance of infliximab therapy is less immunogenic than episodic treatments.[50] Concomitant immunosuppression with infliximab (2-dose induction followed by every 12 weeks, which is more consistent with episodic dosing than standard 3-dose induction and scheduled every 8-week dosing) reduced immunogenicity and increased trough serum levels.[51] Alternatively, in a randomized controlled trial of steroid-dependent patients who underwent a forced steroid taper over 14 weeks, there was no difference between methotrexate in combination with regularly scheduled infliximab or infliximab alone, suggesting that there is no need for immunosuppression in patients receiving regularly scheduled infliximab monotherapy.[52] In contrast to the Van Assche study[51], in which patients had a form of episodic treatment defined as not receiving 3-dose induction and not receiving anti-TNFα therapy every 8 weeks, combination treatment with immunosuppression did seem to be associated with higher trough levels and reduced immunogenicity. Based on the difference in immunogenicity (antibodies to infliximab formation) in the scheduled versus episodic arms of the maintenance trials in Crohn's disease, it was suggested that 1) episodically treated infliximab patients be pretreated with steroids as well as immunomodulators to reduce immunogenicity and 2) controlled trials evaluating 3-dose induction followed by scheduled maintenance with or without immunomodulators be conducted.[53,54]

MOVE TOWARD MONOTHERAPY: REEVALUATION OF COMBINATION STRATEGIES (2005 TO 2008)

Immunogenicity of anti-TNFα therapy may be diminished, and serum concentrations may be increased[51] with combination immunomodulators and anti-TNFα agents in episodically (less than 3-dose induction for infliximab and more than every 8 weeks maintenance infliximab) treated regimens. However, the risk of combination in light of hepatosplenic T-cell lymphomas has led to a recent reevaluation of combination therapy with anti-TNFα agents in patients who have been chronically exposed to steroids and immunomodulators.[55-57] The use of 6-mercaptopurine or azathioprine alone or in combination with infliximab has been associated with non-Hodgkins lymphoma.[58]

An excess risk of lymphoproliferative disorders has been observed in patients receiving long-term azathioprine with a fatal outcome in almost half of the cases and frequent association with Epstein-Barr virus. These patients were not exposed to infliximab.[59] Hepatosplenic T-cell lymphoma has been associated with azathioprine alone or in combination with azathioprine and infliximab or adalimumab in young male adolescents and young adults.[56] Patients with IBD who receive long-standing cumulative dosing of combination immunosuppression and/or biologic therapies may react like posttransplant patients with increased risk for developing Epstein-Barr virus–positive lymphoma.[60]

In the context of the risk of lymphoproliferative disorders in long-standing Crohn's disease with steroids and thiopurine therapy, the need for combination anti-TNFα therapy and immunomodulators was reevaluated. When infliximab 5 mg/kg was administered as regularly scheduled 3-dose induction with maintenance every 8 weeks, the rates of immunogenicity with and without immunomodulators were similar: 4.2 and 12.5, respectively.[61]

Adalimumab induction followed by regularly scheduled dosing also showed similar low rates of immunogenicity with or without concomitant use of immunomodulators, 0 and 3.9%, respectively.[62] Rates of immunogenicity for regularly scheduled certolizumab were also similar with or without concomitant immunomodulators: 4% and 10%, respectively, in the Precise I study and 2% and 12%, respectively, in the Precise II study.[30,63] There was no difference between methotrexate in combination with infliximab or infliximab alone in steroid-dependent patients with a forced steroid taper over 14 weeks, suggesting that with regularly

scheduled infliximab monotherapy, there is no added benefit for methotrexate immunosuppression.[52] These studies and the concern regarding lymphoma in patients with long-standing disease exposed to long-term combination therapy suggested that it may be reasonable to administer biologic agents as monotherapy to optimize the risk-benefit ratio.[55] The key is that we consider monotherapy in patients with long-standing disease who are taking long-term cumulative doses of immunomodulators and steroids. In contrast, early intervention with limited (up to 1 year) combination anti-TNFα and immunomodulator therapy may be more effective and associated with less long-term toxicity.[64]

Another reason to consider monotherapy in select patients with long-standing disease and immunomodulator therapy is the concern about progressive multifocal leukoencephalopathy (PML) that was associated with combination therapy in natalizumab. The drug has been associated with 3 cases of PML in clinical trials. The cases occurred in 2 patients with multiple sclerosis who were receiving combination therapy with natalizumab and interferon β-1a and 1 natalizumab-treated 60-year-old male patient with Crohn's disease and prior exposure to high cumulative dosing of azathioprine and steroids, long-standing underlying disease, as well as an atypical underlying lymphopenia.[65-67] Because PML was associated with combination therapy in patients taking natalizumab, the Food and Drug Administration (FDA) approved this therapy as monotherapy in patients with CD. Some additional cases have been reported in multiple sclerosis patients receiving natalizumab as monotherapy, and, therefore, the duration of the natalizumab cumulative dose needs to be evaluated. In addition, the introduction of natalizumab in the background of long-standing disease where patients have been sequentially and simultaneously exposed to other immunomodulators may be a risk factor.

COMPARATIVE ANTI-TNFα THERAPIES (2006 TO PRESENT)

Although there are no head-to-head analyses of anti-TNFα agents, the comparative infliximab, adalimumab, and certolizumab trials were of similar design. Each randomized controlled maintenance trial of these anti-TNFα agents selected and randomized responders of induction therapy to either maintenance or placebo arms for 6 to 12 months. Adalimumab is approved for inducing and maintaining clinical remission in adult patients with moderate to severe Crohn's disease who have had an inadequate response to conventional therapy and for inducing remission in these patients if they also have lost response or are intolerant to infliximab. Adalimumab, a fully humanized anti-TNFα antibody, was demonstrated to be superior to placebo for the induction of remission in patients with moderate to severe CD who were naïve to anti-TNFα therapy[68] and to maintain clinical remission for up to 56 weeks in these patients.[62] Furthermore, among patients who were intolerant or did not respond to infliximab therapy, adalimumab was shown to induce remission more frequently than placebo.[69] Among patients who initially responded to adalimumab, Colombel et al reported significantly higher rates of remission with adalimumab versus placebo at 1 year.[21] In patients with CD for less than 2 years, approximately 50% remained in steroid-free remission more than 1 year after receiving 40 mg of adalimumab subcutaneously every other week or every week.[70] Anti-TNFα–naïve patients had a 36% remission rate after induction with 160 mg adalimumab at week 0 and 80 mg adalimumab at week 2, compared to a remission rate of only 21% in patients who had previously received infliximab therapy.[67]

Certolizumab pegol is a pegylated Fab fragment of a humanized monoclonal antibody that neutralizes TNFα. Like infliximab and adalimumab, this agent is approved for the treatment of patients with CD who have had an inadequate response to conventional therapy. A phase III, randomized, double-blind, multicenter study that assessed the efficacy and tolerability of certolizumab in patients with moderate to severe CD showed a modest improvement in response rates, as compared with placebo but no significant improvement in remission rates.[71] In addition, patients who had a response to induction therapy with certolizumab were more likely to have maintained response and remission at 26 weeks with continued treatment compared with a switch to placebo.[30]

PRECiSE 2 revealed more than 50% remission at 6 months in patients receiving certolizumab pegol 3-dose induction (400 mg at 0, 2, and 4 weeks followed by 400 mg every 4 weeks) compared with remission rates of only one third in patients who had received previous infliximab therapy.[30] In the anti-TNFα patients who received just the induction dose, one third of patients were in remission at 6 months, suggesting that even the 3-dose induction resulted in a significant remission over a 6-month period. Nearly 70% of patients with recent-onset Crohn's disease (less than 1 year) treated with subcutaneous monthly certolizumab pegol after induction dose were in remission at 6 months compared with only 44% of treated patients with disease duration of greater than 5 years.[72] In contrast, approximately 50% of patients treated with adalimumab induction 80 mg/40 mg followed by adalimumab 40 mg weekly or every other week were in remission and off of steroids at 2 years compared with only one third of patients treated similarly who had a disease duration of more than 5 years.[21] No significant difference occurred with infliximab, adalimumab, or certolizumab with or without immunomodulators if they were administered with standard loading induction doses followed by regularly scheduled doses.[30,61,62,71]

The results from the induction phase of the PRECiSE 2 trial compared favorably with other monoclonal anti-TNFα induction studies. The 6-week response rates of approximately 66% of patients in the study and remission rates of 40% were unaffected by concomitant immunosuppressants or corticosteroids.[73] Long-term data of certolizumab (at 52 and 54 weeks) suggest that 400-mg subcutaneous injections given monthly are well tolerated with low anti-double–stranded DNA—3.2% in PRECiSE 3 and 2.7% in PRECiSE 4—possibly because of the low apoptosis rates associated with certolizumab. In more than 900 patients treated with certolizumab for 1 year, the incidence of infections and malignancy is similar to other anti-TNFα agents.[74] Nearly 66% of patients in the WELCOME study who had lost response or were intolerant to infliximab responded to induction with certolizumab at 0, 2, and 4 weeks with maintenance every 2 or 4 weeks. In addition, almost 40% of those patients achieved remission on certolizumab.[75]

EARLY TREATMENT WITH COMBINATION THERAPY VERSUS MONOTHERAPY: STEROID-EXPOSED, IMMUNOMODULATOR, AND ANTI-TNFα NAÏVE CROHN'S DISEASE PATIENTS

In evaluating the anti-TNFα maintenance trials,[20,21,30,76] there is a trend toward more robust remission and response rates in the subgroup of patients treated early, within 2 years of onset of disease. Although the cumulative steroid dosing is difficult to quantify, many patients in these trials have been treated with steroids, immunomodulators, and in some cases previous anti-TNFα therapies.[21,30,70] The role of regularly scheduled maintenance anti-TNFα therapy in combination with immunomodulators has not been clearly elucidated in many of the maintenance trials.

In contrast, the SONIC trial—a definitive large head-to-head prospective randomized controlled trial evaluating early intervention with 1 year of regularly scheduled infliximab and azathioprine in steroid-exposed moderate-to-severe Crohn's disease patients with evidence of inflammation (elevated C-reactive protein [CRP] level and endoscopic lesions)—showed that infliximab/azathioprine combination therapy is superior to infliximab monotherapy and azathioprine monotherapy in achieving steroid-free remission at 1 year (50%, 42%, and 23%, respectively).[65] Post hoc subanalysis showed that, in patients without evidence of inflammation (normal CRP and no endoscopic lesions), there was no statistical difference between azathioprine and infliximab monotherapy and marginal superiority with combination therapy in steroid-free remission rates (35%, 40%, and 50%, respectively, in patients with a CRP of less than 0.8 mg/dL).

Most gastroenterologists prescribe 6-mercaptopurine (6-MP) and azathioprine as a steroid-sparing therapy for patients with moderate Crohn's disease. However, fewer are using weight-based 6-MP or azathioprine at the time of steroid induction—6-MP/azathioprine top-down therapy. An examination of 6-MP/azathioprine maintenance of remission trials in the context of current prescribing patterns and the new SONIC data, which showed that azathioprine was consistently less effective than infliximab monotherapy or infliximab combination therapy, is instructive. A small head-to-head randomized controlled trial evaluating 6-MP in newly diagnosed Crohn's disease included 27 patients with moderate Crohn's disease who were treated with combination weight-based 6-MP 1.5 mg/kg and steroids versus 28 patients treated with steroids alone. At the end of 1.5 years, only 9% relapsed in the early intervention 6-MP combination group, and more than 95% did not require repeat steroids.[77] In contrast, in the 28 patients treated with steroids alone, nearly two thirds required repeat steroids, and almost 50% relapsed. This trial is so small that the point estimates of efficacy have wide confidence intervals, and the safety of the 2 regimens cannot be adequately assessed. In addition, the trial was conducted in children and does not provide strong evidence for the basis of clinical practice.

Alternatively, Candy et al found that when azathioprine weight-based 2.5 mg/kg was initiated in patients with long-standing disease, only 42% were in remission at 15 months, which compared favorably with only 7% in the placebo group (steroid taper without azathioprine maintenance).[7] However, this underscores the problem with maintenance azathioprine in steroid-exposed patients; fully 60% were not in remission at the end of 15 months. Furthermore, Costes et al found that long-term 4-year follow-up of steroid-dependent (> 6 months of steroid exposure) moderate Crohn's disease patients showed that approximately 85% of patients treated with 6-MP or azathioprine alone or 6-MP/azathioprine in combination with 3-dose induction infliximab as a bridge strategy relapsed at 4 years.[78] Although the SONIC data are less robust in the Crohn's disease patients with less evidence of inflammation, maintenance studies[7,78] suggest that 6-MP/azathioprine does not maintain long-term clinical remission in the majority of moderate Crohn's disease patients previously treated with at least 6 months of steroids. This finding is also supported by the SONIC trial, which showed that azathioprine was not effective in a large study. Furthermore, cost-benefit analyses of steroids in terms of pharmacoeconomic modeling show that patients who have had more than 3 months of steroids have increased costs to society in terms of time out of work and hospitalizations.[9] In contrast, 6-MP/azathioprine top-down therapy initiated in newly diagnosed Crohn's disease patients simultaneously with steroids was successful in achieving steroid-free remission in the majority of patients.[77] The study is too small to form the basis of clinical practice, however. In addition, in the context of SONIC, which showed less efficacy with azathioprine, it may not even be warranted to conduct a large prospective trial evaluating azathioprine/steroid top-down therapy.

SONIC data suggest that even in Crohn's disease without evidence of inflammation, combination therapy for 1 year initiated early in the disease course is more effective than azathioprine monotherapy in achieving steroid-free remission (50% vs 35%, respectively).[65] Likewise, the rates of steroid-free remission with azathioprine monotherapy were low in the Candy et al and Costes et al trials (42% at 15 months and 15% at 4 years, respectively).[7,78]

SONIC is the first definitive randomized controlled trial evaluating 1-year regularly scheduled infliximab and azathioprine as early intervention in steroid-exposed moderate-to-severe Crohn's disease patients. The SONIC trial also included patients who failed to respond to mesalamine. Though infliximab and azathioprine combination therapy was superior to monotherapy in moderate-to-severe Crohn's disease of short duration, patients with severe disease and evidence of inflammation (elevated CRP and endoscopic lesions) had the most significant improvement with combination treatment. In patients with moderate-to-severe disease and evidence of inflammation (elevated CRP and endoscopic lesions), infliximab monotherapy was superior to azathioprine monotherapy, and combination therapy was more effective than either forms of monotherapy.

In conclusion, SONIC is important because it is the first large prospective head-to-head trial supporting the tectonic shift toward early intervention with anti-TNFα therapy and away from unlimited steroid use in moderate-to-severe Crohn's disease with evidence of inflammation (elevated CRP and endoscopic lesions). The superiority of combination therapy may reflect the synergistic effect of 2 effective drugs rather than reduced immunogenicity. Serious adverse events were similar in each of the 3 arms of the SONIC trial. Although the study is not designed to evaluate combination therapy beyond 1-year duration and did not evaluate combination therapy in patients with long-standing Crohn's disease treated with long-standing sequential or simultaneous steroids, immunomodulators, or anti-TNFα and biologic agents or in male adolescents and young adults, it is still the best large randomized controlled prospective head-to-head trial evaluating infliximab and azathioprine. It clearly demonstrates the superiority of infliximab monotherapy and combination therapy in the treatment of moderate-to-severe Crohn's disease with evidence of inflammation (elevated CRP and endoscopic lesions). The study also underscores the importance of determining the extent and severity of inflammation in patients with Crohn's disease prior to embarking on biologic therapy. The SONIC trial provides strong evidence for early infliximab therapy and challenges not only ending the steroid era but also reevaluating the immunomodulator era.

EARLY INTERVENTION WITH COMBINATION THERAPY VERSUS MONOTHERAPY: STEROID, IMMUNOMODULATOR, AND ANTI-TNFα NAÏVE CROHN'S DISEASE PATIENTS

In steroid-naïve patients with short disease duration, early induction with combination therapy (infliximab with weight-based azathioprine) is superior to standard step-up therapy with steroids and the addition of immunomodulators.[12] Early combination infliximab as a bridge to weight-based azathioprine was steroid avoiding at the end of 2 years and was associated with nearly three quarters of patients achieving mucosal healing compared with less than one third mucosal healing in the conventional step-up steroid group. In addition, 41% in the top-down group did require at least 1 additional infliximab dose, underscoring the importance of 6-month to 1-year combination therapy in early intervention.[77] Though this study compared top-down early combination therapy with weight-based azathioprine and 3-dose infliximab induction contrasted with standard steroid escalation therapy, it did not compare top-down early steroid therapy combined with weight-based azathioprine.[77] This randomized controlled trial evaluating 6-MP and top-down steroid therapy was so small that the point estimates of efficacy have wide confidence intervals, and the safety of the 2 regimens cannot be adequately assessed.[77] In addition, the trial was conducted on children and does not provide strong evidence for the basis of clinical practice.

MUCOSAL HEALING

Mucosal healing in Crohn's disease has been strongly correlated with decreased hospitalizations and intestinal resection.[13-17] In contrast, symptomatic improvement is weakly correlated with mucosal healing. Therefore, endoscopic monitoring to assess mucosal healing may emerge as an important outcome in order to establish therapeutic efficacy. Furthermore, endoscopic lesions are evidence of inflammation and may be helpful in identifying select patients who are more likely to respond to early anti-TNFα immunotherapy or combination therapy.[64]

Only one third of steroid-exposed Crohn's disease patients achieve mucosal healing.[79] Steroid sparing with thiopurine 6-MP/azathioprine or methotrexate achieves clinical efficacy, but mucosal healing is achieved in only approximately one third of patients.[10,11] Methotrexate-associated mucosal healing was greater than 40% in 2 small series.[80,81] More than 50% of patients on 6-MP maintenance therapy relapse after 1 year of therapy.[7,8] In contrast, durable mucosal healing occurs after only 4 weeks of infliximab therapy in steroid and immunomodulator refractory patients.[34] A post hoc analysis of ACCENT I reported mucosal healing in nearly one half of 26 patients receiving regularly scheduled infliximab.[13] Early intervention with combination anti-TNFα and azathioprine in steroid-naïve moderate Crohn's disease results in mucosal healing in up to three quarters of patients.[12] In steroid-exposed, azathioprine- and infliximab-naïve moderate Crohn's disease of short duration, patients receiving combination infliximab and azathioprine had more than 40% mucosal healing.[64] Mucosal healing, normal Crohn's Disease Endoscopic Index of Severity (CDEIS) scores, and low CRP were more likely to maintain clinical remission.[82]

At 10 weeks, a significant improvement in CDEIS score, endoscopic remission rates, histologic Crohn's disease score, and mucosal healing from baseline was found with certolizumab.[14] Adalimumab achieves and maintains mucosal healing in moderate-to-severe Crohn's disease. The first results of extended trial mucosal healing occurred in one quarter of patients at the end of 1 year and occurred as early as 12 weeks.[83] An area of concern is endoscopic ulcerations that occur in the postoperative period and predict postoperative recurrence.[84] Three years after surgery, the endoscopic recurrence rate increased to 85%, and symptomatic recurrence was noted in 34% of patients. Those in whom diffuse, deep new ileal recurrences developed within 1 year tended to experience early symptoms and complications. Postoperative infliximab significantly lowered endoscopic recurrence at 1 year in complex fistulizing CD.[85] Adverse events were similar in the infliximab and placebo groups. Only 9% of patients who had undergone an ileocolonic resection had documented endoscopic recurrence after 1 year of postoperative infliximab (3-dose induction followed every 8 weeks for 1 year). The findings underscore the importance of early aggressive therapy in achieving mucosal healing, which in this case was linked to clinical remission. Further prospective trials evaluating mucosal healing with early intervention in steroid-naïve patients will be important in defining the role of endoscopic and histologic mucosal healing in selecting patients for early intervention and for assessing and monitoring the efficacy of early intervention.

As we introduce immunosuppressants and/or biologic agents at an earlier stage (as induction and maintenance therapy in steroid-naïve patients or after short-term steroids), we may see fewer adverse events[64,85,86] than when we layer immunosuppressants and biologics on top of prolonged steroids.[87,88] Until steroid use is limited, adding immunosuppressants and biologics puts a small group of patients at risk for IBD-associated immune deficiency. Clear guidelines for preventing opportunistic infections and registries for documenting lymphoma and cancer risk in patients with moderate to severe IBD need to be established.[89]

SYMPTOMS AND EVIDENCE OF INFLAMMATION

Moving away from treating symptoms to proactively targeting molecules will help to change the natural history of Crohn's disease and arguably prevent progression of disease. Until we can identify molecular signatures and genotyping to stratify therapeutic responses, evidence of inflammation is increasingly important in patient selection for early intervention with biologic therapy either alone or in combination. Anti-TNFα monotherapy may be preferred to combination therapy in patients with long-term disease, the elderly, or male adolescents and young adults. In the absence of inflammation, refractory Crohn's disease may in fact be pseudorefractory due to bile acid diarrhea, celiac disease, lactose intolerance, overlap with irritable bowel syndrome, bacterial overgrowth, adhesions, or intestinal infections (eg, *Salmonella* species, *Shigella* species, *Clostridium difficile*, and *Giardia* species). In addition, intestinal obstruction due to stricture, lymphoma, or carcinoma may be a cause of moderate-to-severe Crohn's disease without evidence of inflammation. These factors may coexist and ought to be evaluated and assessed in patients who do not have evidence of mucosal inflammation, elevated sedimentation rate, or elevated CRP prior to considering anti-TNFα therapy. Fibrotic strictures or even fistulizing disease is cause for surgical evaluation prior to initiating anti-TNFα therapy. In addition, before surgical evaluation in these select patients, it is important to evaluate the extent of disease prior to embarking on anti-TNFα therapy. In contrast, in the presence of inflammation with elevated CRP, endoscopic lesions, or radiographic evidence of ulceration, and active disease, early intervention with anti-TNFα therapy in combination with immunomodulators appears to be most efficacious. In the future, molecular signatures and genotyping will allow for more targeted approaches and make therapies safer. Until that time, evidence of inflammation (eg, elevated CRP, endoscopic lesions, and fecal calprotectin) may help in patient selection for early intervention.[53]

ADVERSE EVENTS

We will now review evidence of toxicity. Assessment of tuberculosis exposure with a purified protein derivative (PPD) skin test and chest x-ray prior to the initiation of anti-TNFα agents will rule out reactivation and prevent against reactivation of latent tuberculosis.[55,90] Infectious complications with other pathogens such as coccidioidomycosis and histoplasmosis will also be identified on chest x-ray. Despite the fact that PPD is recommended, close to two thirds of patients will be anergic, underscoring the importance of the chest x-ray.[91] The TREAT (Crohn's

Therapy, Resource, Evaluation, and Assessment Tool) registry provides evidence that patients on prolonged steroid therapy have an increased risk for serious infection.[87,92] In this prospective patient registry designed to study the long-term safety of therapies for CD, the only medications independently associated with serious infections were prednisone (odds ratio [OR] 2.21; 95% confidence interval [CI] 1.46-3.33; $P < 0.001$) and narcotics (OR 2.11; 95% CI 1.10-4.05; $P = 0.024$).

Treatment with infliximab is generally well tolerated; however, delayed hypersensitivity (serum sickness-like) infusion reactions have been described and anti-double-stranded DNA antibodies have been recognized.[43] In episodic infliximab-treated patients, antibodies to infliximab were correlated with increased risk of infusion reaction and shorter duration of response.[49] Acute infliximab infusion reactions also occurred in episodically treated patients and are characterized by headache, dyspnea, chest pain, pruritis, flushing, fever, and chills and may be controlled by discontinuing the infliximab regimen, administering diphenhydramine 50 mg intravenously (IV), and restarting the infliximab infusion at a slower rate. Pretreatment with acetaminophen, corticosteroids, and/or diphenhydramine is recommended in episodically treated infliximab patients or patients with prior reactions.

Delayed infusion reactions usually occur within 2 weeks of infliximab infusion, again predominantly in episodically treated patients. Patients may experience myalgias, arthralgias, or more rarely may have symptoms such as pruritis, dysphagia, urticaria, and headaches. These symptoms usually respond to a short course (approximately 2 weeks) of corticosteroids.[93] Development of symptomatic lupus in association with antibodies to double-stranded DNA is rare, and no patients developed systemic manifestations such as renal toxicity or CNS involvement associated with positive antinuclear antibody test.[94] Certolizumab has been associated with significantly lower antibodies to DNA.[70,71]

As already discussed, rare postmarketing cases of hepatosplenic T-cell lymphoma have been reported with both infliximab and adalimumab; all of the cases occurred in patients on concomitant treatment with azathioprine or 6-MP. Updated TREAT registry data found no increased risk with infliximab for CD.[56,87] In addition, long-term follow-up of approximately 2000 Crohn's disease patients in the ENCORE registry underscores the TREAT registry findings that steroids, not infliximab, pose increased risk for serious infections.[95,96]

In August 2009, the FDA completed an analysis of anti-TNFα agents and concluded these agents are linked to an increased risk of lymphoma and other cancers associated with the use of these drugs in children and adolescents.[57] This new safety information is now being added to the Boxed Warning for these products. In addition, the FDA is requiring labeling changes to the Warnings and Adverse

Event sections of these agents that will now describe reported cases of leukemia and new-onset psoriasis in patients treated with TNFα blockers.

CONCLUSION

The impact of anti-TNFα therapy on old strategies has moved treatment in a more proactive, personalized direction toward targeting molecules and risk assessment, rather than treating symptoms. The advent of anti-TNFα therapy has established the role of maintenance, mucosal healing, and decreased hospitalization and surgical resection rates in moderate-to-severe Crohn's disease. Although an accurate assessment of the history of symptoms will give the correct diagnosis in more than 90% of cases, assessing evidence of inflammation by CRP and endoscopic lesions is increasingly important, and, in the future, assessing biomarkers and molecular signatures will predict response and make selection of therapy safer. SONIC is an important head-to-head large randomized controlled trial evaluating the role of infliximab and azathioprine in moderate-to-severe Crohn's disease with inflammation. The trial identified patients with evidence of inflammation (elevated CRP and endoscopic lesions) as those who would benefit the most from combination treatment with infliximab and azathioprine or infliximab monotherapy. If patients have symptoms but no evidence of inflammation, it is important to challenge the diagnosis of Crohn's disease and consider overlap with lactose intolerance; celiac disease; irritable bowel syndrome; bacterial overgrowth; bile acid diarrhea; or intercurrent infections such as *Salmonella* species, *Shigella* species, *Clostridium difficile*, and *Giardia* species. The importance of lack of evidence of inflammation with symptoms suggests that there may be evidence of pseudorefractory Crohn's disease, and a more aggressive differential diagnostic approach should be embarked on prior to considering anti-TNFα therapy. It is also possible that without evidence of inflammation patients may have several coexisting conditions.[53]

In select patients with moderate-to-severe disease, an earlier aggressive approach will be indicated; in other patients with mild-to-moderate disease, stepping back and challenging the diagnosis, de-escalating medication dose, and stressing adherence to therapeutic regimens are in order. Identifying immunologically vulnerable subsets of patients with emerging serologic markers, biomarkers, and ultimately genotyping may allow for stratification of therapeutic responses and personalized medicine.

Decoding the human genome is redefining the science of individuality, reminding us that less than 0.1% of our DNA is responsible for disease susceptibility and therapeutic response.[97-99] Though we are poised to recognize the potential for genotyping informing our therapeutic options, we are not yet using genotyping as routine in selection of optimal therapies. We are at a threshold for genotyping both individual patients and bacteria,[25] which will lead to a greater understanding of the pathobiology of IBD and improving clinical outcomes.[100]

Until the science of the human genome and microbiome translates into personalized medicine, predicting and preventing the outcome of disease progression may be achieved by identifying patients with evidence of inflammation who are likely to respond to early intervention with anti-TNFα therapy and by limiting steroid and thiopurine therapies. In contrast, in patients without evidence of inflammation, the diagnosis of refractory Crohn's disease ought to be challenged, and pseudorefractory Crohn's disease due to overlap with intercurrent or coexisting conditions ought to be considered. There has been a tectonic shift toward early biologic and/or immunosuppressive therapy aimed at steroid-free remission and mucosal and histologic healing. Identifying select patients with evidence of inflammation (elevated CRP and endoscopic lesions) in moderate-to-severe Crohn's disease for early intervention will make current therapies safer and may move treatment from symptom-oriented step-up strategies to prevention-oriented strategies more likely to favorably alter the natural history of IBD.

REFERENCES

1. Truelove SC, Witts LJ. Cortisone in ulcerative colitis: final report on a therapeutic trial. *Br Med J.* 1955;2:1041-1048.

2. Truelove SC, Witts LJ. Cortisone and corticotrophin in ulcerative colitis. *Br Med J.* 1959;1:387-394.

3. Lennard-Jones JE, Misiewicz JJ, Connell AM, Baron JH, Jones FA. Prednisone as maintenance treatment for ulcerative colitis in remission. *Lancet.* 1965;1:188-189.

4. Faubion WA Jr, Loftus EV Jr, Harmsen WS, Zinsmeister AR, Sandborn WJ. The natural history of corticosteroid therapy for inflammatory bowel disease: a population-based study. *Gastroenterology.* 2001;121:255-260.

5. Munkholm P, Langholz E, Davidsen M, Binder V. Frequency of glucocorticoid resistance and dependency in Crohn's disease. *Gut.* 1994;35:360-362.

6. Beaugerie L, Seksik P, Nion-Larmurier I, Gendre JP, Cosnes J. Predictors of Crohn's disease. *Gastroenterology.* 2006;130:650-656.

7. Candy S, Wright J, Gerber M, Adams G, Gerig M, Goodman R. A controlled double blind study of azathioprine in the management of Crohn's disease. *Gut.* 1995;37:674-678.

8. Lémann M, Zenjari T, Bouhnik Y, et al. Methotrexate in Crohn's disease: long-term efficacy and toxicity. *Am J Gastroenterol.* 2000;95:1730-1734.

9. Feagan BG, Loftus EV, Kamm MA, Chao J, Mulani P. Impact of steroid discontinuation on health care resource utilization in Crohn's disease [abstract]. *Am J Gastroenterol.* 2007;102(suppl 2):S445.

10. D'Haens G, Geboes K, Rutgeerts P. Endoscopic and histologic healing of Crohn's (ileo-) colitis with azathioprine. *Gastrointest Endosc.* 1999;50:667-671.

11. Kozarek RA, Patterson DJ, Gelfand MD, et al. Methotrexate induces clinical and histologic remission in patients with refractory inflammatory bowel disease. *Ann Intern Med.* 1989;110:353-356.

12. D'Haens G, Baert F, van Assche G, et al. Early combined immuno-suppression or conventional management in patients with newly diagnosed Crohn's disease: an open randomised trial. *Lancet.* 2008;371:660-667.

13. Rutgeerts P, Diamond RH, Bala M, et al. Scheduled maintenance treatment with infliximab is superior to episodic treatment for the healing of mucosal ulceration associated with Crohn's disease. *Gastrointest Endosc.* 2006;63:433-442.

14. Colombel J, Hebuterne X. Endoscopic mucosal improvement in patients with active Crohn's disease treated with certolizumab pegol: first results of the MUSIC clinical trial. *Am J Gastroenterol.* 2008;103(suppl 1):S432.

15. Taxonera C, Rodrigo L, Casellas F, et al. Infliximab maintenance therapy decreases the use of non-pharmacological resources in patients with Crohn's disease [abstract]. *Gastroenterology.* 2008;134.

16. Yoshimura N, Kawaguchi T, Sako M, Takazoe M. Clinical efficacy of infliximab in the management of postsurgical recurring Crohn's disease [abstract]. *Gastroenterology.* 2008;134:A-472.

17. Lichtenstein GR, Yan S, Bala M, Blank M, Sands BE. Infliximab maintenance treatment reduces hospitalizations, surgeries, and procedures in fistulizing Crohn's disease. *Gastroenterology.* 2005; 128:862-869.

18. Targan SR, Hanauer SB, van Deventer SJ, et al. A short-term study of chimeric monoclonal antibody cA2 to tumor necrosis factor alpha for Crohn's disease. Crohn's Disease cA2 Study Group. *N Engl J Med.* 1997;337:1029-1035.

19. Present DH, Sandborn WJ, Rutgeerts PJ, et al. Infliximab treatment for ulcerative colitis: clinical response, clinical remission, and mucosal healing in patients with moderate or severe disease in the active ulcerative colitis trials (ACT1 & ACT2) [abstract]. *Gastroenterology.* 2008;134:A-493.

20. Hanauer SB, Feagan BG, Lichtenstein GR, et al. Maintenance infliximab for Crohn's disease: the ACCENT I randomised trial. *Lancet.* 2002;359:1541-1549.

21. Colombel JF, Sandborn WJ, Rutgeerts P, et al. Adalimumab for maintenance of clinical response and remission in patients with Crohn's disease: the CHARM trial. *Gastroenterology.* 2007;132:52-65.

22. Panaccione R, Colombel JF, Sandborn WJ, et al. Adalimumab maintains long-term remission in moderately to severely active Crohn's disease. *Gastroenterology.* 2008;s134(suppl 1a):a134.

23. Sandborn WJ, Colombel JF, Enns R, et al. Natalizumab induction and maintenance therapy for Crohn's disease. *N Engl J Med.* 2005;353:1912-1925.

24. Podolsky DK. Inflammatory bowel disease. *N Engl J Med.* 2002; 347:417-429.

25. Slack E, Hapfelmeier S, Stecher B, et al. Innate and adaptive immunity cooperate flexibly to maintain host-microbiota mutualism. *Science.* 2009;325:617-620.

26. Van Deventer SJ. Tumour necrosis factor and Crohn's disease. *Gut.* 1997;40:443-448.

27. Scallon BJ, Moore MA, Trinh H, Knight DM, Ghrayeb J. Chimeric anti-TNF-alpha monoclonal antibody cA2 binds recombinant transmembrane TNF-alpha and activates immune effector functions. *Cytokine.* 1995;7:251-259.

28. Van Deventer SJ. Transmembrane TNF-alpha, induction of apoptosis, and the efficacy of TNF-targeting therapies in Crohn's disease. *Gastroenterology.* 2001;121:1242-1246.

29. Osterman MT, Lichtenstein GR. Current and future anti-TNF therapy for inflammatory bowel disease. *Curr Treat Options Gastroenterol.* 2007;10:195-207.

30. Schreiber S, Khaliq-Kareemi M, Lawrance IC, et al, and the PRECiSE 2 Study Investigators. Maintenance therapy with certolizumab pegol for Crohn's disease. *N Engl J Med.* 2007;357:239-250.

31. Sandborn WJ, Hanauer SB, Katz S, et al. Etanercept for active Crohn's disease: a randomized, double-blind, placebo-controlled trial. *Gastroenterology.* 2001;121:1088-1094.

32. Caprilli R, Viscido A, Guagnozzi D. Review article: biological agents in the treatment of Crohn's disease. *Aliment Pharmacol Ther.* 2002;16:1579-1590.

33. Stern M, Herrmann R. Overview of monoclonal antibodies in cancer therapy: present and promise. *Crit Rev Oncol Hematol.* 2005;54:11-29.

34. Podolsky DK. Inflammatory bowel disease. *N Engl J Med.* 2002; 347:417-429.

35. Brown SJ, Mayer L. The immune response in inflammatory bowel disease. *Am J Gastroenterol.* 2007;102:2058-2069.

36. Feagan BG, Greenberg GR, Wild G, et al. Treatment of active Crohn's disease with MLN0002, a humanized antibody to the alpha4beta7 integrin. *Clin Gastroenterol Hepatol.* 2008;6:1370-1377.

37. Keshav S, Johnson D, Bekker P, Schall TJ. PROTECT-1 study demonstrated efficacy of the intestine-specific chemokine receptor antagonist CCX282-B (Traficet-EN) in treatment of patients with moderate to severe Crohn's disease. *Gastroenterology.* 2009; 5(suppl 1):a392.

38. van Dullemen HM, van Deventer SJ, Hommes DW, et al. Treatment of Crohn's disease with anti-tumor necrosis factor chimeric monoclonal antibody (cA2). *Gastroenterology.* 1995;109:129-135.

39. Targan SR, Hanauer SB, van Deventer SJ, et al. A short-term study of chimeric monoclonal antibody cA2 to tumor necrosis factor alpha for Crohn's disease. Crohn's Disease cA2 Study Group. *N Engl J Med.* 1997;337:1029-1035.

40. Present DH, Rutgeerts P, Targan S, et al. Infliximab for the treatment of fistulas in patients with Crohn's disease. *N Engl J Med.* 1999;340:1398-1405.

41. Summers RW, Switz DM, Sessions JT Jr, et al. National Cooperative Crohn's disease study: results of drug treatment. *Gastroenterology.* 1979;77(4 pt 2):847-869.

42. Malchow H, Ewe K, Brandes JW, et al. European Cooperative Crohn's Disease Study (ECCDS): results of drug treatment. *Gastroenterology.* 1984;86:249-266.

43. Rutgeerts P, Van Assche G, Vermeire S. Optimizing anti-TNF treatment in inflammatory bowel disease. *Gastroenterology.* 2004; 126:1593-1610.

44. Sands BE, Anderson FH, Bernstein CN, et al. Infliximab maintenance therapy for fistulizing Crohn's disease. *N Engl J Med.* 2004; 350:876-885.

45. Hyams J, Crandall W, Kugathasan S, et al. Induction and maintenance infliximab therapy for the treatment of moderate-to-severe Crohn's disease in children. *Gastroenterology.* 2007;132:863-873.

46. Smolen JS, Han C, Bala M, et al. Evidence of radiographic benefit of treatment with infliximab plus methotrexate in rheumatoid arthritis patients who had no clinical improvement: a detailed subanalysis of data from the anti-tumor necrosis factor trial in rheumatoid arthritis with concomitant therapy study. *Arthritis Rheum.* 2005;52:1020-1030.

47. Maini R, St Clair EW, Breedveld F, et al. Infliximab (chimeric anti-tumour necrosis factor alpha monoclonal antibody) versus placebo in rheumatoid arthritis patients receiving concomitant methotrexate: a randomised phase III trial. ATTRACT Study Group. *Lancet.* 1999;354:1932-1939.

48. Rutgeerts P, D'Haens G, Targan S, et al. Efficacy and safety of retreatment with anti-tumor necrosis factor antibody (infliximab) to maintain remission in Crohn's disease. *Gastroenterology.* 1999;117:761-769.

49. Baert F, Noman M, Vermeire S, et al. Influence of immunogenicity on the long-term efficacy of infliximab in Crohn's disease. *N Engl J Med.* 2003;348:601-608.

50. Hanauer SB, Wagner CL, Bala M, et al. Incidence and importance of antibody responses to infliximab after maintenance or episodic treatment in Crohn's disease. *Clin Gastroenterol Hepatol*. 2004; 2:542-553.

51. Van Assche G, Magdelaine-Beuzelin C, D'Haens G, et al. Withdrawal of immunosuppression in Crohn's disease treated with scheduled infliximab maintenance: a randomized trial. *Gastroenterology*. 2008;134:1861-1968.

52. Feagan BG, McDonald JWD, Panaccione R, et al. A randomized trial of methotrexate in combination with infliximab for the treatment of Crohn's disease. *Gastroenterology*. 2008;135:294-295.

53. Rutgeerts P, Feagan BG, Lichtenstein GR, et al. Comparison of scheduled and episodic treatment strategies of infliximab in Crohn's disease. *Gastroenterology*. 2004;126:402-413.

54. Farrell RJ, Alsahli M, Jeen YT, Falchuk KR, Peppercorn MA, Michetti P. Intravenous hydrocortisone premedication reduces antibodies to infliximab in Crohn's disease: a randomized controlled trial. *Gastroenterology*. 2003;124:917-924.

55. Lichtenstein GR, Hanauer SB, Sandborn WJ, and the Practice Parameters Committee of American College of Gastroenterology. Management of Crohn's disease in adults. *Am J Gastroenterol*. 2009;104:465-483.

56. Rosh JR, Gross T, Mamula P, Griffiths A, Hyams J. Hepatosplenic T-cell lymphoma in adolescents and young adults with Crohn's disease: a cautionary tale? *Inflamm Bowel Dis*. 2007;13:1024-1030.

57. Food and Drug Administration. Information for healthcare professionals: tumor necrosis factor (TNF) blockers (marketed as Remicade, Enbrel, Humira, Cimzia, and Simponi). FDA Alert, August 4, 2009. Available at http://www.fda.gov/Drugs/DrugSafety/ PostmarketDrugSafetyInformationforPatientsandProviders/Dr ugSafetyInformationforHeathcareProfessionals/ucm174474.htm. Accessed May 6, 2010.

58. Kandiel A, Fraser AG, Korelitz BI, Brensinger C, Lewis JD. Increased risk of lymphoma among inflammatory bowel disease patients treated with azathioprine and 6-mercaptopurine. *Gut*. 2005;54:1121-1125.

59. Beaugerie L, Carrat F, Bouvier AM, et al, for the CESAME Study group. Excess risk of lymphoproliferative disorders (LPD) in inflammatory bowel diseases (IBD): interim results of the CESAME cohort [abstract]. *Gastroenterology*. 2008;134(4 suppl 1): A116.

60. Schwartz LK, Kim MK, Coleman M, Lichtiger S, Chadburn A, Scherl E. Case report: lymphoma arising in an ileal pouch anal anastomosis after immunomodulatory therapy for inflammatory bowel disease. *Clin Gastroenterol Hepatol*. 2006;4:1030-1034.

61. Sandborn W, Wagner C, Fasanmade A, et al. Effects of immunomodulators on pharmacokinetics and immunogenicity of infliximab administered as 3-dose induction followed by systematic maintenance therapy in IBD. *Gastroenterology*. 2007;132: A504-A505.

62. Sandborn WJ, Hanauer SB, Rutgeerts P, et al. Adalimumab for maintenance treatment of Crohn's disease: results of the CLASSIC II trial. *Gut*. 2007;56:1232-1239.

63. Sandborn WJ, Feagan BG, Stoinov S, et al. Certolizumab pegol for the treatment of Crohn's disease. *N Engl J Med*. 2007;357:228-238.

64. Sandborn WJ, Rutgeerts PJ, Reinisch W, et al. One year data from the SONIC Study: a randomized, double-blind trial comparing infliximab and infliximab plus azathioprine to azathioprine in patients with Crohn's disease naive to immunomodulators and biologic therapy [abstract]. Presented at: Digestive Diseases Week 2009; June 2, 2009; Chicago, IL.

65. Kleinschmidt-DeMasters BK, Tyler KL. Progressive multifocal leukoencephalopathy complicating treatment with natalizumab and interferon beta-1a for multiple sclerosis. *N Engl J Med*. 2005;353:369-374.

66. Langer-Gould A, Atlas SW, Green AJ, Bollen AW, Pelletier D. Progressive multifocal leukoencephalopathy in a patient treated with natalizumab. *N Engl J Med*. 2005;353:375-381.

67. Van Assche G, Van Ranst M, Sciot R, et al. Progressive multifocal leukoencephalopathy after natalizumab therapy for Crohn's disease. *N Engl J Med*. 2005;353:362-368.

68. Hanauer SB, Sandborn WJ, Rutgeerts P, et al. Human anti-tumor necrosis factor monoclonal antibody (adalimumab) in Crohn's disease: the CLASSIC-I trial. *Gastroenterology*. 2006;130:323-333.

69. Sandborn WJ, Rutgeerts P, Enns R, et al. Adalimumab induction therapy for Crohn disease previously treated with infliximab: a randomized trial. *Ann Intern Med*. 2007;146:829-838.

70. Schreiber S, Reinisch W, Colombel JF, et al. Early Crohn's disease shows high levels of remission to therapy with adalimumab: subanalysis of CHARM [abstract]. *Gastroenterology*. 2007;132(4 suppl 1):A147.

71. Sandborn WJ, Feagan BG, Stoinov S, et al, and the PRECiSE 1 Study Investigators. Certolizumab pegol for the treatment of Crohn's disease. *N Engl J Med*. 2007;357:228-238.

72. Sandborn WJ, Colombel JF, Panes J, Scholmerich J, McColm JA, Schreiber S. Higher remission and maintenance of response rates with subcutaneous monthly certolizumab pegol in patients with recent-onset Crohn's disease: data from PRECiSE 2 [abstract]. *Am J Gastroenterol*. 2006;101:S454-S455.

73. Thomsen OO, Schreiber S, Khaliq-Kareemi M, Hanauer SB, Bloomfield R, Sandborn WJ. Rapid onset of response and remission to subcutaneous certolizumab pegol and lack of influence of concomitant baseline medications in active Crohn's disease: results from the open-label induction phase of the PRECiSE 2 study [abstract]. *Gastroenterology*. 2007;132(4 suppl 1):A505.

74. Colombel JF, Schreiber S, Hanauer SB, Rutgeerts P, Sandborn WJ. Long-term tolerability of subcutaneous certolizumab pegol in active Crohn's disease: results from PRECiSE 3 and 4 [abstract]. *Gastroenterology*. 2007;132(4 suppl 1):A503.

75. Vermeire S, Abreu MT, D'Haens G, et al. Efficacy and safety of certolizumab pegol in patients with active Crohn's disease who previously lost response or were intolerant to infliximab: open label induction preliminary results of the WELCOME study [abstract]. *Gastroenterology*. 2008;134(4 suppl 1):A67.

76. Sands B, van Deventer S, Bernstein C, et al. Long-term treatment of fistulizing Crohn's disease: response to infliximab in the ACCENT II trial through 54 weeks. *Gastroenterology*. 2002;122:A81.

77. Markowitz J, Grancher K, Kohn N, Lesser M, Daum F. A multicenter trial of 6-mercaptopurine and prednisone in children with newly diagnosed Crohn's disease. *Gastroenterology*. 2000;119:895-902.

78. Costes L, Colombel J-F, Mary J-Y, et al. Long term follow-up of a cohort of steroid-dependent Crohn's disease patients included in a randomized trial evaluating short term infliximab combined with azathioprine [abstract]. *Gastroenterology*. 2008;134:A-134.

79. Olaison G, Sjödahl R, Tagesson C. Glucocorticoid treatment in ileal Crohn's disease: relief of symptoms but not of endoscopically viewed inflammation. *Gut*. 1990;31:325-328.

80. Panaccione R. The use of methotrexate is associated with mucosal healing in Crohn's disease. *Gastroenterology*. 2005;128(suppl):A49.

81. Mañosa M, Naves JE, Leal C, et al. Does methotrexate induce mucosal healing in Crohn's disease? *Inflamm Bowel Dis*. 2010;16:377-378.

82. Louis E, Vernier-Massouille G, Grimaud JC, et al. Infliximab discontinuation in Crohn's disease patients in stable remission on combined therapy with immunosuppressors: a prospective ongoing cohort study [abstract]. *Gatroenterology*. 2009;136:A-146.

83. Rutgeerts P, D'Haens G, Van Assche G. Adalimumab induces and maintains mucosal healing in patients with moderate to severe ileocolonic Crohn's disease—first results of the extend trial [abstract]. *Gastroenterology*. 2009;136:A-116.

84. Rutgeerts P, Geboes K, Vantrappen G, Beyls J, Kerremans R, Hiele M. Predictability of the postoperative course of Crohn's disease. *Gastroenterology.* 1990;99:956-963.

85. Regueiro M, Schraut W, Baidoo L, et al. Infliximab prevents Crohn's disease recurrence after ileal resection. *Gastroenterology.* 2009;136:441-450.

86. Sandborn WJ, Rutgeerts P, Reinisch W, et al. SONIC: a randomized, double-blind, controlled trial comparing infliximab and infliximab plus azathioprine in patients with Crohn's disease naïve to immunomodulators and biologic therapy [abstract]. *Am J Gastroenterol.* 2008;103(suppl 1):S436.

87. Lichtenstein GR, Cohen RD, Feagan BG, et al. Safety of infliximab and other Crohn's disease therapies: TREAT registry data with 24,575 patient-years of follow-up [abstract]. *Am J Gastroenterol.* 2008;103(suppl 1):S436.

88. Toruner M, Loftus EV Jr, Harmsen WS, et al. Risk factors for opportunistic infections in patients with inflammatory bowel disease. *Gastroenterology.* 2008;134:929-936.

89. Sands BE, Cuffari C, Katz J, et al. Guidelines for immunizations in patients with inflammatory bowel disease. *Inflamm Bowel Dis.* 2004;10:677-692.

90. Keane J, Gershon S, Wise RP, et al. Tuberculosis associated with infliximab, a tumor necrosis factor alpha-neutralizing agent. *N Engl J Med.* 2001;345:1098-1104.

91. Mow WS, Abreu-Martin MT, Papadakis KA, et al. High incidence of anergy in inflammatory bowel disease patients limits the usefulness of PPD screening before infliximab therapy. *Clin Gastroenterol Hepatol.* 2004;2:309-313.

92. Lichtenstein GR, Feagan BG, Cohen RD, et al. Serious infections and mortality in association with therapies for Crohn's disease: TREAT registry. *Clin Gastroenterol Hepatol.* 2006;4:621-630.

93. Cheifetz A, Smedley M, Martin S, et al. The incidence and management of infusion reactions to infliximab: a large center experience. *Am J Gastroenterol.* 2003;98:1315-1324.

94. Nancey S, Blanvillain E, Parmentier B, et al. Infliximab treatment does not induce organ-specific or nonorgan-specific autoantibodies other than antinuclear and anti-double-stranded DNA autoantibodies in Crohn's disease. *Inflamm Bowel Dis.* 2005;11:986-991.

95. D'Haens G, Colombel J-F, Hommes D, et al. Corticosteroids pose an increased risk for serious infection: an interim safety analysis of the ENCORE registry [abstract]. *Gastroenterology.* 2008;134:A-140.

96. Colombel JF, Prantera C, Rutgeerts PJ, et al. No new safety signals identified in Crohn's disease patients treated with infliximab in an interim review of the ENCORE registry [abstract]. *Gastroenterology.* 2008;134:A-472.

97. Lander ES, Linton LM, Birren B, et al. Initial sequencing and analysis of the human genome. *Nature.* 2001;409:860-921.

98. Venter JC, Adams MD, Myers EW, et al. The sequence of the human genome. *Science.* 2001;291:1304-1351.

99. Jasny BR, Roberts L. Building on the DNA revolution. *Science.* 2003;300:277-296.

100. Kevles D, Hood L, eds. *The Code of Codes: Scientific and Social Issues in the Human Genome Project.* Cambridge, MA: Harvard University Press; 1992:3-363.

NOVEL BIOLOGICAL THERAPIES FOR CROHN'S DISEASE

Iris Dotan, MD and Daniel Rachmilewitz, MD

The biologic approach to inflammatory bowel disease (IBD) therapy has been developed in recent years based on better understanding of specific immunopathological processes in intestinal inflammation. Thus, drugs that target one molecule, one cell, or one immunological process have been developed; contrasting with the drugs in current use, most of which are small molecules aimed at generally decreasing the immune response.

The most effective biologic therapy that is currently known and approved for commercial use is Remicade (infliximab), the chimeric monoclonal antibody targeting tumor necrosis factor alpha (TNFα) with a remission induction rate of 50% to 60% in active CD[1] and response rate of 50% in fistulizing CD.[2,3] This is the most effective treatment for active moderate to severe CD and shows promise also in maintenance of remission.[4,5] The patient subpopulation that does not respond to this treatment, as well as the patients who lose response or develop side effects, requires an alternative solution. Thus, in parallel to additional TNFα-neutralizing strategies, other biologics are assessed in CD patients. Those will be the focus of this chapter.

Progress in developing biologic drugs was facilitated due to 2 major advancements in basic research. One is the ability to focus on and dissect immunopathologies in the intestinal mucosa up to the level of single molecules. The best example of such progress is the generation of sophisticated experimental models of IBD. Thus, to the armamentarium of chemical models of colitis were added knock-out laboratory (and to a lesser number of models, transgenic) animals in which experimental colitis is being exacerbated or ameliorated because of the lack (or overexpression) of a single gene. The protein that is encoded by that gene is identified

as a key player in mucosal immunology, and treatment strategies to decrease/neutralize or increase the concentration or effect of that protein can be taken. Other models, such as the immunologically manipulated ones where T cell subsets or bone marrow precursors are administered into immunodeficient recipients or the spontaneous models in which chronic inflammation similar to CD develops without any apparent trigger, enable the assessment of the role of lymphocyte subsets and critical processes (such as apoptosis) so that the processes or cells could be suggested as targets for treatment in human CD (animal models reviewed in Sartor's article[6]).

In parallel, advances in biotechnology now enable one to insert genes into viral vectors so that targeted delivery of cytokines is possible, and antisense oligonucleotides can be designed to hybridize with target RNAs; thus, the expression of specific molecules can be decreased, commercial amounts of growth factors can be generated, and humanized antibodies creating less immunogenicity can be engineered.

There are several categories of biologic therapies that are relevant to CD: 1) monoclonal antibodies, receptor fusion proteins, and soluble receptor antagonists, 2) recombinant cytokines, 3) nucleic acid-based therapies, 4) hormones and growth factors, 5) gene therapy, and 6) cell neutralization strategies, leukacytapheresis.

Inherently, as usually large peptides or protein-based drugs, biological therapies are biotechnological products administered parenterally; are aimed at a single molecule, cell, or process; are usually harder to manufacture; and are more expensive than conventional IBD therapy. Unfortunately, this does not render them necessarily safer or more effective.

TABLE 19-1

BIOLOGICAL TREATMENT FOR CROHN'S DISEASE*†

TYPE	BIOLOGIC	ROUTE	EFFECTS	COMMENTS/REFS
Anti-proinflammatory cytokines	Anti-IL-12/23	SC	Induces clinical response in a subgroup of patients with moderate to severe Crohn's disease who are nonresponsive to infliximab	24
	Anti-IFN-γ (Fontolizumab)	IV	Possible effect of high dose (4 mg/kg) in patients with high CRP	33
	Anti-IL6R (MRA)	IV	MRA biweekly, effective in inducing response/remission	16, 17
Regulatory cytokines	IL-10 (Tenovil)	SC/IV	Systemic administration ineffective in most studies	38 to 41 (Local administration seems promising in experimental models)
	IL-11 (Oprelvekin)	SC	Possible effect only of high-dose	53, 54
Anti-adhesion molecules	Natalizumab (Antegren)	IV	Early and sustained efficacy found with natalizumab as induction therapy in patients with elevated C-reactive protein and active Crohn's disease	68, 69
			Effective as maintenance therapy	
			Induces remission at 2 mg/kg	70
	LDP-02 (MLN02)	IV	Possible effect of high-dose (300 to 350 mg 3 times weekly for 4 weeks) in remission induction	105, 106
	ISIS2302 (Alicaforsen)	IV		85
Hormones	Growth hormone (Somatropin)	SC	Daily treatment for 4 months decreases CDAI vs placebo	88
Growth factors	G-CSF (Filgrastim) GM-CSF (Sargamostim)	SC SC	Decreases CDAI in active CD and may be effective for fistulous disease	90 to 93
Apheresis	Leukocyte-apheresis (Cellsorba, Adacolumn)	IV	Did not demonstrate efficacy for induction of clinical remission or response in patients with moderate to severe UC	103

*The table contains information about the major strategies and preparations that were described, and in the eyes of the authors seem promising near future treatments. Further information is included in the text.
†SC indicates subcutaneous; IFN, interferon; IV, intravenous; CRP, C-reactive protein; MRA, monoclonal receptor antibody; CDAI, Crohn's disease activity index.

This chapter focuses on biological therapies from all the above categories that were or are currently assessed for the treatment of Crohn's disease. The topic of biological therapies in IBD has been reviewed in recent years in several publications.[7-12] Here, we chose to focus on therapies that have been used in clinical trials in CD, some of which may be approved for commercial daily use within the near future (Table 19-1).

NEUTRALIZING PROINFLAMMATORY CYTOKINES

Triggered by the success of anti-TNFα neutralizing strategy for the treatment of active CD, various pro-inflammatory cytokines believed to be significant in intestinal inflammation were chosen as targets for neutralization by monoclonal antibodies, a relatively simple strategy where the potential major problem in general is the immunogenicity of the introduced antibodies, as has been the experience with the chimeric anti-TNFα monoclonal antibodies.[13,14]

MONOCLONAL ANTIBODIES

ANTI-IL-6R

The rationale of neutralizing IL-6 in CD is based upon its immunoregulatory potential and on the observations that the serum concentrations of IL-6 and its soluble receptor (IL-6R) are increased in CD and correlate with disease activity. It has also been demonstrated that the administration of the soluble IL-6R ameliorates experimental colitis.[15]

A randomized, placebo-controlled trial was reported in which a humanized monoclonal antibody against the IL-6 receptor (monoclonal receptor antibody [MRA]) was administered to patients with refractory CD in 2 treatment protocols (biweekly infusions of MRA or placebo or alternate biweekly MRA/placebo for 12 weeks at 8 mg/kg). The MRA biweekly protocol was significantly better than placebo in inducing response and remission in contrast to the MRA every 4 weeks. Thus, a therapeutic potential was demonstrated and awaits larger scale supportive trials.[16,17]

IL-12/23 BLOCKING ANTIBODY

IL-12/23 is a key cytokine in the proinflammatory TH1 response that is observed in the intestinal mucosa of patients with CD.[18-21] Thus, it may be a pivotal target for neutralization when planning CD treatment strategies, and anti-IL-12/23 treatment has been demonstrated to ameliorate experimental colitis.[22,23] In addition, ustekinumab—a monoclonal antibody against the p40 subunit of IL-12/23—has induced clinical response in a subgroup of patients with moderate to severe Crohn's disease who are nonresponsive to infliximab.[24]

IL-12/23 p40 protein fused to immunoglobulin (Ig)G2b was assessed for the ex vivo modulation of active CD. In a study that was performed on mucosal samples from patients with CD, the fusion protein decreased inflammatory activity of lamina propria mononuclear cells from IBD versus non-IBD patients, specifically decreasing IL-12-induced interferon (IFN)-γ secretion and proliferation and increasing apoptosis. Whether these effects hold true when administered in vivo to patients remains to be determined in clinical trials.[25]

IFN-γ NEUTRALIZING ANTIBODIES

FONTOLIZUMAB

The rationale of treating CD with interferon-γ neutralizing antibodies is its central role in TH1 polarization,[26,27] its increased secretion by CD mucosa, and the role that it may have in dysregulating the mucosal immune response, as well as the regression of experimental colitis when IFN-γ is neutralized.[28-33] Fontolizumab is an anti-IFN-γ monoclonal Ab humanized through recombinant DNA technology. A preliminary report on its effects when administered intravenously demonstrated an advantage over placebo in the high-dose (4 mg/kg) subgroup of patients with high C-reactive protein (CRP) when administered twice (days 0, 28). Further studies are needed.[34] It is of interest that the opposite approach, ie, administration of interferon-γ to CD patients, has also been assessed in smaller, uncontrolled trials. Low dose (daily administration of 12 million IU intravenously or 45,000 IU/kg x 3/week subcutaneously) was not associated with disease exacerbation, as might have been expected.[35,36]

BOOSTING IMMUNOREGULATORY CYTOKINES

IL-10

This is a regulatory cytokine with antiinflammatory properties that downregulates the production of Th1 cytokines, mainly IL-2 and IFN-γ.[37] The antiinflammatory effects of IL-10 were demonstrated in experimental colitis where its administration ameliorated inflammation in the IL-10 knock-out (KO) mouse model, where severe colitis develops when the mice are not kept in a germ-free facility.[33,38] Systemic administration of IL-10, whether intravenously or subcutaneously, seemed to be beneficial in early studies[39]; however, larger-scale studies failed to show such an effect.[40,41] IL-10 was also not better than placebo in preventing the recurrence of postoperative CD.[42]

Recently, sophisticated local delivery systems enable high IL-10 concentration in the intestinal mucosa without high systemic exposure, thus modulating inflammation locally and avoiding systemic side effects. This promising strategy has been studied in murine models whether using engineered bacteria[43] further modified so that human, not bacterial, IL-10 will be delivered[44] or sustained-release gelatin microspheres containing IL-10 and given rectally to decrease colitis in IL-10 KO mice.[45] Genetic manipulations aimed at local IL-10 delivery also include the use of human adenovirus bearing IL-10 gene[46] or local adenoviral vectors encoding IL-10 (AdvmuIL-10)[47] that decreased inflammation in murine colitis and the engineering of human CD4+T cells to produce IL-10[48] that were effective in preventing colitis in the CD45Rb[high] model.[49] Whether local IL-10 treatment will be effective in human disease and its role in treating active disease versus maintenance of remission (as reviewed in Li and He's article[50]) remains to be determined.

IL-11 (OPRELVEKIN)

This cytokine is produced mainly by mesenchymal cells, and among its biological effects is the ability to enhance intestinal barrier function[51,52] and to ameliorate experimental colitis.[53] Recombinant human IL-11 produced by *Escherichia coli* and differing from native IL-11 in only 1 amino acid (the last one, proline) was administered subcutaneously to 76 patients with active CD at several doses (5, 16, or 40 µg/kg/week) versus placebo. Although no significant benefit was demonstrated, there was a trend towards a positive effect in the 16-µg/kg dose administered in a 2- or 5-day/week protocol.[54] When administered at 15 µg/kg once a week or 7.5 µg/kg twice weekly versus placebo for 6 weeks to 148 steroid-naïve patients, only the 15 µg/kg group had a significant advantage over the placebo group in achieving remission;[55] however, further studies were not completed due to disappointing interim analysis results.

IFN-α

This cytokine is produced in response to viral infection by the infected cells. Recombinant human IFN-α-2a was administered to mildly to moderately active CD patients in an uncontrolled trial, demonstrating a 50% response.[56] Similar response rates (33% to 50%) were demonstrated when IFN-α-2b was used in CD.[57,58] The modest efficacy and side effects associated with IFN-α therapy precluded further assessment of these agents for the treatment of CD patients.

IFN-β AND RECOMBINANT IFN-βIA

This cytokine, produced by virally infected cells, is an effective treatment for multiple sclerosis (MS), where downregulation of inflammatory cytokines and upregulation of IL-10 was demonstrated.[59,60]

A pilot study had demonstrated improvement in 5 patients with CD.[61] An open long-term study of 46 steroid refractory patients with active UC suggested that IFN-β may be effective in both the induction and maintenance of remission in this population.[62] The results of a phase IIb trial have not been published yet.

ANTIBODIES AGAINST T LYMPHOCYTES

CD4+ T lymphocytes are increased in the lamina propria of patients with Crohn's disease and have been the "immediate suspects" in contributing to disease perpetuation. These cells are obvious targets to neutralize when treating IBD. Further support came from the observation that improvement and remission of CD occurred when concurrent acquired immunodeficiency syndrome (AIDS) progressed to low CD4+ counts.[63] Preliminary reports of the use of monoclonal antibodies against CD4+ T cells to treat Crohn's disease were published in the early 1990s[64] and were followed by small clinical trials using several preparations that showed nonsignificant improvements in some disease indices and reasonable tolerability; however, no follow-up placebo-controlled trials were published.

B-F5

This is a murine anti-human CD4+ T cell-specific mAb of the IgG1 isotype that was infused to 12 patients with active CD in doses ranging from 0.5 to 1 mg/kg/day for 7 consecutive days. The results were disappointing, with no significant improvement in disease indices and no sustained CD4+ T cell depletion. A partial explanation was the heterogeneity of the group and severity of the disease, and no further data exist for this drug in CD.[65]

CM-T412

Another anti-CD4 antibody is CM-T412. This is a human-mouse (75%/25% respectively) chimeric depleting anti-CD4 IgG1κ mAb that was used to treat active CD. In a small, open-label, phase I, dose-finding study, a total dose of 70, 210, or 700 mg was infused to patients over the course of 7 consecutive days. The treatment was associated with nonsignificant decreases in Crohn's disease activity index (CDAI) and CD4+ T cell counts and was well tolerated; however, it had no effect on the endoscopic appearance. It was associated with significant decreases in CD4+ T cell counts compared with baseline without significant increase in opportunistic infection. The concern that opportunistic infections may occur combined with its modest efficacy prevented further use of this agent.[66]

ANTI-ADHESION MOLECULES

Selective adhesion molecules blockade is a novel, promising strategy in the therapy of CD. It is aimed at interfering with the recruitment and migration of inflammatory cells to the intestinal mucosa. The relative specificity of the interference is possible due to the recognition of recruitment processes that are unique to the gut-associated lymphoid tissue (such as the interaction of α4β7 molecules on lymphocytes with mucosal addressin cell adhesion molecule-1 (MadCAM-1) on endothelial cells).

BLOCKING THE α4 INTEGRIN PATHWAY

ANTIBODIES TO α4 INTEGRINS

NATALIZUMAB

This is a humanized monoclonal antibody to α4-integrin, in which the variable region of a murine α4-integrin antibody has been inserted into a human IgG4 molecule. The rationale of using α4-integrin blockade in CD is the importance of the interactions between these molecules, expressed on the surface of most leukocytes, and adhesion molecules that are upregulated at sites of chronic inflammation on vascular endothelium (eg, vascular cell adhesion molecule-1 and MAdCAM-1) as do interactions between α4 integrin and extracellular matrix molecules within the inflamed tissue.[67] Two pilot studies in IBD patients followed. In the first pilot study, 30 patients with active Crohn's disease received a 3 mg/kg infusion of natalizumab (n = 18) or placebo (n = 12) by double-blind randomization. At week 2, a significant decrease of a disease activity score was noted. Seven (39%) natalizumab-treated patients achieved remission at week 2, compared with 1 (8%) treated with placebo. In contrast, 4 (33%) of the placebo-treated patients required rescue medication by week 2, compared with 2 (11%) of the natalizumab-treated patients. Adverse effects were similar in the treatment and placebo group.[68]

The results of a large, double-blind, placebo-controlled trial of natalizumab in 248 patients with moderate to severe CD were recently published. Patients were randomly assigned to 1 of 4 treatment arms: 2 infusions of placebo; 1 infusion of 3 mg/kg natalizumab followed by placebo; 2 infusions of 3 mg/kg natalizumab; or 2 infusions of 6 mg/kg natalizumab. Infusions were given 4 weeks apart. The group given 2 infusions of 6 mg/kg did not have a significantly higher rate of clinical remission than the placebo group at week 6. However, both groups that received 2 infusions of natalizumab had higher remission rates than the placebo group at weeks 4, 6, 8, and 12. The highest remission rate was 44%, and the highest response rate was 71% at week 6 in the group given 2 infusions of 3 mg/kg. The rates of adverse events were similar in all 4 groups.[69] The results of a phase III induction trial involving 905 CD patients worldwide (ENACT I) showed no difference in response rates between patients in the treatment and placebo arms.[70] However, 339 CD patients in whom clinical response/remission was achieved by natalizumab in the ENACT 1 study were included in the ENACT 2 trial, in which 300 mg of natalizumab versus placebo were infused monthly (for up to 12 months). Significant superiority of natalizumab versus placebo in sustaining response and remission was demonstrated during the 6-month period.[71] Based upon the current data, it might have seemed that the role of natalizumab is more in maintenance of remission than in controlling active disease; however, the active-disease data deserve further assessment, especially due to possible confounding factors (such as the high placebo response observed in that trial).

Post hoc subgroup analyses of the ENACT 2 and ENCORE maintenance trials found consistently higher induction remission rates for nearly 25% of patients with short duration CD (< 3 years).[72] In the ENCORE trial, 38% of patients who failed to respond to infliximab achieved a sustained response through weeks 8 and 12, compared with 17% of those on placebo.[73] Remission rates at 12 weeks were unaffected by concomitant immunosuppressants for nearly 40% of patients.

Natalizumab has been associated with 3 cases of progressive multifocal leukoencephalopathy (PML) in clinical trials.[74-76] The cases occurred in 2 patients with MS who were receiving combination therapy with natalizumab and interferon beta-1a and 1 patient with CD with prior exposure to azathioprine and steroids and an underlying lymphopenia. A recent report suggested a risk for PML of roughly 1 in 1000 patients treated with natalizumab for a mean of 17.9 months.[77] Currently, more than 25,000 patients (mostly with MS) have been treated, with no new cases of PML reported; however, liver abnormalities have been reported.

ANTIBODIES TO α4β7 INTEGRINS

α4β7 is expressed on activated peripheral blood T and B lymphocytes. The rationale for blocking α4β7 interactions in CD is its role in gut homing of memory CD4+, CD8+, and B lymphocytes where they bind to MAdCAM-1 that is expressed on gut endothelium[78] and on microvilli.

MLN02 (LDP02)

MLN02 (LDP02) is a humanized monoclonal IgG1 antibody against α4β7, constructed by grafting the complementary determining region of mouse anti-α4β7 into a human IgG framework. Feagan et al investigated 181 patients with active UC who were randomized to intravenous MLN02 (0.5 or 2.0 mg/kg) or placebo on day 1 and day 29.[79] Eligible patients also received concomitant mesalamine or no other treatment for colitis. Clinical remission rates at week 6 were significantly higher in the 0.5 mg/kg and 2.0 mg/kg groups (34% and 32%, respectively) compared with the placebo group (14%; P = 0.03).

A dose-dependent effect of MLN02 was found in a more recent randomized controlled study by Feagan et al.[80] A total of 185 patients with CD were randomized to MLN02 (0.5 or 2.0 mg/kg) or placebo on day 1 and day 29. This study evaluated response and remission rates at day 57. The treatment groups showed a similar response rate at day 57 (53%, 49%, and 41% in the 2.0 mg/kg, 0.5 mg/kg, and placebo groups) but a significantly greater remission rate in the 2.0 mg/kg group compared with placebo (37%, 30%, and 21%, respectively; $P = 0.04$). The most common serious adverse event was worsening of CD, and 1 infusion-related hypersensitivity reaction was reported.

BLOCKING THE β2 INTEGRIN PATHWAY

The rationale for interfering with β2 integrin pathways in CD is that these molecules are involved in several leukocyte-vascular/leukocyte-epithelial cell adhesion processes, where β2 integrins (such as αLβ2 integrin, or lymphocyte function associated antigen-1 [LFA-1]) that are expressed on leukocytes as well as on intestinal epithelial cells of UC and CD patients interact with intercellular adhesion molecule-1 (ICAM-1) that is differentially expressed in CD and UC.[81]

ICAM-1 ANTISENSE OLIGONUCLEOTIDE (ALICAFORSEN, ISIS-2302)

This is a 20-base pair complementary nucleotide chain that hybridizes with ICAM-1 mRNA that is thus degraded by RNAse-H, and the message and the expression of ICAM-1 is therefore decreased.[82] The effect of Alicaforsen, whether administered intravenously or subcutaneously, was not significantly better than placebo in treating active or steroid-dependent CD.[83,84] In a later study, patients treated with higher doses (300 to 350 mg infused 3 times weekly for 4 weeks) seemed to have higher serum levels and to benefit from the drug; however, there was no placebo group, and further details are needed in order to evaluate the significance of LFA-1/ICAM-1 blockade for the treatment of active CD.[85]

GROWTH HORMONE

In addition to its well-known effects on growth and metabolism, growth hormone (GH) has multiple effects on the intestine, where it stimulates growth and differentiation of rat small bowel mucosa, is involved in ion transport processes,[86] and ameliorates experimental colitis. The rationale to use GH as a therapeutic agent in Crohn's disease is based on the experimental data mentioned as well as on the motivation to reverse the catabolic effects associated with inflammation. The growth retardation and poor nutritional state seen in a significant number of CD patients have been traditionally attributed to chronic steroid use. However, evidence exists for disturbed GH-IGF axis in chronic diseases and decreased insulin-like growth factor (IGF)-1 in the serum of CD patients.[87] GH has the potential to increase the expression of IGF-1. Thirty-seven patients with moderate to severe CD were treated with daily subcutaneous (sc) injections of growth hormone (somatro-pin; Humatrope, Eli Lilly, Indianapolis, IN) or placebo for 4 months, in addition to their other CD medications and a high protein diet.[88] A significantly greater decrease in CDAI was demonstrated in the treatment versus placebo group after 4 months. Of note was the diagnosis of tumors in 2 patients in the treatment group and 1 in the placebo group that may interfere with the use of this therapeutic strategy, if indeed it will show benefit in larger scale and longer studies (which have not been published yet).

COLONY-STIMULATING FACTORS

A major goal of treatment for CD is suppressing an overreactive mucosal immune response. However, recently, an alternative theory has been suggested[89] emphasizing several points of similarity between CD and immunodeficiency, specifically neutrophil dysfunction states. A case report on the treatment of fistulizing CD with granulocyte colony stimulating factor (G-CSF) was published in 1999.[90] Several uncontrolled small studies were published later on demonstrating a significant decrease in CDAI in patients with inflammatory as well as fistulous CD that were treated with G-CSF (filgrastim) and GM-CSF (sargamostim).[91-93]

Of note, GM-CSF treatment, administered sc at a dose of 4 to 8 mg/kg for 8 weeks was associated with a significant decrease in CDAI with relatively minor side effects such as injection site irritation and bone pain, in addition to the shift in blood counts that is expected when this preparation is used.

EXTRACORPOREAL IMMUNOMODULATION

Though colony-stimulating factors aim at increasing immune cell numbers and possibly modifying their behavior to treat CD, an approach that is opposite in rationale is represented by extra corporeal immunomodulation based on leukapheresis techniques. Early reports on the benefit of lymphocyte apheresis to treat CD were published in the late 1980s, describing selective extracorporeal T cell depletion by ultracentrifugation in 54 patients with active CD, the majority of whom went into long-lasting remission and decreased steroid use to zero.[94] A later controlled study of a group of 28 patients with steroid-induced remission of CD who were assigned to lymphocytapheresis or no treatment in order to maintain remission did not show a meaningful benefit. Aiming at more specific targets, 2 strategies that decrease specific lymphocyte subpopulations were developed in Japan. One technique is a leukocyte removal filter column: Cellsorba (Asahi Medical, Tokyo, Japan). All leukocyte subpopulations, 99% of granulocytes and macrophages, and 40% to 60% of lymphocytes as well as platelets are trapped within the filter made of polyester fibers.[95] In preliminary studies in CD, an intensive induction protocol of leukocytapheresis every week for 5 weeks followed by a maintenance phase of leukocytapheresis every month for 5 months was used to treat 18 patients with active disease.[96] Fifty percent of the patients were in remission at the end of the intensive phase. The responding patients had significantly higher baseline CD4+CD45+ cells and IL-2 production by peripheral blood leukocytes at baseline. Interestingly, in preliminary studies, IBD patients responding to leukocytapheresis had higher CRP, erythrocyte sedimentation rate (ESR), and human leukocyte antigen-DR at baseline.[97]

An alternative leukocytapheresis method, Adacolumn (Japan Immunoresearch Laboratories, Takasaki, Japan), uses a column adsorbing granulocytes and monocytes/macrophages to a 2-mm diameter of cellulose acetate beads without significantly adsorbing lymphocytes.[98] Several trials demonstrated a positive effect of the column in active UC.[99,100] Its effects on CD patients were evaluated in much smaller studies. Seven refractory CD patients were treated with 5 to 6, 1-hour, 30-mL/min weekly sessions. Five of the patients went into remission. Interestingly, it seemed to be that patients with colonic disease and high inflammatory activity had a better chance to respond, reminiscent of the beneficial effects that the Adacolumn had in UC patients.[101] No significant side effects of the treatment were reported in IBD patients.[102]

In a randomized, double-blind, sham-controlled study involving more than 200 patients, the Adacolumn system did not demonstrate efficacy for induction of clinical remission or response in patients with moderate to severe UC.[103] Clinical remission rates were 17% and 11% for the granulocyte/monocyte apheresis and sham treatment groups, respectively, and the rate of clinical response was 44% and 39%, respectively. Of note, strictly speaking, the columns are not biological treatments as no biological is administered into the patients. They are included in this chapter because the concept of using them is based on biological approach-depleting activated cells that may contribute to the inflammatory process in the intestinal mucosa. By this, they are actually similar to the cell-depleting strategies that use monoclonal antibodies. It is of interest to wait for further results from studies in CD patients and see whether using the columns would be more beneficial than the results of studies in which the anti-CD4+ depletion is achieved by monoclonal antibodies.

SUMMARY AND FUTURE DIRECTIONS

SUMMARY

Biological treatments differ from current CD therapy in several aspects: They are usually peptides or proteins; are administered parenterally; target specific molecules, cells, or processes; and their manufacture is more sophisticated and more expensive than the small molecules that are used

for CD therapy. The development of biological treatments is based on better understanding of mucosal intestinal processes in homeostasis and uncontrolled inflammation and is possible due to great biotechnological progress such as genetic engineering and development of novel vehicles.

Among the various biological treatments that were described in this chapter, several directions seem to be promising near-future strategies to treat Crohn's disease.

TARGETING PROINFLAMMATORY CYTOKINES

Based on the success of anti-TNFα neutralization strategies, targeting other proinflammatory cytokines, specifically IL-12 and possibly IL-18, is a reasonable approach to treat CD. This could be achieved by monoclonal antibodies to the cytokines themselves, a technique that, depending on the structure of the antibody, might be associated with side effects associated with immunogenicity. More sophisticated techniques that are already assessed in animal models include recombinant viral vectors expressing cytokine antisense under viral promoter to decrease the expression and biological function of IL-18.[104]

BOOSTING REGULATORY CYTOKINES

In this category, increasing the expression and function of IL-10 deserves a second chance after the systemic administration strategy seems to have failed. Local IL-10 delivery systems using various gene therapy techniques hold promise in several animal models according to recently published studies, and human studies seem to be justified.

SELECTIVE ADHESION MOLECULES TARGETING

Interfering with the recruitment and migration of inflammatory cells to the intestinal mucosa is an exciting treatment modality that integrates our better understanding of inflammatory processes specific to this distinct milieu. The monoclonal antibodies against α4 integrins would probably be the next biological modality joining TNFα neutralization, and their role in maintenance of remission of CD has already been demonstrated. The use of antisense to ICAM-1 to treat CD had modest results so far; however, other modes of interfering with adhesion molecules interactions in the gut mucosa are, in the opinion of these authors, a most promising strategy.

EFFECTOR CELLS

It has long been the notion that in IBD an overactive effector arm drives perpetuation of inflammation. Decreasing the number or the biological function of inflammatory cells, specifically activated leukocytes, is assessed once again in recent years. As appealing as this approach may seem, it still remains to be determined which cell subpopulation is most appropriate to target in CD so that the clinical benefit would much overcome possible cytopenia-associated side effects. Leukacytapheresis that has been working quite efficiently in UC was studied in only small numbers of CD patients; however, if beneficial, the lack of foreign proteins introduced into the patients would be appealing to both physicians and patients. A more innovative, yet less-explored, approach may be to boost the number or, even better, the effect of regulatory cells. These cells, whether of the CD4+ or CD8+ subpopulations, were demonstrated to exist, usually in small numbers (but probably great regulatory potential), in animal models and in humans. Introducing these cells into colitic animals ameliorates inflammation by contact or regulatory cytokine secretion (depending on the regulatory cell subtype). After establishing the existence and specific role of such cells in the intestinal mucosa and further defining their phenotypic characteristics as well as mechanisms of action and, more importantly, their potential stimulation pathways, boosting these cells may rebalance the uncontrolled inflammation in IBD tissues.

REFERENCES

1. Targan SR, Hanauer SB, van Deventer SJ, et al. A short-term study of chimeric monoclonal antibody cA2 to tumor necrosis factor alpha for Crohn's disease. Crohn's Disease cA2 Study Group. N Engl J Med. 1997;337:1029-1035.

2. Present DH, Rutgeerts P, Targan S, et al. Infliximab for the treatment of fistulas in patients with Crohn's disease. N Engl J Med. 1999;340:1398-1405.

3. Sands BE, Anderson FH, Bernstein CN, et al. Infliximab maintenance therapy for fistulizing Crohn's disease. N Engl J Med. 2004; 350:876-885.

4. Hanauer SB, Feagan BG, Lichtenstein GR, et al, and the ACCENT I Study Group. Maintenance infliximab for Crohn's disease: the ACCENT I randomised trial. Lancet. 2002;359:1541-1549.

5. Rutgeerts P, D'Haens G, Targan S, et al. Efficacy and safety of retreatment with anti-tumor necrosis factor antibody (infliximab) to maintain remission in Crohn's disease. Gastroenterology. 1999;117:761-769.

6. Sartor RB. Animal models of intestinal inflammation. In Sartor RB, Sandborn WJ, eds. Kirsner's Inflammatory Bowel Diseases. 6th ed. Philadelphia, PA: WB Saunders; 2004:120-137.

7. van Deventer SJ. New biological therapies in inflammatory bowel disease. Best Pract Res Clin Gastroenterol. 2003;17:119-130.

8. van Deventer SJ. New therapeutic drugs for inflammatory bowel disease. In Sartor RB, Sandborn WJ, eds. Kirsner's Inflammatory Bowel Diseases. 6th ed. Philadelphia, PA: WB Saunders; 2004:574-584.

9. Sandborn WJ, Targan SR. Biologic therapy of inflammatory bowel disease. Gastroenterology. 2002;122:1592-1608.

10. Lim WC, Hanauer SB. Emerging biologic therapies in inflammatory bowel disease. Rev Gastroenterol Disord. 2004;4:66-85.

11. Papachristou GI, Plevy S. Novel biologics in inflammatory bowel disease. Gastroenterol Clin North Am. 2004;33:251-269, ix.

12. Rutgeerts P, Van Deventer S, Schreiber S. Review article: the expanding role of biological agents in the treatment of inflammatory bowel disease: focus on selective adhesion molecule inhibition. Aliment Pharmacol Ther. 2003;17:1435-1450.

13. Su CG, Lichtenstein GR. Influence of immunogenicity on the long-term efficacy of infliximab in Crohn's disease. Gastroenterology. 2003;125:1544-1546.

14. Baert F, Noman M, Vermeire S, et al. Influence of immunogenicity on the long-term efficacy of infliximab in Crohn's disease. N Engl J Med. 2003;348:601-608.

15. Yamamoto M, Yoshizaki K, Kishimoto T, Ito H. IL-6 is required for the development of Th1 cell-mediated murine colitis. J Immunol. 2000;164:4878-4882.

16. Ito H, Takazoe M, Fukuda Y, et al. Effective treatment of active Crohn's disease with humanized monoclonal antibody MRA to interleukin-6 receptor: a randomized placebo-controlled trial. Gastroenterology. 2003;124:A25.

17. Ito H, Takazoe M, Fukuda Y, et al. A pilot randomized trial of a human anti-interleukin-6 receptor monoclonal antibody in active Crohn's disease. Gastroenterology. 2004;126:989-996.

18. Monteleone G, Biancone L, Marasco R, et al. Interleukin 12 is expressed and actively released by Crohn's disease intestinal lamina propria mononuclear cells. Gastroenterology. 1997;112:1169-1178.

19. Parronchi P, Romagnani P, Annunziato F, et al. Type 1 T-helper cell predominance and interleukin-12 expression in the gut of patients with Crohn's disease. Am J Pathol. 1997;150:823-832.

20. Berrebi D, Besnard M, Fromont-Hankard G, et al. Interleukin-12 expression is focally enhanced in the gastric mucosa of pediatric patients with Crohn's disease. Am J Pathol. 1998;152:667-672.

21. Matsuoka K, Inoue N, Sato T, et al. T-bet up-regulation and subsequent interleukin 12 stimulation are essential for induction of Th1 mediated immunopathology in Crohn's disease. Gut. 2004;53:1303-1308.

22. Fuss IJ, Marth T, Neurath MF, Pearlstein GR, Jain A, Strober W. Anti-interleukin 12 treatment regulates apoptosis of Th1 T cells in experimental colitis in mice. Gastroenterology. 1999;117:1078-1088.

23. Neurath MF, Fuss I, Kelsall BL, Stuber E, Strober W. Antibodies to interleukin 12 abrogate established experimental colitis in mice. J Exp Med. 1995;182:1281-1290.

24. Sandborn WJ, Feagan BG, Fedorak RN, et al. A randomized trial of ustekinumab, a human interleukin-12/23 monoclonal antibody, in patients with moderate-to-severe Crohn's disease. Gastroenterology. 2008;135:1130-1141.

25. Stallmach A, Marth T, Weiss B, et al. An interleukin 12 p40-IgG2b fusion protein abrogates T cell mediated inflammation: anti-inflammatory activity in Crohn's disease and experimental colitis in vivo. Gut. 2004;53:339-345.

26. Parkin J, Cohen B. An overview of the immune system. Lancet. 2001;357:1777-1789.

27. Romagnani S. Th1/Th2 cells. Inflamm Bowel Dis. 1999;5:285-294.

28. Camoglio L, Te Velde AA, Tigges AJ, Das PK, Van Deventer SJ. Altered expression of interferon-gamma and interleukin-4 in inflammatory bowel disease. Inflamm Bowel Dis. 1998;4:285-290.

29. Plevy SE, Landers CJ, Prehn J, et al. A role for TNF-alpha and mucosal T helper-1 cytokines in the pathogenesis of Crohn's disease. J Immunol. 1997;159:6276-6282.

30. Strober W, Kelsall B, Fuss I, et al. Reciprocal IFN-gamma and TGF-beta responses regulate the occurrence of mucosal inflammation. Immunol Today. 1997;18:61-64.

31. Fuss IJ, Neurath M, Boirivant M, et al. Disparate CD4+ lamina propria (LP) lymphokine secretion profiles in inflammatory bowel disease. Crohn's disease LP cells manifest increased secretion of IFN-gamma, whereas ulcerative colitis LP cells manifest increased secretion of IL-5. J Immunol. 1996;157:1261-1270.

32. Powrie F, Leach MW, Mauze S, Menon S, Caddle LB, Coffman RL. Inhibition of Th1 responses prevents inflammatory bowel disease in scid mice reconstituted with CD45RBhi CD4+ T cells. Immunity. 1994;1:553-562.

33. Berg DJ, Davidson N, Kuhn R, et al. Enterocolitis and colon cancer in interleukin-10-deficient mice are associated with aberrant cytokine production and CD4(+) TH1-like responses. *J Clin Invest.* 1996;98:1010-1020.

34. Hommes D, Mikhajlova T, Stoinov S, et al. Fontolizumab (Huzaf), a humanized anti-IFN-gamma antibody, has clinical activity and excellent tolerability in moderate to severe Crohn's disease. *Gastroenterology.* 2004;127:332.

35. Yoshida T, Higa A, Sakamoto H, et al. Immunological and clinical effects of interferon-gamma on Crohn's disease. *J Clin Lab Immunol.* 1988;25:105-108.

36. Debinski H, Forbes A, Kamm MA. Low dose interferon gamma for refractory Crohn's disease. *Ital J Gastroenterol Hepatol.* 1997; 29:403-406.

37. Fiorentino DF, Bond MW, Mosmann TR. Two types of mouse T helper cell. IV. Th2 clones secrete a factor that inhibits cytokine production by Th1 clones. *J Exp Med.* 1989;170:2081-2095.

38. Kuhn R, Lohler J, Rennick D, Rajewsky K, Muller W. Interleukin-10-deficient mice develop chronic enterocolitis. *Cell.* 1993;75:263-274.

39. van Deventer SJ, Elson CO, Fedorak RN. Multiple doses of intravenous interleukin 10 in steroid-refractory Crohn's disease. Crohn's Disease Study Group. *Gastroenterology.* 1997;113:383-389.

40. Fedorak RN, Gangl A, Elson CO, et al. Recombinant human interleukin 10 in the treatment of patients with mild to moderately active Crohn's disease. The Interleukin 10 Inflammatory Bowel Disease Cooperative Study Group. *Gastroenterology.* 2000; 119:1473-1482.

41. Schreiber S, Fedorak RN, Nielsen OH, et al. Safety and efficacy of rhuIL-10 in chronic active CD. *Gastroenterology.* 2000;119:1461-1472.

42. Colombel JF, Rutgeerts P, Malchow H, et al. Interleukin 10 (Tenovil) in the prevention of postoperative recurrence of Crohn's disease. *Gut.* 2001;49:42-46.

43. Steidler L, Hans W, Schotte L, et al. Treatment of murine colitis by *Lactococcus lactis* secreting interleukin-10. *Science.* 2000;289:1352-1355.

44. Steidler L, Neirynck S, Huyghebaert N, et al. Biological containment of genetically modified *Lactococcus lactis* for intestinal delivery of human interleukin 10. *Nat Biotechnol.* 2003;21:785-789.

45. Nakase H, Okazaki K, Tabata Y, et al. New cytokine delivery system using gelatin microspheres containing interleukin-10 for experimental inflammatory bowel disease. *J Pharmacol Exp Ther.* 2002;301:59-65.

46. Barbara G, Xing Z, Hogaboam CM, Gauldie J, Collins SM. Interleukin 10 gene transfer prevents experimental colitis in rats. *Gut.* 2000;46:344-349.

47. Lindsay JO, Ciesielski CJ, Scheinin T, Brennan FM, Hodgson HJ. Local delivery of adenoviral vectors encoding murine interleukin 10 induces colonic interleukin 10 production and is therapeutic for murine colitis. *Gut.* 2003;52:981-987.

48. Montfrans C, Hooijberg E, Rodriguez Pena MS, et al. Generation of regulatory gut-homing human T lymphocytes using ex vivo interleukin 10 gene transfer. *Gastroenterology.* 2002;123:1877-1888.

49. Van Montfrans C, Rodriguez Pena MS, Pronk I, Ten Kate FJ, Te Velde AA, Van Deventer SJ. Prevention of colitis by interleukin 10-transduced T lymphocytes in the SCID mice transfer model. *Gastroenterology.* 2002;123:1865-1876.

50. Li MC, He SH. IL-10 and its related cytokines for treatment of inflammatory bowel disease. *World J Gastroenterol.* 2004;10:620-625.

51. Du X, Williams DA. Interleukin-11: review of molecular, cell biology, and clinical use. *Blood.* 1997;89:3897-3908.

52. Keith JC Jr, Albert L, Sonis ST, Pfeiffer CJ, Schaub RG. IL-11, a pleiotropic cytokine: exciting new effects of IL-11 on gastrointestinal mucosal biology. *Stem Cells.* 1994;12(suppl 1):79-89, discussion 89-90.

53. Qiu BS, Pfeiffer CJ, Keith JC Jr. Protection by recombinant human interleukin-11 against experimental TNB-induced colitis in rats. *Dig Dis Sci.* 1996;41:1625-1630.

54. Sands BE, Bank S, Sninsky CA, et al. Preliminary evaluation of safety and activity of recombinant human interleukin 11 in patients with active Crohn's disease. *Gastroenterology.* 1999;117:58-64.

55. Sands BE, Winston BD, Salzberg B, et al, and the RHIL-11 Crohn's Study group. Randomized, controlled trial of recombinant human interleukin-11 in patients with active Crohn's disease. *Aliment Pharmacol Ther.* 2002;16:399-406.

56. Hanauer S, Baert F, Robinson M. Interferon treatment in mild to moderate active Crohn's disease: preliminary results of an open label pilot study. *Gastroenterology.* 1994;106:A696.

57. Davidsen B, Munkholm P, Schlichting P, Nielsen OH, Krarup H, Bonnevie-Nielsen V. Tolerability of interferon alpha-2b, a possible new treatment of active Crohn's disease. *Aliment Pharmacol Ther.* 1995;9:75-79.

58. Gasche C, Reinisch W, Vogelsang H, et al. Prospective evaluation of interferon-alpha in treatment of chronic active Crohn's disease. *Dig Dis Sci.* 1995;40:800-804.

59. Kieseier BC, Hartung HP. Current disease-modifying therapies in multiple sclerosis. *Semin Neurol.* 2003;23:133-146.

60. Ozenci V, Kouwenhoven M, Teleshova N, Pashenkov M, Fredrikson S, Link H. Multiple sclerosis: pro- and antiinflammatory cytokines and metalloproteinases are affected differentially by treatment with IFN-beta. *J Neuroimmunol.* 2000;108:236-243.

61. Vantrappen G, Coremans G, Billiau A, De Somer P. Treatment of Crohn's disease with interferon. A preliminary clinical trial. *Acta Clin Belg.* 1980;35:238-242.

62. Musch E, Andus T, Malek M, Chrissafidou A, Schulz M. Successful treatment of steroid refractory active ulcerative colitis with natural interferon-beta: an open long-term trial. *J Gastroenterol.* 2007; 45:1235-1240.

63. Yoshida EM, Chan NH, Herrick RA, et al. Human immunodeficiency virus infection, the acquired immunodeficiency syndrome, and inflammatory bowel disease. *J Clin Gastroenterol.* 1996;23:24-28.

64. Emmrich J, Seyfarth M, Fleig WE, Emmrich F. Treatment of inflammatory bowel disease with anti-CD4 monoclonal antibody. *Lancet.* 1991;338:570-571.

65. Canva-Delcambre V, Jacquot S, Robinet E, et al. Treatment of severe Crohn's disease with anti-CD4 monoclonal antibody. *Aliment Pharmacol Ther.* 1996;10:721-727.

66. Stronkhorst A, Radema S, Yong SL, et al. CD4 antibody treatment in patients with active Crohn's disease: A phase 1 dose finding study. *Gut.* 1997;40:320-327.

67. von Andrian UH, Engelhardt B. Alpha4 integrins as therapeutic targets in autoimmune disease. *N Engl J Med.* 2003;348:68-72.

68. Targan SR, Feagan BG, Fedorak RN, et al, and the International Efficacy of Natalizumab in Crohn's Disease Response and Remission (ENCORE) Trial Group. Natalizumab for the treatment of active Crohn's disease: results of the ENCORE Trial. *Gastroenterology.* 2007;132:1672-1683.

69. Ghosh S, Goldin E, Gordon FH, Malchow HA, et al, and the Natalizumab Pan-European Study Group. Natalizumab for active Crohn's disease. *N Engl J Med.* 2003;348:24-32.

70. Sandborn WJ, Colombel JF, Enns R, et al. Natalizumab induction and maintenance therapy for Crohn's disease. *N Engl J Med.* 2005;353:1912-1925.

71. Sandborn W, Colombel JF, Enns R, et al. A phase III, double blind, placebo-controlled study of the efficacy, safety, and tolerability of antegren (Natalizumab) in maintaining clinical response and remission in Crohn's disease (ENACT-2). *Gastroenterology.* 2004;127:332.

72. Schreiber S, Targan SR. Efficacy of natalizumab in Crohn's patients with disease duration less than three years [abstract]. *Gastroenterology.* 2007;132(4 suppl 1):A509.

73. Present D, Feagan BG, Fedorak RN, et al. Natalizumab induces sustained response and remission in Crohn's patients after previous infliximab failure: results from the ENCORE trial [abstract]. *Gastroenterology.* 2007;132(4 suppl 1):A507.

74. Langer-Gould A, Atlas SW, Green AJ, Bollen AW, Pelletier D. Progressive multifocal leukoencephalopathy in a patient treated with natalizumab. *N Engl J Med.* 2005;353:375-381.

75. Kleinschmidt-DeMasters BK, Tyler KL. Progressive multifocal leukoencephalopathy complicating treatment with natalizumab and interferon beta-1a for multiple sclerosis. *N Engl J Med.* 2005; 353:369-374.

76. Van Assche G, Van Ranst M, Sciot R, et al. Progressive multifocal leukoencephalopathy after natalizumab therapy for Crohn's disease. *N Engl J Med.* 2005;353:362-368.

77. Yousry TA, Major EO, Ryschkewitsch C, et al. Evaluation of patients treated with natalizumab for progressive multifocal leukoencephalopathy. *N Engl J Med.* 2006;354:924-933.

78. Berlin C, Berg EL, Briskin MJ, et al. Alpha 4 beta 7 integrin mediates lymphocyte binding to the mucosal vascular address in MAdCAM-1. *Cell.* 1993;74:185-195.

79. Feagan BG, Greenberg GR, Wild G, et al. Treatment of ulcerative colitis with a humanized antibody to the alpha-4 beta-7 integrin. *N Engl J Med.* 2005;352:2499-2507.

80. Feagan BG, Greenberg GR, Wild G, et al. Treatment of active Crohn's disease with MLN0002, a humanized antibody to the alpha-4 beta-7 integrin. *Clin Gastroenterol Hepatol.* 2008;6:1370-1377.

81. Vainer B, Nielsen OH, Horn T. Comparative studies of the colonic in situ expression of intercellular adhesion molecules (ICAM-1, -2, and -3), beta-2 integrins (LFA-1, Mac-1, and p150,95), and PECAM-1 in ulcerative colitis and Crohn's disease. *Am J Surg Pathol.* 2000;24:1115-1124.

82. Bennett CF, Condon TP, Grimm S, Chan H, Chiang MY. Inhibition of endothelial cell adhesion molecule expression with antisense oligonucleotides. *J Immunol.* 1994;152:3530-3540.

83. Yacyshyn BR, Chey WY, Goff J, et al, and the ISIS 2302-CS9 Investigators. Double blind, placebo controlled trial of the remission inducing and steroid sparing properties of an ICAM-1 antisense oligodeoxynucleotide, alicaforsen (ISIS 2302), in active steroid dependent Crohn's disease. *Gut.* 2002;51:30-36.

84. Schreiber S, Nikolaus S, Malchow H, et al. Absence of efficacy of subcutaneous antisense ICAM-1 treatment of chronic active Crohn's disease. *Gastroenterology.* 2001;120:1339-1346.

85. Yacyshyn BR, Barish C, Goff J, et al. Dose ranging pharmacokinetic trial of high-dose alicaforsen (intercellular adhesion molecule-1 antisense oligodeoxynucleotide) (ISIS 2302) in active Crohn's disease. *Aliment Pharmacol Ther.* 2002;16:1761-1770.

86. Chow JY, Carlstrom K, Barrett KE. Growth hormone reduces chloride secretion in human colonic epithelial cells via EGF receptor and extracellular regulated kinase. *Gastroenterology.* 2003; 125:1114-1124.

87. Street ME, de'Angelis G, Camacho-Hubner C, et al. Relationships between serum IGF-1, IGFBP-2, interleukin-1 beta and interleukin-6 in inflammatory bowel disease. *Horm Res.* 2004;61:159-164.

88. Slonim AE, Bulone L, Damore MB, Goldberg T, Wingertzahn MA, McKinley MJ. A preliminary study of growth hormone therapy for Crohn's disease. *N Engl J Med.* 2000;342:1633-1637.

89. Korzenik JR, Dieckgraefe BK. Is Crohn's disease an immunodeficiency? *Dig Dis Sci.* 2000;45:1121-1129.

90. Vaughan D, Drumm B. Treatment of fistulas with granulocyte colony-stimulating factor in a patient with Crohn's disease. *N Engl J Med.* 1999;340:239-240.

91. Korzenik JR, Dieckgraefe BK. An open-labeled study of granulocyte colony-stimulating factor in the treatment of active Crohn's disease. *Aliment Pharmacol Ther.* 2005;21:391-400.

92. Korzenik JR, Dieckgraefe BK, Valentine JF, et al. Sargramostim for active Crohn's disease. *N Engl J Med.* 2005;352:2193-2201.

93. Dieckgraefe BK, Korzenik JR. Treatment of active Crohn's disease with recombinant human granulocyte-macrophage colony-stimulating factor. *Lancet.* 2002;360:1478-1480.

94. Bicks RO, Groshart KD. The current status of T-lymphocyte apheresis (TLA) treatment of Crohn's disease. *J Clin Gastroenterol.* 1989;11:136-138.

95. Sawada K, Ohnishi K, Kosaka T, et al. Leukocytapheresis therapy performed with leukocyte removal filter for inflammatory bowel disease. *J Gastroenterol.* 1995;30:322-329.

96. Kosaka T, Sawada K, Ohnishi K, et al. Effect of leukocytapheresis therapy using a leukocyte removal filter in Crohn's disease. *Intern Med.* 1999;38:102-111.

97. Sawada K, Ohnishi K, Fukui S, et al. Leukocytapheresis therapy performed with leukocyte removal filter for inflammatory bowel disease. *J Gastroenterol.* 1995;30:322-329.

98. Ohara M, Saniabadi AR, Kokuma S, et al. Granulocytapheresis in the treatment of patients with rheumatoid arthritis. *Artif Organs.* 1997;21:989-994.

99. Shimoyama T, Sawada K, Hiwatashi N, et al. Safety and efficacy of granulocyte and monocyte adsorption apheresis in patients with active ulcerative colitis: a multicenter study. *J Clin Apheresis.* 2001;16:1-9.

100. Suzuki Y, Yoshimura N, Saniabadi AR, Saito Y. Selective granulocyte and monocyte adsorptive apheresis as a first-line treatment for steroid naive patients with active ulcerative colitis: a prospective uncontrolled study. *Dig Dis Sci.* 2004;49:565-571.

101. Matsui T, Nishimura T, Matake H, Ohta T, Sakurai T, Yao T. Granulocytapheresis for Crohn's disease: a report on seven refractory patients. *Am J Gastroenterol.* 2003;98:511-512.

102. Sakata H, Kawamura N, Horie T, et al. Successful treatment of ulcerative colitis with leukocytapheresis using non-woven polyester filter. *Ther Apher Dial.* 2003;7:536-539.

103. Sands BE, Sandborn WJ, Feagan B, et al. A randomized, double-blind, sham-controlled study of granulocyte/monocyte apheresis for active ulcerative colitis. *Gastroenterology.* 2008;135:400-409.

104. Wirtz S, Neurath MF. Gene transfer approaches for the treatment of inflammatory bowel disease. *Gene Ther.* 2003;10:854-860.

Novel Nonbiologic Therapy for Crohn's Disease

Masayuki Fukata, MD, PhD and Maria T. Abreu, MD

BACKGROUND

Crohn's disease is a chronic inflammatory bowel disease (IBD) whose etiology remains elusive. The first gene, CARD15/NOD2, associated with susceptibility to CD was identified in 2001.[1,2] CARD15/NOD2 encodes a cytoplasmic protein expressed by monocyte/macrophages[3] and Paneth cells.[4] More recently, a second set of genes previously known as IBD5 and now recognized as organic cation transporters have also been identified as CD-susceptibility genes.[5] Carriage of mutations in both CARD15/NOD2 and OCTN increases the risk of CD greatly. Through the advances in our understanding of CD pathogenesis, novel therapies have been developed for CD or old therapies have been resurrected and improved. In this chapter, we will discuss novel compounds that are nonbiologic such as small molecules and chemical compounds with immunomodulatory properties. Biologic agents include monoclonal antibodies, recombinant cytokines or growth factors, and vaccines. Although biologic agents have had dramatic, beneficial effects on patients with CD, there remain limitations to this type of approach including immunogenicity and difficulty of administration.[6]

CD is characterized by chronic intestinal inflammation in the absence of a known pathogen. Patients frequently express antimicrobial antibodies that correlate with disease manifestations such as fibrostenotic or perforating disease but also highlight a fundamental dysregulation in immunologic tolerance to the commensal flora.[7] The immune cascade in patients with CD is characterized by an increase in expression of IL-12 or IL-23 by antigen-presenting cells and a shift towards Th1 cytokine production such as interferon (IFN)-α and tumor necrosis factor alpha (TNFα). These cytokines can initiate or perpetuate disturbed barrier function permitting exposure of the lamina propria to luminal bacteria and pathogen-associated molecular patterns such as lipopolysaccharide (LPS).

Current disease management guidelines include the use of antiinflammatory agents, aminosalicylates, and corticosteroids. Our new expectation as clinicians should be to get closer to the root of the problem, at least to the level of the immunologic players involved in CD pathogenesis. In so doing, there is a better chance of changing the natural history of disease. The best example of this to date is the mucosal healing seen with infliximab and the trend towards a reduction in surgeries for CD.[8]

Clearly, more agents are desirable along more points in the inflammatory cascade. Table 20-1 summarizes novel nonbiologic therapies for CD discussed in this chapter. Because CD is a heterogeneous disorder with diverse clinical manifestations, the choice of agent must be tailored to the patient. At present, the choice of therapy may be based on such patient characteristics as disease location, presence or absence of complications, and response to previous treatment. In the near future, we may use biomarkers, genetic markers, and serologic markers. In addition, the choice of agent should be based on its efficacy relative to safety and cost. Finally, these novel nonbiologic therapies should enhance the quality of life of patients with CD.

TABLE 20-1

NONBIOLOGIC THERAPIES FOR CD*

ANTI-TNFα STRATEGIES

Thalidomide

Thalidomide analogues

Small molecules

- Doramapimod/BIRB-796

- CNI-1493

Pentoxifylline

- TACE inhibitors

OTHER CYTOKINE MEDIATORS

Pralnacasan

Granulocyte and granulocyte-macrophage colony-stimulating factor

PEROXISOME PROLIFERATOR-ACTIVATED RECEPTOR AGONISTS

HORMONAL THERAPY

Growth hormone

Medroxyprogesterone acetate/CBP-1101

Dehydroepiandrosterone

Coherin

NOVEL GLUCOCORTICOIDS

Budesonide

ANTIMETABOLITES

Azathioprine/6-mercaptopurine

Methotrexate

Mycophenolate mofetil

6-Thioguanine

Leflunomide

Cyclophosphamide

CALCINEURIN INHIBITORS

Cyclosporine

Tacrolimus

MISCELLANOUS THERAPIES UNDER INVESTIGATION

Fish oils and omega-3 fatty acids

Neuroimmunomodulation

Hyperbaric oxygen

*TNFα indicates tumor necrosis factor alpha; TACE, TNFα converting enzyme.

ANTI-TNFα STRATEGIES

Several strategies to block TNFα activity have been developed (Figure 20-1). Some of these have already demonstrated great potential for translation to the bedside and confirm the important role of TNFα in CD pathogenesis.

THALIDOMIDE

Thalidomide is an inhibitor of TNFα and IL-12 production by monocytes and has anti-angiogenic properties.[9,10] Its specific effect on TNFα production is to reduce the stability of mRNA.[11] In addition to reducing TNFα mRNA and therefore TNFα protein, it can also inhibit nuclear factor (NF)-kB activation in response to TNFα.[12] Given its ability to reduce circulating TNFα levels, it is predicted to have a beneficial effect on CD. Decreased production of TNFα and IL-12 by colonic lamina propria mononuclear cells and decreased TNFα production in peripheral blood monocytes have been reported in patients with CD during treatment with thalidomide and is dose dependent.[13]

In 1999, we reported the results of an open-label study of a low dose (50 or 100 mg daily) of thalidomide in 12 patients with moderate to severe, steroid-dependent CD.[14] In this study, the response rates were 58% and 70%, and the corresponding remission rates were 17% and 20% at 4 weeks and 12 weeks, respectively. In addition, steroid withdrawal was achieved in 40% of the patients. In another study, 9 patients with luminal CD and 13 with fistulas were given 200 or 300 mg daily of thalidomide for 12 weeks.[15] The findings were a response rate of 33% at 4 weeks and 56% at 12 weeks. The remission rates were 33% at both 4 and 12 weeks. In addition to induction of remission, maintenance of remission for almost 2 years was seen in a small group ($n = 4$) of pediatric patients with medically refractory CD-given thalidomide (1.5 to 2 mg/kg/day).[16] Steroid withdrawal was also achieved within 1 to 3 months in those patients. Finally, thalidomide has been used in patients with obscure gastrointestinal bleeding, 3 with CD and 3 without.[17] Bleeding stopped or slowed down in these within a few weeks of starting. These small studies suggest that thalidomide may be useful in the treatment of patients with refractory CD.

Given its effect to inhibit TNFα, investigators have examined the effect of thalidomide in patients who had previously responded to infliximab.[18] Patients entered the study in an infliximab-induced remission. The remission rates were 92%, 83%, and 83% at 3, 6, and 12 months following the last infliximab infusion, respectively. Since the time of this study, it is apparent that maintenance therapy with infliximab is very effective for the group achieving response. Anecdotally, some patients respond to thalidomide who have not responded to infliximab, suggesting that the effects of thalidomide are not only related to its effect on TNFα but are immunologically broader.

Thalidomide, however, has important limitations that will never permit its widespread use. The most infamous of these side effects is its teratogenicity. Thalidomide causes phocomelia, a severe shortening of the limbs wherein the long bones are shorter than normal and more proximal elements are lost. In extreme cases, the hand or fingers are attached directly to the shoulder.[19,20] Not only is the danger for women conceiving or continuing the medication during pregnancy, but the drug can also be found in spermatic fluid, leading to the theoretical risk of intrauterine exposure of a pregnant woman by a man taking the drug. Appropriately, patients of childbearing age are asked to use 2 forms of contraception and participate in an educational program about the risks. The drug was initially marketed as a sedative and therefore causes significant sedation in at least 50% of patients.[14,15] It should be administered at bedtime. Peripheral neuropathy occurred in 25% to 42% of patients receiving thalidomide.[14,15] This is especially true with use over 6 months. Other adverse effects included rash (6% incidence), constipation (9%), and seborrhea (6%).

THALIDOMIDE ANALOGUES

Given the potential therapeutic benefit of thalidomide, investigators have tried to develop thalidomide analogues that retain or improve upon its biologic effect while reducing its side effects and eliminating teratogenicity.[9,21] Selective cytokine inhibitory drugs (SelCIDs) have greatly improved TNFα inhibitory activity, and immunomodulatory drugs (IMiDs) are structural analogues of thalidomide.[22] Most SelCIDs are phosphodiesterase type 4 inhibitors. Intracellular cyclic adenosine monophosphate (cAMP) elevation inhibits TNFα production in activated monocytes and peripheral blood mononuclear cells (PBMC).[23] Cellular levels of cAMP can be controlled by phosphodiesterases (PDEs) as well as adenylate cyclase. PDE4 is the major enzyme found in monocytes and plays a crucial role in regulation of various cellular activities by degrading cAMP.[24] Inhibition of PDE4 results in elevated camp concentrations and thereby inhibits TNFα production in activated monocytes and PBMC. Not only have these compounds received attention for immunologic disorders but also for their anticancer effects—especially in multiple myeloma.[25,26]

CC-1069 is a thalidomide analogue and phosphodiesterase IV inhibitor, which has been reported to have an inhibitory effect on TNFα and IL-2 secretion in vitro.[27] The effect of CC-1069 on monocytes is stronger than that observed with thalidomide. CC-3052 offers certain advantages compared with other thalidomide analogues. In particular, CC-3052 is water soluble and appears to be nontoxic, nonmutagenic, and nonteratogenic and is more stable in human plasma.[28] CC-3052 has been reported to be 200-fold more potent at inhibiting LPS-induced TNFα production than thalidomide. In addition, CC-3052 stimulates IL-10 mRNA and protein production by whole blood cultures upon LPS stimulation, suggesting that it may have multiple immunomodulatory effects.[28]

CC-1088 inhibits PDE4 and TNFα and is being studied as a potential treatment of inflammatory diseases in phase I/II clinical trials. It decreases intracellular IL-6 and vascular endothelial growth factor levels in human umbilical vein cells co-cultured with myeloma cells. The efficacy of CC-1088 in patients with steroid-dependent CD is currently under investigation.

A double-blind, placebo-controlled, pilot-phase I/II trial of CC-1088 demonstrated clinical improvement in 6 out of 11 patients with moderate to severe CD (54%) after a 12-week treatment with either 800 mg or 1200 mg of CC-1088 (http://www.prnewswire.com/cgi-bin/stories.pl?ACCT=105&STORY=/www/story/01-07-2003/0001867098). CC-1088 was well tolerated. A metallic taste (71%) and headache (29%) were observed as the most common adverse events in this pilot trial.

OPC-6535 (tetomilast) is another novel phosphodiesterase IV inhibitor that has been tested in clinical trials of IBD. It was initially identified by a screen for compounds that inhibited superoxide production by human neutrophils but was subsequently found to inhibit neutrophil chemotaxis and adhesion to endothelial cells.[29] Like the other compounds discussed, it causes a dose-dependent inhibition of LPS-mediated TNFα production by monocytes. In animal models of IBD, it reduces intestinal inflammation in response to 2-, 4-, and 6-trinitrobenzenesulfonic acid (TNBS). In a phase II study by Schreiber et al, 186 patients with mild to moderate active UC were randomized to receive an oral, once-daily dose of placebo or tetomilast 25 mg or 50 mg for 8 weeks.[30] There was no significant difference between groups in the primary outcome of improvement as defined by reduction in Disease Activity Index (DAI) ≥ 3 at week 8 or in remission rates. A post hoc analysis focusing on patients with high activity scores (baseline DAI 7-11) suggested possible benefit of tetomilast that will require further investigation.

SMALL MOLECULE INHIBITORS OF TNFα SIGNALING

In recent years, the focus of attention in CD research is shifting from known intercellular signals such as TNFα, IL-10, IFN-g, and IL-12 toward the intracellular molecules that transduce their signals. Two important intracellular signaling cascades have been identified in the pathogenesis of CD. The first inflammatory signal transduction route found to play a role in inflammatory bowel disease is the NF-kB pathway (Figure 20-1, number 2). The second signal transduction cascade to be implicated in CD consists of the mitogen-activated protein kinase (MAPK) family (Figure 20-1, number 1). This group of signal transduction proteins is involved in the intracellular transmission and interpretation of signals due to inflammation and stress.

DORAMAPIMOD/BIRB 796

BIRB 796 is a specific inhibitor of p38 mitogen-activated protein (MAP) kinase.[31] Activation of p38 is found in activated T cells in the lamina propria of CD patients.[32-34]

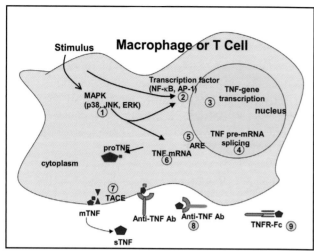

FIGURE 20-1. Steps in TNFα signal transduction. A cell such as a lymphocyte or monocyte receives an external signal through a receptor-ligand interaction (eg, LPS binding to toll-like receptor 4), which results in the activation of the mitogen-activated protein (MAP) kinase pathway. This in turn results in phosphorylation (eg, c-jun) and/or nuclear translocation (eg, NF-kB) of transcription factors that turn on the transcription of RNA for TNFα. All RNA requires splicing to messenger RNA, which exits the nucleus and is translated into the TNFα protein. At the 3' end of mRNA are AU-rich regions, which stabilize mRNA. Certain agents may destabilize the mRNA, resulting in lower levels and thus less to be translated into protein. The promolecule of TNFα is anchored to the cell membrane and requires the action of TACE to release it as soluble TNFα. Nonbiologic antagonists may be directed at multiple steps along this process (Papadakis KA, Targan SR. Tumor necrosis factor: biology and therapeutic inhibitors. *Gastroenterology.* 2000; 119(4):1148-1157). TNFα indicates tumor necrosis factor alpha; LPS, lipopolysaccharide; NF, nuclear factor; TACE, TNFα converting enzyme; MAPK, mitogen-activated protein kinase; JNK, jun-N-terminal kinase; ERK, extracellular-signal-regulated kinase; AP, activator protein.

It has been reported that the 600-mg dose of BIRB 796 strongly inhibited LPS-induced activation of the coagulation cascade and cytokine production (TNFα, IL-6, IL-10, and IL-1R antagonist).[35,36]

In a multicenter, multinational trial, 284 patients with moderate to severe CD were randomized to receive placebo, or 10, 20, 30, or 60 mg of BIRB 796 twice daily for 8 weeks.[37] The findings showed no benefit of BIRB 796 on the primary endpoint of clinical remission or in secondary endpoints including clinical response, Inflammatory Bowel Disease Questionnaire, and Crohn's Disease Endoscopic Index of Severity.

CNI-1493

CNI-1493 is a small molecule that inhibits jun-N-terminal kinase (JNK) and p38 MAP kinase, which are involved in transducing the intracellular response to TNFα within a cell. CNI-1493 inhibits the production of several proinflammatory cytokines and nitric oxide. The safety and efficacy of this agent has been assessed in 12 patients with moderate to severe refractory CD.[38] Six of these patients had received prior therapy with infliximab. Two intravenous doses 8 and 25 mg/m² were studied. Clinical response was seen in 67% of patients at 4 weeks and 58%

at 8 weeks. Clinical remission was observed in 25% of patients at week 4 and 42% at week 8. In addition, response was seen in 3 of 6 infliximab failures, 2 of whom achieved remission. Fistula healing occurred in 4 of 5 patients, and steroids were tapered in 89% of patients. Colonic biopsies displayed decreased p38 MAPK and JNK activity as well as diminished TNFα production. No serious adverse events were noted in the study, but 2 patients discontinued the study drug because of asymptomatic increase in liver enzymes. This approach is being explored with additional compounds.

PENTOXIFYLLINE

Pentoxifylline is a phosphodiesterase IV inhibitor that results in an increase in intracellular cAMP concentration.[39] It also reduces TNFα production of LPS-stimulated monocytes. Pentoxifylline is approved in the United States for use in peripheral vascular disease. In a study of its subclinical effect in CD and UC, pentoxifylline inhibited the release of TNFα by PBMCs and the secretion of TNFα and IL-1b by cultures of mucosal biopsies.[40] An open-label study in 16 chronic to active, steroid-dependent CD patients for 4 weeks at a dose of 400 mg/day failed to demonstrate significant benefit.[41] The failure of pentoxifylline in this study is likely due to its weak TNFα inhibitory properties and would therefore be replaced by more potent inhibitors.

TACE INHIBITION

The release of TNFα by monocytes and T lymphocytes is mediated by a specific metalloprotease termed the *TNFα converting enzyme* (TACE).[42] TACE is required for the release of soluble TNFα from its membrane-bound precursor (Figure 20-1, number 7). If TACE is inactivated, TNFα cannot be secreted.[42,43] The obvious disadvantage of this approach is the continued presence of membrane-bound TNFα, which is still locally bioactive. Dual inhibitors of TACE and matrix metalloproteases (MMP) have the ability to decrease secretion of soluble TNFα and also decrease the ability of LPS-stimulated cells to shed p55 and p75 TNFα receptors, l-selectin, Fas ligand, IL-6 receptor, IL-1 decoy receptor, and epidermal growth factor. One such compound, GW3333, did not completely inhibit inflammation in an animal model of arthritis, raising the possibility that it may have some proinflammatory effects that may be related to accumulation of membrane-bound TNFα.[44] No studies have been done in CD patients at present.

OTHER CYTOKINE MEDIATORS

PRALNACASAN

Pralnacasan is a selective interleukin converting enzyme (ICE, caspase 1) inhibitor that causes reduction in IL-1 beta and IL-18 production.[45] ICE is the primary protease responsible for the proteolytic cleavage of proinflammatory cytokines IL-1 beta and IL-18 from their inactive precursors. In the murine dextran sodium sulfate–induced colitis model of IBD, pralnacasan reduced colonic inflammation and the levels of IFN-γ expressing cells in lymph nodes draining the intestines and isolated splenocytes. The phase I and early phase II clinical programs have confirmed that pralnacasan is well absorbed from oral solutions and tablet formulations and achieves plasma levels sufficient to inhibit the production of IL-1b in an ex vivo assay.[45]

GRANULOCYTE AND GRANULOCYTE MACROPHAGE COLONY-STIMULATING FACTOR

One alternative hypothesis for the pathogenesis of CD is that impaired neutrophil and/or monocyte function results in CD.[46] In this model, a defect in neutrophil function may result in a failure to clear microbes, and this inefficiency might be enough to trigger an inflammatory cascade and result in an adaptive immune response against commensal organisms. Patients with glycogen storage disease 1b have neutrophil dysfunction and chronic intestinal inflammation.[47] The first report of granulocyte colony-stimulating factor (G-CSF) treatment for CD was that of refractory fistulas responding to G-CSF treatment.[48] Following this report, an open-label study of granulocyte macrophage colony-stimulating factor (GM-CSF) in patients with moderate to severe CD resulted in remission in 8 of 15 patients.[49] The caveats are, however, the incidence of injection site reactions and the need for daily administration. A recent placebo-controlled trial also showed beneficial effects.

The mechanism of action of G-CSF or GM-CSF is thought to be an increase in neutrophil number and function resulting in bacterial eradication.[46] A second explanation by which G-CSF and GM-CSF may mediate their beneficial effect in CD is by biasing the adaptive immune response away from a proinflammatory (Th1-type) towards a Th2-type of response. In addition, it is possible that the treatment of CD with GM-CSF might actually promote expansion of dendritic cells, which in turn might promote differentiation or expansion of regulatory T cells that suppress intestinal inflammation.

PEROXISOME PROLIFERATOR-ACTIVATED RECEPTOR GAMMA LIGANDS

Peroxisome proliferator-activated receptor gamma (PPARγ) is a nuclear receptor that was initially identified as a major regulator of adipocyte differentiation but also is a pivotal receptor for inflammatory signals.[50,51] Recently,

PPARγ has attracted attention because PPARγ is highly expressed in the colonic epithelium[52] and a ligand for PPARγ was shown to attenuate inflammation in an animal model of colitis.[53,54] Though the physiological function of PPARγ receptor in the colon is unknown, it has been shown that activation of PPARγ causes inhibition of the signal transducers and activators of transcription protein (STAT) and activator protein 1 (AP-1) signaling pathways, leading to reduction of IL-2, IL-6, IL-8, TNFα, IL-12, and metalloproteinase release.[55,56] Based on promising data in animal models, a small open-label study of rosiglitazone (4 mg bid po) was performed in 15 patients with mild to moderate active UC. The results were encouraging. Furthermore, a multicenter, randomized, double-blind, placebo-controlled clinical trial by Lewis et al compared the efficacy of the PPARγ rosiglitazone 4 mg orally twice daily versus placebo twice daily for 12 weeks in 105 patients with mild to moderate active UC.[57] The findings showed that patients in the rosiglitazone group had significantly higher rates of clinical response ($P = 0.04$) and remission ($P = 0.01$) Studies in CD have not been performed.[58] Concern has been raised regarding possible adverse cardiovascular events associated with rosiglitazone. However, a meta-analysis of data from 42 clinical trials showed a 43% increase in relative risk of myocardial infarction among type 2 diabetics treated with rosiglitazone.[59] In contrast, no cases of myocardial infarction were found in the study by Lewis et al.

HORMONAL THERAPY

GROWTH HORMONE

Growth hormone therapy does not directly target a specific cytokine or inflammatory mediator. Growth hormone enhances the uptake of amino acids and electrolytes by the intestine, decreases intestinal permeability, and increases intestinal protein synthesis in animals. It has a modest effect on short gut syndrome.

In a preliminary study of 37 patients with moderate to severe active CD, growth hormone at a dose of 5 mg/day was administered subcutaneously for 1 week followed by 1.5 mg/day for 4 months.[60] In this trial, 74% of treated patients had a decrease in the Crohn's disease activity index (CDAI) by more than 90 points.[60] Steroid treatment and immunomodulators were discontinued in some patients. Side effects included edema (in 10 patients) and headache (in 5) and usually resolved within the month of treatment. Stricture formation after ulcer healing may be a concern because growth hormone has been suspected to cause strictures by inducing collagen synthesis mediated by insulin-like growth factor.[61] The other theoretical concern is the use of a trophic agent in patients with a premalignant condition such as CD.

MEDROXYPROGESTERONE ACETATE/CBP-1011

CBP-1011 is a drug originally developed in 1997 for the therapy of immune thrombocytopenic purpura (ITP) and inflammatory bowel disorders.[62] CBP-1011 is a medroxyprogesterone compound, which has an effect as a progesterone agonist and has been thought to exert antiinflammatory effects by inhibiting proinflammatory mediators such as IL-6 and TNFα. An open-label, multicenter, phase II trial in patients with mild to moderate CD (baseline CDAI between 200 and 400) who had been resistant to other treatments including corticosteroids and 6-mercaptopurine (6-MP) has been done. CBP-1011 was administered orally 4 g/day for the first 2 days, followed by a daily maintenance dose of 1000 mg (500 mg every 12 hours) for up to 2 months. Seventy-three percent of the patients responded after 4 weeks, with a remission rate of 64%. Some patients experienced transient elevations of serum transaminases, but values returned to normal while patients remained on therapy. One patient dropped out because of fatigue. Otherwise, no serious adverse events occurred during the study period.

DEHYDROEPIANDROSTERONE

Dehydroepiandrosterone (DHEA) and dehydroepiandrosterone sulphate (DHEAS) are endogenous steroid hormones whose concentrations have been shown to be decreased in IBD.[63] DHEA inhibits the activation of NF-kB and IL-6 and IL-12 expression via the activation of peroxisome proliferator-activated receptor alpha. A phase II pilot trial has been reported on 7 CD patients with a mean CDAI of 242 who were treated with 200 mg/day of dehydroepiandrosterone for 56 days.[64] In this trial, 6 patients went into remission within this period. Intermittent nausea, upper respiratory symptoms, herpes labialis, perioral dermatitis, subjective feelings of aggressiveness, and intermittent hoarseness were observed as adverse effects. There was no clinical evidence of masculinization during the treatment period.

COHERIN

Coherin is bovine hormone derived from the pituitary gland.[65] Coherin has an effect on gut motility but its limited availability has not permitted large-scale trials.[66-68] In a provocative study of 19 patients with CD, Hiatt and Goodman found patients refractory to other forms of therapy, mostly corticosteroids, could improve and discontinue or reduce their steroid dose.[69] The most prominent effect was on diarrhea. The exact immunologic effects of coherin are not known but if this peptide can be manufactured synthetically it deserves to be tested in CD.

A retrospective open-label trial involving 62 patients with Crohn's disease given coherin (0.25 to 0.35 mL subcu-

taneously twice daily) for 6 to 24 months was performed.[70] After 4 months of treatment, 34% of patients ($P < 0.05$) achieved clinical remission, and 48% ($P < 0.05$) achieved clinical response. Of 21 patients who achieved remission, 19 were still in remission at 24 months. Improvements in well-being, control of abdominal pain, bowel frequency, and composite index were observed throughout the course of the 24-month study.

NOVEL GLUCOCORTICOSTEROIDS

Corticosteroids continue to be used to control acute inflammation in CD. Novel glucocorticosteroid compounds have focused on enhancing antiinflammatory potency while limiting systemic effects. Of the several available compounds, budesonide has undergone the most testing in CD and is the only one approved in the United States for this indication.

BUDESONIDE

Budesonide, a locally active glucocorticosteroid widely used for inhalation treatment of allergic rhinitis and asthma, has also been approved for treatment of mild to moderate active CD involving the ileum and/or ascending colon.[71] Ileal-release budesonide is coated in an ethylcellulose matrix that results in time-dependent release in the distal ileum and proximal colon. It has high topical activity but once absorbed undergoes extensive first-pass metabolism in the liver. As a result, there is substantial reduction in side effects compared with traditional steroids. It also results in less suppression of the hypothalamic-pituitary-adrenal axis. Significantly less bone loss occurs with budesonide than prednisolone following a year of therapy in previously steroid-naïve patients.[72]

Budesonide has been investigated for the treatment of both active CD and for maintenance of remission in CD, where it has been proven to be almost as good as predonisolone and significantly better than placebo.[73-76] In active CD, budesonide has similar efficacy to prednisolone and is more effective than mesalamine or placebo.[73,74,76] The result of a randomized placebo-controlled study in the United States in patients with mild to moderate CD demonstrated that remission was achieved in 48%, 53%, and 33% with 9 mg once daily, 4.5 mg bid, or placebo, respectively.[76] Although the remission rate was higher in predonisolone (40 mg/day) than budesonide (9 mg/day) in a 10-week trial (predonisolone 66%, budesonide 53%), adverse events were significantly less in the budesonide-treated group than prednisolone.[74] In addition, maintenance therapy with oral budesonide 6 mg/day showed prolonged duration in remission during year 1 but did not reach statistical significance by year 2.[75,77] Thus, budesonide should be considered for a subset of patients with mild to moderate symptoms of ileal CD. Long-term, however, patients should still be transitioned to therapy with immunomodulators to achieve mucosal healing and steroid-sparing.

ANTI-METABOLITE IMMUNOMODULATORS

AZATHIOPRINE AND 6-MERCAPTOPURINE

Following their introduction in the setting of solid organ transplantation, clinicians usurped the use of azathioprine (AZA) and 6-MP to treat other immunologic disorders including UC and CD. Recent data demonstrate that the mechanism of action of AZA/6-MP is likely to be induction of apoptosis of activated T cells by the active metabolite of AZA/6-MP, 6-thioguanine.[78] The metabolism of AZA/6-MP is shown in Figure 20-2.

The efficacy of AZA/6-MP has been evaluated in a variety of contexts for CD. First, it is effective for the treatment of mild to moderate active disease[79-81] and for maintenance of remission.[79,82] It is effective as a steroid-sparing agent in approximately 65% of patients in 3 to 6 months.[79,83,84] In a systematic review on the subject, a steroid-sparing effect was seen with an odds ratio of 3[86] (confidence interval [CI] 2.14-6.96), which corresponds to a number needed to treat of about 3 to observe steroid-sparing in 1 patient.[85] In children, early initiation of AZA/6-MP greatly reduces steroid exposure.[86] Modest activity is seen in fistulizing disease, although this indication has largely been replaced by anti-TNFα strategies.[87] Most recently, it has been used as an immunomodulator to suppress the immunogenicity associated with murine protein-containing biologic agents.[88] Overall, the favorable clinical experience with AZA/6-MP is greater than the weight of well-done clinical trials.

The use of these drugs, however, is limited by their slow onset of action; intravenous administration does not speed up their effectiveness.[89] Although AZA and 6-MP have fewer side effects than corticosteroids, idiosyncratic side effects including pancreatitis, hepatitis, fever, and rash can develop in about 5% of patients, usually within the first weeks of taking the drug.[90] Neutropenia and thrombocytopenia can potentially develop in about 3.8% and 2% of cases, respectively, depending on the dose (even after long-term use).[91] Particularly, severe neutropenia can develop in patients with inherited mutations in the critical catabolic enzyme TPMT (erythrocyte thiopurine methyltransferase).[92] TPMT enzyme activity should be assessed before initiation of therapy to identify patients with low or absent TMPT activity. Even patients with normal TMPT activity, however, must be monitored for hematopoietic toxicity because delayed bone marrow suppression can occur, possibly due to intercurrent viral infections.[93] Because the majority of the population, over 85%, have intact TPMT activity, these individuals can generate high levels of the 6-

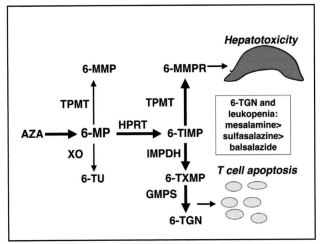

FIGURE 20-2. AZA/6-MP mechanism of action. AZA is nonenzymatically converted to 6-MP. The active metabolite 6-thioguanine nucleotides are generated by IMPDH and GMPS. High levels of 6-MMP generated by TPMT may result in hepatotoxicity (Lowry PW, Franklin CL, Weaver AL, et al. Measurement of thiopurine methyltransferase activity and azathioprine metabolites in patients with inflammatory bowel disease. *Gut.* 2001;49(5):665-670; Dubinsky[94]; Tiede[78]). AZA indicates azathioprine; 6-MP, 6-mercaptopurine; IMPDH, Inosine-5'-monophosphate dehydrogenase; GMPS, guanosine monophosphate synthetase; 6-MMP, 6-methylmercaptopurine; TPMT, thiopurine methyltransferase; HPRT, hypoxanthineguanine-phosphoribosyl-transferase; 6-TXMP, 6-thioxanthosine 5'-monophosphate; 6-TGN, 6-thioguanine nucleotides; 6-MMPR, 6-methylmercaptopurine ribonucleotide; 6-TIMP, 6-thioinosine-5'-monophosphate.

MMPR metabolite, resulting in a dose-related elevation in transaminases.[94] Therefore, regular monitoring is recommended during treatment.

Another dimension of the use of AZA/6-MP that has recently emerged is the utility of metabolite testing to assess blood levels of the 6-TGN and 6-MMPR metabolites. In particular, 6-TGN levels have been found in several studies to correlate with efficacy of the drug.[94-96] Cuffari et al found that patients with higher levels of 6-TGN in the maintenance phase of their IBD were more likely to be in continuous remission compared with those who had lower levels (Figure 20-3). Although the exact cutoff for optimal 6-TG levels is likely to be an individual measurement, levels between 230 and 300 are generally required to achieve and maintain remission.

METHOTREXATE

Methotrexate (MTX) is a folic acid antagonist with proven anti-inflammatory properties due to its inhibition of de novo synthesis of purines and pyrimidines. This originally led to its use in the therapy of some rheumatic and dermatological inflammatory disorders but more recently has been usurped for the treatment of IBD as well. MTX affects both T and B cell function, and methotrexate inhibits production of cytokines induced by T cell activation including IL-4, IL-13, IFN-γ, TNFα, and GM-CSF.[97]

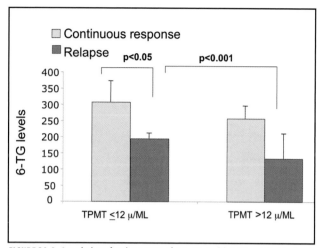

FIGURE 20-3. Correlation of maintenance of response with 6-TG metabolite levels and TMPT activity. In patients with either high or low TMPT activity, remission is associated with higher levels of 6-TG.[96] 6-TG indicates 6-thioguanine; TMPT, thiopurine methyltransferase.

In addition, it has been shown to increase local adenosine concentrations in inflamed sites, resulting in diminished neutrophil chemoattraction.[98]

Several studies have documented the efficacy of MTX in the treatment of CD. An open-label study of MTX for the treatment of active refractory CD was initially reported and led to further studies.[99] In a randomized, placebo-controlled study of 141 patients with active CD, MTX 25 mg given intramuscularly each week allowed steroid withdrawal and induced remission in 39% of steroid-dependent patients, compared with 19% given placebo injections.[100] As a follow-up to the initial study, patients who went into remission using MTX were continued on 15 mg of MTX once per week.[101] This strategy was effective in the maintenance of remission, decreasing the clinical relapse rates and prednisolone use among patients on MTX compared to placebo. Methotrexate may work more rapidly than AZA/6-MP.[100] Therefore, this agent is a good option for patients with CD who are dependent on corticosteroids and who have not responded to AZA/6-MP or who cannot tolerate these drugs. As with AZA/6-MP, MTX may be used in combination with biologics and may suppress immunogenicity against murine-containing biologics. The COMMIT trial showed that in steroid-dependent patients with a forced steroid taper over 14 weeks, there was no difference between methotrexate in combination with infliximab or infliximab alone, suggesting that with regularly scheduled infliximab monotherapy, there is no need for immunosuppression.[102]

In a retrospective series, MTX was effective at improving fistula drainage in approximately half of patients.[103]

Toxicity is an important issue that limits methotrexate use in many patients. Side effects are most commonly flu-like symptoms, nausea, vomiting, fatigue, and diarrhea. Patients must be advised to take concurrent high-dose folate. MTX has classically been feared to cause hepatotoxicity consisting of fibrosis and eventual cirrhosis especially in patients with psoriasis[104] but appears to confer a low and acceptable risk in patients with rheumatoid arthritis.[105] It appears that the risk of hepatoxicity is increased in patients consuming alcohol and those with baseline liver disease, including nonalcoholic steatohepatitis. In IBD patients, the risk appears to be low in the absence of underlying liver disease.[106] MTX pneumonitis is rare, but patients should be aware of the presenting symptoms of dyspnea: nonproductive cough and fever that may begin a few days to several weeks after initiation of therapy and, in rare cases, a few months or years later.[107] Methotrexate causes fetal death and congenital abnormalities and cannot be used by women with child-bearing potential without appropriate contraception. Like all drugs, careful monitoring and patient education will reduce risk and result in a favorable outcome.

MYCOPHENOLATE MOFETIL

Mycophenolate mofetil is a potent, selective inhibitor of inosine monophosphate dehydrogenase (IMPDH) and therefore inhibits the de novo pathway of guanosine nucleotide synthesis without incorporation into DNA like AZA/6-MP metabolites. Because T and B lymphocytes are critically dependent for their proliferation on de novo synthesis of purines, mycophenolate mofetil inhibits proliferative responses of T and B lymphocytes.[108] Although in a theoretical sense, mycophenolate mofetil would be predicted to be superior to AZA/6-MP because of its selective targeting of activated T cells, the clinical results with mycophenolate mofetil have not been as promising. In an open-label study of mycophenolate mofetil in patients failing other forms of immunosuppression, we found that only 1 patient in 11 responded.[109] In another unblinded study, mycophenolate mofetil, combined with corticosteroids, was shown to be more effective than azathioprine for chronic, active CD.[110] However, its effect on the maintenance of remission is debatable.[111]

6-THIOGUANINE

6-Thioguanine (6-TG) is a thiopurine analogue that is closely related to AZA and 6-MP. Clinical and basic science research support the idea that 6-TG is the active metabolite of AZA/6-MP.[78] 6-TG was used as an alternative to AZA or 6-MP in patients who did not adequately respond to the latter drugs and in those who were either intolerant or allergic to AZA/6-MP.[112,113] The efficacy appeared to be high with a shortened onset of action compared to AZA/6-MP. Recurrent pancreatitis was not seen in those patients with previous AZA/6-MP pancreatitis. Unfortunately, hepatoxicity prevents its safe use.[114,115] In particular, patients develop nodular hyperplasia often in the absence of abnormal transaminases or alkaline phosphatase. The most sensitive sign was a lowering of the platelet count.

LEFLUNOMIDE

Leflunomide is a pyrimidine analogue that inhibits de novo pyrimidine synthesis. At higher doses, this agent also inhibits the IL-12 signal transduction pathway by blocking tyrosine kinase. Leflunomide is approved for the treatment of rheumatoid arthritis.[116] An open-label experience with leflunomide in refractory CD has been reported.[117] Leflunomide treatment 20 mg/day resulted in a significant reduction in the serologic parameters and Harvey-Bradshaw scores in 8 of 12 patients (67%). A majority of steroid-dependent patients were able to successfully taper following leflunomide initiation. Adverse reactions including worsening of diarrhea, generalized itching and rash, and asymptomatic increase in serum transaminase were found in 4 individual patients. Hepatic injury and severe infection have also been reported but are not dissimilar to MTX.[118] At present, this should be considered on an experimental basis for IBD.

CYCLOPHOSPHAMIDE

Cyclophosphamide is a chemotherapeutic agent that is converted to alkylating metabolites in the liver that interfere with the growth of susceptible, rapidly proliferating malignant cells by cross-linking of DNA. Its immunosuppressive properties are likely related to inhibition of T cell and B cell proliferation. An open-label uncontrolled pilot study of the use of cyclophosphamide for refractory CD has been reported.[119] Cyclophosphamide pulse (750 mg) was administered monthly for 4 to 6 cycles for steroid-resistant CD. Clinical improvement was seen in all patients, and 6 of the 7 patients achieved remission. In addition, remission was maintained for all patients for a median of 18 months but 1 patient needed a second course of cyclophosphamide. Nonserious side effects of candida esophagitis in 2 and uncomplicated urinary tract infection in 3 patients were reported in the study. However, prolonged use of daily cyclophosphamide has been associated with toxic effects such as gonadal dysfunction (approximately 70%) and infertility, bone marrow suppression, hemorrhagic cystitis (17% to 34%), and increased risk of neoplasms.[120] Given that most IBD patients are of child-bearing potential, the risk and benefits of this treatment should be carefully assessed. It remains an option for severe refractory cases.

CALCINEURIN INHIBITORS

CYCLOSPORINE

Cyclosporine (CsA) is a hydrophilic cyclic undecapeptide extracted from a soil fungus. Its primary effect is selective inhibition of cellular immunity by blocking the production of IL-2 and IL-2 receptors by T lymphocytes.

CsA has been extensively used in the field of transplantation. In the setting of CD treatment, CsA has been reported to have a therapeutic advantage over placebo in active CD (response rate 59% in the CsA group and 32% in the placebo group at 3 months) when given at oral doses of 5 to 7.5 mg/kg/day.[121] Subsequent multicenter controlled trials did not find a beneficial effect.[122,123] Open-label studies in which CsA has been used in a fashion similar to CsA for UC, ie, intravenously for the severely active hospitalized patients, have found a beneficial effect in the majority of patients.[124] CsA has been found in several open-label studies to be effective for short-term treatment of fistulas.[125,126] Often, a change to oral CsA results in reopening of fistulas, but this therapy can be used as a bridge to antimetabolites or surgical therapy.

CsA has the advantage of a more rapid onset of action than AZA and 6-MP. However, its side effects include nephrotoxicity, hypertension, seizures, increased susceptibility to infections, and increased risk of lymphomas in the long-term. Some of the infections that have developed in patients on CsA have been serious, even fatal. Some of these side effects are dose dependent, and therefore monitoring of drug levels both in the inpatient and outpatient settings is essential.

TACROLIMUS

Tacrolimus has a mechanism of action similar to cyclosporine.[108,127] It is more effective than cyclosporine in prevention of rejection in renal and liver transplant recipients and therefore has been explored as a treatment option in patients with IBD. A retrospective examination of the efficacy of tacrolimus in severe, luminal CD showed promising results.[128,129] Based on preliminary encouraging results with oral tacrolimus, in combination with AZA/6-MP for fistulizing disease,[130,131] a randomized, placebo-controlled trial of tacrolimus was performed. Tacrolimus at a dose of 0.2 mg/kg/day was effective for fistula improvement but not for maintenance of remission in patients with perianal CD.[132] It was also associated with nephrotoxicity that resulted in frequent dose reduction. Importantly, tacrolimus was effective in a subset of patients for whom infliximab did not work or had lost its efficacy. Thus, for this subgroup of patients with fistulas refractory to infliximab, tacrolimus can be considered as an option.

MISCELLANEOUS THERAPIES UNDER INVESTIGATION

FISH OILS AND OMEGA-3 FATTY ACIDS

Omega-3 fatty acids, such those found in fish oils, are long-chain polyunsaturated fatty acids with a double bond between carbon atoms 3 and 4 proximal to the methyl end of the fatty acid.[133] Omega-3 fatty acids compete in the substrate pool of the lipoxygenase pathway and thus reduce the production of inflammatory leukotrienes. Omega-3 fatty acids have also been shown to suppress the synthesis of other inflammatory cytokines such as IL-1a and IL-1b and TNFα by mononuclear cells.[134,135]

A maintenance study of an enteric-coated fish oil preparation containing 40% eicosapentaenoic acid (1.8 g/day) and 20% docosahexaenoic acid (0.9 g/day) demonstrated a reduction in the rate of relapse among patients with CD who were in clinical remission.[136] But another randomized controlled multicenter trial argued against the use of fish oil for maintenance of remission in patients with CD.[137] Generally speaking, however, it is safe and can be used as an adjunct to other conventional therapies.

Neuroimmunomodulation

Proinflammatory neuropeptides include substance P, vasoactive intestinal peptide, and neuropeptide YY, whereas calcitonin gene-related peptide, somatostatin, and bombesin possess predominantly antiinflammatory effects.[138] Reduced levels of somatostatin in the mucosa of CD and UC patients as well as enhanced expression of somatostatin receptors on intramural veins of inflamed tissues are found in both diseases.[139,140] By immunocytochemistry, investigators have demonstrated that substance P, vasoactive intestinal polypeptide, and somatostatin-containing nerve fibers are in direct contact with the plasma cells, lymphocytes, and other immunocompetent cells, suggesting that they may have a direct immunologic effect.[141] Increased staining of substance P is seen in the lamina propria of UC[142,143] and pouchitis.[144] In addition, patients with CD and UC demonstrate an increase in expression of neurokinin-1 (NK-1) receptor (NK-1R), the receptor for substance P, on epithelial cells and endothelial cells of capillaries and venules.[145] A selective antagonist of NK-1R, CP-96345, which inhibits binding of substance P, attenuates chemically induced colitis and pouchitis in mouse models.[144,146] Others, however, have found that in prolonged colitis, substance P may play a protective role.[147] In the IL-10-/- model of colitis, lamina propria T cells express NK-1R and produce IFN-γ after induction of colitis but not wild-type mice.[148] The NK-1R antagonist reversed the inflammation even after its induction, suggesting that this is a potentially promising therapy for Th1-dependent colitis such as CD. For these reasons, substance P antagonists are being considered in clinical trials for CD.[149,150]

Upstream of substance P, the neuropeptide neurotensin mediates chloride secretion, motility, and cellular growth. It is an important mediator of colonic secretion, mucosal permeability, and histologic damage in animal models in response to *Clostridium difficile*–derived toxin A.[151] Selective inhibition of the neurotensin receptor using neurotensin receptor antagonist SR-48, 692 prevents toxin A damage. These selective antagonists may someday be used

alone or in combination to limit inflammation and its accompanying visceral hyperalgesia.

Hyperbaric Oxygen

Hyperbaric oxygen has been described as an adjunctive therapy for healing of perianal manifestations of CD.[152,153] The possible mode of action includes decreased activity of nitric oxide synthase, inhibition of proinflammatory cytokines, and a bactericidal effect.[154,155]

CONCLUSION

Although a number of different medications have proven effective in treating CD, there is no standard treatment regimen for managing all patients. This stands to reason given the complexity and variability of CD. A number of factors will determine which treatments are appropriate for the individual patient. These include location of disease, presence or absence of complications, severity of symptoms, genetic markers, and serological markers. Treatment must be tailored to each patient's needs.

Many of the therapies described in this chapter have had limited testing. It is likely that in each case there is a subgroup of CD patients who will have a favorable response to 1 medication, eg, leflunomide, when they have not responded to more conventional therapy with AZA/6-MP. Unfortunately, these patients are always underrepresented in clinical trials, leading clinicians to conclude that a certain therapy should not be used in CD. What is needed is careful attention to biomarkers and genetic markers in all clinical trials of potentially promising medications. In this way, it may be possible to cull out differences between responders and nonresponders and preselect patients for their likelihood of response to therapy. Finally, with high through-screening of thousands of compounds simultaneously for very specific cellular effects, there will be many other small molecules to antagonize or enhance specific intracellular pathways in CD.

REFERENCES

1. Ogura Y, Bonen DK, Inohara N, et al. A frameshift mutation in NOD2 associated with susceptibility to Crohn's disease [see comment]. *Nature.* 2001;411:603-606.

2. Hugot JP, Chamaillard M, Zouali H, et al. Association of NOD2 leucine-rich repeat variants with susceptibility to Crohn's disease [see comment]. *Nature.* 2001;411:599-603.

3. Ogura Y, Inohara N, Benito A, Chen FF, Yamaoka S, Nunez G. Nod2, a Nod1/Apaf-1 family member that is restricted to monocytes and activates NF-kappaB. *J Biol Chem.* 2001;276:4812-4818.

4. Lala S, Ogura Y, Osborne C, et al. Crohn's disease and the NOD2 gene: a role for paneth cells. *Gastroenterology.* 2003;125:47-57.

5. Peltekova VD, Wintle RF, Rubin LA, et al. Functional variants of OCTN cation transporter genes are associated with Crohn disease. *Nat Genet.* 2004;36:471-475.

6. Sandborn WJ, Faubion WA. Biologics in inflammatory bowel disease: How much progress have we made? *Gut*. 2004;53:1366-1373.

7. Mow WS, Vasiliauskas EA, Lin Y-C, et al. Association of antibody responses to microbial antigens and complications of small bowel Crohn's disease. *Gastroenterology*. 2004;126:414-424.

8. Rutgeerts P, Feagan BG, Lichtenstein GR, et al. Comparison of scheduled and episodic treatment strategies of infliximab in Crohn's disease. *Gastroenterology*. 2004;126:402-413.

9. Dredge K, Marriott JB, Dalgleish AG. Immunological effects of thalidomide and its chemical and functional analogs. *Crit Rev Immunol*. 2002;22:425-437.

10. Deng L, Ding W, Granstein RD. Thalidomide inhibits tumor necrosis factor-alpha production and antigen presentation by Langerhans cells. *J Invest Derm*. 2003;121:1060-1065.

11. Moreira AL, Sampaio EP, Zmuidzinas A, Frindt P, Smith KA, Kaplan G. Thalidomide exerts its inhibitory action on tumor necrosis factor alpha by enhancing mRNA degradation. *J Exp Med*. 1993;177:1675-1680.

12. Majumdar S, Lamothe B, Aggarwal BB. Thalidomide suppresses NF-kappa B activation induced by TNF and H2O2, but not that activated by ceramide, lipopolysaccharides, or phorbol ester. *J Immunol*. 2002;168:2644-2651.

13. Bauditz J, Wedel S, Lochs H. Thalidomide reduces tumour necrosis factor alpha and interleukin 12 production in patients with chronic active Crohn's disease. *Gut*. 2002;50:196-200.

14. Vasiliauskas EA, Kam LY, Abreu-Martin MT, et al. An open-label pilot study of low-dose thalidomide in chronically active, steroid-dependent Crohn's disease. *Gastroenterology*. 1999;117:1278-1287.

15. Ehrenpreis ED, Kane SV, Cohen LB, Cohen RD, Hanauer SB. Thalidomide therapy for patients with refractory Crohn's disease: an open-label trial. *Gastroenterology*. 1999;117:1271-1277.

16. Facchini S, Candusso M, Martelossi S, Liubich M, Panfili E, Ventura A. Efficacy of long-term treatment with thalidomide in children and young adults with Crohn disease: preliminary results. *J Pediatr Gastroenterol Nutr*. 2001;32:178-181.

17. Bauditz J, Schachschal G, Wedel S, Lochs H. Thalidomide for treatment of severe intestinal bleeding. *Gut*. 2004;53:609-612.

18. Sabate JM, Villarejo J, Lemann M, Bonnet J, Allez M, Modigliani R. An open-label study of thalidomide for maintenance therapy in responders to infliximab in chronically active and fistulizing refractory Crohn's disease. *Aliment Pharmacol Ther*. 2002;16:1117-1124.

19. Lenz W, Knapp K. Thalidomide embryopathy. *Arch Environ Health*. 1962;5:100-105.

20. Stephens TD. Proposed mechanisms of action in thalidomide embryopathy. *Teratology*. 1988;38:229-239.

21. Bartlett JB, Dredge K, Dalgleish AG. The evolution of thalidomide and its IMiD derivatives as anticancer agents. *Nat Rev Cancer*. 2004;4:314-322.

22. Zhu X, Giordano T, Yu QS, et al. Thiothalidomides: novel isosteric analogues of thalidomide with enhanced TNF alpha inhibitory activity. *J Med Chem*. 2003;46:5222-5229.

23. Verghese MW, McConnell RT, Strickland AB, et al. Differential regulation of human monocyte-derived TNF alpha and IL-1 beta by type IV cAMP-phosphodiesterase (cAMP-PDE) inhibitors. *J Pharmacol Exp Ther*. 1995;272:1313-1320.

24. Verghese MW, McConnell RT, Lenhard JM, Hamacher L, Jin SL. Regulation of distinct cyclic AMP-specific phosphodiesterase (phosphodiesterase type 4) isozymes in human monocytic cells. *Mol Pharmacol*. 1995;47:1164-1171.

25. Marriott JB, Clarke IA, Czajka A, et al. A novel subclass of thalidomide analogue with anti-solid tumor activity in which caspase-dependent apoptosis is associated with altered expression of bcl-2 family proteins. *Cancer Res*. 2003;63:593-599.

26. Mitsiades N, Mitsiades CS, Poulaki V, et al. Apoptotic signaling induced by immunomodulatory thalidomide analogs in human multiple myeloma cells: therapeutic implications. *Blood*. 2002;99:4525-4530.

27. Oliver SJ, Freeman SL, Corral LG, Ocampo CJ, Kaplan G. Thalidomide analogue CC1069 inhibits development of rat adjuvant arthritis. *Clin Exp Immunol*. 1999;118:315-321.

28. Marriott JB, Westby M, Cookson S, et al. CC-3052: a water-soluble analog of thalidomide and potent inhibitor of activation-induced TNF alpha production. *J Immunol*. 1998;161:4236-4243.

29. Chihiro M, Nagamoto H, Takemura I, et al. Novel thiazole derivatives as inhibitors of superoxide production by human neutrophils: synthesis and structure-activity relationships. *J Med Chem*. 1995;38:353-358.

30. Schreiber S, Keshavarzian A, Isaacs KL, et al. A randomized, placebo-controlled, phase II study of tetomilast in active ulcerative colitis. *Gastroenterology*. 2007;132:76-86.

31. Regan J, Breitfelder S, Cirillo P, et al. Pyrazole urea-based inhibitors of p38 MAP kinase: from lead compound to clinical candidate. *J Med Chem*. 2002;45:2994-3008.

32. Waetzig GH, Rosenstiel P, Nikolaus S, Seegert D, Schreiber S. Differential p38 mitogen-activated protein kinase target phosphorylation in responders and nonresponders to infliximab [see comment]. *Gastroenterology*. 2003;125:633-634.

33. Waetzig GH, Seegert D, Rosenstiel P, Nikolaus S, Schreiber S. p38 Mitogen-activated protein kinase is activated and linked to TNF alpha signaling in inflammatory bowel disease. *J Immunol*. 2002;168:5342-5351.

34. Beddy DJ, Watson WR, Fitzpatrick JM, O'Connell PR. Critical involvement of stress-activated mitogen-activated protein kinases in the regulation of intracellular adhesion molecule-1 in serosal fibroblasts isolated from patients with Crohn's disease. *J Am Coll Surg*. 2004;199:234-242.

35. Branger J, van den Blink B, Weijer S, et al. Inhibition of coagulation, fibrinolysis, and endothelial cell activation by a p38 mitogen-activated protein kinase inhibitor during human endotoxemia. *Blood*. 2003;101:4446-4448.

36. Branger J, van den Blink B, Weijer S, et al. Anti-inflammatory effects of a p38 mitogen-activated protein kinase inhibitor during human endotoxemia. *J Immunol*. 2002;168:4070-4077.

37. Schreiber S, Feagan B, D'Haens G, et al. Oral p38 mitogen-activated protein kinase inhibition with BIRB 796 for active Crohn's disease: a randomized, double-blind, placebo-controlled trial. *Clin Gastroenterol Hepatol*. 2006;4:325-334.

38. Hommes D, van den Blink B, Plasse T, et al. Inhibition of stress-activated MAP kinases induces clinical improvement in moderate to severe Crohn's disease. *Gastroenterology*. 2002;122:7-14.

39. Strieter RM, Remick DG, Ward PA, et al. Cellular and molecular regulation of tumor necrosis factor-alpha production by pentoxifylline. *Biochem Biophys Res Commun*. 1988;155:1230-1236.

40. Reimund JM, Dumont S, Muller CD, et al. In vitro effects of oxpentifylline on inflammatory cytokine release in patients with inflammatory bowel disease. *Gut*. 1997;40:475-480.

41. Bauditz J, Haemling J, Ortner M, Lochs H, Raedler A, Schreiber S. Treatment with tumour necrosis factor inhibitor oxpentifylline does not improve corticosteroid dependent chronic active Crohn's disease. *Gut*. 1997;40:470-474.

42. Black RA, Rauch CT, Kozlosky CJ, et al. A metalloproteinase disintegrin that releases tumour-necrosis factor-alpha from cells. *Nature*. 1997;385:729-733.

43. Moss M, Jin S, Milla M, et al. Cloning of a desintegrin metalloprotease that processes precursor tumor necrosis factor alpha. *Nature*. 1997;385:733-736.

44. Conway JG, Andrews RC, Beaudet B, et al. Inhibition of tumor necrosis factor-alpha (TNF alpha) production and arthritis in the rat by GW3333, a dual inhibitor of TNF alpha-converting enzyme and matrix metalloproteinases. *J Pharmacol Exp Ther.* 2001;298:900-908.

45. Randle JC, Harding MW, Ku G, Schonharting M, Kurrle R. ICE/caspase-1 inhibitors as novel antiinflammatory drugs. *Expert Opin Invest Drugs.* 2001;10:1207-1209.

46. Wilk JN, Viney JL. GM-CSF treatment for Crohn's disease: a stimulating new therapy? *Curr Opin Invest Drugs.* 2002;3:1291-1296.

47. Dieckgraefe BK, Korzenik JR, Husain A, Dieruf L. Association of glycogen storage disease 1b and Crohn disease: results of a North American survey. *Eur J Pediatr.* 2002;161 (suppl 1):S88-S92.

48. Vaughan D, Drumm B. Treatment of fistulas with granulocyte colony-stimulating factor in a patient with Crohn's disease. *N Engl J Med.* 1999;340:239-240.

49. Dieckgraefe BK, Korzenik JR. Treatment of active Crohn's disease with recombinant human granulocyte-macrophage colony-stimulating factor. *Lancet.* 2002;360:1478-1480.

50. Tontonoz P, Hu E, Spiegelman BM. Stimulation of adipogenesis in fibroblasts by PPAR gamma 2, a lipid-activated transcription factor. *Cell.* 1994;79:1147-1156.

51. Chawla A, Schwarz EJ, Dimaculangan DD, Lazar MA. Peroxisome proliferator-activated receptor (PPAR) gamma: adipose-predominant expression and induction early in adipocyte differentiation. *Endocrinology.* 1994;135:798-800.

52. Fajas L, Auboeuf D, Raspe E, et al. The organization, promoter analysis, and expression of the human PPAR gamma gene. *J Biol Chem.* 1997;272:18779-18789.

53. Su CG, Wen X, Bailey ST, et al. A novel therapy for colitis utilizing PPAR-gamma ligands to inhibit the epithelial inflammatory response. *J Clin Invest.* 1999;104:383-389.

54. Desreumaux P, Dubuquoy L, Nutten S, et al. Attenuation of colon inflammation through activators of the retinoid X receptor (RXR)/peroxisome proliferator-activated receptor gamma (PPARgamma) heterodimer. A basis for new therapeutic strategies. *J Exp Med.* 2001;193:827-838.

55. Chinetti G, Fruchart JC, Staels B. Peroxisome proliferator-activated receptors (PPARs): nuclear receptors at the crossroads between lipid metabolism and inflammation. *Inflamm Res.* 2000;49:497-505.

56. Faveeuw C, Fougeray S, Angeli V, et al. Peroxisome proliferator-activated receptor gamma activators inhibit interleukin-12 production in murine dendritic cells. *FEBS Lett.* 2000;486:261-266.

57. Lewis JD, Lichtenstein GR, Deren JJ, et al. Rosiglitazone for active ulcerative colitis: a randomized placebo-controlled trial. *Gastroenterology.* 2008;134:688-695.

58. Wada K, Nakajima A, Blumberg RS. PPARgamma and inflammatory bowel disease: a new therapeutic target for ulcerative colitis and Crohn's disease. *Trends Mol Med.* 2001;7:329-331.

59. Nissen SE, Wolski K. Effect of rosiglitazone on the risk of myocardial infarction and death from cardiovascular causes. *N Engl J Med.* 2007;356:2457-2471.

60. Slonim AE, Bulone L, Damore MB, Goldberg T, Wingertzahn MA, McKinley MJ. A preliminary study of growth hormone therapy for Crohn's disease. *N Engl J Med.* 2000;342:1633-1637.

61. Sartor RB. New therapeutic approaches to Crohn's disease. *N Engl J Med.* 2000;342:1664-1666.

62. CBP 1011: Colirest, Hematrol. *Drugs R D.* 2003;4:241-242.

63. Straub RH, Vogl D, Gross V, Lang B, Scholmerich J, Andus T. Association of humoral markers of inflammation and dehydroepiandrosterone sulfate or cortisol serum levels in patients with chronic inflammatory bowel disease. *Am J Gastroenterol.* 1998;93:2197-2202.

64. Andus T, Klebl F, Rogler G, Bregenzer N, Scholmerich J, Straub RH. Patients with refractory Crohn's disease or ulcerative colitis respond to dehydroepiandrosterone: a pilot study. *Aliment Pharmacol Ther.* 2003;17:409-414.

65. Goodman I, Hiatt RB. Coherin: a new peptide of the bovine neurohypophysis with activity on gastrointestinal motility. *Science.* 1972;178:419-421.

66. Mendel C, Jaeck D, Grenier JF, Hiatt RB, Goodman I, Sandler B. Action of coherin on the basic electrical rhythm and propagation in the isolated perfused canine jejunum. *J Surg Res.* 1975;19:403-409.

67. Dauchel J, Schang JC, Kachelhoffer J, Eloy R, Grenier JF. Effects of some drugs on electrical activity of the gut in the postoperative period. *Eur Surg Res.* 1976;8:26-38.

68. Hiatt RB, Goodman I. Peptide treatment of postgastrectomy obstruction. *Arch Surg.* 1976;111:997-999.

69. Hiatt RB, Goodman I. Long-term results in the treatment of regional ileitis with coherin. *Am J Gastroenterol.* 1977;67:274-277.

70. Lichtenstein GR, Jacoby HI. Coherin peptides induce clinical response and remission in patients with active Crohn's disease. *Gastroenterol Hepatol.* 2005;1:57-62.

71. Anonymous. Controlled-release budesonide in Crohn's disease. *Drug & Therapeutics Bulletin.* 1997;35:30-31.

72. van Balkom BP, Schoon EJ, Stockbrugger RW, et al. Effects of anti-tumour necrosis factor-alpha therapy on the quality of life in Crohn's disease [comment]. *Aliment Pharmacol Ther.* 2002;16:1101-1107.

73. Greenberg GR, Feagan BG, Martin F, et al. Oral budesonide for active Crohn's disease. Canadian Inflammatory Bowel Disease Study Group [see comment]. *N Engl J Med.* 1994;331:836-841.

74. Rutgeerts P, Lofberg R, Malchow H, et al. A comparison of budesonide with prednisolone for active Crohn's disease. *N Engl J Med.* 1994;331:842-845.

75. Greenberg GR, Feagan BG, Martin F, et al. Oral budesonide as maintenance treatment for Crohn's disease: a placebo-controlled, dose-ranging study. Canadian Inflammatory Bowel Disease Study Group. *Gastroenterology.* 1996;110:45-51.

76. Tremaine WJ, Hanauer SB, Katz S, et al. Budesonide CIR capsules (once or twice daily divided-dose) in active Crohn's disease: a randomized placebo-controlled study in the United States. *Am J Gastroenterol.* 2002;97:1748-1754.

77. Lofberg R, Rutgeerts P, Malchow H, et al. Budesonide prolongs time to relapse in ileal and ileocaecal Crohn's disease. A placebo controlled one year study. *Gut.* 1996;39:82-86.

78. Tiede I, Fritz G, Strand S, et al. CD28-dependent Rac1 activation is the molecular target of azathioprine in primary human CD4+ T lymphocytes. *J Clin Invest.* 2003;111:1133-1145.

79. Present DH, Korelitz BI, Wisch N, Glass JL, Sachar DB, Pasternack BS. Treatment of Crohn's disease with 6-mercaptopurine. A long-term, randomized, double-blind study. *N Engl J Med.* 1980;302:981-987.

80. Candy S, Wright J, Gerber M, Adams G, Gerig M, Goodman R. A controlled double blind study of azathioprine in the management of Crohn's disease. *Gut.* 1995;37:674-678.

81. Willoughby JM, Beckett J, Kumar PJ, Dawson AM. Controlled trial of azathioprine in Crohn's disease. *Lancet.* 1971;2:944-947.

82. O'Donoghue DP, Dawson AM, Powell-Tuck J, Bown RL, Lennard-Jones JE. Double-blind withdrawal trial of azathioprine as maintenance treatment for Crohn's disease. *Lancet.* 1978;2:955-957.

83. Ewe K, Press AG, Singe CC, et al. Azathioprine combined with prednisolone or monotherapy with prednisolone in active Crohn's disease. *Gastroenterology.* 1993;105:367-372.

84. Pearson DC, May GR, Fick GH, Sutherland LR. Azathioprine and 6-mercaptopurine in Crohn disease. A meta-analysis. *Ann Intern Med.* 1995;123:132-142.

85. Sandborn W, Sutherland L, Pearson D, May G, Modigliani R, Prantera C. Azathioprine or 6-mercaptopurine for inducing remission of Crohn's disease. *Cochrane Database of Systematic Reviews.* 2000:CD000545.

86. Markowitz J, Grancher K, Kohn N, Lesser M, Daum F. A multicenter trial of 6-mercaptopurine and prednisone in children with newly diagnosed Crohn's disease. *Gastroenterology.* 2000;119:895-902.

87. Korelitz BI, Present DH. Favorable effect of 6-mercaptopurine on fistulae of Crohn's disease. *Dig Dis Sci.* 1985;30:58-64.

88. Baert F, Noman M, Vermeire S, et al. Influence of immunogenicity on the long-term efficacy of infliximab in Crohn's disease. *N Engl J Med.* 2003;348:601-608.

89. Sandborn WJ, Tremaine WJ, Wolf DC, et al. Lack of effect of intravenous administration on time to respond to azathioprine for steroid-treated Crohn's disease. North American Azathioprine Study Group [see comments]. *Gastroenterology.* 1999;117:527-535.

90. Present DH, Meltzer SJ, Krumholz MP, Wolke A, Korelitz BI. 6-Mercaptopurine in the management of inflammatory bowel disease: short- and long-term toxicity. *Ann Intern Med.* 1989; 111:641-649.

91. Connell WR, Kamm MA, Ritchie JK, Lennard-Jones JE. Bone marrow toxicity caused by azathioprine in inflammatory bowel disease: 27 years of experience. *Gut.* 1993;34:1081-1085.

92. Lennard L, Van Loon JA, Weinshilboum RM. Pharmacogenetics of acute azathioprine toxicity: relationship to thiopurine methyltransferase genetic polymorphism. *Clin Pharm Ther.* 1989;46:149-154.

93. Colombel JF, Ferrari N, Debuysere H, et al. Genotypic analysis of thiopurine S-methyltransferase in patients with Crohn's disease and severe myelosuppression during azathioprine therapy. *Gastroenterology.* 2000;118:1025-1030.

94. Dubinsky MC, Lamothe S, Yang HY, et al. Pharmacogenomics and metabolite measurement for 6-mercaptopurine therapy in inflammatory bowel disease. *Gastroenterology.* 2000;118:705-713.

95. Cuffari C, Hunt S, Bayless T. Utilisation of erythrocyte 6-thioguanine metabolite levels to optimise azathioprine therapy in patients with inflammatory bowel disease. *Gut.* 2001;48:642-646.

96. Cuffari C, Li DY, Mahoney J, Barnes Y, Bayless TM. Peripheral blood mononuclear cell DNA 6-thioguanine metabolite levels correlate with decreased interferon-gamma production in patients with Crohn's disease on AZA therapy. *Dig Dis Sci.* 2004;49(1):133-137.

97. Gerards AH, de Lathouder S, de Groot ER, Dijkmans BA, Aarden LA. Inhibition of cytokine production by methotrexate. Studies in healthy volunteers and patients with rheumatoid arthritis. *Rheumatology.* 2003;42:1189-1196.

98. Cronstein BN, Naime D, Ostad E. The antiinflammatory mechanism of methotrexate. Increased adenosine release at inflamed sites diminishes leukocyte accumulation in an in vivo model of inflammation. *J Clin Invest.* 1993;92:2675-2682.

99. Kozarek RA, Patterson DJ, Gelfand MD, Botoman VA, Ball TJ, Wilske KR. Methotrexate induces clinical and histologic remission in patients with refractory inflammatory bowel disease. *Ann Intern Med.* 1989;110:353-356.

100. Feagan BG, Rochon J, Fedorak RN, et al. Methotrexate for the treatment of Crohn's disease. The North American Crohn's Study Group Investigators. *N Engl J Med.* 1995;332:292-297.

101. Feagan B. A randomized trial of methotrexate (MTX) in combination with infliximab (IFX) for the treatment of Crohn's disease (CD) [abstract]. Presented at: Digestive Disease Week; May 17-22, 2008; San Diego, CA.

102. Feagan BG, Fedorak RN, Irvine EJ, et al. A comparison of methotrexate with placebo for the maintenance of remission in Crohn's disease. North American Crohn's Study Group Investigators. *N Engl J Med.* 2000;342:1627-1632.

103. Mahadevan U, Marion JF, Present DH. Fistula response to methotrexate in Crohn's disease: a case series. *Aliment Pharmacol Ther.* 2003;18:1003-1008.

104. West SG. Methotrexate hepatotoxicity. *Rheum Dis Clin North Am.* 1997;23:883-915.

105. Kremer JM. Liver toxicity does not have to follow methotrexate therapy of patients with rheumatoid arthritis [see comment]. *Am J Gastroenterol.* 1997;92:194-196.

106. Te HS, Schiano TD, Kuan SF, Hanauer SB, Conjeevaram HS, Baker AL. Hepatic effects of long-term methotrexate use in the treatment of inflammatory bowel disease. *Am J Gastroenterol.* 2000;95:3150-3156.

107. Hasan F, Mark E. A 28-year-old man with increasing dyspnea, dry cough, and fever after chemotherapy for lymphoma. *N Engl J Med.* 1990;323:737-747.

108. Gerber DA, Bonham CA, Thomson AW. Immunosuppressive agents: recent developments in molecular action and clinical application. *Transplant Proc.* 1998;30:1573-1579.

109. Hassard PV, Vasiliauskas EA, Kam LY, Targan SR, Abreu MT. Efficacy of mycophenolate mofetil in patients failing 6-mercaptopurine or azathioprine therapy for Crohn's disease. *Inflamm Bowel Dis.* 2000;6:16-20.

110. Neurath MF, Wanitschke R, Peters M, Krummenauer F, Meyer zum Buschenfelde KH, Schlaak JF. Randomised trial of mycophenolate mofetil versus azathioprine for treatment of chronic active Crohn's disease. *Gut.* 1999;44:625-628.

111. Fellermann K, Steffen M, Stein J, et al. Mycophenolate mofetil: lack of efficacy in chronic active inflammatory bowel disease. *Aliment Pharmacol Ther.* 2000;14:171-176.

112. Dubinsky MC, Hassard PV, Seidman EG, et al. An open-label pilot study using thioguanine as a therapeutic alternative in Crohn's disease patients resistant to 6-mercaptopurine therapy. *Inflamm Bowel Dis.* 2001;7:181-189.

113. Dubinsky MC, Feldman EJ, Abreu MT, Targan SR, Vasiliauskas EA. Thioguanine: a potential alternate thiopurine for IBD patients allergic to 6-mercaptopurine or azathioprine. *Am J Gastroenterol.* 2003;98:1058-1063.

114. Dubinsky MC, Vasiliauskas EA, Singh H, et al. 6-thioguanine can cause serious liver injury in inflammatory bowel disease patients. *Gastroenterology.* 2003;125:298-303.

115. Geller SA, Dubinsky MC, Poordad FF, et al. Early hepatic nodular hyperplasia and submicroscopic fibrosis associated with 6-thioguanine therapy in inflammatory bowel disease. *Am J Surg Pathol.* 2004;28:1204-1211.

116. Sanders S, Harisdangkul V. Leflunomide for the treatment of rheumatoid arthritis and autoimmunity. *Am J Med Sci.* 2002;323:190-193.

117. Prajapati DN, Knox JF, Emmons J, Saeian K, Csuka ME, Binion DG. Leflunomide treatment of Crohn's disease patients intolerant to standard immunomodulator therapy. *J Clin Gastroenterol.* 2003;37:125-128.

118. Suissa S, Ernst P, Hudson M, Bitton A, Kezouh A. Newer disease-modifying antirheumatic drugs and the risk of serious hepatic adverse events in patients with rheumatoid arthritis. *Am J Med Sci.* 2004;117:87-92.

119. Stallmach A, Wittig BM, Moser C, Fischinger J, Duchmann R, Zeitz M. Safety and efficacy of intravenous pulse cyclophosphamide in acute steroid refractory inflammatory bowel disease. *Gut.* 2003;52:377-382.

120. Baker GL, Kahl LE, Zee BC, Stolzer BL, Agarwal AK, Medsger TA Jr. Malignancy following treatment of rheumatoid arthritis with cyclophosphamide. Long-term case-control follow-up study. *Am J Med.* 1987;83:1-9.

121. Brynskov J, Freund L, Norby Rasmussen S, et al. Final report on a placebo-controlled, double-blind, randomized, multicentre trial of cyclosporin treatment in active chronic Crohn's disease. *Scand J Gastroenterol.* 1991;26:689-695.

122. Stange EF, Modigliani R, Pena AS, Wood AJ, Feutren G, Smith PR. European trial of cyclosporine in chronic active Crohn's disease: a 12-month study. The European Study Group. *Gastroenterology.* 1995;109:774-782.

123. Feagan BG, McDonald JW, Rochon J, et al. Low-dose cyclosporine for the treatment of Crohn's disease. The Canadian Crohn's Relapse Prevention Trial Investigators. *N Engl J Med.* 1994;330:1846-1851.

124. Sandborn WJ, Tremaine WJ, Lawson GM. Clinical response does not correlate with intestinal or blood cyclosporine concentrations in patients with Crohn's disease treated with high-dose oral cyclosporine. *Am J Gastroenterol.* 1996;91:37-43.

125. Hanauer SB, Smith MB. Rapid closure of Crohn's disease fistulas with continuous intravenous cyclosporin A. *Am J Gastroenterol.* 1993;88:646-649.

126. Present DH, Lichtiger S. Efficacy of cyclosporine in treatment of fistula of Crohn's disease. *Dig Dis Sci.* 1994;39:374-380.

127. Flanagan WM, Corthesy B, Bram RJ, Crabtree GR. Nuclear association of a T-cell transcription factor blocked by FK-506 and cyclosporin A. *Nature.* 1991;352:803-807.

128. Sandborn WJ. Preliminary report on the use of oral tacrolimus (FK506) in the treatment of complicated proximal small bowel and fistulizing Crohn's disease. *Am J Gastroenterol.* 1997;92:876-879.

129. Ierardi E, Principi M, Francavilla R, et al. Oral tacrolimus long-term therapy in patients with Crohn's disease and steroid resistance. *Aliment Pharmacol Ther.* 2001;15:371-377.

130. Lowry PW, Weaver AL, Tremaine WJ, Sandborn WJ. Combination therapy with oral tacrolimus (FK506) and azathioprine or 6-mercaptopurine for treatment-refractory Crohn's disease perianal fistulae. *Inflamm Bowel Dis.* 1999;5:239-245.

131. Ierardi E, Principi M, Rendina M, et al. Oral tacrolimus (FK 506) in Crohn's disease complicated by fistulae of the perineum. *J Clin Gastroenterol.* 2000;30:200-202.

132. Sandborn WJ, Present DH, Isaacs KL, et al. Tacrolimus for the treatment of fistulas in patients with Crohn's disease: a randomized, placebo-controlled trial. *Gastroenterol.* 2003;125:380-388.

133. Endres S, De Caterina R, Schmidt EB, Kristensen SD. n-3 Polyunsaturated fatty acids: update 1995. *Eur Clin Invest.* 1995;25:629-638.

134. Endres S, Sinha B, Eisenhut T. Omega 3 fatty acids in the regulation of cytokine synthesis. *World Rev Nutr Diet.* 1994;76:89-94.

135. Endres S, Eisenhut T, Sinha B. n-3 Polyunsaturated fatty acids in the regulation of human cytokine synthesis. *Biochem Soc Trans.* 1995;23:277-281.

136. Belluzzi A, Brignola C, Campieri M, Pera A, Boschi S, Miglioli M. Effect of an enteric-coated fish-oil preparation on relapses in Crohn's disease. *N Engl J Med.* 1996;334:1557-1560.

137. Lorenz-Meyer H, Bauer P, Nicolay C, et al. Omega-3 fatty acids and low carbohydrate diet for maintenance of remission in Crohn's disease. A randomized controlled multicenter trial. Study Group Members (German Crohn's Disease Study Group). *Scand J Gastroenterol.* 1996;31:778-785.

138. Reinshagen M, Flamig G, Ernst S, et al. Calcitonin gene-related peptide mediates the protective effect of sensory nerves in a model of colonic injury. *J Pharma Exp Ther.* 1998;286:657-661.

139. Koch TR, Carney JA, Morris VA, Go VL. Somatostatin in the idiopathic inflammatory bowel diseases. *Dis Colon Rectum.* 1988;31:198-203.

140. Reubi JC, Mazzucchelli L, Laissue JA. Intestinal vessels express a high density of somatostatin receptors in human inflammatory bowel disease. *Gastroenterology.* 1994;106:951-959.

141. Feher E, Kovacs A, Gallatz K, Feher J. Direct morphological evidence of neuroimmunomodulation in colonic mucosa of patients with Crohn's disease. *Neuroimmunomodulation.* 1997;4:250-257.

142. Neunlist M, Aubert P, Toquet C, et al. Changes in chemical coding of myenteric neurones in ulcerative colitis. *Gut.* 2003;52:84-90.

143. Lee CM, Kumar RK, Lubowski DZ, Burcher E. Neuropeptides and nerve growth in inflammatory bowel diseases: a quantitative immunohistochemical study. *Dig Dis Sci.* 2002;47:495-502.

144. Stucchi AF, Shebani KO, Leeman SE, et al. A neurokinin 1 receptor antagonist reduces an ongoing ileal pouch inflammation and the response to a subsequent inflammatory stimulus. *Am J Physiol Gastrointest Liver Physiol.* 2003;285:G1259-1267.

145. Renzi D, Pellegrini B, Tonelli F, Surrenti C, Calabro A. Substance P (neurokinin-1) and neurokinin A (neurokinin-2) receptor gene and protein expression in the healthy and inflamed human intestine. *Am J Pathol.* 2000;157:1511-1522.

146. Stucchi AF, Shofer S, Leeman S, et al. NK-1 antagonist reduces colonic inflammation and oxidative stress in dextran sulfate-induced colitis in rats. *Am J Physiol Gastrointest Liver Physiol.* 2000;279:G1298-1306.

147. Castagliuolo I, Morteau O, Keates AC, et al. Protective effects of neurokinin-1 receptor during colitis in mice: role of the epidermal growth factor receptor. *Br J Pharmacol.* 2002;136:271-279.

148. Weinstock JV, Blum A, Metwali A, Elliott D, Bunnett N, Arsenescu R. Substance P regulates Th1-type colitis in IL-10 knockout mice. *J Immunol.* 2003;171:3762-3767.

149. Moriarty D, Goldhill J, Selve N, O'Donoghue DP, Baird AW. Human colonic anti-secretory activity of the potent NK(1) antagonist, SR140333: assessment of potential anti-diarrhoeal activity in food allergy and inflammatory bowel disease. *Br J Pharmacol.* 2001;133:1346-1354.

150. Anton PA, Shanahan F. Neuroimmunomodulation in inflammatory bowel disease. How far from "bench" to "bedside"? *Ann NY Acad Sci.* 1998;840:723-734.

151. Castagliuolo I, Wang CC, Valenick L, et al. Neurotensin is a proinflammatory neuropeptide in colonic inflammation. *J Clin Invest.* 1999;103:843-849.

152. Lavy A, Weisz G, Adir Y, Ramon Y, Melamed Y, Eidelman S. Hyperbaric oxygen for perianal Crohn's disease. *J Clin Gastroenterol.* 1994;19:202-205.

153. Colombel JF, Mathieu D, Bouault JM, et al. Hyperbaric oxygenation in severe perineal Crohn's disease. *Dis Colon Rectum.* 1995;38:609-614.

154. Rachmilewitz D, Karmeli F, Okon E, Rubenstein I, Better OS. Hyperbaric oxygen: a novel modality to ameliorate experimental colitis. *Gut.* 1998;43:512-518.

155. Weisz G, Lavy A, Adir Y, et al. Modification of in vivo and in vitro TNF alpha, IL-1, and IL-6 secretion by circulating monocytes during hyperbaric oxygen treatment in patients with perianal Crohn's disease. *J Clin Immunol.* 1997;17:154-159.

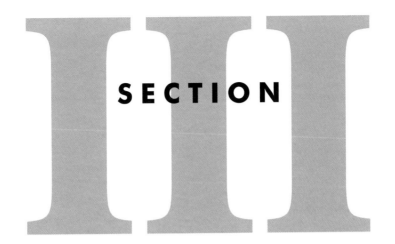

SECTION III

SPECIFIC CLINICAL SCENARIOS

ASSESSMENT OF DISEASE ACTIVITY IN CROHN'S DISEASE

Alain Bitton, MD, FRCP(C)

Crohn's disease is a chronic relapsing inflammatory bowel disorder characterized by periods of remission punctuated by acute episodes of symptomatic recurrence. Determining the extent and activity of CD remains the cornerstone of the medical and surgical management of this condition. Defining disease activity permits doctors to assess severity of illness, to monitor response to therapy, and possibly to predict the clinical course. Disease activity is best defined by the presence of active intestinal mucosal inflammation. Endoscopy and histology that provide direct evaluation of the mucosa are reliable indicators of gut inflammatory activity. However, endoscopy with or without biopsy is an invasive procedure, it is not always technically possible, and it does not permit the complete visualization of the small bowel. In addition, as a means to monitor disease activity, it is too costly and impractical. The ideal parameter of disease activity must be highly sensitive, be specific for gut inflammation, reflect disease severity and extent, be simple and rapid, be reproducible, and be available at a low cost. To date, no single parameter fulfills all these criteria.

A problem that arises when defining disease activity is the discrepancy between presence of bowel inflammation and patient well-being. Biologic, endoscopic, histologic, or radiologic indicators of inflammation that reflect ongoing intestinal disease activity may be heightened in patients who systemically feel otherwise well. The significance of these indicators in the context of subclinical disease is unclear although their increase may herald an impending clinical relapse. Furthermore, whether the normalization of these parameters (even if related to subclinical disease) should be a goal of therapy and whether this will alter the natural history of CD remains to be determined. Endoscopy (mucosal healing) has been associated with better outcomes such as decreased surgeries and hospitalizations in CD.

PARAMETERS OF DISEASE ACTIVITY

Various parameters have been evaluated as potential markers of disease activity (Table 21-1). It is difficult to navigate through the myriad parameters that have been assessed, given the heterogeneity of studies (different design, patient population, statistical and technical methodologies) and the sometimes conflicting results that are reported. Essentially, parameters of disease activity can be categorized as clinical, endoscopic, histologic, biologic, and radiologic. Many of these are intercorrelated, and all have advantages and disadvantages for use in clinical practice.

In this chapter, to be consistent, when referring to disease activity, the implication is that there is active intestinal mucosal inflammation. Most of the reports in the literature discussing CD activity have focused mainly on luminal CD. Perianal disease activity, to a lesser degree, has also been studied. This chapter will review evaluation of activity of both luminal and perianal CD.

LUMINAL DISEASE

CLINICAL PARAMETERS

Clinical parameters to be considered when evaluating CD activity include those relating to the inflammatory (ie, diarrhea, abdominal pain) and transmural nature (ie, obstruction, fistulas, phlegmon/abscess) of CD as well as extraintestinal manifestations and general well-being. A major difficulty when relying on clinical features is the nonspecificity of symptoms that can result from noninflammatory disorders. Irritable bowel syndrome (IBS) can occur in CD and can be responsible for a clinical picture compatible

Lichtenstein GR, ed.
Crohn's Disease: The Complete Guide to Medical Management (pp 251-266).
© 2011 SLACK Incorporated

TABLE 21-1

PARAMETERS USED TO ASSESS CROHN'S DISEASE ACTIVITY*

LUMINAL

CLINICAL INDICES

CDAI

Van Hees Index

Harvey-Bradshaw Index

Cape Town Index

Pediatric CDAI

ENDOSCOPIC INDICES

CDEIS

SES-CD

Postoperative CDEIS

HISTOLOGIC MARKERS

BIOLOGIC MARKERS

Serum

- C-reactive protein
- Erythrocyte sedimentation rate
- Orosomucoid
- B$_2$ microglobulin
- Soluble IL-2r, IL-6, TNFα

Fecal

- Calprotectin
- Lactoferrin
- α-1 Antitrypsin
- Indium-111

Intestinal permeability

RADIOLOGIC

Barium studies (SBFT, enteroclysis, enema)

Ultrasound/Doppler

Helical CT scan (abdominal, enteroclysis/enterography, colonography)

Magnetic resonance (abdominal, enteroclysis/enterography, colonography)

Leukocyte scintigraphy: Technetium-99m, Indium-111

PERIANAL

CLINICAL INDICES

PDAI

Fistula drainage score

RADIOLOGIC

Endoanal ultrasound

Magnetic resonance

*CDAI indicates Crohn's disease activity index; CDEIS, Crohn's disease endoscopic index of severity; SES-CD, Simple endoscopic score CD; PDAI, Perianal disease activity index; TNFα, tumor necrosis factor alpha; SBFT, small bowel follow-through ; CT, computed tomography

with active CD.[1] Superimposed carbohydrate intolerance, bacterial overgrowth, malabsorption, bile salt diarrhea, and fibrotic strictures can also all contribute to symptoms. Several clinical CD activity indices have been developed but are subject to a lack of sensitivity and specificity.

CLINICAL INDICES

The repeated attempts to develop clinical indices that quantify CD activity underscores the importance of having an accurate measure for the clinical management of CD patients. In the late 1970s and early 1980s, various indices reflecting CD activity were developed. Importantly, they have remained in use but mainly as efficacy outcomes for therapeutic clinical trials. These clinical indices, however, are subject to limitations. They are subject to interobserver variation when being calculated.[2] They were not developed for patients with ileostomies, colostomies, and extensive bowel resections. They consist in varying degrees of subjective parameters. In addition, these indices often show weak correlation when compared to surrogate markers of inflammation (serum or fecal) or to endoscopic or radiologic findings of disease activity.

CROHN'S DISEASE ACTIVITY INDEX

The Crohn's Disease Activity Index (CDAI) is an index that uses several clinical parameters to assess disease activity (Table 21-2). It was initially developed for and validated by the National Cooperative Crohn's Disease Study.[3,4] Data on 18 predictor variables were collected prospectively from 187 visits of 112 patients. Physicians recorded their overall evaluation of the patient's clinical status at each visit. Multiple regression analysis was used to derive an equation with 8 predictor variables of physicians' overall ratings: the CDAI. It consists of 8 items measured daily over the preceding 7 days. These include self-report of daily symptoms (ie, abdominal pain, diarrhea, well-being), extraintestinal manifestations, use of antidiarrheals, presence of an abdominal mass, hematocrit, and body weight. Each item is attributed a score. A global score is then computed. A score of less than 150 is considered remission and >450 severely active disease. Scores between 150 and 250 and between 250 and 400 correspond to mild to moderate and moderately active disease, respectively. A change of 70 points is considered to be clinically significant.[3] The CDAI coefficients were later rederived from 1058 patient visits and did not differ significantly from the original CDAI.[5]

The CDAI has several pitfalls. For the clinician, it may not be practical to arrange for patients to record information for 7 days prior to their office visit, and during a visit it may be too time consuming to collect the data and compute the score. Second, it consists of several subjective parameters that may be influenced by many factors other than inflammatory disease activity (eg, previous bowel resection, concurrent medication, patient's perception of well-being). CD patients may have concurrent irritable bowel syndrome, which contributes to an elevation of the CDAI score. In fact, patients with IBS alone may score above the remission score, based on their symptomatology. Patients with fibrostenotic disease may score high despite having no or minimal active inflammation. The CDAI may also be unreliable to detect recurrence following bowel resection.[6] Bile salt diarrhea and mucosal recurrence preceding symptomatic recurrence contribute to the lack of specificity and sensitivity in this setting. Despite these limitations, almost 35 years after its development, the CDAI remains the most widely used index in clinical trials.

A validated CDAI has also been developed to quantify CD activity in the pediatric population. The Pediatric Crohn's Disease Activity Index (PCDAI) assesses clinical parameters including abdominal pain, loose stools, general well-being, weight, height, abdominal exam, perirectal disease, extraintestinal manifestations, and laboratory parameters (including erythrocyte sedimentation rate (ESR), hematocrit, and albumin).[7]

HARVEY-BRADSHAW INDEX (THE SIMPLE INDEX)

The Harvey-Bradshaw Index (HBI) was derived from the CDAI and is the simplest of all indices. It consists of 5 clinical variables occurring within the previous 24 hours of an office visit (Table 21-3). These include well-being, abdominal pain, number of daily liquid stools, abdominal mass, and extraintestinal complications. The HBI correlates highly with the CDAI.[8]

CAPE TOWN INDEX

The Cape Town Index (CTI) was developed as a simple index that was not heavily driven by a single item such as diarrhea.[9] It consists of 10 items including symptoms, signs, and laboratory data (Table 21-4). Unlike the CDAI or HBI, items are not scored using absolute values but rather by ranking of the items. Each item is attributed a score of 0 to 3, with an overall score ranging from 0 to 30. The CTI, CDAI, and HBI correlate with each other.

VAN HEES INDEX

The Van Hees Index (VHI) was developed in follow-up to the CDAI in view of quantifying inflammatory activity based on more objective variables (Table 21-5).[10] Eighteen predictor variables were evaluated to determine which ones correlated best with physicians' overall evaluations of disease activity. Multiple stepwise regression analysis identified 9 variables. The VHI includes ESR, albumin, Quetelet Index, presence of abdominal mass, gender, fever, stool consistency, resection, and extraintestinal manifestations. Each item is attributed a score, and a global score is given. Scores less than 100 reflect inactive disease and greater than 210 indicate severe to very severe disease activity. Scores of 100 to 150 and 150 to 210 indicate mild and moderate inflammatory activity, respectively. The initial study by Van Hees et al[10] showed only moderate correlation between VHI and CDAI. This was explained by the fact that the VHI was based mainly on objective variables, whereas subjective variables weighed heavily in the CDAI.

HEALTH-RELATED QUALITY OF LIFE

Measuring health-related quality of life (HRQOL) is important in determining the effect of inflammatory bowel disease (IBD) and its treatment on patients' overall well-being. IBD patients' subjective perceptions of HRQOL may be affected compared to the general population. Clinical indices do not reflect well certain aspects

TABLE 21-2

CROHN'S DISEASE ACTIVITY INDEX (CDAI): FORMAT FOR HAND CALCULATION*

	Days	Sum	x	Factor	=	Subtotal
	1 2 3 4 5 6 7					
1. Number of liquid or very soft stools	— — — — — — —	_____	x	2	=	_____
2. Abdominal pain rating (0 = none, 1 = mild, 2 = moderate 3 = severe)	— — — — — — —	_____	x	5	=	_____
3. General well being (0 = gen. well, 1 = slightly under par, 2 = poor, 3 = very poor, 4 = terrible)	— — — — — — —	_____	x	7	=	_____
4. Number of 6 listed categories patient now has		_____	x	20	=	_____

Arthritis/arthralgia

Iritis/uveitis

Erythema nodosum/pyoderma/gangrenosum/aphthous stomatitis

Anal fissure, fistula, or abscess

Other fistula

Fever >100° F during the past week

		Sum	x	Factor	=	Subtotal
5. Taking lomotil/opiates for diarrhea (0=no, 1=yes)		_____	x	30	=	_____
6. Abdominal mass (0=none, 2=questionable, 5=definite)		_____	x	10	=	_____
7. Hematocrit: _____	Males (47-crit) Female (42-crit) Subtotal	_____	x	6	=	_____
8. Body weight:_____ Standard weight: _____ units (1 = lbs, 2 = kg): _____						
Percent below standard weight (nomogram):		_____	x	1	=	_____
Add (underweight) or subtract (overweight) by sign, to give CDAI					=	_____

*Adapted from Best WR, Becktel JM, Singleton JW, Kern F Jr. Development of a Crohn's disease activity index. National Cooperative Crohn's Disease Study. *Gastroenterology.* 1976;70:439-444.

TABLE 21-3

HARVEY-BRADSHAW INDEX (SIMPLE INDEX)*

A. General well-being   0 = very well,   1 = slightly below par,   2 = poor,   3 = very poor,   4 = terrible

B. Abdominal pain: 0 = none,   1 = mild,   2 = moderate,   3 = severe

C. Number of liquid stools per day

D. Abdominal mass: 0 = none,   1 = dubious,   2 = definite,   3 = definite and tender

E. Complications: Arthralgia, uveitis, erythema nodosum, aphthous ulcers, pyoderma gangrenosum, anal fissure, new fistula, abscess   (Score 1 per item)

(Sum of all item scores = overall score)

*Adapted from Harvey RF, Bradshaw JM. A simple index of Crohn's-disease activity. *Lancet*. 1980;1:514.

TABLE 21-4

THE CAPE TOWN INDEX (SOUTH AFRICAN INDEX)*

ITEM	SCORE			
	0	1	2	3
Diarrhea (# stools/day)	None	≤ 4	5	≥ 6
Abdominal pain	None	Mild	Moderate	Severe
Well-being	Normal	Below par	Unwell	Terrible
Complications				
Local	None	Skin tag	Sinus	Fistula
Systemic	None	Stomatitis Iritis	Arthralgia	Arthritis Iritis Erythema nodosum
Fever (°C)	Normal (≤ 37)	≤ 38	≤ 39	> 39
Weight vs last weight	No change	No change	< 95%	< 90%
Abdominal exam				
Mass	None	None	Indefinite	Certain
Tenderness	None	Mild	Moderate	Severe
Hemoglobin (g/L)	≥ 120	< 120	< 110	< 100
†ESR (mm/first hour)	≤ 15	> 15	> 25	> 40

*Adapted with permission from Wright JP, Marks IN, Parfitt A. A simple clinical index of Crohn's disease activity—the Cape Town index. *S Afr Med J*. 1985;68:502-503.

†Common indicator of inflammation but not included in the original index.

TABLE 21-5

VAN HEES ACTIVITY INDEX*†

VARIABLE		
X_1	Serum albumin	g/L
X_2	ESR	mm after first hour
X_3	Quetelet index	W/H2‡
X_4	Abdominal mass	1 = absent, 2 = dubious, 3 = diameter <6 cm, 4 = diameter 6 to 12 cm, 5 = diameter > 12 cm
X_5	Gender	1 = male, 2 = female
X_6	Temperature	Mean daily (°C) of last week
X_7	Stool consistency	1 = well-formed, 2 = soft, variable, 3 = watery
X_8	Resection	1 = no, 2 = yes
X_9	Extraintestinal lesions	1 = no, 2 = yes

Total score = $-209 - 5.48(X_1) + 0.29(X_2) - 0.22(X_3) + 7.83(X_4) - 1.23(X_5) + 16.4(X_6) + 8.46(X_7) - 9.17(X_8) + 10.7(X_9)$

*ESR indicates erythrocyte sedimentation rate.

†Adapted from Van Hees PA, Van Elteren PH, Van Lier HJ, van Tongeren JH. An index of inflammatory activity in patients with Crohn's disease. *Gut.* 1980;21:279-286.

‡Weight (kg) x 10, Height (cm^2)

that define quality of life (ie, psychological and social). Several generic questionnaires assessing HRQOL exist. A validated disease-specific Inflammatory Bowel Disease Questionnaire (IBDQ) has been designed to appraise quality of life in IBD patients.[11,12] It is commonly used in clinical trials as a secondary outcome when assessing a drug's efficacy. The IBDQ is a 32-item tool that asks questions in 4 domains (social, emotional, bowel, and systemic). Each item is scored from 1 to 7, with a maximum total score of 224. High scores correspond to better quality of life. The IBDQ was not developed to measure inflammatory activity of CD but rather to quantify a patient's perception of health and function.

ENDOSCOPIC PARAMETERS

Endoscopy with biopsies remains the gold standard for assessing mucosal inflammatory activity in CD. The inaccessibility to small bowel segments and the inability to assess transmural and extraluminal involvement are limitations of endoscopy. The advent of wireless capsule endos-

copy provides a complete evaluation of the small bowel, potentially overcoming the problem of inaccessibility.

ILEOCOLONOSCOPY

Whereas the primary goal of CD therapy has long been symptom relief, better understanding of the importance of mucosal lesions is shifting the therapeutic goal toward one of complete mucosal healing. It is therefore important to have a standardized and reproducible means of quantifying endoscopic activity. An endoscopic index of CD severity in patients with colonic involvement was developed and validated prospectively by the Groupes D'Etudes Thérapeutiques des Affections Inflammatoires du Tube Digestif (GETAID) group.[13] The authors collected prospective endoscopic (using fiberoptic colonoscopies) findings in 75 patients and assessed 9 preselected lesions in various colonic segments and in the ileum. Data on extent of disease were also obtained. A stepwise multiple regression selected independent variables that were correlated with the endoscopists' global evaluation of lesion severity.

TABLE 21-6

POSTOPERATIVE CROHN'S DISEASE ENDOSCOPIC INDEX OF SEVERITY*

GRADE	LESIONS
0	None
1	≤ 5 Aphthous lesions
2	> 5 Aphthous lesions with normal mucosa between, or skip areas of larger lesions or lesions confined to ileocolonic anastomosis (<1 cm in length)
3	Diffuse aphthous ileitis with diffusely inflamed mucosa
4	Diffuse ileitis with large ulcers, nodules, and/or narrowing

*For endoscopic lesions in the neoterminal ileum. Adapted from Rutgeerts P, Geboes K, Vantrappen G, Beyls J, Kerremans R, Hiele M. Predictability of the postoperative course of Crohn's disease. Gastroenterology. 1990;99:956-963.

The Crohn's Disease Endoscopic Index of Severity (CDEIS) consists of 6 weighted item scores. These include mucosal abnormalities of superficial and deep ulcerations, ulcerated and nonulcerated stenosis, and estimates of surface involved by the disease and involved by ulcerations only. This index may be too time consuming to calculate in regular clinical practice but serves as an outcome measure in clinical trials. A simpler, validated endoscopic score of severity, the Simple Endoscopic Score (SES-CD), has been developed. It is highly correlated with the CDEIS and lends itself better to clinical use.[14]

POSTOPERATIVE ILEOCOLONOSCOPY

In the postoperative setting, the CDAI may not accurately reflect CD disease activity.[6] Endoscopy remains the best parameter to assess postsurgical mucosal activity. The postoperative CDEIS was developed to quantify the severity of endoscopic recurrence in patients who had undergone ileal/ileocolic resection with ileocolic anastomosis (Table 21-6).[15] This index has been used commonly in postoperative maintenance drug trials in which endoscopic recurrence served as an outcome. Grade 2 to 4 endoscopic grade has been shown to be predictive of earlier clinical relapse.[15]

SMALL BOWEL ENDOSCOPY, WIRELESS CAPSULE ENDOSCOPY

The small bowel has long been an area of the gastrointestinal tract not readily amenable to complete endoscopic visualization. Push and sonde enteroscopy are invasive with a risk of perforation and often provide incomplete visualization of the small bowel. Intraoperative enteroscopy introduces risks of laparotomy and general anesthesia. Wireless capsule endoscopy (WCE) represents an important technological advancement that allows for live imaging of the small intestine with a video capsule. Patients with suspected small bowel strictures are excluded from study with WCE. Small trials have shown its superiority in detecting extent of active CD over barium studies, push enteroscopy, and computed tomography (CT) enteroclysis.[16-18] One study in patients with known CD reported a strong correlation between WCE and small bowel follow-through (SBFT), with neither of these correlating with clinical (Harvey-Bradshaw Index) or biological indices (C-reactive protein [CRP], erythrocyte sedimentation rate [ESR], fecal alpha-1 antitrypsin) of disease activity.[19] A recent meta-analysis reported a significantly higher diagnostic yield in patients with established CD, when compared to CT enterography, push enteroscopy, or SBFT.[20] Larger prospective studies comparing WCE with clinical activity indices, conventional SBFT, or enteroclysis, CT or MR enterography, or ileoscopy are needed to define the role of WCE in assessing disease activity. Nonetheless, in well-established CD, WCE will likely have an important role in determining extent of small bowel involvement and assessing for activity in symptomatic patients whose radiologic tests or ileoscopy are negative or show minimal disease. A WCE index of severity that can quantify small bowel involvement has recently been developed.[21]

HISTOLOGIC ACTIVITY

Histologic abnormalities can persist despite endoscopic normalization of mucosa following medical therapy.[22] This suggests that histology may be a more sensitive marker of mucosal inflammatory activity; however, mucosal biopsies may not reliably reflect disease activity because of the focality and inhomogeneous involvement of tissue in CD. In addition, CD (being a disease characterized primarily by ulceration) may be better evaluated by endoscopy. A histologic score for CD colitis showed no correlation with clinical or laboratory indices.[23] A histologic scoring system of severity of mucosal biopsies in the neoterminal ileum following resective surgery for CD has been used and requires further validation.[24]

BIOLOGIC MARKERS

There is a constellation of biologic markers that have been proposed as indicators of inflammatory disease activity. These markers are attractive because they are minimally invasive and in some instances not costly. However, they are subject to limitations. They may not adequately reflect disease severity in the subgroup of patients with primarily fibrostenotic disease. They do not specifically reflect the degree of inflammation at the mucosal level, although those measured in stool may better reflect this. They often poorly correlate with each other and with endoscopy.[23] Finally, they may not be readily available to clinicians. Acute phase proteins, markers of immune activation, intestinal permeability, and fecal markers have been studied.

ACUTE PHASE PROTEINS

Acute phase proteins are synthesized by the liver in response to an acute inflammatory stimulus and as such are not specific to inflammatory bowel disease. Nonetheless, their role as markers of disease activity has been studied.

C-REACTIVE PROTEIN

C-reactive protein (CRP) has been used as a parameter of activity in various conditions including IBD, autoimmune diseases, rheumatological diseases, and cardiovascular disease. Although not specific, it has been used reliably as a marker of disease activity in CD when compared to standard clinical indices including the CDAI.[25,26] Patients in clinical remission who have higher CRPs have been shown to be at increased risk of earlier clinical relapse.[27] Thus, CRP can help monitor disease activity and predict clinical course. CRP remains an attractive marker because it is simple to measure, inexpensive, and widely available to clinicians.

OROSOMUCOID (α-1 ACID GLYCOPROTEIN) AND SERUM AMYLOID A

Serum orosomucoid and serum amyloid A are acute phase proteins that, like CRP, are nonspecific for IBD but have been reported to correlate with CD activity as evaluated by standard clinical indices.[28-31]

ERYTHROCYTE SEDIMENTATION RATE

Erythrocyte sedimentation rate (ESR) has been used for many years as a marker of IBD activity. However, studies evaluating the usefulness of ESR as such are inconsistent. Two studies reported a positive correlation with active large but not small bowel CD, whereas other studies showed no correlation with disease activity.[28,32-34] These conflicting reports make ESR a less reliable marker of disease activity.

β_2 MICROGLOBULIN

β_2 microglobulin is a low-molecular-weight protein released from activated lymphocytes. It has been assessed as a marker of disease activity. Early studies reported conflicting results with positive[35,36] and negative correlations[37] between circulating levels of β_2 microglobulin and CD activity. A more recent study showed levels of β_2 microglobulin correlated with activity and extent of CD.[38]

MARKERS OF IMMUNE ACTIVATION

Crohn's disease is characterized by a heightened activation of T cells and an increase in inflammatory cells in the intestinal mucosa. Traditionally, CD has been viewed as a type 1 T-helper cell (Th-1)-mediated immune response with an increase in proinflammatory cytokines. Much research has focused on the role of cytokines in the pathogenesis of CD. The possibility that serum cytokines may be more specific and better reflect CD activity has led to their evaluation as markers of disease activity.

Tumor necrosis factor alpha (TNFα) is a proinflammatory cytokine secreted by activated macrophages and monocytes that plays a pivotal role in the immunopathogenesis of CD. Both serum levels and fecal excretion of TNFα have been reported to correlate with CD activity, but this has been inconsistent.[39-41] Urinary excretion of soluble TNFα receptors p55 and p75 shows promise as an indicator of CD activity but requires further study.[42]

Soluble interleukin-2 receptor (sIL-2R) is an indicator of systemic immune activation and may indirectly reflect intestinal inflammation. Some studies have shown correlation between serum sIL-2R and disease activity when compared to standard clinical indices.[43-45]

Serum levels of interleukin-6 (IL-6), a proinflammatory cytokine, are elevated in active CD.[46,47] Interleukin-6 was found to correlate with patients who had a primarily inflammatory type of CD behavior.[47] Interleukin-6 is involved in the acute phase response to inflammation, so it is highly correlated with CRP.[46,47] Much like CRP, it is not specific for bowel inflammation. Given its correlation with CRP, it would likely not provide any additional information as a parameter of disease activity.

Adhesion molecules are important for the adherence and trafficking of leukocytes into areas of tissue inflammation. Serum soluble intercellular adhesion molecule-1 (sICAM-1) concentrations have been reported to be increased in active CD and to correlate with serum orosomucoid and CRP levels.[48,49] One study, however, showed a negative correlation between sICAM-1 and CD activity.[50]

FECAL MARKERS

Fecal markers have been assessed as surrogate markers of intestinal inflammation. They may be useful when differentiating IBS from IBD. They have been evaluated as indicators of gut inflammation and seem to correlate with CD activity. Several markers studied to date appear to be sensitive but not necessarily specific for CD given their increase in non-IBD inflammatory conditions such as infections. Stool markers may also be useful in predicting the clinical course in patients with medically or surgically induced clinical remissions. They may also be useful for monitoring response to medical therapy. They are noninvasive and may prove to be cost effective.[51]

FECAL LEUKOCYTES

Microscopic examination of stool for leukocytes has been studied mainly to detect infectious causes of diarrhea; nonetheless, they may reflect active IBD.[52]

FECAL CALPROTECTIN

Calprotectin is a calcium-binding protein found in the cytoplasm of neutrophils. Its presence in stool reflects an inflammatory bowel process. In IBD, it correlates well with fecal excretion of indium-111 labeled leukocytes.[53] Calprotectin can be measured using a commercially available enzyme-linked immunosorbent assay (ELISA) kit on a spot stool sample. High levels in CD patients correlate with disease activity as defined by standard clinical indices.[54] Fecal calprotectin has been shown to correlate with endoscopic disease activity as measured by the CDEIS and SES-CD.[55-57] Furthermore, elevated fecal calprotectin levels seem to predict subsequent relapse in patients with quiescent CD.[58]

FECAL α_1-ANTITRYPSIN AND LACTOFERRIN

Fecal clearance of α_1-antitrypsin (AAT) reflects protein loss from the gut and indirectly indicates ongoing bowel inflammation.[59] Random fecal concentration or fecal clearance of AAT (fecal volume x fecal AAT concentration ÷ by serum AAT) are increased in active CD as defined by CDAI.[60-62] Stool AAT may also correlate with anatomic extent of disease and predict relapse in asymptomatic patients with ileal CD.[63,64]

Lactoferrin, a neutrophil-derived protein, may also be a useful measure of intestinal inflammation. One study reported a correlation between fecal lactoferrin and CD activity as evaluated by the HBI.[65] As with calprotectin, fecal lactoferrin has been shown to correlate well with the CDEIS and SES-S and may be useful as a predictor of clinical relapse in quiescent CD.[55-57,66]

ANTI-SACCHAROMYCES CEREVISIAE ANTIBODY

Anti-*Saccharomyces cerevisiae* antibody (ASCA) is an antibody to baker's and brewer's yeast used as a potential diagnostic marker for CD. The sensitivity of ASCA for CD ranges from 41% to 76% and can vary based on the type of assay used.[67] There is no clear correlation between serum titers of ASCA and disease activity, although a recent pediatric study reported such a correlation.[68] Because of its relatively low sensitivity for CD, it will have a limited role, if any, in providing information on disease activity.

INTESTINAL PERMEABILITY

A primary or secondary defect in intestinal permeability (IP) has been proposed as a mechanism contributing to the pathogenesis of IBD. An abnormal intestinal epithelial barrier may lead to entrance of noxious antigens into the gut wall, which in turn trigger and perpetuate the inflammatory response. A variety of probes have been used to measure IP including lactulose, polyethylene glycol 400, and (51)Cr-labelled ethylenediaminetetraacetic acid (CrEDTA).[51] IP has been associated with active disease and in some instances has been shown to predict CD relapse.[69-73] Measuring intestinal permeability is a somewhat complex test for the patient who must follow strict instructions (ie, avoiding alcohol, nonsteroidal antiinflammatory drugs [NSAIDs]), drink the test solution, and collect an overnight urine. It also requires a laboratory familiar with the methodology for the measurements. For these reasons, it is unlikely to gain wide use in monitoring for disease activity.

RADIOLOGIC MARKERS

Several radiologic modalities have been used to help diagnose and define CD activity and extent (Table 21-7). Traditionally, barium studies of the small and large bowel were the main modalities used to assess mucosal CD. Advances and refinements in ultrasonography, CT, magnetic resonance imaging (MRI), and leukocyte scintigraphy provide enhanced imaging of transmural and extramural CD. Conventional radiologic exams and cross-sectional imaging are complementary and as such are better suited to assess disease activity.[74]

BARIUM STUDIES

Barium contrast studies including upper gastrointestinal series, SBFT, enteroclysis, and barium enema have been the mainstay of diagnostic imaging in CD for many years, providing information on mucosal abnormalities, disease extent, and location. Findings in CD include ulceration, cobblestoning, presence of fistula, and strictures. Enteroclysis, in which barium followed by methylcellulose or air is administered via a nasojejunal tube, as well as double-contrast barium enema may provide more information on mucosal detail than standard SBFT and single-contrast barium enema, respectively. Barium studies, however, do not reliably reflect disease activity as assessed by ileocolonoscopy or clinical parameters.[75-77] In addition, the use of barium exams is limited due to their inability to detect mural and extraluminal complications and their inability to differentiate fibrotic from inflammatory disease activity.

CONVENTIONAL, DOPPLER, AND CONTRAST-ENHANCED ULTRASONOGRAPHY

Bowel wall thickness and length of involvement determined by conventional ultrasound (US) have been used as an indirect measure of disease activity and extent. Bowel wall thickness seems to be unreliable, showing weak or no concordance with clinical (CDAI) or laboratory parameters (CRP, ESR)[78,79] of disease activity. This may be due to the inability to differentiate wall thickness due to inflammation from fibrosis.[80] However, combining conventional US with Doppler may be more accurate in identifying active CD.[80]

TABLE 21-7

RADIOLOGIC MODALITIES FOR ASSESSING LUMINAL (SMALL AND LARGE BOWEL) CROHN'S DISEASE ACTIVITY*

	FINDINGS	ADVANTAGES	DISADVANTAGES
Barium studies	• Ulceration, cobblestoning • Strictures, fistula • Fold thickening • Peristalsis, distensibility	• Inexpensive	• Radiation exposure • Operator-dependent
Small bowel follow-through (SBFT)	—	—	—
Barium enteroclysis	—	• Superior to SBFT for mucosal details and stricture	• More invasive than SBFT • Greater radiation exposure
Barium enema (double contrast)	—	—	—
Ultrasound	• Thickened bowel wall • Phlegmon, abscess	• Inexpensive • No radiation • Readily available	• Operator-dependent • No mucosal detail
Doppler	• Hyperdynamic SMA flow parameters • Bowel wall vascularity	• Inexpensive • No radiation • Readily available	• Operator-dependent • No mucosal detail
Ultrasound and Doppler combined	—	• Superior to either modality alone	—
Contrast enhanced	• Quantitative measurement of bowel wall vascularity	• Better correlation with endoscopy	• IV contrast exposure
Helical CT scan/magnetic resonance imaging	• Bowel wall thickening • Wall contrast enhancement • Strictures, fistula • Mesenteric fibrofatty proliferation, adenopathy, and hypervascularity • Phlegmon, abscess	• Detects mural, extramural disease • Can assess large and small bowel • MRI avoids radiation	• Cost • Radiation and IV contrast exposure with HCT • Not possible in all patients and restricted availability for MRI
HCT/MRI enteroclysis/enterography	—	• Luminal distension allows better delineation of diseased bowel • May detect mucosal changes	• Enteroclysis more invasive than enterography with oral contrast
HCT/MRI colonography		• Detects strictures and intraluminal elevations	• Will not reliably detect mild colonic inflammation

*SMA indicates superior mesenteric artery; CT, computed tomography; IV, intravenous; HCT, helical CT scan; MRI, magnetic resonance imaging.

Doppler ultrasonography takes advantage of the hyperdynamic and neohypervascularization state that occurs with IBD. Superior mesenteric artery (SMA) blood flow quantified by Doppler was shown to be increased in active CD as determined by standard clinical scores[81,82] and in 1 small study correlated with enteroclysis.[83] Superior mesenteric artery flow, however, was found to correlate poorly with endoscopic findings in 1 trial.[82] A subsequent prospective study suggested that SMA Doppler was an unreliable tool to assess disease activity because of the overlap of flow parameters in active and inactive CD and should not be used routinely in clinical practice.[84]

Highly sensitive color Doppler, which assesses bowel wall vascularization, is another ultrasonographic tool that may prove useful in determining CD activity. This modality combined with ultrasonography was found to correlate well with ileocolonoscopic findings in CD.[85]

Small intestine contrast ultrasonography in which a patient is given oral contrast may improve the diagnostic accuracy of US, but its correlation with disease activity remains to be determined.[74] More recently, the addition of IV contrast to ultrasonography has provided quantitative measurements of the microvascularity of the bowel wall with good correlation with CT, MR enterography, and severity of endoscopy.[86,87] In a small series, contrast-enhanced ultrasonography correlated well with CDAI and showed greater sensitivity than conventional ultrasound or power Doppler ultrasound for detecting CD inflammatory activity.[88]

COMPUTED TOMOGRAPHY

Standard and helical CT scanning of the abdomen have been used in CD to detect mural and extramural complications such as abscesses or phlegmons. Post-IV contrast wall enhancement and mesenteric abnormalities (fibrofatty proliferation, hypervascularity, adenopathy) seem to be the most reliable indicators of inflammatory activity.[89] Bowel wall thickening may reflect disease activity less well, although 1 study demonstrated a correlation between patterns of bowel wall thickening and laboratory activity.[90] Another study in CD reported a sensitivity of 68% and specificity of 100% for detection of active CD inflammation using endoscopy and surgery as the gold standard.[91] Correlation between CT and surgery-endoscopy for segmental inflammation in CD was high in this study.[91]

More recently, helical CT-enteroclysis (HCTE) has been used for diagnosis and detection of active small bowel CD. The procedure consists of a helical CT combined with contrast administered through a nasojejunal tube placed under fluoroscopy. This provides distension and opacification of the small bowel so that HCTE can better delineate diseased bowel wall segments than CT alone. One study of 39 patients with established or suspected ileal CD who underwent HCTE and ileocolonoscopy[92] reported a sensitivity and specificity for detecting ileal CD with HCTE

of 86.7% and 100%, respectively, in patients without prior surgery. Post-IV contrast wall density was significantly correlated with clinical severity. CT enterography in which patients ingest oral contrast avoids the use of a nasojejunal tube making the examination more tolerable. CT enterography seems as effective as HCTE in identifying active small bowel CD.[93] CT colonography, which assesses the colon by sectional volume imaging data with the added possibility of reconstructing 3D models using specific computer software, has proven useful for detection of polyps. When compared to endoscopy, CT colonography has a similar sensitivity for elevated lesions but poorly detects mucosal ulcerations.[94]

MAGNETIC RESONANCE IMAGING

The ability to view the small and large bowel, to obtain dynamic and coronal images, and to detect transmural and extramural involvement while avoiding radiation exposure make MRI an attractive radiologic alternative in IBD. Most MRI studies of the small bowel are performed with oral contrast for bowel opacification (MRI enterography). The main parameters used to assess disease activity on MRI include length and thickness of inflamed bowel wall, mesenteric involvement, and mural contrast enhancement.[95-97] Good correlation of CDAI, SBFT, endoscopy, and leukocyte scintigraphy with MRI of the large and small bowel was reported in 1 study.[98] Small studies have shown a positive correlation between bowel wall contrast enhancement on MRI and histologic and endoscopic evaluations of CD activity.[99,100] One study reported a significant correlation between CDIES of bowel segments and MR findings.[101] MRI enterograph following oral ingestion of a 2.5% mannitol solution correlated poorly with CDAI and CRP in a prospective study but was useful in differentiating fibrotic from inflammatory strictures.[102] Recent small prospective studies have reported similar sensitivities for MR and CT enterography in detecting active small bowel CD.[103,104] MRI enteroclysis is also being evaluated in CD. Presence of deep ulceration, small bowel wall thickening, and enhancement of mesenteric lymph nodes were reported as the best indicators of CD activity as assessed by CDAI.[105] Virtual MR colonography has also been assessed. When compared to conventional colonoscopy, MR colonography was able to detect severe but not mild CD inflammation with an overall sensitivity for CD per segment of colon of 31.6%.[106]

LEUKOCYTE SCINTIGRAPHY

Nuclear scintigraphy with radiolabeled leukocytes has been used to quantify CD inflammatory activity.[107] This technique may also be useful in locating the site of disease. Indium-111 (In-111) and technetium-99m (Tc-99) hexamethyl propylene amine oxime (HMPAO) are commonly used radionuclides. These agents accumulate at sites of inflammation that are demonstrated on nuclear scans. Fecal excretion of In-111 may be a more sensitive

TABLE 21-8

PERIANAL CROHN'S DISEASE ACTIVITY INDEX*

ITEM	SCORE
1. Discharge	0 = none, 1 = minimal mucous, 2 = moderate mucous/purulent, 3 = substantial, 4 = fecal soiling
2. Pain/restriction of activities	0 = none/none, 1 = mild/none, 2 = moderate/some, 3 = marked/marked, 4 = severe/severe
3. Restriction of sexual activity	0 = none, 1 = slight, 2 = moderate, 3 = marked, 4 = unable to engage in sexual activity
4. Type of perianal disease	0 = none/skin tags, 1 = fissure/mucosal tear, 2 = < 3 fistulae, 3 = $\geq$ 3 fistulae, 4 = anal sphincter ulceration/fistulae with significant skin undermining
5. Degree of induration	0 = none, 1 = minimal, 2 = moderate, 3 = substantial, 4 = gross fluctuance/abscess

*Adapted with permission from Irvine EJ. Usual therapy improves perianal Crohn's disease as measured by a new disease activity index. McMaster IBD Study Group. *J Clin Gastroenterol.* 1995;20:27-32.

indicator of inflammatory disease activity.[108] It correlates well with endoscopy and histology but is a more laborious technique.[109] Studies have shown good correlation between leukocyte scintigraphy and endoscopy in CD, although this correlation may be highest with more severe endoscopic lesions.[110,111] Scintigraphy can also identify abscesses and usually can differentiate these from inflamed bowel wall.[112] Sensitivities and specificities for detecting active CD of 76% to 95% and 80% to 100%, respectively, have been reported with Tc-99 scanning.[110,113,114] Although noninvasive, scintigraphy has its limitations, including cost, availability, and radiation exposure.

PERIANAL DISEASE

Perianal complications of CD include anal ulcers, fissures, fistulas, and abscesses. Exam under general anesthesia has long been considered the standard for evaluation of perianal disease. Both clinical and radiologic modalities have been used to describe and quantify the severity of perianal disease.

PERIANAL DISEASE ACTIVITY INDEX

The presence of a perianal fistula is one of the parameters used in the calculation of the CDAI; however, the CDAI does not provide information on the severity of this perianal complication and therefore cannot be used to assess fistula activity. A perianal disease activity index (PDAI) has been developed but not evaluated in clinical studies.[115] The instrument assesses 5 categories relating to fistulas including discharge, pain/restriction of activities, restriction of sexual activity, type of perianal disease, and degree of duration (Table 21-8). Each category has a score ranging from 0 to 4. Higher scores reflect more severe disease. The absolute score defining perianal disease remission has not been clearly determined. There is poor correlation between the PDAI and CDAI.[115] Recently, the fistula drainage assessment was developed and used in 2 therapeutic drug trials in fistulizing CD.[116,117] This classification describes fistulas as closed or opened and draining.

RADIOLOGY: MRI, CT SCAN, AND ANORECTAL ENDOSONOGRAPHY

Advances in radiologic imaging have contributed to the improved evaluation of perianal disease and to monitoring response to therapy. Endoscopic ultrasound (EUS), helical CT scan, and MRI are radiologic modalities used commonly in the evaluation of perianal CD.[118,119] EUS and MRI are superior to CT scan for the delineation of perianal fistula. EUS offers a clear depiction of fistulous tracts; however, it is operator dependent. EUS may be more sensitive and specific than MRI for anal abscesses and complex fistulas.[120] One study on MRI, EUS, and exam under general anesthesia reported that the combination of 2 of these 3 modalities was the best approach to assessing perianal fistulas.[121]

CONCLUSION

Accurately defining CD activity is crucial to initiating a therapeutic strategy and to monitoring response to treatment. It is not always sufficient to rely on clinical indices to quantify disease activity, because of their lack of sensitivity and specificity to detect bowel inflammation. The

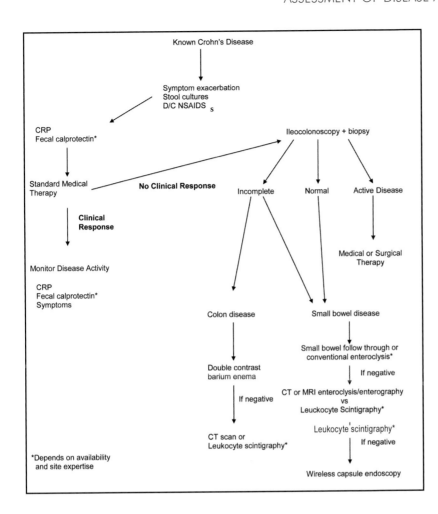

FIGURE 21-1. Proposed algorithm for evaluation of disease activity in the management of Crohn's disease. NSAIDs indicates nonsteroidal antiinflammatory drugs; CRP, C-reactive protein; CT, computed tomography; MRI, magnetic resonance imaging.

patient with established CD who has ongoing symptoms that do not improve with standard therapy proves challenging and requires an approach that will lead to a clear appraisal of disease activity (Figure 21-1). Mucosal evaluation by endoscopy and histology should be considered the gold standard for assessing and monitoring inflammatory disease activity but is not always possible and practical. A large number of biomarkers, both in the serum and in the stool, may be helpful. Fecal excretion of markers may have the theoretical advantage of directly reflecting gut inflammation. Refinements in ultrasonography with Doppler, MRI, and CT scanning add to the armamentarium of tools that can be employed in assessing disease activity. Overall, the accurate assessment of CD activity has remained a challenge due to the plethora of parameters that have been studied and that often weakly correlate with each other. A simple, standardized, and reproducible means of accurately determining CD activity encompassing clinical, biologic, radiologic, and endoscopic parameters is needed. Advances in technology and insight into the pathogenesis of CD will render this objective realizable in the near future.

REFERENCES

1. Minderhoud IM, Oldenburg B, Wismeijer JA, van Berge Henegouwen GP, Smout AJ. IBS-like symptoms in patients with inflammatory bowel disease in remission; relationships with quality of life and coping behavior. *Dig Dis Sci.* 2004;49:469-474.

2. De Dombal FT, Softley A. IOIBD report no 1: observer variation in calculating indices of severity and activity in Crohn's disease. International Organisation for the Study of Inflammatory Bowel Disease. *Gut.* 1987;28:474-481.

3. Best WR, Becktel JM, Singleton JW, Kern F Jr. Development of a Crohn's disease activity index. National Cooperative Crohn's Disease Study. *Gastroenterology.* 1976;70:439-444.

4. Summers RW, Switz DM, Sessions JT Jr, et al. National Cooperative Crohn's Disease Study: results of drug treatment. *Gastroenterology.* 1979;77:847-869.

5. Best WR, Becktel JM, Singleton JW. Rederived values of the eight coefficients of the Crohn's Disease Activity Index (CDAI). *Gastroenterology.* 1979;77:843-846.

6. Viscido A, Corrao G, Taddei G, Caprilli R. "Crohn's disease activity index" is inaccurate to detect the post-operative recurrence in Crohn's disease. A GISC study. Gruppo Italiano per lo Studio del Colon e del Retto. *Ital J Gastroenterol Hepatol.* 1999;31:274-279.

7. Hyams JS, Ferry GD, Mandel FS, et al. Development and validation of a pediatric Crohn's disease activity index. *J Pediatr Gastroenterol Nutr.* 1991;12:439-447.

8. Harvey RF, Bradshaw JM. A simple index of Crohn's-disease activity. *Lancet.* 1980;1:514.

9. Wright JP, Marks IN, Parfitt A. A simple clinical index of Crohn's disease activity—the Cape Town index. *S Afr Med J.* 1985;68:502-503.

10. Van Hees PA, Van Elteren PH, Van Lier HJ, van Tongeren JH. An index of inflammatory activity in patients with Crohn's disease. *Gut.* 1980;21:279-286.

11. Guyatt G, Mitchell A, Irvine EJ, et al. A new measure of health status for clinical trials in inflammatory bowel disease. *Gastroenterology*. 1989;96:804-810.

12. Irvine EJ, Feagan B, Rochon J, et al. Quality of life: a valid and reliable measure of therapeutic efficacy in the treatment of inflammatory bowel disease. Canadian Crohn's Relapse Prevention Trial Study Group. *Gastroenterology*. 1994;106:287-296.

13. Mary JY, Modigliani R. Development and validation of an endoscopic index of the severity for Crohn's disease: a prospective multicentre study. Groupe d'Etudes Therapeutiques des Affections Inflammatoires du Tube Digestif (GETAID). *Gut*. 1989;30:983-989.

14. Daperno M, D'Haens G, Van Assche G, et al. Development and validation of a new, simplified endoscopic activity score for Crohn's disease: the SES-CD. *Gastrointest Endosc*. 2004;60(4):505-512.

15. Rutgeerts P, Geboes K, Vantrappen G, Beyls J, Kerremans R, Hiele M. Predictability of the postoperative course of Crohn's disease. *Gastroenterology*. 1990;99:956-963.

16. Eliakim R, Suissa A, Yassin K, Katz D, Fischer D. Wireless capsule video endoscopy compared to barium follow-through and computerised tomography in patients with suspected Crohn's disease—final report. *Dig Liver Dis*. 2004;36:519-522.

17. Voderholzer WA, Beinhoelzl J, Rogalla P, et al. Small bowel involvement in Crohn's disease: a prospective comparison of wireless capsule endoscopy and computed tomography enteroclysis. *Gut*. 2005;54:369-373.

18. Chong AK, Taylor A, Miller A, Hennessy O, Connell W, Desmond P. Capsule endoscopy versus push enteroscopy and enteroclysis in suspected small-bowel Crohn's disease. *Gastrointest Endosc*. 2005; 61:255-261.

19. Buchman AL, Miller FH, Wallin A, Chowdhry AA, Ahn C. Videocapsule endoscopy versus barium contrast studies for the diagnosis of Crohn's disease recurrence involving the small intestine. *Am J Gastroenterol*. 2004;99:2171-2177.

20. Dionisio PM, Gurudu SR, Leighton JA, et al. Capsule endoscopy has a significantly higher diagnostic yield in patients with suspected and established small-bowel Crohn's disease: a meta-analysis. *Am J Gastroenterol*. 2010;105(6):1240-1248.

21. Gal E, Geller A, Fraser G, et al. Assessment and validation of the new capsule endoscopy Crohn's disease activity index (CECDAI). *Dig Dis Sci*. 2008;53:1933-1937.

22. Korelitz BI, Sommers SC. Response to drug therapy in Crohn's disease: evaluation by rectal biopsy and mucosal cell counts. *J Clin Gastroenterol*. 1984;6:123-127.

23. Gomes P, du BC, Smith CL, Holdstock G. Relationship between disease activity indices and colonoscopic findings in patients with colonic inflammatory bowel disease. *Gut*. 1986;27:92-95.

24. D'Haens GR, Geboes K, Peeters M, Baert F, Penninckx F, Rutgeerts P. Early lesions of recurrent Crohn's disease caused by infusion of intestinal contents in excluded ileum. *Gastroenterology*. 1998;114:262-267.

25. Andre C, Descos L, Vignal J, Gillon J. C-reactive protein as a predictor of relapse in asymptomatic patients with Crohn's disease. *Scott Med J*. 1983;28:26-29.

26. Fagan EA, Dyck RF, Maton PN, et al. Serum levels of C-reactive protein in Crohn's disease and ulcerative colitis. *Eur J Clin Invest*. 1982;12:351-359.

27. Bitton A, Dobkin PL, Edwardes MD, et al. Predicting relapse in Crohn's disease: a biopsychosocial model. *Gut*. 2008;57:1386-1392.

28. Wright JP, Young GO, Tigler-Wybrandi N. Predictors of acute relapse of Crohn's disease. A laboratory and clinical study. *Dig Dis Sci*. 1987;32:164-170.

29. Andre C, Descos L, Landais P, Fermanian J. Assessment of appropriate laboratory measurements to supplement the Crohn's disease activity index. *Gut*. 1981;22:571-574.

30. Andre C, Descos L, Andre F, Vignal J, Landais P, Fermanian J. Biological measurements of Crohn's disease activity—a reassessment. *Hepatogastroenterology*. 1985;32:135-137.

31. Niederau C, Backmerhoff F, Schumacher B, Niederau C. Inflammatory mediators and acute phase proteins in patients with Crohn's disease and ulcerative colitis. *Hepatogastroenterology*. 1997;44:90-107.

32. Sachar DB, Smith H, Chan S, Cohen LB, Lichtiger S, Messer J. Erythrocytic sedimentation rate as a measure of clinical activity in inflammatory bowel disease. *J Clin Gastroenterol*. 1986;8:647-650.

33. Sachar DB, Luppescu NE, Bodian C, Shlien RD, Fabry TL, Gumaste VV. Erythrocyte sedimentation as a measure of Crohn's disease activity: opposite trends in ileitis versus colitis. *J Clin Gastroenterol*. 1990;12:643-646.

34. Cooke WT, Prior P. Determining disease activity in inflammatory bowel disease. *J Clin Gastroenterol*. 1984;6:17-25.

35. Descos L, Andre C, Beorghia S, Vincent C, Revillard JP. Serum levels of beta-2-microglobulin—a new marker of activity in Crohn's disease. *N Engl J Med*. 1979;301:440-441.

36. Manicourt DH, Orloff S. Serum levels of beta 2-microglobulin in Crohn's disease. *N Engl J Med*. 1980;302:696.

37. Kruis W, Fateh-Mogadam A, Sandel P. Serum levels of beta 2-microglobulin: A new marker of activity in Crohn's disease. *N Engl J Med*. 1979;301:1348.

38. Zissis M, Afroudakis A, Galanopoulos G, et al. B2 microglobulin: is it a reliable marker of activity in inflammatory bowel disease? *Am J Gastroenterol*. 2001;96:2177-2183.

39. Sategna-Guidetti C, Pulitano R, Fenoglio L, Bologna E, Manes M, Camussi G. Tumor necrosis factor/cachectin in Crohn's disease. Relation of serum concentration to disease activity. *Recenti Prog Med*. 1993;84:93-99.

40. Nielsen OH, Brynskov J, Bendtzen K. Circulating and mucosal concentrations of tumour necrosis factor and inhibitor(s) in chronic inflammatory bowel disease. *Dan Med Bull*. 1993;40:247-249.

41. Braegger CP, Nicholls S, Murch SH, Stephens S, MacDonald TT. Tumour necrosis factor alpha in stool as a marker of intestinal inflammation. *Lancet*. 1992;339:89-91.

42. Hadziselimovic F, Emmons LR, Gallati H. Soluble tumour necrosis factor receptors p55 and p75 in the urine monitor disease activity and the efficacy of treatment of inflammatory bowel disease. *Gut*. 1995;37:260-263.

43. Williams AJ, Symons JA, Watchet K, Duff GW. Soluble interleukin-2 receptor and disease activity in Crohn's disease. *J Autoimmun*. 1992;5:251-259.

44. Crabtree JE, Juby LD, Heatley RV, Lobo AJ, Bullimore DW, Axon AT. Soluble interleukin-2 receptor in Crohn's disease: relation of serum concentrations to disease activity. *Gut*. 1990;31:1033-1036.

45. Louis E, Belaiche J, Van KC, Schaaf N, Mahieu P, Mary JY. Soluble interleukin-2 receptor in Crohn's disease. Assessment of disease activity and prediction of relapse. *Dig Dis Sci*. 1995;40:1750-1756.

46. Holtkamp W, Stollberg T, Reis HE. Serum interleukin-6 is related to disease activity but not disease specificity in inflammatory bowel disease. *J Clin Gastroenterol*. 1995;20:123-126.

47. Reinisch W, Gasche C, Tillinger W, et al. Clinical relevance of serum interleukin-6 in Crohn's disease: single point measurements, therapy monitoring, and prediction of clinical relapse. *Am J Gastroenterol*. 1999;94:2156-2164.

48. Nielsen OH, Langholz E, Hendel J, Brynskov J. Circulating soluble intercellular adhesion molecule-1 (sICAM-1) in active inflammatory bowel disease. *Dig Dis Sci*. 1994;39:1918-1923.

49. Jones SC, Banks RE, Haidar A, et al. Adhesion molecules in inflammatory bowel disease. *Gut*. 1995;36:724-730.

50. Goke M, Hoffmann JC, Evers J, Kruger H, Manns MP. Elevated serum concentrations of soluble selectin and immunoglobulin

type adhesion molecules in patients with inflammatory bowel disease. *J Gastroenterol.* 1997;32:480-486.

51. Vaishnavi C, Bhasin DK, Singh K. Fecal lactoferrin assay as a cost-effective tool for intestinal inflammation. *Am J Gastroenterol.* 2000;95:3002-3003.

52. Seva-Pereira A, Franco AO, de Magalhaes AF. Diagnostic value of fecal leukocytes in chronic bowel diseases. *Sao Paulo Med J.* 1994; 112:504-506.

53. Roseth AG, Schmidt PN, Fagerhol MK. Correlation between faecal excretion of indium-111-labelled granulocytes and calprotectin, a granulocyte marker protein, in patients with inflammatory bowel disease. *Scand J Gastroenterol.* 1999;34:50-54.

54. Tibble JA, Bjarnason I. Fecal calprotectin as an index of intestinal inflammation. *Drugs Today (Barc).* 2001;37:85-96.

55. Jones J, Loftus EV Jr, Panaccione R, et al. Relationships between disease activity and serum and fecal biomarkers in patients with Crohn's disease. *Clin Gastroenterol Hepatol.* 2008;6:1218-1224.

56. Schoepfer AM, Beglinger C, Straumann A, et al. Fecal calprotectin correlates more closely with the Simple Endoscopic Score for Crohn's disease (SES-CD) than CRP, blood leukocytes, and the CDAI. *Am J Gastroenterol.* 2010;105:162-169.

57. Vieira A, Fang CB, Rolim EG, et al. Inflammatory bowel disease activity assessed by fecal calprotectin and lactoferrin: correlation with laboratory parameters, clinical, endoscopic, and histological indexes. *BMC Res Notes.* 2009;2:221.

58. Tibble JA, Sigthorsson G, Bridger S, Fagerhol MK, Bjarnason I. Surrogate markers of intestinal inflammation are predictive of relapse in patients with inflammatory bowel disease. *Gastroenterology.* 2000;119:15-22.

59. Desmazures C, Giraudeaux V, Florent C, L'Hirondel C, Bernier JJ. Intestinal clearance of alpha 1 anti-trypsin: a simple technique for diagnosis of protein losing enteropathy (author's transl). *Nouv Presse Med.* 1980;9:1691-1694.

60. Arndt B, Schurmann G, Betzler M, Herfarth C, Schmidt-Gayk H. Assessment of Crohn's disease activity and alpha 1-antitrypsin in faeces. *Lancet.* 1992;340:1037.

61. Becker K, Frieling T, Haussinger D. Quantification of fecal alpha 1-antitrypsin excretion for assessment of inflammatory bowel diseases. *Eur J Med Res.* 1998;3:65-70.

62. Miura S, Yoshioka M, Tanaka S, et al. Faecal clearance of alpha 1-antitrypsin reflects disease activity and correlates with rapid turnover proteins in chronic inflammatory bowel disease. *J Gastroenterol Hepatol.* 1991;6:49-52.

63. Meyers S, Lichtiger S, Feuer EJ, Lahman EA, Janowitz HD. Fecal alpha 1-antitrypsin as a measure of Crohn's disease activity. The effect of therapy and anatomical extent of disease. *J Clin Gastroenterol.* 1988;10:491-497.

64. Biancone L, Fantini M, Tosti C, Bozzi R, Vavassori P, Pallone F. Fecal alpha 1-antitrypsin clearance as a marker of clinical relapse in patients with Crohn's disease of the distal ileum. *Eur J Gastroenterol Hepatol.* 2003;15:261-266.

65. Kane SV, Sandborn WJ, Rufo PA, et al. Fecal lactoferrin is a sensitive and specific marker in identifying intestinal inflammation. *Am J Gastroenterol.* 2003;98:1309-1314.

66. Gisbert JP, Bermejo F, Pérez-Calle JL, et al. Fecal calprotectin and lactoferrin for the prediction of inflammatory bowel disease relapse. *Inflamm Bowel Dis.* 2009;15:1190-1198.

67. Vermeire S, Joossens S, Peeters M, et al. Comparative study of ASCA (Anti-Saccharomyces cerevisiae antibody) assays in inflammatory bowel disease. *Gastroenterology.* 2001;120:827-833.

68. Canani RB, Romano MT, Greco L, et al. Effects of disease activity on anti-*Saccharomyces cerevisiae* antibodies: implications for diagnosis and follow-up of children with Crohn's disease. *Inflamm Bowel Dis.* 2004;10:234-239.

69. Andre F, Andre C, Emery Y, Forichon J, Descos L, Minaire Y. Assessment of the lactulose-mannitol test in Crohn's disease. *Gut.* 1988;29:511-515.

70. Pironi L, Miglioli M, Ruggeri E, et al. Relationship between intestinal permeability to [51Cr]EDTA and inflammatory activity in asymptomatic patients with Crohn's disease. *Dig Dis Sci.* 1990;35:582-588.

71. D'Inca R, Di LV, Corrao G, et al. Intestinal permeability test as a predictor of clinical course in Crohn's disease. *Am J Gastroenterol.* 1999;94:2956-2960.

72. Tibble JA, Sigthorsson G, Bridger S, Fagerhol MK, Bjarnason I. Surrogate markers of intestinal inflammation are predictive of relapse in patients with inflammatory bowel disease. *Gastroenterology.* 2000;119:15-22.

73. Hilsden RJ, Meddings JB, Hardin J, Gall DG, Sutherland LR. Intestinal permeability and postheparin plasma diamine oxidase activity in the prediction of Crohn's disease relapse. *Inflamm Bowel Dis.* 1999;5:85-91.

74. Carucci LR, Levine MS. Radiographic imaging of inflammatory bowel disease. *Gastroenterol Clin North Am.* 2002;31:93-117, ix.

75. Freeny PC. Crohn's disease and ulcerative colitis. Evaluation with double-contrast barium examination and endoscopy. *Postgrad Med.* 1986;80:139-146.

76. Tribl B, Turetschek K, Mostbeck G, et al. Conflicting results of ileoscopy and small bowel double-contrast barium examination in patients with Crohn's disease. *Endoscopy.* 1998;30:339-344.

77. Goldberg HI, Caruthers SB Jr, Nelson JA, Singleton JW. Radiographic findings of the National Cooperative Crohn's Disease Study. *Gastroenterology.* 1979;77:925-937.

78. Maconi G, Parente F, Bollani S, Cesana B, Bianchi PG. Abdominal ultrasound in the assessment of extent and activity of Crohn's disease: clinical significance and implication of bowel wall thickening. *Am J Gastroenterol.* 1996;91:1604-1609.

79. Mayer D, Reinshagen M, Mason RA, et al. Sonographic measurement of thickened bowel wall segments as a quantitative parameter for activity in inflammatory bowel disease. *Z Gastroenterol.* 2000;38:295-300.

80. Neye H, Voderholzer W, Rickes S, Weber J, Wermke W, Lochs H. Evaluation of criteria for the activity of Crohn's disease by power Doppler sonography. *Dig Dis.* 2004;22:67-72.

81. Van Oostayen JA, Wasser MN, Griffioen G, van Hogezand RA, Lamers CB, de Roos A. Activity of Crohn's disease assessed by measurement of superior mesenteric artery flow with Doppler ultrasound. *Neth J Med.* 1998;53:S3-S8.

82. Ludwig D, Wiener S, Bruning A, Schwarting K, Jantschek G, Stange EF. Mesenteric blood flow is related to disease activity and risk of relapse in Crohn's disease: a prospective follow-up study. *Am J Gastroenterol.* 1999;94:2942-2950.

83. Van Oostayen JA, Wasser MN, Griffioen G, van Hogezand RA, Lamers CB, de Roos A. Diagnosis of Crohn's ileitis and monitoring of disease activity: value of Doppler ultrasound of superior mesenteric artery flow. *Am J Gastroenterol.* 1998;93:88-91.

84. Byrne MF, Farrell MA, Abass S, et al. Assessment of Crohn's disease activity by Doppler sonography of the superior mesenteric artery, clinical evaluation and the Crohn's disease activity index: a prospective study. *Clin Radiol.* 2001;56:973-978.

85. Parente F, Greco S, Molteni M, et al. Oral contrast enhanced bowel ultrasonography in the assessment of small intestine Crohn's disease. A prospective comparison with conventional ultrasound, x-ray studies, and ileocolonoscopy. *Gut.* 2004;53:1652-1657.

86. Girlich C, Jung EM, Iesalnieks I, et al. Quantitative assessment of bowel wall vascularisation in Crohn's disease with contrast-enhanced ultrasound and perfusion analysis. *Clin Hemorheol Microcirc.* 2009;43:141-148.

87. Ripollés T, Martínez MJ, Paredes JM, et al. Crohn disease: correlation of findings at contrast-enhanced US with severity at endoscopy. *Radiology.* 2009;253:241-248.

88. Migaleddu V, Scanu AM, Quaia E, et al. Contrast-enhanced ultrasonographic evaluation of inflammatory activity in Crohn's disease. *Gastroenterology.* 2009;137:43-52.

89. Del CL, Arribas I, Valbuena M, Mate J, Moreno-Otero R. Spiral CT findings in active and remission phases in patients with Crohn disease. *J Comput Assist Tomogr.* 2001;25:792-797.

90. Tomei E, Diacinti D, Marini M, Boirivant M, Paoluzi P. Computed tomography of bowel wall in patients with Crohn's disease: relationship of inflammatory activity to biological indices. *Ital J Gastroenterol.* 1996;28:487-492.

91. Kolkman JJ, Falke TH, Roos JC, et al. Computed tomography and granulocyte scintigraphy in active inflammatory bowel disease. Comparison with endoscopy and operative findings. *Dig Dis Sci.* 1996;41:641-650.

92. Hassan C, Cerro P, Zullo A, Spina C, Morini S. Computed tomography enteroclysis in comparison with ileoscopy in patients with Crohn's disease. *Int J Colorectal Dis.* 2003;18:121-125.

93. Wold PB, Fletcher JG, Johnson CD, Sandborn WJ. Assessment of small bowel Crohn disease: noninvasive peroral CT enterography compared with other imaging methods and endoscopy—feasibility study. *Radiology.* 2003;229:275-281.

94. Ota Y, Matsui T, Ono H, et al. Value of virtual computed tomographic colonography for Crohn's colitis: comparison with endoscopy and barium enema. *Abdom Imaging.* 2003;28:778-783.

95. Schunk K. Small bowel magnetic resonance imaging for inflammatory bowel disease. *Top Magn Reson Imaging.* 2002;13:409-425.

96. Gourtsoyiannis N, Papanikolaou N, Grammatikakis J, Prassopoulos P. MR enteroclysis: technical considerations and clinical applications. *Eur Radiol.* 2002;12:2651-2658.

97. Koh DM, Miao Y, Chinn RJ, et al. MR imaging evaluation of the activity of Crohn's disease. *Am J Roentgenol.* 2001;177:1325-1332.

98. Madsen SM, Thomsen HS, Munkholm P, et al. Inflammatory bowel disease evaluated by low-field magnetic resonance imaging. Comparison with endoscopy, 99mTc-HMPAO leucocyte scintigraphy, conventional radiography and surgery. *Scand J Gastroenterol.* 2002;37:307-316.

99. Shoenut JP, Semelka RC, Magro CM, Silverman R, Yaffe CS, Micflikier AB. Comparison of magnetic resonance imaging and endoscopy in distinguishing the type and severity of inflammatory bowel disease. *J Clin Gastroenterol.* 1994;19:31-35.

100. Shoenut JP, Semelka RC, Silverman R, Yaffe CS, Micflikier AB. Magnetic resonance imaging in inflammatory bowel disease. *J Clin Gastroenterol.* 1993;17:73-78.

101. Rimola J, Rodriguez S, Garcia-Bosch O, et al. Magnetic resonance for assessment of disease activity and severity in ileocolonic Crohn's disease. *Gut.* 2009;58:1113-1120.

102. Schunk K, Kern A, Oberholzer K, et al. Hydro-MRI in Crohn's disease: appraisal of disease activity. *Invest Radiol.* 2000;35:431-437.

103. Siddiki HA, Fidler JL, Fletcher JG, et al. Prospective comparison of state-of-the-art MR enterography and CT enterography in small-bowel Crohn's disease. *Am J Roentgenol.* 2009;193:113-121.

104. Lee SS, Kim AY, Yang SK, et al. Crohn disease of the small bowel: comparison of CT enterography, MR enterography, and small-bowel follow-through as diagnostic techniques. *Radiology.* 2009;251:751-761.

105. Gourtsoyiannis N, Papanikolaou N, Grammatikakis J, Papamastorakis G, Prassopoulos P, Roussomoustakaki M. Assessment of Crohn's disease activity in the small bowel with MR and conventional enteroclysis: preliminary results. *Eur Radiol.* 2004;14:1017-1024.

106. Schreyer AG, Rath HC, Kikinis R, et al. Comparison of magnetic resonance imaging colonography with conventional colonoscopy for the assessment of intestinal inflammation in patients with inflammatory bowel disease: a feasibility study. *Gut.* 2005;54:250-256.

107. Weldon MJ, Lowe C, Joseph AE, Maxwell JD. Review article: quantitative leucocyte scanning in the assessment of inflammatory bowel disease activity and its response to therapy. *Aliment Pharmacol Ther.* 1996;10:123-132.

108. Becker W, Fischbach W, Weppler M, Mosl B, Jacoby G, Borner W. Radiolabelled granulocytes in inflammatory bowel disease: diagnostic possibilities and clinical indications. *Nucl Med Commun.* 1988;9:693-701.

109. Saverymuttu SH, Camilleri M, Rees H, Lavender JP, Hodgson HJ, Chadwick VS. Indium 111-granulocyte scanning in the assessment of disease extent and disease activity in inflammatory bowel disease. A comparison with colonoscopy, histology, and fecal indium 111-granulocyte excretion. *Gastroenterology.* 1986;90:1121-1128.

110. Sciarretta G, Furno A, Mazzoni M, Basile C, Malaguti P. Technetium-99m hexamethyl propylene amine oxime granulocyte scintigraphy in Crohn's disease: diagnostic and clinical relevance. *Gut.* 1993;34:1364-1369.

111. Heresbach D, Bretagne JF, Raoul JL, et al. Indium scanning in assessment of acute Crohn's disease. A prospective study of sensitivity and correlation with severity of mucosal damage. *Dig Dis Sci.* 1993;38:1601-1607.

112. Wheeler JG, Slack NF, Duncan A, Whitehead PJ, Russell G, Harvey RF. The diagnosis of intra-abdominal abscesses in patients with severe Crohn's disease. *Q J Med.* 1992;82:159-167.

113. Arndt JW, Grootscholten MI, van Hogezand RA, Griffioen G, Lamers CB, Pauwels EK. Inflammatory bowel disease activity assessment using technetium-99m-HMPAO leukocytes. *Dig Dis Sci.* 1997;42:387-393.

114. Molnar T, Papos M, Gyulai C, et al. Clinical value of technetium-99m-HMPAO-labeled leukocyte scintigraphy and spiral computed tomography in active Crohn's disease. *Am J Gastroenterol.* 2001;96:1517-1521.

115. Irvine EJ. Usual therapy improves perianal Crohn's disease as measured by a new disease activity index. McMaster IBD Study Group. *J Clin Gastroenterol.* 1995;20:27-32.

116. Sandborn WJ, Present DH, Isaacs KL, et al. Tacrolimus for the treatment of fistulas in patients with Crohn's disease: a randomized, placebo-controlled trial. *Gastroenterology.* 2003;125:380-388.

117. Present DH, Rutgeerts P, Targan S, et al. Infliximab for the treatment of fistulas in patients with Crohn's disease. *N Engl J Med.* 1999;340:1398-1405.

118. Schratter-Sehn AU, Lochs H, Vogelsang H, Schurawitzki H, Herold C, Schratter M. Endoscopic ultrasonography versus computed tomography in the differential diagnosis of perianorectal complications in Crohn's disease. *Endoscopy.* 1993;25:582-586.

119. Borley NR, Mortensen NJ, Jewell DP. MRI scanning in perianal Crohn's disease: an important diagnostic adjunct. *Inflamm Bowel Dis.* 1999;5:231-233.

120. Orsoni P, Barthet M, Portier F, Panuel M, Desjeux A, Grimaud JC. Prospective comparison of endosonography, magnetic resonance imaging and surgical findings in anorectal fistula and abscess complicating Crohn's disease. *Br J Surg.* 1999;86:360-364.

121. Schwartz DA, Wiersema MJ, Dudiak KM, et al. A comparison of endoscopic ultrasound, magnetic resonance imaging, and exam under anesthesia for evaluation of Crohn's perianal fistulas. *Gastroenterology.* 2001;121:1064-1072.

GENERAL PRINCIPLES OF MEDICAL THERAPY OF CROHN'S DISEASE

Denis Franchimont, MD, PhD and Gary Wild, MD

Crohn's disease runs a chronic intermittent or continuous clinical course that is characterized by a marked impairment of health-related quality of life. Because curative treatments remain to be defined, the current therapeutic goals are focused on the induction of remission in the clinical setting of acute onset or reactivation of symptoms and the maintenance of remission. Maintenance therapies are aimed at preventing relapses (or recurrences), complications, the need for surgery, and ultimately at modifying the natural history of the disease. When considering the various therapeutic modalities available for the treatment of patients with CD, the physician bases his or her treatment decisions on integrating a three-dimensional vectorial approach as defined by the patient profile, disease profile, and medication profile (Figure 22-1). The physician will then assess the disease activity and decide upon the most appropriate treatment regimen in the context of attainable therapeutic goals. The subsequent evaluation of the patient's clinical response will further direct the physician's decisions across the recommended therapeutic algorithms. Specific considerations will also be given to treat (or prevent) osteoporosis, extraintestinal manifestations, or specific complications such as anemia.

SELECTING A TREATMENT PLAN

PATIENT PROFILE

An accurate definition of the patient profile is a critical step in the evaluation of patients with CD as it affords the opportunity to rule out concomitant disease, identify aggravating or precipitating factors, catalog the patient's therapeutic history (including surgery), assess the patient's adherence and psychological profile, and predict the disease phenotype. Crohn's disease onset or relapse is often associated with diarrhea, abdominal pain, and sometimes fatigue, fever, and weight loss. These symptoms can, however, be misleading as they can also reflect a concomitant disease. Thus, efforts must be made to exclude other causes of their symptoms such as gastroenteritis, irritable bowel syndrome (IBS), bacterial overgrowth, bile salt wastage, secondary lactase deficiency, short bowel syndrome, or medication-induced diarrhea.[1] Though only a small number of patients with active disease will go into remission without specific treatment, recent double-blind controlled trials of patients with moderately active CD clearly demonstrated that a third of the patients will go into remission on placebo.[2] This emphasized that brain-gut interactions may give rise to IBS-related symptoms that may alter the clinical picture.[3] Environmental factors such as smoking, nonsteroidal antiinflammatory drug (NSAID) use, and high fiber diets can be potentially very deleterious to CD by triggering disease recurrences or worsening existing disease activity.[4] For example, smoking is more frequent in CD than in the general population and is associated, especially in women, with a more severe disease course, increased need for immunosuppressive therapies, increased indications for surgery, and a higher postoperative recurrence.[5-8]

THE DISEASE HISTORY

Patient disease history may help in understanding the evolution and aggressive character of the disease. After a surgically induced remission, the most important predic-

Lichtenstein GR, ed.
Crohn's Disease: The Complete Guide to Medical Management (pp 267-282).
© 2011 SLACK Incorporated

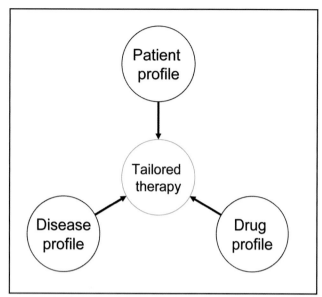

FIGURE 22-1. A three-dimensional vectorial approach to treatment decisions.

tor of relapse is the duration a patient has been in remission before the initiation of maintenance therapy.[9,10] Age at onset, previous surgery, extraintestinal manifestations, and history of perianal manifestations help distinguish disease behaviors. Age at onset not only documents disease duration but is associated with several clinical parameters.[11] For example, younger patients at diagnosis are more likely to have a positive family history, small bowel disease, a stricturing phenotype, and a higher frequency of surgery. Older patients at diagnosis are less likely to have a positive family history (sporadic case) and more likely to have colonic disease and inflammatory phenotype.[9-14] Surgery for complications of CD (ie, fistula and abscess) or previous surgery for CD increased the risk of recurrence. Extraintestinal manifestations are usually associated with the *inflammatory* phenotype.[15] A recent large cohort study showed that initial requirement for steroid use, an age below 40 years, and the presence of perianal disease were independent early predictors at diagnosis for future subsequent disabling disease.[16]

THE TREATMENT HISTORY

Inquiring about the therapeutic history aids in defining the patient's response to a given medication as well as previous intolerance or adverse reactions to medications. The history alone often allows the clinician to discriminate between corticosteroid sensitivity, dependence, and resistance.[17-19] Patients with a 2- to 3-year history of exposure to 6-mercaptopurine (6-MP) or azathioprine (AZA) may relate a similar pattern of disease course, suggesting either a poor drug response or problems with medication adherence.[20] Shorter duration of response with infliximab may suggest loss of response.[21,22] Poor medical adherence is associated with significant morbidity and should be

investigated in every patient with a suboptimal medical outcome.[23]

Finally, the physical exam should be targeted at identifying clinical signs of toxicity (ie, fever, dehydration, hypotension, and tachycardia), looking at CD complications, and evaluating nutritional status.

DISEASE PROFILE

Defining the disease profile helps predict the natural history of the disease and select the best treatment choice for the patient. Whereas disease phenotypes were first recognized by Farmer et al,[24] the more recent Vienna and Montreal classifications help distinguish these using a schematic grading score (Table 22-1).[24-26]

DISEASE LOCATION

Crohn's disease is first defined by its anatomical location: ileal only (L1), colonic only (L2), ileocolonic (L3), and upper gastrointestinal tract (L4). Maximum extent of disease is defined as the degree of involvement at any time point prior to the first resection. Minimum involvement for a specific anatomical location is defined as any aphthous lesion or ulceration. Mucosal erythema and edema are excluded. For classification purposes, examination of at least the small and large bowel is required.[25-27]

L1 includes disease limited to the terminal ileum with or without spillover into the caecum. *L2* includes any colonic location between the caecum and rectum with no small bowel or upper gastrointestinal involvement. *L3* includes disease of the terminal ileum with or without spillover into the caecum and any location between the ascending colon and rectum. Finally, *L4* represents any disease location proximal to the terminal ileum (excluding the mouth), regardless of additional involvement of the terminal ileum or colon. L4 is now considered as a modifier in the Montreal classification.[26]

Patients with involvement of multiple segments are more likely to relapse.[28] As well, a higher rate of postoperative recurrence is observed in patients with ileocolonic disease and is correlated with disease extent before surgery.[9,10,14] Disease location should be assessed in every patient before initiating medical treatment because of the different sites of drug delivery, especially when topical administration is contemplated, such as with left-sided CD colitis. Whereas sulfasalazine is delivered primarily to the colon, the 5-aminosalicylic acid (5-ASA) derivatives can be released throughout the ileum and colon or in the colon only. Budesonide mostly targets the small bowel and right colon.

Disease behavior is a more complex notion and is defined as either inflammatory (or nonstricturing nonpenetrating, B1), fibrostenotic (or stricturing, B2), or fistulizing (or penetrating, B3).[25-27] Combinations of disease behavior are often encountered and reflect the continuum of the clinical course of the disease that evolves from the inflammatory to stricturing and penetrating phenotypes.[29,30] Nonetheless, pure stricturing and penetrating phenotypes at diagnosis can remain stable over time. To the same extent, some patients will always present with an inflammatory phenotype without stricturing or penetrating complications.[29,30] Thus, the Vienna and Montreal classifications provide a useful clinical taxonomy of CD, without providing information on disease evolution and aggressiveness.

The *inflammatory disease* (nonstricturing nonpenetrating) (B1) is defined by the absence of complications at any time during the course of disease.[25-27] This phenotype is not transmurally aggressive, is associated with more frequent clinical relapses (chronic active) with steroid dependence or resistance, is more easily suppressed with antiinflammatory and immunosuppressive drugs, and may better respond to prophylactic therapies after surgery.

The *stricturing disease* (B2) is defined as the occurrence of constant luminal narrowing demonstrated by radiological, endoscopic, or surgical-pathological methods, with prestenotic dilatation or obstructive signs/symptoms without the presence of penetrating disease at any time in the course of disease.[25-27] The stricturing phenotype more frequently involves the small bowel location only, but may also be observed in the colon. The evolution is usually insidious and may only give rise to clinical symptoms many years after disease onset or previous resection. Fistulization or perforation with abscess development may occur secondarily to the presence of stenotic obstruction.

The penetrating disease (B3) is defined as the occurrence of intraabdominal fistulae, inflammatory masses, and/or abscesses at any time in the course of disease. Excluded are postoperative intraabdominal complications.[25-27] The penetrating behavior reflects a transmural aggressive disease within the first few years after the diagnosis. The ileocolon is the usual site; occasional perforation is seen in the left colon. Postoperative recurrences are similar in character with early recurrence of fistula and/or abscess.

Perianal disease (*p*) includes perianal fistula or abscess but is not part of the (ie, does not enter in the definition of) penetrating B3 disease per se and is considered as a modifier for the behavior in the Montreal classification.[26] Perianal ulcers are also included, but skin tags are not considered as perianal disease. Indeed, perianal disease can be associated with B1 or B2 diseases, and its course may be independent from the disease course of the small bowel and/or colon. Having perianal disease is associated with steroid-resistant disease and, when present at diagnosis, has been shown to be an independent predictor of future disabling disease.[16,31]

Disease behavior guides clinicians in their choice of therapeutic modalities. Although all therapies demonstrate some variable degree of efficacy in inflammatory CD; corticosteroids, budesonide, and 5-ASA are of unproven clinical benefit in the management of patients with fistulizing disease. As well, there is no specific medical treatment for purely fibrostenotic disease.

MEDICATION PROFILE

Many of the medications that comprise the therapeutic mainstay for the management of CD are associated with a significant set of short- and long-term adverse reactions. Thus, conventional wisdom dictates that the drugs used in the treatment of CD should only be prescribed if they show therapeutic efficacy as demonstrated by the highest level of evidence derived from randomized, double-blinded clinical trials.[32] The risk-benefit ratio should always be taken into account, such that first-line therapy will remain safe and effective enough to induce remission. On the other hand, second- and third-line agents are often chosen for their efficacy if remission must be met despite the broader adverse event profile that accompanies the use of these medications.[33] There is a considerable effort to refine therapeutic choices that are based on patient and disease profiles and incorporate the use of serological (ie, anti-saccharomyces cerevisiae antibody/anti-neutrophil cytoplasmic antibody [ASCA/ANCA], OmpC, I2, Cbir1, etc) and pharmacogenomic (ie, 6-thioguanine nucleotides [6-TGN] for 6-MP/AZA therapy) and genetic markers (ie, thiopurine methyltransferase [TPMT] genotyping for 6-MP/AZA therapy) (see following discussion). This focused approach relies on establishing an individual's genotypic and phenotypic composite in order to better target patients (or patient subgroups), hence improving the efficacy and the safety of the treatment. Importantly, there are parameters associated with the patient and disease profiles that can be predictive factors for safety and/or efficacy.

PREDICTIVE FACTORS OF EFFICACY

Smoking habit and colonic disease have been shown to be associated with steroid dependence.[18] Prior bowel resection, perianal disease, and high Crohn's Disease Activity Index (CDAI) are predictive of steroid resistance.[31] Patients with perianal CD, age ≥40 years, with recently diagnosed perianal disease (<22 months) without fistulae were the best responders to azathioprine.[34] AZA appears to be more effective in the treatment of patients with colonic involvement.[35] Nonsmokers and patients treated with concomitant immunosuppressive agents are more likely to respond to infliximab.[36] High C-reactive protein (CRP) levels and/or colonic disease alone also appear to be good predictors of response to infliximab.[36-38] Early use of biologics such as infliximab, adalimumab, or certoluzimab in the course of the disease in naïve patients appears to be associated with a better response and remission to these biologics.[39-41]

PREDICTIVE FACTORS OF SAFETY

The toxicity profile of the current therapeutic agents in CD is now well recognized. However, it is noteworthy that predictive factors for toxicity are lacking, such as with the use of steroids. A main concern when starting a patient on infliximab is the occurrence and development of antibodies against infliximab. These antibodies are thought to be responsible for a small subset of all patients who develop infusion reactions and shorter duration of response.[21] The ACCENT I trial together with a prospective cohort study suggests that scheduled maintenance treatment is associated with less formation of antibodies and fewer infusion reactions than episodic retreatment.[21,42-44] Immunosuppressive therapies also prevent antibody formation (especially during episodic treatment) and, hence, infusion reactions.[21,42-44] In the same line, both scheduled treatment and immunosuppressive therapies were found to prevent loss of response to infliximab[35-37] in a small subset of patients. Thus, we initially thought that immunosuppressive therapies should always be initiated together with infliximab if not already administered. Combination of immunosuppressive therapies can be associated with serious and opportunistic infections and likely lymphoma, however.[45-47] We currently agree that scheduled treatment should always be preferred over episodic treatment. Immunosuppressive therapies with AZA and methotrexate may not be needed if scheduled treatment with infliximab is contemplated. Indeed, a recent study suggests that discontinuation of AZA after 6 months in patients

on scheduled treatment with infliximab was not associated with a higher rate of loss of response at 2 years compared to patients who continued AZA combined with scheduled treatment with infliximab.[48] Continuation of immunosuppressive therapies beyond 6 months did not offer a clear benefit over scheduled infliximab monotherapy, yet it was associated with higher median infliximab trough and decreased CRP levels, suggesting a better control of the disease and infliximab availability (in those patients who did not have 3-dose induction and who tended to have 12-week interval infusion rather than every 8 weeks). Prophylactic treatment with hydrocortisone appears to prevent the formation of antibodies and may prevent infusion reactions in patients who have had intermittent or episodic infliximab.[22] Although the measurement of these antibodies is not routinely available at this time, elevated antibody titers could be indicative of only 40% of the total of infusion reactions in ACCENT 1.[44] Hepatosplenic T cell lymphomas have been described largely in patients who have received combination infliximab and adalimumab with long-term AZA. Data from the CESAME trial showed a 4.5-fold increased risk of lymphomas in patients on long-term AZA[49]; clearly, all of the patients treated with infliximab in this study were also on long-term AZA. However, a recent study (SONIC) showed that short-term combination of infliximab and AZA (<6 months) in patients with a short duration of disease (<2.5 years) was more effective than either drug alone and was not associated with an increased risk of adverse events.[50] Thus, short-term combination therapy in patients with short-duration disease may prove to be of less risk than long-term combination therapy in patients with long-term disease.

Recently, pharmacogenomic studies have been carried out with AZA/6-MP, examining its metabolism based on TPMT genotypes and the pharmacokinetic properties of its active metabolites, 6-TGN, in CD patient responders and nonresponders to AZA/6-MP.[51] 6-TGN is responsible for both the therapeutic efficacy and the risk of myelotoxicity. Based on TPMT phenotypes, patients are subdivided into normal (NM), medium (MM), or low metabolizers (LM). TPMT-deficient homozygotes or LM patients (0.3%) with high 6-TGN levels are at high risk of developing myelotoxicity and sometimes aplasia. Though most of leukopenia is independent of TPMT status, 30% of leukopenia appears to be related to TPMT phenotypes, especially when this occurs early on in treatment. TPMT phenotyping is currently recommended before starting AZA/6-MP.[52] TPMT phenotyping also helps the physician achieve a clinical response above the 6-TGN threshold level with lower doses of AZA/6-MP.[53] 6-TGN seems to be a reliable marker for drug response, and a therapeutic threshold has emerged when comparing responders and nonresponders to AZA/6-MP.[51,54] However, intraindividual variability remains high, and multiple sampling is needed to obtain a patient's accurate level.[55] As well, the measurement of 6-TGN levels provides an important tool to assess patient adherence. For example, CD patients treated with AZA who demonstrate undetectable 6-TGN levels may not be adherent to the prescribed therapeutic regimen. Despite these advantages, the routine use of 6-TGN monitoring remains difficult to apply and translate to daily clinical practice.[56]

Combination of immunosuppressive treatments is significantly associated with a higher rate of serious and/or opportunistic infections. Thus, appropriate vaccination is recommended, and monotherapy should always be preferred when immunosuppressive treatments are contemplated, especially in older patients.[47,57]

ESTABLISHING THERAPEUTIC GOALS AND ASSESSING DISEASE ACTIVITY AND TREATMENT RESPONSES

The establishment of therapeutic goals is a critical step in the clinical management of patients with CD. The main therapeutic goals are inducing and maintaining a symptom-free disease state and the tapering of steroids in the setting of steroid dependency. The impressive action of infliximab on mucosal healing has challenged the clinician in considering achieving ultimate mucosal remission as a therapeutic endpoint, which may redefine the future of our current clinical approach to the treatment of CD.[58] In order to decide upon the optimal therapeutic goals for a particular patient, the severity of the disease must be evaluated together with the patient and disease profiles and the profile of medication if already selected (see previous discussion). Assessing disease activity and/or therapeutic response is largely based on symptoms. This remains a complex issue because the 3 disease behaviors of CD have to be selectively considered, especially if present within the same patient. For example, a severe inflammatory disease phenotype is associated with diarrhea and fever, whereas a severe fibrostenotic disease phenotype is best defined by several episodes of small bowel obstruction. Measuring the severity of disease and the subsequent treatment response/remission based solely on symptoms can be misleading because it does not always reflect the magnitude of inflammation or fibrosis because of interfering concomitant disease (see previous). This may explain in part the high placebo rate of response and remission reported in recent clinical trials.[2] Indeed, the CDAI is mostly based on a grading score of various symptoms, such as pain, diarrhea, and general well-being and thus has a large subjective component.[59]

THE INFLAMMATORY DISEASE

Despite the need for a better grading system of severity and therapeutic response, the CDAI is well accepted and is considered the most reliable of indices for the assessment of disease activity. Though it is used in clinical trials, its use is rather cumbersome in day-to-day clinical practice. A CDAI of less than 150 points represents quiescent disease, 200 to 450 indicates moderately active disease, and over 450 signifies severe disease.[60] Because the CDAI is a symptom score that is independent of the severity of the mucosal lesions or biological activity, there is not always an association between clinical improvement and endoscopic healing in patients with CD.[61] In view of these observations, the serial monitoring of endoscopic disease activity in patients who receive medical therapy for CD is not recommended. Nevertheless, a Crohn's Disease Endoscopic Index of Severity (CDEIS) has been developed but is equally difficult to use in routine clinical practice. However, a simpler score has been recently described that not only correlates with CDEIS but also significantly correlates with biological markers such as C-reactive protein.[62] The use of an endoscopic scoring system is reinforced today by the positive influence of mucosal healing on the course of the disease and the recognition of deep ulcers as clinical markers of poor disease outcome and the need for surgery.[63] Recent studies have shown that mucosal healing following infliximab administration is associated with decreased number and duration of hospitalizations, decreased need for surgery, and lower recurrence rate.[64] This striking observation brings into question the poor therapeutic effect on mucosal healing when considering other conventional agents such as steroids and the aminosalicylate compounds or the modest degree of mucosal healing observed with AZA therapy.[52] Disease activity has been better defined by the resurgence of interest in the major liver-derived acute-phase protein, specifically the CRP.[65] When abscess formation or infections are ruled out, the level of serum CRP represents an excellent biological marker of response for patients with elevated CRP whether with active luminal or fistulizing disease. The therapeutic action of some of the newer biologics is more striking upon stratification of the treatment response by serum CRP levels. Importantly, this more objective and scientific parameter of disease activity has drastically decreased the placebo response. There are new biological markers of disease activity of which fecal calprotectin appears to be the most promising but needs further investigation and is not routinely used at the present time.[66]

The conventional therapeutic strategy, based on the "step-up" sequential use of more potent antiinflammatory and immunosuppressive agents related to the severity of the disease, has been recently challenged by a novel approach already explored by rheumatologists. The "top-down" strategy consists of the very early use of aggressive treatments, immunosuppressive therapies, and/or biologics in naïve patients with newly diagnosed Crohn's disease. In rheumatoid arthritis, in the BEST and PREMIER studies, combined immunosuppression has been shown to better control disease activity and prevent progressive joint destruction than conventional treatment and, therefore, improve long-term outcomes.[67,68] Similarly, in CD, a higher and faster remission rate (without steroids and surgery) was associated with early combined aggressive treatment (infliximab induction and episodic maintenance) and AZA compared with conventional treatment (sequential use of steroids; ie, 2 cycles: AZA and infliximab) in naïve newly diagnosed Crohn's disease patients.[69] Such approach is further supported by the observation in clinical trials of a better response and remission rate to biologics when use in naïve and newly diagnosed patients.[39-41] The strong rationale advocating for the top-down strategy is the marked efficacy on mucosal healing and remission of biologics that, when used early on, will prevent deleterious tissue remodeling and prevent the development of complications such as strictures and fistula. This is well illustrated with the decreased hospitalization rate and surgery need in patients treated with infliximab.[64] Thus, early aggressive treatment with biologics could ultimately change the natural course of the disease. A major concern is the increased risk of serious/opportunistic infections and lymphoma that severely outweigh the benefits of the top-down strategy in this category of young, naïve, and newly diagnosed patients.[45-47] Identifying patients with future disabling disease from the beginning of their disease who will benefit from an early aggressive treatment is the correct answer to the aforementioned ethical and pharmaco-economic issues. In fact, only a third of the patients might need early aggressive treatment; if 60% of patients will need corticosteroid treatment in the course of their disease, 40% of patients will do well without steroids. In the 60% of patients who will require steroids, only 50% will become steroid dependent or steroid resistant and require immunosuppressive treatment and/or biologics (these figures may change depending on definitions and type of studies).[16-19] Although the term *disabling disease* is still to be defined, a recent study showed that initial requirement for steroid use, an age below 40 years, and the presence of perianal disease were independent early predictors at diagnosis for future subsequent disabling disease.[16] Some serological markers, such as ASCA, have been associated with a complicated course and the need for early surgery.[70-72] Yet, collaborative efforts in translational research should attempt characterizing the population of patients at risk for disabling disease to be treated early on with immunosuppressive therapies and/or biologics.

The Fistulizing Disease

In fistulizing disease, the therapeutic goals are to stop the draining of fistula and, ultimately, close the fistula. Patients with fistulizing Crohn's disease may have internal or external fistulas that may be open (actively draining) or closed. External (enterocutaneous) fistulas may involve the perianal region or the abdominal wall. Internal fistulas may involve adjacent loops of bowel (enteroenteric), the vagina

(enterovaginal, rectovaginal), the bladder (enterovesical), or the peritoneal cavity (intraabdominal abscess).[60] The Perianal Disease Activity Index (PDAI) is a complex measurement tool that was used in earlier clinical trials to assess treatment response in fistulizing disease.[60] More recently, the assessment of fistula response and remission was defined in the ACCENT II study.[73] Briefly, clinical remission was defined as closure of individual fistulas (ie, no fistula drainage despite gentle finger compression). Remission was further defined as closure of all fistulas that were draining at baseline for at least 2 consecutive visits (ie, at least 4 weeks). Clinical response or improvement was defined as closure of individual fistulas, defined as no fistula drainage despite gentle finger compression. Improvement is defined as a decrease from baseline in the number of open draining fistulas of $\geq 50\%$ for at least 2 consecutive visits (ie, at least 4 weeks).[74]

SELECTING THE TREATMENT REGIMEN

Selecting the treatment regimen must be based on the highest level of published evidence. However, the limitations of data derived from randomized controlled trials (RCTs) must be recognized when treating individual patients.[32] The study populations reported in RCTs may be either too heterogeneous or too homogeneous. Indeed, disease location is often overshadowed by disease activity indexes. Only a minor percentage of patients enrolled in RCTs are reflective of the types of CD patients seen in routine clinical practice. Primary objectives and, hence, treatment goals may vary from one study to another. RCT outcomes can be affected by type II errors because of statistical power issues. Most maintenance therapies are evaluated for 12 to 18 months only. Thus, choosing a treatment regimen must not only rely on evidence-based medicine but on clinical reasoning. The dosage, administration route, and duration of treatment are shown in Table 22-2.

Inflammatory Disease

Acute Intermittent Disease

The acute intermittent disease relapses only a few times a year.

Induction Therapy

Because of its benign course, first-line therapies are usually sufficient to induce remission in mild to moderate disease (Figure 22-2). First-line therapies include budesonide for ileal and right-sided colonic disease location and sulfasalazine for purely colonic location. Medications are usually prescribed for 3 months. Sulfasalazine is more effective than placebo for inducing remission in patients with mildly

TABLE 22-2

DOSAGE, ADMINISTRATION ROUTE, AND DURATION OF TREATMENT*

	DOSE	ROUTE	DURATION
ANTIBIOTICS			
Ciprofloxacin	500 mg	PO	7 days
Metronidazole	10 to 20 mg/kg	PO	10 days
MESALAMINE	3 to 4 g/day	PO	12 weeks
BUDESONIDE	3 to 9 mg/day	PO	12 weeks
PREDNISONE	0.5 to 1 mg/day	PO or IV	6 to 12 weeks
AZATHIOPRINE	2 to 2.5 mg/kg	PO	N/A
6-MP	1 to 1.5 mg/kg	PO	N/A
METHOTREXATE			
Induction	25 mg/week	IM	3 months
Maintenance	15 mg/week	IM	N/A
INFLIXIMAB			
Induction	5 mg/kg	IV	At 0, 2, and 6 weeks
Maintenance	5 mg/kg	IV	Q8 weeks or on demand
ADALIMUMAB			
Induction	160 to 80 (w0) or 80 to 40 mg (w2)	SC	At 0 and 2 weeks
Maintenance	40 mg	SC	Q2 wks or Q1 week

*PO indicates orally; IV, intravenous; 6-MP, 6-mercaptopurine; IM, intramuscular; N/A, not applicable; Q, every; SC, subcutaneous.

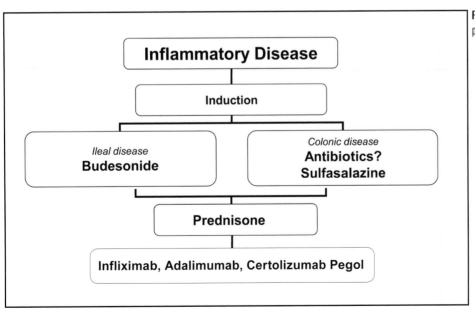

FIGURE 22-2. Treatment algorithm for patients with active Crohn's disease.

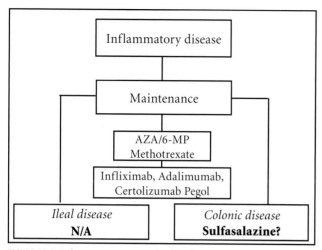

FIGURE 22-3. Maintenance treatment algorithm for patients with Crohn's disease.

to moderately active CD,[75-78] especially in patients with Crohn's colitis or ileocolitis. Budesonide is more effective than placebo for inducing remission in patients with mildly to moderately active CD.[79-84] The role of the 5-ASA derivatives (ie, mesalamine) has been widely debated, with many recent RCTs demonstrating its lack of efficacy in Crohn's disease.[85-90] Though the therapeutic benefit of antibiotics (metronidazole and/or ciprofloxacin) remains uncertain, they are usually preferred in patients with colonic disease, because 2 studies demonstrated a modest increase in therapeutic gain in patients with Crohn's colitis.[91-97] In mildly to moderately active Crohn's disease, prednisone is more effective than placebo[76,78,98] and more effective than sulfasalazine[100] and perhaps budesonide[80,81,100,101] and is thus preferred as a second-line therapy. However, the use of prednisone in addition to sulfasalazine in patients with active Crohn's disease results in a significantly faster initial improvement, with a similar remission rate compared to sulfasalazine alone.[99] Population studies have shown that more than 60% of patients receiving steroids for the first time will become steroid dependent or resistant and 38% will require surgery within 1 year.[19] Thus, the need for prednisone heralds the transition from an acute intermittent disease to a chronic active disease state in more than 50% of patients and therefore must be handled as such (see following discussion).

MAINTENANCE THERAPY

In acute intermittent disease, induction therapy is not always followed by maintenance therapy (Figure 22-3). Although sulfasalazine is not more effective than placebo for the maintenance of medically induced remission in patients with Crohn's disease,[76,78,102] it is recommended that, if patients have responded to therapy with sulfasalazine, this clinical response can be maintained with sulphasalazine, especially if patients suffer from CD-associated spondylarthropathy or ankylosing spondylar-

thropathy. Budesonide maintains remission up to 6 months without apparent further therapeutic benefits beyond this point.[103-106] Interestingly, maintenance therapy with a variable dose of budesonide maintains symptomatic remission.[107] Also, budesonide allows steroid tapering and maintains remission in steroid-dependent patients.[108] The 5-ASA derivatives no longer have a role for this indication, as highlighted by a meta-analysis demonstrating the relatively poor efficacy of mesalamine in this clinical setting.[109-119]

CHRONIC ACTIVE DISEASE

Patients with chronic active disease usually relapse several times a year or suffer from a continuously active disease throughout the year. Induction therapy is always followed by maintenance therapy.

INDUCTION THERAPY

Prednisone is considered the first-line therapy in this indication per os or IV if needed (see Figure 22-2).[76,78,98] A chronic active disease is often steroid dependent and can be steroid resistant. Though the definition has always been fuzzy and may vary depending on the authors, steroid dependence is best defined as 2 successive relapses at dose tapering or within 1 or 2 months after complete weaning from steroid therapy. The role of AZA/6-MP in this clinical setting has been examined as induction therapy.[76,120-125] The most recent Cochrane analysis reports a number needed to treat for 1 patient to respond was 5, with a pooled odds ratio (OR) for response of 2.36 (confidence interval [CI] 1.57-3.53).[126,127] However, it must be emphasized that the onset of action of AZA/6-MP is markedly slow (3 to 6 months) relative to steroids or infliximab, both of which are associated with a more rapid clinical response. Methotrexate may, however, be used as an induction therapy, although induction is generally slower than infliximab and steroids.[32,128] In patients with chronic active disease, infliximab is an effective second-line therapy in steroid-dependent or -resistant patients currently receiving prednisone and/or in patients with serious adverse effects to steroids and/or in patients who failed to respond to maintenance therapy with 6-MP/AZA or methotrexate. Infliximab is more effective than placebo at inducing remission in moderate to severe disease.[43,74,129] Similarly, adalimumab is effective in inducing clinical response and remission in moderate to severe disease.[40,130]

MAINTENANCE THERAPY

6-MP and AZA are widely used as front-line maintenance therapies (see Figure 22-3).[49] Also, a large controlled trial showed that methotrexate is superior to placebo in maintaining remission.[131] Five controlled trials demonstrated that AZA/6-MP were more efficient than placebo at maintaining remission; only 1 controlled trial did not.[76,120,124,132-134] The Cochrane analysis reported a

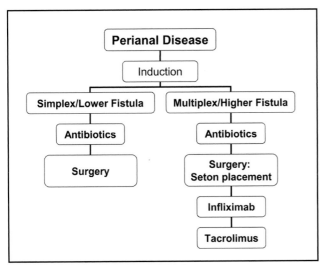

FIGURE 22-4. Induction therapy for perianal disease.

pooled OR for response to AZA of 2.16 (CI 1.35-3.47), and the number needed to treat to prevent 1 recurrence was 7, which was in agreement with earlier reports published by Pearson and coworkers.[126,135] The Cochrane analysis also reported the steroid-sparing effects of these agents with a pooled OR of 3.86 (CI 2.14-6.96) and a number needed to treat (ie, spare from steroids) of 3.[126,135] When patients do not respond or develop side effects to 6-MP/AZA, either methotrexate, infliximab, or adalimumab is indicated. Mounting evidence suggests starting the maintenance therapy together with the induction therapy.[134] Evidence regarding the optimal duration of maintenance therapy with 6-MP/AZA is lacking, but long-term use is recommended because of high relapse rates when the medication is stopped.[35,136,137] When patients fail to respond to 6-MP/AZA or methotrexate, maintenance therapy with infliximab or adalimumab is indicated. Infliximab and adalumimab are more effective than placebo at maintaining remission in moderate to severe disease.[40,43,138] Scheduled treatment appears to be more beneficial than episodic retreatment.[42] The duration of maintenance therapy with infliximab and adalumimab beyond 54 weeks (ACCENT I study and CHARM) remains to be defined. Finally, the use of infliximab as bridge therapy until a clinical response is seen with the purine analogs is commonplace in clinical practice.

FISTULIZING DISEASE

PERIANAL FISTULA

The therapeutic goals are to stop the draining of fistulas (clinical response) and close the fistulas (clinical remission).[139] Diagnosis of perianal fistula is best achieved using high-resolution imaging, such as endoscopic ultrasound or magnetic resonance, and examination under

anesthesia.[140] The combination of 2 modalities yields a 100% diagnostic accuracy.[139] A recent population-based study revealed that the cumulative incidence of fistula is 21% and 26% at 10 and 20 years, and 33% of patients will develop recurrent perianal fistulas.[141] Lower simplex fistulas have a low rate of recurrence, are best treated surgically, and do not require maintenance therapy. In contrast, higher complex fistulas have an increased risk of recurrence and require a combination of medical and surgical therapy.[142] When an abscess is diagnosed, surgery is always required, whether the fistula is situated upper or lower in the pelvis.

LOWER SIMPLEX FISTULA

INDUCTION THERAPY

First-line therapy is surgery together with antibiotics such as metronidazole, ciprofloxacin, or amoxicillin/clavulinic acid (Figure 22-4). These antibiotics have been evaluated in uncontrolled, open-label studies.[143-148]

MAINTENANCE THERAPY

Maintenance treatment is required only if a high rate of recurrence is observed during follow-up (see Figure 22-3). Maintenance therapy with metronidazole is often associated with peripheral sensory neuropathies, metallic taste, and gastrointestinal intolerance.[145] Maintenance therapy with AZA can be used in this clinical setting.[120,122,123,126,132,149] The 5-ASA derivatives and steroids (including budesonide) are not indicated and are possibly even contraindicated.

UPPER COMPLEX FISTULA

INDUCTION THERAPY

The management of upper complex fistulas benefits from a multidisciplinary approach requiring an accurate diagnosis and location of the fistula tracts and abscess (see Figure 22-4). Optimal drainage and prevention of abscess development is required before starting aggressive medical therapy. This is achieved by the placement of setons and the empiric use of prophylactic antibiotics.[139,142] Thus, surgery and antibiotics represent the first-line therapy. Infliximab is then administered as a second-line therapy with antibiotics. Infliximab is more effective than placebo at inducing remission in fistulizing disease.[71,150] The 3-dose regimen at 0, 2, and 6 weeks is preferred to achieve rapid remission and closure of fistula.[151] In addition, adalimumab and certolizumab have demonstrated efficacy for fistulizing Crohn's disease based upon post-hoc analyses.[152,153] When one encounters severe perianal disease, total parenteral nutrition may be required for bowel rest, as the fecal stream represents a continuous trigger and does not allow fistula to stop draining and close. However, even if clinical remission is obtained, the fistulous tract always persists as demonstrated by a recent cohort study using magnetic resonance imaging (MRI).[154] External fistulas in general

FIGURE 22-5. Maintenance therapy for perianal disease.

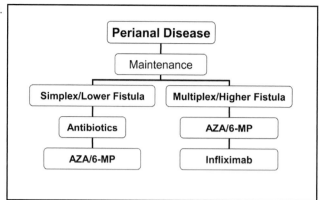

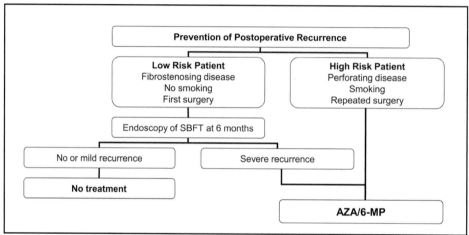

FIGURE 22-6. Prevention of anastomotic recurrence after ileocecal resection.

and perianal fistulas in particular have a higher rate of closure in response to infliximab compared to other types of fistulas such as rectovaginal fistulas.[36,155,156] If infliximab fails to induce clinical response or remission, tacrolimus can be considered as a third-line therapy, as demonstrated by 1 controlled trial.[157]

MAINTENANCE THERAPY

Maintenance therapy must always be started together with the induction therapy because of the high rate of recurrence of upper complex fistulas (Figure 22-5). 6-MP/AZA has been shown to be effective and represents the first-line maintenance in perianal Crohn's disease.[120,122,123,126,132,149] The Cochrane analysis from a few controlled trials reported a response rate of 55% for therapy and 29% for placebo and a pooled OR of 4.58 (CI 0.49-42.82) favoring, although not significantly, fistula healing.[127] Because of the delayed action of 6-MP/AZA, scheduled infliximab maintenance therapy is recommended at least as a bridge therapy. Infliximab is more effective than placebo at maintaining remission in fistulizing disease.[73,158] The optimal duration of infliximab therapy awaits definition.

INTERNAL FISTULA

Internal or intraabdominal fistulas are represented by enteroenteric fistulas, enterocolonic fistulas, entero-vesi-

cal fistulas, recto-vaginal fistulas, and entero-cutaneous fistulas.[142] Though treatment of internal fistulas has not been specifically addressed, the ACCENT II subgroup analysis and recent reports suggest variable response to antibiotics, AZA, and infliximab.[73] Enteroenteric or colonic fistulas can remain asymptomatic and do not always require immediate surgery, whereas entero-vesical fistulas will require surgery. Tolerance and discomfort arising from recto-vaginal fistulas is highly variable, and surgery must be carefully discussed with the patient. Internal abscesses require transabdominal drainage or surgery. Transabdominal drainage only delays surgery because of the high rate of recurrence.[142]

FIBROSTENOTIC DISEASE

INDUCTION THERAPY

Induction therapy of fibrostenosis diseases is surgical resection or stricturoplasty.[158] However, the inflammatory component of some strictures can be treated medically with some degree of therapeutic gain in patients with fibrostenotic disease presenting with small bowel obstruction. Alternative treatment to surgery also includes endoscopic treatment with balloon dilatation for strictures not longer than 4 cm.[159]

Maintenance Therapy

Maintenance therapy (Figure 22-6) in this setting is prevention of anastomotic recurrence after ileocecal resection with disease-free section margins.[160,161] Though both metronidazole and ornidazole prevent recurrence in controlled trials, they are associated with a significant rate of adverse reactions such as metallic taste, gastrointestinal intolerance, and peripheral neuropathy.[162,163] The 5-ASA derivatives fail to prevent symptomatic recurrence as shown by 4 controlled trials,[118,164-166] with modest benefits reported in 2 studies.[167,168] A meta-analysis reported that the number needed to treat to prevent symptomatic recurrence in 1 patient was 8, with a 13% reduction of risk of recurrence for a 2- to 3-year treatment period.[119] One controlled trial demonstrated the possible benefit,[169] whereas 2 failed to show the efficacy of sulfasalazine on postoperative recurrence.[170,171] A recent controlled trial suggested that AZA may represent a potential promise for disease prevention[172] and therefore may be indicated for patients at a high risk of relapse. Patients, mostly women who smoke, with ileocolonic disease, chronic active inflammatory, and/or fistulizing behaviors, and previous surgeries are high-risk patients and are more likely to benefit from a maintenance therapy with an agent such as AZA. Low- and intermediate-risk patients who do not smoke and suffer from a limited ileal and fibrostenotic disease with no previous surgery may not require maintenance therapy.

REFERENCES

1. Papadakis KA, Tabibzadeh S. Diagnosis and misdiagnosis of inflammatory bowel disease. *Gastrointest Endosc Clin N Am.* 2002; 12:433-449.

2. Su C, Lichtenstein GR, Krok K, et al. A meta-analysis of the placebo rates of remission and response in clinical trials of active Crohn's disease. *Gastroenterology.* 2004;126:1257-1269.

3. Minderhoud IM, Oldenburg B, Wismeijer JA, et al. IBS-like symptoms in patients with inflammatory bowel disease in remission; relationships with quality of life and coping behavior. *Dig Dis Sci.* 2004;49:469-474.

4. Timmer A. Environmental influences on inflammatory bowel disease manifestations. Lessons from epidemiology. *Dig Dis.* 2003; 21:91-104.

5. Somerville KW, Logan RF, Edmond M, et al. Smoking and Crohn's disease. *Br Med J (Clin Res Ed).* 1984;289:954-956.

6. Cottone M, Rosselli M, Orlando A, et al. Smoking habits and recurrence in Crohn's disease. *Gastroenterology.* 1994;106:643-648.

7. Cosnes J, Carbonnel F, Beaugerie L, et al. Effects of cigarette smoking on the long-term course of Crohn's disease. *Gastroenterology.* 1996;110:424-431.

8. Cosnes J. Tobacco and IBD: relevance in the understanding of disease mechanisms and clinical practice. *Best Pract Res Clin Gastroenterol.* 2004;18:481-496.

9. Rutgeerts P, Geboes K, Vantrappen G, et al. Predictability of the postoperative course of Crohn's disease. *Gastroenterology.* 1990;99:956-963.

10. D'Haens GR, Gasparaitis AE, Hanauer SB. Duration of recurrent ileitis after ileocolonic resection correlates with presurgical extent of Crohn's disease. *Gut.* 1995;36:715-717.

11. Polito JM 2nd, Childs B, Mellits ED, et al. Crohn's disease: influence of age at diagnosis on site and clinical type of disease. *Gastroenterology.* 1996;111:580-586.

12. Colombel JF, Grandbastien B, Gower-Rousseau C, et al. Clinical characteristics of Crohn's disease in 72 families. *Gastroenterology.* 1996;111:604-607.

13. Michelassi F, Balestracci T, Chappell R, et al. Primary and recurrent Crohn's disease. Experience with 1379 patients. *Ann Surg.* 1991;214:230-238; discussion 8-40.

14. Heimann TM, Greenstein AJ, Lewis B, et al. Prediction of early symptomatic recurrence after intestinal resection in Crohn's disease. *Ann Surg.* 1993;218:294-298; discussion 8-9.

15. Greenstein AJ, Janowitz HD, Sachar DB. The extra-intestinal complications of Crohn's disease and ulcerative colitis: a study of 700 patients. *Medicine (Baltimore).* 1976;55:401-412.

16. Beaugerie L, Seksik P, Nion-Larmurier I, et al. Predictors of Crohn's disease. *Gastroenterology.* 2006;130:650-656.

17. Munkholm P, Langholz E, Davidsen M, et al. Frequency of glucocorticoid resistance and dependency in Crohn's disease. *Gut.* 1994; 35:360-362.

18. Franchimont DP, Louis E, Croes F, et al. Clinical pattern of corticosteroid dependent Crohn's disease. *Eur J Gastroenterol Hepatol.* 1998;10:821-825.

19. Faubion WA Jr, Loftus EV Jr, Harmsen WS, et al. The natural history of corticosteroid therapy for inflammatory bowel disease: a population-based study. *Gastroenterology.* 2001;121:255-260.

20. Louis E, Belaiche J. Optimizing treatment with thioguanine derivatives in inflammatory bowel disease. *Best Pract Res Clin Gastroenterol.* 2003;17:37-46.

21. Baert F, Noman M, Vermeire S, et al. Influence of immunogenicity on the long-term efficacy of infliximab in Crohn's disease. *N Engl J Med.* 2003;348:601-608.

22. Farrell RJ, Alsahli M, Jeen YT, et al. Intravenous hydrocortisone premedication reduces antibodies to infliximab in Crohn's disease: a randomized controlled trial. *Gastroenterology.* 2003;124:917-924.

23. Husain A, Triadafilopoulos G. Communicating with patients with inflammatory bowel disease. *Inflamm Bowel Dis.* 2004;10:444-450; discussion 51.

24. Farmer RG, Hawk WA, Turnbull RB Jr. Clinical patterns in Crohn's disease: a statistical study of 615 cases. *Gastroenterology.* 1975;68:627-635.

25. Gasche C, Scholmerich J, Brynskov J, et al. A simple classification of Crohn's disease: report of the Working Party for the World Congresses of Gastroenterology, Vienna 1998. *Inflamm Bowel Dis.* 2000;6:8-15.

26. Silverberg MS, Satsangi J, Ahmad T, et al. Toward an integrated clinical, molecular and serological classification of inflammatory bowel disease: report of a Working Party of the 2005 Montreal World Congress of Gastroenterology. *Can J Gastroenterol.* 2005; 19:5-36.

27. Gasche C, Grundtner P. Genotypes and phenotypes in Crohn's disease: do they help in clinical management? *Gut.* 2005;54:162-167.

28. Lock MR, Farmer RG, Fazio VW, et al. Recurrence and reoperation for Crohn's disease: the role of disease location in prognosis. *N Engl J Med.* 1981;304:1586-1588.

29. Louis E, Collard A, Oger AF, et al. Behaviour of Crohn's disease according to the Vienna classification: changing pattern over the course of the disease. *Gut.* 2001;49:777-782.

30. Cosnes J, Cattan S, Blain A, et al. Long-term evolution of disease behavior of Crohn's disease. *Inflamm Bowel Dis.* 2002;8:244-250.

31. Gelbmann CM, Rogler G, Gross V, et al. Prior bowel resections, perianal disease, and a high initial Crohn's disease activity index are associated with corticosteroid resistance in active Crohn's disease. *Am J Gastroenterol.* 2002;97:1438-1445.

32. Feagan BG, McDonald JW, Koval JJ. Therapeutics and inflammatory bowel disease: a guide to the interpretation of randomized controlled trials. *Gastroenterology.* 1996;110:275-283.

33. Navarro F, Hanauer SB. Treatment of inflammatory bowel disease: safety and tolerability issues. *Am J Gastroenterol.* 2003;98:S18-S23.

34. Lecomte T, Contou JF, Beaugerie L, et al. Predictive factors of response of perianal Crohn's disease to azathioprine or 6-mercaptopurine. *Dis Colon Rectum.* 2003;46:1469-1475.

35. Fraser AG, Orchard TR, Jewell DP. The efficacy of azathioprine for the treatment of inflammatory bowel disease: a 30 year review. *Gut.* 2002;50:485-489.

36. Arnott ID, McNeill G, Satsangi J. An analysis of factors influencing short-term and sustained response to infliximab treatment for Crohn's disease. *Aliment Pharmacol Ther.* 2003;17:1451-1457.

37. Parsi MA, Achkar JP, Richardson S, et al. Predictors of response to infliximab in patients with Crohn's disease. *Gastroenterology.* 2002;123:707-713.

38. Vermeire S, Louis E, Carbonez A, et al. Demographic and clinical parameters influencing the short-term outcome of anti-tumor necrosis factor (infliximab) treatment in Crohn's disease. *Am J Gastroenterol.* 2002;97:2357-2363.

39. Costes L, Colombel J-F. Long term follow-up of a cohort of steroid-dependent Crohn's disease patients included in a randomized trial evaluating short term infliximab combined with azathioprine. *Gastroenterology.* 2008;134:A134.

40. Colombel JF, Sandborn WJ, Rutgeerts P, et al. Adalimumab for maintenance of clinical response and remission in patients with Crohn's disease: the CHARM trial. *Gastroenterology.* 2007;132:52-65.

41. Sandborn WJ, Feagan BG, Stoinov S, et al. Certolizumab pegol for the treatment of Crohn's disease. *N Engl J Med.* 2007;357:228-238.

42. Rutgeerts P, Feagan BG, Lichtenstein GR, et al. Comparison of scheduled and episodic treatment strategies of infliximab in Crohn's disease. *Gastroenterology.* 2004;126:402-413.

43. Hanauer SB, Feagan BG, Lichtenstein GR, et al. Maintenance infliximab for Crohn's disease: the ACCENT I randomised trial. *Lancet.* 2002;359:1541-1549.

44. Hanauer SB, Wagner CL, Bala M, et al. Incidence and importance of antibody responses to infliximab after maintenance or episodic treatment in Crohn's disease. *Clin Gastroenterol Hepatol.* 2004;2:542-553.

45. Lichtenstein GR, Feagan BG, Cohen RD, et al. Serious infections and mortality in association with therapies for Crohn's disease: TREAT registry. *Clin Gastroenterol Hepatol.* 2006;4:621-630.

46. Mackey AC, Green L, Liang LC, et al. Hepatosplenic T cell lymphoma associated with infliximab use in young patients treated for inflammatory bowel disease. *J Pediatr Gastroenterol Nutr.* 2007; 44:265-267.

47. Viget N, Vernier-Massouille G, Salmon-Ceron D, et al. Opportunistic infections in patients with inflammatory bowel disease: prevention and diagnosis. *Gut.* 2008;57:549-558.

48. Van Assche G, Magdelaine-Beuzelin C, D'Haens G, et al. Withdrawal of immunosuppression in Crohn's disease treated with scheduled infliximab maintenance: a randomized trial. *Gastroenterology.* 2008;8:8.

49. Beaugerie L, Carrat F, Bouvier A-M, et al. Excess risk of lymphoproliferative disorders in inflammatory bowel disease: interim results of the Cesame cohort [abstract]. *Gastroenterology.* 2008;134:A-116.

50. Colombel JF, Sandborn WJ, Reinisch W, et al. Infliximab, azathioprine, or combination therapy for Crohn's disease. *N Engl J Med.* 2010;362:1383-1395.

51. Dubinsky MC. Azathioprine, 6-mercaptopurine in inflammatory bowel disease: pharmacology, efficacy, and safety. *Clin Gastroenterol Hepatol.* 2004;2:731-743.

52. Dubinsky MC. Optimizing immunomodulator therapy for inflammatory bowel disease. *Curr Gastroenterol Rep.* 2003;5:506-511.

53. Kaskas BA, Louis E, Hindorf U, et al. Safe treatment of thiopurine S-methyltransferase deficient Crohn's disease patients with azathioprine. *Gut.* 2003;52:140-142.

54. Lichtenstein GR. Use of laboratory testing to guide 6-mercaptopurine/azathioprine therapy. *Gastroenterology.* 2004;127:1558-1564.

55. Wright S, Sanders DS, Lobo AJ, et al. Clinical significance of azathioprine active metabolite concentrations in inflammatory bowel disease. *Gut.* 2004;53:1123-1128.

56. Goldenberg BA, Rawsthorne P, Bernstein CN. The utility of 6-thioguanine metabolite levels in managing patients with inflammatory bowel disease. *Am J Gastroenterol.* 2004;99:1744-1748.

57. Toruner M, Loftus EV Jr, Harmsen WS, et al. Risk factors for opportunistic infections in patients with inflammatory bowel disease. *Gastroenterology.* 2008;134:929-936.

58. D'Haens G, Van Deventer S, Van Hogezand R, et al. Endoscopic and histological healing with infliximab anti-tumor necrosis factor antibodies in Crohn's disease: a European multicenter trial. *Gastroenterology.* 1999;116:1029-1034.

59. Best WR, Becktel JM, Singleton JW, et al. Development of a Crohn's disease activity index. National Cooperative Crohn's Disease Study. *Gastroenterology.* 1976;70:439-444.

60. Sandborn WJ, Feagan BG, Hanauer SB, et al. A review of activity indices and efficacy endpoints for clinical trials of medical therapy in adults with Crohn's disease. *Gastroenterology.* 2002;122:512-530.

61. Modigliani R, Mary JY, Simon JF, et al. Clinical, biological, and endoscopic picture of attacks of Crohn's disease. Evolution on prednisolone. Groupe d'Etude Therapeutique des Affections Inflammatoires Digestives. *Gastroenterology.* 1990;98:811-818.

62. Daperno M, D'Haens G, Van Assche G, et al. Development and validation of a new, simplified endoscopic activity score for Crohn's disease: the SES-CD. *Gastrointest Endosc.* 2004;60:505-512.

63. Allez M, Lemann M, Bonnet J, et al. Long term outcome of patients with active Crohn's disease exhibiting extensive and deep ulcerations at colonoscopy. *Am J Gastroenterol.* 2002;97:947-953.

64. Lichtenstein GR, Yan S, Bala M, et al. Remission in patients with Crohn's disease is associated with improvement in employment and quality of life and a decrease in hospitalizations and surgeries. *Am J Gastroenterol.* 2004;99:91-96.

65. Vermeire S, Van Assche G, Rutgeerts P. C-reactive protein as a marker for inflammatory bowel disease. *Inflamm Bowel Dis.* 2004; 10:661-665.

66. Tibble JA, Sigthorsson G, Bridger S, et al. Surrogate markers of intestinal inflammation are predictive of relapse in patients with inflammatory bowel disease. *Gastroenterology.* 2000;119:15-22.

67. Breedveld FC, Weisman MH, Kavanaugh AF, et al. The PREMIER study: a multicenter, randomized, double-blind clinical trial of combination therapy with adalimumab plus methotrexate versus methotrexate alone or adalimumab alone in patients with early, aggressive rheumatoid arthritis who had not had previous methotrexate treatment. *Arthritis Rheum.* 2006;54:26-37.

68. Goekoop-Ruiterman YP, de Vries-Bouwstra JK, Allaart CF, et al. Clinical and radiographic outcomes of four different treatment strategies in patients with early rheumatoid arthritis (the BeSt study): a randomized, controlled trial. *Arthritis Rheum.* 2005; 52:3381-3390.

69. D'Haens G, Baert F, van Assche G, et al. Early combined immunosuppression or conventional management in patients with newly diagnosed Crohn's disease: an open randomised trial. *Lancet.* 2008;371:660-667.

70. Sands BE, Arsenault JE, Rosen MJ, et al. Risk of early surgery for Crohn's disease: implications for early treatment strategies. *Am J Gastroenterol.* 2003;98:2712-2718.

71. Dubinsky MC, Lin YC, Dutridge D, et al. Serum immune responses predict rapid disease progression among children with Crohn's disease: immune responses predict disease progression. *Am J Gastroenterol.* 2006;101:360-367.

72. Odes S, Friger M, Vardi H, et al. Role of ASCA and the NOD2/CARD15 mutation Gly908Arg in predicting increased surgical costs in Crohn's disease patients: a project of the European Collaborative Study Group on Inflammatory Bowel Disease. *Inflamm Bowel Dis.* 2007;13:874-881.

73. Sands BE, Anderson FH, Bernstein CN, et al. Infliximab maintenance therapy for fistulizing Crohn's disease. *N Engl J Med.* 2004; 350:876-885.

74. Targan SR, Hanauer SB, van Deventer SJ, et al. A short-term study of chimeric monoclonal antibody cA2 to tumor necrosis factor alpha for Crohn's disease. Crohn's Disease cA2 Study Group. *N Engl J Med.* 1997;337:1029-1035.

75. Anthonisen P, Barany F, Folkenborg O, et al. The clinical effect of salazosulphapyridine (Salazopyrin r) in Crohn's disease. A controlled double-blind study. *Scand J Gastroenterol.* 1974;9:549-554.

76. Summers RW, Switz DM, Sessions JT Jr, et al. National Cooperative Crohn's Disease Study: results of drug treatment. *Gastroenterology.* 1979;77:847-869.

77. Van Hees PA, Van Lier HJ, Van Elteren PH, et al. Effect of sulphasalazine in patients with active Crohn's disease: a controlled double-blind study. *Gut.* 1981;22:404-409.

78. Malchow H, Ewe K, Brandes JW, et al. European Cooperative Crohn's Disease Study (ECCDS): results of drug treatment. *Gastroenterology.* 1984;86:249-266.

79. Greenberg GR, Feagan BG, Martin F, et al. Oral budesonide for active Crohn's disease. Canadian Inflammatory Bowel Disease Study Group. *N Engl J Med.* 1994;331:836-841.

80. Rutgeerts P, Lofberg R, Malchow H, et al. A comparison of budesonide with prednisolone for active Crohn's disease. *N Engl J Med.* 1994;331:842-845.

81. Campieri M, Ferguson A, Doe W, et al. Oral budesonide is as effective as oral prednisolone in active Crohn's disease. The Global Budesonide Study Group. *Gut.* 1997;41:209-214.

82. Bar-Meir S, Chowers Y, Lavy A, et al. Budesonide versus prednisone in the treatment of active Crohn's disease. The Israeli Budesonide Study Group. *Gastroenterology.* 1998;115:835-840.

83. Tremaine WJ, Hanauer SB, Katz S, et al. Budesonide CIR capsules (once or twice daily divided-dose) in active Crohn's disease: a randomized placebo-controlled study in the United States. *Am J Gastroenterol.* 2002;97:1748-1754.

84. Thomsen OO, Cortot A, Jewell D, et al. A comparison of budesonide and mesalamine for active Crohn's disease. International Budesonide-Mesalamine Study Group. *N Engl J Med.* 1998;339:370-374.

85. Rasmussen SN, Lauritsen K, Tage-Jensen U, et al. 5-Aminosalicylic acid in the treatment of Crohn's disease. A 16-week double-blind, placebo-controlled, multicentre study with Pentasa. *Scand J Gastroenterol.* 1987;22:877-883.

86. Mahida YR, Jewell DP. Slow-release 5-amino-salicylic acid (Pentasa) for the treatment of active Crohn's disease. *Digestion.* 1990;45:88-92.

87. Singleton JW, Hanauer SB, Gitnick GL, et al. Mesalamine capsules for the treatment of active Crohn's disease: results of a 16-week trial. Pentasa Crohn's Disease Study Group. *Gastroenterology.* 1993; 104:1293-1301.

88. Singleton J. Second trial of mesalamine therapy in the treatment of active Crohn's disease. *Gastroenterology.* 1994;107:632-633.

89. Tremaine WJ, Schroeder KW, Harrison JM, et al. A randomized, double-blind, placebo-controlled trial of the oral mesalamine (5-ASA) preparation, Asacol, in the treatment of symptomatic Crohn's colitis and ileocolitis. *J Clin Gastroenterol.* 1994;19:278-282.

90. Harrell LE, Hanauer SB. Mesalamine derivatives in the treatment of Crohn's disease. *Gastroenterol Clin North Am.* 2004;33:303-317, ix-x.

91. Blichfeldt P, Blomhoff JP, Myhre E, et al. Metronidazole in Crohn's disease. A double blind cross-over clinical trial. *Scand J Gastroenterol.* 1978;13:123-127.

92. Ambrose NS, Allan RN, Keighley MR, et al. Antibiotic therapy for treatment in relapse of intestinal Crohn's disease. A prospective randomized study. *Dis Colon Rectum.* 1985;28:81-85.

93. Sutherland L, Singleton J, Sessions J, et al. Double blind, placebo controlled trial of metronidazole in Crohn's disease. *Gut.* 1991; 32:1071-1075.

94. Prantera C, Kohn A, Zannoni F, et al. Metronidazole plus ciprofloxacin in the treatment of active, refractory Crohn's disease: results of an open study. *J Clin Gastroenterol.* 1994;19:79-80.

95. Colombel JF, Lemann M, Cassagnou M, et al. A controlled trial comparing ciprofloxacin with mesalazine for the treatment of active Crohn's disease. Groupe d'Etudes Therapeutiques des Affections Inflammatoires Digestives (GETAID). *Am J Gastroenterol.* 1999;94:674-678.

96. Arnold GL, Beaves MR, Pryjdun VO, et al. Preliminary study of ciprofloxacin in active Crohn's disease. *Inflamm Bowel Dis.* 2002; 8:10-15.

97. Steinhart AH, Feagan BG, Wong CJ, et al. Combined budesonide and antibiotic therapy for active Crohn's disease: a randomized controlled trial. *Gastroenterology.* 2002;123:33-40.

98. Chun A, Chadi RM, Korelitz BI, et al. Intravenous corticotrophin vs. hydrocortisone in the treatment of hospitalized patients with Crohn's disease: a randomized double-blind study and follow-up. *Inflamm Bowel Dis.* 1998;4:177-181.

99. Rijk MC, van Hogezand RA, van Lier HJ, et al. Sulphasalazine and prednisone compared with sulphasalazine for treating active Crohn disease. A double-blind, randomized, multicenter trial. *Ann Intern Med.* 1991;114:445-450.

100. Levine A, Weizman Z, Broide E, et al. A comparison of budesonide and prednisone for the treatment of active pediatric Crohn disease. *J Pediatr Gastroenterol Nutr.* 2003;36:248-252.

101. Escher JC. Budesonide versus prednisolone for the treatment of active Crohn's disease in children: a randomized, double-blind, controlled, multicentre trial. *Eur J Gastroenterol Hepatol.* 2004; 16:47-54.

102. Lennard-Jones JE. Sulphasalazine in asymptomatic Crohn's disease. A multicentre trial. *Gut.* 1977;18:69-72.

103. Greenberg GR, Feagan BG, Martin F, et al. Oral budesonide as maintenance treatment for Crohn's disease: a placebo-controlled, dose-ranging study. Canadian Inflammatory Bowel Disease Study Group. *Gastroenterology.* 1996;110:45-51.

104. Lofberg R, Rutgeerts P, Malchow H, et al. Budesonide prolongs time to relapse in ileal and ileocaecal Crohn's disease. A placebo controlled one year study. *Gut.* 1996;39:82-86.

105. Gross V, Andus T, Ecker KW, et al. Low dose oral pH modified release budesonide for maintenance of steroid induced remission in Crohn's disease. The Budesonide Study Group. *Gut.* 1998; 42:493-496.

106. Ferguson A, Campieri M, Doe W, et al. Oral budesonide as maintenance therapy in Crohn's disease: results of a 12-month study. Global Budesonide Study Group. *Aliment Pharmacol Ther.* 1998;12:175-183.

107. Green JR, Lobo AJ, Giaffer M, et al. Maintenance of Crohn's disease over 12 months: fixed versus flexible dosing regimen using budesonide controlled ileal release capsules. *Aliment Pharmacol Ther.* 2001;15:1331-1341.

108. Cortot A, Colombel JF, Rutgeerts P, et al. Switch from systemic steroids to budesonide in steroid dependent patients with inactive Crohn's disease. *Gut.* 2001;48:186-190.

109. Coated oral 5-aminosalicylic acid versus placebo in maintaining remission of inactive Crohn's disease. International Mesalazine Study Group. *Aliment Pharmacol Ther.* 1990;4:55-64.

110. Brignola C, Iannone P, Pasquali S, et al. Placebo-controlled trial of oral 5-ASA in relapse prevention of Crohn's disease. *Dig Dis Sci.* 1992;37:29-32.

111. Prantera C, Pallone F, Brunetti G, et al. Oral 5-aminosalicylic acid (Asacol) in the maintenance treatment of Crohn's disease. The Italian IBD Study Group. *Gastroenterology.* 1992;103:363-368.

112. Gendre JP, Mary JY, Florent C, et al. Oral mesalamine (Pentasa) as maintenance treatment in Crohn's disease: a multicenter placebo-controlled study. The Groupe d'Etudes Therapeutiques des Affections Inflammatoires Digestives (GETAID). *Gastroenterology.* 1993;104:435-439.

113. Bresci G, Parisi G, Banti S. Long-term therapy with 5-aminosalicylic acid in Crohn's disease: is it useful? Our four years experience. *Int J Clin Pharmacol Res.* 1994;14:133-138.

114. Arber N, Odes HS, Fireman Z, et al. A controlled double blind multicenter study of the effectiveness of 5-aminosalicylic acid in patients with Crohn's disease in remission. *J Clin Gastroenterol.* 1995;20:203-206.

115. Thomson AB, Wright JP, Vatn M, et al. Mesalazine (Mesasal/Claversal) 1.5 g b.d. vs. placebo in the maintenance of remission of patients with Crohn's disease. *Aliment Pharmacol Ther.* 1995;9:673-683.

116. Modigliani R, Colombel JF, Dupas JL, et al. Mesalamine in Crohn's disease with steroid-induced remission: effect on steroid withdrawal and remission maintenance, Groupe d'Etudes Therapeutiques des Affections Inflammatoires Digestives. *Gastroenterology.* 1996;110:688-693.

117. de Franchis R, Omodei P, Ranzi T, et al. Controlled trial of oral 5-aminosalicylic acid for the prevention of early relapse in Crohn's disease. *Aliment Pharmacol Ther.* 1997;11:845-852.

118. Sutherland LR, Martin F, Bailey RJ, et al. A randomized, placebo-controlled, double-blind trial of mesalamine in the maintenance of remission of Crohn's disease. The Canadian Mesalamine for Remission of Crohn's Disease Study Group. *Gastroenterology.* 1997;112:1069-1077.

119. Camma C, Giunta M, Rosselli M, et al. Mesalamine in the maintenance treatment of Crohn's disease: a meta-analysis adjusted for confounding variables. *Gastroenterology.* 1997;113:1465-1473.

120. Willoughby JM, Beckett J, Kumar PJ, et al. Controlled trial of azathioprine in Crohn's disease. *Lancet.* 1971;2:944-947.

121. Rhodes J. Azathioprine in the treatment of Crohn's disease. *Br J Surg.* 1972;59:819-821.

122. Klein M, Binder HJ, Mitchell M, et al. Treatment of Crohn's disease with azathioprine: a controlled evaluation. *Gastroenterology.* 1974;66:916-922.

123. Present DH, Korelitz BI, Wisch N, et al. Treatment of Crohn's disease with 6-mercaptopurine. A long-term, randomized, double-blind study. *N Engl J Med.* 1980;302:981-987.

124. Candy S, Wright J, Gerber M, et al. A controlled double blind study of azathioprine in the management of Crohn's disease. *Gut.* 1995;37:674-678.

125. Ewe K, Press AG, Singe CC, et al. Azathioprine combined with prednisolone or monotherapy with prednisolone in active Crohn's disease. *Gastroenterology.* 1993;105:367-372.

126. Pearson DC, May GR, Fick GH, et al. Azathioprine and 6-mercaptopurine in Crohn disease. A meta-analysis. *Ann Intern Med.* 1995;123:132-142.

127. Sandborn W, Sutherland L, Pearson D, et al. Azathioprine or 6-mercaptopurine for inducing remission of Crohn's disease. *Cochrane Database Syst Rev.* 2000:CD000545.

128. Oren R, Moshkowitz M, Odes S, et al. Methotrexate in chronic active Crohn's disease: a double-blind, randomized, Israeli multicenter trial. *Am J Gastroenterol.* 1997;92:2203-2209.

129. Rutgeerts P, D'Haens G, Targan S, et al. Efficacy and safety of retreatment with anti-tumor necrosis factor antibody (infliximab) to maintain remission in Crohn's disease. *Gastroenterology.* 1999;117:761-769.

130. Hanauer SB, Sandborn WJ, Rutgeerts P, et al. Human anti-tumor necrosis factor monoclonal antibody (adalimumab) in Crohn's disease: the CLASSIC-I trial. *Gastroenterology.* 2006;130:323-333; quiz 591.

131. Feagan BG, Fedorak RN, Irvine EJ, et al. A comparison of methotrexate with placebo for the maintenance of remission in Crohn's disease. North American Crohn's Study Group Investigators. *N Engl J Med.* 2000;342:1627-1632.

132. Rosenberg JL, Levin B, Wall AJ, et al. A controlled trial of azathioprine in Crohn's disease. *Am J Dig Dis.* 1975;20:721-726.

133. O'Donoghue DP, Dawson AM, Powell-Tuck J, et al. Double-blind withdrawal trial of azathioprine as maintenance treatment for Crohn's disease. *Lancet.* 1978;2:955-957.

134. Markowitz J, Grancher K, Kohn N, et al. A multicenter trial of 6-mercaptopurine and prednisone in children with newly diagnosed Crohn's disease. *Gastroenterology.* 2000;119:895-902.

135. Pearson DC, May GR, Fick G, et al. Azathioprine for maintaining remission of Crohn's disease. *Cochrane Database Syst Rev.* 2000:CD000067.

136. Bouhnik Y, Lemann M, Mary JY, et al. Long-term follow-up of patients with Crohn's disease treated with azathioprine or 6-mercaptopurine. *Lancet.* 1996;347:215-219.

137. Lemann M, Mary JY, Colombel JF, et al. A randomized, double-blind, controlled withdrawal trial in Crohn's disease patients in long-term remission on azathioprine. *Gastroenterology.* 2005;128:1812-1818.

138. Rutgeerts P. Budesonide led to a greater remission rate and fewer severe adverse events than did mesalamine in Crohn's disease. *Gut.* 1999;45:13-14.

139. Schwartz DA, Pemberton JH, Sandborn WJ. Diagnosis and treatment of perianal fistulas in Crohn disease. *Ann Intern Med.* 2001;135:906-918.

140. Sandborn WJ, Fazio VW, Feagan BG, et al. AGA technical review on perianal Crohn's disease. *Gastroenterology.* 2003;125:1508-1530.

141. Schwartz DA, Loftus EV Jr, Tremaine WJ, et al. The natural history of fistulizing Crohn's disease in Olmsted County, Minnesota. *Gastroenterology.* 2002;122:875-880.

142. Lichtenstein GR. Treatment of fistulizing Crohn's disease. *Gastroenterology.* 2000;119:1132-1147.

143. Ursing B, Alm T, Barany F, et al. A comparative study of metronidazole and sulfasalazine for active Crohn's disease: The cooperative Crohn's disease study in Sweden. II. Result. *Gastroenterology.* 1982;83:550-562.

144. Bernstein LH, Frank MS, Brandt LJ, et al. Healing of perineal Crohn's disease with metronidazole. *Gastroenterology.* 1980;79:357-365.

145. Brandt LJ, Bernstein LH, Boley SJ, et al. Metronidazole therapy for perineal Crohn's disease: a follow-up study. *Gastroenterology.* 1982;83:383-387.

146. Jakobovits J, Schuster MM. Metronidazole therapy for Crohn's disease and associated fistulae. *Am J Gastroenterol.* 1984;79:533-540.

147. Irvine EJ. Usual therapy improves perianal Crohn's disease as measured by a new disease activity index. McMaster IBD Study Group. *J Clin Gastroenterol.* 1995;20:27-32.

148. Dejaco C, Harrer M, Waldhoer T, et al. Antibiotics and azathioprine for the treatment of perianal fistulas in Crohn's disease. *Aliment Pharmacol Ther.* 2003;18:1113-1120.

149. Rhodes J, Bainton D, Beck P, et al. Controlled trial of azathioprine in Crohn's disease. *Lancet.* 1971;2:1273-1276.

150. Present DH, Rutgeerts P, Targan S, et al. Infliximab for the treatment of fistulas in patients with Crohn's disease. *N Engl J Med.* 1999;340:1398-1405.

151. Sandborn WJ, Hanauer SB. Infliximab in the treatment of Crohn's disease: a user's guide for clinicians. *Am J Gastroenterol.* 2002; 97:2962-2972.

152. Colombel JF, Schwartz DA, Sandborn WJ, et al. Adalimumab for the treatment of fistulas in patients with Crohn's disease. *Gut.* 2009;58:940-948.

153. Schreiber S, Khaliq-Kareemi M, Lawrance IC, et al. Maintenance therapy with certolizumab pegol for Crohn's disease. *N Engl J Med.* 2007;357:239-250.

154. Van Assche G, Vanbeckevoort D, Bielen D, et al. Magnetic resonance imaging of the effects of infliximab on perianal fistulizing Crohn's disease. *Am J Gastroenterol.* 2003;98:332-339.

155. Miehsler W, Reinisch W, Kazemi-Shirazi L, et al. Infliximab: lack of efficacy on perforating complications in Crohn's disease. *Inflamm Bowel Dis.* 2004;10:36-40.

156. Sands BE, Blank MA, Patel K, et al. Long-term treatment of rectovaginal fistulas in Crohn's disease: response to infliximab in the ACCENT II Study. *Clin Gastroenterol Hepatol.* 2004;2:912-920.

157. Sandborn WJ, Present DH, Isaacs KL, et al. Tacrolimus for the treatment of fistulas in patients with Crohn's disease: a randomized, placebo-controlled trial. *Gastroenterology.* 2003;125:380-388.

158. McLeod RS. Surgery for inflammatory bowel diseases. *Dig Dis.* 2003;21:168-179.

159. Erkelens GW, van Deventer SJ. Endoscopic treatment of strictures in Crohn's disease. *Best Pract Res Clin Gastroenterol.* 2004;18:201-207.

160. Van Assche G, Rutgeerts P. Medical management of postoperative recurrence in Crohn's disease. *Gastroenterol Clin North Am.* 2004;33:347-360, x.

161. Rutgeerts P. Strategies in the prevention of post-operative recurrence in Crohn's disease. *Best Pract Res Clin Gastroenterol.* 2003; 17:63-73.

162. Rutgeerts P, Hiele M, Geboes K, et al. Controlled trial of metronidazole treatment for prevention of Crohn's recurrence after ileal resection. *Gastroenterology.* 1995;108:1617-1621.

163. Rutgeerts P, Van Assche G, Vermeire S, et al. Ornidazole for prophylaxis of postoperative Crohn's disease recurrence: a randomized, double-blind, placebo-controlled trial. *Gastroenterology.* 2005;128:856-861.

164. Brignola C, Cottone M, Pera A, et al. Mesalamine in the prevention of endoscopic recurrence after intestinal resection for Crohn's disease. Italian Cooperative Study Group. *Gastroenterology.* 1995;108: 345-349.

165. Florent C, Cortot A, Quandale P, et al. Placebo-controlled clinical trial of mesalazine in the prevention of early endoscopic recurrences after resection for Crohn's disease. Groupe d'Etudes Therapeutiques des Affections Inflammatoires Digestives (GETAID). *Eur J Gastroenterol Hepatol.* 1996;8:229-233.

166. Lochs H, Mayer M, Fleig WE, et al. Prophylaxis of postoperative relapse in Crohn's disease with mesalamine: European Cooperative Crohn's Disease Study VI. *Gastroenterology.* 2000;118:264-273.

167. McLeod RS, Wolff BG, Steinhart AH, et al. Prophylactic mesalamine treatment decreases postoperative recurrence of Crohn's disease. *Gastroenterology.* 1995;109:404-413.

168. Caprilli R, Andreoli A, Capurso L, et al. Oral mesalazine (5-aminosalicylic acid; Asacol) for the prevention of post-operative recurrence of Crohn's disease. Gruppo Italiano per lo Studio del Colon e del Retto (GISC). *Aliment Pharmacol Ther.* 1994;8:35-43.

169. Ewe K, Herfarth C, Malchow H, et al. Postoperative recurrence of Crohn's disease in relation to radicality of operation and sulfasalazine prophylaxis: a multicenter trial. *Digestion.* 1989;42:224-232.

170. Bergman L, Krause U. Postoperative treatment with corticosteroids and salazosulphapyridine (Salazopyrin) after radical resection for Crohn's disease. *Scand J Gastroenterol.* 1976;11:651-656.

171. Wenckert A, Kristensen M, Eklund AE, et al. The long-term prophylactic effect of salazosulphapyridine (Salazopyrin) in primarily resected patients with Crohn's disease. A controlled double-blind trial. *Scand J Gastroenterol.* 1978;13:161-167.

172. Hanauer SB, Korelitz BI, Rutgeerts P, et al. Postoperative maintenance of Crohn's disease remission with 6-mercaptopurine, mesalamine, or placebo: a 2-year trial. *Gastroenterology.* 2004;127:723-729.

23

MEDICAL MANAGEMENT OF SEVERE CROHN'S DISEASE

Themistocles Dassopoulos, MD and Theodore M. Bayless, MD

In the absence of a "gold standard" indicator for the activity of Crohn's disease, experienced inflammatory bowel disease (IBD) clinicians assess and synthesize a number of parameters to make a global assessment of disease severity. This assessment is clearly subjective. In clinical trials, the Crohn's Disease Activity Index (CDAI) has been the most widely used instrument to measure disease severity. The CDAI was developed and validated against the physician's global assessment and contains 8 weighted variables. Scores range from 0 to approximately 600. Remission and very severe disease are defined as CDAI scores below 150 and above 450 points, respectively. Subsequent investigators arbitrarily labeled CDAI scores of 150 to 219 as mildly active disease and scores of 220 to 450 as moderately severe disease (Table 23-1).[1] All clinical trials have excluded patients with very severe disease (CDAI > 450), and only 1 randomized trial studied hospitalized patients,[2] so that management of these patients relies on experience rather than on evidence.

The CDAI system has several limitations, including high interobserver variability and lack of accuracy in patients with stenosing CD or concomitant irritable bowel syndrome (IBS). Several randomized controlled trials of biologic agents in active CD have hinted at the limitations of the CDAI. Post hoc analyses showed that subjects in the placebo arms with normal C-reactive protein (CRP) levels had pronounced improvements in their CDAI scores. These findings suggest that concomitant conditions such as IBS, short bowel syndrome, cholerrheic diarrhea, small bowel bacterial overgrowth, and partial intestinal obstruc-

tion may raise the CDAI, leading to a false impression of more severe CD.

The American College of Gastroenterology (ACG) has implemented "working definitions" of CD activity[3] (Table 23-2). In the ACG guidelines, mild to moderate CD applies to ambulatory patients without dehydration, toxicity, abdominal tenderness, painful mass, obstruction, or >10% weight loss. Moderate to severe disease applies to nonhospitalized patients who failed to respond to treatment for mild to moderate disease or those with more prominent symptoms of fever, significant weight loss, abdominal pain or tenderness, intermittent nausea or vomiting (without obstructive findings), or significant anemia. Severe to fulminant disease refers to patients with persisting symptoms despite the introduction of steroids as outpatients or to individuals presenting with high fever, persistent vomiting, as well as evidence of intestinal obstruction, rebound tenderness, cachexia, or abscess. Using these definitions, patients who have had partial response or no response to oral steroids and can be treated as outpatients with infliximab are classified as having moderately severe disease.

In this chapter, we review the management of severe CD. We define severe CD as disease that is moderately severe (CDAI of 220 to 450) or very severe (CDAI > 450) or that necessitates hospitalization. These patients may have uncomplicated inflammatory CD or CD complicated by intestinal obstruction, abscess, severe gastrointestinal bleeding, or toxic megacolon. Some of these complications can be managed medically, whereas others will require urgent radiologic and/or surgical interventions. Optimal

TABLE 23-1

CROHN'S DISEASE SEVERITY BY CROHN'S DISEASE ACTIVITY INDEX

Remission	< 150
Mildly active disease	150 to 219
Moderately severe disease	220 to 450
Very severe disease	> 450

TABLE 23-2

CROHN'S DISEASE SEVERITY: WORKING DEFINITIONS OF THE PRACTICE PARAMETERS COMMITTEE OF THE AMERICAN COLLEGE OF GASTROENTEROLOGY*

MILD TO MODERATE DISEASE

Mild to moderate Crohn's disease applies to ambulatory patients able to tolerate oral alimentation without manifestations of dehydration, toxicity (high fevers, rigors, prostration), abdominal tenderness, painful mass, obstruction, or >10% weight loss.

MODERATE TO SEVERE DISEASE

Moderate to severe disease applies to patients who have failed to respond to treatment for mild to moderate disease or those with more prominent symptoms of fevers, significant weight loss, abdominal pain or tenderness, intermittent nausea or vomiting (without obstructive findings), or significant anemia.

SEVERE TO FULMINANT DISEASE

Severe to fulminant disease refers to patients with persisting symptoms despite the introduction of steroids as outpatients or individuals presenting with high fever, persistent vomiting, evidence of intestinal obstruction, rebound tenderness, cachexia, or evidence of an abscess.

*Lichtenstein GR, Hanauer SB, Sandborn WJ, and the Practice Parameters Committee of American College of Gastroenterology. Management of Crohn's disease in adults. *Am J Gastroenterol.* 2009;104:465-483.

preoperative and postoperative medical management is critical in ensuring good outcomes.

SEVERE INFLAMMATORY CROHN'S DISEASE

CLINICAL PRESENTATION

Patients with severe inflammatory CD present with abdominal pain and tenderness, inflammatory masses, diarrhea, fever, weight loss, malaise, extraintestinal manifestations, and significant anemia but without evidence of obstruction or abscess.

As with all patients experiencing flares of inflammatory bowel disease, the clinician must inquire about possible precipitants, such as the use of aspirin and nonsteroidal antiinflammatory drugs (NSAIDs) (including the cyclooxygenase-2 [COX-2] inhibitors),[4-6] antibiotic use pre-disposing to *Clostridium difficile*, travel history, exposure to food pathogens, or nonadherence.[7] We have encountered several patients who developed fulminant disease or intestinal perforation after abrupt cessation of immunomodulator therapies. Absent or very low levels of the 6-thioguanine and 6-methylmercaptopurine nucleotide metabolites indicate nonadherence to azathioprine (AZA) and 6-mercaptopurine (6-MP) therapy.[8] Infectious pathogens are frequently responsible for CD flares in both inpatients and outpatients. A British study[9] found an enteric infection in 10.5% of IBD relapses. *Clostridium difficile* toxin was the most common organism, detected in slightly more than half of the relapses. A variety of other organisms (*Campylobacter* species, *Entamoeba histolytica*, *Salmonella* species, *Plesiomonas shigelloides*, *Strongyloides stercoralis*, and *Blastocystis hominis*) were also found.[9] There was a significant association between infection and the need for hospital admission.[9] A high index of suspicion is also required to recognize *Cytomegalovirus* and *Aeromonas*.

In addition to fever and dehydration, the physical exam in the severely ill patient may reveal rebound tenderness and an abdominal mass, most frequently in the right lower quadrant. Laboratory evaluation demonstrates anemia (iron deficiency and/or anemia of chronic disease), leukocytosis (sometimes with elevated bands), electrolyte and renal disturbances, and hypoalbuminemia. We routinely measure the erythrocyte sedimentation rate and CRP in all our hospitalized patients, because normal values call into question the presence of severe inflammatory CD. However, it should be recognized that some individuals with documented, severe CD may have a normal CRP. Computed tomography findings include thickened bowel walls that enhance after intravenous (IV) contrast injection, fibrofatty proliferation, increased mesenteric vascularity, mesenteric adenopathy, and/or an inflammatory mass (phlegmon), usually in the right lower quadrant. Phlegmons are radiologically distinguished from abscesses by the absence of air bubbles.

SUPPORTIVE THERAPY

Supportive or resuscitative therapy with fluid and electrolytes is indicated for dehydrated patients, and transfusions may be necessary in the setting of anemia and active hemorrhage. Severely ill patients are treated with bowel rest and parenteral nutritional support. Oral feedings are usually continued, as tolerated, for patients without severe abdominal pain or obstruction. Although elemental, peptide, and polymeric diets appear effective as primary therapies for active CD,[10-14] they are less effective than corticosteroids,[15] and most patients relapse upon resumption of a normal diet.[11] Their high cost and poor palatability have also limited their use in adults. Enteral feedings are still used in the pediatric population where they promote growth.

CORTICOSTEROIDS

CORTICOSTEROIDS FOR MODERATELY SEVERE CROHN'S DISEASE

Oral corticosteroids are the mainstay therapy in outpatients with moderately severe CD. In the prednisone arm of the National Cooperative Crohn's Disease Study,[16] prednisone was dosed at 0.75 mg/kg/day for subjects with CDAI > 300 and at 0.5 mg/kg/day for those with a CDAI of 150 to 300. At 17 weeks, 47% of the prednisone-treated patients were in remission (CDAI < 150), compared with 26% in the placebo group, 38% in the sulfasalazine group, and 36% in the AZA group. In the European Cooperative Crohn's Disease Study,[17] patients with active CD (CDAI ≥150, $n = 215$) were treated for 6 weeks with a methylprednisolone taper (48 mg/day tapered to 12 mg/day), sulfasalazine (3 g/day), methylprednisolone/sulfasalazine combined, or placebo. Remission rates were 83%, 50%, 79%, and 38%, respectively. In a prospective, uncontrolled study from France (Groupe d'Etude Therapeutique des

Affections Inflammatoires Digestives, GETAID),[18] 92% of 142 patients with active Crohn's colitis or ileocolitis achieved clinical remission within 7 weeks of treatment with oral prednisolone (1 mg/kg/day).

Five trials have compared budesonide to conventional steroids in patients with moderately severe CD.[19-23] The study populations included some patients with mild CD (CDAI 150 to 220). Three studies enrolled patients with CDAI scores > 200 (mean CDAI scores of 275 to 280,[20,23] and 240 to 270[21]), and 2 studies enrolled patients with CDAI scores > 150 (mean CDAI scores of 265[19] and 262[22]). Remission rates at 8 weeks varied between 51% and 60% for budesonide and between 52.5% and 72.7% for conventional steroids. Two studies assessed response based on the baseline CDAI.[20,22] In the study by Campieri,[20] out of the patients with a CDAI < 300, remission was achieved in 62% in the budesonide arm versus 50% in the prednisolone arm. In the patients with a CDAI ≥ 300, remission was achieved in 23% and 54% of the budesonide and prednisolone groups, respectively. Disease activity was a prognostic factor that significantly ($P = 0.0007$) influenced the remission rates.[20] In the study by Gross,[22] remission rates on budesonide in patients with a baseline CDAI ≥ 300 and < 300 were 40% and 62.5% (not significant, NS). The corresponding rates in the prednisone arm were 60% and 78.3% (NS).[22] A Cochrane review of these 5 trials ($n = 667$) found that budesonide was inferior to conventional steroids for the induction of remission at 8 weeks (pooled odds ratio [OR] 0.69, 95% confidence interval [CI] 0.51-0.95; number needed to treat [NNT] = 12).[24] However, budesonide was associated with fewer steroid-related adverse events (pooled OR 0.38, 95% CI 0.28-0.53).[24]

In a randomized trial of budesonide (Entocort, AstraZeneca, DE) 9 mg/day versus mesalamine (Pentasa) 4 g/day in patients with mild-moderate CD (CDAI 200 to 400, mean CDAI 272), the rates of clinical remission at 8 weeks were 69% and 45% ($P = 0.001$).[25] The rates of remission were lower in patients with more severe disease (CDAI > 300), 41% and 11% in the budesonide and mesalamine groups, respectively ($P = 0.001$).[25] There have been 2 placebo-controlled trials of budesonide in active CD. In the study by Greenberg et al[26] (CDAI > 200, mean CDAI 285 to 296), remission rates at 8 weeks were 51% and 20% for the budesonide 9 mg/day and the placebo groups, respectively ($P < 0.001$). In the study by Tremaine et al[27] (CDAI 200 to 450, mean CDAI 271 to 280), remission at 8 weeks was achieved in 48%, 53%, and 33% of the budesonide 9 mg/day, budesonide 4.5 mg bid, and placebo groups, respectively (NS).

CORTICOSTEROIDS FOR VERY SEVERE CROHN'S DISEASE

Parenteral corticosteroids have been the mainstay of therapy for severe inflammatory CD. In a retrospective study of 49 patients with severe CD (relapsed disease, $n = 35$; or an acute initial presentation, $n = 14$) who were treated with intravenous prednisolone (16 mg qid), 76% achieved immediate remission.[28] No dose-ranging studies have been performed to define the optimal dose or schedule of administration. Most clinicians administer parenteral corticosteroids equivalent to 40 to 60 mg of prednisone in divided doses or as a continuous infusion (hydrocortisone 300 mg/day, methylprednisolone 40 mg/day). Intravenous adrenocorticotropic hormone [ACTH] can be used instead of intravenous corticosteroids, but is potentially complicated by adrenal hemorrhage.[29] In a randomized, double-blind trial of continuous IV infusion of ACTH 120 U/day of versus hydrocortisone 300 mg/day in hospitalized patients, the rates of response after 10 days of therapy were 82% and 93%, respectively (NS).[2] Parenteral corticosteroids are continued until abdominal pain, fever, and diarrhea resolve. Oral feedings are started at that time and are advanced as tolerated. If the patient is able to tolerate a full diet, oral steroids are then begun.

In 1 uncontrolled study from an era before computed tomography and ultrasonography were available, parenteral corticosteroids were safe and effective in 24 patients with inflammatory masses.[30] In 15 patients, the mass resolved completely, and in another 9, it decreased in size by at least 50%. Fourteen patients eventually required resection for persistence or recurrence of disease activity (with or without the abdominal mass), but the operation was performed electively in all of them. At least 8 patients never required resection during a mean follow-up period of 40 months. In 13 patients, the mass was later shown to actually contain an abscess cavity. No complications attributable to steroid therapy were seen in either the operative or nonoperative group.[30] We avoid corticosteroids when we suspect an abscess on the basis of a high fever or suspicious imaging findings. We administer IV antibiotics to patients with inflammatory masses and carefully monitor for the development of abscess.

PREDICTORS OF RESPONSE TO CORTICOSTEROIDS

To date, there are no clinical, laboratory, or endoscopic features that reliably predict refractoriness to corticosteroids.[18,31] In the largest study to date, a high initial CDAI, prior bowel resection, and perianal disease predicted resistance to corticosteroids in CD.[32] Steroid-resistant patients had a significantly higher initial CDAI than responders (346.5 ± 90.5 versus 301.2 ± 80.6, $P = 0.009$). None of the laboratory parameters examined (erythrocyte sedimentation rate, C-reactive protein, hematocrit, hemoglobin, leukocyte count, platelet count, total protein, and albumin) showed a significant difference in initial values in responders compared to steroid-resistant or steroid-dependent patients, and information on cigarette smoking was not available.[32] In a French study, no clinical, biological, or endoscopic parameters predicted clinical response to prednisolone.[18] The molecular and cellular mechanisms for steroid resistance are under active investigation.[31,33-37]

INFLIXIMAB

INFLIXIMAB FOR MODERATELY SEVERE CROHN'S DISEASE

The pivotal trial of infliximab in active luminal CD[38] enrolled outpatients who had moderately severe disease (CDAI 220 to 450) despite therapy with aminosalicylates, steroids, or immunomodulators. The study excluded patients who had received parenteral corticosteroids or ACTH in the previous 4 weeks. The mean baseline CDAI was 307 ± 55 points. Patients were randomized to a single IV infusion of placebo ($n = 25$) or infliximab at doses of 5, 10, or 20 mg/kg ($n = 27$, 27, and 28, respectively). The primary endpoint of clinical response (reduction of 70 points in the CDAI) at 4 weeks was observed in 81% of the 5 mg/kg group, 50% of the 10 mg/kg group, 64% of the 20 mg/kg group, and 17% of the placebo group. No dose-response relation was seen, and the overall clinical response in the 3 infliximab groups combined was 65% (risk ratio [RR] 4.1, 95% CI 1.6-10.1).[38,39] Clinical remission (CDAI < 150) was achieved by 33% of the infliximab-treated patients versus 4% of the placebo-treated patients (RR 8.1, 95% CI 1.2-56.9; NNT 4; 95% CI 3-9).[38,39] Clinical response after 12 weeks was 41% in the combined infliximab-treated patients versus 12% in the placebo group, but the difference in clinical remission was no longer statistically significant. This trial confirmed the efficacy of infliximab in the treatment of moderate to severe CD, with the 5-mg/kg dose showing the best results. A subsequent subgroup analysis of this pivotal trial found that the mean CD Endoscopic Index of Severity decreased significantly in the infliximab group (13.0 ± 7.1 to 5.3 ± 4.4; $P < 0.001$), but not in the placebo group.[40]

The ACCENT I maintenance trial[41] also enrolled patients with moderately severe disease (CDAI 220 to 450). Half of the patients were on steroids, and a quarter were on immunosuppressants. Of 573 patients given infliximab 5 mg/kg, 335 (58%) responded at week 2. These 335 responders were randomly assigned to repeat infusions of placebo at weeks 2 and 6 and then every 8 weeks thereafter until week 46 (group 1), repeat infusions of 5 mg/kg infliximab at the same time points (group 2), or 5 mg/kg infliximab at weeks 2 and 6 followed by 10 mg/kg every 8 weeks (group 3). The baseline median CDAI score was 299 (range 264 to 342). At week 30 (primary endpoint), 21% of group 1 was in remission, compared with 39% of group 2 ($P = 0.003$) and 45% of group 3 ($P = 0.0002$). At week 54, the corresponding rates of remission were 9%, 24%, and 32%. The median time to loss of response was 38 weeks and > 54 weeks for groups 2 and 3, respectively, compared with 19 weeks for group 1 ($P = 0.002$ and 0.0002, respectively). By week 54, 29% of patients in groups 2 and 3 combined were off corticosteroids and in clinical remission, compared with 9% of patients in group 1 (OR 4.2, 95% CI 1.5-11.5; $P = 0.004$). In open label studies, 40% to 73% of patients discontinued steroids.[42-44]

ANTIBODIES TO INFLIXIMAB AND INFUSION REACTIONS

Infliximab induction therapy can be associated with the development of antibodies to infliximab (ATI), particularly among patients who receive episodic retreatment.[41] ATI in turn are associated with acute and delayed infusion reactions, lower infliximab concentrations,[45,46] and decreased duration of response.[45] Many patients require higher doses and/or more frequent infusions because of an attenuated response, whereas some lose their response altogether. In the ACCENT I trial, 30% of patients in the 5 mg/kg arm and 26% in the 10 mg/kg arm crossed over to episodic treatment with 10 mg/kg and 15 mg/kg respectively because of lack of response.[41] In another study, 27 of 56 (48%) patients on long-term infliximab required an increase in dosage and/or frequency of infusions to maintain response.[47] Surprisingly, these dosage and frequency adjustments were required despite a high frequency of concomitant AZA and methotrexate use in 82% of the patients.[47]

To maintain efficacy and tolerance to infliximab, induction therapy is followed by maintenance therapy.[41] Premedication with steroids and concomitant immunosuppressants are additional approaches to enhance efficacy and reduce ATI and infusion reactions. In a randomized, placebo-controlled trial of hydrocortisone premedication (200 mg IV), ATI developed in 26% of hydrocortisone-treated patients versus 42% of placebo-treated patients (P = 0.06).[48] Several trials and open-label studies have suggested that concomitant immunosuppressants increase the efficacy of infliximab,[41,43,49-54] reduce ATI,[41,45,48] and decrease infusion reactions.[41,45]

In the ACCENT I study,[41] there was a nonsignificant trend towards higher response rates in patients on concomitant immunosuppressants. Fifty percent of patients who received a concomitant baseline immunosuppressant maintained clinical response at week 54 compared with 41% of those who were not receiving these drugs. Over the course of the trial, the frequency of infusion reactions among patients receiving both steroids and immunomodulators was 8%, compared with 20% of patients receiving only immunomodulators, 23% of patients receiving steroids alone, and 32% of patients on no steroids/immunomodulators. Acute infusion reactions occurred in 61 of 993 (6%) and 45 of 1033 (4%) group 2 and 3 infliximab infusions, respectively, compared with 23 of 837 (3%) of group 1 infusions. Of the patients receiving both steroids and immunomodulators at baseline, 6% developed ATI. In contrast, the frequency of ATI was 17% in patients receiving steroids alone (at baseline), 10% in patients receiving immunomodulators alone, and 18% in patients on no steroids/immunomodulators.

In a subsequent analysis of ACCENT I data collected through week 72, ATI developed in 18% of patients not taking immunomodulators and in 10% of those on immunomodulators (OR 0.50; 95% CI 0.28-0.91; P = 0.02).[46]

The effect of concomitant immunomodulator use on ATI development was much greater for patients in the placebo arm (38% versus 16%; P = 0.003) than it was for patients in either maintenance arms (5 mg/kg group, 11% versus 7%, P = 0.42; and 10 mg/kg group, 8% versus 4%, P = 0.42).[46] Across all treatment groups, there was a reduced incidence of infusion reactions for patients receiving concomitant immunomodulators (3% of infusions, 38/1174) relative to patients not receiving 6-MP, AZA, or methotrexate (6%, 171/2666; P < 0.001). Serious infusion reactions, infusion reactions leading to discontinuation of infliximab therapy, and serum sickness-like reactions were similarly distributed across the 3 treatment groups. In summary, the ACCENT I trial demonstrated that concomitant immunomodulator(s) reduce the incidence of ATI (especially in patients treated episodically), as well as the incidence of infusion reactions. Despite an association between the induction of ATI and the occurrence of infusion reactions, ATI are poorly predictive of these events, with a positive predictive value of 36%.[46]

In a Belgian cohort of 125 CD patients who received episodic infliximab infusions, ATI predicted a higher risk of acute infusion reactions.[45] Infusion reactions were associated with lower infliximab concentrations at 4 weeks and a decreased duration of clinical response (median duration of response of 38.5 days versus 65 days among patients who did not have an infusion reaction; P < 0.001). Concomitant immunosuppressive therapy was predictive of lower titers of ATI and higher concentrations of infliximab 4 weeks after an infusion. On multivariate analysis, ATI (but not immunosuppressants or infliximab concentrations) predicted a shorter duration of response (35 days versus 71 days in patients with concentrations ≥ 8.0 µg/mL and < 8.0 µg/mL; P < 0.001).[45]

SAFETY OF INFLIXIMAB

Acute infusion reactions consist of fever, chills, flushing, pruritus, urticaria, palpitations, diaphoresis, chest pain, dyspnea, hypotension or hypertension, and, rarely, anaphylaxis. In all the clinical trials, acute reactions occurred in approximately 20% of infliximab-treated patients compared with 10% of placebo-treated patients.[55] Delayed infusion reactions may develop 2 to 14 days after infusion and consist of polyarthralgias, myalgias, fever, rash, and malaise. Delayed reactions are uncommon, occurring in 2% to 2.8% of patients,[41,56] but these patients often cannot tolerate subsequent infusions.[56] Most acute reactions can be treated by slowing or stopping the infusion and administering acetaminophen, antihistamines, steroids, and/or epinephrine.[57] Acute and delayed reactions can be lessened by instituting immunomodulators for at least 4 to 6 weeks before the next infusion, premedicating with steroids, slowing the rate of infusion, and administering acetaminophen and antihistamines.[57]

Sepsis, pneumonia, and reactivation of tuberculosis (frequently disseminated or extrapulmonary) have occurred in patients receiving infliximab. Patients should be evaluated for latent tuberculosis (TB) with a skin test and a chest x-ray. Treatment of latent TB infection should be initiated prior to therapy with infliximab. Because TB has developed in patients who were negative on the tuberculin skin test, we carefully monitor all patients (including those with negative skin tests) for signs and symptoms of TB. In the United States, the clinician must also weigh the benefits and risks of infliximab in patients who have resided in regions endemic for histoplasmosis (ie, central United States) and coccidioidomycosis (ie, southwest United States). A number of other opportunistic infections have also been reported in infliximab-treated patients, including pneumocystosis, varicella-zoster virus and cytomegalovirus infections, listeriosis, aspergillosis, cryptococcosis, and systemic candidiasis.

Other serious toxicities linked to infliximab include drug-induced lupus, worsening heart failure, demyelinating syndromes (multiple sclerosis and optic neuritis), hematologic toxicity (leukopenia, neutropenia, thrombocytopenia, and pancytopenia), lymphoma, and hepatotoxicity (reactivation of hepatitis B and acute liver failure). Decreases in leukocyte counts can occur in AZA- or 6-MP-treated patients who embark on infliximab therapy. The mechanism may be infliximab-mediated mucosal healing that leads to enhanced thiopurine bioavailability. In a prospective study of 32 patients receiving AZA who required infliximab for ileocolonic or anoperineal CD, mean 6-thioguanine nucleotide (6-TGN) concentrations and mean corpuscular volume increased significantly within 1 to 3 weeks after the first infusion, whereas leukocyte counts decreased significantly.[58] These parameters reverted to baseline 3 months after the infusion. In all our patients, we obtain hepatitis B virus (HBV) serologies before treatment (HBsAg, HBcAb, HbsAb), and we monitor blood counts, aminotransferases, and antinuclear antibodies.

INFLIXIMAB FOR VERY SEVERE CROHN'S DISEASE

There are no data from randomized controlled trials on the efficacy of infliximab in the treatment of very severe CD (CDAI > 450) or CD that necessitates hospitalization. However, the potential role of infliximab in this setting is supported by its rapid onset of action, with median times to clinical response and remission after the initial infusion of 8 days (range 5 to 35 days) and 9 days (range 6 to 91 days), respectively.[43] There have been no comparisons of infliximab and IV corticosteroids in very severe CD. Because infliximab is approved for patients with moderate to severe CD and an inadequate response to conventional therapy,[55] its use in severe CD was initially limited to patients who were refractory to IV corticosteroids or had contraindications to steroids. However, we have begun to use infliximab as first-line therapy (with or without IV steroids) in some patients hospitalized with very severe CD.

PREDICTORS OF RESPONSE TO INFLIXIMAB

A number of clinical, biochemical, serologic, and genetic predictors of response to infliximab have been investigated. As noted previously, several trials and open-label studies have suggested that concomitant immunosuppressants increase the efficacy of infliximab, particularly among patients with inflammatory (rather than perianal fistulizing) disease and patients who receive episodic (rather than scheduled) infliximab infusions.[41,43,49-54] This effect is mediated by a reduction in the frequency and titer of ATI.[45] Potential negative response predictors include cigarette smoking, isolated ileal disease, prior surgery for CD, and presence of intestinal strictures.[59] Isolated colonic disease may be associated with higher response.[52,53] Gender, race, and duration of disease do not seem to predict response.[59] Neither the pivotal induction trial[38] nor the ACCENT I study[41] analyzed outcomes according to baseline CDAI score or duration of disease. In 2 open-label studies of patients with mildly to moderately severe CD (CDAI 150 to 400), the baseline CDAI did not predict likelihood of response.[54,60] With regard to laboratory parameters, levels of CRP predicted response in 1 study.[61] Platelet counts and albumin are not predictive.[59] A serological profile of pANCA$^+$ASCA$^-$ may be associated with a poorer response, whereas *NOD2/CARD15* genotype does not influence response.[59] A single report has suggested that genetic polymorphism of the FcγRIIIa receptor (important in antibody-dependent, cell-mediated cytotoxicity of tumor necrosis factor alpha (TNFα)–expressing macrophages and natural killer cells) influences response to infliximab, but this finding requires confirmation.[62] In initial infliximab responders, mechanisms of attenuated response or loss of response include ATI and, possibly, the emergence of immune cells resistant to infliximab-mediated apoptosis, increased activity of non–TNFα inflammatory pathways, and development of strictures.

CYCLOSPORINE

Patients with severe CD unresponsive to parenteral steroids have been treated with intravenous cyclosporine. Several small, open-label studies have suggested that intravenous cyclosporine (4 to 5 mg/kg/day) may be effective in some of these patients.[63-66] In a study from the Mayo Clinic, 4 out of 9 patients with refractory inflammatory CD treated with IV cyclosporine (4 mg/kg/day) had a partial response, which they maintained during oral therapy. After discontinuing oral cyclosporine, all patients relapsed, probably because of inadequate duration of overlap with AZA or 6-MP therapy.[63] However, there are no controlled or dose-response data for IV cyclosporine in patients with severe inflammatory CD. Although IV cyclosporine may be useful in this setting, its use has been largely superseded by the advent of biologic anti-TNFα therapies. Nonetheless, cyclosporine remains a second-line agent in patients refractory to IV corticosteroids. In this setting, as in severe UC, cyslosporine is deemed as "bridge" therapy until maintenance therapy with AZA, 6-MP, or methotrexate becomes effective. Careful monitoring is required to prevent the numerous complications of cyclosporine therapy. Because of concerns for severe immunosuppression, we avoid cyclosporine in patients who are less than 12 weeks past treatment with infliximab or have infliximab detectable in their serum.

Low-dose oral cyclosporine (5 mg/kg/day) has also been studied in outpatients with moderately severe CD. A randomized clinical trial that stratified subjects according to disease activity (CDAI $\geq$ 150) showed that low-dose cyclosporine (5 mg/kg/day adjusted to a whole-blood trough concentration of 200 ng/mL; Sandimmune, Sandoz) added to conventional treatment for CD did not improve symptoms or reduce requirements for other forms of therapy.[67] Cyclosporine was not beneficial in the subgroup of patients with high CD activity (mean CDAI 230). Two other trials also found no statistically significant benefit for clinical improvement or induction of remission for low-dose cyclosporine compared to placebo.[68,69] The European trial[68] stratified subjects according to CDAI ($\leq$200) and found no difference in clinical efficacy overall, within the 2 strata, or within a small group of patients with very active CD (CDAI > 300). The single positive study,[70] which used high-dose cyclosporine (median 7.6 mg/kg/day), has been criticized for its small size, unvalidated grading scale, and lack of efficacy in the induction of clinical remission. A recent meta-analysis concluded that low-dose oral cyclosporine is ineffective for the induction of remission of CD.[71]

Tacrolimus, which has a mechanism of action similar to cyclosporine, has anecdotally been effective in severe CD[72,73] but has not been subjected to randomized trials in this setting.

OTHER THERAPIES

Numerous biologic agents are being studied, and several appear promising in patients with moderately severe CD (CDAI 220 to 450). Adalimumab, a recombinant, fully humanized immunoglobulin (Ig)G1 anti-TNFα monoclonal antibody (mAb), represents a conceptually attractive option in patients with an attenuated response or hypersensitivity to infliximab. Like infliximab, adalimumab induces apoptosis of activated immune cells.[74] As well, adalimumab has the theoretical advantage of less immunogenicity and lack of cross-reactivity with ATI directed against murine sequences (but not with ATI directed against human IgG1 sequences). In the CLASSIC I trial,[75] 299 patients with moderately severe CD (CDAI 220 to 450; mean standard deviation [SD] CDAI 298 [57]) and without previous exposure to TNFα antagonists were randomized to 1 of 4 treatments administered subcutaneously at weeks 0 and 2: Adalimumab 160 mg/80 mg, 80 mg/40 mg, 40 mg/20 mg, or placebo/placebo. The primary endpoint of

clinical remission (CDAI < 150 at week 4) was achieved in 30% of patients in the combined 160/80 and 80/40 groups, versus 12% in the placebo arm (P = 0.004). There was a clear dose response for both clinical remission and clinical response (CDAI decreases of 70 and 100). The most common adverse event was injection site reactions.[75] In the CHARM maintenance trial,[76] patients with active CD received adalimumab 80 mg subcutaneously (SQ) at week 0 and 40 mg SQ at week 2. At week 4, subjects were randomized to adalimumab 40 mg every other week, adalimumab 40 mg weekly, or placebo and continued treatment through week 56. Of the 854 subjects who received open-label adalimumab induction, 58% responded and 25% were in complete remission at week 4.

Adalimumab has proved effective in two 56-week-long maintenance trials, CLASSIC II[77] and the previously mentioned CHARM.[76] In the CLASSIC II trial, antibodies to adalimumab and antinuclear antibody (ANA) developed in 2.6% and 19% of patients, respectively.[77] Antibodies to adalimumab and ANA were not measured in the CHARM trial. Although longer studies are needed, data to date suggest that the safety profile of adalimumab is not different from that of infliximab in Crohn's disease or that of adalimumab in rheumatoid arthritis.

Several small studies reported that adalimumab was effective in patients who had developed allergy or intolerance to infliximab or had experienced an attenuated response or loss of response.[78-80] A recent, randomized, double-blind, placebo-controlled trial assessed the short-term efficacy of adalimumab in patients with active Crohn's disease (mean CDAI 313) who had become intolerant to infliximab or had previously responded to infliximab and then lost response.[81] Twenty-one percent (34 of 159) of patients in the adalimumab group versus 7% (12 of 166) of those in the placebo group achieved remission at week 4 (P < 0.001).[81] Adalimumab appears efficacious for patients with active CD and no previous exposure to TNFα antagonists or intolerance or attenuated response to infliximab. In view of the similar structure and function shared by infliximab and adalimumab, one may predict that patients who are primary infliximab failures will also fail adalimumab, but this remains to be shown.

Preliminary reports suggest that certolizumab pegol (CDP870), the pegylated Fab' fragment of a humanized anti-TNFα mAb, may have efficacy in moderately severe CD.[82,83] In an initial phase II trial of a single IV dose of certolizumab (n = 92; CDAI 220 to 450; mean CDAI 310), the proportion of patients achieving the primary endpoint of clinical response (CDAI decrease 100 points at 4 weeks) was comparable across all treatment groups (56.0%, 60.0%, 58.8%, and 47.8% for placebo, certolizumab 5, 10, and 20 mg/kg, respectively).[82] Remission (CDAI < 150) at week 2 was achieved in 47.1% of patients in the certolizumab 10 mg/kg group versus 16.0% in the placebo group (P = 0.041).[82]

In a larger phase II placebo-controlled dose-response study, 292 patients with moderate to severe CD (CDAI 220 to 450; mean CDAI not given) received SQ certolizumab 100, 200, or 400 mg, or placebo at weeks 0, 4, and 8.[83] The primary endpoint was the percentage of patients with a clinical response at week 12 (defined as a CDAI decrease of 100 points or remission, CDAI 150). All certolizumab doses were superior to placebo at week 2: placebo, 15.1%; certolizumab 100 mg, 29.7% (P = 0.033); 200 mg, 30.6% (P = 0.026); 400 mg, 33.3% (P = 0.010). At all time points, the clinical response rates were highest for certolizumab 400 mg, greatest at week 10 (certolizumab 400 mg, 52.8%; placebo, 30.1%; P = 0.006), but not significant at week 12 (certolizumab 400 mg, 44.4%; placebo, 35.6%; P = 0.278). Patients with baseline CRP levels of 10 mg/L or greater (n = 119) showed clearer separation between active treatment and placebo (week 12 clinical response: certolizumab 400 mg, 53.1%; placebo, 17.9%; P = 0.005; post hoc analysis) due to a lower placebo response rate than patients with CRP levels of less than 10 mg/L. The 2 certolizumab studies failed to meet their primary endpoints, although secondary endpoints were achieved, suggesting efficacy of the drug. The high placebo response rates likely influenced study results.

The design of 2 subsequent large trials took into account the apparent importance of baseline CRP in certolizumab response. In the PRECISE 1 trial (Pegylated Antibody Fragment Evaluation in Crohn's Disease: Safety and Efficacy 1),[84] 662 adults with moderate to severe Crohn's disease (mean CDAI 299) were randomized to 400 mg of certolizumab or placebo subcutaneously at weeks 0, 2, and 4 and then every 4 weeks. The co-primary endpoints were induction of a response at week 6 and a response at both weeks 6 and 26 in the stratum with a baseline serum CRP concentration of at least 10 mg/L. At week 6, response rates were 37% and 26% in the certolizumab and placebo groups, respectively (P = 0.04). At both weeks 6 and 26, the corresponding values were 22% and 12%, respectively (P = 0.05). In the overall population, response rates at week 6 were 35% in the certolizumab group and 27% in the placebo group (P = 0.02); at both weeks 6 and 26, the response rates were 23% and 16%, respectively (P = 0.02). Remission rates did not differ significantly at weeks 6 and 26. In the certolizumab group, antibodies to the drug developed in 8% of patients: in 4% of subjects on concomitant immunomodulators and in 10% of subjects who did not receive immunomodulators. ANA were present in 1.1% and 1.8% of the placebo and certolizumab groups, respectively. The corresponding numbers for anti-dsDNA were 0.7% and 1.4%.[84]

The PRECISE 2 trial[85] evaluated the efficacy of certolizumab as maintenance therapy in adults with moderate to severe Crohn's disease (mean CDAI 304). Responders to certolizumab open-label inductive therapy (400 mg SQ at weeks 0, 2, and 4) were stratified according to their baseline CRP levels and were randomly assigned to 400 mg of certolizumab or placebo every 4 weeks through week 24. At week 6 (after three 400-mg doses of certolizumab), 43% of patients (289 of 668) had a remission, and 64% (428 of 668) had a response. Among the responders, the response was maintained through week 26 in 62% of patients with a baseline CRP level of at least 10 mg/L (the primary endpoint) who were receiving certolizumab versus 34% of those receiving placebo (P < 0.001). In the overall population, response rates at 26 weeks were 63% and 36% in the certolizumab and placebo groups, respectively (P < 0.001). Nine percent of patients had detectable antibodies against certolizumab at some point during the study. Maintenance therapy with certolizumab (8% versus 18% on placebo) and concomitant immunomodulators (12% versus 24% in patients not on immunomodulators) were associated with lower rates of positivity to antibodies. New antinuclear antibodies developed in 8% (16 of 192) of patients receiving certolizumab and in 1% (2 of 178) of patients receiving placebo.[85]

Data to date suggest that the safety profile of certolizumab is similar to that of infliximab and adalimumab.

Other biologic agents under study are the recombinant granulocyte-macrophage colony-stimulating factor Sargramostim[86,87]; the humanized, anti-α_4 integrin mAb natalizumab[88,89]; the humanized, anti-IL-12 mAb ABT-874[90]; the humanized anti-interferon antibody fontolizumab[91]; and the humanized anti-IL-6 receptor antibody MRA.[92] Leukocyte apheresis is also under investigation.[93] [Addendum: Since submission of this chapter, adalimumab and certolizumab have received FDA approval for CD, and natalizumab has received approval for limited use in CD.]

INTESTINAL OBSTRUCTION

Intestinal obstruction in CD can occur as a result of acute active inflammation superimposed on a stenotic bowel segment or as a result of an adjacent phlegmon or abscess with mass effect. However, obstruction is more commonly due to intraabdominal adhesions in the setting of prior abdominal surgery or dietary indiscretion, namely consumption of poorly digestible solids, in the setting of an underlying stricture. As such, intestinal obstruction is usually treated conservatively with cessation of oral intake, nasogastric aspiration, correction of fluid and electrolyte disturbances, and avoidance of narcotics. We frequently consult an experienced surgeon. IV steroids are not routinely indicated and are associated with numerous side effects. We reserve steroid therapy for the patient with symptoms and signs of systemic inflammation (fever, night sweats, arthralgias, elevated erythrocyte sedimentation rate [ESR] and CRP). Repeated episodes of intestinal obstruction due to fibrostenotic CD are an indication for surgery. Strictured ileocolic anastomoses can occasionally be treated with endoscopic balloon dilation.[94-96]

TABLE 23-3

MEDICAL MANAGEMENT OF SEVERE INFLAMMATORY CROHN'S DISEASE*

ASSESSMENT OF DISEASE ACTIVITY, LOCATION, AND COMPLICATIONS

1. HISTORY

a. Rule out precipitants, such as use of aspirin and NSAIDs (including the COX-2 inhibitors), and abrupt cessation or nonadherence to immunomodulatory therapies

2. PHYSICAL EXAMINATION

a. Fever

b. Dehydration

c. Rebound tenderness

d. Abdominal mass

3. LABORATORY EVALUATION

a. Complete blood count

b. Electrolytes and renal function

c. ESR and CRP

d. Rule out enteric infection: *Clostridium difficile, Campylobacter* species, *Salmonella* species, *Aeromonas hydrophila, Plesiomonas shigelloides, Entamoeba histolytica, Strongyloides stercoralis, Cytomegalovirus*

4. IMAGING STUDIES

a. Plain films of the abdomen

b. CT of abdomen and pelvis

THERAPY

1. SUPPORTIVE THERAPIES

a. Fluid resuscitation

b. Electrolyte replacement

c. Transfusions in the setting of anemia and active hemorrhage

d. DVT prophylaxis

e. Oral feedings as tolerated for patients without obstructive manifestations or severe abdominal pain

f. Bowel rest and parenteral nutritional support for more severely ill patients or those with evidence of obstruction

2. SPECIFIC THERAPIES

a. Antibiotics

b. Corticosteroids

c. Infliximab

*NSAID indicates nonsteroidal antiinflammatory drug; COX-2, cyclooxygenase-2; ESR, erythrocyte sedimentation rate; CRP, C-reactive protein; CT, computed tomography; DVT, deep vein thrombosis.

ABSCESS

The immediate management of abscesses in CD obeys the principles of drainage, treatment with antibiotics, and supportive therapies. Oral feedings are stopped, and parenteral nutrition, IV fluids, and electrolytes are provided. These measures, along with avoidance of corticosteroids, optimize the patient's status prior to definitive surgical repair. Traditionally, most abscesses were drained operatively; however, with advances in interventional radiological techniques, percutaneous drainage has been increasingly used. Gervais and colleagues reviewed 32 patients with CD who underwent percutaneous drainage from 1985 to 1999.[97] Drainage was technically successful in 96% of patients. Short-term success, defined as avoidance of surgery within 60 days of drainage, was possible in 50% of patients. Nine of 16 short-term successes and 5 of 15 short-term failures eventually required surgery (NS). Recurrent abscesses occurred in 7 (22%) patients, a rate comparable to that with surgical abscess drainage; 4 (44%) of 9 cases of redrainage were successful.

Because abscesses in CD result from fistulization through transmurally diseased bowel, definitive surgical therapy is almost always the rule after the initial management. In a recent American study, 51 patients with CD and an abdominal abscess managed at 1 institution during a 10-year period were retrospectively identified.[98] Fewer patients developed recurrent abscesses after initial surgical drainage and bowel resection (12%) than patients treated with medical therapy only or percutaneous drainage (56%) ($P = 0.016$). One half of the patients treated nonoperatively ultimately required surgery, whereas only 12% of those treated with initial surgery required reoperation during the follow-up period ($P = 0.010$).[98]

SEVERE GASTROINTESTINAL BLEEDING

Acute, severe gastrointestinal bleeding is a rare complication of CD. Most patients have known CD, whereas others may present with acute bleeding as the initial symptom of CD.[99,100] Bleeding is more frequent among patients with colonic involvement than among those with small bowel disease alone.[101,102] Localization of the bleeding site is not easy, as colonoscopy and angiography do not always identify the source. If the patient does not immediately require surgery, specific medical therapy of CD, endoscopic treatment, and/or angiography are applied. Bleeding may subside but frequently recurs, and surgery is required in 20% to 50% of cases.[99-103] There are case reports of patients with severe bleeding treated successfully with infliximab.[104,105]

OTHER SCENARIOS

Crohn's colitis, like ulcerative colitis, can be complicated by toxic megacolon.[106] Management is similar to that in ulcerative colitis, which is reviewed in another chapter. Superimposed infection with cytomegalovirus and *Clostridium difficile* can also occur and should be ruled out in all hospitalized CD patients. The risk of thrombosis (particularly deep vein thrombosis [DVT] and pulmonary emboli) is increased in IBD, especially in active disease.[107] We institute DVT prophylaxis in all of our patients hospitalized with severe inflammatory CD, obstruction, or abscess.

REFERENCES

1. Sandborn WJ, Feagan BG, Hanauer SB, et al. A review of activity indices and efficacy endpoints for clinical trials of medical therapy in adults with Crohn's disease. *Gastroenterology*. 2002;122:512-530.

2. Chun A, Chadi RM, Korelitz BI, et al. Intravenous corticotrophin vs. hydrocortisone in the treatment of hospitalized patients with Crohn's disease: a randomized double-blind study and follow-up. *Inflamm Bowel Dis*. 1998;4:177-181.

3. Lichtenstein GR, Hanauer SB, Sandborn WJ, and the Practice Parameters Committee of American College of Gastroenterology. Management of Crohn's disease in adults. *Am J Gastroenterol*. 2009;104:465-483.

4. Mahadevan U, Loftus EV Jr, Tremaine WJ, Sandborn WJ. Safety of selective cyclooxygenase-2 inhibitors in inflammatory bowel disease. *Am J Gastroenterol*. 2002;97:910-914.

5. Reinisch W, Miehsler W, Dejaco C, et al. An open-label trial of the selective cyclo-oxygenase-2 inhibitor, rofecoxib, in inflammatory bowel disease-associated peripheral arthritis and arthralgia. *Aliment Pharmacol Ther*. 2003;17:1371-1380.

6. Biancone L, Tosti C, Geremia A, et al. Rofecoxib and early relapse of inflammatory bowel disease: an open-label trial. *Aliment Pharmacol Ther*. 2004;19:755-764.

7. Sewitch MJ, Abrahamowicz M, Barkun A, et al. Patient non-adherence to medication in inflammatory bowel disease. *Am J Gastroenterol*. 2003;98:1535-1544.

8. Dubinsky MC. Azathioprine, 6-mercaptopurine in inflammatory bowel disease: pharmacology, efficacy, and safety. *Clin Gastroenterol Hepatol*. 2004;2:731-743.

9. Mylonaki M, Langmead L, Pantes A, Johnson F, Rampton DS. Enteric infection in relapse of inflammatory bowel disease: importance of microbiological examination of stool. *Eur J Gastroenterol Hepatol*. 2004;16:775-778.

10. Gonzalez-Huix F, de Leon R, Fernandez-Banares F, et al. Polymeric enteral diets as primary treatment of active Crohn's disease: a prospective steroid controlled trial. *Gut*. 1993;34:778-782.

11. Gorard DA, Hunt JB, Payne-James JJ, et al. Initial response and subsequent course of Crohn's disease treated with elemental diet or prednisolone. *Gut*. 1993;34:1198-1202.

12. Mansfield JC, Giaffer MH, Holdsworth CD. Controlled trial of oligopeptide versus amino acid diet in treatment of active Crohn's disease. *Gut*. 1995;36:60-66.

13. Rigaud D, Cosnes J, Le Quintrec Y, Rene E, Gendre JP, Mignon M. Controlled trial comparing two types of enteral nutrition in treatment of active Crohn's disease: elemental versus polymeric diet. *Gut*. 1991;32:1492-1497.

14. Verma S, Brown S, Kirkwood B, Giaffer MH. Polymeric versus elemental diet as primary treatment in active Crohn's disease: a randomized, double-blind trial. *Am J Gastroenterol*. 2000;95:735-739.

15. Zachos M, Tondeur M, Griffiths AM. Enteral nutritional therapy for inducing remission of Crohn's disease. *Cochrane Database Syst Rev*. 2001:CD000542.

16. Summers RW, Switz DM, Sessions JT Jr, et al. National Cooperative Crohn's Disease Study: results of drug treatment. *Gastroenterology*. 1979;77:847-869.

17. Malchow H, Ewe K, Brandes JW, et al. European Cooperative Crohn's Disease Study (ECCDS): results of drug treatment. *Gastroenterology*. 1984;86:249-266.

18. Modigliani R, Mary JY, Simon JF, et al. Clinical, biological, and endoscopic picture of attacks of Crohn's disease. Evolution on prednisolone. Groupe d'Etude Therapeutique des Affections Inflammatoires Digestives. *Gastroenterology*. 1990;98:811-818.

19. Bar-Meir S, Chowers Y, Lavy A, et al. Budesonide versus prednisone in the treatment of active Crohn's disease. The Israeli Budesonide Study Group. *Gastroenterology*. 1998;115:835-840.

20. Campieri M, Ferguson A, Doe W, Persson T, Nilsson LG. Oral budesonide is as effective as oral prednisolone in active Crohn's disease. The Global Budesonide Study Group. *Gut*. 1997;41:209-214.

21. Escher JC. Budesonide versus prednisolone for the treatment of active Crohn's disease in children: a randomized, double-blind, controlled, multicentre trial. *Eur J Gastroenterol Hepatol.* 2004;16:47-54.

22. Gross V, Andus T, Caesar I, et al. Oral pH-modified release budesonide versus 6-methylprednisolone in active Crohn's disease. German/Austrian Budesonide Study Group. *Eur J Gastroenterol Hepatol.* 1996;8:905-909.

23. Rutgeerts P, Lofberg R, Malchow H, et al. A comparison of budesonide with prednisolone for active Crohn's disease. *N Engl J Med.* 1994;331:842-845.

24. Otley A, Steinhart AH. Budesonide for induction of remission in Crohn's disease. *Cochrane Database Syst Rev.* 2005:CD000296.

25. Thomsen OO, Cortot A, Jewell D, et al. Budesonide and mesalazine in active Crohn's disease: a comparison of the effects on quality of life. *Am J Gastroenterol.* 2002;97:649-653.

26. Greenberg GR, Feagan BG, Martin F, et al. Oral budesonide for active Crohn's disease. Canadian Inflammatory Bowel Disease Study Group. *N Engl J Med.* 1994;331:836-841.

27. Tremaine WJ, Hanauer SB, Katz S, et al. Budesonide CIR capsules (once or twice daily divided-dose) in active Crohn's disease: a randomized placebo-controlled study in the United States. *Am J Gastroenterol.* 2002;97:1748-1754.

28. Shepherd HA, Barr GD, Jewell DP. Use of an intravenous steroid regimen in the treatment of acute Crohn's disease. *J Clin Gastroenterol.* 1986;8:154-159.

29. Felder JB, Mendelsohn RA, Korelitz BI. Adrenocorticotropin-induced adrenal hemorrhage. *J Clin Gastroenterol.* 1991;13:111-112.

30. Felder JB, Adler DJ, Korelitz BI. The safety of corticosteroid therapy in Crohn's disease with an abdominal mass. *Am J Gastroenterol.* 1991;86:1450-1455.

31. Gelbmann CM. Prediction of treatment refractoriness in ulcerative colitis and Crohn's disease—do we have reliable markers? *Inflamm Bowel Dis.* 2000;6:123-131.

32. Gelbmann CM, Rogler G, Gross V, et al. Prior bowel resections, perianal disease, and a high initial Crohn's disease activity index are associated with corticosteroid resistance in active Crohn's disease. *Am J Gastroenterol.* 2002;97:1438-1445.

33. Farrell RJ, Kelleher D. Glucocorticoid resistance in inflammatory bowel disease. *J Endocrinol.* 2003;178:339-346.

34. Farrell RJ, Murphy A, Long A, et al. High multidrug resistance (P-glycoprotein 170) expression in inflammatory bowel disease patients who fail medical therapy. *Gastroenterology.* 2000;118:279-288.

35. Honda M, Orii F, Ayabe T, et al. Expression of glucocorticoid receptor beta in lymphocytes of patients with glucocorticoid-resistant ulcerative colitis. *Gastroenterology.* 2000;118:859-866.

36. Bantel H, Domschke W, Schulze-Osthoff K, Kaskas B, Gregor M. Abnormal activation of transcription factor NF-kappaB involved in steroid resistance in chronic inflammatory bowel disease. *Am J Gastroenterol.* 2000;95:1845-1846.

37. Rogler G, Meinel A, Lingauer A, et al. Glucocorticoid receptors are down-regulated in inflamed colonic mucosa but not in peripheral blood mononuclear cells from patients with inflammatory bowel disease. *Eur J Clin Invest.* 1999;29:330-336.

38. Targan SR, Hanauer SB, van Deventer SJ, et al. A short-term study of chimeric monoclonal antibody cA2 to tumor necrosis factor alpha for Crohn's disease. Crohn's Disease cA2 Study Group. *N Engl J Med.* 1997;337:1029-1035.

39. Akobeng AK, Zachos M. Tumor necrosis factor-alpha antibody for induction of remission in Crohn's disease. *Cochrane Database Syst Rev.* 2004:CD003574.

40. D'Haens G, Van Deventer S, Van Hogezand R, et al. Endoscopic and histological healing with infliximab anti-tumor necrosis factor antibodies in Crohn's disease: a European multicenter trial. *Gastroenterology.* 1999;116:1029-1034.

41. Hanauer SB, Feagan BG, Lichtenstein GR, et al. Maintenance infliximab for Crohn's disease: the ACCENT I randomised trial. *Lancet.* 2002;359:1541-1549.

42. Farrell RJ, Shah SA, Lodhavia PJ, et al. Clinical experience with infliximab therapy in 100 patients with Crohn's disease. *Am J Gastroenterol.* 2000;95:3490-3497.

43. Cohen RD, Tsang JF, Hanauer SB. Infliximab in Crohn's disease: first anniversary clinical experience. *Am J Gastroenterol.* 2000; 95:3469-3477.

44. Ricart E, Panaccione R, Loftus EV, Tremaine WJ, Sandborn WJ. Infliximab for Crohn's disease in clinical practice at the Mayo Clinic: the first 100 patients. *Am J Gastroenterol.* 2001;96:722-729.

45. Baert F, Noman M, Vermeire S, et al. Influence of immunogenicity on the long-term efficacy of infliximab in Crohn's disease. *N Engl J Med.* 2003;348:601-608.

46. Hanauer SB, Wagner CL, Bala M, et al. Incidence and importance of antibody responses to infliximab after maintenance or episodic treatment in Crohn's disease. *Clin Gastroenterol Hepatol.* 2004; 2:542-553.

47. Shih CE, Bayless TM, Harris ML. Maintenance of long term response to infliximab over 1 to 5 years in Crohn's Disease including shortening dosing intervals or increasing dosage [abstract]. *Gastroenterology.* 2004;126:A-631.

48. Farrell RJ, Alsahli M, Jeen YT, Falchuk KR, Peppercorn MA, Michetti P. Intravenous hydrocortisone premedication reduces antibodies to infliximab in Crohn's disease: a randomized controlled trial. *Gastroenterology.* 2003;124:917-924.

49. Rutgeerts P, D'Haens G, Targan S, et al. Efficacy and safety of retreatment with anti-tumor necrosis factor antibody (infliximab) to maintain remission in Crohn's disease. *Gastroenterology.* 1999;117:761-769.

50. Mortimore M, Gibson PR, Selby WS, Radford-Smith GL, Florin TH. Early Australian experience with infliximab, a chimeric antibody against tumour necrosis factor-alpha, in the treatment of Crohn's disease: is its efficacy augmented by steroid-sparing immunosuppressive therapy? The Infliximab User Group. *Intern Med J.* 2001;31:146-150.

51. Laharie D, Salzmann M, Boubekeur H, et al. Predictors of response to infliximab in luminal Crohn's disease. *Gastroenterol Clin Biol.* 2005;29:145-149.

52. Parsi MA, Achkar JP, Richardson S, et al. Predictors of response to infliximab in patients with Crohn's disease. *Gastroenterology.* 2002;123:707-713.

53. Arnott ID, McNeill G, Satsangi J. An analysis of factors influencing short-term and sustained response to infliximab treatment for Crohn's disease. *Aliment Pharmacol Ther.* 2003;17:1451-1457.

54. Vermeire S, Louis E, Carbonez A, et al. Demographic and clinical parameters influencing the short-term outcome of anti-tumor necrosis factor (infliximab) treatment in Crohn's disease. *Am J Gastroenterol.* 2002;97:2357-2363.

55. Remicade [package insert]. Malvern, PA: Centocor Ortho Biotech; 2006.

56. Colombel JF, Loftus EV Jr, Tremaine WJ, et al. The safety profile of infliximab in patients with Crohn's disease: the Mayo clinic experience in 500 patients. *Gastroenterology.* 2004;126:19-31.

57. Sandborn WJ, Hanauer SB. Infliximab in the treatment of Crohn's disease: a user's guide for clinicians. *Am J Gastroenterol.* 2002;97:2962-2972.

58. Roblin X, Serre-Debeauvais F, Phelip JM, Bessard G, Bonaz B. Drug interaction between infliximab and azathioprine in patients with Crohn's disease. *Aliment Pharmacol Ther.* 2003;18:917-925.

59. Su C, Lichtenstein GR. Are there predictors of Remicade treatment success or failure? *Adv Drug Deliv Rev.* 2005;57:237-245.

60. Ardizzone S, Colombo E, Maconi G, et al. Infliximab in treatment of Crohn's disease: the Milan experience. *Dig Liver Dis.* 2002;34:411-418.

61. Louis E, Vermeire S, Rutgeerts P, et al. A positive response to infliximab in Crohn disease: association with a higher systemic inflammation before treatment but not with -308 TNF gene polymorphism. *Scand J Gastroenterol.* 2002;37:818-824.

62. Louis E, El Ghoul Z, Vermeire S, et al. Association between polymorphism in IgG Fc receptor IIIa coding gene and biological response to infliximab in Crohn's disease. *Aliment Pharmacol Ther.* 2004;19:511-519.

63. Egan LJ, Sandborn WJ, Tremaine WJ. Clinical outcome following treatment of refractory inflammatory and fistulizing Crohn's disease with intravenous cyclosporine. *Am J Gastroenterol.* 1998;93:442-448.

64. Santos JV, Baudet JA, Casellas FJ, Guarner LA, Vilaseca JM, Malagelada JR. Intravenous cyclosporine for steroid-refractory attacks of Crohn's disease. Short- and long-term results. *J Clin Gastroenterol.* 1995;20:207-210.

65. Mahdi G, Israel DM, Hassall E. Cyclosporine and 6-mercaptopurine for active, refractory Crohn's colitis in children. *Am J Gastroenterol.* 1996;91:1355-1359.

66. Hermida-Rodriguez C, Cantero Perona J, Garcia-Valriberas R, Pajares Garcia JM, Mate-Jimenez J. High-dose intravenous cyclosporine in steroid refractory attacks of inflammatory bowel disease. *Hepatogastroenterology.* 1999;46:2265-2268.

67. Feagan BG, McDonald JW, Rochon J, et al. Low-dose cyclosporine for the treatment of Crohn's disease. The Canadian Crohn's Relapse Prevention Trial Investigators. *N Engl J Med.* 1994;330:1846-1851.

68. Stange EF, Modigliani R, Pena AS, Wood AJ, Feutren G, Smith PR. European trial of cyclosporine in chronic active Crohn's disease: a 12-month study. The European Study Group. *Gastroenterology.* 1995;109:774-782.

69. Jewell DP, Lennard-Jones JE, Lowes J, Dalton HR, Shaffer JL, Littlewood A. Oral cyclosporine for chronic active Crohn's disease: A multicenter controlled trial. *Eur J Gastroenterol Hepatol.* 1994;6:499-505.

70. Brynskov J, Freund L, Rasmussen SN, et al. A placebo-controlled, double-blind, randomized trial of cyclosporine therapy in active chronic Crohn's disease. *N Engl J Med.* 1989;321:845-850.

71. McDonald JW, Feagan BG, Jewell D, Brynskov J, Stange EF, Macdonald JK. Cyclosporine for induction of remission in Crohn's disease. *Cochrane Database Syst Rev.* 2005:CD000297.

72. Ierardi E, Principi M, Francavilla R, et al. Oral tacrolimus long-term therapy in patients with Crohn's disease and steroid resistance. *Aliment Pharmacol Ther.* 2001;15:371-377.

73. Sandborn WJ. Preliminary report on the use of oral tacrolimus (FK506) in the treatment of complicated proximal small bowel and fistulizing Crohn's disease. *Am J Gastroenterol.* 1997;92:876-879.

74. Shen C, Assche GV, Colpaert S, et al. Adalimumab induces apoptosis of human monocytes: a comparative study with infliximab and etanercept. *Aliment Pharmacol Ther.* 2005;21:251-258.

75. Hanauer SB, Sandborn WJ, Rutgeerts P, et al. Human anti-tumor necrosis factor monoclonal antibody (adalimumab) in Crohn's disease: the CLASSIC-I trial. *Gastroenterology.* 2006;130:323-333; quiz 591.

76. Colombel JF, Sandborn WJ, Rutgeerts P, et al. Adalimumab for maintenance of clinical response and remission in patients with Crohn's disease: the CHARM trial. *Gastroenterology.* 2007;132:52-65.

77. Sandborn WJ, Hanauer SB, Rutgeerts P, et al. Adalimumab for maintenance treatment of Crohn's disease: results of the CLASSIC II trial. *Gut.* 2007;56:1232-1239.

78. Papadakis KA, Shaye OA, Vasiliauskas EA, et al. Safety and efficacy of adalimumab (D2E7) in Crohn's disease patients with an attenuated response to infliximab. *Am J Gastroenterol.* 2005;100:75-79.

79. Youdim A, Vasiliauskas EA, Targan SR, et al. A pilot study of adalimumab in infliximab-allergic patients. *Inflamm Bowel Dis.* 2004;10:333-338.

80. Sandborn WJ, Hanauer S, Loftus EV Jr, et al. An open-label study of the human anti-TNF monoclonal antibody adalimumab in subjects with prior loss of response or intolerance to infliximab for Crohn's disease. *Am J Gastroenterol.* 2004;99:1984-1989.

81. Sandborn WJ, Rutgeerts P, Enns R, et al. Adalimumab induction therapy for Crohn disease previously treated with infliximab: a randomized trial. *Ann Intern Med.* 2007;146:829-838.

82. Winter TA, Wright J, Ghosh S, Jahnsen J, Innes A, Round P. Intravenous CDP870, a PEGylated Fab' fragment of a humanized antitumour necrosis factor antibody, in patients with moderate-to-severe Crohn's disease: an exploratory study. *Aliment Pharmacol Ther.* 2004;20:1337-1346.

83. Schreiber S, Rutgeerts P, Fedorak RN, et al. A randomized, placebo-controlled trial of certolizumab pegol (CDP870) for treatment of Crohn's disease. *Gastroenterology.* 2005;129:807-818.

84. Sandborn WJ, Feagan BG, Stoinov S, et al. Certolizumab pegol for the treatment of Crohn's disease. *N Engl J Med.* 2007;357:228-238.

85. Schreiber S, Khaliq-Kareemi M, Lawrance IC, et al. Maintenance therapy with certolizumab pegol for Crohn's disease. *N Engl J Med.* 2007;357:239-250.

86. Korzenik JR, Dieckgraefe BK, Valentine JF, Hausman DF, Gilbert MJ. Sargramostim for active Crohn's disease. *N Engl J Med.* 2005;352:2193-2201.

87. Dieckgraefe BK, Korzenik JR. Treatment of active Crohn's disease with recombinant human granulocyte-macrophage colony-stimulating factor. *Lancet.* 2002;360:1478-1480.

88. Ghosh S, Goldin E, Gordon FH, et al. Natalizumab for active Crohn's disease. *N Engl J Med.* 2003;348:24-32.

89. Sandborn WJ, Colombel JF, Enns R, et al. Natalizumab induction and maintenance therapy for Crohn's disease. *N Engl J Med.* 2005;353:1912-1925.

90. Mannon PJ, Fuss IJ, Mayer L, et al. Anti-interleukin-12 antibody for active Crohn's disease. *N Engl J Med.* 2004;351:2069-2079.

91. Hommes DW, Mikhajlova TL, Stoinov S, et al. Fontolizumab, a humanised anti-interferon-gamma antibody, demonstrates safety and potential clinical activity in patients with moderate-to-severe Crohn's disease. *Gut.* 2006;55:1131-1137.

92. Ito H, Takazoe M, Fukuda Y, et al. A pilot randomized trial of a human anti-interleukin-6 receptor monoclonal antibody in active Crohn's disease. *Gastroenterology.* 2004;126:989-996; discussion 947.

93. Fukuda Y, Matsui T, Suzuki Y, et al. Adsorptive granulocyte and monocyte apheresis for refractory Crohn's disease: an open multicenter prospective study. *J Gastroenterol.* 2004;39:1158-1164.

94. Thomas-Gibson S, Brooker JC, Hayward CM, Shah SG, Williams CB, Saunders BP. Colonoscopic balloon dilation of Crohn's strictures: a review of long-term outcomes. *Eur J Gastroenterol Hepatol.* 2003;15:485-488.

95. Morini S, Hassan C, Cerro P, Lorenzetti R. Management of an ileocolic anastomotic stricture using polyvinyl over-the-guidewire dilators in Crohn's disease. *Gastrointest Endosc.* 2001;53:384-386.

96. Sabate JM, Villarejo J, Bouhnik Y, et al. Hydrostatic balloon dilatation of Crohn's strictures. *Aliment Pharmacol Ther.* 2003;18:409-413.

97. Gervais DA, Hahn PF, O'Neill MJ, Mueller PR. Percutaneous abscess drainage in Crohn disease: technical success and short- and long-term outcomes during 14 years. *Radiology.* 2002;222:645-651.

98. Garcia JC, Persky SE, Bonis PA, Topazian M. Abscesses in Crohn's disease: outcome of medical versus surgical treatment. *J Clin Gastroenterol.* 2001;32:409-412.

99. Veroux M, Angriman I, Ruffolo C, et al. Severe gastrointestinal bleeding in Crohn's disease. *Ann Ital Chir.* 2003;74:213-215; discussion 216.

100. Kostka R, Lukas M. Massive, life-threatening bleeding in Crohn's disease. *Acta Chir Belg.* 2005;105:168-174.

101. Robert JR, Sachar DB, Greenstein AJ. Severe gastrointestinal hemorrhage in Crohn's disease. *Ann Surg.* 1991;213:207-211.

102. Belaiche J, Louis E, D'Haens G, et al. Acute lower gastrointestinal bleeding in Crohn's disease: characteristics of a unique series of 34 patients. Belgian IBD Research Group. *Am J Gastroenterol.* 1999;94:2177-2181.

103. Pardi DS, Loftus EV Jr, Tremaine WJ, et al. Acute major gastrointestinal hemorrhage in inflammatory bowel disease. *Gastrointest Endosc.* 1999;49:153-157.

104. Papi C, Gili L, Tarquini M, Antonelli G, Capurso L. Infliximab for severe recurrent Crohn's disease presenting with massive gastrointestinal hemorrhage. *J Clin Gastroenterol.* 2003;36:238-241.

105. Belaiche J, Louis E. Severe lower gastrointestinal bleeding in Crohn's disease: successful control with infliximab. *Am J Gastroenterol.* 2002;97:3210-3211.

106. Sankaran SK, Veitch PC. Crohn's disease presenting as toxic megacolon in an elderly man. *Aust N Z J Med.* 1995;25:539-540.

107. Koutroubakis IE. Therapy insight: vascular complications in patients with inflammatory bowel disease. *Nat Clin Pract Gastroenterol Hepatol.* 2005;2:266-272.

MEDICAL MANAGEMENT OF ENTERIC FISTULAE IN CROHN'S DISEASE

Mamoon Raza, MD and Charles N. Bernstein, MD

Enteric fistulae are an important and well-known complication of Crohn's disease. Their association dates back to the original report[1] by Crohn in 1932 and predates the description of perianal fistulae. Since that time, a wide range of locations, symptoms, and extraintestinal organ involvements (including skin, vagina, and urinary bladder) have been described. Generally, fistulae are categorized into internal (bowel to bowel, bowel to bladder, bowel to vagina, bowel to urethra or prostate) (Figure 24-1) and external (entero-cutaneous, perianal) (Figure 24-2) or abdominal and perianal. Regardless of their location, Crohn's fistulae pose a particular challenge in terms of diagnosis and treatment. As symptoms may be nonspecific or mimic luminal disease, diagnosis often relies upon a high index of suspicion or is realized as an incidental finding. Routine diagnostic imaging studies may be too insensitive to pick up many enteric fistulae, and specialized techniques are not available at all centers. Even when the diagnosis is established, medical therapy is limited by the paucity of randomized placebo-controlled trials designed specifically for the treatment of enteric fistulae. As a result, this complication has typically been treated by the surgeon's knife with varied success. However, as the clinician's armamentarium grows, so does the endeavor to provide medical management. The aim of this chapter is to review the epidemiology, pathogenesis, imaging, and medical management of enteric fistulae.

EPIDEMIOLOGY

Reports of the incidence of enteric fistulae in Crohn's disease vary widely. Table 24-1 presents a summary of the published literature with a breakdown of incidence by type of enteric fistula. It is important to be cognizant of the group of patients reported and the methods of fistula detection used in these reports. For instance, in 1 surgical series of 639 patients with Crohn's disease, 34.7% were found to have a total of 290 intraabdominal fistulae.[2] Only 154 patients (24%) had fistulae clinically apparent preoperatively by a combination of history and physical exam, radiography, and endoscopic procedures. Of these patients, only 9% (14/154) had surgery primarily for the management of their fistula (6.3% of all patients in the series) because either 1) the fistula was draining to the exterior and was a cause for personal discomfort or embarrassment, 2) the fistula communicated with the genitourinary system, or 3) the fistula produced a functional or anatomic bypass of a major intestinal segment with consequent malabsorption and/or profuse diarrhea. In the remainder, fistulae were found intraoperatively (60/639, 9%) or after examination of the resected specimen (8/639, 1%). In the subgroup of patients who presented with an abdominal mass or abscess, 41.8% were found to have fistulae. Therefore, in this series of patients, the incidence of abdominal fistula varied based on preoperative diagnosis (24%), surgical findings (35%), or by presentation with mass or abscess (42%).

Lichtenstein GR, ed.
Crohn's Disease: The Complete Guide to Medical Management (pp 297-304).
© 2011 SLACK Incorporated

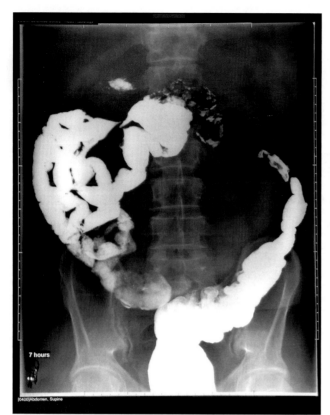

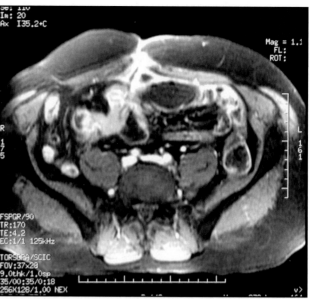

FIGURE 24-2. MRI of a patient with small bowel Crohn's disease. There is a distended loop of small bowel in the lower abdomen, which is adherent to the anterior abdominal wall. This loop has an asymmetrically thickened wall. There is a small fistula extending to the abdominal wall and skin. The bowel distal to this is collapsed in comparison. MRI indicates magnetic resonance imaging.

FIGURE 24-1. Small bowel follow-through of a patient with small bowel Crohn's disease. There is a fistulous communication noted between a loop of distal small bowel and the rectosigmoid. Contrast appears in the rectum before the transverse colon is visualized.

In a population-based study of 169 patients with known CD in Olmsted County, Minnesota, the incidence of all fistulizing disease was 35%, of which only 20% of the entire study population had perianal fistulae.[3] In another review, the incidence of internal and entero-cutaneous fistulae was 34%, 17%, and 16% in those with ileocolonic, small bowel, and colonic disease, respectively ($P < 0.0001$).[4] This relationship between site of disease activity and incidence of enteric fistulae was confirmed in another study of 569 patients where, although the overall incidence for internal fistulae was 16.3%, in those with colonic, small bowel, or ileocolonic patterns, the incidence varied between 8.3%, 9.0%, and 23.2%, respectively.[5] In the same group, the incidence of enterocutaneous fistulae (excluding perianal) also varied from 5.3% of the overall group, to 5% of those with colonic involvement, to 1.9% of those with small bowel involvement, and to 7.7% of those with ileocolonic disease. In an older series, the incidence of enteric fistulae varied from 17% to 48%; however, the inclusion or exclusion of perianal fistulae was not always made clear.[6]

In a recent report from a population-based IBD registry in Manitoba, 5.5% of 1289 patients with CD were found to have internal fistulae, and another 3% had both internal and perianal fistulae.[7]

The incidence of individual types of enteric fistulae has also been reported. In 1 review, 11.4% of patients with CD presented with enterocutaneous fistulae, and 3.8% required surgery for this complication.[8] Enterovesical fistulae occur at a frequency of 2% to 5% and were first reported in 1936.[9] Between 1937 and 1997, only 32 cases of gastrocolic Crohn's fistulae had ever been published.

PATHOGENESIS

The precise mechanism by which fistula formation occurs has not been well described. Transmural inflammation is considered to be a prerequisite, along with enhanced fibrolysis. A recent report described a genetic predisposition in some patients.[10] Among 97 patients with CD, 18 of 23 (78%) who had a c-insertion mutation of the NOD2 gene had fistulae compared to 37 of 74 (50%) who did not have the mutation ($P = 0.029$). Recent studies have helped to delineate the role of matrix metalloproteinases (MMPs), a structurally related class of at least 20 zinc-dependent proteases, and tissue inhibitors of metalloproteinases (TIMPs), which are secreted by the same cells and help regulate MMP activity. Severe inflammation leads to release and activation of MMPs by cells of the inflammatory infiltrate and degrades the extracellular matrix in areas with active inflammation. Fistula formation occurs when there is an absence of a rapid compensatory fibrogenic response to fill up the defect. Specific MMPs, namely MMP-3 and MMP-9, have been found to be markedly upregulated specifically in patients with fistulizing disease along with a paucity of TIMP-1, TIMP-2, and TIMP-3.[11]

TABLE 24-1

INCIDENCE OF ABDOMINAL FISTULAE*

Study	Type of Patients	Total	Enteroduodenal	Enteroenteric	Enterocolonic	Enterosigmoid	Enterovesical	Colosigmoid	Enterosalpingeal	Enterocutaneous	Enterovaginal
Michelassi et al[2]	S	34.7%	5%	18%	29%	17%	12%	2%	16%	4%	17%
Yamamoto et al[9]	C	NR	NR	NR	NR	NR	2-5%	NR	NR	NR	NR
Steinberg et al[6]	C	17%	5%	5%	5%	5%	5%	5%	5%	11%	11%
Schwartz et al[3]	C	NR	2%	2%	2%	2%	2%	NR	NR	3%	5%
Tang et al[7]	C	8.46%	NR	7%	NR	NR	2%	NR	NR	2%	3%

*C indicates combined medical/surgical; M, medical, NR, not reported; S, surgical.

Immunohistochemistry data suggest that the cellular response in CD fistulae differ from non-Crohn's fistulae. In a retrospective comparison of 84 Crohn's fistulae with 13 controls (non-Crohn's fistulae), CD fistulae presented with central infiltration by CD45R0+ T cells followed by a small band of CD68+ macrophages and dense accumulation of CD20+ B cells.[12] In contrast, those with non-Crohn's fistulae (the control group) had a dense infiltration with CD68+ macrophages with only a few CD20+ B cells and CD45R0+ T cells. The difference in cellular response highlights the different roles of the various cell types in Crohn's fistulae. Based on these and other histological nuances, the authors hypothesized the following succession in the formation and maturation of Crohn's fistulae: 1) initially, a stimulus in combination with a proinflammatory response leads to deep tissue destruction, which may be perpetuated in the base of the fistula by intruding luminal antigens/bacteria; 2) myofibroblasts migrate or divide in the vicinity of the lesion; 3) they become organized by development of gap junctions and adherens and, in trying to protect the body from the contents within the intestinal lumen, form a basement membrane; and 4) epithelial cells migrate from the surrounding of the inner lumen of the fistula onto the freshly formed basement membrane, therefore leading to an epithelialized fistula. It is necessary to further understand the molecular mechanisms and cellular interplay that are responsible for the formation and differences between CD and non-Crohn's fistulae. This might lead to better therapeutic strategies.[12]

There is a strong association between strictures and enteric fistulae formation.[13] In a study of surgical specimens from 42 consecutive patients with CD, fistulae were found in 27 (64.3%). Eleven (40.7%) were found within a stricture, 15 (55.6%) at the proximal end of a stricture, and in only 1 (3.7%) was no stricture observed.[14] Interestingly, in 26% of cases, a blood vessel was identified adjacent to a fistula traversing the muscularis propria. In another 22%, a paravascular path for fistulae through the muscular layer was suggested. This raises the possibility that increased intraluminal pressure plays an important role in the formation of enteric fistulae and that perforating vessels act as lead point for their development. This is further evidenced by the fact that fistulae almost exclusively form at the mesenteric border, an area where the largest blood vessels are found.

IMAGING

Ultrasound (US), computed tomography (CT), and barium x-ray studies are widely used in the diagnosis and staging of CD. Their clinical applicability in a wide range of scenarios has been studied, including accuracy in detecting luminal disease, strictures, and abscesses. Unfortunately, the accuracy of these imaging studies in detecting internal enteric fistulae is not well reported. Most data are reported in retrospective series. In the absence of an established gold standard imaging test, intraoperative findings have been used to calculate sensitivities—allowing for a potential selection bias of patients with advanced and severe fistulae. Thus, reported literature may overestimate the true accuracy of radiology in detecting internal fistulae.

In one of the largest prospective series to date comparing CT, US, and contrast radiology in the detection of internal fistulae, no statistical difference was detected between each of these modalities.[15] However, the combination of barium x-ray and US increased sensitivities to 90% from 69% for x-ray and 71% for US individually. All 3 modalities were highly specific. The number or type of fistulae in each patient did not alter sensitivities significantly.

During the past decade, the use of magnetic resonance imaging (MRI) in the diagnosis and staging of CD has been increasing.[16-19] In some reports, MRI was superior in detecting abdominal fistulae over other modalities. In 1 study with 27 Crohn's patients, a contrast-enhanced MRI was performed after enteroclysis.[20] Surgically compared sensitivities for fistula detection were 83.3% and 16.7% for MRI and enteroclysis, respectively.

In most centers, the preferential imaging modality is determined by physician preference, resources, and local expertise as much as it is by comparative data.

MANAGEMENT

Prior to the era of biologics, medical therapy for enteric fistulae achieved less than modest gains, and most patients ultimately required surgical management. In a retrospective review, records from 87 patients with active Crohn's fistulae were analyzed for healing rate, number of therapeutic trials administered during the study period, mean time to healing, and proportion requiring surgical intervention.[21] Among those with enteric fistulae (35%), 12 of 12 with internal fistulae (enteroenteric, enterourethral, enterovesical, enteroprostatic), 15 of 20 with enterocutaneous, and 22 of 27 with rectovaginal fistulae achieved healing at the end of the study period. Medical therapy (antibiotics, azathioprine [AZA], enteral and parenteral nutrition) was credited with being responsible for healing in only a minority (internal 8%, enterocutaneous 7%, rectovaginal 13.5%). The remainder required simple or complex surgery in order to achieve fistula resolution. The number of treatments required prior to healing of abdominal wall (median 2, range 1 to 4), rectovaginal (median 3, range 1 to 7), and internal fistulae (median 1, range 1 to 9) varied. Relapse rates after initial healing were highest in those with rectovaginal fistulae.

Disappointing results such as these have prompted interest in the development of newer therapies to improve outcomes in patients with abdominal fistulae; however, there are few studies in which there are large numbers of patients with enteric fistulae, and in reviewing many trials, it is often difficult to categorize patients with perianal fistulae from those with isolated enteric fistulae.

AMINOSALICYLATES

There are no clinical data to support the use of 5-aminosalicylic acid (5-ASA) or sulfasalazine in either promoting or maintaining enteric fistula closure.

CORTICOSTEROIDS

The use of corticosteroids in fistulizing CD has been associated with an increased incidence of surgical resection in 2 large uncontrolled clinical trials.[22,23] No trials have demonstrated efficacy in the treatment of enteric fistulae.

ANTIBIOTICS

There are no controlled trials evaluating the use of either metronidazole or ciprofloxacin in the treatment specifically of abdominal Crohn's fistulae. Metronidazole has been evaluated in several small and uncontrolled clinical trials for the treatment of perianal fistulae.[24-26] Ciprofloxacin alone has not been evaluated in controlled clinical trials; however, it has demonstrated efficacy in combination with metronidazole for perianal fistulae.[27]

6-MERCAPTOPURINE/AZATHIOPRINE

A follow-up study to a randomized, placebo-controlled trial[28] evaluating the utility of 6-mercaptopurine (6-MP) in active CD was published to highlight this agent's effect specifically on Crohn's fistulae.[29] Although in the original report 6-MP achieved a superior response rate to placebo (31% versus 6%, closure), small numbers prevented this difference from achieving statistical significance. Twenty-seven patients from the original study, as well as 7 others with CD fistulae who were treated with 6-MP, were analyzed in the subsequent report. Of 41 total fistulae in the study, 23 (56%) had enteric fistulae. Although the proportion responding to treatment, defined as closure or improvement, varied in the study population, the most impressive rates were achieved in patients with enteroenteric (86%) and abdominal wall fistulae (75%). Patients with rectovaginal, vulval, and perianal fistulae also showed improvement (56%, 56%, and 50%, respectively). The mean time to response was 3.1 months, and 45% of responders improved within 2 months of therapy, whereas 95% had responded by 6 months. All 10 patients who remained on 6-MP did not show any evidence of recurrence for a period ranging from 1 to 5 years. All 8 patients in whom the drug was withdrawn relapsed, and all 6 patients who were placed back on 6-MP achieved subsequent reclosure. Among the responders, only 1 patient required surgical intervention for the treatment of fistula.

In addition to facilitating fistula closure, 6-MP may be of benefit in preventing recurrence postoperatively. In a more recent trial comparing 6-MP 50 mg/day with mesalamine 3 g/day and placebo in patients undergoing an ileocolic resection, 6-MP was found to be superior to placebo in preventing clinical recurrence at the anastomotic site (50% versus 77%, $P = 0.045$).[30] On subgroup analysis, 6-MP showed a benefit in the avoidance of endoscopic recurrence in the perforating-type disease subgroup ($P = 0.03$). Incidentally, perforating-type disease was also found to be an independent predictor of subsequent clinical recurrence. Further sufficiently powered studies are required to more definitively determine the benefit of AZA/6-MP in closing enteric fistulae for prolonged periods.

METHOTREXATE

Methotrexate is a folate analogue and inhibitor of dihydrofolate reductase, which is involved in several reactions of purine and pyrimidine synthesis.[31] Although its use in the induction and maintenance of remission in luminal CD is well established,[32,33] its effect on Crohn's fistulae has been less well studied.

A recent case series suggests that methotrexate may have a role in a subgroup of patients with Crohn's fistulae.[34] Of the 16 patients in the report, 7 had enteric fistulae. The overall response rate was 56% (25% complete closure, 31% partial response) in patients who had failed or were intolerant to 6-MP therapy. Four (25%) had also failed trials with cyclosporine; however, of the 4 patients who had failed both 6-MP and cyclosporine, only 1 (25%) showed a partial response to methotrexate, whereas the other 3 (75%) failed completely. Prospective randomized, placebo-controlled trials are needed to further evaluate the efficacy of methotrexate for enteric fistulae.

CYCLOSPORINE A

Data on the use of cyclosporine A (CyA) in fistulous CD are limited. Its efficacy specifically in enteric fistulae is even less well established. In 1 report of 18 patients with refractory CD, all patients were treated with IV cyclosporine at a dose of 4 mg/kg/day.[35] Of the 9 patients in the study with fistulizing disease, 7 showed a partial response. Responders were then placed on oral cyclosporine, and 6 out of 7 maintained remission, only to recur when taken off oral therapy. Only 2 of the 9 fistulizing patients had enteric fistulae (both enterocutaneous).

In another report of 5 patients with 12 fistulae (5 enterovaginal, 3 perianal, 3 enterocutaneous, 1 enterovesical) unresponsive to previous surgery, steroids, antibiotics, total parenteral nutrition, or 6-MP/AZA, patients were treated with 6 to 10 days of intravenous (IV) CyA at a dose of 4 mg/kg/day.[36] Patients were then given oral dosing at 8 mg/kg/day to maintain serum levels between 100 and 200 ng/mL. Complete resolution was seen in 10 of 12 fistulae after a mean of 7.9 days. Initial response was seen as early as 2 days (mean 3.6). Therapy was continued for a mean of 6.2 months. Relapses while on therapy (2 perianal, 2 enterovaginal, 1 enterocutaneous) usually correlated with low serum levels or the development of fibrostenotic disease. These reports are on such a few patients that the efficacy of CyA for enteric fistulae can be described as anecdotal at best.

TACROLIMUS

Tacrolimus is a fungus (*Streptomyces*)-derived macrolide antibiotic that inhibits the transcription of interleukin 2 in T-helper lymphocytes. It has been proven effective in the prevention of hepatic allograft rejection. Case reports and uncontrolled retrospective series have suggested efficacy for the treatment of fistulizing CD.[37,38] These included perianal, small bowel, and pouch-vaginal fistulae. Success in early uncontrolled experiences with this agent prompted the development of a randomized, placebo-controlled trial in patients with fistulizing disease.[39] In this trial of 48 patients treated with tacrolimus for 10 weeks, only 4 patients had enteric fistulae, of whom 3 were in the placebo arm. As a result, any indication of efficacy in this group can only be extrapolated from the underwhelming effect of tacrolimus in the treatment of perianal disease.

MYCOPHENOLATE MOFETIL

Mycophenolate mofetil is another potent inhibitor of lymphocyte proliferation. It acts by blocking the synthesis of guanosine nucleotide in T cells. The only controlled trials using this agent are in those with steroid refractory CD. However, there are case series or small open-label trials reporting its efficacy in the treatment of internal fistulae.[40]

INFLIXIMAB

Infliximab is a genetically constructed immunoglobulin (Ig)G1 murine-human chimeric monoclonal antibody that binds to both the soluble subunit and the membrane-bound precursor of human tumor necrosis factor alpha (TNFα).[41,42] It is felt that its effect in inflammatory bowel disease (IBD) is a result of binding to the transmembrane TNFα and causing a reduction in the number of lamina propria T lymphocytes.[43]

There are 2 reports on the efficacy of infliximab in the treatment of fistulizing CD.[44,45] In both trials, the majority of the study population was comprised of patients with perianal fistulae; however, both also incorporated patients with enterocutaneous and other types of enteric fistulae, albeit in small numbers.

In the first trial, 94 patients with Crohn's fistulae (9 of whom had enterocutaneous location, the remainder were perianal) were randomized to 1 of 3 arms consisting of 3-dose induction therapy (0, 2, and 6 weeks) of infliximab 5 mg/kg, 10 mg/kg, or placebo.[44] The primary endpoint was induction of remission defined as a reduction in the number of draining fistulas by greater than 50% of baseline. Although results were not presented in a manner that differentiated perianal from enteric fistula, the primary endpoint was reached in 68% and 56% of those receiving infliximab 5 mg/kg and 10 mg/kg, respectively, as compared to 26% of those receiving placebo (5 mg/kg versus placebo, $P = 0.002$, 10 mg/kg versus placebo, $P = 0.02$; 5 mg/kg versus 10 mg/kg, $P = 0.35$). Although induction of remission was achieved quickly and in a larger proportion than previous therapies, the mean time to relapse was only 3 months. A need for sustained response and the concern over a higher prevalence of antibody formation with episodic therapy[46,47] led to a trial investigating maintenance therapy with infliximab. This trial included 306 patients with enteric or perianal fistulae who were given induction therapy with 5 mg/kg of infliximab via 3 IV infusions at 0, 2, and 6 weeks. Responders and nonresponders were then randomized to placebo or 5 mg/kg of infliximab every 8 weeks and followed until week 54. In this study population, 54/306 had enteric fistulae. Among initial responders, the time to recurrence was significantly shorter in those randomized to maintenance with placebo (14 weeks versus 40 weeks, $P < 0.001$). The proportion of patients who maintained response at the end of the study period (54 weeks) was greater in those receiving infliximab (46% versus 23%, $P = 0.001$). Among those who did not respond to the 3-dose induction regimen, there was no difference in rate of subsequent fistula closure between those receiving placebo or infliximab (16% versus 21%, $P = 0.6$). Based on these data, some expert panels recommend 3-dose induction (at 0, 2, and 6 weeks) followed by 8 weekly maintenance infusions indefinitely;[48] however, as 1- or 2-dose induction has never been evaluated in a published clinical trial, it is not known if this approach is equally effective. Also, considering the cost and potential side effects, some clinicians advocate frequent follow-up and individualizing the interval of maintenance infusions based on the patient's symptoms.

In order to help elucidate whether non-perianal fistulae respond as well as perianal fistulae, 60 consecutive patients with Crohn's fistulae were evaluated after 3 doses of infliximab.[49] Patients were grouped according to type (internal $n = 16$, external $n = 35$, mixed $n = 9$) and location (abdominal wall $n = 8$, perianal $n = 27$, rectovaginal $n = 14$, enterovesical $n = 2$), and response rates were compared. Those with external fistula had a greater complete response rate than those with internal fistulae (69% versus 13%, $P = 0.001$). Those with perianal fistulae had the greatest response (78%), followed by the abdominal wall (38%) and rectovaginal (14%) groups. Both patients with enterovesical fistulae had only a partial response. Another reason for caution in treating patients with enteric fistulae with infliximab is the concern that clinical healing may not correlate with MRI findings and that unresolved fistulous tracts and clinically silent sepsis may persist.[50]

A fully humanized monoclonal antibody to TNFα, CDP571, has been studied as a maintenance agent after induction with infliximab in order to avoid human antichimeric antibody (HACAs) formation.[51] In a study of 396 patients with active CD that included 86 with perianal or enterocutaneous fistulizing disease, no statistical benefit was achieved in the rate of fistula closure when compared to placebo.

NUTRITION

The role of nutritional therapy in complex fistulas has not been clearly evaluated. No controlled studies have examined the role of total parenteral nutrition (TPN) or enteral nutrition in fistulizing CD. Some reports of case series have demonstrated fistula closure in patients receiving exclusively TPN or enteral feeding.[52] Although TPN and bed rest have been established as ineffective therapies for active disease,[53] its role in promoting fistula closure in CD is not well known. Based on anecdotal evidence and expert opinion, a trial of TPN with bed rest may be tried for those with proximal or medically refractory fistulae.

CONCLUSION

Enteric fistulae are a serious and difficult complication in Crohn's disease. Aside from causing symptoms related to their site of involvement, they have been associated with intraabdominal abscesses[54] and the development of squamous cells and adenocarcinoma.[55,56] Although in the past treatment was considered to be primarily surgical, the advent of newer biologics has enabled clinicians and patients to delay or avoid bowel resections for this indication. Important considerations when assessing a patient suspected of harboring an enteric fistula are to define the anatomy, treat any septic or infective complications, and eradicate the fistulous tract using medical or surgical therapy.

REFERENCES

1. Crohn BB, Ginzburg L, Oppenheimer GD. Regional ileitis: A pathologic and clinical entity. *JAMA.* 1932;99:1323-1329.

2. Michelassi F, Stella M, Balestracci T, et al. Incidence, diagnosis, and treatment of enteric and colorectal fistulae in patients with Crohn's disease. *Ann Surg.* 1993;218:660-666.

3. Schwartz DA, Loftus EV, Tremaine WJ, et al. The natural history of fistulizing Crohn's disease in Olmsted County, Minnesota. *Gastroenterology.* 2002;122:875-880.

4. Farmer RG, Hawk WA, Turnbull RB. Clinical patterns in Crohn's disease: a statistical study of 615 cases. *Gastroenterology.* 1975; 68:627-635.

5. Rankin GB, Watts DH, Melnyk CS, et al. National Cooperative Crohn's Disease Study: extraintestinal manifestations and perianal complications. *Gastroenterology.* 1979;77:914-920.

6. Steinberg DM, Trevor Cooke W, Alexander-Williams J. Abscess and fistulae in Crohn's disease. *Gut.* 1973;14:865-869.

7. Tang YL, Rawsthorne P, Bernstein CN. Does perianal disease correlate with luminal fistulizing Crohn's disease? A population based study [abstract]. *Gastroenterology.* 2006;4:1130-1134.

8. Ozdil S, Demir K, Boztas G, et al. Crohn's disease: analysis of 105 patients. *Hepatogastroenterology.* 2003;50(suppl 2):cclxxxvii-ccxci.

9. Yamamoto T, Keighley MRB. Enterovesical fistulas complicating Crohn's disease: clinicopathological features and management. *Int J Colorectal Dis.* 2000;15:211-215.

10. Radlmayr M, Torok, HP, Martin K, Folwanczny C. The c-insertion mutation of the NOD2 gene is associated with fistulizing and fibrostenotic phenotypes in Crohn's disease. *Gastroenterology.* 2002;122:2091-2095.

11. Kirkegaard T, Hansen A, Bruun E, Brynskov J. Expression and localization of matrix metalloproteinases and their natural inhibitors in fistula of patients with Crohn's disease. *Gut.* 2004;53:701-709.

12. Bataille F, Rummele P, Schroeder J, et al. Morphological characterization of Crohn's disease fistulae. *Gut.* 2004;53:1314-1321.

13. Kelly JK, Preshaw RM. Origin of fistulas in Crohn's disease. *J Clin Gastroenterol.* 1989;11:193-196.

14. Oberhuber G, Stangl PC, Vogelsang H, et al. Significant association of strictures and internal fistula formation in Crohn's disease. *Virchows Arch.* 2000;437:293-297.

15. Maconi G, Sampietro GM, Parente F, et al. Contrast radiology, computed tomography and ultrasonography in detecting internal fistulas and intra-abdominal abscesses in Crohn's disease: a prospective comparative study. *Am J Gastroenterol.* 2003;98:1545-1555.

16. Shoenut JP, Semelka RC, Magro CM, et al. Comparison of magnetic resonance imaging and endoscopy in distinguishing the type and severity of inflammatory bowel disease. *J Clin Gastroenterol.* 1994;19:31-35.

17. Kettritz U, Isaaks K, Warshauer DM, et al. Crohn's disease, pilot study comparing MRI of the abdomen with clinical evaluation. *J Clin Gastoenterol.* 1995;21:249-253.

18. Rieber A, Wruk D, Nuessle K, et al. MRI of the abdomen compared with enteroclysis in Crohn's disease using oral and intravenous Gd-DTPA. *Radiologe.* 1998;38:23-28.

19. Rollandi GA, Martinolli C, Conzi R, et al. Magnetic resonance imaging of the small intestine and colon in Crohn's disease. *Radiol Med Torino.* 1996;91:81-85.

20. Rieber A, Aschoff A, Nussle K, et al. MRI in the diagnosis of small bowel disease: use of positive and negative oral contrast media in combination with enteroclysis. *Eur Radiol.* 2000;10:1377-1382.

21. Bell SJ, Williams AB, Wiesel P, et al. The clinical course of fistulating Crohn's disease. *Aliment Pharmacol Ther.* 2003;17:1145-1151.

22. Sparberg M, Kirsner JB. Long term corticosteroid therapy for regional enteritis: an analysis of 58 courses in 54 patients. *Am J Dig Dis.* 1966;11:865-880.

23. Jones JH, Lennard-Jones JF. Corticosteroids and corticotropin in the treatment of Crohn's disease. *Gut.* 1966;7:181-187.

24. Ursing B, Kamme C. Metronidazole for Crohn's disease. *Lancet.* 1975;1:775-777.

25. Bernstein LH, Frank MS, Brandt LJ, et al. Healing of perianal Crohn's disease with metronidazole. *Gastroenterology.* 1980;79:357-365.

26. Brandt LJ, Bernstein LH, Boley SJ, et al. Metronidazole therapy for perianal Crohn's disease: a follow-up study. *Gastroenterology.* 1982;83:383-387.

27. Solomon M, McLeod R, O'Connor B, et al. Combination ciprofloxacin and metronidazole in severe perianal Crohn's disease. *Can J Gastroenterol.* 1993;7:571-573.

28. Present DH, Korelitz BI, Wisch N, et al. Treatment of Crohn's disease with 6-mercaptopurine. *N Engl J Med.* 1980;302:981-987.

29. Korelitz BI, Present DH. Favorable effect of 6-mercaptopurine on fistulae of Crohn's disease. *Dig Dis Sci.* 1985;30:58-64.

30. Hanauer SB, Korelitz BI, Rutgeerts P, et al. Postoperative maintenance of Crohn's disease remission with 6-mercaptopurine, mesalamine, or placebo: a 2-year trial. *Gastroenterology.* 2004;127:723-729.

31. Cutulo M, Sulli A, Pizzorni, et al. Anti-inflammatory mechanisms of methotrexate in rheumatoid arthritis. *Ann Rheum Dis.* 2001;60:729-735.

32. Feagan BG, Rochon J, Fedorak RN, et al. Methotrexate for the treatment of Crohn's disease. The North American Crohn's Study Group Investigators. *N Engl J Med.* 1995;332:292-297.

33. Feagan BG, Fedorak RN, Irvine EJ. A comparison of methotrexate with placebo for the maintenance of remission in Crohn's disease. The North American Crohn's Study Group Investigators. *N Engl J Med.* 2000;342:1627-1632.

34. Mahadevan U, Marion JF, Present DH. Fistula response in Crohn's disease: a case series. *Aliment Pharmacol Ther.* 2003;18:1003-1008.

35. Egan LJ, Sandborn WJ, Tremaine WJ. Clinical outcome following treatment of refractory inflammatory and fistulizing Crohn's disease with intravenous cyclosporine. *Am J Gastroenterol.* 1998;93:442-448.

36. Hanauer SB, Smith MB. Rapid closure of Crohn's fistulas with continuous intravenous cyclosporine A. *Am J Gastroenterol.* 1993;88:646-649.

37. Lowry PW, Weaver AL, Tremaine WJ, et al. Combination therapy with oral tacrolimus (FK506) and azathioprine or 6-mercaptopurine for treatment-refractory Crohn's disease perianal fistulae. *Inflamm Bowel Dis.* 1999;5:239-245.

38. Sandborn WJ. Preliminary report on the use of oral tacrolimus (FK506) in the treatment of complicated proximal small bowel and fistulizing Crohn's disease. *Am J Gastroenterol.* 1997;92:876-879.

39. Sandborn WJ, Present DH, Isaacs KL, et al. Tacrolimus for the treatment of fistulas in patients with Crohn's disease: a randomized, placebo-controlled trial. *Gastroenterology.* 2003;125:380-388.

40. Levy C, Tremaine WJ. Management of internal fistulas in Crohn's disease. *Inflamm Bowel Dis.* 2002;8:106-111.

41. Knight DM, Trinh H, Le J, et al. Construction and initial characteristics of a mouse-human chimeric anti-TNF antibody. *Mol Immunol.* 1993;30:1443-1453.

42. Scallon BJ, Moore MA, Trinh H, et al. Chimeric anti-TNF alpha monoclonal antibody cA2 binds recombinant transmembrane TNF-alpha and activates immune effector functions. *Cytokine.* 1995;7:251-259.

43. Sabatino AD, Ciccocioppo R, Cinque B, et al. Defective mucosal T cell death is sustainably reverted by infliximab in a caspase dependent pathway in Crohn's disease. *Gut.* 2004;53:70-77.

44. Present DH, Rutgeerts P, Targan S, et al. Infliximab for the treatment of fistulas in patients with Crohn's disease. *N Engl J Med.* 1999;340:1398-1405.

45. Sands BE, Anderson FH, Bernstein CN, et al. Infliximab maintenance therapy for fistulizing Crohn's disease. *N Engl J Med.* 2004;350:876-885.

46. Hanauer SB, Wagner CL, Bala M, et al. Incidence and importance of antibody responses to infliximab after maintenance or episodic treatment in Crohn's disease. *Clin Gastroenterol Hepatol.* 2004;2:542-553.

47. Rutgeerts P, Feagan BG, Lichtenstein GR, et al. Comparison of scheduled and episodic treatment strategies of infliximab in Crohn's disease. *Gastroenterology.* 2004;126:402-413.

48. Panaccione R, Fedorak RN, Aumais G, et al. Canadian Association of Gastroenterology Clinical Practice Guidelines: the use of infliximab in Crohn's disease. *Can J Gastroenterol.* 2004;18:503-508.

49. Parsi MA, Lashner BA, Achkar J, et al. Type of fistula determines response to infliximab in patients with fistulous Crohn's disease. *Am J Gastroenterol.* 2003;12:445-448.

50. Bell SJ, Halligan S, Windsor CJ, et al. Response of fistulating Crohn's disease to infliximab treatment assessed by magnetic resonance imaging. *Aliment Pharmacol Ther.* 2003;17:387-393.

51. Sandborn WJ, Feagan BG, Radford-Smith G, et al. CDP571, a humanized monoclonal antibody to tumour necrosis factor alpha, for moderate to severe Crohn's disease: a randomized, double blind, placebo controlled trial. *Gut.* 2004;53:1485-1493.

52. Rombeau JL, Rolandelli RH. Enteral and parenteral nutrition in patients with enteric fistulas and short bowel syndrome. *Surg Clin North Am.* 1987;67:551-571.

53. Greenberg GR, Fleming CR, Jeejeebhoy KN, et al. Controlled trial of bowel rest and nutritional support in the management of Crohn's disease. *Gut.* 1988;29:1309-1315.

54. Yamaguchi A, Matsui T, Sakura T, et al. The clinical characteristics and outcomes of intraabdominal abscess in Crohn's disease. *J Gastroenterol.* 2004;39:441-448.

55. Church JM, Weakley FL, Fazio VW, et al. The relationship between fistulas in Crohn's disease and associated carcinoma. *Dis Colon Rectum.* 1985;28:361-366.

56. Ying LT, Hurlbut DJ, Depew WT, et al. Primary adenocarcinoma in an entero-cutaneous fistula associated with Crohn's disease. *Can J Gastroenterol.* 1998;12:265-269.

25

MANAGEMENT OF REFRACTORY CROHN'S DISEASE

Herbert Tilg, MD and Arthur Kaser, MD

BACKGROUND

REFRACTORY DISEASE

A common and challenging problem is the patient who, regardless of disease location, remains symptomatic despite adequate doses of steroids (steroid-resistant), 5-aminosalicylic acid (5-ASA) agents, and antibiotics or the patient who flares once corticosteroids are decreased or stopped (steroid-dependent). Currently, the main therapeutic options for those patients are immunosuppressants such as azathioprine (AZA) or 6-mercaptopurine (6-MP). Chapters 15 and 16 cover all details regarding immunosuppressive treatment, and therefore these aspects are covered only briefly. This section will summarize recommendations that have to be taken into consideration and how patients with refractory Crohn's disease should be managed.

TREATMENT STRATEGIES IN PATIENTS WITH REFRACTORY DISEASE

IMMUNOSUPPRESSANTS—AZATHIOPRINE AND 6-MERCAPTOPURINE

For most refractory patients, the major alternatives are AZA or its active metabolite 6-MP.[1,2] The response rate to these medications is 60% to 70% in both small bowel and colonic disease. Treatment can be initiated with either drug at a dose of 50 mg/day; within 1 to 2 weeks, the dose can

be increased to a maximum of 2 mg/kg/day for 6-MP and 2.5 mg/kg/day for AZA as indicated by clinical response and lack of bone marrow depression. A response to these medications will usually be seen within 3 to 6 months. During this period, patients often require concomitant steroid therapy with a gradual reduction in the steroid dose after 1 to 2 months of treatment with AZA or 6-MP. Patients receiving these drugs require regular monitoring for toxicity (blood cell counts, liver function tests, serum amylase). Testing for metabolites as well as susceptibility to toxicity (by measuring thiopurine-methyltransferase activity) is available, although such testing is not recommended routinely.

METHOTREXATE

Methotrexate is an alternative for the patient who does not tolerate or is unresponsive to AZA or 6-MP and may be used in preference to AZA or 6-MP in patients with complicated CD-related arthropathy. The drug should be given initially intramuscularly at a dose of 25 mg per week, and a response is anticipated within 1 to 2 months. For those patients on steroid therapy, the drug should be continued during this period with a gradual lowering of the corticosteroid dose. Once a response to intramuscular methotrexate is achieved, the patient can be switched to oral methotrexate with an attempt to lower the dose gradually over several months.

Concomitant therapy with folic acid 1 mg/day may reduce adverse effects to methotrexate. Optimal strategies for surveillance liver biopsies in these patients have not been established. However, clinical experience to date suggests that the incidence of hepatotoxicity is low and

Lichtenstein GR, ed.
Crohn's Disease: The Complete Guide to Medical Management (pp 305-316).
© 2011 SLACK Incorporated

surveillance liver biopsies based upon the cumulative methotrexate dose may not be necessary.

ANTI-TUMOR NECROSIS FACTOR AGENTS—INFLIXIMAB

In recent years, tumor necrosis factor alpha (TNFα) has been identified as a key cytokine with proinflammatory properties. In the 1990s, the central role of TNFα in CD became clearer.[3] Increased levels of TNFα are found in the stool of patients with CD, and it can be detected immunohistochemically in the intestine with inflammatory changes. Infliximab is a so-called chimeric immunoglobulin (Ig)G1-monoclonal antibody that consists of 75% human and 25% murine sequences. Infliximab neutralizes the biological activity of TNFα and thus prevents TNFα from binding to its receptors. However, the effectiveness of this substance is presumably mainly due to its ability to induce apoptosis of activated T cells in the afflicted section of the bowel.[3-5] Apoptosis of disease-mediating T cells is rapid and explains the often rapid onset of the effect of infliximab in clinical practice.

The administration of infliximab results in an improvement of clinical condition and quality of life, accompanied by a decrease in endoscopic and histological activity scores.[6] The half-life of this substance is about 10 days, therefore, infliximab does not accumulate with applications at weeks 0, 2, and 6.

Infliximab is approved for reducing signs and symptoms and inducing and maintaining clinical remission in pediatric patients with moderate to severe active CD who have had an inadequate response to conventional therapy. The first publication that investigated infliximab in CD was published in 1995.[7] In this study, van Dullemen et al showed that infliximab produced a rapid, dramatic clinical improvement in patients with CD that was accompanied by endoscopic improvement. The first placebo-controlled, randomized study was published in the *New England Journal of Medicine* in 1997.[8] Of the 108 patients given a single dose of infliximab (5 mg/kg, 10 mg, or 20 mg/kg body weight), 22 of 27 (81%) patients who received 5 mg/kg body weight showed clinical improvement (decrease in Crohn's Disease Activity Index [CDAI], CDAI > 70 points) after 4 weeks. In the group receiving 10 mg/kg body weight, 14 of 28 (50%) patients showed an improvement; and in the group receiving 20 mg/kg body weight, 18 of 28 (64%) showed an improvement (placebo: 4 of 24; 17%). Clinical remission (CDAI < 150) was achieved in 33% of patients treated with infliximab, compared with only 4% of patients in the placebo group. Clinical improvement was maintained for 12 weeks in 41% of patients (placebo: 12%). Interestingly enough, the concomitant medication

(immunosuppressive agents, aminosalicylates, steroids) and disease localization did not have any influence on therapy response, and the dosage of 5 mg/kg body weight was the most effective.[8] Moreover, the first studies clearly showed that infliximab results both in endoscopic healing and in a marked histological improvement.[9]

In the ACCENT I Study, a single dose of infliximab was compared with a triple induction regimen at weeks 0, 2, and 6 (infliximab 5 mg/kg body weight). The clinical response reported in the earlier studies was confirmed, whereby the triple application proved significantly more effective, although the differences at week 10 were still minor.[10] Another finding from this study that is important for clinical practice was the fact that if there is no response to the second infusion (evaluation at week 4), response to the third infusion is unlikely. Conversely, it appears to be relevant that up to 60% of patients do not respond until after the second infusion. Thus, this regimen, namely 2 applications at weeks 0 and 2 followed by clinical evaluation, can also be implemented in daily practice.

Adalimumab is now Food and Drug Administration (FDA)-approved for inducing and maintaining clinical remission in adult patients with moderate to severe CD who have had an inadequate response to conventional therapy and for inducing remission in these patients if they have also lost response to or are intolerant to infliximab. Adalimumab, a fully humanized anti-TNFα antibody, was demonstrated to be superior to placebo for the induction of remission in patients with moderate to severe CD who were naïve to anti-TNFα therapy[11] and to maintain clinical remission for up to 56 weeks in these patients.[12] Among patients who were intolerant or did not respond to infliximab therapy, adalimumab was shown to induce remission more frequently than placebo.[13]

Certolizumab pegol is a pegylated Fab' fragment of a humanized monoclonal antibody that neutralizes TNFα. A phase III, randomized, double-blind, multicenter study that assessed the efficacy and tolerability of certolizumab in patients with moderate to severe CD showed a modest improvement in response rates, as compared with placebo, but no significant improvement in remission rates.[14] In addition, patients who had a response to induction therapy with certolizumab were more likely to have maintained response and remission at 26 weeks with continued monthly subcutaneous injection compared to those who switched to placebo.[15] Certolizumab pegol is currently FDA approved for the treatment and maintenance of response in adults with moderate to severe Crohn's disease who had an inadequate response to conventional therapy.

The results from the induction phase of the PRECiSE 2 trial compared favorably to other monoclonal anti-TNFα induction studies. The 6-week response rates of approximately two thirds of patients in the study and remission rates of 40% were unaffected by concomitant immunosuppressants or corticosteroids.[16]

ROLE OF ANTI-TNFα AND NOVEL BIOLOGICS IN THE MAINTENANCE THERAPY OF CROHN'S DISEASE: EPISODICAL VS CONTINUOUS APPLICATION

This aspect is probably the most important and, at the same time, the most critical area of infliximab therapy today. Initial study data on repeated administration were first published in 1999.[17] The therapeutic effectiveness of a single infliximab dose without parallel immunosuppressive therapy is present in less than one third of patients after 3 months. The above-mentioned ACCENT I study investigated continuous therapy. In 2004, Rutgeerts et al published the central results from this study, which give us important information for our daily patient management.[18] In this study, all 573 patients receiving infliximab episodically or regularly (every 8 weeks) over a period of 54 weeks within the scope of maintenance treatment have been analyzed. Episodical therapy ("on demand") means that all patients treated with placebo whose disease became clinically active during the study were able to receive treatment with infliximab 5 mg/kg body weight. In both infliximab groups (5 and 10 mg/kg) with regular administration, the dosage could be increased by 5 mg/kg if there was no further response to infliximab ("rescue therapy"). However, the patients did not have access to on-demand or rescue therapy until after study week 14. At certain times in the course of the study, regular therapy was superior to episodical treatment in certain clinical aspects (clinical remission, response, quality of life, use of steroids). This superiority was observed mainly in the group receiving 10 mg/kg infliximab and less at the dose authorized for maintenance therapy of 5 mg/kg. It must be emphasized that the rate of hospital stays ($P = 0.047$) and intraabdominal surgery ($P = 0.04$) was lower in the group receiving 5 mg/kg infliximab than in the group receiving episodical treatment. It may well be concluded from current data that on-demand therapy (in this study a mean number of 2.2 infusions over a period of 46 weeks) is slightly inferior to regular therapy and therefore probably not a treatment modality of choice.[18,19]

Long-term data of certolizumab (at 52 and 54 weeks) suggest that 400-mg subcutaneous injections given monthly are well tolerated with low anti-double-stranded DNA—3.2% in PRECiSE 3 and 2.7% in PRECiSE 4—possibly because of the low apoptosis rates associated with certolizumab. In more than 900 patients treated with certolizumab for 1 year, the incidence of infections and malignancy is similar to other anti-TNFα agents.[20] In the WELCOME study, nearly two thirds of patients who had lost response or were intolerant to infliximab responded to induction with certolizumab at 0, 2, and 4 weeks, with maintenance every 2 or 4 weeks. In addition, almost 40% of those patients achieved remission on certolizumab.[21]

Patients who went into remission during CLASSIC I were randomized to receive placebo, adalimumab 40 mg every other week, or adalimumab 40 mg every week. Patients who did not go into remission with adalimumab were then given open-label adalimumab 40 mg every other week. Among patients who initially responded to adalimumab, significantly higher rates of remission were found with adalimumab versus placebo at 1 year.[22] In patients with CD for less than 2 years, approximately 50% remained in remission more than 1 year after receiving 40 mg of adalimumab subcutaneously every other week or weekly, again arguing for earlier aggressive treatment.[23] The results of a phase III induction trial involving 905 CD patients worldwide (ENACT I) showed no difference in response rates between patients in the natalizumab treatment and placebo arms.[24] However, 339 CD patients in whom clinical response/remission was achieved by natalizumab in the ENACT 1 study were included in the ENACT 2 trial, in which 300 mg of natalizumab versus placebo were infused monthly (for up to 12 months). Post hoc subgroup analyses of the ENACT 2 and ENCORE maintenance trials found consistently higher induction remission rates for nearly 25% of patients with short-duration CD (< 3 years).[25] Furthermore, two thirds of patients given natalizumab in ENACT 2 were able to discontinue steroids within 10 weeks of initiating a steroid taper, and they maintained remission over 1 year.[24] In an open-label extension trial of patients in the ENACT 2 trial, the mean CDAI score over 24 months of continuous treatment showed that nearly three quarters of patients were in clinical remission.[26]

INFLIXIMAB IN FISTULIZING CROHN'S DISEASE

FISTULAE

The transmural inflammatory nature of Crohn's disease predisposes to the formation of fistulae, a complication that may dominate the clinical picture. Infliximab 5 mg/kg administered at weeks 0, 2, and 6, and AZA 2 to 2.5 mg/kg or 6-MP 1 to 1.5 mg/kg are the drugs with the best-established roles for the medical treatment of active Crohn's fistulous disease.[27-30] Infliximab should be considered for all Crohn's patients with active draining fistulas. Although traditionally antibiotics such as metronidazole have been used for perianal fistulas, no evidence from controlled trials supports this practice.

Before initiating infliximab and AZA or 6-MP therapy for perianal fistulous disease, it is important to establish a thorough understanding of the anatomic site of the fistula tract(s), to exclude abscesses, and to evaluate for the presence of inflammation of the rectal mucosa. This may entail endoscopy and, frequently, a combination of magnetic resonance imaging (MRI) of the pelvis, endorectal ultrasound (US), and/or examination under anesthesia with appropriate surgical and radiological treatment of abscess cavities and fistula tracts.

Whereas antibiotics are often administered as monotherapy for simple fistulas (defined as superficial, low intersphinctal, or low trans-sphinctal course; singular fistula opening; no perianal pain and fluctuations; and absence of rectovaginal fistulas, anorectal strictures, and active inflammation of the rectal mucous), the range of treatments for complex fistulas also includes AZA (6-MP),[30] cyclosporine (CyA), tacrolimus, and now infliximab. However, despite these general recommendations, there are no controlled studies with the endpoint of fistula occlusion to date, either with antibiotics or with AZA and 6-MP.[1]

Meanwhile, 2 controlled studies with infliximab are available, in which the chosen endpoint was fistula occlusion. In the first study,[27] 94 patients with fistulating CD (85 patients had perianal fistulas) were treated. The patients received infliximab at weeks 0, 2, and 6 (5 mg/kg versus 10 mg/kg) or placebo. Occlusion of all fistulas was reported in 13% of patients on placebo, in 55% of patients on 5 mg/kg infliximab, and in 38% of patients on 10 mg/kg infliximab. The median duration of remission was 3 months. Eleven percent of patients on infliximab developed a perianal abscess.

In the second major recent study (ACCENT II), 306 patients were initially included with 5 mg/kg infliximab at weeks 0, 2, and 6.[28] Responders subsequently received placebo or 5 mg/kg infliximab at 8-week intervals from week 14 until the end of the study at week 54. At week 14, 195/306 patients (69%) showed a response to the infliximab induction therapy with occlusion of at least 50% of the fistulas. The primary endpoint of this study, the largest fistula study performed to date, was "time until loss of response to the therapy." The median time until this event was 14 weeks on placebo and > 40 weeks on infliximab. In week 54, which appears to be the significant point in time, 39% of patients on infliximab and only 19% of patients on placebo showed occlusion of all fistulas ($P = 0.009$). It should also be mentioned that a part of the patients who did not respond to 5 mg/kg or experienced loss of effect benefited from a dosage increase to 10 mg/kg. In ACCENT II, unlike the first study, an increased incidence of fistula-associated abscesses was not observed.[29] However, proper surgical drainage of all retentions prior to planned infliximab therapy would appear to be important for successful therapy. On the other hand, it was observed that even after so-called healing (ie, cessation of secretion) the fistula ducts still remained visible on MRI scans.[31-33] Internal fistulas do not appear to benefit from infliximab administration[34]; here, surgical treatment is indicated.

EXTRAINTESTINAL MANIFESTATIONS

Extraintestinal manifestations occur in more than 20% of all CD patients (skin, joints, eyes, etc), and they often represent a major therapeutic challenge, frequently requiring an aggressive therapy approach, such as the use of CyA in case of pyoderma gangrenosum. In a prospective open study, infliximab showed good effectiveness for arthritis/arthralgia within the scope of CD.[35] There are numerous case reports on the treatment of pyoderma gangrenosum with infliximab, some of which describe the effectiveness very impressively.[6] Moreover, infliximab also shows good response in other dermatological manifestations such as vasculitis or ulcerations of the oral cavity.[6]

SIDE EFFECTS OF INFLIXIMAB

This topic is covered extensively in chapter 17.

INFLIXIMAB AND MORTALITY

The infliximab mortality rate reported in the periodical Centocor safety reports has been relatively stable between 0.61 and 1.21/1000 patient-years since the first reports in August 1998, most recently 0.94/1000 patient-years in Periodic Safety Update Report 8. An increased mortality during infliximab therapy cannot be concluded from randomized studies or from a comparison with the expected number of deaths. Nonetheless, an older patient population with substantial comorbidity would appear to have an increased mortality rate.[36] There are also other reports on deaths possibly associated with infliximab. Andus et al recently published a small series of 8 patients with lethal infections and a possible association with infliximab.[37] In a study conducted throughout Austria, 2/153 CD patients treated with infliximab died within 2 years; an association with infliximab was classified as possible.[38] However, 1 of these patients suffered from myelodysplastic syndrome, which was ultimately the cause of death. These case reports must all be taken seriously, and they ultimately show that the indications are the decisive factor for such a potent substance. Last but not least, it must be pointed out that the first major controlled studies with steroids reported deaths in cases of CD and that every immunosuppressive therapy is associated with the risk of lethal infections.

PRACTICAL RECOMMENDATIONS FOR THE ADMINISTRATION OF INFLIXIMAB

DOSAGE

The recommended infliximab dosage for all CD indications is 5 mg/kg body weight, administered by IV infusion over a period of 2 hours. The treatment must be administered under the supervision and control of a specialized physician, with emergency equipment for severe infusion reactions at the ready. A follow-up observation period of 1 to 2 hours is recommended.

The following listing gives practical recommendations for the administration of infliximab.

1. Treatment of severe, active CD in patients who have not responded despite complete and adequate therapy with a corticosteroid and an immunosuppressive agent (therapy resistant) or who cannot receive such therapies due to intolerance or medical contraindications (therapy intolerant)

   a. For induction therapy, the administration of infliximab at weeks 0 and 2 is recommended; the patient should be controlled again after 4 weeks at the site at which the indication for infliximab was determined. In case of nonresponse after 2 infusions, a third infusion is not recommended. In case of response, a further infusion at week 6 is recommended.

   b. Further treatment with immunosuppressive agents is recommended despite therapy resistance, in order to reduce the development of antibodies to infliximab (ATIs) and infusion reactions; moreover, this could prevent the potential loss of effectiveness of infliximab.

   c. In case of intolerance of immunosuppressive agents, these should be discontinued or a change to the immunosuppressive agent of second choice (ie, change from AZA/6-MP to methotrexate) is recommended. There are no study data on the simultaneous treatment of therapy with infliximab and an immunosuppressive agent in the sense of bridging until the latter takes effect, although the rationale exists.

   d. Weaning of concomitant steroid therapy: If patients on infliximab achieve remission, weaning of concomitant steroid therapy is recommended (over 20 mg prednisolone: 5 to 10 mg prednisolone/week; under 20 mg prednisolone: 2.5 to 5 mg/kg prednisolone/week).

   e. Active nicotine abuse results in less response and a significantly shorter duration of effect of infliximab.[39] This should be discussed with the patient, and nicotine abstinence should be aimed for prior to any infliximab therapy.

2. In maintenance therapy, if there was initial response to infliximab (study data over a period of 54 weeks available)

   a. Episodical administration of infliximab is inferior to regular therapy at 8-week intervals in some clinical endpoints; lower ATI rates, fewer hospital stays, and fewer operations speak in favor of regular administration of infliximab, especially in patients who cannot receive concomitant immunosuppressive therapy due to intolerance. Ultimately, a clear final recommendation with regard to episodical versus continuous therapy, especially for patients treated with immunosuppressive agents, is not possible on the basis of the data available to date. In episodical infliximab therapy, premedication with steroids appears to be beneficial.[6] This can be provided either with 50 mg prednisolone orally on the day before or intravenously on the same day as the infliximab administration (75 to 100 mg prednisolone). In terms of toxicity, there are no significant differences between regular and episodical therapy. In the case of a loss of effect of infliximab in terms of a clinical exacerbation during regular 8-week administration, the intervals between doses should be shortened in accordance with the authorization for 5 mg/kg. Shortening the intervals to less than 4 weeks is not recommended. Alternatively, a dosage increase by 5 mg/kg could be considered.

3. Treatment of CD with fistulas in patients who have not responded despite complete and adequate therapy with conventional treatments (including antibiotics, drainage, and immunosuppressive therapy)

   a. A first infusion of 5 mg/kg is followed by further infusions of the same dosage at weeks 2 and 6. Despite the data available from the comprehensive ACCENT II study, many questions are still unanswered, including the question whether the success achieved with continuous infliximab therapy would stand up to comparison with combined standard therapy with antibiotics, AZA, and surgery. It remains to be seen whether infliximab is more expedient as a bridging therapy or as continuous therapy.

   b. A wide variety of fistula types were included in the ACCENT II study. It is still unclear which type of fistula is the primary indication for infliximab (simple, complex, enterocutaneous, rectovaginal). Concomitant immunosuppressive therapy during continuous infliximab therapy is recommended, especially in complex fistula cases. The administration of infliximab for internal fistulas is not recommended. Prior to the administration of infliximab, an exact clarification of the fistula anatomy is required (clinical examination possibly with anesthesia, endosonography, MRI) in order to exclude abscessing. Abscesses must be drained adequately prior to treatment with infliximab. Seton drains should not be removed prior to the second infliximab infusion in order to avoid retentions. It must be pointed out that cessation of the fistula secretion during infliximab therapy relates to the persistence of fistula ducts and therefore does not mean actual healing.

4. Strictures

   a. Patients with intestinal strictures usually do not respond as well to infliximab treatment.[40] Although no indications of an increased intestinal stricture formation were found in the ACCENT I study, special attention should be paid to patients with preexisting strictures and/or clinical signs.

5. Extraintestinal manifestations are not included in the authorized indications, but numerous case reports confirm effectiveness.

   a. Infliximab is suitable for the treatment of therapy-resistant extraintestinal manifestations of CD, although there are no data from controlled studies available.

6. Safety

   a. The main risk of infliximab therapy is reactivation of tuberculosis (TB). Therefore, a skin test (Mendel-Mantoux, 5 standard purified protein derivative (PPD) tuberculin units injected strictly intradermally) and a chest x-ray are recommended. The skin test should be assessed after 48 to 72 hours based on the induration in millimeters. Basically, an induration ≥5 mm must be interpreted as positive and the patient regarded as having latent TB. The positive predictive value of this skin test in populations with a low TB rate (at least in Western countries) is only approximately 50%. The false-negative rates correlate with the degree of immunosuppression. Since the average infliximab patient has usually been treated with steroids and immunosuppressive agents already, the false-negative result could represent the main problem in our patient collective.[41] Therefore, the skin test is unreliable and does not replace a comprehensive medical history (exposure or contact with *Mycobacterium tuberculosis*) and chest x-ray. Patients with a positive skin test should be treated with isonazide (INH) 300 mg for 9 months or rifampicin 600 mg for 4 months. The duration of this therapy prior to administration of infliximab has not been established or investigated; depending on the clinical situation, however, infliximab therapy should not be considered until after 1 to 2 months of INH/rifampicin therapy.[42] Active TB is an absolute contraindication. It is always recommendable to review the infliximab indication strictly and to contact a pulmonologist in cases of positive skin test or suspected TB. Against the background of anergy in immunosuppressed patients,[41] we recommend repeating the chest x-ray at 6-month intervals during maintenance therapy with infliximab in order to detect any reactivation of latent tuberculosis as early as possible.

7. Contraindications

   a. Infliximab is contraindicated in patients with tuberculosis and other serious infections, such as sepsis; undrained abscesses within the past 2 months; opportunistic infections, such as Herpes zoster, cytomegalovirus, or *Pneumocystis carinii* within the past 2 months; moderate to severe heart failure (New York Heart Association class III/IV); and known hypersensitivity to infliximab, other murine proteins, or any of the excipients. Special care must be taken in patients with demyelizing disorders, malignomas, and lymphomas. Infliximab should not be administered to patients over the age of 70.

8. Pregnancy

   a. The available data allow the cautious conclusion that infliximab exposure around the time of conception is not associated with an increased rate of deformities. Nonetheless, infliximab is contraindicated during pregnancy, and a contraceptive should be used. An abortion due to infliximab treatment is not justified based on the available information. There are no reliable data available on breastfeeding and infliximab.

PRACTICAL RECOMMENDATIONS: WHEN TO USE INFLIXIMAB IN CROHN'S DISEASE

- Treatment of severe, active CD in patients who have not responded despite complete and adequate therapy with a corticosteroid and an immunosuppressive agent (therapy resistant) or patients who cannot receive such therapies due to intolerance or medical contraindications (therapy intolerant)

- In maintenance therapy, if there was initial response to infliximab (study data over a period of 54 weeks available)

- Treatment of CD with fistulas in patients who have not responded despite complete and adequate therapy with conventional treatments (including antibiotics, drainage, and immunosuppressive therapy)

CAVEATS REGARDING USE OF INFLIXIMAB IN CROHN'S DISEASE

- Check for contraindications (Evidence of malignancy? Heart failure? Hypersensitivity?)
- Careful history regarding infections
- Tuberculosis history
- Evidence of strictures
- Smoking history

CONTINUED DISEASE RESISTANCE

There are 2 medical approaches to patients who continue to have chronic active symptoms of their Crohn's disease despite therapy with 5-ASA agents, antibiotics, immunomodulators, and infliximab: chronic low-dose steroid therapy and total parenteral nutrition (TPN).

Some of these patients can achieve a relative degree of remission only with low-dose corticosteroids. Such patients should be maintained on the lowest dose that is necessary for maintenance of decreased symptoms; alternate-day therapy can be tried for maintenance to minimize toxicity.

This approach should be considered only in patients who have failed a trial of immunomodulator therapy, because maintenance corticosteroids have not been proven to reduce the rate of relapse and are associated with many side effects.[1] Patients receiving long-term corticosteroids should be monitored for cataract formation and should be given a regimen to minimize bone loss.

An alternative for steroid-resistant or steroid-refractory Crohn's disease is TPN or enteral feeding with an elemental or polymeric diet. In a retrospective study of 100 patients treated with TPN and complete bowel rest, 77 achieved clinical remission.[43] The remission rate was similar in patients with subacute bowel obstruction, an inflammatory mass, and uncomplicated severe active disease; approximately 60% of these patients remained in remission at 1 year. A lower initial response rate (63%) and 1-year remission rate (36%) were seen with fistulae.

There are, however, potential problems with bowel rest in addition to relapse when regular feedings are resumed. Many patients will not tolerate enteral feedings, and long-term TPN carries the risk of line sepsis and thrombophlebitis. Nevertheless, these nutritional approaches should be considered in refractory patients and can be lifesaving in those with short bowel syndrome.

OTHER FACTORS CONTRIBUTING TO REFRACTORY DISEASE

SMOKING

Sommerville et al were the first to observe the association between smoking and CD.[44] In a case-control study including 82 patients with CD and matched control subjects, they found that patients with CD were significantly more likely to be smokers than the control subjects, and the association was stronger for smoking habit before the onset of the disease than for current smoking. In a large meta-analysis performed by Calkins of 7 CD studies, the association between smoking and CD was found to be remarkably consistent.[45] Persson et al postulated that the effect of smoking on CD might be more pronounced in women, with a 5-fold increased risk for current female smokers of acquiring CD compared with their nonsmoking female counterparts, whereas male smokers had only a slightly increased risk.[46]

INFLUENCE ON DISEASE BEHAVIOR AND CLINICAL COURSE

Holdstock et al were the first to report that smokers with CD colitis experienced more relapses and more severe pain than their nonsmoking counterparts and that smokers with small bowel CD tended to have a higher probability for hospitalization and the need for surgery than did nonsmokers.[47] There is now substantial information on the detrimental effect of smoking on the clinical course of CD. Smokers have reported significantly more days troubled by symptoms than nonsmokers, and women smokers documented a lower quality of life than those of women not consuming tobacco.[48,49]

In terms of the risk of recurrence or relapse, a deleterious effect of smoking has consistently been observed. Cottone et al found smoking to be an independent risk factor for the development of clinical, surgical, and endoscopic recurrence in a large group of patients who had undergone surgery for CD over a period of almost 20 years.[50] A recent study emphasized the importance of smoking cessation to reduce the risk of reoperation for recurrent CD.[51] Very importantly, smoking adversely affects the need for corticosteroid and immunosuppressive therapy.[52-54] Besides the deleterious effects already mentioned, smoking was found to be an independent risk factor for osteoporosis in women with inflammatory bowel disease (IBD).[55,56]

The mechanisms by which smoking influences disease presentation and clinical course yet remain to be elucidated. Special emphasis should be put on smoking cessation in the postoperative setting to reduce the risk of reoperation, as it is probably in this case that smoking cessation is the most beneficial. Regarding these results as well as the general health hazards induced by smoking, and considering the fact that patients with CD seem to be unaware of the risk that smoking has on their disease, smoking cessation should be emphasized as a major component in the management of CD.

NONSTEROIDAL ANTI-INFLAMMATORY DRUGS

A number of published reports indicate a link between use of nonsteroidal antiinflammatory drugs (NSAIDs) and either initial onset of IBD or flares of quiescent disease. Most of these studies are based on case reports or retrospective studies of patients hospitalized for flare-ups of CD. The mechanisms by which NSAIDs might cause these exacerbations have not been clarified, although inhibition of colonic prostaglandin synthesis might be a factor. NSAIDs inhibit both cyclooxygenase-1 and cyclooxygenase-2 isoforms, and cyclooxygenase-1 is expressed in many tissues, including the gastrointestinal mucosa, maintaining mucosal integrity. Also, the frequencies of such exacerbations by NSAIDs and the circumstances under which they might occur are not known.

Evans et al[57] found an increased odds ratio (OR) of 1.77 for current and 1.93 for recent use of NSAIDs among hospital submissions for colitis due to IBD. Although the time course of flare-ups of IBD after NSAID use is unclear, some reports suggest that this should occur within a few days. The Evans et al study, however, assessed NSAID use within 6 months, and data therefore have to be seen critically.[57] Evidence for a potential association of NSAID use and disease exacerbation in IBD also comes from a study by Felder et al.[58] They found a significantly higher use of NSAIDs among patients with IBD within 1 month compared to a control group consisting of patients with irritable bowel disease (25% versus 2%). Some other authors have not found a relationship between NSAID use and IBD flares. A retrospective review of IBD patients through an HMO database found a hazard ratio of only 0.93 for use of NSAIDs within 3 months of a flare.[59]

Bonner and colleagues recently, however, demonstrated that the use of low-doses of NSAIDs was not associated with an increase in disease activity in patients with both CD and UC.[60] Use of high doses of NSAIDs was associated with a higher numerical disease activity index score among CD patients with colonic involvement, but this was not reflected by an increase in significant disease flares. Unfortunately, this study does not provide a clear answer regarding the risk of NSAID use for IBD patients. For CD patients with colonic involvement, there has been a clear association of higher level of disease activity but not an obvious increase in clinically significant flares. Therefore,

discussion about the clinical relevance of NSAIDs and their effects on disease exacerbation has now been reopened, and further prospective studies are needed to clarify whether NSAIDs indeed activate and worsen human IBD. This is of critical importance, as many IBD patients, especially with extraintestinal disease manifestation, are in urgent need of respective pain treatment. In the interim, low-dose NSAID use might be safe for IBD patients; however, high-dose use might carry the risk of activating disease activity at least in certain patient subgroups.

STRICTURES

Intestinal fibrostenosis is a frequent and debilitating complication of CD, not only resulting in small bowel obstruction but eventually in repeated bowel resection and short bowel syndrome. More than one third of patients with CD have a clear stenosing disease phenotype, often in the absence of luminal inflammatory symptoms. Intestinal fibrosis is a consequence of chronic transmural inflammation in CD. As in other organs and tissues, phenotypic transformation and activation of resident mesenchymal cells, such as fibroblasts and smooth muscle cells, underlie fibrogenesis in the gut. The molecular mechanisms and growth factors involved in this process have not been identified. However, it is clear that inflammatory mediators may have effects on mesenchymal cells in the submucosa and the muscle layers that are profoundly different from their action on leukocytes or epithelial cells. Transforming growth factor-beta (TGF-β), for instance, has profound anti-inflammatory activity in the mucosa and probably serves to keep physiologic inflammation at bay, but at the same time it appears to be driving the process of fibrosis in the deeper layers of the gut. Tumor necrosis factor, on the other hand, has antifibrotic bioactivity, and pharmacologic inhibition of this cytokine carries a theoretical risk of enhanced stricture formation. Endoscopic management of intestinal strictures with balloon dilation is an accepted strategy to prevent or postpone repeated surgery, but careful patient selection is of paramount importance to ensure favorable long-term outcomes. Specific medical therapy aimed at preventing or reversing intestinal fibrosis is not yet available, but candidate molecules are emerging from research in the liver and in other organs.

MEDICAL THERAPY FOR STRICTURES IN CD

Obviously, controlling disease activity and preventing postoperative recurrence will have a major role in the prevention of stricture formation. Nevertheless, rapid mucosal repair by powerful drugs such as anti-TNFα agents may not be beneficial for the fibrosis in deeper mesenchymal layers; therefore, unraveling the very mechanisms of fibrogenesis may open new therapeutic perspectives for the future.

ENDOSCOPIC BALLOON DILATION AND ANTIFIBROTIC THERAPY

Through-the-scope (TTS) balloon dilation is a well-established technique in the upper gastrointestinal tract, but in the past 15 years this procedure has also come to age in the management of CD-related ileocolonic strictures.[61] TTS balloons can be introduced through the stenosis under full endoscopic guidance, thus eliminating the need for fluoroscopy. Careful patient selection is of paramount importance to optimize the outcomes of both endoscopic and surgical stricturoplasty. Therefore, a carefully performed barium meal with good visualization of the ileocolonic anastomosis is mandatory to allow a proper prediction of successful outcome. Endoscopic balloon dilation is indicated for relatively short, symptomatic strictures of the ileocolonic anastomosis. These postoperative strictures are generally easily accessible. Several series have been published in the past 10 years with immediate success rates varying between 71% and 100%.[62] The long-term success rates are lower and also more variable between different series. Symptom recurrence has been reported in 13% to 100% of patients; however, not all of these patients need surgery. Repeated dilation is an option. This will imply each time that the patient is brought under general anesthesia, and the length of the symptom-free interval will be the main parameter used to decide between surgery and repeat endoscopic dilation.

Because of suboptimal long-term outcomes of endoscopic balloon dilation, adjuvant techniques have been studied. In 1 series, unsuccessful balloon dilation was supplemented by carving the stricture with a sphincterotome.[63] The incisions with the sphincterotome did not result in extra complications. Also, more recently, endoscopic stenting of ileocolonic stenoses has been reported in a limited number of patients, with beneficial outcome.[64] Also, the role of intramural or topical corticosteroids in preventing restenosis has been reported. Unfortunately, no prospective randomized study has ever been published. Ramboer et al reported a 100% immediate success rate in 13 patients with endoscopic dilation and intramural injection of corticosteroids after the procedure.[65] Unfortunately, no follow-up data were provided. More recently, Lavy [66] and Brooker et al[67] reported on intramural triamcinolone injection in 10 and 14 patients, respectively. Both studies were retrospective, and the long-term outcomes did compare with reports on dilation alone. Therefore, placebo-controlled studies are needed. Preliminary data from Raedler et al indicated that patients receiving budesonide along with azathioprine after dilation are more likely to have a good long-term outcome than patients receiving azathioprine alone.[68]

CLOSTRIDIUM DIFFICILE INFECTION

Clostridium difficile infection is the most common infectious complication in IBD. Recurrent *Clostridium difficile*–associated disease is also common and a difficult treatment problem. The importance of this issue is highlighted by the fact that each infectious agent is able to activate and induce disease and flare-ups. Therefore, treatment is mandatory in each situation as soon as infection is documented.[69] Antibiotics are indicated, either metronidazole or vancomycin. In case of recurrent infection, tapering and pulsing the antibiotic dose after a 10-day standard course decreases the incidence of recurrences compared with abruptly stopping antibiotics after a simple 10-day course. There is also a role for probiotics in the treatment of recurrent infection; *Saccharomyces boulardii* has been shown to decrease recurrences by about 50%, especially when combined with high-dose vancomycin. Such data, however, have so far not been reported specifically in the IBD setting. Altogether, *Clostridium difficile* infection is a common and serious clinical issue in IBD patients that is often overlooked and contributes to refractory disease.[70-72]

IRRITABLE BOWEL SYNDROME

Functional symptoms occur in IBD probably more than in the general population. Existing disease indices rely heavily on symptoms that may be organic or functional. This may explain inconsistencies between therapeutic trials in IBD. Clinically, misinterpretation can lead to overtreatment of functional symptoms with potent agents (even immunosuppressants) and to undertreatment of IBD when inflammatory features are more subtle.[73] Recent data suggest that Crohn's and IBS patients have a similar rate of functional features. Therefore, it would be of high clinical relevance to develop scores in the future that better identify functional complaints and identify the patient with true inflammation, which is not always the case in typical scores such as the CDAI. Currently, we have to emphasize and recognize the overall importance of functional gastrointestinal complaints in Crohn's patients and the major consequences in either treatment direction (ie, over- and undertreatment).

NONADHERENCE

Besides the previously discussed clinical aspects in each chronic disease, patient noncompliance (or nonadherence, as it is more currently called) has to be considered in refractory disease. This chronic and often devastating disease is a great challenge for every patient and is often accompanied by depression, frustration, and inability to accept the chronic nature of the disease. Therefore, and for various other reasons, patients with refractory disease especially need adequate psychologic counseling and supportive psychiatric treatments.

FACTORS CONTRIBUTING TO REFRACTORY DISEASE

- Smoking
- Nonsteroidal antiinflammatory drugs (NSAIDs)
- Strictures
- *Clostridium difficile* infection
- Irritable bowel syndrome (IBS)
- Nonadherence

CONCLUSION AND FUTURE DIRECTIVES

Refractory CD is an important clinical challenge in the management of patients with this disease. A priori steroid refractoriness appears in at least one third of treated patients and requires treatment intensification such as the use of immunosuppressants and infliximab. Whereas nowadays a refractory patient is defined by nonresponding to steroids, in the future, such a definition should or could include a patient being refractory to immunosuppressive treatment and in need of more aggressive therapy, such as anti-TNFα agents. In case such patients still present disease activity, low-dose steroid treatment and enteral nutritional therapy might be considered. Even more importantly, however, other major clinical aspects have to be taken into consideration. These aspects include clinical features such as smoking, NSAIDs, infection with *Clostridium difficile*, nonadherence, and the presence of IBS. Only when these complications/features are well taken, a practical and adequate management of these complex patients might be possible.

REFERENCES

1. Dubinsky MC. Azathioprine, 6-mercaptopurine in inflammatory bowel disease: pharmacology, efficacy, and safety. *Clin Gastroenterol Hepatol.* 2004;2:731-743.

2. Reinisch W, Dejaco C, Knoflach P, Petritsch W, Vogelsang H, Tilg H. Immunsuppressiva in der therapie chronisch-entzündlicher Darmerkrankungen. *Z Gastroenterol.* 2004;42:1-13.

3. ten Hove T, van Montfrans C, Peppelenbosch MP, van Deventer SJ. Infliximab treatment induces apoptosis of lamina propria T lymphocytes in Crohn's disease. *Gut.* 2002;50:206-211.

4. Ten Hove T, van Montfrans C, Peppelenbosch MP, van Deventer SJ. Infliximab treatment induces apoptosis of lamina propria T lymphocytes in Crohn's disease. *Gut.* 2002;50:206-211.

5. Lugering A, Schmidt A, Lugering N, Pauels HG, Domschke W, Kucharzik T. Infliximab induces apoptosis in monocytes from patients with chronic active Crohn's disease by using a caspase-dependent pathway. *Gastroenterology.* 2001;121:1145-1157.

6. Di Sabatino A, Ciccocioppo R, Cinque B, et al. Defective mucosal T cell death is sustainably reverted by infliximab in a caspase dependent pathway in Crohn's disease. *Gut.* 2004;53:70-77.

7. Van Dullemen HM, van Deventer SJ, Hommes DW, et al. Treatment of Crohn's disease with anti-tumor necrosis factor chimeric monoclonal antibody (cA2). *Gastroenterology.* 1995;109:129-135.

8. Targan SR, Hanauer SB, van Deventer SJ, et al. A short-term study of chimeric monoclonal antibody cA2 to tumor necrosis factor alpha for Crohn's disease. Crohn's Disease cA2 Study Group. *N Engl J Med.* 1997;337:1029-1035.

9. D'Haens G, van Deventer SJ, van Hogezand R, et al. Endoscopic and histological healing with infliximab anti-tumor necrosis factor antibodies in Crohn's disease: a European multicenter trial. *Gastroenterology.* 1999;116:1029-1034.

10. Rutgeerts P, van Assche G, Vermeire S. Optimizing anti-TNF treatment in inflammatory bowel disease. *Gastroenterology.* 2004;126:1593-1610.

11. Hanauer SB, Feagan BG, Lichtenstein GR, et al. Maintenance infliximab for Crohn's disease: the ACCENT I randomised trial. *Lancet.* 2002;359:1541-1549.

12. Hanauer SB, Sandborn WJ, Rutgeerts P, et al. Human anti-tumor necrosis factor monoclonal antibody (adalimumab) in Crohn's disease: the CLASSIC-I trial. *Gastroenterology.* 2006;130:323-333.

13. Sandborn WJ, Hanauer SB, Rutgeerts P, et al. Adalimumab for maintenance treatment of Crohn's disease: results of the CLASSIC II trial. *Gut.* 2007;56:1232-1239.

14. Sandborn WJ, Feagan BG, Stoinov S, et al, and the PRECiSE 1 Study Investigators. Certolizumab pegol for the treatment of Crohn's disease. *N Engl J Med.* 2007;357:228-238.

15. Schreiber S, Khaliq-Kareemi M, Lawrance IC, et al, and the PRECiSE 2 Study Investigators. Maintenance therapy with certolizumab pegol for Crohn's disease. *N Engl J Med.* 2007;357:239-250.

16. Thomsen OO, Schreiber S, Khaliq-Kareemi M, Hanauer SB, Bloomfield R, Sandborn WJ. Rapid onset of response and remission to subcutaneous certolizumab pegol and lack of influence of concomitant baseline medications in active Crohn's disease: results from the open-label induction phase of the PRECiSE 2 study [abstract]. *Gastroenterology.* 2007;132(4 suppl 1):A505.

17. Rutgeerts P, D'Haens G, Targan S, et al. Efficacy and safety of retreatment with anti-tumor necrosis factor antibody (infliximab) to maintain remission in Crohn's disease. *Gastroenterology.* 1999;117:761-769.

18. Rutgeerts P, Feagan BG, Lichtenstein GR, et al. Comparison of scheduled and episodic treatment strategies of infliximab in Crohn's disease. *Gastroenterology.* 2004;126:402-413.

19. Sartor RB. Episodic retreatment versus scheduled maintenance therapy for Crohn's disease with infliximab: not so far apart. *Gastroenterology.* 2004;126:598-600.

20. Colombel JF, Schreiber S, Hanauer SB, Rutgeerts P, Sandborn WJ. Long-term tolerability of subcutaneous certolizumab pegol in active Crohn's disease: results from PRECiSE 3 and 4 [abstract]. *Gastroenterology.* 2007;132(4 suppl 1):A503.

21. Vermeire S, Abreu MT, D'Haens G, et al. Efficacy and safety of certolizumab pegol in patients with active Crohn's disease who previously lost response or were intolerant to infliximab: open-label induction preliminary results of the WELCOME study [abstract]. *Gastroenterology.* 2008;134(4 suppl 1):A67.

22. Colombel JF, Sandborn WJ, Rutgeerts P, et al. Adalimumab for maintenance of clinical response and remission in patients with Crohn's disease: the CHARM trial. *Gastroenterology.* 2007;132:52-65.

23. Schreiber S, Reinisch W, Colombel JF, et al. Early Crohn's disease shows high levels of remission to therapy with adalimumab: sub-analysis of CHARM [abstract]. *Gastroenterology.* 2007;132(4 suppl 1):A147.

24. Sandborn WJ, Colombel JF, Enns R, et al. Natalizumab induction and maintenance therapy for Crohn's disease. *N Engl J Med.* 2005;353:1912-1925.

25. Schreiber S, Targan SR. Efficacy of natalizumab in Crohn's patients with disease duration less than three years [abstract]. *Gastroenterology.* 2007;132(4 suppl 1):A509.

26. Panacione R, Colombel J-F, Enns R, et al. Natalizumab maintains remission in patients with moderately to severely active Crohn's disease for up to 2-years: results from an open-label extension study [abstract]. *Gastroenterology.* 2006;130:A-111.

27. Present DH, Rutgeerts P, Targan S, et al. Infliximab for the treatment of fistulas in patients with Crohn's disease. *N Engl J Med.* 1999;340:1398-1405.

28. Sands BE, Anderson FH, Bernstein CN, et al. Infliximab maintenance therapy for fistulizing Crohn's disease. *N Engl J Med.* 2004; 350:876-885.

29. Fiocchi C. Closing fistulas in Crohn's disease—Should the accent be on maintenance or safety? *N Engl J Med.* 2004;350:934-936.

30. Pearson DC, May GR, Fick GH, Sutherland LR. Azathioprine and 6-mercaptopurine in Crohn's disease. A meta-analysis. *Ann Intern Med.* 1995;123:132-142.

31. Van Bodegraven AA, Sloots CE, Felt-Bersma RJ, Meuwissen SG. Endosonographic evidence of persistence of Crohn's disease-associated fistulas after infliximab treatment, irrespective of clinical response. *Dis Colon Rectum.* 2002;45:39-45.

32. Van Assche G, Vanbeckevoort D, Bielen D, et al. Magnetic resonance imaging of the effects of infliximab on perianal fistulizing Crohn's disease. *Am J Gastroenterol.* 2003;98:332-339.

33. Poritz LS, Rowe WA, Koltun WA. Remicade does not abolish the need for surgery in fistulizing Crohn's disease. *Dis Colon Rectum.* 2002;45:771-775.

34. Miehsler W, Reinisch W, Kazemi-Shirazi L, et al. Infliximab: lack of efficacy on perforating complications in Crohn's disease. *Inflamm Bowel Dis.* 2004;10:36-40.

35. Herfarth H, Obermeier F, Andus T, et al. Improvement of arthritis and arthralgia after treatment with infliximab in a German prospective, open-label, multi-centre trial in refractory Crohn's disease. *Am J Gastroenterol.* 2002;97:2688-2690.

36. Colombel J-F, Loftus EV, Tremaine WJ, et al. The safety profile of infliximab in patients with Crohn's disease: the Mayo clinic experience in 500 patients. *Gastroenterology.* 2004;126:19-31.

37. Andus T, Stange EF, Höffler D, Keller-Stanislawski B. Verdachtsfälle schwerwiegender Nebenwirkungen nach Infliximab aus Deutschland. *Med Klin.* 2003;98:429-436.

38. Wenzl H, Reinisch W, Kirchgatterer A, Vogelsang H, Tilg H, Petritsch W. Austrian infliximab experience in Crohn's disease: a nation-wide cooperative study with long term follow up. *Eur J Gastroenterol Hepatol.* 2004;16:767-773.

39. Arnott IDR, McNeill G, Satsangi J. An analysis of factors influencing short-term and sustained response to infliximab treatment for Crohn's disease. *Aliment Pharmacol Ther.* 2003;17:1451-1457.

40. Lichtenstein GR, Stein R, Lewis JD, Deren J. The presence of intestinal strictures is associated with poorer responses for active or fistulizing Crohn's disease. *Am J Gastroenterol.* 1999;94:2676-2681.

41. Mow WS, Abreu-Martin MT, Papadakis KA, Pitchon HE, Targan SR, Vasiliauskas EA. High incidence of anergy in inflammatory bowel disease patients limits the usefulness of PPD screening before infliximab therapy. *Clin Gastroenterol Hepatol.* 2004;4:309-313.

42. Gardam MA, Keystone EC, Menzies R, et al. Anti-tumour necrosis factor agents and tuberculosis risk: mechanisms of action and clinical management. *Lancet Infect Dis.* 2003;3:148-155.

43. Ostro MJ, Greenberg GR, Jeejeebhoy KN. Total parenteral nutrition and complete bowel rest in the management of Crohn's disease. *J Parenter Enteral Nutr.* 1985;9:280-287.

44. Sommerville KW, Logan RFA, Edmond M, et al. Smoking and Crohn's disease. *BMJ.* 1984;289:954-956.

45. Calkins BM. A meta-analysis of the role of smoking in inflammatory bowel disease. *Dig Dis Sci.* 1989;34:1841-1854.

46. Persson PG, Ahlbom A, Hellers G. Inflammatory bowel disease and tobacco smoke—a case-control study. *Gut.* 1990;31:1377-1381.

47. Holdstock G, Savage D, Harman M, et al. Should patients with inflammatory bowel disease smoke? *BMJ.* 1984;288:362.

48. Kurata JH, Kantor-Fish S, Frankl H, et al. Crohn's disease among ethnic groups in a large health maintenance organization. *Gastroenterology.* 1992;102:1940-1948.

49. Russel MG, Nieman FH, Bergers JM, et al. Cigarette smoking and quality of life in patients with inflammatory bowel disease: South Limburg IBD Study Group. *Eur J Gastroenterol Hepatol.* 1996;8:1075-1081.

50. Cottone M, Rosselli M, Orlando A, et al. Smoking habits and recurrence in Crohn's disease. *Gastroenterology.* 1994;106:643-648.

51. Ryan WR, Allan RN, Yamamoto T, et al. Crohn's disease patients who quit smoking have a reduced risk of reoperation for recurrence. *Am J Surg.* 2004;187:219-225.

52. Cosnes J, Carbonnel F, Beaugerie L, et al. Effects of cigarette smoking on the long-term course of Crohn's disease. *Gastroenterology.* 1996;110:424-431.

53. Cosnes J, Beaugerie L, Carbonnel F, et al. Smoking cessation and the course of Crohn's disease: an intervention study. *Gastroenterology.* 2001;120:1093-1099.

54. Russel MG, Volovics A, Schoon EJ, et al. Inflammatory bowel disease: is there any relation between smoking status and disease presentation? European Collaborative IBD Study Group. *Inflamm Bowel Dis.* 1998;4:182-186.

55. Buchman AL. Bones and Crohn's: problems and solutions. *Inflamm Bowel Dis.* 1999;5:212-217.

56. Silvennoinen JA, Lehtola JK, Niemela SE. Smoking is a risk factor for osteoporosis in women with inflammatory bowel disease. *Scand J Gastroenterol.* 1996;31:367-371.

57. Evans JMM, McMahon AD, Murray FE, et al. Non-steroidal anti-inflammatory drugs are associated with emergency admission to hospital for colitis due to inflammatory bowel disease. *Gut.* 1997; 40:619-622.

58. Felder JB, Korelitz BI, Rajapakse R, et al. Effects of nonsteroidal anti-inflammatory drugs on inflammatory bowel disease: a case-control study. *Am J Gastroenterol.* 2000;95:1949-1954.

59. Dominitz JA, Koepsell TD, Boyko EJ. Association between analgesic use and inflammatory bowel disease (IBD) flares: a retrospective cohort study. *Gastroenterology.* 2000;118:A581.

60. Bonner GF, Walczak M, Kitchen L, et al. Tolerance of nonsteroidal anti-inflammatory drugs in patients with inflammatory bowel disease. *Am J Gastroenterol.* 2000;95:1946-1948.

61. Blomberg B, Rolny P, Jarnerot G. Endoscopic treatment of anastomitic strictures in Crohn's disease. *Endoscopy.* 1991;23:195-198.

62. Couckuyt H, Gevers AM, Coremans G, et al. Efficacy and safety of hydrostatic balloon dilatation of ileocolonic Crohn's strictures: a prospective longterm analysis. *Gut.* 1995;36:577-580.

63. Bedogni G, Ricci E, Pedrazzoli C, et al. Endoscopic dilation of anastomotic colonic stenosis by different techniques: an alternative to surgery? *Gastrointest Endosc.* 1987;33:21-24.

64. Matsuhashi N, Nakajima A, Suzuki A, et al. Long-term outcome of non-surgical strictureplasty using metallic stents for intestinal strictures in Crohn's disease. *Gastrointest Endosc.* 2000;52:343-345.

65. Ramboer C, Verhamme M, Dhondt E, et al. Endoscopic treatment of stenosis in recurrent Crohn's disease with balloon dilation combined with local corticosteroid injection. *Gastrointest Endosc.* 1995;42:252-255.

66. Lavy A. Triamcinolone improves outcome in Crohn's disease strictures. *Dis Colon Rectum.* 1997;40:184-186.

67. Brooker JC, Beckett CC, Saunders BP, et al. Long-acting steroid injections after endoscopic dilation of anastomotic Crohn's strictures may improve outcome: a retrospective case series. *Endoscopy.* 2003;35:333-337.

68. Raedler A, Peters I, Schreiber S. Treatment with azathioprine and budesonide prevents reoccurrence of ileocolonic stenoses after endoscopic dilatation in Crohn's disease. *Gastroenterology.* 1997;112:A1067.

69. Surawicz CM. Treatment of recurrent *Clostridium difficile*-associated disease. *Nat Clin Pract Gastroenterol Hepatol.* 2004;1:32-38.

70. Gerding DN, Muto CA, Owens RC Jr. Treatment of *Clostridium difficile* infection. *Clin Infect Dis.* 2008;46 (suppl 1):S32-S42.

71. Issa M, Ananthakrishnan AN, Binion DG. *Clostridium difficile* and inflammatory bowel disease. *Inflamm Bowel Dis.* 2008;14:1432-1442.

72. Kelly CP, LaMont JT. *Clostridium difficile*—more difficult than ever. *N Engl J Med.* 2008;359:1932-1940.

73. Barratt HS, Kalantzis C, Polymeros D, Forbes A. Functional symptoms in inflammatory bowel disease and the potential influence in misclassification of clinical status. *Aliment Pharmacol Ther.* 2005;15:141-147.

Medical Management of Postoperative Recurrence of Crohn's Disease

Geert D'Haens MD, PhD and David N. Moskovitz MD, FRCP(C)

The vast majority of patients with Crohn's disease will develop recurrence of their condition following curative resection. After ileocolonic resection, new lesions almost invariably appear in the previously unaffected mucosa of the neoterminal ileum. Several medical therapies to prevent postoperative recurrence have been studied and will be discussed. The definition of postoperative disease recurrence can be based on clinical, endoscopic, radiologic, or surgical criteria. Clinical recurrence of Crohn's disease is observed in 10% to 20% of all patients undergoing resection per year postoperatively.[1,2] Olaison and colleagues reported clinical recurrence in one third of their patients as early as 3 months after surgery.[3] Clinical recurrence is, however, ill defined; it is unclear whether the clinical parameter Crohn's Disease Activity Index (CDAI) can be used reliably in the postoperative setting.

Endoscopic recurrence occurs early after ileocolonic anastomosis. By means of ileocolonoscopy, endoscopic recurrence can be diagnosed in 50% to 75% of patients at 3 months and in 50% to 90% at 12 months after surgery.[3-5] Rutgeerts et al developed an endoscopic scoring system to assess postoperative lesions. The score varies from i0 to i4 (*i* for *ileal*) and assesses the severity of the lesions in the proximity of the ileocolonic anastomosis.[6] Several trials have demonstrated that the clinical disease course correlated well with endoscopic appearance at a given point.[7] It is unclear why postoperative recurrence of Crohn's disease typically develops in the ileum proximal to the ileocolonic anastomosis. At a microscopic level, the inflammatory events in recurrent Crohn's disease begin within the first days following resection with ileocolonic anastomosis. As long as the fecal stream is diverted, the mucosa in the neoterminal ileum remains unaffected. Within 8 days of exposure to ileal fluid, however, massive influx of inflammatory cells into the mucosal compartment of the neoterminal ileum begins, accompanied by villous architectural changes, patchy surface epithelial cell damage, and necrosis. In an earlier study, it was demonstrated that recurrent Crohn's lesions in the neoterminal ileum did not appear as long as the fecal stream was diverted. The majority of patients develop mucosal lesions 6 months after intestinal continuity has been restored.[8]

SMOKING

Smoking has a significant influence on the course of inflammatory bowel disease (IBD), particularly cigarette smoking. Active smoking is associated with poor outcome in Crohn's disease. Cigarette use increases the frequency of disease relapse and the need for surgery in patients with Crohn's disease. Moreover, discontinuation of cigarettes improves the disease course.[9] The mechanisms underlying the differential effect of smoking in CD or UC are unknown, but it has been demonstrated that smoking affects systemic and mucosal immunity.[10] Among its many effects, smoking alters the ratio of T helper to T suppressor cells, modulates apoptosis, reduces T cell proliferation, and decreases serum and mucosal immunoglobulin levels. Smoking enhances small bowel permeability and colonic mucus production. The effects of smoking have been studied in postoperative Crohn's disease. Most studies report active smoking as a risk factor for early recurrence. In 1994, Cottone et al reported that 6 years after surgery 60% of nonsmokers, 41% of ex-smokers, and 27% of active smokers were in clinical remission.[11] Sutherland demonstrated that repeat surgery was performed in 20% of nonsmokers and in 36% of smokers.[12] At 10 years, the figures rose to 41% and 70%, respectively. In this study, female smokers with small bowel disease were at highest risk for recurrence. An interventional study by the French GETAID group demonstrated that smoking cessation resulted in a less aggressive disease course.[13]

5-AMINOSALICYLATES (MESALAMINE)

The largest number of recurrence prevention trials has been performed with 5-aminosalicylic acid (5-ASA) products. Medications in this class are considered safe and well tolerated. The benefit of this class of drugs as maintenance agents for Crohn's disease, however, has recently been questioned.[14] Sandborn and Feagan recently reviewed the efficacy and safety data of conventional corticosteroids, mesalamine, sulfasalazine, budesonide, and antibiotics for inducing remission of mild to moderate Crohn's disease from randomized controlled trials and proposed an evidence-based treatment approach.[15] With respect to the 5-ASA class of drugs, they concluded that sulfasalazine demonstrated modest efficacy when Crohn's disease is confined to the colon, whereas mesalamine had no clear benefit over placebo in treating active Crohn's disease. Camma and colleagues performed a meta-analysis of all the controlled clinical trials with 5-ASA for maintenance of remission in Crohn's disease and demonstrated that the benefit was rather marginal.[16] The authors selected randomized clinical trials using the MEDLINE (1986-1997) database, reference lists from published articles, or reviews. Fifteen randomized, controlled trials of mesalamine maintenance therapy involving a total of 2097 patients were selected. The trials included both postoperative trials and trials where patients were randomized after medical induction of remission. Therapy with mesalamine significantly reduced the risk of symptomatic relapse (risk difference, −6.3%; 95% confidence interval [CI] −10.4% to −2.1%). The risk difference was significant in the postsurgical setting (−13.1%; 95% CI −21.8% to −4.5%) but *not* in the medical setting (−4.7%; 95% CI −9.6% to −2.8%). Multifactorial analysis revealed that mesalamine therapy reduced the risk of symptomatic relapse by an average of 6%, with the best results in the postsurgical setting in patients with ileal disease and with prolonged disease duration. Possible explanations of why not all trials with 5-ASA preparations have led to positive results could be sought in the different pharmacological preparations that were used, differences in dosing schedules, and the time point when postoperative treatment was initiated (from immediate start-up to 12 weeks following surgery). Another explanation is that

postoperative prevention studies with 5-ASA have been heterogeneous in design, endpoints, and patient populations. Some studies focused on clinical recurrence as an endpoint, whereas others looked at endoscopic or radiological signs of recurrent inflammation.

SULFASALAZINE

BACKGROUND

Sulfasalazine possesses both antiinflammatory (5-ASA) and antibacterial (sulfapyridine) properties. The drug is partially absorbed in the jejunum after oral ingestion. The remainder of the drug then passes into the colon where it is reduced by the bacterial enzyme azoreductase to sulfapyridine and 5-ASA. Coliform bacteria split the relatively inactive parent drug into its active moieties. As a result, sulfasalazine has its greatest effect in patients with colonic disease. Side effects of sulfasalazine include nausea, headache, fever, rash, and male infertility. Agranulocytosis is one of the most severe, adverse reactions to sulfasalazine occurring within the first 2 months of therapy. A dose of 2 to 4 g/day (preferably of an enteric-coated preparation) is tolerated without headache or nausea by the majority of patients; some are even able to tolerate up to 6 g/day.

CLINICAL TRIALS TO PREVENT RECURRENCE WITH SULFASALAZINE

Three studies have looked at the effect of sulfasalazine initiated early after resection.[17-19] The study of Bergman and Krause evaluated 97 patients with Crohn's disease.[17] All underwent a radical excision of the inflamed parts of the bowel. Patients were randomly divided into 2 groups, 1 treated for 33 weeks postoperatively by corticosteroids and sulfasalazine and the other without any postoperative treatment. Patients were followed up for 3 years with an annual x-ray of the bowel. Thirteen patients were excluded. After 1, 2, or 3 years of observation time a statistically significant difference in the number of recurrences between the 2 groups of patients could not be observed. However, there was a statistically significant longer time between diagnosis and operation in the group of patients with recurrences than in patients with no recurrences. The authors concluded that patients with Crohn's disease undergoing an early operation might have a lower risk of developing recurrences.

Though Wenckert et al showed no benefit of sulfasalazine over placebo,[18] Ewe and colleagues found different results in a multicenter trial.[19] The study looked at the effect of radical or nonradical surgery and of sulfasalazine prophylaxis versus placebo on postoperative recurrence. Two hundred and thirty-two patients with Crohn's disease at 16 medical and surgical centers participated in the study.

At 7 of the centers, patients underwent "radical" resections; at 9 other centers, "nonradical" procedures were performed. The follow-up period was 3 years. Drug treatment was randomized and double blinded. Recurrence was significantly less frequent and occurred later in patients who were operated on nonradically. Patients on sulfasalazine prophylaxis (3 g/day) had a better prognosis than patients on placebo. This effect achieved statistical significance only during the first 2 years of treatment. Both strategies were additive: nonradical operation and sulfasalazine led to the best prognosis, radical operation and placebo to the worst. The authors concluded that that postoperative recurrence is best prevented by nonradical resection and prescribing 3 g of sulfasalazine daily for at least 2 years.

MESALAMINE

ASACOL

BACKGROUND

Asacol is characterized by a Eudragit-S-coating and drug release at pH 7. As a consequence, the drug is released more in the right side of the colon than in the terminal ileum. In theory, therefore, Asacol is designed to treat patients with predominantly colonic disease.

CLINICAL TRIALS TO PREVENT RECURRENCE

Dr. Caprilli and colleagues studied the effects of the 5-ASA formulation Asacol in 2 large studies, of which only the second one was blinded.[20] In the first study, 47 patients were randomized to receive mesalamine therapy, 2.4 g of Asacol per day for 2 years following their first intestinal resection. This cohort was compared to a group of 48 control patients who received no therapy at all, not even placebo. All patients underwent an ileocolonoscopy at 6, 12, and 24 months following surgery with scoring of the lesions as normal, mild, or severe recurrence. Patients were followed clinically to detect signs of clinical recurrence. All patients in the Asacol group were taking more than 80% of the tablets. Two patients had to discontinue therapy because of severe adverse events (skin rash, epigastric pain, vomiting). In the untreated group, endoscopic recurrence was observed in 29% of patients at 6 months, 56% at 1 year, and 85% at 2 years, similar to what had been observed in earlier observational studies. The cumulative proportion of patients with endoscopic recurrence at 24 months in mesalamine-treated patients was only 52% and of symptomatic recurrence 18%, versus 41% symptomatic recurrence in untreated patients ($P = 0.006$). The authors concluded that Asacol prevented 39% of all recurrences and 55% of the severe recurrences after 2 years. Recurrence rates did not differ among patients operated on for fibrostenotic or for perforating disease. The major problem with this trial was, of course, the absence of a proper placebo treatment.

In the second trial by the same group, the effect of Asacol 4.0 g/day was compared with 2.4 g/day of the same drug in the prevention of both endoscopic and clinical postoperative recurrence of Crohn's disease.[21] The study was a double-blind, randomized, multicenter, prospective and controlled clinical trial. Two hundred and six patients, submitted to first or second intestinal resection for Crohn's disease limited to the terminal ileum with or without involvement of the cecum/ascending colon, were enrolled (101 allocated to 4 g/day of Asacol, 105 to 2.4 g/day starting 2 weeks after surgery). Endoscopic recurrence, the primary outcome, was defined as scores >0, >1, and >2 by the Rutgeerts' score. The secondary outcome was clinical recurrence, defined as a CDAI of more than 150 points or an increase in the CDAI index of 100 points or more. Eighty-four patients (83%) in the 4.0 g group and 81 patients (77%) in the 2.4 g group were evaluable by endoscopy. Endoscopic recurrence of >0 was significantly higher in the 2.4 g/day group than in the 4.0 g/day group (62% versus 46%; $P < 0.04$), but no difference was observed with regard to the other 2 endoscopic outcomes (>1 and >2) and clinical recurrence. These results led the authors to conclude that a 4.0 g/day regimen of mesalamine does not offer a clinically significant advantage over a 2.4 g/day regimen in the prevention of postoperative endoscopic and clinical recurrence of Crohn's disease at 1 year of follow-up.

RESIN-COATED MESALAMINE WITH pH-DEPENDENT RELEASE (COLITOFALK, SALOFALK, CLAVERSAL)

CLINICAL TRIALS TO PREVENT RECURRENCE

In an early Belgian trial, Claversal (SmithKline Beecham), an Eudragit-coated mesalamine formulation, was given in a dose of 3 g/day starting 3 months after resection. The results have only been published in abstract form.[22] Clinical and radiological criteria were used to establish the presence of recurrence. A significant difference in the clinical relapse rates or severity of radiological lesions at 1 year in the 37 patients (19 on placebo and 18 on 5-ASA) who completed the trial could not be established. The major drawbacks of this study were the time point at which the therapy was introduced (only 3 months postoperatively), the rather small patient population, and the endpoint of clinical recurrence after only 1 year. Many studies have shown that recurrence begins to develop already within these first months, which would mean that antiinflammatory therapy has to be started early. On the other hand, clinical symptoms most often appear after several years and not after 1 year, which renders the endpoints in this trial rather weak.

A French trial, which was carefully designed and performed by the GETAID (Groupe d'Etudes Thérapeutiques des Affections Inflammatoires Digestives), also used the Claversal 5-ASA preparation 1 g 3 times daily or placebo for 12 weeks, starting as soon as oral feeding was resumed. At week 12, a colonoscopy was performed. Sixty-one patients were included in the 5-ASA group and 61 in the placebo group. Forty-two percent of the patients treated with Claversal had no signs of recurrence versus 34% with placebo, a difference that was not statistically significant. In conclusion, this 5-ASA drug did not affect the presence of endoscopic recurrence or its severity. Patients who had never smoked had a lower recurrence rate.

A much larger Canadian multicenter trial was finally able to demonstrate benefit of mesalamine in the prevention of postoperative recurrence in 163 patients who underwent a surgical resection and had no evidence of residual disease. The patients were randomized to receive active treatment (1.5 g mesalamine twice per day) or placebo within 8 weeks after surgery, with a follow-up period up to 72 months. Symptomatic recurrence, the primary endpoint in this trial, was confirmed by endoscopic and/or radiological techniques. The proportion of patients with symptomatic recurrence amounted to 31% in the 5-ASA treatment group versus 41% in the control group ($P = 0.031$). The relative risk of developing recurrent disease was 0.628 (90% CI 0.40-0.97) in the active treatment group ($P = 0.039$; one-tailed test) using an intention-to-treat analysis and 0.532 (90% CI 0.32-0.87) using an efficacy analysis. Endoscopic and radiologic recurrences were also significantly decreased with relative risks of 0.654 (90% CI 0.47-0.91) in the effectiveness analysis and 0.635 (90% CI 0.44-0.91) in the efficacy analysis. The most important limitation of this study was that therapy was initiated 8 weeks after surgery, a time when some patients undoubtedly already had microscopic (and endoscopic) signs of Crohn's recurrence. Based on the placebo results in this study, one could argue that 53% of the patients received unnecessary treatment for 3 years.[23]

Pentasa

BACKGROUND

The Pentasa formulation of mesalamine is unique because of the granules that gradually release the active compound in the small and large intestine.

Six randomized, double-blind, placebo-controlled studies have been conducted using the Pentasa formulation of mesalamine in patients with mild to moderately active Crohn's disease.[24-29] These trials were all heterogeneous with varying doses and lengths of treatment. Singleton[27] compared 3 doses of Pentasa (1, 2, or 4 g daily) with placebo in a 16-week trial. The group found a significant difference between the 4 g/day mesalamine group and placebo.

Since then, 4 g has been the recommended dose for active Crohn's disease. Pentasa has also been compared with corticosteroids, including budesonide, in the treatment of active mild to moderate Crohn's disease. Thomsen et al compared budesonide 9 mg/day with 2 g of Pentasa twice daily for 16 weeks.[30] At 8, 12, and 16 weeks, budesonide was significantly more effective than mesalamine at inducing remission of Crohn's disease.

CLINICAL TRIALS TO PREVENT POSTOPERATIVE RECURRENCE

The first trial with Pentasa for this indication was performed by an Italian group of investigators led by Brignola.[31] Treatment consisted of 3 g/day of this drug, initiated within 1 month following resection with ileocolonic anastomosis. The endpoint was endoscopic and radiologic recurrence at 12 months. Severe recurrence was observed in 56% of the placebo patients and in 21% of the Pentasa-treated patients ($P < 0.001$).

The Pentasa formulation was also used in a large multicenter trial in Austria, Germany, Denmark, Norway, and Switzerland named the "European Cooperative Crohn's Disease Study VI."[32] The investigators tried to optimize outcome with 3 measures:

1. Therapy was initiated within 2 weeks after surgery.

2. They chose the 5-ASA formulation with the highest drug release in the small bowel (ie, Pentasa).

3. They used the highest dose of 5-ASA ever studied at a large scale in active Crohn's disease, namely 4 g/day.

Only 70% of the eligible patients were randomized, 154 to Pentasa and 170 to placebo. Treatment was continued for 18 months, with clinical relapse as the primary outcome measure. Relapse was defined as a CDAI score above 250 or an increase in this score of at least 60 points above the lowest postoperative value *and* a value > 200. Endoscopic evaluation was only recommended at week 6 and month 18 after the start of therapy or at the time of clinical relapse but was not mandatory. The intent-to-treat analysis demonstrated that the cumulative clinical relapse rates after 18 months amounted to 24.5 ± 3.6% in the Pentasa group and 31.4 ± 3.7% in the placebo group (not significant [NS]). In a subgroup analysis, relapse rates were recalculated in patients with ileal resection alone (ie, no colonic involvement). In this group of 124 patients, clinical relapse rates were significantly lower in Pentasa- than in placebo-treated patients (21.8 ± 5.6% versus 39.7 ± 6.1%, $P = 0.002$). Variables leading to earlier recurrence included duration of the disease and age of the patient. Unfortunately, only 97 patients were included in the colonoscopy substudy at week 6 and 133 at month 18. A correlation between the severity of the endoscopic lesions and the presence of symptoms could not be established. The incidence of endoscopic recurrence was not significantly lower in Pentasa-treated patients (66% versus 50% with placebo). The authors concluded that the study failed to demonstrate a protective effect of Pentasa on the development of clinical recurrence but that patients operated on for small bowel disease alone may benefit from this treatment nonetheless. An important number of patients never made it into the study in the first weeks after surgery due to complications. One could argue that exactly these patients, with more complicated and possibly more aggressive disease, would have the greatest benefit from antiinflammatory therapy. Sutherland added the ECCDS IV trial to the meta-analysis of all 5-ASA recurrence prevention trials, which led to a number needed to treat (NNT) of 25. When the trial by Caprilli, which had not used a placebo drug, was withdrawn from the analysis, the NNT became 100.[33]

A Canadian prevention study treated patients with both medically and surgically induced remission (the latter comprising 26% of the study population) with Pentasa 750 mg 4 times per day or placebo for 48 weeks.[34] Patients were examined at regular intervals, with CDAI calculations on every occasion. Patients whose remission was induced by a bowel resection had a lower relapse rate than patients who had a medically induced remission ($P = 0.003$). For unclear reasons, the effect of mesalamine was more pronounced in women than in men and in patients with ileocolitis. No benefit could be demonstrated in patients with ileal disease alone. Although conventional statistical significance could not be achieved, the proportion of patients that relapsed within 2 years was lower with mesalamine (25%) than with placebo (36%, $P = 0.056$). When only the patients with surgical remission were analyzed, the results became insignificant, probably due to the small sample size that was left.

Hanauer et al[35] randomized patients to receive Pentasa 3 g/day, 6-mercaptopurine (6-MP) 50 mg/day, or placebo. The details of the trial are discussed below. The endpoints selected for this trial included clinical, endoscopic, and radiographic recurrence of disease. Clinical recurrence rates by life table analysis for Pentasa were 58% (95% CI 41%-75%) versus 77% (95% CI 61%-91%) for placebo ($P = 0.123$); endoscopic recurrence rates were 63% (95% CI, 47%-79%) for Pentasa versus 64% (95% CI 46%-81%) for placebo ($P = 0.458$); and radiographic recurrence rates were 46% (95% CI 29%-66%) for Pentasa versus 49% (95% CI 30%-72%) ($P = 0.19$). The authors concluded that mesalamine was not more effective than placebo at reducing the rates of clinical and endoscopic recurrence of Crohn's disease.

ANTIBIOTICS

BACKGROUND

In a study from Oxford in which ileal fluid was infused into defunctioned colon previously affected by Crohn's disease,[36] no signs of recurrent inflammation developed when this ileal effluent was first ultrafiltrated. This observation suggested that intact bacteria or large dietary particles (> 0.22 μ) had to be responsible for the induction of inflammation.[37] Among potential infective candidates, *Bacteroides* species seem particularly important, given their markedly increased concentrations in Crohn's disease ileal resection specimens.[38] This indirect evidence suggests a potential role of bacteria or bacterial molecules most likely from anaerobic bacteria in the induction of Crohn's disease recurrence. The idea that antibiotics might be useful in the prevention of recurrent Crohn's disease became particularly attractive. Earlier on, several trials had already demonstrated the efficacy of nitro-imidazole antibiotics in fistulizing and active Crohn's disease. Besides its antibacterial properties, metronidazole also interferes with the immunologic system including the interference of leukocyte endothelial adhesion and inhibition of the transmigration of inflammatory cells.[39]

The data supporting the use of antibiotics in patients who have not received an operation are based on case controlled, nonrandomized, controlled trails. In a study by Ursing and Kamme,[40] 5 patients with Crohn's disease were treated with metronidazole. Four of them improved after 2 to 4 weeks of treatment. In 3 of the patients, corticosteroids and sulphasalazine could be withdrawn. In 3 patients, metronidazole could be discontinued after 4 to 6 months of treatment. Two of them had no signs or symptoms of relapse 3 and 6 months later. Evidence has also supported a role for ciprofloxacin in active Crohn's disease.[41-43] Although ciprofloxacin has some effect in active CD, the drug has not been tested in postoperative recurrence. Furthermore, the low activity of fluoroquinolones against anaerobes may implicate that this antibiotic is not the best choice to prevent postoperative recurrence.

CLINICAL TRIALS TO PREVENT RECURRENCE WITH ANTIBIOTICS

Rutgeerts and colleagues[44] performed a controlled trial with metronidazole 20 mg/kg/day or placebo started within a week after resection for 12 weeks. After this therapy, 75% of the patients in the placebo group had recurrent mucosal lesions in the neoterminal ileum versus 52% in the metronidazole group. Metronidazole also reduced the clinical recurrence rates at 1 year (4% versus 25%), but this benefit was not sustained at 2 and 3 years.[44] A significant proportion of patients developed metallic taste (7/30), paresthesias and polyneuropathy (5/30), gastrointestinal intolerance (5/30), leukopenia (2/30), abnormal liver function tests (1/30), and psychosis (1/30). In a randomized controlled trial by D'Haens et al, 3 months of metronidazole combined with 12 months of azathioprine (AZA) was linked to significantly lower recurrence rates and a significantly greater proportion of patients with no endoscopic lesions at 12 months compared with metronidazole plus placebo.[45]

A similar beneficial effect with respect to endoscopic recurrence was demonstrated with ornidazole (Tiberal) 500 mg twice daily given for a full year after surgery. Ornidazole is a drug that resembles metronidazole but is believed to have fewer side effects. This was not confirmed, however, in a 1-year recurrence prevention trial with ornidazole. Ornidazole significantly reduced the clinical recurrence rate at 1 year from 15/40 (37.5%) in the placebo group to 3/38 patients (7.9%) in the ornidazole group ($P = 0.0046$). Ornidazole reduced endoscopic recurrence at 12 months from 26/33 (79%) in the placebo group to 15/28 (53.6%) in the ornidazole group ($P = 0.037$). Significantly more patients ($P = 0.041$) dropped out from the study due to side effects in the ornidazole group. The most frequent adverse events with ornidazole included gastrointestinal intolerance, metallic taste, paresthesias, and disturbed liver function tests, all occurring in 10% to 15% of the patients.[46] For this reason, the prolonged use of metronidazole or ornidazole is unfortunately often limited because of toxicity. As a consequence, metronidazole or ornidazole treatment will often be limited to the first 3 months after surgery.

PROBIOTICS

BACKGROUND

Modification of the microbial environment through the use of antibiotics was soon followed by the use of probiotics for similar purposes. The beneficial effects of probiotics are attributed to intestinal colonization and inhibition of pathogen growth, as well as to enhancement of the host immune response and barrier function through interactions with epithelial and immune cells.[47] The immune system can be modulated by bacterial strains in the intestine. Immune cells are continually sampling and responding to intestinal microflora.[48] Different bacterial strains can signal through pattern-recognition receptors, thereby modulating various intracellular signaling pathways.[49,50] Fedorak outlined 5, likely interrelated, probiotic mechanisms of action relative to therapy for IBD 47: (1) receptor competition, whereby probiotics compete with microbial pathogens for a limited number of receptors present on the surface epithelium; (2) immunomodulation and/or stimulation of immune function of gut-associated lymphoid and epithelial cells; (3) probiotic-induced suppression of pathogen growth through release of antimicrobial fact, such as lactic and acetic acid, hydrogen peroxide, and bacteriocins; (4) probiotic-induced enhancement of mucosal barrier function; and (5) induction of T cell apoptosis in the lamina propria.[45]

CLINICAL TRIALS FOR RECURRENCE PREVENTION

Two Italian trials studied the role of probiotics in preventing postoperative recurrence of Crohn's disease. In the first study, so far only published as an abstract in 2000, the use of VSL#3 as probiotic therapy following induction with antibiotics was superior to mesalamine.[48] Prantera and colleagues, however, found no difference between placebo and *Lactobacillus GG* 6 x 10[9] colony-forming units twice daily given for 12 months and started within 10 days from surgery.[49] Forty-five patients were enrolled in a trial with adequate follow-up. For unclear reasons, patients with a high recurrence risk were excluded from the trial. Nine (60%) out of 15 patients in the probiotic group and 6 of 17 in the placebo group had endoscopic recurrence (NS). Clinical recurrence was observed in 17% of probiotics-treated and in 10.5% of placebo-treated patients (NS). The difference between the 2 trials may lie in the type of probiotic preparations, as well as in a longer duration of treatment in the trial using VSL #3. Furthermore, the sample size in both trials did not power the studies to detect subtle differences between groups. Though the use of probiotics is appealing, there is not enough evidence to draw conclusions on their efficacy.

CORTICOSTEROIDS

BACKGROUND

The first controlled studies with enteric-coated budesonide in Crohn's disease showed that 9 mg of budesonide was equally effective as conventional glucocorticosteroids in patients with ileocecal inflammation.[50-52] Side effects were significantly reduced with budesonide, in particular the suppression of plasma cortisol. Dose-finding studies have indicated that 9 mg is the optimal dose.[53] A comparison of 9 mg of budesonide with 4 g of 5-ASA demonstrated a better response with budesonide.[54] When budesonide was used to maintain clinical remission, 2 studies showed a delay of relapse using 6 mg/day of budesonide compared with placebo, but at the end of 1 year, the proportion of patients suffering relapse with budesonide was comparable to the group treated with placebo.[55,56]

CLINICAL TRIALS FOR RECURRENCE PREVENTION

In spite of the disappointing maintenance results, a collaborative, double-blind, placebo-controlled European trial was set up and included 129 patients to be randomized to budesonide 6 mg/day or placebo started within 2 weeks following surgery and continued for 52 weeks.[57] Endoscopic and clinical recurrence rates were not different between both groups at 3 and 12 months. A subanalysis showed a significant reduction in endoscopic lesions with budesonide (12 months: 32% versus 65% for placebo, $P < 0.05$) in patients operated on for inflammatory luminal disease, not in patients with fibrostenosis as the indication for surgery. A comparable trial was performed by a group of German investigators, which used 3 x 1 mg oral pH-modified release budesonide or placebo for 1 year.[58] Of the 88 randomized patients, 83 patients were included in the efficacy analysis (budesonide $n = 43$, placebo $n = 40$).

Treatment was started within 2 weeks after surgery; colonoscopy was performed 3 and 12 months postoperatively. The recurrence rate after 1 year (endoscopic and/or clinical) was 57% in the budesonide group and 70% in the placebo group (NS). Mean time to failure was 196 days under budesonide and 154 days under placebo (NS). Steroid-related side effects were reported more frequently in the placebo than in the budesonide group (32% versus 17%); (NS). Although the effect of budesonide was altogether positive in almost all variables studied in this trial, the differences were small and the power for detecting differences versus placebo was too low to be statistically significant. Based on these trials, there is currently no evidence to support the systematic use of budesonide for postoperative management.

IMMUNOSUPPRESSIVES

BACKGROUND

Immunosuppression is an effective maintenance strategy for luminal Crohn's disease. In addition, retrospective studies have reported mucosal healing with the use of AZA.[59,60] Since these initial trials, there has been an increased use of endoscopic healing as a surrogate marker for disease remission. Regarding safety, reported adverse effects with immunosuppressives in adults include significant infection (7% to 10%), pancreatitis (3% to 5%), neoplasm, bone marrow suppression, allergy, and drug-induced hepatitis. Many studies with years of data suggest there is little probability that immunomodulatory therapy might increase the risk of malignancy in patients with Crohn's disease.

CLINICAL TRIALS FOR RECURRENCE PREVENTION

The well-defined immunological changes taking place in the early postoperative phase prompted the use of immunomodulators to prevent postoperative recurrence. Furthermore, AZA and 6-MP are the most effective agents in the maintenance treatment of established CD. It was therefore logical to study the benefit of these agents to prevent postsurgical recurrence. Cuillerier and colleagues performed a retrospective analysis of 38 patients treated with azathioprine between 1987 and 1996 following subtotal colectomy with ileorectal anastomosis ($n = 12$), ileocolonic resection ($n = 18$), coloproctectomy with ileoanal anastomosis ($n = 4$), or segmental ileal or colonic resection.[61] Twelve patients were already taking AZA prior to surgery and continued the medication, and 26 started to take it within 2 months after surgery. With a mean duration of follow-up of 29 months, recurrence rates amounted to 9%, 16%, and 28% at 1, 2, and 3 years, respectively. The authors

concluded that these numbers were lower than what would be expected in untreated patients and recommended further investigation of azathioprine in this indication.

In a Spanish study, 39 patients were treated with mesalamine 3 g/day ($n = 21$) or with azathioprine 50 mg/day ($n = 17$).[62] After 2 years, no significant differences between both groups were observed in terms of clinical or endoscopic recurrence. This study had a number of serious shortcomings, however: the sample size was too small to allow reliable conclusions, the dose of AZA was suboptimal (generally doses of 2 to 2.5 mg/kg/day are recommended), and the study was not appropriately randomized and controlled.

Hanauer et al[35] randomized 131 patients to receive 6-MP (fixed dose of 50 mg/day), mesalamine (Pentasa 3 g/day), or placebo daily in a double-blind, double-dummy trial. Patients had clinical assessments at 7 weeks and then every 3 months, with colonoscopies at 6, 12, and 24 months and small bowel series at 12 and 24 months. Endpoints were clinical, endoscopic, and radiographic recurrence rates at 24 months. Clinical recurrence rates at 24 months were 50% (95% CI 34%-68%), 58% (95% CI 41%-75%), and 77% (95% CI 61%-91%) in patients receiving 6-MP, mesalamine, and placebo, respectively. Endoscopic recurrence rates were 43% (95% CI 28%-63%), 63% (95% CI 47%-79%), and 64% (95% CI 46%-81%), and radiographic recurrence rates were 33% (95% CI 19%-54%), 46% (95% CI 29%-66%), and 49% (95% CI 30%-72%), respectively. Concerns resulting from this trial include a high clinical relapse rate (77%) observed in the placebo group at 2 years, which was higher than the endoscopic recurrence rate. This finding likely reflects the lack of a valid assessment of disease activity. Moreover, 20% of the patients in the trial were not assessed for clinical or endoscopic outcomes. It could be argued that a higher dose of 6-MP (up to 1 to 1.5 mg/kg/day) may have led to more convincing results.

In a simultaneously published paper, Ardizzone et al prospectively randomized 142 patients to receive AZA (2 mg/kg/day) or mesalamine (3 g/day) for 24 months after surgery.[63] Clinical recurrence was defined as the presence of symptoms with a CDAI score > 200 and surgical relapse as the presence of symptoms refractory to medical treatment or complications requiring surgery. After 24 months, the risk of clinical relapse was comparable in the azathioprine and mesalamine groups (odds ratio [OR] 2.04, 95% CI 0.89-4.67). No difference was observed with respect to surgical relapse at 24 months between the 2 groups. In a subgroup analysis, AZA was more effective than mesalamine in preventing clinical relapse in patients with previous intestinal resections (OR 4.83, 95% CI 1.47-15.8). The authors concluded that AZA is more effective in those patients who have undergone previous intestinal resection.

In conclusion, it remains somewhat unclear what the optimal use of immunomodulators in the postoperative setting would consist of. It is often recommended that patients with an important disease history who have been put on immunomodulators before surgery be continued on these drugs. Whether immunomodulator-naïve patients should be started on it is unclear. In patients with a high-risk profile for recurrence such as smokers, patients with multiple resections in the past, and patients with an aggressive disease course, it is probably beneficial to institute AZA/6-MP in normal therapeutic doses. The randomized controlled trial by D'Haens et al underscores the efficacy of concomitant use of metronidazole and AZA in prevention postoperative recurrence.[45] The trial evaluated 3 months of metronidazole combined with either AZA or placebo and showed a significant improvement in the combination treatment group. In addition, metronidazole in both treatment arms showed efficacy in endoscopic healing.

BIOLOGIC AGENTS

BACKGROUND

Early intestinal inflammation is characterized by a disturbance in the balance of mucosal cytokines. The inflamed mucosa of Crohn's disease is characterized by a typical T helper 1 (Th1)-pattern of cytokines with abundance of tumor necrosis factor alpha (TNFα), interleukin-1 (IL-1), and interferon-γ (IFN-γ). This pattern is in contrast to the one observed in early ileal Crohn's lesions, where low levels of IFN-γ and high levels of interleukin-4 (IL-4, a typical immunoregulatory Th2 cytokine) are dominant.[64] IL-4 attenuates the barrier function of the intestinal epithelium, resulting in the potential enhanced penetration of noxious agents. Incubation of monocytes/macrophages with IL-4 stimulates IL-12, and TNFα production by these cells may explain a switch from a Th2 towards a more typical Th1 response.[65] Most recently, it has been revealed that low mucosal levels of interleukin-10 (IL-10), a typical anti-inflammatory cytokine, were correlated with severe postoperative recurrence.[66]

IL-10 has indeed been shown to display numerous inhibitory effects on mediator synthesis by T and B cells, monocytes-macrophages, neutrophils, mast cells, and eosinophils.[67] Animal models of inflammatory bowel disease have provided most of the evidence for a role of IL-10 in CD. Pretreatment with IL-10 completely prevented arthritis and significantly attenuated intestinal inflammation in the peptidoglycan-polysaccharide granulomatous enterocolitis model.[68,69] One of the leading theories as to the development of CD is the interaction of one's genetic composition with environmental factors, resulting in a dysregulation of the immune response.[70] One immunoregulatory mechanism of the immune system is the balance of cytokines. In vitro, IL-10 diminished both Th1 and Th2 cell activity.

CLINICAL TRIALS

One multicenter trial investigated patients with Crohn's disease who underwent curative ileal or ileocolonic resection and primary anastomosis.[71] Patients were randomized within 2 weeks after surgery to receive subcutaneous IL-10 (Tenovil) 4 µg/kg/day (QD) ($n = 22$); or 8 µg/kg twice weekly (TIW) ($n = 21$); or placebo (QD or TIW; $n = 22$). At 12 weeks, 11 of 21 patients (52%) in the placebo group had recurrent lesions compared with 17 of 37 patients (46%) in the Tenovil group (NS). The incidence of severe endoscopic recurrence was similar in both groups (9%). The trial showed no benefit over placebo for preventing postoperative recurrence of disease.

Although biologic agents, such as the anti-tumor necrosis factor antibody infliximab, are now widely used in treatment of refractory Crohn's disease, no data are available on their efficacy to prevent postsurgical relapse. These expensive drugs should therefore not be used in this setting until further trials have been performed.

Infliximab has been shown in a small randomized controlled trial to prevent postoperative recurrence when administered after intestinal resective surgery.[72] Infliximab, when administered for the first year post-ileal resection, significantly decreased endoscopic, histologic, and clinical CD recurrence. At the end of 1 year, 90% of patients given infliximab (5 mg/kg given at 0, 2, and 6 weeks, then every 8 weeks for 1 year) were in clinical and endoscopic remission compared with only 15.4% of patients in the placebo group. Clinical remission rates were similar between infliximab and placebo groups (66.7% versus 53.8%, respectively). The discrepancy between endoscopic remission and clinical remission underscores the importance of postoperative colonoscopy to assess risk for recurrence.

OMEGA-3 FATTY ACIDS

Certain lipid compounds such as n-3 polyunsaturated fatty acids have been shown to exert anti-inflammatory effects.[73] N-3 polyunsaturated fatty acids reduce the production of proinflammatory metabolites in the arachidonic acid cascade, such as leukotrienes, and also the production of proinflammatory cytokines. Lorenz and colleagues published the first controlled trial in 1989 with n-3 fatty acids in Crohn's disease in which patients received placebo (olive oil) or 3.2 g of omega-3 fatty acids.[74] The clinical disease activity did not improve, however, with either treatment. A larger controlled trial by Lorenz-Meyer was reported in 1996.[75] Patients were treated with omega-3 fatty acids following induction of remission with classic therapy; however, the treatment did not prolong remission. Belluzzi et al used a new enteric-coated fish oil preparation in a trial to maintain remission in Crohn's disease. After 1 year of treatment, 59% of patients treated with active omega-3 fatty acids were still in remission versus 26% of the placebo group.[76] Although the results of this trial were quite promising, a subsequent trial by Feagan et al demonstrated no efficacy over placebo when used in the prevention of relapse in patients with Crohn's disease.[77] As a result of the published data, omega-3 fatty acids have not been used systematically for prevention of postoperative recurrence.

CONCLUSION

Based on the available evidence, some useful guidelines can be proposed. This was also the purpose of a consensus conference held by the European Crohn's and Colitis Organization (ECCO), which was held in Prague in September 2004. It is beyond any doubt that one of the most useful measures to prevent recurrence is to quit smoking, so all patients who smoke should be encouraged to quit. The decision on whether or not to treat with prophylactic medical therapy needs to be answered on a case-by-case basis. In the presence of high-risk factors such as multiple previous resections, young age, or perforating disease, the initiation or continuation of immunomodulatory therapy with AZA/6-MP is strongly recommended. For this indication, most likely "classic doses" (AZA 2 to 2.5 mg/kg/day and 6-MP 1 to 1.5 mg/kg/day) should be used. In patients intolerant to these drugs, 3 months of metronidazole treatment may be beneficial. It is clear that the combination of immunomodulators and metronidazole offers an even more potent protection; hence, the combination therapy should be considered. An equally useful approach may consist of an ileocolonoscopy 6 to 12 months post-resection and then initiate therapy based on the endoscopic findings: if severe ulcerative lesions are found, immunomodulators must be started; in the absence of lesions or the presence of minor lesions such as aphthous ulcerations, no therapy or aminosalicylates should be considered. Aminosalicylates can be used as primary prophylaxis at doses of at least 2 g/day, but the overall benefit of this approach is rather limited. The start of the prophylactic treatment is recommended within 2 weeks after operation on the basis of pathophysiological considerations, although it has not been proven that earlier start is superior. The duration of prophylaxis should be at least 2 years. Longer treatment is probably useful, but evidence of efficacy is lacking. The symptomatic patient should have a colonoscopy and has to be treated as any patient with active disease.

If endoscopy is used as a marker of Crohn's recurrence, it should be focused at the neoterminal ileum proximal to the ileocolonic anastomosis, where most early lesions first appear. Mild lesions are not associated with an increased risk of clinical recurrence; therefore, no induction or change of therapy is recommended in asymptomatic patients. Symptomatic patients with mild lesions can be treated with aminosalicylates. Severe lesions are associated with a high risk of clinical recurrence. In this situation, the start of AZA/6-MP must be considered.

REFERENCES

1. Lee ECG, Papaioannou N. Recurrences following surgery for Crohn's disease. *Clin Gastroenterol.* 1980;9:419-438.

2. Kyle J. Prognosis after ileal resection for Crohn's disease. *Br J Surg.* 1971;58:735-737.

3. Olaison G, Smedh K, Sjödahl R. Natural course of Crohn's disease after ileocolic resection: endoscopically visualised ileal ulcers preceding symptoms. *Gut.* 1992;33:331-335.

4. McLeod RS, Wolff B, Steinhart H, et al. Risk and significance of endoscopic/radiological evidence of recurrent Crohn's disease. *Gastroenterology.* 1997;113:1823-1827.

5. Florent C, Cortot A, Quandale P, et al. Placebo-controlled clinical trial of mesalazine in the prevention of early endoscopic recurrences after resection for Crohn's disease. *Eur J Gastroenterol Hepatol.* 1996;8:229-233.

6. Rutgeerts P, Geboes K, Vantrappen G, et al. Predictability of the postoperative course of Crohn's disease. *Gastroenterology.* 1990;99:956-963.

7. D'Haens G, Geboes K, Peeters M, et al. Early lesions of recurrent Crohn's disease caused by infusion of intestinal contents in excluded ileum. *Gastroenterology.* 1998;114:262-267.

8. Rutgeerts P, Goboes K, Peeters M. Effect of faecal stream diversion on recurrence of Crohn's disease in the neoterminal ileum. *Lancet.* 1991;338(8770):771-774.

9. Rubin DT, Hanauer SB. Smoking and inflammatory bowel disease. *Eur J Gastroenterol Hepatol.* 2000;12:855-862.

10. Sopori M. Effects of cigarette smoke on the immune system. *Nat Rev Immunol.* 2002;2:372-377.

11. Cottone M, Rosselli M, Orlando A, et al. Smoking habits and recurrence in Crohn's disease. *Gastroenterology.* 1994;106:643-648.

12. Sutherland LR, Ramcharan S, Bryant H, Fick G. Effect of cigarette smoking on recurrence of Crohn's disease. *Gastroenterology.* 1990;98:1123-1128.

13. Cosnes J, Carbonnel F, Beaugerie L, et al. Effects of cigarette smoking on the long-term course of Crohn's disease. *Gastroenterology.* 1996;110:424-431.

14. Camma C, Giunta M, Roselli M, et al. Mesalamine in the maintenance treatment of Crohn's disease: a meta-analysis adjusted for confouding variables. *Gastroenterology.* 1997;113:1465-1473.

15. Sandborn WJ, Feagan BG. Review article: mild to moderate Crohn's disease—defining the basis for a new treatment algorithm. *Aliment Pharmacol Ther.* 2003;18:263-277.

16. Camma C, Giunta M, Roselli M, et al. Mesalamine in the maintenance treatment of Crohn's disease: a meta-analysis adjusted for confounding variables. *Gastroenterology.* 1997;113:1465-1473.

17. Bergman L, Krause U. Postoperative treatment with corticosteroids and salazosulphapyridine (Salazopyrin). *Scand J Gastroenterol.* 1976;11:651-656.

18. Wenckert A, Kristensen M, Eklund AE, et al. The long term prophylactic effect of salazosulphapyridine (Salazopyrin) in primary resected patients with Crohn's disease. *Scand J Gastroenterol.* 1978;13:161-167.

19. Ewe K, Herfarth HC, Malchow WH, Jesdinsky HJ. Postoperative recurrence of Crohn's disease in relation to radicality of operation and sulphasalazine prophylaxis. *Digestion.* 1989;42:224-232.

20. Caprilli R, Andreoli A, Capurso L, et al. Oral mesalazine (Asacol) for the prevention of postoperative recurrence of Crohn's disease. *Eur J Gastroenterol Hepatol.* 1994;8:35-43.

21. Caprilli R, Cottone M, Tonelli F, et al. Two mesalazine regimens in the prevention of the post-operative recurrence of Crohn's disease: a pragmatic, double-blind, randomized controlled trial. *Aliment Pharmacol Ther.* 2003;17:517-523.

22. Fiasse R, Fontaine F, Vanheuverzwyn R. Prevention of Crohn's disease recurrences after intestinal resection with Eudragit-L-coated 5-ASA. *Gastroenterology.* 1991;100:A208.

23. McLeod RS, Wolff BG, Steinhart AH, et al. Prophylactic mesalamine treatment decreases postoperative recurrence of Crohn's disease. *Gastroenterology.* 1995;109:404-413.

24. Rasmussen SN, Lauritsen K, Tage-Jensen U, et al. 5-Aminosalicylic acid in the treatment of Crohn's disease. A 16-week double-blind, placebo-controlled, multicentre study with Pentasa. *Scand J Gastroenterol.* 1987;22:877-883.

25. Mahida YR, Jewell DP. Slow-release 5-amino-salicylic acid (Pentasa) for the treatment of active Crohn's disease. *Digestion.* 1990;45:88-92.

26. Singleton JW, Hanauer SB, Gitnick GL, et al. Mesalamine capsules for the treatment of active Crohn's disease: results of a 16-week trial. Pentasa Crohn's Disease Study Group. *Gastroenterology.* 1993;104:1293-1301.

27. Singleton J. Second trial of mesalamine therapy in the treatment of active Crohn's disease. *Gastroenterology.* 1994;107:632-633.

28. Tremaine WJ, Schroeder KW, Harrison JM, et al. A randomized, double-blind, placebo-controlled trial of the oral mesalamine (5-ASA) preparation, Asacol, in the treatment of symptomatic Crohn's colitis and ileocolitis. *J Clin Gastroenterol.* 1994;19:278-282.

29. Hanauer SB, Stromberg U. Efficacy of oral Pentasa 4 g/day in treatment of active Crohn's disease: a meta-analysis of double-blind, placebo-controlled trials [abstract]. *Gastroenterology.* 2001;120:A453.

30. Thomsen OÖ, Cortot A, Jewell D, et al. A comparison of budesonide and mesalamine for active Crohn's disease. International Budesonide-Mesalamine Study Group. *N Engl J Med.* 1998;339:370-374.

31. Brignola C, Cottone M, Pera A, et al. Mesalamine in the prevention of endoscopic recurrence after intestinal resection for Crohn's disease. Italian Cooperative Study Group. *Gastroenterology.* 1995;108:345-349.

32. Lochs H, Mayer M, Fleig WE, et al. Prophylaxis of postoperative relapse in Crohn's disease with mesalazine (Pentasa): European Cooperative Crohn's Disease Study VI. *Gastroenterology.* 2000;118:264-273.

33. Sutherland LR. Mesalamine for the prevention of postoperative recurrence: is nearly being there the same as being there? *Gastroenterology.* 2000;118:436-438.

34. Sutherland LR, Martin F, Bailey RJ, et al. A randomized, placebo-controlled, double-blind trial of mesalamine in the maintenance of remission of Crohn's disease. The Canadian Mesalamine for Remission of Crohn's Disease Study Group. *Gastroenterology.* 1997;112(4):1069-1077.

35. Hanauer SB, Korelitz BI, Rutgeerts P, et al. Postoperative maintenance of Crohn's disease remission with 6-mercaptopurine, mesalamine, or placebo: a 2-year trial. *Gastroenterology.* 2004;127:723-729.

36. Fasoli R, Kettlewell MGW, Mortensen N, et al. Response to fecal challenge in defunctioned colonic Crohn's disease: prediction of long-term response. *Br J Surg.* 1990;77:616-617.

37. Harper PH, Lee ECG, Kettlewell MGW, et al. Role of fecal stream in the maintenance of Crohn's colitis. *Gut.* 1985;26:279-284.

38. Keighly MR, Arabi Y, Dimock F, et al. Influence of inflammatory bowel disease on intestinal microflora. *Gut.* 1978;19:1099-1104.

39. Ursing B, Kamme C. Metronidazole for Crohn's disease. *Lancet.* 1975;1:775-777.

40. Ursing B, Kamme C. Metronidazole for Crohn's disease. *Lancet.* 1975;1:775-777.

41. Arnold GL, Beaves MR, Pryjdun VO, Mook WJ. Preliminary study of ciprofloxacin in active Crohn's disease. *Inflamm Bowel Dis.* 2002;8:10.

42. Prantera, C, Zannoni, F, Scribano, ML, et al. An antibiotic regimen for the treatment of active Crohn's disease: a randomized, controlled clinical trial of metronidazole plus ciprofloxacin. *Am J Gastroenterol.* 1996;91:328.

43. Steinhart AH, Feagan BG, Wong CJ, et al. Combined budesonide and antibiotic therapy for active Crohn's disease: a randomized controlled trial. *Gastroenterology.* 2002;123:33.

44. Rutgeerts P, Hiele M, Geboes K, et al. Controlled trial of metronidazole treatment for prevention of Crohn's recurrence after ileal resection. *Gastroenterology.* 1995;108:1617-1621.

45. D'Haens GR, Vermeire S, Van Assche G, et al. Therapy of metronidazole with azathioprine to prevent postoperative recurrence of Crohn's disease: a controlled randomized trial. *Gastroenterology.* 2008;135:1123-1129.

46. Rutgeerts P, Van Assche G, D'Haens G, et al. Ornidazol for prophylaxis of postoperative Crohn's disease: final results of a double blind placebo controlled trial. *Gastroenterology.* 2002;122:A666.

47. Fedorak RN, Madsen KL. Probiotics and the management of inflammatory bowel disease. *Inflamm Bowel Dis.* 2004;10:286-299.

48. Campieri M, Rizello F, Venturi A, et al. Combination of antibiotic and probiotic treatment is efficacious in prophylaxis of postoperative recurrence of Crohn's disease: a randomized controlled study vs mesalamine. *Gastroenterology.* 2000;118:A781.

49. Prantera C, Scribano ML, Falasco G, Andreoli A, Luzi C. Ineffectiveness of probiotics in preventing recurrence after curative resection for Crohn's disease: a randomised controlled trial with *Lactobacillus GG.* Gut. 2002;51:405-409.

50. Rutgeerts P, Löfberg R, Malchow H, et al. A comparison of budesonide with prednisolone for active Crohn's disease. *N Engl J Med.* 1994;331:842-845.

51. Gross V, Andus T, Caesar I, et al. Oral pH-modified release budesonide versus 6-methylprednisolone in active Crohn's disease. German/Austrian Budesonide Study Group. *Eur J Gastroenterol Hepatol.* 1996;8:905-909.

52. Bar-Meir S, Chowers Y, Lavy A, et al. Oral budesonide is as effective as oral budesonide versus prednisone in the treatment of active Crohn's disease. The Israeli Budesonide Study Group. *Gastroenterology.* 1998:835-840.

53. Greenberg GR, Feagan BG, Martin F, et al. Oral budesonide for active Crohn's disease. Canadian Inflammatory Bowel Disease Study Group. *N Engl J Med.* 1994;331:836-841.

54. Ostergaard-Thomsen O, Cortot A, Jewell D, et al. A comparison of budesonide and mesalamine for active Crohn's disease. International Budesonide-Mesalamine Study Group. *N Engl J Med.* 1998;399:370-374.

55. Gross V, Andus T, Ecker KW, et al. Low dose oral pH modified release budesonide for maintenance of steroid induced remission in Crohn's disease. The Budesonide Study Group. *Gut.* 1998;42:493-496.

56. Greenberg GR, Feagan BG, Martin F, et al. Oral budesonide as maintenance treatment for Crohn's disease: a placebo-controlled, dose-ranging study. Canadian Inflammatory Bowel Disease Study Group. *Gastroenterology.* 1996;110:45-51.

57. Hellers G, Cortot A, Jewell D, et al. Oral budesonide for prevention of postsurgical recurrence in Crohn's disease. *Gastroenterology.* 1999;116:294-300.

58. Ewe K, Bottger T, Buhr HJ, Ecker KW, Otto HF. Low-dose budesonide treatment for prevention of postoperative recurrence of Crohn's disease: a multicentre randomized placebo-controlled trial. German Budesonide Study Group. *Eur J Gastroenterol Hepatol.* 1999;11:277-282.

59. D'Haens G, Geboes K, Ponette E, Penninckx F, Rutgeerts P. Healing of severe recurrent ileitis with azathioprine therapy in patients with Crohn's disease. *Gastroenterology.* 1997;112:1475-1481.

60. D'Haens G, Geboes K, Rutgeerts P. Endoscopic and histologic healing of Crohn's (ileo-) colitis with azathioprine. *Gastrointest Endosc.* 1999;50:667-671.

61. Cuillerier E, Lemann M, Bouhnik Y. Azathioprine for prevention of postoperative recurrence in Crohn's disease. *Eur J Gastroenterol Hepatol.* 2001;13:1291-1296.

62. Nos P, Hinojosa J, Aguilera V, et al. Azathioprine and 5-ASA in the prevention of postoperative recurrence of Crohn's disease. *Gastroenterol Hepatol.* 2000;23:374-378.

63. Ardizzone S, Maconi G, Sampietro GM, et al. Azathioprine and mesalamine for prevention of relapse after conservative surgery for Crohn's disease. *Gastroenterology.* 2004;127:730-740.

64. Desreumaux P, Brandt E, Gambiez L, et al. Distinct cytokine patterns in early and chronic ileal lesions of Crohn's disease. *Gastroenterology.* 1997;113:118-126.

65. D'Andrea A, Ma X, Aste-Amezaga M, et al. Stimulatory and inhibitory effects of interleukin-4 and IL-13 on the production of cytokines by human peripheral blood mononuclear cells: priming for IL-12 and TNF production. *J Exp Med.* 1995;181:537-546.

66. Meresse B, Rutgeerts P, Malchow H, et al. Low ileal interleukin 10 concentrations are predictive of endoscopic recurrence in patients with Crohn's disease. *Gut.* 2002;50:25-28.

67. Mac Donald TT. Effector and regulatory lymphoid cells and cytokines in mucosal sites. *Curr Top Microbiol Immunol.* 1999;236:113-135.

68. Herfarth HH, Mohanty SP, Rath HC, et al. Interleukin-10 suppresses chronic granulomatous inflammation induced by bacterial cell wall polymers in a rat model. *Gut.* 1996;39:836-845.

69. Herfarth HH, Böcker U, Janardhanam R, et al. Subtherapeutic corticosteroids potentiate the ability of interleukin 10 to prevent chronic inflammation in rats. *Gastroenterology.* 1998;115:856-865.

70. Pretolani M, Goldman M. Il-10: a potential therapy for allergic inflammation. *Immunol Today.* 1997;18:277-280.

71. Colombel JF, Rutgeerts P, Malchow H, et al. Interleukin 10 (Tenovil) in the prevention of postoperative recurrence of Crohn's disease. *Gut.* 2001;49:42-46.

72. Regueiro M, Schraut W, Baidoo L, et al. Infliximab prevents Crohn's disease recurrence after ileal resection. *Gastroenterology.* 2009;136:441-450.

73. Endres S, von Schacky C. n-3 Polyunsaturated fatty acids and human cytokine synthesis. *Curr Opin Lipidol.* 1996;7:48-52.

74. Lorenz R, Weber PC, Szimnau P, Heldwein W, Strasser T, Loeschke K. Supplementation with n-3 fatty acids from fish oil in chronic inflammatory bowel disease—a randomized, placebo-controlled, double-blind cross-over trial. *J Intern Med.* 1989;225(suppl):225-232.

75. Lorenz-Meyer H, Bauer P, Nicolay C, et al. Omega-3 fatty acids and low carbohydrate diet for maintenance of remission in Crohn's disease. A randomized controlled multicenter trial. Study Group Members (German Crohn's Disease Study Group). *Scand J Gastroenterol.* 1996;31:778-785.

76. Belluzzi A, Brignola C, Campieri M, Pera A, Boschi S, Miglioli M. Effect of an enteric-coated fish-oil preparation on relapses in Crohn's disease. *N Engl J Med.* 1996;334:1557-1560.

77. Feagan BG, Sandborn WJ, Mittmann U, et al. Omega-3 free fatty acids for the maintenance of remission in Crohn disease: the EPIC Randomized Controlled Trials. *JAMA.* 2008;299:1690-1697.

MANAGEMENT OF STEROID-
UNRESPONSIVE CROHN'S DISEASE

Sarathchandra I. Reddy, MD, MPH and Robert Burakoff, MD, MPH, FACG, FACP

The use of steroids often represents an important inflection point in the history of a patient with Crohn's disease. Glucocortioid resistance and dependence are commonly seen in patients with CD. Dr. Munkholm and colleagues found that among patients with CD in a population-based cohort analysis, glucocorticoid resistance was seen in 20% of patients, usually within the first month of therapy. In this same study, 45% of patients either relapsed after steroids were tapered or were unable to taper off of treatment within a year.[1] Therefore, for a substantial proportion of patients with CD, additional therapies will be required to achieve clinical response and remission. In this chapter, we will examine the clinical evidence for several medical treatments that are presently available for steroid unresponsive CD and outline a general approach to the management of these patients.

In the patient with persistent symptoms suggestive of refractory Crohn's disease, additional evaluation may be necessary to exclude other conditions that may be responsible for the symptoms (Table 27-1). Before attributing symptoms to refractory CD, it is necessary to rule out infection with bacterial and parasitic pathogens. Enteric infections may contribute to flares of otherwise controlled disease or can mimic clinical inflammatory bowel disease (IBD). *Clostridium difficile* infection has also been associated with exacerbations of IBD. In 1 series of patients with IBD flares, 19% of patients had *Clostridium difficile* infection, and most improved with antibiotic therapy.[2]

In addition to bacterial and parasitic pathogens, cytomegalovirus (CMV) infection should be considered in refractory cases of IBD. CMV infection occurs more commonly in patients being treated with corticosteroids and other immunosuppressive agents but has been noted even in the absence of immunosuppressive therapy. CMV infection is estimated to occur in between 19% and 36% of steroid-resistant patients and is diagnosed by biopsy obtained at the time of colonoscopy. Recognition of CMV colitis and treatment with antiviral therapy can result in dramatic clinical improvement.[3,4]

It is also important to exclude use of other environmental factors, such as use of nonsteroidal anti-inflammatory drugs (NSAIDs), that may contribute to flares of IBD.[5] Cigarette smoking is also a significant cause of refractory Crohn's disease, and smoking cessation represents an important component of the management of patients with CD.[6]

Patients with extensive small bowel disease with areas of stricturing and prestenotic dilatation are at increased risk of bacterial overgrowth and may benefit from empiric antibiotic therapy or hydrogen breath test to formally assess for the presence of bacterial overgrowth as the cause for refractory symptoms.

Another common condition that should be considered is lactose intolerance, which can be assessed by hydrogen breath testing or clinical response to a dairy-free diet. Finally, given the high prevalence of concomitant IBS in patients with CD, it is important to differentiate symptoms of IBS from refractory CD.

Prior to labeling a patient as *steroid refractory*, it is important to obtain additional laboratory, radiologic, or endoscopic evaluation that will help to determine the degree of disease activity and exclude other etiologies for a patient's symptoms. Laboratory assessment may include the erythrocyte sedimentation rate and C-reactive protein, which are nonspecific but may provide some insight

TABLE 27-1

THERAPEUTIC OPTIONS IN THE TREATMENT
OF STERIOD-UNRESPONSIVE CROHN'S DISEASE*

THERAPY	STUDIES	DOSE	SIDE EFFECTS/CONSIDERATIONS
6-Mercaptopurine	Present et al, 1980	1 to 1.5 mg/kg	Leukopenia
Azathioprine	Korelitz et al, 1993	2 to 2.5 mg/kg	Pancreatitis
	Markowitz et al, 2000		Periodic monitoring of CBC and LFTs
			Determination of TPMT enzyme activity, 6-TG, and 6-MMP levels to optimize dosing
Infliximab	Targan et al, 1997	5 to 10 mg/kg	Infusion reactions
	Hanauer et al, 2002		Infections
			Disseminated TB
			Regular dosing and concomitant 6-MP/AZA therapy to reduce immunogenicity
Methotrexate	Feagan et al, 1995	25 mg	Hepatotoxicity
	Kozarek et al, 1989	IM/SC/week	Pneumonitis
Cyclosporine	Brynskov et al, 1989	7.6 mg/kg/day	Nephrotoxicity
			Infections
Tacrolimus	Sandborn et al, 2003	0.2 mg/kg/day	Paresthesias
			Nephrotoxicity
Mycophenolate	Neurath et al, 1999	15 to 20 mg/kg	Nausea/vomiting
			Infection
Thalidomide	Ehrenpreis et al, 1999	100 to 300 mg/kg	Sedative effects
	Vasiliauskas et al, 1999		Peripheral neuropathy
			Teratogenicity

CBC, complete blood count; LFTs, liver function tests; TPMT, thiopurine methyltransferase; 6-TG, 6-thioguanine; 6-MMP, 6-methylmercaptopurine; TB, tuberculosis; 6-MP, 6-mercaptopurine; AZA, azathioprine; IM, intramuscular; SC, subcutaneous.

into presence of inflammatory activity particularly when compared to a patient's baseline. Stool studies for infectious pathogens and *Clostridium difficile* toxin should be obtained. Small bowel radiographic assessment by follow-through study, computed tomography (CT), or magnetic resonance imaging (MRI) enterography may help assess the degree and extent of disease and presence of strictures contributing to obstructive symptoms. Endoscopic testing is often necessary, and colonoscopy and ileoscopy is often the best method to assess extent and severity of disease.

In addition, newer imaging modalities such as video capsule endoscopy may be more sensitive than other radiologic modalities in assessing disease activity in the small bowel.[7] Data from several studies have demonstrated that video capsule endoscopy may help to evaluate for the presence of small bowel CD in patients with strong clinical evidence of CD but nondiagnostic small bowel radiographs. These studies demonstrated a mean diagnostic yield of 65%, which was superior to small bowel radiographs.[7-9] Therefore, this modality may be used to assess the presence and severity of disease activity in patients with small bowel CD and to guide decisions regarding medical therapy.

IMMUNOMODULATOR THERAPY

There are a number of immunomodulatory drugs that have been studied in the treatment of CD and are so named for the diverse mechanisms in which they may regulate immune responses and hence inflammatory activity. The mainstays of immunomodulatory therapy in patients with steroid unresponsive CD are azathioprine (AZA) and 6-mercaptopurine (6-MP). Classified as thiopurines, AZA and 6-MP are metabolized to purine analogues, which results in the inhibition of ribonucleotide synthesis, nucleic acid metabolism, and cytotoxic effects on lymphoid cells, thereby resulting in immunosuppression. These agents were initially used in the treatment of childhood leukemias but were later recognized as having immunosuppressive properties.

AZA and 6-MP are widely regarded as effective in the treatment of CD. Indications for use of these agents in patients with CD include induction of remission, maintenance of remission, and treatment of fistulizing disease. A meta-analysis of 8 randomized, placebo-controlled trials including 425 patients revealed that these agents were superior to placebo in the treatment of patients with active CD; 54% of patients treated with 6-MP or AZA exhibited clinical improvement or achieved remission in comparison to 33% of patients treated with placebo.[10,11]

6-MP and AZA are commonly prescribed for patients who are steroid-dependent. Several controlled and uncontrolled trials have shown that immunomodulator therapies permit withdrawal of steroid therapy and increase the likelihood of attaining remission.[12-15] A randomized, placebo-controlled trial showed that 75% of patients receiving 6-MP were able to achieve reduction in their steroid dose in comparison to 36% of patients receiving placebo.[15] In this study, dose reduction was defined as successful withdrawal of steroids or reduction in the dose to less than 10 mg/day with control of symptoms. Korelitz et al reported the results of 20 years of clinical experience in 148 patients with steroid-unresponsive Crohn's disease and found that steroids were eliminated in 66% of the patients.[16] Thus, these agents offer a strategy for withdrawing steroids in patients with steroid-dependent CD.

Several controlled trials have demonstrated that AZA is effective in the maintenance of remission in patients with CD. A meta-analysis of 5 placebo-controlled studies including 319 patients found that 67% of patients receiving AZA maintained remission in comparison to 53% of patients receiving placebo.[10,14] In a prospective placebo-controlled study involving pediatric patients with newly diagnosed Crohn's disease, use of 6-MP was linked to a significantly reduced need for prednisone and improved maintenance of remission over 18 months.[17] Though only this 1 trial to date has specifically evaluated 6-MP for maintenance of remission in CD, its similar pharmacologic properties support its use interchangeably with AZA for the maintenance of remission in CD.

The typical dose range for 6-MP is 1.0 to 1.5 mg/kg and for AZA is 2.0 to 2.5 mg/kg. The 6-MP dose can be increased gradually while monitoring the white blood cell (WBC) count. A typical starting dose of 50 mg can be increased gradually every few weeks until the goal dose is achieved. Alternatively, it is also possible to start at the target dose immediately when using 6-MP. The metabolism of 6-MP is mediated primarily by the enzyme thiopurine methyltransferase (TPMT) resulting in several metabolites, such as 6-methylmercaptopurine (6-MMP), 6 thioguanine (6-TG), and 6 methyl thioinosine 5'-monophosphate. Variations in the activity of TPMT enzyme activity can alter the relative proportion of resulting metabolites. Approximately 1 in 300 patients are deficient in TPMT and are therefore at an increased risk for developing leukopenia with thiopurine treatment.[18] Assessment of TPMT enzyme activity can help determine a patient's risk of developing leukopenia and permits more rapid increases in dose to attain the goal dose.

Whether or not leukopenia is required for induction of response remains controversial. The measurement of 6-TG permits some optimization of 6-MP dosing. Though a wide range of 6-TG levels are correlated with clinical response, a study of 131 patients with IBD on long-term AZA therapy found that patients who remained in clinical remission had a mean 6-TG level of 236 in comparison to a mean 6-TG level of 175 in the group of patients who developed active disease.[19] Thus, it has been said by some investigators that monitoring of the 6-TG level in patients without adequate clinical response, in spite of weight-based dosing, permits optimization of 6-MP and AZA dosing.[18]

Though generally well-tolerated, possible side effects include bone marrow suppression, allergic reactions, hepatotoxicity, and pancreatitis. Fatigue, nausea, and loss of appetite are also common side effects. More serious side effects such as pancreatitis occur in 3% to 7% of patients. Pancreatitis is an idiosyncratic reaction and often occurs during the first month of therapy. In the event that a patient develops pancreatitis, medication should be discontinued immediately; furthermore, any attempt to rechallenge with this medication is likely to result in recurrent pancreatitis. Elevated liver enzymes may occur in up to 9% of patients and is associated with high levels of 6-MMP. More serious hepatitis is rare, occurring in 1% of patients. Bone marrow suppression manifested by significant leukopenia (WBC < 3000) occurred in 3.8% of patients in a 27-year retrospective study assessing more than 700 patients treated with AZA.[20] The latter 2 side effects are usually dose related and respond to dose reduction. Assessment of 6-TG and 6-MMP can provide additional confirmation that an adjustment in dose may be required. Therefore, close monitoring of CBC and liver function tests is required upon introduction of therapy or changes in medication dosing.

METHOTREXATE

Another agent with proven efficacy in Crohn's disease is methotrexate, an agent that has been used for many years to treat conditions such as rheumatoid arthritis and psoriasis. Methotrexate inhibits the enzyme dihydrofolate reductase and thereby impairs DNA synthesis. Though the anti-inflammatory effects of methotrexate are not well understood, they are believed to involve suppression of cytokine synthesis (IL-1, IL-2, IL-6, and IL-8), apoptosis of cytotoxic T cells, and reduction in neutrophil activity. Methotrexate can be administered orally, intramuscularly, or subcutaneously, but dosing is most reliable when the agent is administered parenterally. Unlike 6-MP and AZA, the therapeutic effects of methotrexate are seen more quickly, and therefore methotrexate may be a useful alternative to these immunomodulators if more rapid therapeutic effects are required.

Two studies have demonstrated the efficacy of methotrexate in patients with moderate or severe steroid-unresponsive Crohn's disease. A double-blind, placebo-controlled trial including 141 patients showed that methotrexate administered by intramuscular injection at a dose of 25 mg/week for 16 weeks led to a greater rate of withdrawal from prednisone compared to patients who were treated with placebo. After 16 weeks, 39% of patients who had received methotrexate were in remission compared with 19% of the placebo group.[21,22] A follow-up study by the same group demonstrated that patients who had achieved remission on methotrexate were more likely to maintain remission if treated with methotrexate 15 mg intramuscular (IM) weekly compared to placebo. In this study, after 40 weeks of follow-up, 65% of the patients in the methotrexate-treated group were in remission versus 39% of patients in the group treated with placebo.[23]

Potential toxicities of methotrexate include stomatitis, nausea, diarrhea, and hair loss. More serious side effects include leukopenia and hepatic fibrosis, which necessitate periodic monitoring of CBC and liver-associated chemistries. It should be noted, however, that serum transaminase elevation does not often correlate with hepatic fibrosis. Though liver biopsy has been recommended in patients undergoing treatment with methotrexate for psoriasis, the role of liver biopsy in patients with IBD remains unclear. Though liver function tests should be monitored while on therapy, the role of liver biopsy in assessing hepatotoxicity or fibrosis has not been clearly established. Other factors that can increase the risk of fibrosis include obesity and alcohol use. Although rare, hypersensitivity pneumonitis can be a serious complication. Methotrexate should not be used in women of child-bearing age due to its known teratogenicity.

CYCLOSPORINE

Cyclosporine has been studied in refractory Crohn's disease. The mechanism of the drug involves inhibition of T cell-mediated response through inhibition of IL-2 production by helper T cells and blocking additional cytokines such as IL-3, IL-4, and tumor necrosis factor alpha (TNFα) in the inflammatory pathway. In comparison to other modulators such as 6-MP, AZA, and methotrexate, cyclosporine achieves its therapeutic effects more rapidly. There have been 3 large controlled trials of low-dose oral cyclosporine (4.8 mg to 5.0 mg/kg/day) in the treatment of CD. These studies did not show any difference in treatment response or remission rates.[24-26] Numerous uncontrolled studies and 1 controlled trial have shown the efficacy of higher doses of cyclosporine in induction and maintenance of remission. Brynskov et al[27] studied 71 patients with active Crohn's disease randomized to either oral cyclosporine 7.6 mg/kg/day or to placebo and followed for a 3-month period. The study found that 59% of patients in the treatment group went into remission compared with 32% in the placebo group. It should be pointed out that corticosteroid use was not restricted by the study, and patients receiving concomitant corticosteroids appeared to have a greater response compared with patients receiving cyclosporine alone.[27] Uncontrolled trials suggest that oral cyclosporine may have good short-term response rates but relatively poor long-term remission rates. In their analysis of numerous uncontrolled trials involving 227 patients, Loftus et al found that the overall mean response rate in these studies was 64%. Furthermore, the effect of cyclosporine is usually rapid and occurred within 3 weeks; in contrast to a favorable short-term response, analysis of these studies indicated a long-term response rate of only 29%.[28] In many studies, immunomodulator therapy was not used consistently, and additional studies are needed to assess whether using cyclosporine as a bridge to other immunomodulators as maintenance therapy results in better long-term response rates.

Use of cyclosporine as either long- or short-term therapy is associated with a wide range of side effects and toxicities. Sandborn[29] assessed adverse effects of high-dose cyclosporine in the treatment of 343 IBD patients in 27 trials. Common side effects observed included paresthesias, hypertrichosis, hypertension, tremor, nausea and vomiting, seizures, nephrotoxicity, and hepatotoxicity. Many of these adverse effects were dose related and reversed with reduction in the cyclosporine dose. Seizures occur in 1% of patients, and the risk of seizures increases if the serum cholesterol is less than 120 mg/dL. Perhaps the most serious concern regarding cyclosporine therapy is the risk of nephrotoxicity. This has been observed in patients with various autoimmune diseases treated with long-term cyclosporine, particularly at doses greater than 8 mg/kg/day. Up to a 20% reduction in glomerular filtration rates (GFR) can occur without significant change in serum creatinine, and histologic evidence of nephrotoxicity may be seen in 21% of patients.[28,29] Furthermore, the risk of serious opportunistic infections is higher in patients treated with cyclosporine. This risk is higher in patients on concomitant therapy with corticosteroids and other immunomodulators. Therefore, trimethoprim/sulfamethoxazole prophylaxis should be prescribed during cyclosporine therapy.

TACROLIMUS

Tacrolimus is a macrolide antibiotic that is similar to cyclosporine in terms of immunomodulatory effects. In the only randomized controlled trial utilizing this agent, Sandborn et al[30] studied 48 patients with CD and draining fistula who were randomized to oral tacrolimus at a dose of 0.2 mg/kg/day or placebo for 10 weeks. In this study, the primary endpoints were fistula improvement as well as fistula closure. Fistula improvement was higher in patients treated with tacrolimus compared to placebo, whereas there was no difference in fistula remission.[30] Additionally, 5 uncontrolled studies have demonstrated the beneficial effects of tacrolimus with response rates in the range of 75% to 85% among patients with Crohn's disease.[28] The primary adverse effects of tacrolimus include nephrotoxicity, which occurred in 38% of patients in Sandborn's study. Based on the limited data available, tacrolimus should be considered a treatment option in patients with fistulizing Crohn's disease who have not responded to or not tolerated other therapies including antibiotics, 6-MP, AZA, and infliximab. Additional studies and controlled trials are necessary to fully evaluate the role of tacrolimus in patients with nonfistulizing CD.

MYCOPHENOLATE MOFETIL

Mycophenolate mofetil is the prodrug form of mycophenolic acid, which is an inhibitor of inosine monophosphate dehydrogenase, which is involved in purine synthesis.

Two randomized trials and several smaller uncontrolled studies with mycophenolate mofetil have shown that this drug may have a role in the treatment of patients with inflammatory bowel disease. Neurath et al[31] reported their experience treating 70 patients with Crohn's disease randomized to either mycophenolate or azathioprine in combination with tapering doses of prednisone. The study found that patients with severe disease treated with mycophenolate had a more pronounced decline in disease activity as assessed by the Crohn's Disease Activity Index (CDAI) in comparison to patients in the AZA group. These differences were not observed in patients with moderate CD as there was no difference in decline in disease activity observed between the 2 groups.[31] Additionally, several uncontrolled trials involving 56 patients with Crohn's disease have demonstrated an overall response rate of 52% among patients with Crohn's disease.[28]

Adverse effects with mycophenolate mofetil are common and occurred in 20% of patients who have received this agent for treatment of IBD. In these studies, 95 patients discontinued therapy due to side effects. Observed adverse effects include nausea and vomiting, rash, medication-related diarrhea, bone marrow suppression, and various infections.[28]

Though mycophenolate may have a role in patients intolerant to or refractory to other immunomodulator therapy, additional studies are required to determine the optimal dosing and to better assess the efficacy and safety of this agent.

INFLIXIMAB

Infliximab is the first in the category of biologic therapies approved for the treatment of luminal and fistulizing CD. Infliximab is a chimeric monoclonal antibody to TNFα, which plays a role in various inflammatory pathways involved in IBD. These effects include decrease in IL-2 expression, interferon gamma, and other cytokines.[32]

Infliximab is indicated in patients with moderate to severe Crohn's disease who fail to respond to conventional therapy with steroids and immunosuppressive agents. Infliximab is also indicated for treatment of fistulizing disease. The efficacy of infliximab in treating patients with both fistulizing and luminal disease has been demonstrated in several randomized, placebo-controlled trials. The agent has displayed impressive results with regard to endoscopic and mucosal healing in patients with CD.[33] A study of 108 patients with CD who were refractory to other treatments demonstrated that a single infusion of infliximab resulted in significant clinical response at 4 weeks compared to placebo. Among patients treated with a dose of 5 mg/kg, the clinical response rate at 4 weeks was 81% in the treatment group, compared with 17% in the placebo group.[34] Infliximab also yielded impressive results in patients with fistulizing disease. Present et al studied the efficacy of infliximab in patients with abdominal and perianal fistulas and found that 68% of patients receiving a dose of 5 mg/kg had a clinical response defined as 50% reduction in number of draining fistulas compared with 26% in the placebo group.[35] These clinical trials revealed that infliximab can yield significant benefits in patients with refractory luminal disease and those with concomitant fistulizing disease.

Clinical trials have also established that infliximab may also be utilized as maintenance therapy in patients with either fistulizing or luminal disease.[36,37] The ACCENT I study (A Crohn's disease Clinical trial Evaluating infliximab in a New long-term Treatment regimen) evaluated 573 patients with CD who received infliximab infusions at doses of either 5 mg/kg or 10 mg/kg every 8 weeks compared with a single infusion.[37] Patients receiving maintenance therapy with infliximab were more likely to display a clinical response in comparison to patients who received a single infusion followed by placebo infusions (28% and 38% versus 14%). Patients receiving scheduled therapy had fewer Crohn's disease-related hospitalizations and surgeries. Furthermore, maintenance therapy with infliximab demonstrated a more potent steroid-sparing effect, as 28% of patients in the 5 mg/kg group and 32% of patients in the 10 mg/kg group were successfully tapered off of steroids in comparison to 9% of patients in the single infusion group.[37]

A strategy employing regular infusions of infliximab is preferable to a strategy of on-demand or episodic usage. Rutgeerts et al analyzed patients treated in the ACCENT I study and found that those who had been randomized to receive regular infusions had a lower incidence of antibodies to infliximab, higher rates of mucosal healing, and fewer Crohn's disease-related hospitalizations and surgeries. These findings were most pronounced in those patients receiving regular infusions of 10 mg/kg every 8 weeks as maintenance therapy.[38]

Based on the data from these clinical trials, infliximab can be administered at a dose of 5 mg/kg for the induction of remission with 3 doses administered at 0, 2, and 6 weeks.[34,35] In patients requiring maintenance therapy, 5 mg/kg may be administered every 8 weeks, and, if clinical response becomes attenuated over time, the dose may be increased to 10 mg/kg every 8 weeks.

Long-term and episodic use of infliximab is associated with the development of antibodies to infliximab (HACA, ATI), which are associated with increased risk of infusion reactions and decreased treatment response. ATI may develop in up to 13% of patients with CD. The development of ATI may result in delayed hypersensitivity reactions characterized by polyarthralgias, urticaria, rash, and facial edema occurring between 3 and 12 days following infliximab infusion.[39]

Studies demonstrate that patients receiving episodic infusions are more likely to develop antibodies to infliximab compared to patients receiving infusions every 8 weeks. Concomitant immunomodulator therapy may also decrease the risk of developing antibodies to infliximab. Patients treated with induction regimens consisting of 3 doses administered at 0, 2, and 6 weeks may be less likely to develop antibodies to infliximab and experience infusion reactions. It is hypothesized that a 3-dose induction regimen results in some form of immunologic tolerance to infliximab.[40]

Common side effects of infliximab include fever, fatigue, and headache. However, more serious side effects including invasive opportunistic infections and fungal infections have been described. In a study assessing experience with infliximab among 500 patients, serious adverse events attributable to infliximab were observed in 6% of patients. Acute infusion reactions occurred in 3.8% of patients, and serum sickness reactions occurred in 2.8%. Serious infec-

tions were reported in 20 patients including fatal sepsis, pneumonia, viral infections, abdominal abscess, and histoplasmosis.[41]

Disseminated tuberculosis (TB) is another serious complication of infliximab therapy, and there are 117 reported cases of disseminated TB. Thus, it is advised that prior to infliximab therapy, all patients should be evaluated by protein purified derivative (PPD) and chest x-ray.[42]

A newer biologic agent, adalimumab, is a humanized antibody to TNFα that may offer therapeutic benefits of infliximab while reducing the risk of infusion reactions. Youdim et al assessed the use of adalimumab in 7 patients who were steroid dependent and had serious reactions to infliximab preventing further use of the drug. The study demonstrated that 6 out of 7 patients tolerated infliximab without reaction, and there was significant clinical improvement in these patients as assessed by reduction in Harvey-Bradshaw Index.[43]

Adalimumab is now Food and Drug Administration (FDA) approved for inducing and maintaining clinical remission in adult patients with moderate to severe CD who have had an inadequate response to conventional therapy and for inducing remission in these patients if they have also lost response to or are intolerant to infliximab. Adalimumab, a fully humanized anti-TNFα antibody, was demonstrated to be superior to placebo for the induction of remission in patients with moderate to severe CD and naïve to anti-TNFα therapy[44] and to maintain clinical remission for up to 56 weeks in these patients.[45] Among patients who were intolerant or did not respond to infliximab therapy, adalimumab was shown to induce remission more frequently than placebo.[46] Among patients who initially responded to adalimumab, Colombel et al reported significantly higher rates of remission with adalimumab versus placebo at 1 year.[47] In patients with CD for less than 2 years, approximately 50% remained in remission more than 1 year after receiving 40 mg of adalimumab subcutaneously every other week or weekly, again arguing for earlier aggressive treatment.[48]

Certolizumab pegol is a pegylated Fab' fragment of a humanized monoclonal antibody that neutralizes TNFα. A phase III, randomized, double-blind, multicenter study that assessed the efficacy and tolerability of certolizumab in patients with moderate to severe CD showed a modest improvement in response rates as compared with placebo but no significant improvement in remission rates.[49] In addition, patients who had a response to induction therapy with certolizumab were more likely to have maintained response and remission at 26 weeks with continued monthly subcutaneous injection compared to those who switched to placebo.[50]

The results from the induction phase of the PRECiSE 2 trial compared favorably to other monoclonal anti-TNFα induction studies. The 6-week response rates of approximately two thirds of patients in the study and remission rates of 40% were unaffected by concomitant immunosuppressants or corticosteroids.[51] Long-term data of certolizumab (at 52 and 54 weeks) suggest that 400-mg subcutaneous injections given monthly are well tolerated with low anti-doublestranded DNA—3.2% in PRECiSE 3 and 2.7% in PRECiSE 4—possibly because of the low apoptosis rates associated with certolizumab. In more than 900 patients treated with certolizumab for 1 year, the incidence of infections and malignancy is similar to other anti-TNFα agents.[52] In the WELCOME study, nearly two thirds of patients who had lost response or were intolerant to infliximab responded to induction with certolizumab at 0, 2, and 4 weeks, with maintenance every 2 or 4 weeks. In addition, almost 40% of those patients achieved remission on certolizumab.[53]

In the SONIC trial—a randomized, double-blind controlled trial comparing infliximab and infliximab plus AZA to AZA alone in CD patients of short duration who were naïve to biologics and immunomodulators—patients with elevated C-reactive protein (CRP) and ulcerations at baseline colonoscopy had a particularly strong benefit from early infliximab, with similar safety outcomes in all 3 arms.[54] In these patients, corticosteroid remission-free survival rates at 26 weeks were 28% with AZA monotherapy, 56.9% with infliximab monotherapy, and 68.8% with combination therapy.

Natalizumab, a humanized immunoglobulin (Ig)-G4 monoclonal antibody against #4-integrin also used to treat multiple sclerosis (MS), has demonstrated some improvement in response and remission rates in patients with CD[55]; however, the drug has been associated with 3 cases of progressive multifocal leukoencephalopathy (PML) in clinical trials.[56-58] The cases occurred in 2 patients with MS who were receiving combination therapy with natalizumab and interferon beta-1a, and 1 natalizumab-treated patient with CD with prior exposure to AZA and steroids, and an underlying lymphopenia. Subsequently, no new cases of PML were identified in patients treated with natalizumab in clinical trials, and a recent report suggested a risk for PML of roughly 1 in 1000 patients treated with natalizumab for a mean of 17.9 months.[59] Currently, more than 25,000 patients (mostly with MS) have been treated, with no new cases of PML reported. However, there have been some reports of liver abnormalities.

A recent randomized, placebo-controlled trial of natalizumab induction therapy in patients with CD reported response and remission at week 8 that persisted through week 12; both response and remission rates were superior to those in patients taking placebo at weeks 4, 8, and 12 of the study, demonstrating an early and sustained efficacy of natalizumab as induction therapy.[60] Natalizumab was well tolerated in this study.

THALIDOMIDE

Another anti-TNFα agent that has shown promising results in CD is thalidomide. The reputation of thalidomide was linked to birth defects in the 1950s where it was prescribed as a sedative and antiemetic. Its resurrection for use in therapy for CD results from its activity in reducing TNFα levels. In addition to its activity against TNFα, thalidomide is believed to have other effects, including altering expression of nuclear factor (NF)κB, which regulates expression of a number of cytokines.

Though there have been no randomized, controlled trials utilizing thalidomide, several case reports and open-labeled trials have demonstrated clinical benefit of thalidomide in CD. Ehrenpreis et al studied thalidomide at doses of 200 and 300 mg in 22 patients for 14 weeks. In this study, 9 out of 22 patients achieved complete remission, and clinical improvement was observed in 64% of patients.[61] Vasiliauskas et al studied thalidomide at lower doses of 50 to 100 mg in 12 patients with steroid-unresponsive Crohn's disease. Twenty percent of patients in the trial achieved remission, and 44% were able to taper off of steroids.[62]

Side effects observed with thalidomide therapy include excessive sedation, peripheral neuropathy, rash, and hypertension. With higher doses of thalidomide, sedation is commonly observed. Though the sedative effects are reduced with lower doses, even in the lower dose study, excessive sedation was observed in 7 out of 12 patients.[62] Though concern over pregnancy remains the preeminent issue with thalidomide, these other side effects are likely to be significant and will inhibit the use of thalidomide in the treatment of steroid-refractory CD.

Other agents with anti-TNFα activity that have been studied in CD but have not shown significant clinical response include pentoxifylline, etanercept, and CDP-571 (a humanized anti-TNFα monoclonal antibody). Although touted as an alternative to infliximab with reduced side effects due to a reduced number of murine peptide sequences (5% versus 25%), CDP-571 has yielded results far less impressive than infliximab in clinical trials. In a large trial of 193 patients, CDP 571 was not shown to be effective in induction or maintenance of remission.[63] As a result of these disappointing results, its development was terminated.

Another anti-TNFα agent that may hold greater promise is CDP-870, which is a pegylated humanized anti-TNFα antibody. The pegylation increases the plasma half-life of the drug. There have been 2 controlled trials of this agent in the treatment of CD. Neither trial has yet been published, but initial results are promising for the use of this agent in the treatment of CD. A placebo-controlled trial including 292 adults with active CD studied several doses of the drug or placebo given subcutaneously at weeks 0, 4, and 8. The primary endpoint was the proportion of patients achieving

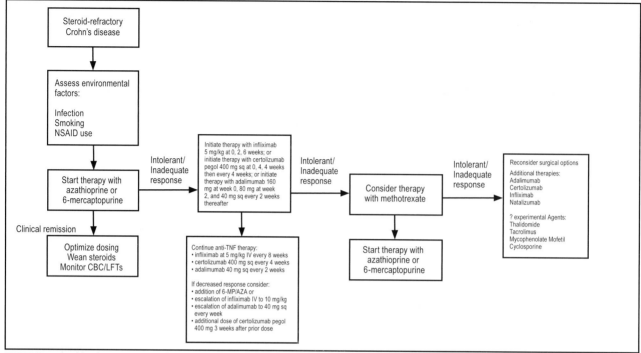

FIGURE 27-1. Algorithm for management of steroid-refractory Crohn's disease.

a clinical response or remission at week 12. Though the primary endpoint of benefit at week 12 was not achieved, the highest clinical response was observed in the 400-mg group and 53% of patients treated with this dose had a clinical response at week 10 versus 30% in the placebo group. Patients with CRP levels greater than 10 mg/dL had better response rates.[64] Additional studies will be required to determine the efficacy and safety of this agent in the treatment of CD.

Anti-IL-12/IL-23 is another mechanism that is currently under investigation for the treatment of steroid-refractory CD. This agent, known as ABT-874, mediates anti-inflammatory effects through regulation of the Th1 pathway. A double-blind, placebo-controlled trial involving 79 patients with active CD found that when administered subcutaneously at a dose of 3 mg/kg/week for 7 weeks, anti-IL-12/IL-23 resulted in clinical improvement in 75% of the treatment cohort compared with 25% in the placebo group and resulted in clinical remission in 38% of the treatment cohort compared with 0% in the placebo group. Furthermore, the beneficial effects of treatment were durable, lasting through the 18 weeks of follow-up. This promising study suggests that anti-IL-12 therapy may offer a novel approach to treating CD.[65] There are now phase 3 studies ongoing.

Another agent that works by inhibition of the IL-12/23 pathway, ustekinumab (previously known as CNTO 1275), is effective in primary anti-TNFα nonresponders. In a randomized, double-blind crossover trial involving 104

patients with moderate to severe CD, clinical response rates were significantly higher with ustekinumab at weeks 4 and 6 (53% versus 30% with placebo) but were not significantly different at week 8 (49% and 40%, respectively).[66] However, among primary anti-TNFα nonresponders (ie, patients who did not respond to an induction dose of infliximab, adalimumab, or certolizumab) clinical response to ustekinumab was significantly greater than response to placebo ($p < 0.05$) through week 8.

Natalizumab, a humanized IgG4 monoclonal antibody directed against α-4 integrin, is also effective for anti-TNFα nonresponders. This agent is FDA approved for the induction and maintenance of clinical response and remission in adult patients with moderate to severe CD in patients with evidence of inflammation who have had an inadequate response to, or are unable to tolerate, conventional CD therapies and anti-TNFα inhibitors.

GENERAL APPROACH TO THE MANAGEMENT OF PATIENTS WITH STEROID-REFRACTORY CROHN'S DISEASE

Once a patient has demonstrated dependence on corticosteroids or refractory symptoms in spite of prednisone use without attaining remission, it is reasonable to utilize various therapies in step-wise fashion. An algorithm for

TESTS IN THE EVALUATION OF STEROID-UNRESPONSIVE CROHN'S DISEASE

- Stool studies for infectious pathogens
- Histology for cytomegalovirus infection
- C-reactive protein/erythrocyte sedimentation rate
- Small bowel radiography
- Colonoscopy
- Capsule endoscopy

management of steroid-refractory CD is provided in Figure 27-1. Agents that have been evaluated for treatment of steroid-refractory CD in controlled trials, recommended dose ranges, and major side effects are listed in Table 27-2.

As they have been extensively studied, 6-MP or AZA should first be utilized in patients with moderate refractory disease activity. As these agents may require 8 to 12 weeks to attain clinical effectiveness, during that period, steroids should be continued. Assessment of TPMT activity can help guide how rapidly the dose of medications are increased. Most patients will attain therapeutic levels when dosed between 1 and 1.5 mg/kg for 6-MP and 2 and 2.5 mg/kg for AZA. In patients who continue with symptoms in spite of these doses, it is reasonable to check 6-MP metabolites to further guide dose increases.

In patients with more severe disease, concomitant use of infliximab can be utilized for more rapid induction. Patients should be dosed with infusions at 0, 2, and 6 weeks and then every 8 weeks. After 3 to 4 months, consideration can be given to discontinuing infliximab and maintaining the patient on immunomodulator therapy alone.

In patients who are either refractory or intolerant to 6-MP and AZA, maintenance therapy with infliximab infusions every 8 weeks is a reasonable approach. Adalimumab and certolizumab are effective treatments for patients who are intolerant to or who have lost response to infliximab and have also been shown to be effective in infliximab-naïve patients. However, for primary anti-TNFα nonresponders, the class of anti-TNFs needs to be changed to anti-Il 12/23 (ABT-874 or ustekinumab) or natalizumab. Natalizumab is an effective agent for both inducing and maintaining steroid-free remission in patients who are primary anti-TNFα nonresponders or have lost response to or are intolerant of anti-TNFα agents.

If patients become refractory or intolerant to infliximab, other therapeutic modalities such as methotrexate should be utilized given the more extensive experience with that agent as well as extensive clinical experience in treating other conditions with this agent. Methotrexate can be dosed at 25 mg IM and continued every other week.

Although additional data are required for use of other agents, in the patient with diffuse small bowel disease or who is not a candidate for surgery, other modalities that can be considered for treatment of Crohn's disease include cyclosporine, tacrolimus, mycophenolate mofetil, and thalidomide. However, the side effect profiles of these agents and lack of large placebo-controlled trials should render them as therapeutic choices only when all other modalities have failed and surgery is not an option for the patient.

REFERENCES

1. Munkholm P, Langhola E, Davidsen M, et al. Frequency of glucocorticoid resistance and dependency in Crohn's disease. *Gut.* 1994;35:360-362.

2. Meyer AM, Ramzan NN, Loftus EV, et al. The diagnostic yield of stool studies during relapses of inflammatory bowel disease [abstract]. *Gastroenterology.* 2002;122(4 suppl 1):A-219.

3. Papadakis KA, Tung JK, Binder SW, et al. Outcome of CMV infections in patients with inflammatory bowel disease. *Am J Gastroenterol.* 2001;96:2137-2142.

4. Vega R, Bertran X, Menacho M, et al. Cytomegalovirus in patients with inflammatory bowel disease. *Am J Gastroenterol.* 1999;94:1053-1056.

5. Felder JB, Korelitz BI, Rajapakse R, et al. Effects of nonsteroidal anti-inflammatory drugs on inflammatory bowel disease: a case control study. *Am J Gastroenterol.* 2000;95:1949-1954.

6. Cosnes J, Carbonnel F, Beaugerie L, et al. Effects of cigarette smoking on the long-term course of Crohn's disease. *Gastroenterology.* 1996;110:424-431.

7. Eliakim R, Fischer D, Suissa A, et al. Wireless capsule video endoscopy is a superior diagnostic tool in comparison to barium follow-through and computerized tomography in patients with suspected Crohn's disease. *European J Gastroenterol Hepatol.* 2003;15:363-367.

8. Mascarenhas-Saraiva M, Lopes L, Mascarenhas-Saraiva A. Wireless capsule endoscopy is applicable in diagnosis and monitoring of small bowel Crohn's disease. *Gut.* 2002;51S:A69.

9. Fireman Z, Mahajna E, Broide E, et al. Diagnosing small bowel Crohn's disease with wireless capsule endoscopy. *Gut.* 2003;52(3):390-392.

10. Su C, Lichtenstein GR. Treatment of inflammatory bowel disease with azathioprine and 6-mercaptopurine. *Gastroenterol Clin N Am.* 2004;33:209-234.

11. Sandborn W, Sutherland L, Pearson D, et al. Azathioprine or 6-mercaptopurine for inducing remission of Crohn's disease. *Cochrane Database Syst Rev.* 2000;2:CD000545.

12. Candy S, Wright J, Gerber M, et al. A controlled double blind study of azathioprine in the management of Crohn's disease. *Gut.* 1995;37:674-678.

13. Markowitz J, Grancher K, Kohn N, et al. A multicenter trial of 6-mercaptopurine and prednisone in children with newly diagnosed Crohn's disease. *Gastroenterology.* 2000;119:895-902.

14. Pearson DC, May GR, Fick GH, et al. Azathioprine and 6-mercaptopurine in Crohn's disease: a meta-analysis. *Ann Intern Med.* 1995;123(2):132-142.

15. Present DH, Korelitz BI, Wisch N, et al. Treatment of Crohn's disease with 6-mercaptopurine. A long term, randomized, double blind study. *N Engl J Med.* 1980;302:981-987.

16. Korelitz BI, Adler DJ, Mendelsohn RA, et al. Long term experience with 6-mercaptopurine in the treatment of Crohn's disease. *Am J Gastroenterol.* 1993;88(8):1198-1205.

17. Markowitz J, Grancher K, Kohn N, Lesser M, Daum F. A multicenter trial of 6-mercaptopurine and prednisone in children with newly diagnosed Crohn's disease. *Gastroenterology.* 2000;119:895-902.

18. Dubinsky MC, Lamothe S, Yang HY, et al. Pharmacogenomics and metabolite measurement for 6-mercaptopurine therapy in inflammatory bowel disease. *Gastroenterology.* 2000;118:705.

19. Wright S, Sanders DS, Lobo AJ, Lennard L. Clinical significance of azathioprine metabolite concentrations in inflammatory bowel disease. *Gut.* 2004;53(8):1123-1128.

20. Connell WR, Kamm MA, Ritchie JK, et al. Bone marrow toxicity caused by azathioprine in inflammatory bowel disease: 27 years of experience. *Gut.* 1993;34:1081-1085.

21. Feagan BG, Rochon J, Fedorak RN. Methotrexate for the treatment of Crohn's disease. The North American Crohn's Study Group Investigators. *N Engl J Med.* 1995;332:292-297.

22. Kozarek RA, Patterson DJ, Gelfand MD, et al. Methotrexate induces clinical and histologic remission in patients with refractory inflammatory bowel disease. *Ann Intern Med.* 1989;110:353-356.

23. Feagan BG, Fedorak RN, Irvine EJ, et al. A comparison of methotrexate with placebo for the maintenance of remission in Crohn's disease. North American Crohn's Study Group Investigators. *N Engl J Med.* 2000;342:1627-1632.

24. Jewell DP, Lennard-Jones JE. Oral cyclosporine for chronic active Crohn's disease: a multicentre controlled trial. *European Journal Gastroenterol Hepatol.* 1994;6:499-505.

25. Feagan BG, McDonald JW, Rochon J, et al. Low dose cyclosporine for the treatment of Crohn's disease. The Canadian Crohn's Relapse Prevention Trial Investigators. *N Engl J Med.* 1994;330:1846-1851.

26. Stange EF, Modigliani R, Pena AS, et al. European trial of cyclosporine in chronic active Crohn's disease: a 12 month study. *Gastroenterology.* 1995;109:774-782.

27. Brynskov J, Freund L, Rasmussen SN, et al. A placebo controlled double-blind randomized trial of cyclosporine therapy in active Crohn's disease. *N Engl J Med.* 1989;321:845-850.

28. Loftus CG, Egan LJ, Sandborn WJ. Cyclosporine, tacrolimus, and mycophenolate mofetil in the treatment of inflammatory bowel disease. *Gastroenterol Clin N Am.* 2004;33:141-169.

29. Sandborn WJ. A critical review of cyclosporine therapy in inflammatory bowel disease. *Inflamm Bowel Dis.* 1995;1:48-63.

30. Sandborn WJ, Present DH, Isaccs KL, et al. Tacrolimus for the treatment of fistulas in patients with Crohn's disease: a randomized placebo controlled trial. *Gastroenterology.* 2003;125:380-388.

31. Neurath MF, Wanitschke R, Peters M, et al. Mycophenolate mofetil versus azathioprine for treatment of chronic active Crohn's disease. *Gut.* 1999;44:625-628.

32. Plevy SE, Landers CS, Prehn J, et al. A role for TNF alpha and mucosal T helper-1 cytokines in the pathogenesis of Crohn's disease. *J Immunol.* 1997;159:6276-6282.

33. D'Haens G, Deventer SV, Hogezand RV, et al. Endoscopic and histological healing with infliximab anti-tumor necrosis factor antibodies in Crohn's disease: a European Multicenter Trial. *Gastroenterology.* 1999;116:1029.

34. Targan SR, Hanauer SB, van Deventer SJ, et al. A short term study of chimeric monoclonal antibody cA2 to tumor necrosis factor alpha for Crohn's disease. Crohn's Disease cA2 Study Group. *N Engl J Med.* 1997;337:1029-1035.

35. Present DH, Rutgeerts P, Targan S, et al. Infliximab for the treatment of fistulas in patients with Crohn's disease. *N Engl J Med.* 1999;340:1398-1405.

36. Hyams J, Crandall W, Kugathasan S, et al. Induction and maintenance infliximab therapy for the treatment of moderate-to-severe Crohn's disease in children. *Gastroenterology.* 2007;132(3):863-873.

37. Hanauer SB, Feagan BG, Lichtenstein GR, et al. Maintenance infliximab for Crohn's disease: the ACCENT I randomized trial. *Lancet.* 2002;359:1541-1549.

38. Rutgeerts P, Feagan BG, Lichtenstein GR, et al. Comparison of scheduled and episodic treatment strategies of infliximab in Crohn's disease. *Gastroenterology.* 2004;126:402-413.

39. Hanauer SB, Rutgeerts PJ, D'Haens G, et al. Delayed hypersensitivity to infliximab reinfusion after 2-4 year interval without treatment. *Gastroenterology.* 1999;116:A731.

40. Sandborn WJ, Hanauser SB. Infliximab in the treatment of Crohn's disease: a user's guide for clinicians. *Am J Gastroenterol.* 2002;97(2):2962-2972.

41. Colombel JF, Loftus EV Jr, Tremaine WJ, et al. The safety profile of infliximab in patients with Crohn's disease: the Mayo Clinic experience in 500 patients. *Gastroenterology.* 2004;126(1):19-31.

42. Mow WS, Abreu-Martin MT, Papadakis KA, et al. High incidence of anergy in inflammatory bowel disease patients limits the usefulness of PPD screening before infliximab therapy. *Clin Gastroenterol Hepatol.* 2004;2(4):309-313.

43. Youdim A, Vasiliauskas EA, Targan SR, et al. A pilot study of adalimumab in infliximab-allergic patients. *Inflamm Bowel Dis.* 2004;10(4):333-338.

44. Hanauer SB, Sandborn WJ, Rutgeerts P, et al. Human anti-tumor necrosis factor monoclonal antibody (adalimumab) in Crohn's disease: the CLASSIC-I trial. *Gastroenterology.* 2006;130(2):323-333.

45. Sandborn WJ, Hanauer SB, Rutgeerts P, et al. Adalimumab for maintenance treatment of Crohn's disease: results of the CLASSIC II trial. *Gut.* 2007;56(9):1232-1239.

46. Sandborn WJ, Rutgeerts P, Enns R, et al. Adalimumab induction therapy for Crohn disease previously treated with infliximab: a randomized trial. *Ann Intern Med.* 2007;146(12):829-838.

47. Colombel JF, Sandborn WJ, Rutgeerts P, et al. Adalimumab for maintenance of clinical response and remission in patients with Crohn's disease: the CHARM trial. *Gastroenterology.* 2007;132(1):52-65.

48. Schreiber S, Reinisch W, Colombel JF, et al. Early Crohn's disease shows high levels of remission to therapy with adalimumab: sub-analysis of CHARM [abstract]. *Gastroenterology.* 2007;132(4 suppl 1):A147.

49. Sandborn WJ, Feagan BG, Stoinov S, et al, and the PRECiSE 1 Study Investigators. Certolizumab pegol for the treatment of Crohn's disease. *N Engl J Med.* 2007;357(3):228-238.

50. Schreiber S, Khaliq-Kareemi M, Lawrance IC, et al, and the PRECiSE 2 Study Investigators. Maintenance therapy with certolizumab pegol for Crohn's disease. *N Engl J Med.* 2007;357(3):239-250.

51. Thomsen OO, Schreiber S, Khaliq-Kareemi M, Hanauer SB, Bloomfield R, Sandborn WJ. Rapid onset of response and remission to subcutaneous certolizumab pegol and lack of influence of concomitant baseline medications in active Crohn's disease: results from the open-label induction phase of the PRECiSE 2 study [abstract]. *Gastroenterology.* 2007;132(4 suppl 1):A505.

52. Colombel JF, Schreiber S, Hanauer SB, Rutgeerts P, Sandborn WJ. Long-term tolerability of subcutaneous certolizumab pegol in active Crohn's disease: results from PRECiSE 3 and 4 [abstract]. *Gastroenterology.* 2007;132(4 suppl 1):A503.

53. Vermeire S, Abreu MT, D'Haens G, et al. Efficacy and safety of certolizumab pegol in patients with active Crohn's disease who previously lost response or were intolerant to infliximab: open-label induction preliminary results of the WELCOME study [abstract]. *Gastroenterology.* 2008;134(4 suppl 1):A67.

54. Colombel JF, Sandborn WJ, Reinisch W, et al. Infliximab, azathioprine, or combination therapy for Crohn's disease. *N Engl J Med.* 2010;362:1383-1395.

55. Sandborn WJ, Colombel JF, Enns R, et al, and the International Efficacy of Natalizumab as Active Crohn's Therapy (ENACT-1) Trial Group and Evaluation of Natalizumab as Continuous Therapy (ENACT-2) Trial Group. Natalizumab induction and maintenance therapy for Crohn's disease. *N Engl J Med.* 2005;353(18):1912-1925.

56. Langer-Gould A, Atlas SW, Green AJ, Bollen AW, Pelletier D. Progressive multifocal leukoencephalopathy in a patient treated with natalizumab. *N Engl J Med.* 2005;353(4):375-381.

57. Kleinschmidt-DeMasters BK, Tyler KL. Progressive multifocal leukoencephalopathy complicating treatment with natalizumab and interferon beta-1a for multiple sclerosis. *N Engl J Med.* 2005; 353(4):369-374.

58. Van Assche G, Van Ranst M, Sciot R, et al. Progressive multifocal leukoencephalopathy after natalizumab therapy for Crohn's disease. *N Engl J Med.* 2005;353(4):362-368.

59. Yousry TA, Major EO, Ryschkewitsch C, et al. Evaluation of patients treated with natalizumab for progressive multifocal leukoencephalopathy. *N Engl J Med.* 2006;354(9):924-933.

60. Targan SR, Feagan BG, Fedorak RN, et al, Natalizumab for the treatment of active Crohn's disease: results of the ENCORE Trial. *Gastroenterology.* 2007;132:1672-1683.

61. Ehrenpreis ED, Kane SV, Cohen LB, et al. Thalidomide therapy for patients with refractory Crohn's disease: an open label trial. *Gastroenterology.* 1999;117(6):1271-1277.

62. Vasiliauskas EZ, Kam LY, Abreu-Martin MT, et al. An open-label pilot study of low dose thalidomide in chronically active, steroid dependent Crohn's disease. *Gastroenterology.* 1999;117:1278-1287.

63. Sandborn WJ, Feagan BG, Hanauer SB, et al. An engineered human antibody to TNF (CDP 571) for active Crohn's disease: a randomized double blind placebo controlled trial. *Gastroenterology.* 2001;120:1330-1338.

64. Schreiber S, Rutgeerts P, Fedorak R, et al. A randomized, placebo-controlled trial of certolizumab pegol (CDP870) for treatment of Crohn's disease. *Gastroenterology.* 2005;129:807-818.

65. Mannon P, Fuss I, Mayer L, et al. Anti-interleukin-12 antibody for active Crohn's disease. *N Engl J Med.* 2004;351:2069-2079.

66. Sandborn WJ, Feagan BG, Fedorak RN, et al. A randomized trial of ustekinumab, a human interleukin-12/23 monoclonal antibody, in patients with moderate-to-severe Crohn's disease. *Gastroenterology.* 2008;135:1130-1141.

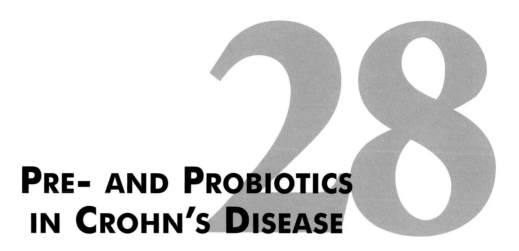

PRE- AND PROBIOTICS
IN CROHN'S DISEASE

Robert M. Penner, BSc, MD, FRCP(C), MSc; Karen L. Madsen, PhD;
and Richard N. Fedorak, MD, FRCP(C)

The currently accepted pathogenic model for inflammatory bowel disease (IBD) is one in which the enteric immune system's interaction with luminal microflora is deranged in a manner leading to unchecked intestinal inflammation. Pre- and probiotics, as modifiers of the enteral bacterial ecosystem, are potentially safe and effective tools to alter the luminal microflora population into one that is relatively beneficial and capable of down regulating or mollifying the intestinal inflammatory response. The rationale for pre- and probiotic use, and their evidence in the treatment of ulcerative colitis and pouchitis, are discussed in Chapter 33. The use of these exciting new therapies in the management of Crohn's disease is the subject of this chapter.

PROBIOTICS

BACKGROUND

As will be seen in Chapter 33, probiotics have been promising in the management of ulcerative colitis-related inflammation, particularly in the setting of pouchitis. Intuitively, CD might offer an even more advantageous setting for the use of probiotics, since the intestinal luminal bacterial population in CD has been previously found to differ more from normal subjects than that of ulcerative colitis, with the affected terminal ileum harboring an even more concentrated population of pathogenic bacteria and a markedly diminished population of probiotic bacteria than seen in ulcerative colitis.[1] Unfortunately, as we will see, the clinical evidence for the use of probiotics in CD is even more limited than in UC.

PHARMACOKINETICS

Pharmacokinetic considerations of probiotic use are considered in Chapter 33.

ADVERSE EVENTS

Because probiotics are bacteria that are normally associated with the human intestine, specific side effects have been rare, and the agents in use clinically are regarded as safe. This subject is considered in more detail in Chapter 33. The safety profile for the use of probiotics in Crohn's disease would be expected to be similar to that seen in UC.

CLINICAL TRIALS

Because of the inhomogeneity of preparations used in clinical research, we approach the evidence for probiotic use by clinical indication. A summary of this evidence is presented in Table 28-1.

ACUTE ACTIVE CROHN'S DISEASE

Gupta et al[2] conducted an open-label pilot trial in children with mildly to moderately active disease (Pediatric Crohn's Disease Activity Index [PCDAI] > 10), in conjunction with concomitant therapy with prednisone and immunomodulatory agents. Patients received a 6-month, open-label evaluation of *Lactobacillus* GG (2 x 10^10 colony-forming units [cfu] per day). Four patients were enrolled in this pilot project. There was significant improvement in the PCDAI 1 week after beginning *Lactobacillus* GG. This improvement was sustained throughout the study, with the

Lichtenstein GR, ed.
Crohn's Disease: The Complete Guide to Medical Management (pp 341-344).
© 2011 SLACK Incorporated

TABLE 28-1

CLINICAL EVIDENCE FOR PROBIOTICS IN CROHN'S DISEASE*

Disease/Setting	Level of Evidence and Probiotic	N	Duration of Probiotic Treatment	Results	Comments
Active Crohn's disease	**1 RCT:**				Promising but uncontrolled results using 2 different probiotic agents; 1 in children, 1 in adults.
	(LrGG)[4]	11	2 weeks	Only 5 of 11 patients completed study (P = ns)	
	2 Open-Label:				
	1) LrGG[2]	4	6 months	PCDAI ↓ 73% from baseline	
	2) Lactobacillus salivarius[3]	25	3 months	CDAI drop 217-150	
Maintenance of medical remission	**2 RCTs:** 1) (EcN)[5]	28	12 months	70% remission with EcN vs. 30% with placebo (P = ns)	Despite a positive trend, negative results for EcN in the only available useful RCT preclude recommendation of probiotics in this setting. Results for SB are encouraging and await a confirmatory RCT.
	2) (LrGG)[4]	11	6 months	n = 5, P = ns only 5 of 11 patients completed the study	
	1 Open-label: SB[6]	32	6 months	SB + Pentasa (2 g/day) 94% remission versus Pentasa (3 g/day) 38% (P = 0.04)	
Maintenance of surgical remission	2 RCTs: 1) LrGG[7]	45	12 months	No difference in clinical or endoscopic recurrence rates, LrGG versus placebo	Available RCTs are inadequate to support the use of any probiotic for postoperative Crohn's maintenance. The VSL#3 RCT remains in abstract form.
	2) VSL#3 (following rifaximin)[8]	40	12 months	Endoscopic remission 80% for VSL#3 versus 60% placebo (P = 0.05)	

*RCT indicates randomized controlled trial; LrGG, *Lactobacillus rhamnosus*; PCDAI, Pediatric Crohn's Disease Activity Index; CDAI, Crohn's Disease Activity Index; EcN, *Escherichia coli Nissle* 1917; SB, *Saccharomyces boulardii*.

median PCDAI 73% lower than baseline. In 3 patients, it was possible to taper the dose of steroids while they were receiving *Lactobacillus* GG. Intestinal permeability, as determined by a double sugar permeability test, improved significantly with the *Lactobacillus* GG. Three patients had relapse of their CD within 4 to 12 weeks of discontinuation of the *Lactobacillus* GG.

An open-label trial using the probiotic *Lactobacillus salivarius* UCC118 has also yielded encouraging results in treating acute active Crohn's disease.[3] Patients with active disease were given the opportunity to receive the probiotic *Lactobacillus salivarius* (1 x 10 cfu per day) instead of corticosteroids. Twenty-five patients enrolled, 4 dropped out with disease exacerbation, and 2 required corticosteroid therapy. Nineteen patients (76%) completed 3 months of treatment and were able to avoid other therapy. In addition,

Crohn's Disease Activity Index (CDAI) in these patients fell from a mean of 217 at entry to a mean of 150 at 3 months (P < 0.05). Controlled trials using this probiotic are currently underway.

Finally, a randomized controlled trial by Schultz and colleagues[4] attempted to examine the effect of *Lactobacillus* GG when used at the conclusion of an induction dose of steroids for induction and maintenance of remission. Because the trial enrolled only 11 patients, and 6 did not complete the study, the results were understandably not significant and, unfortunately, not helpful.

These trials constitute an optimistic beginning for research on probiotics in acute active CD, but as nonrandomized, uncontrolled trials, they can only be regarded as preliminary.

MAINTENANCE OF DRUG-INDUCED REMISSION

Malchow[5] investigated the role of *Escherichia coli* Nissle 1917 (Mutaflor, Ardeypharm, Herdecke, Germany) in a randomized, double-blind, placebo-controlled pilot study of corticosteroid-induced remission. Twenty-eight patients with active colonic Crohn's disease (CDAI > 150) were treated with prednisolone (60 mg/day) in a standard tapering regimen over 14 weeks. At the start of the prednisolone therapy, patients were randomized to receive either *E. coli* Nissle 1917 (5×10^9 cfu once daily) or placebo for 1 year. Using intent-to-treat analysis, the initial remission rate was 92% in the prednisolone and placebo group and 75% in the prednisolone and *E. coli* group (P = ns). Using per-protocol analysis, the results were 92% and 86%, respectively. Once remission was achieved and the prednisolone had been tapered to 0, the percentage of patients that remained in remission at the end of 1 year was 70% in the *E. coli* Nissle 1917 treated group versus 30% in the placebo group (P = ns). The lack of a statistically significant result in this trial is disappointing, but the positive trend that was observed makes further research essential.

Guslandi et al[6] examined the role of *Saccharomyces boulardii* in the maintenance of remission in 32 patients with CD. These patients had been in a medically induced remission for at least 3 months (CDAI < 150). At the time of entry into the study, the patients had been off all medications for at least 3 months. Patients were then randomized to receive mesalamine (Pentasa; 3 g/day in 3 divided doses) or mesalamine (Pentasa; 2 g/day in 2 divided doses) plus a preparation of *Saccharomyces boulardii* (1 g/day) for 6 months. Clinical remission at 6 months was observed in 10 of the 16 patients on mesalamine maintenance and in 15 out of 16 patients receiving mesalamine *Saccharomyces boulardii* (P = 0.04). Despite this encouraging result, no further studies with *Saccharomyces boulardii* have been published.

Evidence for the use of probiotics in maintenance of medical remission, as in probiotic research in other settings, is hampered by the fact that different probiotic agents are used at varying dosages, in varying patient populations, and with markedly different clinical trial designs. Furthermore, with only a single trial to support their use, probiotics are unlikely to gain widespread acceptance in this setting. Further research, particularly on *Saccharomyces boulardii*, may impact practice.

MAINTENANCE OF SURGICALLY INDUCED REMISSION

Prantera et al[7] performed a randomized, double-blind, single-centered, placebo-controlled, maintenance of surgical-induced remission trial. Forty-five patients in clinical remission (CDAI < 150) were randomized to receive either *Lactobacillus GG casei* subspecies *rhamnosus* (1.2×10^{10} cfu daily) or placebo within 10 days following surgical resection of their Crohn's disease. After 52 weeks of treatment, 15 patients (83%) treated with *Lactobacillus GG* and 17 patients (89%) treated with placebo remained in clinical remission (P = 0.948). In contrast, endoscopic remission was identified in 6 patients (40%) in the *Lactobacillus GG* group, compared to 11 patients (65%) in the placebo group (P = 0.243). Considering the success of *Lactobacillus GG* in the prevention of antibiotic, *Clostridium difficile*, and childhood diarrhea, the reason for these marked negative results in the maintenance of surgically induced remission in Crohn's disease remains speculative. It may be that, similar to the results seen with pouchitis, treatment with certain single species of probiotics is less effective than combination agents. Whether this represents individual species selection or quantity of bacteria delivered and/or colonized remains to be determined.

Campieri et al[8] reported, in abstract form, that a combination of antibiotic and the probiotic mixture (VSL#3 Yovis, Sigma-Tau, Pomezia, Italy) treatment was efficacious in prevention of the postoperative recurrence of CD when compared to mesalamine. Forty patients were randomized to receive either rifaximin (1.8 g/day) for 3 months followed by VSL#3 (6×10^{11} cfu per day) for 9 months or mesalamine (4 g/day) for 12 months. After 1 year, the antibiotic/VSL#3 group had an endoscopic remission rate of 80% compared to 60% in the mesalamine group ($P < 0.05$). Interestingly, these endoscopic remission rates at 1 year with an antibiotic followed by VSL#3 are similar to those that have been previously described with metronidazole alone.[9] This is an intriguing study into a setting of CD therapy in which no agent has proven consistently reliable. Unfortunately, the study design does not permit us to differentiate between effects of the probiotic preparation versus effects of the initial antibiotic therapy. This is particularly relevant given the postoperative prevention of recurrence demonstrated for antibiotics in the past.[9] As it has not yet been published as a full manuscript, further comment is not yet possible.

Results of probiotic research are again disappointing in the setting of surgically induced maintenance of remission, particularly because this is a setting where clearly effective therapy is not available. Data to date do not support probiotic therapy for this indication. Nevertheless, an international, randomized, placebo-controlled, double-blind clinical trial to assess the effectiveness of VSL#3 in the prevention of postoperative ileal-colonic anastomotic CD recurrence is currently underway.

FUTURE DIRECTIVES

Clearly, these promising early data in the field of probiotics need to be pursued further if effective CD-specific therapeutic agents are to be identified and incorporated into the IBD armamentarium. Rigorous and well-designed randomized controlled trials, confirmatory in duplicate, are a necessity. If they are to impact clinical practice, they must use probiotic agents that can meet the regulatory requirements for manufacturing and consistency of product. In addition to the efficacy question, the clinical trial must also address: (1) single versus combination agents, (2) optimal dosage, (3) timing of administration, (4) colonization, and (5) whether the probiotics need to be living to provide their beneficial therapeutic effects.

Though clinical trials are ongoing, new possibilities are reaching the level of animal experimentation. Specifically, genetically engineered probiotics may provide new therapies. Recently, murine IL-10 synthesis and secretion by genetically modified *Lactococcus lactis* was shown to be an efficient way to deliver high concentrations of this anti-inflammatory cytokine.[10] When these *Lactococcus lactis* were administered to murine experimental models of IBD, IL-10 was delivered to the mucosal surface at a concentration that reduced or prevented the onset of enterocolitis.[11] These studies introduced new and exciting proof of the ability to merge cytokine therapy for IBD with genetic engineering of probiotics. The safety issues related to the genetic modification of this probiotic have been addressed by replacing the thymidylate synthase gene in the *Lactococcus lactis* with a synthetic human IL-10 gene. This thymidylate synthase-negative human IL-10–positive *Lactococcus lactis* strain produces human IL-10. However, when it is deprived of thymidine or thymine, the strain is not viable and is eliminated by the mouse body.[12] Theoretically, this built-in biologic containment system should prevent accumulation of the genetically modified probiotic in the mammalian environment. Currently, a pilot trial involving humans with CD is underway to examine the therapeutic safety and efficacy of this human IL-10-secreting *Lactococcus lactis*. As the understanding of human IBD develops, the use of bacteria as "Trojan horses" to deliver a host of therapeutic agents should provide exciting possibilities.

PREBIOTICS

Though prebiotics may hold the same promise that is being studied in ulcerative colitis (see Chapter 33), to date, there are no human data to support their use in Crohn's disease.

REFERENCES

1. Schultsz C, Van Den Berg FM, Ten Kate FW, Tytgat GN, Dankert J. The intestinal mucus layer from patients with inflammatory bowel disease harbors high numbers of bacteria compared with controls. *Gastroenterology*. 1999;117(5):1089-1097.

2. Gupta P, Andrew H, Kirschner BS, Guandalini S. Is *Lactobacillus* GG helpful in children with Crohn's disease? Results of a preliminary, open-label study. *J Pediatr Gastroenterol Nutr*. 2000;31(4): 453-457.

3. McCarthy J, O'Mahony L, Dunne C, et al. An open trial of a novel probiotic as an alternative to steroids in mild/moderately active Crohn's disease. *Gut*. 2001;49(Suppl III):2447.

4. Schultz M, Timmer A, Herfarth HH, Sartor RB, Vanderhoof JA, Rath HC. *Lactobacillus* GG in inducing and maintaining remission of Crohn's disease. *BMC Gastroenterol*. 2004;4(1):5.

5. Malchow HA. Crohn's disease and *Escherichia coli*. A new approach in therapy to maintain remission of colonic Crohn's disease? *J Clin Gastroenterol*. 1997;25(4):653-658.

6. Guslandi M, Mezzi G, Sorghi M, Testoni PA. *Saccharomyces boulardii* in maintenance treatment of Crohn's disease. *Dig Dis Sci*. 2000;45(7):1462-1464.

7. Prantera C, Scribano ML, Falasco G, Andreoli A, Luzi C. Ineffectiveness of probiotics in preventing recurrence after curative resection for Crohn's disease: a randomized controlled trial with *Lactobacillus* GG. *Gut*. 2002;51(3):405-409.

8. Campieri M, Rizzello F, Venturi A, et al. Combination of antibiotic and probiotic treatment is efficacious in prophylaxis of post-operative recurrence of Crohn's disease: a randomized controlled study vs mesalamine. *Gastroenterology*. 2000;118:A781.

9. Rutgeerts P, Hiele M, Geboes K, et al. Controlled trial of metronidazole treatment for prevention of Crohn's recurrence after ileal resection. *Gastroenterology*. 1995;108(6):1617-1621.

10. Schotte L, Steidler L, Vandekerckhove J, Remaut E. Secretion of biologically active murine interleukin-10 by *Lactococcus lactis*. *Enzyme Microb Technol*. 2000;27(10):761-765.

11. Steidler L, Hans W, Schotte L, et al. Treatment of murine colitis by *Lactococcus lactis* secreting interleukin-10. *Science*. 2000; 289(5483):1352-1355.

12. Steidler L, Neirynck S, Huyghebaert N, et al. Biological containment of genetically modified *Lactococcus lactis* for intestinal delivery of human interleukin 10. *Nat Biotechnol*. 2003;21(7):785-789.

MANAGEMENT OF CROHN'S DISEASE IN THE ILEAL-POUCH ANAL ANASTOMOSIS

Gilaad G. Kaplan MD, FRCP(C) and Remo Panaccione, MD, FRCP(C)

BACKGROUND

Medical therapy for UC is limited to sulfasalazine, 5-aminosalicylic acid (5-ASA), corticosteroids, and azathioprine (AZA). Refractory patients may be hospitalized and treated with IV glucocorticoids and occasionally intravenous (IV) cyclosporine. The latter is associated with a significant toxicity, and the long-term results have been variable. Arguably, the most significant advance in the treatment of UC in the past 2 decades has been the development and expanded use of the proctocolectomy with ileal pouch-anal anastomosis (IPAA) formation.[1] Although most UC patients with an IPAA do remarkably well, postoperatively, there are several treatable complications that may occur. These complications and their management are described in Chapter 36.

Historically, IPAA has been considered a contraindication in CD patients due to poor outcomes. Several studies have been published that outline the poor outcomes associated with an IPAA in CD patients.[2-7] CD in the pouch has been associated with refractory pouchitis, peri-pouch abscess, fistula formation, pouch strictures, and dreaded pouch failure. If surgery is required for pouch failure, pouch excision is associated with subsequent bowel shortening with a loss of 30 cm of ileum required to form the pouch. Table 29-1 highlights the most common complications reported in CD patients with an IPAA, and Figure 29-1 represents the typical pattern of CD recurrence in the ileal pouch.[2-8] Pouch failure, defined as complete excision or diversion, ranges between 30% and 45% in the early studies.[2-7]

However, in a large series from the Cleveland Clinic (n = 1800), 60 patients undergoing an IPAA had their preoperative diagnosis of UC or indeterminate colitis revised to Crohn's disease postoperatively. The overall pouch failure rate was 12%, and only one third of patients developed active CD postoperatively.[8] These studies demonstrate that a portion of CD patients could adequately maintain a functioning pouch for an indefinite period of time (range of follow-up was 17 months to 10 years).[2-8]

The notion that an IPAA is contraindicated in CD patients was recently challenged in 1996 when Panis et al[9] demonstrated that a preselected population of Crohn's patients could have a good outcome with an IPAA. The authors selected 31 CD patients who had no evidence of perianal or small bowel disease for IPAA formation. Two (6%) of these patients lost their pouches because of fistula formation. However, after 5 years of follow-up, there was no significant difference in pouch functioning between CD and UC patients undergoing an IPAA.[9] These results were replicated by Regimbeau et al, who demonstrated pouch failure rates of only 10% in properly selected CD patients.[10] In both of these studies, the Crohn's-related complications outlined in Table 29-1 were reported; however, they were managed medically or with pouch-preserving procedures resulting in overall low pouch failure rates. Despite these results, performing an IPAA in known CD patients is still controversial and not recommended universally.[11]

Combining the results of the previously discussed studies, 3.5% of preoperative diagnoses of UC or indeterminate colitis are revised to CD postoperatively (range 2.5% to 12.5%).[2-8] CD can be easily recognized in patients who

Lichtenstein GR, ed.
Crohn's Disease: The Complete Guide to Medical Management (pp 345-348).
© 2011 SLACK Incorporated

TABLE 29-1

POSTOPERATIVE CD COMPLICATIONS FOLLOWING ILEAL POUCH-ANAL ANASTOMOSIS*

Pouch failure[†]	29%
FUNCTIONING POUCH COMPLICATIONS	
Fistula[‡]	27%
Small bowel obstruction/stricture	15%
Peripouch abscess/sepsis	6%
Ileoanal stenosis/stricture	10%

*The percentage reported is a composite of the results of 7 studies.[2-8]
[†]Defined as either pouch excision or permanent diversion
[‡]Fistuli included perianal, cutaneous, vaginal, enteric, and vesicular

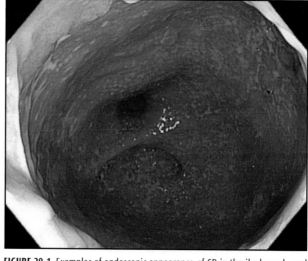

FIGURE 29-1. Examples of endoscopic appearance of CD in the ileal pouch-anal anastomosis. (Courtesy of Douglas Weine, MD.)

have inflammation proximal to the pouch or who develop fistulizing disease outside the pouch that occurs remote to surgery. However, differentiating pouchitis from CD can be difficult in patients with inflammation isolated to the pouch as the endoscopic and histologic features can be similar in both conditions. The presence of a granuloma is pathoneumonic for CD, though this histological presentation is rare. One study that compared the endoscopic and histologic findings of pouchitis and CD of the pouch showed that granulomas in pouch biopsies occurred in only 5% of cases.[12] Furthermore, this study showed that pouchitis and CD shared endoscopic findings of the pouch including erythema, nodularity, ulcerations, and friability.[12] The only predictive endoscopic finding of Crohn's disease was inflammation in the afferent limb.[12] This association was also described in a study showing that afferent limb ulcers were seen in nearly half of CD patients.[13] Fifteen percent of UC patients had afferent limb ulcers; however, none of the UC patients exhibited these lesions when the group was controlled for the use of nonsteroidal anti-inflammatory drugs (NSAIDs).[13] The lack of response of pouchitis to antibiotics should raise the suspicion of CD; however, many of these patients may have refractory pouchitis.[14]

The gastroenterologist and surgeon will be faced with patients who develop CD in an ileal pouch following proctocolectomy with IPAA. The rest of this chapter will highlight the limited evidence that supports the aggressive medical management directed at pouch preservation when CD occurs in the IPAA.

MEDICAL MANAGEMENT

Due to the relative rarity of Crohn's disease following IPAA, there have been no randomized controlled trials

assessing the efficacy of specific medical management. Furthermore, the available literature on this topic is limited to a few case reports and small open-label, noncontrolled studies. The predominant medical therapy for CD will be reviewed with respect to its applicability in treating CD of the pouch. Given the undesirable outcome of pouch failure and possible pouch excision, the authors believe an early aggressive approach following this diagnosis is mandated.

5-ASA

There are sparse reports in the literature describing the use of 5-ASA medications in the treatment of CD of the pouch. The use of 5-ASA products in the management of CD has recently been challenged based on the available literature.[15] Following resection of the bowel with primary anastomosis for CD, mesalamine products have been shown to reduce the risk of recurrence by approximately 10% compared to placebo.[16] However, it is unlikely that these data can be extrapolated to Crohn's patients with an IPAA, as these patients have aggressive disease with high pouch failure rates. Therefore, in this population, the use of 5-ASA drugs would likely fail and is not recommended. In 1 case report, topical mesalamine was tried unsuccessfully to manage CD recurrence in the IPAA.[17]

ANTIBIOTICS

Antibiotics are the mainstay of therapy of acute and recurrent pouchitis;[18] however, adequate analysis of antibiotics' role in the management of CD of the IPAA is not present. Case reports of antibiotic treatment in Crohn's patients with active pouch disease show no response to antibiotics or a loss of initial response.[17,19] This is not surprising, given the lack of evidence supporting a therapeutic effect of antibiotics in the treatment of CD in randomized controlled trials. However, pouchitis can be difficult to distinguish from active CD of the pouch, and the 2 conditions may coexist. Given this possibility, the authors do recommend a course of antibiotics (eg, ciprofloxacin and metronidazole) to treat any coexisting pouchitis, although there is no literature to support this action. In cases where there is a diagnostic uncertainty, the authors will repeat pouch endoscopy following a course of antibiotics in an attempt to clarify the diagnosis.

CORTICOSTEROIDS

Induction of remission in CD with glucocorticoids occurs in 60% to 80% of patients.[20,21] The use of corticosteroids in CD of the pouch is limited, reported primarily in combination with immunomodulator therapy. In 2 cases, high-dose corticosteroids were used to induce remission that was subsequently maintained by AZA (see the following section).[17] Given the fact that it may take several months to appreciate the full therapeutic benefit of purine antimetabolites or methotrexate, the use of a course of corticosteroid while starting an immunomodulator is recommended.

IMMUNOMODULATORS

AZA/6-mercaptopurine (6-MP) has been effective in the induction and maintenance of remission of CD.[22] Likewise, AZA has been applied in the maintenance of remission of Crohn's activity in a pouch following induction with corticosteroids.[17] Two cases have shown the effectiveness of combining prednisone for induction and then AZA for maintenance.[17] Outcome studies of pouch complications in Crohn's patients with IPAA have reported efficacy of AZA as well.[9,10] No case reports were identified for the specific use of 6-MP or methotrexate in CD of the pouch. We would presume that 6-MP has comparable efficacy with AZA, given pharmacodynamic similarities and equivalence in studies. Methotrexate has been shown to be effective in the management of moderate to severe CD,[23] and thus it should be considered in patients who cannot tolerate AZA or 6-MP.

Although AZA is effective in many patients with an IPAA and Crohn's disease, there have been several cases of AZA failures.[19,24]

INFLIXIMAB

Infliximab is a promising treatment for CD of the pouch, which typically manifests aggressively and is refractory to traditional CD medications. In the literature, there are 33 patients with Crohn's recurrence in an IPAA that have been treated with infliximab.[19,24] In the largest open-label, noncontrolled trial, 26 patients with an IPAA and Crohn's activity were treated with induction and maintenance therapy of infliximab. All patients received 3 doses of 5 mg/kg infliximab over 8 weeks for induction; maintenance therapy was variable and at the physician's discretion. Fifteen of the patients had been previously started on an immunomodulator (AZA, 6-MP, methotrexate, or FK-506), and the rest were started concurrently. Eight-five percent of these patients improved clinically on infliximab. Of these patients, 62% had a complete response defined as a resolution of diarrhea and abdominal pain and/or closure of all fistulas. Long-term follow-up (median of 21.5 months) demonstrated pouch failure, excision, or diversion in one third of the patients. In the two thirds of patients ($n = 16$) who kept their pouch at the end of follow-up, 11 were on regular (every 8 weeks) or on-demand infliximab. The fistula closure rate was approximately 50%, which is similar to the response rate reported in maintenance trials of Crohn's patients with fistula without a pouch.[25] Infliximab has also been shown to be effective in children. Four children with an IPAA and Crohn's recurrence refractory to medical management (5-ASA, antibiotics, and immunomodulators) were treated concurrently with an immunomodulator and infliximab at 5 mg/kg at weeks 0, 2, and 6, followed by the medication every 8 weeks. Patients were followed between 1 and 2 years; all had preserved and functioning pouches.[26]

NONMEDICAL MANAGEMENT

In addition to a variety of medical approaches to preserving pouch integrity, there are a number of adjuvant nonmedical procedures. Symptomatic strictures of the inlet or outlet of the pouch are typically refractory to medical management. Nineteen patients with CD of the pouch associated with inlet and/or outlet pouch strictures were treated successfully with endoscopic-guided balloon dilation. After a mean follow-up of 6 months, only 1 patient failed dilation and lost his pouch.[27] Additionally, pouch strictureplasty is an option in patients with a long fibrotic stricture.[28] Patients with medically refractory fistulas can be treated with a seton catheter or a fistulotomy. Ultimately, when the preceding management strategies fail, these patients are treated with an ileostomy.

CONCLUSION

The rarity of IPAA in Crohn's patients has led to few clinical trials investigating the optimal management approach. Available literature is limited to small open-label, noncontrolled trials and case reports. The natural history of Crohn's disease in patients with IPAA is aggressive with high rates of fistula formation, stricturing, and inflammation. These complications lead to pouch failure, requiring excision or diversion of the pouch in a high proportion of these patients. Thus, we recommend an

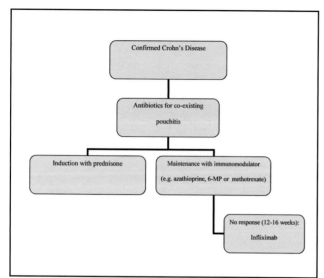

FIGURE 29-2. An approach to the medical management of CD of the ileal pouch-anal anastomosis.

aggressive approach to treating these patients with the goal of pouch preservation (Figure 29-2). A trial of antibiotics (ciprofloxacin and metronidazole) is recommended to treat possible coexisting pouchitis. Patients with an IPAA and endoscopic, radiologic, and/or histologic evidence of CD should be induced with corticosteroids and concurrently treated with AZA for long-term maintenance. Alternatives to AZA include 6-MP or methotrexate. Patients who do not respond to this approach should be escalated to infliximab therapy. Remission should be induced with 5 mg/kg of infliximab at 0, 2, and 6 weeks and then repeated every 8 weeks for maintenance therapy. An immunomodulator should be used concurrently with infliximab. Fibrotic and fistulizing disease refractory to medical management should be treated with balloon dilation or strictureplasty and fistulotomy, respectively. Failure of this approach should be managed with a diverting ileostomy or possible pouch excision.

REFERENCES

1. Parks A, Nicholls RJ. Proctocolectomy without ileostomy for ulcerative colitis. *Br Med J.* 1978;8(2):85-88.

2. Deutsch A, McLeod RS, Cullen J, Cohen Z. Results of the pelvic-pouch procedure in patients with Crohn's disease. *Dis Colon Rectum.* 1991;34:475-477.

3. Hyman NH, Fazio VW, Tuckson WB, et al. Consequences of ileal pouch-anal anastomosis for Crohn's colitis. *Dis Colon Rectum.* 1991;34:653-657.

4. Sagar P, Dozois RR, Wolff BG. Long-term results of ileal pouch-anal anastomosis in patients with Crohn's disease. *Dis Colon Rectum.* 1996;39:893-898.

5. Peyregne V, Francois Y, Gilly F-N, et al. Outcome of ileal pouch after secondary diagnosis of Crohn's disease. *Int J Colorectal Dis.* 2000;15:49-53.

6. Grobler SP, Hosie KB, Affie E, et al. Outcome of restorative proctocolectomy when the diagnosis is suggestive of Crohn's disease. *Gut.* 1993;34:1384-1388.

7. Braveman JM, Schoetz DJ, Marcello PW, et al. The fate of ileal pouch in patients developing Crohn's disease. *Dis Colon Rectum.* 2004;47:1613-1619.

8. Hartley JE, Fazio VW, Remzi FH, et al. Analysis of the outcome of ileal pouch-anal anastomosis in patients with Crohn's disease. *Dis Colon Rectum.* 2004;47:1808-1815.

9. Panis Y, Poupard B, Hautefeuille P, et al. Ileal pouch anal anastomosis for Crohn's disease. *Lancet.* 1996;347:854-857.

10. Regimbeau JM, Panis Y, Pocard M, et al. Long-term results of ileal pouch anal anastomosis for colorectal Crohn's disease. *Dis Colon Rectum.* 2001;44:769-778.

11. Strong SA. Invited editorial. *Dis Colon Rectum.* 2001;44:776-778.

12. Shen B, Fazio V, Remzi FH, et al. Comprehensive evaluation of inflammatory and noninflammatory sequelae of ileal pouch-anal anastomoses. *Am J Gastroenterol.* 2005;100(1):93-101.

13. Wolf JM, Achkar JP, Lashner BA, et al. Afferent limb ulcers predict Crohn's disease in patients with ileal pouch-anal anastomosis. *Gastroenterology.* 2004;126(7):1686-1691.

14. Shen B. Diagnosis and treatment of patients with pouchitis. *Drugs.* 2003;63(5):453-461.

15. Sandborn BJ, Feagan B. Review article: mild to moderate Crohn's disease—defining the basis for a new treatment algorithm. *Aliment Pharmacol Ther.* 2003;18(3):263-277.

16. Camma C, Giunta M, Roseseli M. 5-Aminosalicylic acid in the maintenance of Crohn's disease: a meta-analysis adjusted for confounding variables. *Gastroenterology.* 1997;113:1465-11473.

17. Berrebi W, Chaussade S, Bruhl AL, et al. Treatment of Crohn's disease recurrence after ileoanal anastomosis by azathioprine. *Dig Dis Sci.* 1993;38(8):1558-1560.

18. Achkar JP, Shen B. Medical management of postoperative complications of inflammatory bowel disease: pouchitis and Crohn's disease recurrence. *Curr Gastroenterol Rep.* 2001;3(6):484-490.

19. Ricart E, Panaccione R, Loftus EV, et al. Successful management of Crohn's disease of the ileoanal pouch with infliximab. *Gastroenterology.* 1999;117:429-432.

20. Summers RW, Switz DM, Sessions JT Jr, et al. National Cooperative Crohn's Disease Study: results of drug treatment. *Gastroenterology.* 1979;77(4 Pt 2):847-869.

21. Malchow H, Ewe K, Brandes JW, et al. European Cooperative Crohn's Disease Study (ECCDS): results of drug treatment. *Gastroenterology.* 1984;86(2):249-266.

22. Pearson DC, May GR, Fick G, et al. Azathioprine for maintaining remission of Crohn's disease. *Cochrane Database Syst Rev.* 2000;2: CD000067.

23. Feagan BG, Alfadhli A. Methotrexate in inflammatory bowel disease. *Gastroenterol Clin North Am.* 2004;33(2):407-420, xi.

24. Colombel JF, Ricart E, Loftus EV Jr, et al. Management of Crohn's disease of the ileoanal pouch with infliximab. *Am J Gastroenterol.* 2003;98(10):2239-2244.

25. Sands BE, Anderson FH, Bernstein CN, et al. Infliximab maintenance therapy for fistulizing Crohn's disease. *N Engl J Med.* 2004;350:876-885.

26. Kooros K, Katz AJ. Infliximab therapy in pediatric Crohn's pouchitis. *Inflamm Bowel Dis.* 2004;10(4):417-420.

27. Shen B, Fazio VW, Remzi FH, et al. Endoscopic balloon dilation of ileal pouch strictures. *Am J Gastroenterol.* 2004;99(12):2340-2347.

28. Matzke GM, Kang AS, Dozois EJ, et al. Mid pouch strictureplasty for Crohn's disease after ileal pouch-anal anastomosis: an alternative to pouch excision. *Dis Colon Rectum.* 2004;47(5):782-786.

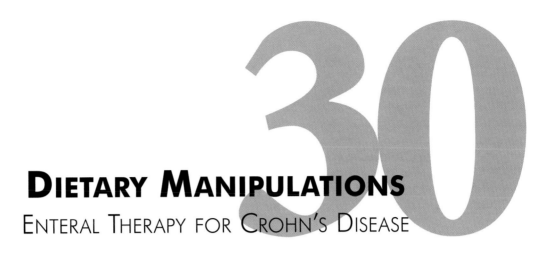

DIETARY MANIPULATIONS
ENTERAL THERAPY FOR CROHN'S DISEASE

Alan L. Buchman, MD, MSPH

ELIMINATION DIETS

ROLE OF REFINED SUGAR, FIBER, AND MARGARINE

Several epidemiological studies from Israel,[1] Italy,[2] Sweden,[3] and the United Kingdom[4-7] have suggested an association between increased sugar and margarine consumption and the development of Crohn's, although a multinational study was able to find only a weak association with mortality risk from CD, but not the actual incidence of disease.[8]

Dietary fiber intake appears to be similar in patients with CD versus age, gender, and socioeconomic background-matched controls.[9,10] However, refined sugar, starch, and total energy intake tend to be greater than controls.[9-15] It is to be noted that patients may change their diet once diagnosed with CD.[16] This may occur on the basis of individual preference or perceived health benefits or advice from family, friends, or professionals.

This association led to interventional studies that tested the use of an unrefined, fiber-rich diet to maintain remission. In a small retrospective study of 32 patients in England prescribed such a diet, the number of hospital admissions and intestinal surgeries over an 18- to 80-month (mean 52 months) period were lower in those that received the dietary recommendations versus matched controls with CD that had no specific prescribed dietary therapy.[17] The diet-treated patients received a mean of 33.4 ± 1.8 g/day of dietary fiber; control data were not reported, although refined sugar intake was 90 ± 7 g/day in controls

versus 39 ± 4 g/day in the diet group ($P < 0.001$). A much larger, multicenter study in the United Kingdom in which 352 patients with CD were randomized to a low refined carbohydrate (white flower and rice) diet with increased unrefined carbohydrate intake or avoidance of unrefined carbohydrates for 2 years. This study found similar, although nonstatistically significant, differences between groups,[18] although the incidence of disease relapse was nearly identical between groups.

Although it has been thought the increased intake of refined sugars in patients with CD may reflect a dietary compensation for decreased overall energy intake or perhaps even ill-conceived advice to avoid roughage, rather than a cause for CD itself,[8] dietary carbohydrate modification might result in a change in enteric bacterial flora that may impact on the natural history of CD. A study of 71 Italian patients randomized to a low residual diet in which legumes, whole grains, nuts, and all fruits and vegetables were excluded or normal diet also showed no benefit from fiber restriction on the maintenance of remission.[19]

ROLE OF DIETARY FAT

It has been suggested that diets with high concentrations of long-chain triglycerides (LCT) may either decrease the effectiveness of dietary therapy for active CD or increase the likelihood of relapse. The theory holds that if there is more linoleic acid in the diet, there is more substrate for metabolism to proinflammatory prostaglandins (see discussion of fish oils following). Middleton et al showed that remission rate in patients who received enteral nutritional support (see following discussion) was negatively correlated with the amount of energy derived from LCT.[20] This

Lichtenstein GR, ed.
Crohn's Disease: The Complete Guide to Medical Management (pp 349-360).
© 2011 SLACK Incorporated

was confirmed ($r = -0.63$, $P = 0.006$) in a meta-analysis of 11 studies in which the fat constituents of the enteral formula were available.[20] A modest negative association between remission rate and the amount of dietary linoleic acid was observed, although in the meta-analysis the effect was lost when LCT intake exceeded 15% of dietary energy; a significant decline in the efficacy of enteral nutrition in terms of disease remission occurred when the percentage of dietary LCT exceed 15%. After 4 weeks of feeding using an elemental formula that varied in fat content only, Japanese investigators found remission of CD occurred in 80% of patients ($n = 10$ per group) who received a low-fat diet containing 3.1 g/day, 40% in those who received 16.7 g/day, and only 25% in those who received 30.1 g/day, although biochemical indices of inflammation exhibited a variable response.[21] In contrast, Leiper et al found no difference in remission rates (26% for low LCT feeds and 33% for high LCT feeds) among a group of 54 patients with active CD who were fed by mouth or nasogastric tube (NGT).[22] Both formulas were polymeric. A recent study reported by Gassull et al found that an enteral formulation containing a similar amount of LCT but a higher concentration of n6 polyunsaturated fats (high linoleate, low oleate) was significantly more effective for induction of remission than a formula containing a relatively higher concentration of monounsaturated fatty acids (high oleate, low linoleate) in a randomized study of 62 patients (52% versus 20% remission rate after 2 weeks of therapy), although treatment with corticosteroids (prednisone 1 mg/kg/day) was the most effective regimen (remission rate of 79%).[23] These observations contrast with those of Middleton et al[20] and suggest that qualitative changes in dietary fat may be as important as, if not more important than, total dietary fat content, although changes in a single fatty acid concentration may be of limited significance.

Medium-chain triglycerides (MCT) modulate the expression of adhesion molecules and cytokines, in addition to linoleic fatty acid metabolism.[24-27] Higher remission rates in studies of enteral diets have been achieved when such diets have a high percentage of MCT.[20,28] However, other studies have suggested the amount of MCT in the formula appears to have little importance in so far as remission of CD is concerned.[29]

FOOD INTOLERANCES

Shortly after CD was initially described, Collins et al reported a patient who improved clinically with an elimination diet.[30] Other clinicians reported similar cases. Data from Alun Jones et al support the hypothesis that diet may have a primary role in the cause of CD.[31] These investigators found that certain foods, when eliminated from the diet, caused symptoms consistent with CD in 20 consecutive patients with active disease. When the items were added back to the diet 1 by 1 in a controlled fashion, symptoms

recurred. Interestingly, the majority of food intolerance was to wheat (an excellent stool-bulking agent), dairy products, and vegetables (including mustard greens, corn, and tomatoes) that contain a significant amount of biomass, subject to bacterial degradation. Tap water was also listed as a food intolerance by 8 patients. A multicenter study of 136 patients who were successfully treated for a relapse of CD with an elemental diet (31% refused to continue for a sufficient treatment period with the elemental diet) were then randomized to an elimination diet and placebo or a regular diet with corticosteroids followed by corticosteroid taper.[32] Common food intolerances included corn, wheat, milk, yeast, egg, potato, rye, tea, and coffee. Seventy-nine percent of patients in the corticosteroid group relapsed versus 62% in the diet group, although 25% of the diet group patients were withdrawn due to nonadherence. Decreases in C-reactive protein (CRP) and erythrocyte sedimentation rate (ESR) were observed in both groups, although both remained elevated in most patients. This may have been a marker for impending clinical relapse. Median remission times were 7.5 months for those who were assigned the elimination diet versus 3.8 months for those on a regular diet. Elimination diets may have some role in the maintenance of remission in CD, but their use must be balanced against nonadherence, as well as what may amount to a nutritionally inadequate diet if staple foods must be avoided.

The "fast food" diet (hamburger or hotdog with mustard or ketchup, together with french fries or creamed potatoes and a soft drink) has also been associated with the development of CD. A study in Stockholm found the risk for development of CD was 3.4 times greater for those who had at least 2 fast food meals weekly,[13] although this finding may have reflected a particular patient lifestyle. These investigators also observed an association between increased sucrose intake and risk for CD. It must be observed, however, that control individuals for many studies were often selected from hospital outpatient clinics and therefore may not have been appropriate normal controls. It is also possible that current reported dietary habits may not reflect even lengthy past behavior and, in fact, given the frequent delay in diagnosis of CD, individuals may have consciously changed their diet based on their undiagnosed symptoms. In addition, proof of association is not necessarily proof of a cause-and-effect relationship as multiple dietary variables may be associated with various lifestyles, including smoking, sedentary behavior, occupational exposure, education level, frequency of physician visits, etc.

A low oxalate diet may be required in those patients who have had their terminal ileum resected or who have significant fat malabsorption and still have part of their colon remaining. These patients have a propensity for oxalate kidney stones.

DIETARY SUPPLEMENTS

FISH OILS

Omega-3 fatty acids are so named because of a double bond that is located between the third and fourth carbon atom from the methyl end of the fatty acid chain. These fatty acids are an insignificant part of the Western diet. In vivo data have suggested that omega-3 (n3) fatty acids have antiinflammatory properties; neutrophil aggregation, neutrophil chemotaxis, neutrophil adherence to epithelial cells, and mononuclear cell IL-1 and tumor necrosis factor synthesis are all decreased.[33-35] Eicosanoids are released from membrane phospholipids during cellular activation and competitively inhibit arachidonic acid (omega-6; n6) metabolism. Eicosanoid metabolites have diminished inflammatory effects when compared to arachidonic acid metabolites.[36] Dietary fatty acid composition affects tissue fatty acid composition. Dietary supplementation with Ω-6 fatty acids (cod liver oil or perilla oil) was provided to rats that where subsequently administered trinitrobenzene sulphonic acid enemas. A blunted rise in luminal PGE_2, TXB_2, and LTB_4 was observed, and significantly less severe colitis was observed when compared with animals that received dietary supplementation with either safflower or sunflower oil (omega-3 fatty acids).[36,37] A clinical study of 78 patients reported by Belluzzi et al found 2.7 g (3 capsules tid) of n-3 fatty acids administered as an enteric-coated fish oil preparation maintained 59% of Crohn's patients in remission after 1 year compared to 26% in the placebo group ($P = 0.003$).[38] However, another study by Lorenz-Meyer in 204 patients failed to show a difference in remission rates compared to placebo after 1 year of therapy.[39] In each study, large doses of fish oil were administered; this may be unpalatable for most people, although the enteric-coated preparation used in the Belluzzi study led to diarrhea in a small minority of patients, and no one reported fish odor objections. A Cochrane Collaborative report that included 6 randomized, placebo-controlled trials concluded fish oil supplementation was ineffective for the maintenance of remission of CD.[40]

GLUTAMINE

Glutamine is a nonessential amino acid synthesized from glutamate and glutamic acid by the enzyme glutamine synthetase. It stimulates crypt cell proliferation of ileal and colonic and therefore presumably of jejunal epithelial cells as well in vitro.[41] Although previous investigations found that glutamine was the preferred fuel for the small intestine,[42] more recent studies have demonstrated that glutamate is interchangeable with glutamine as an intestinal fuel.[43] Glutamine may also be oxidized as a fuel and can be a primary energy substrate for enterocytes and lymphocytes. In rats, it has generally been found that

intestinal villus hypoplasia increased intestinal permeability to macromolecules, decreased immunoglobulin (Ig) A production, and induced changes in the amount of gut-associated lymphoid tissue (GALT). Decreases in intestinal mucus gel secretion occur when animals experience systemic injury such as major trauma or sepsis or are provided with glutamine-free total parenteral nutrition (TPN) as an exclusive means of nutritional support.[43-53]

Four studies (1 open-label) have been performed with glutamine supplementation in patients with CD. No benefit from glutamine supplementation in patients who received 21 g/day ($n = 16$ with placebo), 21 g/day ($n = 38$ with placebo), 15 g/day ($n = 13$ with crossover), 42% of amino acid intake as glutamine versus 4% in the control group ($n = 18$), or 12 g/day of glutamine ($n = 9$) was observed on disease activity, intestinal permeability, or nutritional parameters,[54-57] although in the preliminary open-label study of Zoli et al, a significant decrease in intestinal permeability was described.[56] However, the pretreatment intestinal permeability in the patients studied was greater than in virtually any other study of such, and the clinical significance of this observation is unclear. Such observations have not been replicated by others.[57]

The metabolism of glutamine to nitric oxide may actually increase intestinal and colonic inflammation rather than decrease it. In addition, glutamine supplementation stimulates T cell function, which may also lead to increased inflammation. For example, Shinozaki et al observed significantly increased colonic inflammation in a rodent model of UC in those animals that received a diet supplemented with 24% glutamine.[58] The least inflammation was observed in animals that had received the least amount of glutamine. These data suggest the possibility that inflammatory bowel disease (IBD) could potentially worsen in patients who receive supplemental glutamine. Consistent with that theory is a study in children with CD where the Pediatric CD Activity Index (PCDAI) actually improved more in the control group than in the glutamine-supplemented group.[57]

A study that included 11 UC patients with pouchitis following total colectomy, IPAA, and glutamine suppositories (1 g/day for 21 days) resulted in significant clinical improvement in 6 patients. However, the follow-up period may have been too brief for this conclusion to have validity.[59]

VITAMINS AND MINERALS

Vitamin B_{12} deficiency is probably the most common vitamin deficiency encountered in patients with CD.[60] Because this vitamin is absorbed only in the terminal ileum, and the majority of patients with Crohn's have involvement of the terminal ileum, vitamin B_{12} status should be monitored and sublingual, intramuscular injection or intranasal supplementation initiated to correct

TABLE 30-1

ENTERAL FEEDING IN CROHN'S DISEASE

Author and Series	No. of Patients	Short-Term Remission (%)	Long-Term Remission (%)	Length of Follow-Up
Prospective, Uncontrolled Studies				
O'Morain (1980)	27	24 (89)	18 (67)	6 months
Lochs (1984)	25	15 (60)	12 (48)	6-24 months
O'Brien (1991)	16	10 (62)	4 (25)	12 months

a deficiency or prevent recurrent depletion. In addition, patients with > 60 cm of resected ileum should receive vitamin B_{12} routinely. Sulfasalazine is a competitive inhibitor of folate absorption.[61,62] Folate deficiency is relatively uncommon in patients with CD but may result in macrocytic anemia and/or peripheral neuropathy.[63-65] Patients who are treated with sulfasalazine should receive a dietary folate supplement.[62] Folate supplementation may be useful for the prevention of dysplasia and colon cancer in patients with Crohn's colitis.[66,67] Other water-soluble vitamin deficiencies are rare.

Fat-soluble vitamin deficiency may develop in patients with significant or long-standing steatorrhea. Vitamin A deficiency and night vision difficulty have been described in patients with CD.[68,69] Vitamin D deficiency is not uncommon in patients with CD and may be associated with calcium malabsorption and osteomalacia.[70-72] Vitamin D supplementation may help prevent osteoporosis in patients with CD,[73] although that remains controversial.[74] Vitamin E deficiency is uncommon in CD,[69-71] and low plasma concentrations may be related solely to decreased total plasma lipid concentration.[75]

Because of diarrheal losses, both zinc and selenium deficiencies may occur in CD.[76-80] Zinc deficiency has been associated with growth abnormalities, immunologic abnormalities, skin rash, and increased diarrhea. More recently, sperm dysfunction and dysmotility has been described in zinc-deficient patients with CD.[76] Selenium deficiency may be associated with neuropathy, myopathy, cardiomyopathy, and pseudoalbinism.

ENTERAL NUTRITIONAL SUPPORT

In the absence of bowel obstruction, proximal fistula, or toxic megacolon, enteral nutrition is the preferred form of nutritional support, provided that the patient will consent to placement of a nasoenteric feeding tube. Oral supplementation is generally not useful because of patient nonadherence. Enteral nutritional support may be provided to patients as *adjunctive* therapy, to promote growth and to correct and/or prevent malnutrition.

Studies have shown that the provision of enteral formula given either orally or via a feeding tube may have potential benefit as primary treatment in Crohn's patients. The composite data suggest that the administration of either an elemental (free amino acid-based), peptide-based (di- or tripeptide-based), or polymeric (intact protein) diet for 3 to 6 weeks will achieve a remission rate of approximately 68%, which is similar to the remission rate reported with TPN and bowel rest (Table 30-1).

So-called elemental diets were originally developed for the space program in the early 1960s. The idea was that consumption of a predigested diet would result in less effluent, an obvious concern in a tiny space capsule. Such dietary formulas utilize small-chain peptides and/or free amino acids as a protein source. Despite these significant differences, these products are often considered together. In the absence of intact protein, such formulas are "hypoallergenic." Many uncontrolled, anecdotal, and retrospective reports have emerged over the past 30 years that support the use of these formulas in the successful primary treatment of CD. Such reports must be tempered by the fact that many had extremely small numbers of patients, and the placebo response rate in CD often approaches 35% to 40%.[81] More recently, prospective, randomized, controlled trials have been undertaken, comparing elemental formulas to medication and polymeric (standard formula) diets. Many of these subsequent studies were also plagued by small numbers of patients. Virtually all studies have grouped patients with CD afflicting varying locations (ie, small bowel, ileocolonic, isolated colon) together. The data of Lochs et al suggest there is limited impact of dietary therapy in patients with colon involvement.[82-85] In many cases, power test calculations to estimate the necessary sample size were not performed, or many patients failed to tolerate the feeding devices or simply would not drink the formula.

Several studies either evaluated elemental diets prospectively, but without controls, or compared elemental diets and TPN (Table 30-2). O'Morain et al studied 27 patients, 24 of whom achieved short-term remission with Vivonex, although the follow-up was only 6 months.[86] O'Brien et al

TABLE 30-2

ELEMENTAL DIETS IN CROHN'S DISEASE

AUTHOR AND SERIES	NO. OF PATIENTS	SHORT-TERM REMISSION (%)		LONG-TERM REMISSION (%)		LENGTH OF FOLLOW-UP
PROSPECTIVE, UNCONTROLLED STUDIES						
		Steroids	Enteral	Steroids	Enteral	
O'Morain (1984)	21	8/10 (88)	9/11 (82)	7/10 (70)	8/11 (73)	3 months
Saverymuttu (1985)*	37	16/16 (100)	15/21 (71)			
Sanderson (1987)	17	7/8 (88)	8/9 (89)			
Malchow (1990)	95	32/44 (73)	21/51 (41)	32/44 (73)	21/51 (41)	3 months
Lochs (1991)†	107	41/52 (79)	29/55 (53)	5/8 (63)‡		
Lindor (1992)	19	7/10 (70)	3/9 (33)			

*Diet also included antibiotics
†Peptide
‡Diet + steroids

found that an elemental diet induced remission in 62% of 16 corticosteroid-refractory and corticosteroid-dependent patients, although only 25% remained in remission after 1 year.[87] Lochs et al studied 25 patients, of whom 15 (60%) achieved short-term remission with a peptide-based formula delivered via a nasogastric tube, although there was no control group.[82] Of the 7 patients who had no therapy after the tube feeding, 3 had recurrences after 6 months. Alun Jones found that 22 out of 23 patients achieved remission after a mean of 9 days following the institution of enteral feeding with Vivonex.[88] Results were similar to TPN. Cravo et al, however, achieved remission in only 50% of patients assigned to a low residual diet or an elemental diet, versus 75% with TPN.[89]

Only one study has compared an enteral formula, in this case, a peptide-based formula, to a true control—a regular hospital diet.[90] Munkholm Larsen et al reported that feeding with Pepti 2000 (Nutricia) resulted in a 30% remission rate (*n* = 9) after 2 weeks of feeding. This was the same as those who received a normal diet and is also similar to the placebo effect observed in many clinical trials.[90]

Several studies compared a free amino acid-based formula with steroids (Table 30-3). An initial small study suggested corticosteroid therapy was superior.[91] O'Morain et al found that 9 out of 11 patients who received Vivonex achieved remission at 4 weeks versus 8 out of 10 corticosteroid-treated (prednisolone 0.75 mg/kg/day) patients.[92] Remission rates at 3 months were similar in both groups. Saverymuttu et al randomized 37 patients with active CD to a normal diet and prednisolone 0.5 mg/kg/day or Vivonex (1800 to 2400 mL/day via a nasogastric tube) with nonabsorbable oral antibiotics and found that virtually all patients in both groups achieved remission.[93] However,

despite the title of the article, there was no control group for comparison. Seidman et al found that 8 out of 10 pediatric patients who received the formula (Vivonex, 50 to 80 kcal/kg/day via nasogastric tube) achieved short-term remission (at 3 weeks), although only 6 achieved long-term remission (9 weeks).[94] All corticosteroid-treated (prednisone 1 mg/kg/day) patients achieved long-term remission. The time to relapse was also significantly less in the formula-treated group (0.8 versus 1.2 years). Gorard et al found that only 11 out of 22 (50%) patients who received Vivonex achieved short-term remission.[95] Only 3 of these patients maintained long-term remission (6 months). More than 40% were intolerant of the diet. Nineteen out of 22 steroid-treated (prednisolone 0.75 mg/kg/day) patients achieved short-term remission, and 13 remained in long-term remission at 6 months.

Several studies compared peptide-based formulas and steroids (Table 30-4). Seidman et al found that 26 out of 34 (76%) pediatric patients who received Vital HN achieved short-term remission (by 4 weeks) compared to 31 out of 34 (90%) corticosteroid-treated (1 mg/kg/day) patients.[96] Long-term remission rates were not reported. Prednisone was significantly better, however, in patients with relapsed disease (versus new onset). Lindor et al found that 6 out of 9 patients who received Vital HN (40 kcal/kg/day) achieved remission at 4 weeks versus 7 out of 10 who received prednisone (0.75 mg/kg/day) and 6 out of 8 who received both.[97] Several patients could not tolerate Vital HN. After 3 months, 1 out of 2 patients in the Vital HN group relapsed, compared with 4 out of 7 prednisone-treated patients. Engelman et al reported on a small study of 11 patients with active ileocolonic CD who were randomized to receive either Peptamen (Nestle Nutrition, Minnetonka, MN) or

TABLE 30-3

DIET VS STEROIDS IN CROHN'S DISEASE

Author and Series	No. of Patients	Short-Term Remission (%)		Long-Term Remission (%)		Length of Follow-Up
Prospective, Controlled Studies						
		Steroids	**Elemental**	**Steroids**	**Elemental**	
O'Keefe (1989)	6	2/3 (67)	1/3 (33)			
Seidman (1991)	19	6/9 (67)	8/10 (80)	9/9 (100)	6/10 (60)	2.5 months
		Steroids	**Peptide**	**Steroids**	**Peptide**	
Engelman (1993)	11	4/4 (100)	7/7 (100)	4/4 (100)	7/7 (100)	6.5 months
Seidman (1993)	68	31/34 (90)	26/34 (76)			
Gorard (1993)	42	19/22 (86)	11/22 (50)	13/19 (67)	3/11 (28)	6 months
		Steroids	**Polymeric**	**Steroids**	**Polymeric**	
Ruuska (1994)	20	8/9 (89)	9/10 (90)	7/9 (78)	8/10 (80)	5 months

TABLE 30-4

ENTERAL DIETS IN CROHN'S DISEASE

Author and Series	No. of Patients	Short-Term Remission (%)		Long-Term Remission (%)		Length of Follow-Up
Prospective, Controlled Studies						
		TPN	**Elemental**	**TPN**	**Elemental**	
Alun-Jones (1987)	36	17/19 (89)	15/17 (88)			
Cravo (1991)	39	18/24 (75)	11/15 (73)	12/23 (52)	4/22 (18)	34 months
		Peptide	**Elemental**	**Peptide**	**Elemental**	
Middleton (1991)	29	11/15 (73)	11/14 (79)			
Royall (1994)	40	15/21 (71)	16/19 (84)	6/21 (29)	5/19 (26)	12 months
Mansfield (1995)	44	8/22 (36)	8/22 (36)			
		Polymeric	**Elemental**	**Polymeric**	**Elemental**	
Gaiaffer (1990)	30	5/14 (36)	12/16 (75)	8/17 (47)	8/17 (47)	6 months
Rigaud (1991)	30	11/15 (73)	10/15 (67)	4/15 (27)	3/15 (20)	12 months
Raouf (1991)	24	8/11 (73)	9/13 (69)	9/24 (38)	9/24 (38)	3 to 9 months
Park (1991)	14	5/7 (71)	2/7 (29)	1/7 (14)	0/7 (0)	12 months
Verma (2000)	21	6/11 (55)	8/10 (80)			
		Peptide	**Hospital Diet**	**Peptide**	**Hospital Diet**	
Munkholm-Larsen (1989)	19	6/11 (55)	8/10 (80)			0.5 month

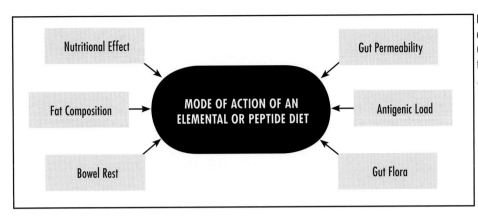

FIGURE 30-1. Mode of action of enteral diets in Crohn's disease. (Adapted from O'Sullivan MA, O'Morain CA. Nutritional therapy in Crohn's disease. *Inflamm Bowel Dis.* 1998;4:45-53.)

prednisolone (0.5 mg/kg/day).[98] All patients in both groups achieved remission after 2 weeks of therapy, and all had maintained remission at 6 months. Malchow et al randomized 95 patients in a multicenter European trial to either a peptide diet (Survimed, Fresenius) or 6-mercaptopurine (6-MP) and sulfasalazine.[99] After 6 weeks of therapy, the remission rate was significantly greater in the medication group. The results were affected by a significant dropout in the diet group because of intolerance to the product. That problem was corrected in a subsequent multicenter European trial by using nasoenteric feeding.[83] However, the results remained essentially the same. Forty-one out of 52 patients in the medication group (48 mg/day 6-MP) achieved remission after 6 weeks versus 29/55 in the diet group. In addition, time to remission was significantly longer in the diet group (31 versus 8 days).

One question that arises is whether it is necessary to use peptide and/or free amino acid-based formulas. Studies from 20 years ago indicated no efficacy of elemental diets in patients with short bowel syndrome because the nitrogen and fat from standard formula were nearly completely absorbed in the first 60 to 100 cm of the intestine. The limited data suggest that both peptide and free amino acid-based formulas may be similarly useful for the induction of short term remission, but neither is useful for sustaining long-term remission (Figure 30-1). Royall et al randomized 40 patients to receive either Vivonex TEN (elemental) or Peptamen (peptide) formula via a nasogastric tube.[100] A similar majority in each group attained remission, although this was relatively brief. Mansfield randomized patients to receive either amino acid-based or peptide-based formulas administered via NGT.[101] Some patients were corticosteroid refractory and others were not. Some patients had disease localized to the small intestine, others to the colon, and still others to both large and small bowel. Despite these shortcomings, the groups were well matched, but only 8 out of 22 patients in each group attained even short-term remission. However, despite the title "controlled trial," there was no control group with which to compare. Interestingly, superior results have been obtained in some trials with polymeric formulas, which are significantly less expensive and more palatable when compared with corticosteroid therapy.[102,103] Although polymeric formulas present an antigenic load to the gastrointestinal tract, the protein is usually of a single source, and therefore the dietary protein intake is still substantially different from a patient's usual dietary intake. The reason patients with active CD may respond to polymeric enteral formulas, but not an ad-lib regular oral diet, is unclear but may be related to the lipid composition of the enteral formula. Diets high in LCTs and polyunsaturated fats may be risk factors for the relapse of CD.

All of these studies suffered from small number of subjects and the lumping of all patients, regardless of disease location. Raouf et al randomized 24 (including 9 with ileal, 11 with ileocolonic, and 4 with colonic disease) patients to orally consume a free amino acid-based formula (E-028, Scientific Hospital Supplies, Liverpool, UK) or a polymeric formula.[104] Nine out of 13 patients who received the elemental diet achieved remission, compared to 8 out of 11 who received the polymeric formula. Zero out of 6 patients who were crossed over to the polymeric diet relapsed within 3 weeks, compared to 3 out of 7 patients who crossed over to the amino acid-based formula. Nearly 50% of all responders relapsed within 3 to 9 months, however. Verma et al reported the results of a small study in which 8 out of 10 (80%) patients who received an elemental formula via a nasogastric tube achieved remission after 4 weeks of therapy versus only 55% of a group of patients who received a polymeric formula, although the difference was not statistically different.[105] Rigaud et al randomized 30 patients to receive either Vivonex HN (elemental) or Realmentyl (Sopharga) or Nutrison (Nutricia; peptide) formula via a nasogastric tube.[106] A similar majority in each group attained remission, although this was relatively brief. Giaffer found that elemental formulas were significantly more efficacious in achieving short-term remission, but the subjects in the polymeric group were much sicker to start with (eg, lower hemoglobin, albumin and higher platelet count, and alpha-acid glycoprotein), and twice the number of patients in the Vivonex group had disease involving the small intestine that may be more responsive to nutritional therapy than colonic disease.[107] In addition, the polymeric formula was a milk-based diet. There is evidence that milk may exacerbate symptoms of CD.[108]

Five published meta-analyses, a meta-analysis of trials involving only children, and 2 *Cochrane Database Systemic Reviews* have been published of randomized controlled trials of enteral feeding in patients with CD.[109-115] Inherent in such meta-analyses is that the various formulations studied differed by nitrogen source, type and amount of fat, and MCT content. In addition, safety profiles of enteral nutrition versus corticosteroids were not compared. Enteral nutrition compares favorably with corticosteroids in this respect.[116] Dearl et al found that patients who were treated with enteral nutrition and other noncorticosteroid modalities had greater bone mineral density that those treated predominantly with corticosteroids.[117] It appears that, although formula diets may not be as effective as steroids in inducing remission in CD, the data indicate that such formula diets have a role not only in nutritional rehabilitation of these patients but as primary therapy as well given the approximately 60% of patients who achieved remission. That figure includes patients who withdrew from the therapy due to intolerance. The mechanism for this effect remains unclear. Perhaps it is simply the consumption of a sterile diet that is most important. Whether or not this relates to a bacterial cause (including bacterial remnants) for CD remains the subject of intense speculation.

Two studies from Japan have suggested a role for an elemental diet in the maintenance of remission of CD. Yamamoto et al found significantly lower mucosal cytokine concentrations and less of an increase in endoscopic disease activity scoring in 20 patients who received an elemental formula nightly via a self-inserted nasogastric tube with an infusion pump in a prospective, but nonrandomized trial.[118] Consumption of 50% of daily energy requirements via an elemental formula (vs unrestricted meals) was associated with nearly a 50% decreased rate of relapse at 1 year.[119]

The proposed mechanisms by which enteral nutrition may result in clinical remission in CD include the fact that the formula is sterile; hence, there is a decreased dietary bacterial load. Formulas using peptides or free amino acids as their nitrogen source rather than intact protein eliminate dietary protein antigens, although there are currently no data available to support a mucosal immunologic down regulation. The provision of adequate nutrition itself may have an effect on systemic immunity and/or mucosal immune function. Formulas low in fats, or specific fats, may further modulate the systemic and mucosal immune systems. In any event, these diets are not as efficacious as standard pharmacologic therapy; however, the fact that the clinical response is significantly better than placebo with these diets suggests some degree of efficacy. Although patient adherence as well as expense may be issues, it is reasonable to attempt enteral nutritional therapy with con-comitant pharmacologic therapy, although specific data to support or contradict such a combination approach are lacking, aside from a small group included in the Lindor et al study.[97] The available data do, however, suggest that less expensive and more palatable polymeric formulas are just as efficacious nutritionally as primary or adjunctive therapy as are so-called elemental formulas. Enteral nutritional therapy may be more effective in those patients with small intestinal disease.[120] Clearly, the role of enteral nutrition in the reversal of growth failure in children with CD is important.[121,122]

REFERENCES

1. Silkoff K, Hallak A, Yegena L, et al. Consumption of refined carbohydrates by patients with Crohn's disease in Tel Aviv-Yaffo. *Postgrad Med J.* 1980;56:842-846.

2. Panz E, Bianchi Porro GB. Smoking, sugar, and inflammatory bowel disease [letter]. *Br Med J.* 1985;291:971-972.

3. Jarnerot G, Jarnmark I, Nilsson K. Sugar consumption in Crohn's disease, ulcerative colitis and irritable bowel syndrome. *Scand J Gastroenterol.* 1983;28:L999-L1002.

4. Graham WB, Torrance B, Taylor TV. Breakfast and Crohn's disease (letter). *Br Med J.* 1978;2:768.

5. Thorton JR, Emmett PM, Heaton KW. Diet and Crohn's disease: characteristics of the pre-illness habit. *Br Med J.* 1979;2:762-764.

6. Mayberry JF, Rhodes J, Newcombe RG. Increased sugar consumption in Crohn's disease. *Digestion.* 1980;20:323-326.

7. Mayberry JF, Rhodes J, Allen R, et al. Diet in Crohn's disease: two studies of current and previous habits in newly diagnosed patients. *Dig Dis Sci.* 1981;26:444-448.

8. Sonnenberg A. Geographic and temporal variations of sugar and margarine consumption in relation to Crohn's disease. *Digestion.* 1988;41:161-171.

9. Kasper H, Sommer H. Dietary fiber and nutrient intake in Crohn's disease. *Am J Clin Nutr.* 1979;32:1898-1901.

10. Tragnone A, Valpiani D, Miglio F, et al. Dietary habits as risk factors for inflammatory bowel disease. *Eur J Gastroenterol Hepatol.* 1995;7:47-51.

11. Martini GA, Brandes JW. Increased consumption of refined carbohydrates in patients with Crohn's disease. *Klin Wochenschr.* 1976;54:367-371.

12. Mayberry JF, Rhodes J, Newcombe RG. Increased sugar consumption in Crohn's disease. *Digestion.* 1980;20:323-326.

13. Persson PG, Ahlbom A, Hellers G. Diet and inflammatory bowel disease: A case-control study. *Epidemiology.* 1992;3:47-52.

14. Geerling BJ, Badart-Smook A, Stockbrugger RW, Brummer RJ. Comprehensive nutritional status in recently diagnosed patients with inflammatory bowel disease compared with population controls. *Eur J Clin Nutr.* 2000;54:514-521.

15. Schutz T, Drude C, Paulisch E, et al. Sugar intake, taste changes and dental health in Crohn's disease. *Dig Dis.* 2003;21:252-257.

16. Mayberry JF, Rhodes J, Allan R, et al. Diet in Crohn's disease: two studies of current and previous habits in newly diagnosed patients. *Dig Dis Sci.* 1981;26:444-448.

17. Heaton KW, Thorton JR, Emmett PM. Treatment of Crohn's disease with an unrefined-carbohydrate, fibre-rich diet. *Br Med J.* 1979;2:764-766.

18. Ritchie JK, Wadsworth J, Lennard-Jones JE, Rogers E. Controlled multicentre therapeutic trial of an unrefined carbohydrate, fibre rich diet in Crohn's disease. *Br Med J.* 1987;295:517-520.

19. Levenstein S, Prantera C, Luzi C, D'Ubaldi A. Low residue or normal diet in Crohn's disease: a prospective controlled study in Italian patients. *Gut*. 1985;26:989-993.

20. Middleton SJ, Rucker JT, Kirby GA, et al. Long-chain triglycerides reduce the efficacy of enteral feeds in patients with active Crohn's disease. *Clin Nutr*. 1995;14:229-236.

21. Bamba T, Shimoyama T, Sasaki M, et al. Dietary fat attenuates the benefits of an elemental diet in active Crohn's disease: a randomized, controlled trial. *Eur J Gastroenterol Hepatol*. 2003;15:151-157.

22. Leiper K, Woolner J, Mulan MMC, et al. A randomised controlled trial of high versus low long chain triglyceride whole protein feed in active Crohn's disease. *Gut*. 2001;49:790-794.

23. Gassull MA, Fernandez-Banares F, Cabre E, et al. Fat composition may be a clue to explain the primary therapeutic effect of enteral nutrition in Crohn's disease: results of a double blind randomised multicentre European trial. *Gut*. 2002;51:164-168.

24. Sadeghi S, Wallace FA, Calder PC. Dietary lipids modify cytokine response to bacterial lipopolysaccharide in mice. *Immunology*. 1999;96:404-410.

25. Wanten GJ, Geijtenbeek TBH, Raymakers RAP, et al. Medium chain triglyceride-containing emusions increase human neutrophil β2 integrin expression, adhesion, and degranulation. *JPEN*. 2000;24:228-233.

26. Andoh A, Takaya H, Araki Y, et al. Medium- and long-chain fatty acids differentially modulate interleukin-8 secretion in human fetal intestinal epithelial cells. *J Nutr*. 2000;130:2636-2640.

27. Rodriguez-Palmero M, Kiss S, Fink M, et al. Effects of medium-chain triglycerides on metabolism of linoleic acid in preterm infants [abstract]. *Clin Nutr*. 1999;18:207A.

28. Gonzalez-Huix F, de Leon R, Fernandez-Banares F, et al. Polymeric enteral diets as primary treatment of active Crohn's disease: a prospective steroid controlled trial. *Gut*. 1993;34:778-782.

29. Sakuri T, Matsui T, Yuo T, et al. Short-term efficacy of enteral nutrition in the treatment of active Crohn's disease: a randomized controlled trial comparing nutrient formulas. *JPEN*. 2002;26:98-103.

30. Collins EM, Rowe AR, Uyeyama K. Allergy as a factor in disturbances of the gastrointestinal tract. *Med Clin N Am*. 1938;22:297-317.

31. Alun Jones V, Workman E, Freeman AH, et al. Crohn's disease: maintenance of remission by diet. *Lancet*. 1985;ii:177-181.

32. Riordan AM, Hunter JO, Cowan RE, et al. Treatment of active Crohn's disease by exclusion diet: East Anglian multi-centre controlled trial. *Lancet*. 1993;342:1131-1134.

33. Lee TH, Hoover RL, Williams JD, et al. Effects of dietary enrichment with eicosapentaenoic and docosahexaenoic acids on in vitro neutrophil and monocyte leukotriene generation and neutrophil function. *N Engl J Med*. 1985;312:1217-1224.

34. Mehta JL, Lopez LM, Lawson D, et al. Dietary supplementation with omega-e polyunsaturated fatty acids in patients with stable coronary heart disease. Effects on indices of platelet and neutrophil function and exercise performance. *Am J Med*. 1988;84:45-52.

35. Endres S, Ghorbani R, Kelly VE, et al. The effect of dietary supplementation with −3 polyunsaturated fatty acids on the synthesis of interleukin-1 and tumor necrosis factor by mononuclear cells. *N Engl J Med*. 1989;320:265-271.

36. Vilaseca J, Salas A, Guarner F, et al. Dietary fish oil reduces progression of chronic inflammatory lesions in a rat model of granulomatous colitis. *Gut*. 1990;31:539-544.

37. Shoda R, Matsueda K, Yamato S, Umeda N. Therapeutic efficacy of -3 polyunsaturated fatty acid in experimental Crohn's disease. *J Gastroenterol*. 1995;8:98S-101S.

38. Belluzzi A, Brignola C, Campieri M, et al. Effect of enteric coated fish oil preparations on relapses in Crohn's disease. *N Engl J Med*. 1996;334:1557-1560.

39. Lorenz-Meyer H, Nicolay C, Schulz B, et al. Omega 3 fatty acids and low carbohydrate diet for maintenance of remission in Crohn's disease: a randomized controlled multicenter trial. *Scand J Gastroenterol*. 1996;31:778-785.

40. Turner D, Zlotkin SH, Shan PS, Griffith AM. Omega 3 fatty acids (fish oil) for maintenance of remission in Crohn's disease. *Cochrane Database Syst Rev*. 2009; CD006320.

41. Scheppach W, Loges C, Bartram P, et al. Effect of free glutamine and alanyl-glutamine dipeptide on mucosal proliferation of the human ileum and colon. *Gastroenterology*. 1994;107:429-434.

42. Windmueller HG, Spaeth AE. Metabolism of absorbed aspartate, asparagine, and arginine by rat small intestine in vivo. *Arch Biochem Biophys*. 1976;175:670-676.

43. Reeds PJ, Burrin DG. Glutamine and the bowel. *J Nutr*. 2001; 131:2505S-2508S.

44. Sitren HS, Bryant M, Ellis LM. Species specific differences in TPN-induced intestinal villus atrophy [abstract]. *JPEN*. 1992;16:30S.

45. Bark T, Svenberg T, Theodorsson E, et al. Glutamine supplementation does not prevent small bowel mucosal atrophy after total parenteral nutrition in the rat. *Clin Nutr*. 1994;13:79-84.

46. Scott T, Moellman J. Intravenous glutamine supplementation fails to accelerate gut mucosal recovery following 10Gy abdominal radiation [abstract]. *JPEN*. 1991;15:17S.

47. Wusteman M, Tate H, Weaver L, et al. The effect of enteral glutamine deprivation and supplementation on the structure of rat small-intestine mucosa during a systemic injury response. *JPEN*. 1995;19:22-27.

48. Spaeth G, Gottwald T, Haas W, Holmer M. Glutamine peptide does not improve gut barrier function and mucosal immunity in total parenteral nutrition. *JPEN*. 1993;17:317-323.

49. Marks SL, Cook AK, Reader R, et al. Effects of glutamine supplementation of an amino acid-based purified diet on intestinal mucosal integrity in cats with methotrexate-induced enteritis. *Am J Vet Res*. 1999;60:755-763.

50. Horvath K, Jami M, Hill ID, et al. Short-term effect of a complete but glutamine-free oral diet on the small intestine [abstract]. *Gastroenterology*. 1994;106:A610.

51. Garrel DR, Bernier J, Jobin N. Inhibition of T lymphocyte proliferation after burn injury is abolished by low fat diet but not by glutamine [abstract]. *Clin Nutr*. 1999;18:S6.

52. Vanderhoff JA, Blackwood DJ, Mohammadpour BS, Park JHY. Effects of oral supplementation of glutamine on small intestinal mucosal mass following resection. *J Am Coll Nutr*. 1992;11:223-227.

53. Jacobs DO, Evans A, O'Dwyer ST, et al. Disparate effects of 5-fluorouracil on the ileum and colon of enterally fed rats with protection by dietary glutamine. *Surg Forum*. 1987;38:45-47.

54. Akobeng AK, Miller V, Stanton J, et al. Double-blind randomized controlled trial of glutamine-enriched polymeric diet in the treatment of active Crohn's disease. *J Pediatr Gastroenterol Nutr*. 2000; 30:78-84.

55. Cordum NR, Schloerb P, Sutton D, et al. Oral glutamine supplementation in patients with Crohn's disease with or without glucocorticoid treatment. *Gastroenterology*. 1996;110:A888.

56. Zoli G, Care M, Falco F, et al. Effect of oral glutamine on intestinal permeability and nutritional status in Crohn's disease. *Gut*. 1995; 37:A13.

57. Den Hond E, Hiele M, Peeters M, et al. Effect of long-term oral glutamine supplements on small intestinal permeability in patients with Crohn's disease. *JPEN*. 1999;23:7-11.

58. Shinozaki M, Saito H, Muto T. Excess glutamine exacerbates trinitrobenzenesulfonic acid-induced colitis in rats. *Dis Colon Rectum*. 1997;40:S59-S63.

59. Wischmeyer P, Pemberton JH, Phillips SF. Chronic pouchitis after ileal pouch-anal anastomosis: responses to butyrate and glutamine suppositories in a pilot study. *Mayo Clin Proc.* 1993;68:978-981.

60. Barton R. Macrocytic anaemias. Three fifths of patients with Crohn's disease that have not been operated on have vitamin B12 malabsorption [letter]. *Br Med J.* 1997;314:1552.

61. Selhub J, Dhar GJ, Rosenberg IH. Inhibition of folate enzymes by sulphasalazine. *J Clin Invest.* 1978;61:221-224.

62. Pironi L, Cornia GL, Ursitti MA, et al. Evaluation of oral administration of folic and folinic acid to prevent folate deficiency in patients with inflammatory bowel disease treated with salicylazosulfapyridine. *Int J Clin Pharmacol Res.* 1988;8:143-148.

63. Lossos A, Argov Z, Ackerman Z, Abramsky O. Peripheral neuropathy and folate deficiency as the first sign of Crohn's disease. *J Clin Gastroenterol.* 1991;13:442-444.

64. Elsborg L, Larsen L. Folate deficiency in chronic inflammatory bowel diseases. *Scand J Gastroenterol.* 1979;14:1019-1024.

65. Hoffbrand AV, Stewart JS, Booth CC, Mollin DL. Folate deficiency in Crohn's disease: incidence, pathogenesis, and treatment. *Br Med J.* 1968;2:71-75.

66. Mouzas IA, Papavassiliou E, Koutroubakis I. Chemoprevention of colorectal cancer in inflammatory bowel disease? A potential role for folate. *Ital J Gastroenterol Hepatol.* 1998;30:421-425.

67. Lashner BA, Provencher KS, Seidner DL, et al. The effect of folic acid supplementation on the risk for cancer or dysplasia in ulcerative colitis. *Gastroenterology.* 1997;40:485-491.

68. Main AN, Mills PR, Russell RI, et al. Vitamin A deficiency in Crohn's disease. *Gut.* 1983;24:1169-1175.

69. Bousvaros A, Zurakowski D, Duggan C, et al. Vitamins A and E serum levels in children and young adults with inflammatory bowel disease: effect of disease activity. *J Pediatric Gastroenterol Nutr.* 1998;26:129-135.

70. Harries AD, Brown R, Heatley RV, et al. Vitamin D status in Crohn's disease, association with nutriton and disease activity. *Gut.* 1985;26:1197-1203.

71. Driscoll R, Meredith S, Wagonfeld J, Rosenberg I. Bone histology and vitamin D status in Crohn's disease: assessment of vitamin D therapy [abstract]. *Gastroenterology.* 1977;72:A28.

72. Leichtmann GA, Bengoa JM, Bolt MJ, Sitrin MD. Intestinal absorption of cholecalciferol and 25-hydroxycholecalciferol in patients with both Crohn's disease and intestinal resection. *Am J Clin Nutr.* 1991;54:548-552.

73. Vogelsang H, Ferenci P, Resch H, et al. Prevention of bone mineral loss in patients with Crohn's disease by long-term oral vitamin D supplementation. *Eur J Gastroenterol Hepatol.* 1995;7:609-614.

74. Bernstein CN, Seeger LL, Anton PA, et al. A randomized, placebo-controlled trial of calcium supplementation for decreased bone density in corticosteroid-using patients with inflammatory bowel disease: a pilot study. *Aliment Pharmacol Ther.* 1996;10:777-786.

75. Kuroki F, Iida M, Tominaga M, et al. Is vitamin E depleted in Crohn's disease at initial diagnosis. *Dig Dis.* 1994;12:248-254.

76. El-Tawil AM. Zinc deficiency in men with Crohn's disease may contribute to poor sperm function and male infertility. *Andrologia.* 2003;35:337-341.

77. Brignola C, Belloli C, De Simone G, et al. Zinc supplementation restores plasma concentration of zinc and thymulin in patients with Crohn's disease. *Aliment Pharmacol Ther.* 1993;7:275-280.

78. Hendricks KM, Walker WA. Zinc deficiency in inflammatory bowel disease. *Nutr Rev.* 1988;46:401-408.

79. Kuroki F, Matsumoto T, Iida M. Selenium is depleted in Crohn's disease on enteral nutrition. *Dig Dis.* 2003;21:266-270.

80. Rannem T, Ladefoged K, Hylander E, et al. Selenium status in patients with Crohn's disease. *Am J Clin Nutr.* 1992;56:933-937.

81. Su C, Lichtenstein GR, Krok K, Brensinger CM, Lewis JD. A meta-analysis of the placebo rates of remission and response in clinical trials of active Crohn's disease. *Gastroenterology.* 2004;126:1257-1269.

82. Lochs H, Egger-Schodl AW, Schuh R, et al. Is tube feeding with elemental diets a primary therapy of Crohn's disease? *Klin Wochenschr.* 1984;62:821-825.

83. Lochs H, Steinhardt HJ, Klaus-Wentz B, et al. Comparison of enteral nutrition and drug treatment in active Crohn's disease. *Gastroenterology.* 1991;101:881-888.

84. Sanderson JR, Udeen A, Davies PSW, et al. Remission induced by an elemental diet in small bowel Crohn's disease. *Arch Dis Child.* 1987;61:123-127.

85. Giaffer MH, Cann P, Holdsworth CD. Long-term effects of elemental and exclusion diets for Crohn's disease. *Aliment Pharmacol Ther.* 1991;5:115-125.

86. O'Morain C, Segal AW, Levi AJ. Elemental diets in the treatment of acute Crohn's disease. *Br Med J.* 1980;281:1173-1175.

87. O'Brien CJ, Giaffer MH, Cann PA, Holdsworth CD. Elemental diet in steroid-dependent and steroid-refractory Crohn's disease. *Am J Gastroenterol.* 1991;86:1614-1618.

88. Alun Jones V. Comparison of total parenteral nutrition and elemental diet in induction of remission of Crohn's disease. *Dig Dis Sci.* 1987;32:100S-107S.

89. Cravo M, Camilo ME, Correia JP. Nutritional support in Crohn's disease: which route? *Am J Gastroenterol.* 1991;86:317-321.

90. Munkholm Larsen, Rasmussen D, Ronn B, et al. Elemental diet: a therapeutic approach in chronic inflammatory bowel disease. *J Intern Med.* 1989;225:325-331.

91. O'Keefe SJ, Ogden J, Rund J, Potter P. Steroids and bowel rest versus elemental diet in the treatment of patients with Crohn's disease: the effects on protein metabolism and immune function. *JPEN.* 1989;13:455-460.

92. O'Morain C, Segal AW, Levi AJ. Elemental diet as primary treatment of acute Crohn's disease: a controlled trial. *Br Med J.* 1984;288:1859-1862.

93. Saverymuttu, Hodgson HJF, Chadwick VS. Controlled trial comparing prednisolone with an elemental diet plus non-absorbable antibiotics in active Crohn's disease. *Gut.* 1985;26:994-998.

94. Seidman EG, Lohoues MJ, Turgeon J, et al. Elemental diet versus prednisone as initial therapy in Crohn's disease: early and long term results. *Gastroenterology.* 1991;100:A250.

95. Gorard DA, Hunt JB, Payne-James JJ, et al. Initial response and subsequent course of Crohn's disease treated with elemental diet or prednisolone. *Gut.* 1993;34:1198-1202.

96. Seidman E, Griffiths A, Jones A, et al. Semi-elemental diet vs prednisone in pediatric Crohn's disease. *Gastroenterology.* 1993;104:A778.

97. Lindor KD, Fleming CR, Burnes JU, et al. A randomized prospective trial comparing a defined formula diet, corticostersteroids, and a defined formula diet plus corticosteroids in active Crohn's disease. *Mayo Clin Proc.* 1992;67:394-395.

98. Engelman JL, Black L, Murphy GM, Sladen GE. Comparison of a semi elemental diet with prednisolone in the primary treatment of active ileal Crohn's disease [abstract]. *Gastroenterology.* 1993;104:A697.

99. Malchow H, Steinhardt HJ, Lorenz-Meyer H, et al. Feasibility and effectiveness of a defined-formula diet regimen in treating active Crohn's disease. *Scand J Gastroenterol.* 1990;25:235-244.

100. Royall D, Jeejeebhoy KN, Baker JP, et al. Comparison of amino acid vs peptide based enteral diets in active Crohn's disease: clinical and nutritional outcome. *Gut.* 1994;35:783-787.

101. Mansfield JC, Giaffer MH, Holdsworth CD. Controlled trial of oligopeptide versus amino acid diet in treatment of active Crohn's disease. *Gut.* 1995;36:60-66.

102. Ruuska T, Savilahti E, Maki M, et al. Exclusive whole protein enteral diet versus prednisolone in the treatment of acute Crohn's disease in children. *J Pediatr Gastroenterol Nutr.* 1994;19:175-180.

103. Park RHR, Galloway A, Danesh B, et al. Double blind trial comparing elemental and polymeric diet as primary therapy for active Crohn's disease [abstract]. *Clin Nutr.* 1989;8:79.

104. Raouf AH, Hildrey V, Daniel J, et al. Enteral feeding as sole treatment for Crohn's disease: controlled trial of whole protein vs amino acid based feed and a case study of dietary challenge. *Gut.* 1991;32:702-707.

105. Verma S, Brown S, Kirkwood B, et al. Polymeric versus elemental diet as primary treatment in active Crohn's disease: a randomized, double-blind trial. *Am J Gastroenterol.* 2000;95:735-739.

106. Rigaud D, Cosnes J, Le Quintrec Y, et al. Controlled trial comparing two types of enteral nutrition in treatment of active Crohn's disease: elemental versus polymeric diet. *Gut.* 1991;32:1492-1497.

107. Giaffer MH, North G, Holdsworth CD. Controlled trial of polymeric versus elemental diet in treatment of active Crohn's disease. *Lancet.* 1990;335:816-819.

108. Ginsberg AL, Albert MB. Treatment of patient with severe steroid-dependent Crohn's disease with nonelemental formula diet. *Dig Dis Sci.* 1989;34:1624-1628.

109. Fernandez-Banares F, Cabre E, Esteve-Comas M, Gassull MA. How effective is enteral nutrition in inducing clinical remission in active Crohn's disease? A meta-analysis of the randomized clinical trials. *JPEN.* 1995;19:356-364.

110. Messori A, Trallori G, D'Albasio G, et al. Defined-formula diets versus steroids in the treatment of active Crohn's disease. A meta-analysis. *Scand J Gastroenterol.* 1996;31:267-272.

111. Griffiths AM, Ohlsson A, Sherman PM, Sutherland LR. Meta-analysis of enteral nutrition as a primary treatment of active Crohn's disease. *Gastroenterology.* 1995;108:1056-1067.

112. Heuschkel RB, Menache CC, Megerian JT, et al. Enteral nutrition and corticosteroids in the treatment of acute Crohn's disease in children. *J Pediatr Gastroenterol Nutr.* 2000;31:905-910.

113. Zachos M, Tondeur M, Griffiths AM. Enteral nutritional therapy for inducing remission in Crohn's disease. *Cochrane Database Sys Rev.* 2001;3:CD000542.

114. Zachos M, Tondeur M, Griffiths AM. Enteral nutritional therapy for induction of remission in Crohn's disease. *Cochrane Database Syst Rev.* 2007; CD000542.

115. Dziechciarz P, Horvath A, Shamir R, Szajewska H. Meta-analysis: enteral nutrition in active Crohn's disease in children. *Aliment Pharmacol Ther.* 2007;26:795-806.

116. Buchman AL. Side effects of corticosteroids in inflammatory bowel disease. *J Clin Gastroenterol.* 2001;33:289-294.

117. Dearl KL, Compston JE, Hunter JO. Treatments for Crohn's disease that minimize steroid doses are associated with a reduced risk of osteoporosis. *Clin Nutr.* 2001;20:541-546.

118. Yamamoto T, Nakahigashi M, Saniabadi AR, et al. Impacts of long-term enteral nutrition on clinical and endoscopic disease activities and mucosal cytokines during remission in patients with Crohn's disease: a prospective study. *Inflamm Bowel Dis.* 2007; 13:1493-1501.

119. Takagi S, Utsunomiya K, Kuriyama S, et al. Effectiveness of an 'half elemental diet' as maintenance therapy for Crohn's disease: A randomized-controlled trial. *Aliment Pharmacol Ther.* 2006; 24:1333-1340.

120. Giaffer MH, Cann P, Holdsworth CD. Long-term effects of elemental and exclusion diets for Crohn's disease. *Aliment Pharmacol Ther.* 1991;5:115-125.

121. Morin CL, Roulet M, Roy CC, Weber A. Continuous elemental enteral alimentation in children with Crohn's disease and growth failure. *Gastroenterology.* 1980;79:1205-1210.

122. Motil KJ, Grand RJ, Mathews DE, et al. Whole body leucine metabolism in adolescents with Crohn's disease and growth failure during nutritional supplementation. *Gastroenterology.* 1982;82:1359-1368.

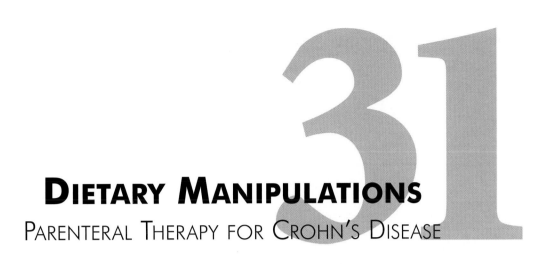

DIETARY MANIPULATIONS
PARENTERAL THERAPY FOR CROHN'S DISEASE

Alan L. Buchman, MD, MSPH

There are few prospective and prospectively controlled trials that have evaluated the use of total parenteral nutrition (TPN) either as clinical observations or compared to medical therapy alone. TPN may also be used as supportive therapy in order to maintain normal nutritional status or to correct undernutrition in patients with severe CD and, much less commonly, severe UC. Indications for TPN as a supportive therapy in patients with CD include intestinal obstruction, bowel perforation, prolonged postoperative ileus, part of a regimen to treat enterocutaneous or entero-enteric fistulae, severe malabsorption from widespread disease, and short bowel syndrome stemming from multiple bowel resections or mesenteric thrombosis related to the hypercoagulable state occasionally encountered in patients with inflammatory bowel disease (IBD).[1] In general, TPN should only be provided when insufficient nutrients and fluid cannot be delivered via the gastrointestinal tract. The use of TPN may result in increased patient charges, although not always cost; it is associated with many complications, each of which may increase morbidity and thereby increase the cost of care.[2] Retrospective observations have suggested that preoperative TPN leads to increased serum albumin concentration and weight gain[3] and decreased postoperative infection risk,[4] but it is unclear whether similar results could have been achieved with enteral feeding.

Whether the combination of complete bowel rest and TPN can be used successfully as *primary therapy* in patients with acute IBD with or without the addition of other medical therapy including diet is controversial. The consensus of the literature would suggest that patients with Crohn's enteritis might be placed into short-term clinical remission with the combination of bowel rest and parenteral nutrition

alone (Table 31-1).[5-10] The composite results suggest *nil per os* and TPN for 3 to 6 weeks will achieve a clinical response rate of 64% in patients with acute CD.[10] These studies were generally retrospective and uncontrolled. In addition, in most studies, prednisone was given simultaneously with TPN, which makes it difficult to discern whether the positive effects observed are the result of bowel rest and TPN or the combined effects of prednisone. A more recent prospective study, presented in preliminary form, in which enteral feeding was compared to parenteral feeding in a group of 25 patients with primarily CD involving the colon, found that those who received TPN had a greater improvement in clinical symptoms as well as endoscopic severity.[11] However, the consensus of the literature would suggest that patients with Crohn's colitis and idiopathic UC do not respond any better to TPN and bowel rest (with or without prednisone) than patients treated with prednisone and diet.[12-15] Although retrospective, some studies have indicated that sole therapy with TPN or TPN in addition to continued corticosteroids at the same dose may result in significant responses.[16,17] For example, 25 of 30 patients in Muller's study achieved sufficient improvement after 12 weeks of TPN so that oral diets could be resumed and the patients could return to work.[16] However, 60% of the patients relapsed after 2 years, and 85% relapsed after 4 years. Other investigators have observed similar long-term relapse rates in retrospective studies.[5,16,18] However, in all of these studies, a few patients did achieve prolonged remission with mild relapse when it occurred. Several relatively small, but prospectively performed, studies have indicated that TPN may be no better or worse than therapy with so-called elemental diets.[8,19,20] No data are available to enable the clinician to discern prospectively

Lichtenstein GR, ed.
Crohn's Disease: The Complete Guide to Medical Management (pp 361-368).
© 2011 SLACK Incorporated

TABLE 31-1

TPN IN CROHN'S DISEASE

Author and Series	No. of Patients	In-Hospital Remission (%)	TPN Duration (Days)	Long-Term Remission	Length of Follow-Up
Prospective Studies					
Elson (1980)	20	13 (65)	36	8 (40)	12 months
Meryn (1983)	25	20 (80)	27		
Muller (1983)	30	25 (83)	21	17 (57)	3-48 months
Prospective, Controlled Studies					
		Medication	**TPN**	**Medication**	**TPN**
Dickinson (1980)	9	3/3 (100)	4/6 (67)	0/3 (0)	1/6 (17)
Lochs (1983)	20	6/10 (60)	6/10 (60)	6/10 (60)	5/10 (50)
McIntyre (1986)	16	5/7 (71)	9/9 (100)	2/7 (29)	3/9 (33)
Alun-Jones (1987)	36	15/17 (88)	17/19 (89)		
Greenberg (1988)	32	9/15 (60)	12/17 (71)	6/15 (40)	8/17 (47)

which patient may benefit from TPN when used as a primary therapy and which patients might experience a prolonged remission without TPN. These data suggest that TPN may have some value for the induction of remission, but its use does not affect the natural history of CD. TPN should generally be reserved for supportive therapy to maintain nutritional reserve, rather than as primary treatment.

Intestinal fistula is one circumstance that is *nil per os*, and bowel rest may serve as primary treatment. A 38% of fistula closure rate has been reported in Crohn's patients.[14] The reported studies lack a non-TPN control group, and there generally was no long-term follow-up reported. If closure is not obvious after 3 months, surgery is usually required. A randomized study comparing TPN plus bowel rest to infliximab in addition to an oral diet is needed. Octreotide should only be used in patients with high output proximal fistulas. Octreotide is not compatible with the lipid emulsion in TPN and therefore should not be added to the solution.

HOME PARENTERAL NUTRITION

Patients may require home parenteral nutrition (HPN) because they have developed short bowel syndrome from multiple bowel resections for CD, have chronically draining enteroenteric or enterocutaneous fistulae, or have become severely malnourished in the face of active disease. Such therapy requires assessment of the home environment for appropriateness and safety, as well as proper training of either the patient or a responsible adult (especially on aseptic catheter care).

Patients with CD represent the largest subgroup of those with short bowel syndrome that require HPN. However, since the advent of surgical strictureplasty as well as medical therapy with infliximab, the incidence of new patients with CD who require HPN because of short bowel syndrome is significantly decreased compared to that encountered in the 1980s and 1990s.

Catheter infection is the most common complication associated with HPN use; however, catheter infection is no greater in the IBD group compared to other patients receiving HPN. Patients with CD have an increased 5-year survival over other groups of patients treated with HPN.[21]

CATHETER-RELATED COMPLICATIONS

The most commonly encountered catheter-related complication is infection. There are 3 types of catheter-related infections: 1) catheter sepsis, the most common[22]; 2) exit site or cuff infection (erythema or purulence at the catheter skin exit site caused by an infection in the subcutaneous cuff that anchors the catheter); and 3) tunnel infections (erythema and tenderness over the subcutaneous catheter tract), the least common.

CATHETER SEPSIS

The diagnosis of early catheter sepsis often requires a high index of suspicion. The patients with catheter-related sepsis may present with fever or shortness of breath only during TPN infusion or flushing of their catheter, prior to development of rigors, hypotension, and other systemic manifestations of sepsis. Blood bacterial and fungal cultures should be obtained from both the catheter as well as from a peripheral vein. Sufficient blood must be obtained for culture (10 to 20 mL).[23] In general, therapy should be initiated in the hospital, although patients may be discharged to home to complete their antimicrobial course as soon as they are stable. Sometimes, if the patient lives close to a medical facility and is otherwise stable, cultures can be obtained by home nurses and empiric antibiotics initiated at home.

A single bacterial count of >100 colony-forming units (cfu)/mL from the catheter or a colony count ratio of 4:1 (central versus peripheral blood) is a reliable identifier of catheter sepsis.[24,25] However, the diagnosis must often be made on a clinical basis when other potential infection sources have been excluded, especially if blood cannot be obtained from the catheter and one is considering an attempt at catheter salvage. A large variety of organisms may cause catheter infections. Most are Gram-positive bacteria, although infections with Gram-negative bacteria or fungi are frequent. Most exit site and tunnel infections are caused by *Staphylococcus* species.

TREATMENT OF CATHETER SEPSIS

TPN should be withheld for 24 hours (longer if the patient is unstable) in order to effect catheter sterilization and to prevent further bloodstream seeding. Intravenous fluids may be infused via a peripheral intravenous (IV). Aggressive initial antimicrobial therapy with broad-spectrum antibiotics such as vancomycin and an aminoglycoside such as gentamicin may be useful in keeping the mortality rate low.[22] Therapy can be adjusted once blood culture results are available.[22] A convenient antimicrobial therapy regimen should be selected that can be administered once or twice daily (eg, before and after the TPN infusion) in order to avoid excessive catheter manipulations, which are inconvenient and potentially invite the risk of yet another infection. Antimicrobial agents should be selected that are compatible with TPN, although vigorous catheter flushing can be done before and after they are infused. It has often been recommended to continue antibiotic treatment for 4 weeks if the catheter remains in situ, although the supporting data are largely anecdotal.[22] Others have used a median of 7 days of IV antibiotic therapy and have reported a <10% recurrence.[26] Scarring may occur to the central vein with catheter removal and insertion and may ultimately lead to venous occlusion. Therefore, given that long-term home TPN patients require life-long venous access, every attempt should be made to treat infections with the catheter in situ. However, catheter salvage should be attempted only for bacterial infections.

A major issue in the treatment of TPN-related infections is catheter removal. Most episodes of catheter sepsis can be treated successfully without catheter removal.[22] The catheter should always be removed with fungemia, septic shock, or failure to defervesce and should otherwise improve within 48 to 72 hours from the start of antibiotic therapy.

Increased mortality may occur in patients for whom catheter removal is delayed when fungemia is present.[27,28] Catheter replacement may be undertaken once the patient has been completely afebrile for 48 to 72 hours. Catheter removal should be followed by a week of appropriate IV antibiotics, although there are few data on optimal treatment duration. Fungal infections generally require a total dose of 100 to 250 mg of Amphotericin B in addition to catheter removal.[22] There has been little experience with fluconazole and other antifungal treatment in this setting.[29]

The antibiotic lock technique, in which a highly concentrated antibiotic solution is instilled into the catheter in a volume sufficient only to fill the catheter, twice daily (eg, before and after TPN infusion) for 1 to 2 weeks has been described more recently for treatment of patients with uncomplicated catheter sepsis.[30-32] Success rates have been reported to be >90%, although treatment of fungemia has not generally been effective.[31] Amikacin (1.5 mg/mL), gentamicin (5 mg/mL), minocycline (0.2 mg/mL), and vancomycin (1.0 to 5.0 mg/mL) have been used. The antibiotic lock technique is much less expensive than the delivery of systemic antibiotics, appears to be more successful (although the currently available data are rather limited), and is more convenient for the patient.

CATHETER CARE

Catheter care technique is arguably the most important determinant of the risk of catheter infection.[22,33] Contamination of the catheter skin exit site[34] and catheter hub[35-37] are the primary sources for infections. Proper cleaning of these sites is essential. Evidence suggests that the nurse's or patient's hand may contaminate both the exit site and catheter hub during catheter manipulations, including connecting or disconnecting TPN.[38] Even a single inoculum may be sufficient to result in catheter sepsis for virulent organisms such as *Pseudomonas aeruginosa*.[39] Endoluminal bacterial seeding begins with hub contamination at the junction between the catheter and infusion line.[37] Luer locks themselves have no antibacterial properties and require strict aseptic manipulation. Improvement in catheter hub care results in significantly decreased infection risk.[37,40] This includes avoidance of 3-way stopcocks because of the risk of hub contamination.[41,42]

EXIT SITE AND TUNNEL INFECTIONS

Most exit site and tunnel infections are caused by skin flora, most notably the *Staphylococcus* species.[22] Purulent drainage from the exit site should be cultured and initial therapy provided with IV vancomycin until culture results are available.[22,43] Neither exit site nor tunnel infections are systemic infections and are rarely associated with fever or leukocytosis. However, delayed treatment may lead to more serious sequelae. Duration of therapy has been recommended for 2 weeks, although the data are largely anecdotal.[22,43] Most exit site infections can be treated successfully without catheter removal[22]; however, antibiotic penetration of the subcutaneous tunnel is suboptimal. Therefore, catheter removal is required for tunnel infections.

CATHETER DRESSINGS AND DRESSING CHANGES

Less frequent dressing changes and the use of gauze rather than transparent polyurethane dressings have been associated with a lower risk for catheter infection.[44-49] Increased bacterial colonization was noted under the transparent dressings. This may result in part from moisture accumulation under such dressings. These data are from inpatient populations. There have been no studies on the optimal frequency for dressing changes in home TPN patients who have tunneled or peripherally inserted central catheters. Similarly, no studies have compared gauze to transparent dressings in home TPN patients. It is unclear whether the results from inpatient studies can be generalized to this patient group.

CATHETER OCCLUSIONS

Occlusions are the second most common catheter-related problem. These may occur because of thrombus, precipitate formation, or mechanical problems.

THROMBOSIS

Thrombosis generally results from disruption of the intimal surface of the vein followed by development of a fibrin sheath around the catheter.[50,51] Although catheter thrombosis is relatively uncommon, if unrecognized and untreated, it may lead to the need for catheter removal and long-term loss of a venous access site. Over time (>10 years in some cases), thrombosed veins may recanalize. The incidence of catheter thrombosis is greater in some patients, such as those with a history of mesenteric venous thrombosis, and the incidence of subclinical catheter thrombosis may be much greater.[52-54] It is unknown whether blood clots found on routine, scheduled catheter checks result in development of clinically significant thromboses.

Very low-dose warfarin (1 to 2 mg daily) does not alter the prothrombin time or activated partial thromboplastin time but may prevent catheter thrombosis.[55] This may be related to incomplete but critical inhibition of vitamin K-dependent factors.[56-59] Patients who develop catheter thrombosis despite low-dose warfarin should be fully anticoagulated as long as they require home TPN.[59,60] Anticoagulation may require increased warfarin for patients who receive more lipid emulsion because vitamin K is intrinsically contained in lipid emulsions.[61] Vitamin K-containing multivitamins should not be used in patients who require warfarin anticoagulation. Long-term heparin use is not recommended because of the risk of osteoporosis,[62] although low-molecular-weight heparin may have less detrimental effects on bone than unfractionated heparin.[63] Intravenous heparin is incompatible with lipid emulsion (which has significance with the increased use of 3-in-1 emulsions),[64] although catheter flushing with heparin 100 µ/mL (0.6 to 3 mL, depending on the catheter volume) is recommended.[65] There are limited data on the use of low-molecular-weight heparin in home TPN patients.

Catheter thrombosis may be treated using urokinase (5000 µ/mL, 2 mL for tunneled catheters and 1 mL for ports)[43,66,67] or tissue plasminogen activator (TPA, 2 mg/mL, 2 mL for tunneled catheters and 1 mL for ports).[68,69] If medical treatment is unsuccessful, removal and replacement in another site is necessary. Thrombosed veins may recanalize over several years, and it may be possible to reuse a former site for catheter placement.

NONTHROMBOTIC OCCLUSION

Up to 50% of nonthrombotic occlusions may be related to mechanical problems with the catheter. These include catheter migration from the superior or inferior vena cava into a smaller vessel, damage to the catheter,[67,70,71] medication-TPN incompatibilities leading to precipitation within the catheter,[72-76] and lipid deposition within the catheter.[77] Hydrochloric acid dissolves some mineral and medication precipitates that form because of low calcium/phosphate solubility in TPN solutions. This occurs most frequently when medications that have a low acid dissociation constant are used in the TPN solutions.[72-76] Sodium hydroxide (0.1 N) may also dissolve some mineral precipitates although it may require up to 6 to 7 hours after instillation into the catheter before any attempt at aspiration can be made.[76] Ethanol may be used to dissolve waxy lipid deposits around the catheter.[75,77]

BILIARY DISEASE

Home TPN patients are at risk for both acalculous and calculous cholecystitis.[78] Acalculous cholecystitis occurs because of decreased food-mediated cholecystokinin (CCK) release, which results in decreased gallbladder function.[79,80] Narcotic use, bile stasis, and increased bile lithogenecity may decrease gallbladder contraction.[79-81] Massive gallbladder dilation may develop; percutaneous cholecystostomy is required for drainage. The gallbladder dysmotility and abnormal emptying during TPN may result in false-positive iminodiacetic (IDA) hepatic scintigraphy,[81-83] although the use of an IV morphine bolus injection may improve scan specificity.[83] Patients should be encouraged to eat on a daily basis, even if they are completely TPN dependent because of severe malabsorption, in order to insure adequate gallbladder emptying and to help prevent development of cholecystitis.

Biliary sludge develops in 50% of patients following 4 to 6 weeks of TPN and in virtually 100% of patients after 6 weeks of TPN.[84,85] Some of these patients will ultimately develop gallstones. However, sludge resolves in virtually all patients following 4 weeks of enteral/oral refeeding.[84]

Gallbladder stasis may be the most important risk factor for the development of gallstones, similar to acalculous cholecystitis.[86,87] However, most gallstones found in patients who receive long-term TPN are calcium-bilirubinate in composition, rather than cholesterol.[88-90] This suggests the possibility that a chronic infectious process involving the biliary tree may play a role in the stone formation, although the exact etiology for pigmented stones is uncertain.[91]

CCK injections have been used to induce gallbladder contraction and reduce the prevalence of biliary sludge.[92-95] However, this treatment is not universally successful and has been associated with cholecystitis, nausea, and flushing in some patients.[92-94] Rapid, high-dose intravenous amino acid infusions (0.3 to 2.1 g/min versus 0.12 to 0.14 g/min for cyclic HPN patients) have also been used to stimulate gallbladder contraction.[96,97] However, this approach is clinically impractical, and lower amino acid infusion rates do not generally stimulate gallbladder contraction.[97] Relatively rapid infusion of lipid emulsion (10% emulsion @ 100 mL/hour for 3 hours) also stimulates gallbladder contraction and may be useful preventative therapy.[98,99] This may be mediated via CCK release,[100] although presumably the effect would be centrally mediated. Intravenous chenodeoxycholate infusion has shown promise in the prairie dog model for the prevention of calcium bilirubinate gallstones, although it has not been studied in humans.[101] The prevention of calculous cholecystitis still remains suboptimal in HPN patients. That has led some to recommend prophylactic cholecystectomy in patients. The best and least expensive means to prevent cholecystitis in HTPN patients is to simply encourage patients to eat.

Renal, hepatic, and bone disease associated with malabsorption and longer-term parenteral nutrition may also occur. These complications have been reviewed elsewhere.[102-105]

REFERENCES

1. Talbot RW, Heppell J, Dozois RR, Beart RW Jr. Vascular complications of inflammatory bowel disease. *Mayo Clin Proc.* 1989;61:140-145.

2. Buchman AL. Complications of home total parenteral nutrition. *Dig Dis Sci.* 2001;46:1-18.

3. Gouzma DJ, von Meyenfeldt MF, Rouflart M, et al. Preoperative total parenteral nutrition in severe Crohn's disease surgery. *Surgery.* 1988;103:648-662.

4. Rombeau JL, Barot LR, Williamson CE, Mullen JL. Preoperative total parenteral nutrition and surgical outcome in patients with inflammatory bowel disease. *Am J Surg.* 1982;143:139-143.

5. Ostro MJ, Greenberg GR, Jeejeebhoy KN. Total parenteral nutrition and complete bowel rest in the management of Crohn's disease. *JPEN.* 1985;9:280-287.

6. Reilly J, Ryan JA, Stole W, et al. Hyperalimentation in inflammatory bowel disease. *Am J Surg.* 1976;131:192-200.

7. Mullen JL, Hargrove WC, Dudrick SJ, et al. Ten years experience with intravenous hyperalimentation and inflammatory bowel disease. *Ann Surg.* 1978;187:523-529.

8. Greenberg GR, Fleming CR, Jeejeebhoy KN. Controlled trial of bowel rest and nutritional support in the management of Crohn's disease. *Gut.* 1988;29:1309-1315.

9. Lochs SH, Meryn S, Marosi L, et al. Does total bowel rest have a beneficial effect in the treatment of Crohn's disease. *Clin Nutr.* 1983;2:61-64.

10. Greenberg GR. Nutritional management of inflammatory bowel disease. *Semin Gastrointest Dis.* 1993;4:69-86.

11. Dickinson RJ, Ashton MG, Axon AT, et al. Controlled trial of intravenous hyperalimentation and bowel rest as an adjunct to routine therapy of acute colitis. *Gastroenterology.* 1980;79:1199-1204.

12. Sitzmann JV, Converse RL, Bayless TM. Favorable response to parenteral nutrition and medical therapy in Crohn's colitis. *Gastroenterology.* 1990;99:1647-1652.

13. Afonso JJ, Rombeau JL. Nutritional care for patients with Crohn's disease. *Hepatogastroenterology.* 1990;37:32-41.

14. Scolapio JS, Fleming CR, Kelly DG, et al. Survival of home parenteral nutrition treated patients: 20 year experience at the Mayo Clinic. *Mayo Clinic Proc.* 1999;74:217-222.

15. Lerebours E, Messing B, Chevalier B, et al. An evaluation of total parenteral nutrition in the management of steroid-dependent and steroid-resistant patients with Crohn's disease. *JPEN.* 1986;10:274-278.

16. Muller JM, Keller HW, Erasmi H, et al. Total parenteral nutrition as the sole therapy in Crohn's disease—a prospective study. *Br J Surg.* 1983;70:40-43.

17. Kushner RF, Shapir J, Sitrin MD. Endoscopic, radiographic, and clinical response to prolonged bowel rest and home parenteral nutrition in Crohn's disease. *JPEN.* 1986;10:568-573.

18. Wright RA, Adler EC. Peripheral parenteral nutrition is no better than enteral nutrition in acute exacerbations of Crohn's disease: a prospective trial. *J Clin Gastroenterol.* 1990;86:317-321.

19. Jones A. Comparison of total parenteral nutrition and elemental diet in induction of remission of Crohn's disease. *Dig Dis Sci.* 1987;32:100S-107S.

20. Rigaud D, Cerf M, Melchlor C, et al. Nutritional assistance and acute attacks of Crohn's disease: efficacy of total parenteral nutrition as compared with elemental and polymeric enteral nutrition [abstract]. *Gastroenterology.* 1989;96:A416.

21. Elson CO, Layden TJ, Nemchausky BA, et al. An evaluation of total parenteral nutrition in the management of inflammatory bowel disease. *Dig Dis Sci.* 1980;25:42-48.

22. Buchman AL, Moukarzel A, Goodson B, et al. Catheter-related infections associated with home parenteral nutrition and predictive factors for the need for catheter removal in their treatment. *JPEN.* 1994;18:297-302.

23. Mermel LA, Maki DG. Detection of bacteremia in adults: consequences of culturing an inadequate volume of blood. *Ann Intern Med.* 1993;119:270-272.

24. Mosca R, Curtas S, Forbes B, Meguid MM. The benefits of isolated cultures in the management of suspected catheter sepsis. *Surgery.* 1987;102:718-723.

25. Capdevilla JA, Planes AM, Palomar M, et al. Value of differential quantitative blood cultures in the diagnosis of catheter-related sepsis. *Eur J Microbiol Infect Dis.* 1992;11:403-407.

26. Rannen T, Ladefofed K, Tvede M, Lorentzen JE, Jarnum S. Catheter-related septicaemia in patients receiving home parenteral nutrition. *Scand J Gastroenterol.* 1986;21:455-460.

27. Lecciones JA, Lee JW, Navarro EE, et al. Vascular catheter-associated fungemia in patients with cancer: analysis of 155 episodes. *Clin Infect Dis.* 1992;14:875-883.

28. Dato VM, Dajani AS. Candidemia in children with central venous catheters: role of catheter removal and amphotericin B therapy. *Pediatr Infect Dis J.* 1990;9:309-314.

29. Rex JH, Bennett JE, Sugar AM, et al. Intravenous catheter exchange and duration of Candidemia. *Clin Infect Dis.* 1995;21:994-996.

30. Messing B, Peitra-Cohen S, Debure A, Beliah M, Bernier JJ. Antibiotic-lock technique: a new approach to optimal therapy for catheter-related sepsis in home-parenteral nutrition patients. *JPEN.* 1988;12:185-189.

31. Benoit JL, Carandang G, Sitrin M, Arnow PM. Intraluminal antibiotic treatment of central venous catheter infections in patients receiving parenteral nutrition at home. *Clin Infect Dis.* 1995;21:1286-1288.

32. Krzywda EA, Andris DA, Edmiston CE Jr, Quebbeman EJ. Treatment of Hickman catheter sepsis using antibiotic lock technique. *Infect Control Hosp Epidemiol.* 1996;16:596-598.

33. Keohane PP, Attrill H, Northover J, Jones BJM, Cribb A, Frost P. Effect of catheter tunneling and a nutrition nurse on catheter sepsis during parenteral nutrition. *Lancet.* 1983;2:1388-1390.

34. O'Keefe SJD, Burnes JU, Thompson RL. Recurrent sepsis in home parenteral nutrition patients: an analysis of risk factors. *JPEN.* 1994;18:256-263.

35. Sitges-Serra A, Linears J, Garau J. Catheter sepsis: the clue is the hub. *Surgery.* 1985;97:355-357.

36. Salzman MB, Rubin LG. Relevance of the catheter hub as a portal for microorganisms causing catheter-related bloodstream infections. *Nutrition.* 1997;13:15S-17S.

37. Stotter AT, Ward H, Waterfield AH, Hilton J, Sim AJW. Junctional care: the key to prevention of catheter sepsis in intravenous feeding. *JPEN.* 1987;11:159-162.

38. De Cicco M, Panarello G, Chiaradia V, et al. Source and route of microbial colonization of parenteral nutrition catheters. *Lancet.* 1989;2:1258-1261.

39. Segura M, Alia C, Valverde J, Franch G, Rodriguez JMT, Sitges-Serra A. Assessment of a new hub design and the semiquantitative catheter culture methods using an in vivo experimental model of catheter sepsis. *J Clin Microbiol.* 1990;28:2551-2554.

40. Sitges-Serra A, Puig P, Linaires J, et al. Hub colonization as the initial step in an outbreak of catheter-related sepsis due to coagulase-negative staphylococci during parenteral nutrition. *JPEN.* 1984;8:668-672.

41. Brismar B, Jordahl L, Nystrom B, Pettersson N. Bacterial contamination of intravenous line side ports of different designs. *Clin Nutr.* 1987;6:31-33.

42. Snydman DR, Murray SA, Kornfield EJ, Majka JA, Ellis CA. Total parenteral nutrition-related infections. *Am J Med.* 1982;73:695-699.

43. Buchman AL. *Practical Nutritional Support Techniques.* 2nd ed. SLACK Incorporated: Thorofare, NJ; 2003:211.

44. Stebbins J, O'Neill M, Steiger E. The effect of decreased catheter care on primary sepsis rate in central venous catheters (CVC) used in parenteral nutrition [abstract]. *JPEN.* 1989;13:16S.

45. Powell C, Regan C, Fabri PJ, Ruberg RL. Evaluation of opsite catheter dressings for parenteral nutrition, a prospective, randomized trial. *JPEN.* 1982;6:43-46.

46. Anderson PT, Herlevsen P, Schaumburg H. A comparative study of "op-site" and "nobecutan gauze" dressings for central venous line care. *J Hosp Infect.* 1986;7:161-168.

47. Conly JM, Grieves K, Peters B. A prospective, randomized study comparing transparent and dry gauze dressings for central venous catheters. *J Infect Dis.* 1989;159:310-319.

48. Hoffman KK, Weber DJ, Samsa GP, Rutala WA. Transparent polyurethane film as an intravenous catheter dressing. *JAMA.* 1992;267:2072-2076.

49. Powell CR, Traetow MJ, Fabri PJ, et al. Op-site dressing study: a prospective randomized study evaluating povidone-iodine ointment and extension set changes with 7-day op-site dressings applied to total parenteral nutrition subclavian sites. *JPEN.* 1985;9:443-446.

50. Hashal VL Jr, Ause RG, Hoskins PA. Fibrin sleeve formation on indwelling subclavian central venous catheters. *Arch Surg.* 1971; 102:353-358.

51. Cassidy FP, Zajko AB, Bron KM, Reilly JJ, Peitzman AB, Steel DL. Noninfectious complications of long-term central venous catheters: radiologic evaluation and management. *Am J Radiol.* 1987;149:671-675.

52. Burt ME, Dunnick NR, Drudy AG, Maher MM, Brennan MF. Prospective evaluation of subclavian vein thrombosis during total parenteral nutrition by contrast venography [abstract]. *Clin Res.* 1981;20:264A.

53. Bozzetti F, Scarpa D, Terno G, et al. Subclavian venous thrombosis due to indwelling catheters: A prospective study on 52 patients. *JPEN.* 1983;7:560-562.

54. Fabri PJ, Mirtalo JM, Ruberg RL, et al. Incidence and prevention of thrombosis of the subclavian vein during total parenteral nutrition. *Surg Gyne Obstet.* 1982;155:238-240.

55. Bern MM, Bothe A, Bistrian BR, Champagne CD, Keane MS, Blackburn GL. Prophylaxis against central venous vein thrombosis with low dose warfarin. *Surgery.* 1986;99:216-221.

56. Bern MM, Lokich JJ, Wallach SR, et al. Very low dose warfarin can prevent thrombosis in central venous catheters. *Ann Intern Med.* 1990;112:423-428.

57. Wessler T, Gittel SN, Bank H, Martinowitz U, Stephenson RC. An assay of the antithrombotic action of warfarin. Its correlation with the inhibition of stasis thrombosis in rabbits. *Thromb Haemost.* 1978;40:486-496.

58. Bertina RM, Westhoek-Kuipers MEJ, Alderkamp GHJ. The inhibitor of prothrombin conversion in plasma of patients on oral anticoagulant treatment. *Thromb Haemost.* 1981;45:237-241.

59. Gittel SN, Wessler S. Dose-dependent antithrombotic effect of warfarin in rabbits. *Blood.* 1983;61:435-438.

60. Veerabagu MP, Tuttle-Newhall J, Maliakkal R, Champagne C, Mascioli EA. Warfarin and reduced central venous thrombosis in home total parenteral nutrition patients. *Nutrition.* 1995;11:142-144.

61. Lutomski DM, Palascak JE, Bower RH. Warfarin resistance associated with intravenous lipid administration. *JPEN.* 1987;11:316-318.

62. Griffith GC, Nichols G, Asher JD, Flanaghan B. Heparin osteoporosis. *JAMA.* 1965;193:85-88.

63. Pettila V, Leinonen P, Markkola A, Hiilesmaa V, Kaaja R. Postpartum bone density in women treated for thromboprophylaxis with unfractionated heparin or LMW heparin. *Thromb Haemost.* 2002;87:182-186.

64. Johnson OL, Washington C, Davis SS, Schaupp K. The destabilization of parenteral feeding emulsions by heparin. *Int J Pharm.* 1989;53:237-240.

65. Moreno JM, Valero MA, Gomis P, Leon-Sanz M. Central venous catheter occlusion in home parenteral nutrition patients [letter]. *Clin Nutr.* 1998;17:35-36.

66. Glynn MFX, Langer B, Jeejeebhoy KN. Therapy for thrombotic occlusion of long-term intravenous alimentation catheters. *JPEN.* 1980;4:387-390.

67. Stephens LC, Haire WD, Kotulak GD. Are clinical signs accurate indicators of the cause of central venous catheter occlusion? *JPEN.* 1995;19:75-79.

68. Atkinson JB, Bagnall HA, Gomperts E. Investigational use of tissue plasminogen activator (t-PA) for occluded central venous catheters. *JPEN.* 1990;14:310-311.

69. Semba CP, Deitcher SR, Li X, Resnansky L, Tu T, McClusky ER. Treatment of occluded central venous catheters with alteplase: results in 1,064 patients. *J Vasc Interv Radiol.* 2002;13:1199-1205.

70. Johnson RL, Lieberman RP, Kaplan PA, Haire WD. Silicone rubber catheter venography using standard angiographic techniques. *Cardiovasc Interventional Radiol.* 1988;11:45-49.

71. Cassidy FP, Zajiko AB, Bron KM, Reilly JJ, Peitzman AB, Stead DL. Noninfectious complications of long-term central venous catheters: radiologic evaluation and management. *Am J Radiol.* 1987;149:671-675.

72. Breaux CW, Duke D, Georgeson KE, Mestre JR. Calcium phosphate crystal occlusion of central venous catheters used for total parenteral nutrition in infants and children: prevention and treatment. *J Pediatr Surg.* 1987;22:829-832.

73. Shulman RJ, Reed T, Pitre D, Laine L. Use of hydrochloric acid to clear obstructed central venous catheters. *JPEN.* 1988;12:509-510.

74. Pennington CR, Pithie AD. Ethanol lock in the management of catheter occlusion. *JPEN.* 1987;11:507-508.

75. Werlin SL, Lausten T, Jessen S, et al. Treatment of central venous catheter occlusions with ethanol and hydrochloric acid. *JPEN.* 1995;19:416-418.

76. Sando K, Fujii M, Tanaka K, et al. Lock method using sodium hydroxide solution to clear occluded central venous access devices. *Clin Nutr.* 1997;16:185-188.

77. Johnston DA, Walker K, Richards J, Pennington CR. Ethanol flush for the prevention of catheter occlusion. *Clin Nutr.* 1992;11:97-100.

78. Roslyn JJ, Pitt HA, Mann LL, Ament ME, DenBesten L. Gallbladder disease in patients on long-term parenteral nutrition. *Gastroenterology.* 1983;84:148-154.

79. Flati G, Flati D, Jonsson PE, et al. Role of cholesterol and calcium bilrubinate crystals in acute postoperative acalculous cholecystitis. *Ital J Surg Sci.* 1984;14:333-336.

80. Deitch EA, Engel JM. Acute acalculous cholecystitis. *Am J Surg.* 1983;142:290-292.

81. Warner BW, Hamilton FN, Silberstein EB, et al. The value of hepatobiliary scans in fasted patients receiving total parenteral nutrition. *Surgery.* 1987;102:595-601.

82. Schuman WP, Gibbs P, Rudd TG, Mack LA. PIPIDA scintigraphy for cholecystitis: false positive in alcoholism and total parenteral nutrition. *Surgery.* 1987;102:595-601.

83. Flancbaum L, Alden SM. Morphine cholescintigraphy. *Surg Gynecol Obstet.* 1990;171:227-232.

84. Messing B, Bories C, Kunstlinger F, Bernier JJ. Does total parenteral nutrition induce gallbladder sludge formation and lithiasis? *Gastroenterology.* 1983;84:1012-1019.

85. Messing B, Aprahamian M, Rautureau M, Baries C, Bisalli A, Stock-Damge S. Gallstone formation during total parenteral nutrition: a prospective study in man [abstract]. *Gastroenterology.* 1984;86:1183.

86. Roslyn JJ, Denbesten L, Pitt HA, Kuchenbecker S, Polarek JW. Effect of cholecystokinin on gallbladder stasis and cholesterol gallstone formation. *J Surg Res.* 1981;30:200-204.

87. Mashako MNK, Cezard JP, Boige N, Chayvialle JA, Bernard C, Navarro J. The effect of artificial feeding on cholestasis, gallbladder sludge and lithiasis in infants: correlation with plasma cholecystokinin levels. *Clin Nutr.* 1991;10:320-327.

88. Allen B, Bernhoft R, Blanckaert N, et al. Sludge is calcium bilirubinate associated with bile stasis. *Am J Surg.* 1981;141:51-56.

89. Pitt HA, Berquist WE, Mann LL, et al. Parenteral nutrition induces calcium bilirubinate gallstones (abstr.). *Gastroenterology.* 1983;84:1274.

90. O'Brien CB, Berman JM, Fleming CR, Malet PF, Soloway RD. Total parenteral nutrition gallstones contain more calcium bilirubinate than sickle cell gallstones [abstract]. *Gastroenterology.* 1986;90:1752.

91. Stewart L, Smith L, Pellegrini CA, Matson RW, Way LW. Pigment gallstones form as a composite of bacterial microcolonies and pigment solids. *Ann Surg.* 1987;206:242-250.

92. Doty JE, Pitt HA, Porter-Fink V, Denbesten L. Cholecystokinin prophylaxis of parenteral nutrition-induced gallbladder disease. *Ann Surg.* 1985;201:76-80.

93. Sitzman JV, Pitt HA, Steinborn PA, Pasha ZR, Sanders RC. Cholecystokinin prevents parenteral nutrition induced biliary sludge in humans. *Surg Gynecol Obstet.* 1990;170:25-31.

94. Apelgren KN, Willard DA, Vargish T. TPN alters gallbladder responsivity to cholecystokinin [abstract]. *JPEN.* 1988;12:11S.

95. Dawes LG, Muldoon JP, Greiner MA, Bertolotti M. Cholecystokinin increases bile acid synthesis with total parenteral nutrition but does not prevent stone formation. *J Surg Res.* 1997;67:84-89.

96. de Boer SY, Masclee AAM, Lam WF, Jansen JBMJ, Lamers CBHW. Intravenous amino acids stimulate gallbladder contraction [abstract]. *Gastroenterology.* 1993;104:A358.

97. Kalfarentzos F, Vagenas C, Michail A, et al. Gallbladder contraction after administration of intravenous amino acids and long-chain triacylglycerols in humans. *Nutrition.* 1991;7:347-349.

98. Doty JE, Pitt HA, Porter-Fink V, Denbesten L. The effect of intravenous fat and total parenteral nutrition on biliary physiology. *JPEN.* 1984;8:263-268.

99. Priori P, Lezzilli R, Panuccio D, Nardi R, Gullo L. Stimulation of gallbladder emptying by intravenous lipids. *JPEN.* 1997;21:350-352.

100. Guedon C, Ducrotte P, Chayvialle JA, Lerebours E, Denis P, Colin R. Effect of intravenous and intraduodenal fat on jejunal motility and on plasma cholecystokinin in man. *Dig Dis Sci.* 1988;33:558-564.

101. Broughton G, Fitzgibbons RJ Jr, Geiss RW, Adrian TE, Anthone G. IV chenodeoxycholate prevents calcium bilirubinate gallstones during total parenteral nutrition in the prairie dog. *JPEN.* 1996;20:187-193.

102. Buchman AL. Complications of home total parenteral nutrition. *Dig Dis Sci.* 2001;46:1-18.

103. Buchman AL, Ament ME, Moukarzel A, et al. The impairment of renal function is associated with long term parenteral nutrition. *JPEN.* 1993;17:438-444.

104. Buchman AL, Moukarzel AA. Metabolic bone disease associated with TPN. *Clin Nutr.* 2000;19:217-231.

105. Buchman AL. Total parenteral nutrition-associated liver disease. *JPEN.* 2002;26:S43-S48.

32

GASTRODUODENAL/PROXIMAL CROHN'S DISEASE

Ellen J. Scherl, MD, FACP, AGAF; Brian P. Bosworth, MD; Felice Schnoll-Sussman, MD; Douglas M. Weine, MD; and Peter H. R. Green, MD

Proximal Crohn's disease involving the stomach, duodenum, and jejunum is becoming increasingly recognized as a result of both better diagnostic tools, such as conventional upper endoscopy, chromoendoscopy, and wireless capsule endoscopy (WCE), as well as improved histologic characterization (eg, focally enhanced gastritis in the absence of *Helicobacter pylori*). CD and colitis may thus be a more proximal disease than previously recognized. As many as 30% to 50% of patients with established CD will have upper gastrointestinal involvement.[1] Though the symptoms of gastroduodenal CD include dyspepsia, epigastric pain, early satiety, nausea, and vomiting, many patients with proximal CD will initially present with abdominal cramping or pain and generalized malaise. Some gastroduodenal Crohn's patients, however, may be entirely asymptomatic and have no upper intestinal complaints.[2,3] In addition to evaluating the impact of medical therapy on proximal CD, diagnosing proximal CD may favorably impact medical therapy for ileitis and colitis.

DEFINITION

CD occurs most frequently either as ileitis, ileocolitis, or colitis alone. Proximal CD occurs less often. The prevalence depends on how proximal CD is defined; ie, clinically radiographically, endoscopically, or histologically.[4] A widely accepted diagnosis of duodenal CD requires (1) histologic presence of noncaseating granulomas and duodenitis with or without documented CD elsewhere and (2) absence of systemic granulomatous disease and radiologic and/or endoscopic diffuse Crohn's-like inflammation of the duodenum.[1] Many patients with meticulous histologic evaluation may meet these criteria even though they are asymptomatic. Symptoms alone should not be used as an indication for upper endoscopy in the diagnostic workup of CD.

Those patients who are symptomatic usually present with atypical epigastric pain, retrosternal pain, eructation, anorexia, weight loss, and cachexia. This definition of proximal CD may be expanded from duodenal involvement to include esophageal, gastric, and jejunal CD.[5] When both a dedicated upper gastrointestinal (GI)/small bowel series as well as an upper endoscopy with multiple biopsies are performed in patients with documented distal Crohn's ileitis, ileocolitis, or colitis, some patients are then found to have proximal disease. A subset of radiographically—*H. pylori* and nonsteroidal anti-inflammatory drug (NSAID)—negative patients with focally enhanced gastritis have proximal CD.[6-10] Upper endoscopy as well as WCE will more accurately define the true prevalence of proximal Crohn's disease.

DIAGNOSTIC MODALITIES

RADIOLOGY

Although the early detection of proximal CD by upper GI/small bowel series has a lower accuracy than either upper endoscopy or WCE, its role in the diagnosis of CD remains helpful.[11-15] Radiologic features of proximal CD include nodularity, cobblestoning, narrowing of the antrum, and slowed gastric emptying. Antroduodenal CD may have

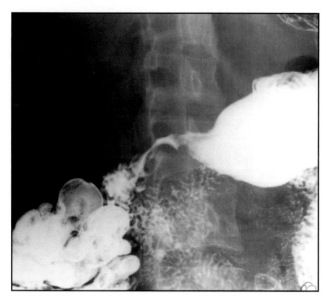

FIGURE 32-1. "Ram's horn" sign of antroduodenal Crohn's disease.

a pathognomonic funnel-like contour, creating a "ram's horn" sign (Figure 32-1).[16] In cases of pyloric obstruction, gastric dilation and delayed gastric emptying is common. A fixed stenotic duodenum may appear as a string sign and occasionally may present with proximal dilation of the duodenum and even megaduodenum (Figure 32-2). An isolated duodenal stricture, without known peptic ulcer disease or NSAID use, raises the question of duodenal CD. This further underscores the importance of performing a dedicated small bowel series and endoscopy to determine the existence of and extent of underlying Crohn's.[17]

Gastrocolic fistulas identified on radiologic imaging are more common than duodenocolic fistulas. Both lesions originate from the bowel in areas with active or inactive colitis (less frequently ileitis), often requiring barium enema for diagnosis. In addition to primary sclerosing cholangitis-associated pancreatitis, duodenal CD has been associated with pancreatitis. Although rare, adenocarcinoma has been reported in patients with longstanding gastroduodenal CD.[18]

ENDOSCOPY

Endoscopic features of proximal CD include multifocal erythema, nodularity, and aphthoid as well as deep serpiginous ulcerations most commonly involving the antrum and duodenum (Figure 32-3). Giant ulcers near the pylorus have also been reported.[19] Conversely, notching of Kerckring's folds may be an isolated pathognomonic finding of duodenal Crohn's disease.[2] Chromoendoscopy using indigo carmine dye has been reported to enhance notching and duodenal fold changes by revealing associated aphthoid ulcerations in a longitudinal skip pattern.[20]

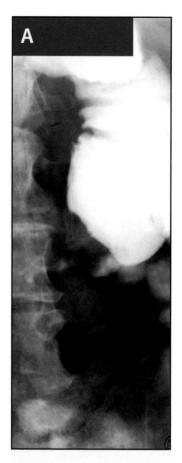

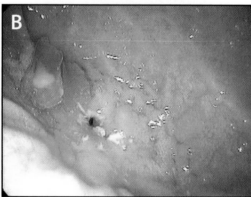

FIGURE 32-2. A fixed stenotic duodenum may appear as a string sign (A UG/small bowel series) and occasionally may present with proximal dilation of the duodenum and even megaduodenum (B endoscopic megaduodenum).

Focally enhanced gastritis in the absence of *H. pylori* occurs more frequently in the antrum and has been identified in up to 76% of established CD patients. The positive predictive value of focal gastritis indicating CD was 94%. However, there was a very poor negative predictive value of 37%.[6,7] Wright and Riddell[8] compared gastric and duodenal biopsies from Crohn's patients with matched controls and found that only 10% of gastroduodenal CD showed the presence of *H. pylori* compared with 71% of the non-CD

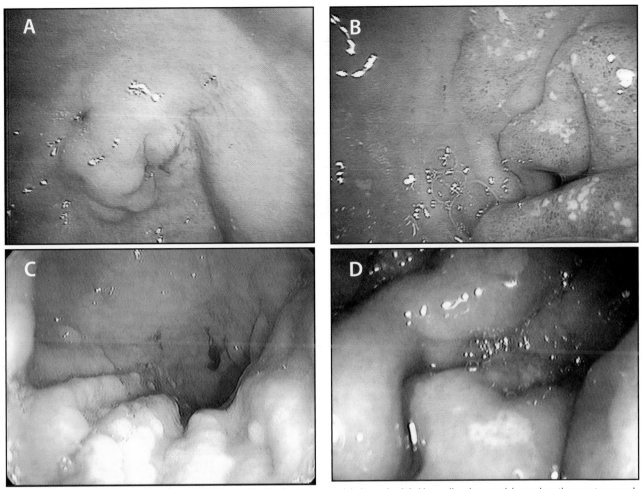

FIGURE 32-3. Endoscopic features of proximal CD include multiple focal erythema, nodularity, and aphthoid as well as deep serpiginous ulcerations most commonly involving the antrum and duodenum.

control population. *H. pylori*-negative focal acute gastro-duodenitis was therefore characteristic of CD—present in 31% of gastric and 40% of duodenal CD compared with only 2% and 8%, respectively, of controls. Additionally, surface intraepithelial neutrophils of the duodenum were present in 25% of Crohn's patients without *H. pylori*, compared with only 4% of controls.[8]

In another study, 48% of CD gastritis patients were *H. pylori* negative, suggesting that *H. pylori*-negative gastritis might be a typical finding in CD.[9] Approximately one-quarter of small bowel series-negative *H. pylori* and NSAID focally enhanced gastroduodenitis will have CD.[10]

WCE is a novel noninvasive technology designed primarily to provide diagnostic imaging of the entire small intestine. Images acquired are of excellent resolution and have a 1:8 magnification, allowing for visualization of individual villi. The capsule (Given Imaging, Ltd, Yoqneam, Israel), now called PillCam SB, was approved by the Food and Drug Administration (FDA) in August 2000. The system includes localization and blood detection software.

Capsule endoscopy seems to be most valuable in diagnosing early CD. Several studies have demonstrated its utility in patients with symptoms suggestive of CD with negative colonoscopies and radiologic studies.[6-10] Early capsule endoscopy features of CD that may be visualized prior to radiologic involvement include aphthous ulcers, large or linear ulcers, vasculitis, abnormal vascularity, circumferential involvement, and cobblestoning (Figure 32-4). Voderholzer et al compared WCE and computed topography (CT) enteroclysis in a consecutive series of patients with CD.[21] The frequency of small intestinal CD found by WCE was double that detected by CT enteroclysis (25 versus 12/41; $P < 0.005$). These findings led to a change in management and clinical improvement in 10 patients.[21]

HISTOLOGY

Lamina propria-associated macrophage aggregates and granulomas were more likely identified in CD patients and were generally absent in controls or UC patients. Focal subepithelial accumulations of macrophages may lead to

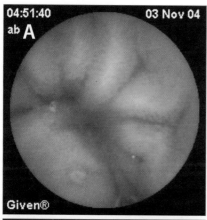
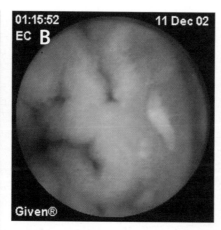
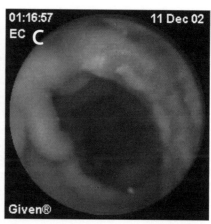

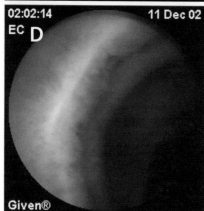

FIGURE 32-4. Capsule endoscopy can demonstrate apthous ulcers, large or linear ulcers, vasculitis, abnormal vascularity, circumferential involvement, and cobblestoning.

the patchy mucosal lesions characteristic of Crohn's.[22,23] One-quarter of patients with negative upper GI/small bowel series and no documented *H. pylori* or history of NSAID use have histologic lesions consistent with CD of the antrum and duodenum. Granulomas were found in only 7% of patients, all from normal-appearing mucosa.[10] Epithelioid granulomas, in the absence of known systemic granulomatous disease, are considered pathognomonic of CD.[24] These patients may be asymptomatic for GI tract disease.[8] In a recent series, 20% of otherwise undiagnosed CD in pediatric cases were confirmed to have CD by upper endoscopy and histology.

The advent of newer endoscopic technologies and evolving serologic profiling may help identify a subset of ileitis and colitis with more proximal disease. WCE and serology may also identify a subset of UC patients with proximal disease who may be at risk for developing CD after ileal pouch anal anastomosis. Proximal CD detected on video capsule endoscopy needs to be distinguished from NSAID-associated aphthous enteropathies or self-limited infectious enteritities, in order to avoid over diagnosis of proximal CD. NOD2/CARD15 mutations have recently been strongly associated with proximal CD.[23,25-27] Further studies evaluating the sensitivity and specificity of upper endoscopy, WCE, and serologic profiling in identifying an immunologically vulnerable subset of asymptomatic small bowel series-negative colitis who may have features of CD are warranted.

CONFOUNDING DIAGNOSES

INFLAMMATORY

Possible complicating inflammatory etiologies include severe peptic ulcer disease (with both strictures and penetrating duodenal ulcers), suture granulomas, sarcoidosis involving the stomach, and granulomatous gastritis, which is distinct from Wegener's granulomatosis and other types of vasculitis.

Often overlooked is an overlap between CD and celiac disease/gluten-sensitive enteropathy. Upper endoscopy with biopsies of the duodenum to exclude celiac are recommended. This is also an emerging additional diagnostic use of WCE.[28,29]

INFECTIOUS

H. pylori gastritis may in fact be difficult to differentiate from CD both endoscopically and histologically, underscoring the importance of staining for the bacteria.[30] Duodenal giardiasis may mimic symptoms of CD and should be excluded by stool cultures and stool *Giardia* antigen testing, as well as by testing duodenal aspirates in select patients.[31]

Tuberculosis typically is an insidious disease presenting with indolent symptoms. When it involves the intestines, masquerading as CD, fistulizing upper esophageal disease may be present. Purified protein derivative (PPD) and chest x-rays, as well as *Mycobacterium tuberculosis* polymerase chain reaction (PCR) will aid in distinguishing this entity from CD. Furthermore, these tests are important as a means of diagnosing tuberculosis in patients with established CD who have been treated with infliximab or other biologic agents. It should be underscored that a PPD, although anergic in up to two thirds of patients with CD, should be performed prior to initiation of infliximab and other novel anti-tumor necrosis factor alpha (TNFα) agents. Intercurrent infections in patients with well-established CD who worsen on anti-TNFα or other biologic therapies should be investigated. Leprosy, actinomycosis, histoplasmosis, syphilis, Whipple's disease, and helminthic infections such as strongyloides should be considered in the differential of suspected duodenal CD.

MALIGNANT

Lymphoma, gastric adenocarcinoma (including linitis plastica and scirrhous carcinoma), and duodenal and pancreatic carcinoma must be excluded before diagnosing proximal CD.

MEDICAL THERAPY/TREATMENT

Though medical therapy is the mainstay of nonobstructing gastroduodenal and proximal CD (including esophageal and jejunal), efficacy has not been studied in randomized clinical trials. Acid suppression therapy is frequently used to diminish pain. The contribution of acid to the immunoinflammatory response of gastroduodenal Crohn's remains unclear.[32] There are no comparative trials evaluating proton pump inhibitors and/or H2 receptor antagonists in gastroduodenal CD. If patients develop increasing diarrhea or constipation with a specific proton pump inhibitor, switching to another medicine in the class may prove helpful. Sucralfate may be effective as a cytoprotective agent in gastroduodenal Crohn's and has been used topically for local symptom relief of oral aphthae.

The effect of aminosalicylates on proximal CD has not been proven, but Pentasa—the slow release, moisture-dependent, pH-independent form of mesalamine encapsulated in ethyl cellulose microgranules—begins releasing in the proximal small intestine. It distributes in solution throughout the small and large intestine and may prove clinically helpful in gastroduodenal as well as jejunal CD. Pentasa has also been helpful in duodenal-jejunal stricturing disease. The induction dose is 1 g 4 times daily and is now available in 500-mg capsules, allowing for an 8-capsule-a-day regimen. This is certainly a welcome change from the previously formulation of 250-mg capsules, which resulted in a 4 capsules 4 times a day schedule for a total of 16 capsules per day. pH-dependent coated mesalamine preparation, Asacol, may accumulate proximal to

strictures. Azo-bonded 5-aminosalicylates—sulfasalazine olsalazine and balsalazide—release primarily in the colon and play little role in the treatment of proximal CD.

Steroids are effective in inducing remission of active CD irrespective of disease location and therefore may be effective in proximal CD. Entocort is a topically active, rapidly metabolized formulation of the steroid budesonide consisting of 1-mm granules containing 3 mg of budesonide and coated with a gelatin, iron oxide, and titanium dioxide capsule that dissolves in a pH > 5.5. The budesonide itself is imbedded in ethyl cellulose, which releases in a pH-independent, moisture/time-dependent manner. More than two thirds of budesonide is absorbed in the ileocecal area and has a high first-pass metabolism in the liver—leading to fewer side effects than conventional oral steroids. The effect of opening Entocort capsules and releasing the ethyl cellulose embedded budesonide has not been studied in proximal CD. Beclomethosone diproprionate, an orally administered topical steroid (usually delivered in corn oil 0.3 mg/cc dispensed as 1 L for a 6-week period of time: 5 cc QID) has been utilized in proximal CD but has not been formally studied.

The use of immunomodulator therapy—azathioprine (AZA) and 6-mercaptopurine (6-MP)—in proximal CD should be similar to the induction and maintenance of remission seen in CD of the ileum and colon.[33] Similarly, methotrexate might be expected to induce and maintain remission.[34] Infliximab would also be expected to induce remission in proximal CD, although its role in stricturing gastroduodenal remains to be defined. In all of the infliximab controlled trials, patients with stricturing and internal fistulizing disease were excluded. In a recent report of open-label use of infliximab in the TREAT Registry, there is no increase in obstruction noted. In addition, the ACCENT 1 and ACCENT 2 maintenance trials of infliximab showed no increase in strictures and, although primary stricturing disease was excluded, the fact that no secondary strictures were noted throughout the maintenance trial is encouraging.[35,36] There is a smaller series reporting a modest increase in small bowel obstruction in patients who had previously documented strictures. Again, patients who have obstructing duodenal strictures ought to be evaluated by surgical colleagues.[37-39]

SURGICAL THERAPY

When medical therapy fails, endoscopic or surgical therapy is indicated, and surgery remains the treatment of choice for obstructing proximal CD. Endoscopic dilation with local steroid injection has been used for patients with intestinal stricturing CD.[40] Few data exist in evaluating endoscopic balloon dilation in gastroduodenal CD (Figure 32-5). In patients with severe obstructive duodenal CD, surgery may be the best option. Laparoscopic gastrojeju-

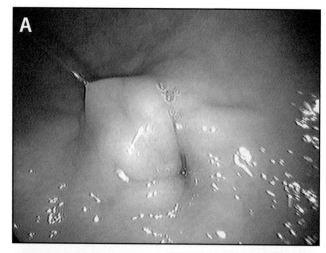

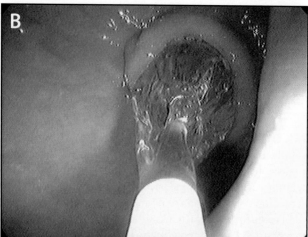

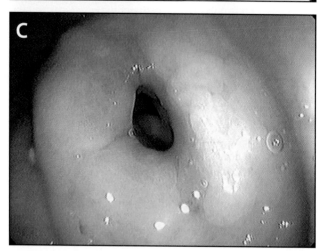

FIGURE 32-5. Endoscopic dilation with local steroid injection has been used for patients with intestinal stricturing.

nostomy should be attempted, and open surgery should be performed only if a laparoscopic approach is not feasible.[41] Duodenal stricturoplasty may be performed in select patients, particularly if proximal to an uninvolved papilla (Figure 32-6). It is debated whether there is a higher

reoperative rate with stricturoplasty compared to bypass surgery.[42-44] The presence of a duodenal-colonic fistula is almost always related to primary colonic and not duodenal CD.[45] When fistulization occurs, closure of the fistula is recommended by resection of the colonic or ileal site of active CD with an accompanied duodenojejunostomy or gastrojejunostomy.[46,47]

CONCLUSION

Proximal CD, involving the stomach, duodenum, and jejunum, is increasingly recognized. Endoscopic evaluations are more accurate than an upper GI/small bowel series. The impact of early diagnosis of proximal CD on therapeutic strategies for managing colitis and distal ileal CD are discussed. The evolution of newer endoscopic and immunologic technologies may allow for identification of previously unrecognized proximal CD. The impact of medical therapies—acid suppression, mesalamine, conventional and rapidly metabolized topicalized steroids, immunomodulators, and biologics such as infliximab—is reviewed in nonobstructing proximal CD. Surgical options are recommended for obstructing disease and medically refractory nonobstructing proximal CD. The early detection of proximal CD may identify a subset of colitis patients who are more likely to relapse, respond to infliximab, or develop CD after ileal pouch anal anastomosis. IBD treatment paradigms will change with accurate characterization of the proximal disease. Newer technologies, both WCE and earlier use of diagnostic upper endoscopy, hold the promise of redefining distal ileitis and colitis as more proximal diseases and changing treatment paradigms accordingly.

REFERENCES

1. Nugent FW, Roy MA. Duodenal Crohn's disease: an analysis of 89 cases. *Am J Gastroenterol.* 1989;84(3):249-254.

2. Wagtmans MJ, van Hogezand RA, Grifioen G, Verspaget HW, Lamers CB. Crohn's disease of the upper gastrointestinal tract. *Neth J Med.* 1997;50(2):S2-S7.

3. Wagtmans MJ, Verspaget HW, Lamers CB, van Hogezand RA. Clinical aspects of Crohn's disease of the upper gastrointestinal tract: a comparison with distal Crohn's disease. *Am J Gastroenterol.* 1997;92(9):1467-1471.

4. van Hogezand RA, Witte AM, Veenendaal RA, Wagtmans MJ, Lamers CB. Proximal Crohn's disease: review of the clinicopathologic features and therapy. *Inflamm Bowel Dis.* 2001;7(4):328-337.

5. Rutgeerts P, Onette E, Vantrappen G, Geboes K, Broeckaert L, Talloen L. Crohn's disease of the stomach and duodenum: a clinical study with emphasis on the value of endoscopy and endoscopic biopsies. *Endoscopy.* 1980;12(6):288-294.

6. Oberhuber G, Hirsch M, Stolte M. High incidence of upper gastrointestinal tract involvement in Crohn's disease. *Virchows Arch.* 1998;432(1):49-52.

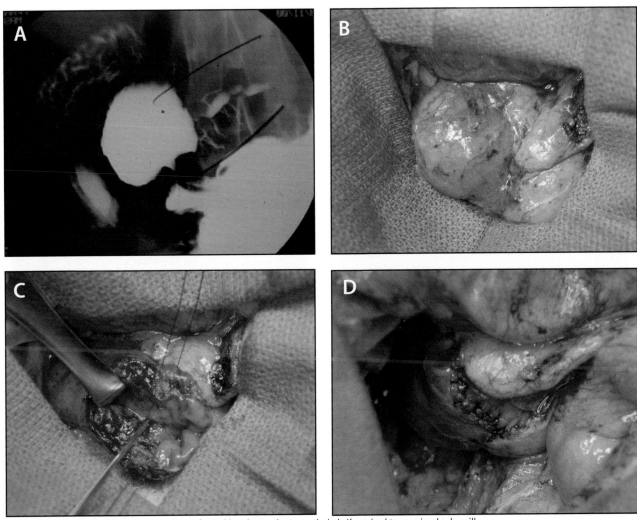

FIGURE 32-6. Duodenal stricturoplasty may be performed in select patients, particularly if proximal to an uninvolved papilla.

7. Oberhuber G, Püspök A, Oesterreicher C, et al. Focally enhanced gastritis: a frequent type of gastritis in patients with Crohn's disease. *Gastroenterology.* 1997;112(3):698-706.

8. Wright CL, Riddell RH. Histology of the stomach and duodenum in Crohn's disease. *Am J Surg Pathol.* 1998;22(4):383-390.

9. Halme L, Kärkkäinen P, Rautelin H, Kosunen TU, Sipponen P. High frequency of helicobacter negative gastritis in patients with Crohn's disease. *Gut.* 1996;38(3):379-383.

10. Korelitz BI, Waye JB, Kreuning J, et al. Crohn's disease in endoscopic biopsies of the gastric antrum and duodenum. *Am J Gastroenterol.* 1981;76(2):103-109.

11. Appleyard M, Fireman Z, Glukhovsky A, et al. A randomized trial comparing wireless capsule endoscopy with push enteroscopy for the detection of small-bowel lesions. *Gastroenterology.* 2000;119(6):1431-1438.

12. Buchman AL, Miller FH, Wallin A, Chowdhry A, Ahn C. Videocapsule endoscopy versus barium contrast studies for diagnosis of Crohn's disease recurrence involving the small intestine. *Am J Gastroenterol.* 2004;99:2171-2177.

13. Costamagna G, Shah SK, Riccioni ME, et al. A prospective trial comparing small bowel radiographs and video capsule endoscopy for suspected small bowel disease. *Gastroenterology.* 2002;123(4):999-1005.

14. Eliakim R, Fischer D, Suissa A, et al. Wireless capsule video endoscopy is a superior diagnostic tool in comparison to barium follow-through and computerized tomography in patients with suspected Crohn's disease. *Eur J Gastroenterol Hepatol.* 2003;15(4):363-367.

15. Triester SL, Leighton JA, Leontiadis GI, et al. A meta-analysis of the yield of capsule endoscopy compared to other diagnostic modalities in patients with non-stricturing small bowel Crohn's disease. *Am J Gastroenterol.* 2006;101:954-964.

16. Farman J, Faegenburg D, Dallemand S, Chen CK. Crohn's disease of the stomach: the "ram's horn" sign. *Am J Roentgenol Radium Ther Nucl Med.* 1975;123(2):242-251.

17. Scherl E, Sachar D. Crohn's disease of the small intestine. In: Schiller L, ed. *Gastroenterology and Hepatology.* Philadelphia, PA: Current Medicine, Inc; 1997:7.1-7.22.

18. Meiselman MS, Ghahremani GG, Kaufman MW. Crohn's disease of the duodenum complicated by adenocarcinoma. *Gastrointest Radiol.* 1987;12(4):333-336.

19. Moonka D, Lichtenstein GR, Levine MS, Rombeau JL, Furth EE, MacDermott RP. Giant gastric ulcers: an unusual manifestation of Crohn's disease. *Am J Gastroenterol.* 1993;88(2):297-299.

20. Hokama A, Kinjo F, Sugama R, et al. Gastrointestinal: duodenal Crohn's disease. *J Gastroenterol Hepatol.* 2003;18(12):1425.

21. Voderholzer WA, Beinhoelzl J, Rogalla P, et al. Small bowel involvement in Crohn's disease: a prospective comparison of wireless capsule endoscopy and computed tomography enteroclysis. *Gut.* 2005;54:369-373.

22. Yao K, Iwashita A, Yao T, et al. Increased numbers of macrophages in noninflamed gastroduodenal mucosa of patients with Crohn's disease. *Dig Dis Sci.* 1996;41(11):2260-2267.

23. Alcántara M, Rodriguez R, Potenciano JL, Carrobles JL, Muñoz C, Gomez R. Endoscopic and bioptic findings in the upper gastrointestinal tract in patients with Crohn's disease. *Endoscopy.* 1993;25(4):282-286.

24. Rotterdam H, Sommers SC. Biopsy diagnosis of the digestive tract. In: Blaustein A, ed. *Biopsy Interpretation Series.* New York, NY: Raven Press; 1981:265-274.

25. Abreu MT, Taylor KD, Lini YC, et al. Mutations in NOD2 are associated with fibrostenosing disease in patients with Crohn's disease. *Gastroenterology.* 2002;123(3):679-688.

26. Marteau P, Daniel F, Seksik P, Jian R. Inflammatory bowel disease: what is new? *Endoscopy.* 2004;36(2):130-136.

27. Mardini HE, Selby L, et al. Upper gasgtrointestinal involvment in patients with Crohn's disease is strongly associated with double dose of the NOD2/CARD15 allelic variants. *Am J Gastroenterol.* 2004;99:S253.

28. Green PH, Murray JA. Routine duodenal biopsies to exclude celiac disease? *Gastrointest Endosc.* 2003;58(1):92-95.

29. Alaedini A, Green PH. Narrative review: celiac disease: understanding a complex autoimmune disorder. *Ann Intern Med.* 2005;142(4):289-298.

30. el-Omar E, Penman I, Cruikshank G, et al. Low prevalence of *Helicobacter pylori* in inflammatory bowel disease: association with sulphasalazine. *Gut.* 1994;35(10):1385-1388.

31. Gunasekaran TS, Hassall E. Giardiasis mimicking inflammatory bowel disease. *J Pediatr.* 1992;120(3):424-426.

32. Witte AM, Veenendaal RA, van Hogezand RA, Verspaget HW, Lamers CB. Crohn's disease of the upper gastrointestinal tract: The value of endoscopic examination. *Scand J Gastroenterol.* 1998;225:100-105.

33. Pearson DC, May GR, Fick GH, Sutherland LR. Azathioprine and 6-mercaptopurine in Crohn disease. A meta-analysis. *Ann Intern Med.* 1995;123(2):132-142.

34. Feagan BG, Rochon J, Fedorak RN, et al. Methotrexate for the treatment of Crohn's disease. The North American Crohn's Study Group Investigators. *N Engl J Med.* 1995;332(5):292-297.

35. Hanauer SB, Feagan BG, Lichtenstein GR, et al. Maintenance infliximab for Crohn's disease: the ACCENT I randomised trial. *Lancet.* 2002;359(9317):1541-1549.

36. Hanauer SB, Wagner CL, Bala M, et al. Incidence and importance of antibody responses to infliximab after maintenance or episodic treatment in Crohn's disease. *Clin Gastroenterol Hepatol.* 2004;2(7):542-553.

37. Lichtenstein GR, Ran S, Bala M, Hanauer S. Remission in patients with Crohn's disease is associated with improvement in employment and quality of life and a decrease in hospitalizations and surgeries. *Am J Gastroenterol.* 2004;99(1):91-96.

38. Di Febo G, Calabrese C, Matassoni F. New trends in non-absorbable antibiotics in gastrointestinal disease. *Ital J Gastroenterol.* 1992;24(9 suppl 2):10-13.

39. Hanauer SB, Smith MB. Rapid closure of Crohn's disease fistulas with continuous intravenous cyclosporin A. *Am J Gastroenterol.* 1993;88(5):646-649.

40. Ranboer C, Verhamme M, Dhondt E, Huys S, Van Eygen K, Vermeire L. Endoscopic treatment of stenosis in recurrent Crohn's disease with balloon dilation combined with local corticosteroid injection. *Gastrointest Endosc.* 1995;42:252-255.

41. Salky B. Severe gastroduodenal Crohn's disease: surgical treatment. *Inflamm Bowel Dis.* 2003;9(2):129-130.

42. Michelassi F. Side-to-side isoperistaltic strictureplasty for multiple Crohn's strictures. *Dis Colon Rectum.* 1996;39(3):345-349.

43. Yamamoto T, Bain IM, Connolly AB, Allan RN, Keighley MR. Outcome of strictureplasty for duodenal Crohn's disease. *Br J Surg.* 1999;86(2):259-262.

44. Worsey MJ, Hull T, Ryland L, Fazio V. Strictureplasty is an effective option in the operative management of duodenal Crohn's disease. *Dis Colon Rectum.* 1999;42(5):596-600.

45. Greenstein AJ, Present DH, Sachar DB, et al. Gastric fistulas in Crohn's disease. Report of cases. *Dis Colon Rectum.* 1989;32(10):888-892.

46. Yamamoto T, Bain IM, Connolly AB, Keighley MR. Gastroduodenal fistulas in Crohn's disease: clinical features and management. *Dis Colon Rectum.* 1998;41(10):1287-1292.

47. Sandborn WJ, Present DH, Isaacs KL, et al. Tacrolimus for the treatment of fistulas in patients with Crohn's disease: a randomized, placebo-controlled trial. *Gastroenterology.* 2003;125(2):380-388.

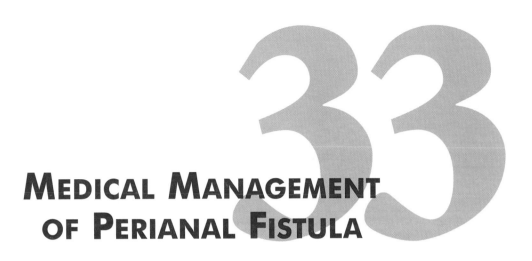

MEDICAL MANAGEMENT
OF PERIANAL FISTULA

Tarun Misra, MD, FRCP(C) and Richard N. Fedorak, MD, FRCP(C)

BACKGROUND

Many of the people who suffer from Crohn's disease, especially when it involves the colon, also have perianal problems. This comorbidity complicates an already difficult disease. Among the manifestations of perianal disease, perianal fistulas are the most common and pose the greatest management challenge. Assessment of functional and psychosocial problems should be a routine undertaking, as patients often are embarrassed to discuss this area and clinicians fail to question and examine thoroughly. However, the identification of perianal fistulas through diagnostic imaging has improved. The advents of magnetic resonance imaging (MRI) and endoscopic ultrasound (EUS) have allowed for easier classification of fistulas. Management with traditional therapies such as antibiotics and immunosuppressives is still common; however, newer biologic therapy has reshaped the management of this disease.

DEFINITION

The strict definition of a *fistula* (Latin for "pipe") is any abnormal anatomic connection between 2 epithelialized surfaces.[1] The abnormal connection may be enterocutaneous (bowel to skin), enterovesical (bowel to bladder), or enteroenteric (bowel to bowel). A perianal fistula, then, is an abnormal connection from an internal opening to the external surface of the perianal skin.

ANATOMY

To understand fistula development and how to identify the extent of the disease, a basic knowledge of perianal anatomy is required (Figure 33-1). Both the internal and external anal sphincters are important in providing fecal continence. They are also used for the classification of perianal fistulas.

The rectum is lined with columnar epithelium, as is the rest of the colon. Towards the distal end of the rectum, the epithelium becomes transitional. The dentate line, located at approximately the midline of the internal sphincter, separates the rectum from the anal canal, which is lined with squamous epithelium. The anal canal is 3 to 4 cm long, and its squamous epithelium is very unlike skin. The lining, also known as *anoderm*, does not contain hair, sebaceous glands, or sweat glands. Innervation above the dentate line is sympathetic and parasympathetic, and thus there is minimal pain sensation in this area. Below the dentate line, however, the innervation is primarily somatic, necessitating the use of anesthesia for biopsies or even for thorough physical examinations.[2]

The rectum consists of circular smooth muscle that extends downward to the anal canal, forming the internal anal sphincter. The internal anal sphincter is under involuntary control. The external anal sphincter, however, consists of skeletal muscle and is, therefore, under voluntary control. This sphincter extends distally from the puborectalis muscle and continues past the internal anal sphincter. A potential space between the 2 sphincters, called the *intersphincteric space*, is helpful for classifying fistulas into proper terms (Figure 33-2). This space can be palpated as a groove during a digital rectal exam.[3]

At the dentate line, anal crypts are present. Anal glands are located at the base of the crypts.[2] Penetration of these anal glands into the intersphincteric space may play a role

Lichtenstein GR, ed.
Crohn's Disease: The Complete Guide to Medical Management (pp 377-394).
© 2011 SLACK Incorporated

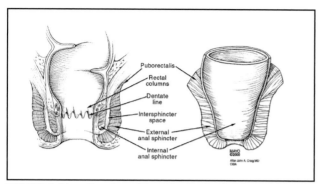

FIGURE 33-1. Schematic anatomy of the perianal region. (Reprinted with permission from Fry RD, Kodner IJ. Anorectal disorders. *Clin Symp.* 1985;37:2-32.)

in the development of perianal fistulas. Also, blockage of one end often leads to perianal abscesses.[4]

CLASSIFICATION

Many classification systems are used for defining the extent of perianal fistulas. A summary is provided in Table 33-1. None are perfect, and therefore clinicians usually choose one and use it for the purposes of describing these abnormalities. Classification of fistulas is important in assisting the communication between clinicians and allowing for easier identification of those patients who might benefit from early surgical intervention.

Many classification systems have been proposed over the years. The simplest and earliest system divided fistulas into a low or high category depending on the fistula's relationship to the dentate line.[5] Those above the dentate line are high, and those below are low. Most colorectal surgeons prefer this simple scheme; however, it is not always anatomically or pathologically accurate.

Because of the association of various other manifestations of perianal disease (anal fissures, anorectal strictures, and anal ulcers) with CD, the Cardiff classification system was developed in 1978 and modified in 1992.[6,7] This system allows for a more precise anatomic and pathologic description of both perianal fistulas and other accompanying perianal clinical manifestations. Each major manifestation of perianal CD (ulceration, fistula, and stricture) is graded on a scale of 0 to 2 (0, absent; 2, severe). Fistulas are also classified as low or high, in relation to the dentate line. The 1992 modifications to the classification system led to the inclusion of other anal conditions (such as hemorrhoids and cancer), the intestinal location of other sites of CD, and a global assessment of the activity of the perianal disease.[7] Although anatomically correct and highly comprehensive, Cardiff classification has never gained much acceptance in clinical practice.[8] Perhaps this is because it has never achieved reproduction or prospective validation in relation to meaningful clinical endpoints.[9]

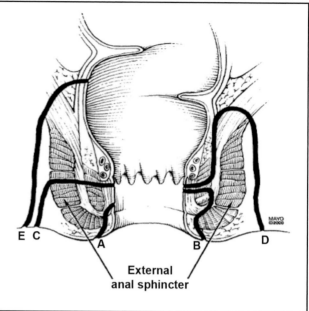

FIGURE 33-2. The Parks classification system. (A) A superficial fistula tracks below both the internal and external anal sphincters. (B) An intersphincteric fistula tracks between the internal and external anal sphincters in the intersphincteric space. (C) A trans-sphincteric fistula tracks from the intersphincteric space through the external anal sphincter. (D) A suprasphincteric fistula leaves the intersphincteric space over the top of the puborectalis and penetrates the levator muscle before tracking down to the skin. (E) An extrasphincteric fistula tracks outside of the external anal sphincter and penetrates the levator muscle into the rectum. (Modified and reprinted with permission from Parks A. The pathogenesis and treatment of fistula-in-ano. *Br Med J.* 1961;1:463.)

The Parks classification system, which uses the external anal sphincter as a point of reference, is the most anatomically precise.[10] Five types of perianal fistulas are described (see Figure 33-2): superficial, intersphincteric, trans-sphincteric, suprasphincteric, and extrasphincteric. Although Parks is used extensively in classifying fistulas, its major limitation is the failure to address the other perianal manifestations of CD.

In a recent American Gastroenterological Association technical review on perianal CD, the authors proposed an empirical approach that is likely to become widely used.[11] For this classification system, careful examination of the perianal area is essential, including identification of anal skin tags, anal fissures, perianal fistulas, suspected perianal abscesses, anorectal strictures, and rectovaginal fistulas. The authors also propose endoscopic evaluation for the presence of macroscopic inflammation of the rectum, although the routine use of this investigative tool is the subject of controversy. Fistulas are divided into simple or complex categories. Simple perianal fistulas are low. These include superficial, low intersphincteric, and low trans-sphincteric fistulas. They have only 1 opening, are not associated with a perianal abscess, have no con-

TABLE 33-1

PROPOSED CLASSIFICATION SYSTEMS FOR PERIANAL FISTULAS

CLASSIFICATION	DEFINING COMPONENTS	COMMENTS
Simple	Earliest and simplest classification system. 1) Low: Fistulas below dentate line 2) High: Fistulas above dentate line	Not anatomically or pathologically correct. Fails to address other perianal manifestations.
Cardiff	Major manifestations of perianal disease (ulceration, fistula, stricture) described accurately and graded on a scale of 0 to 2 (0: not present; 2: severe). Also assesses intestinal disease activity and location.	Comprehensive and precise. Limited clinical relevance. Has never been formally validated.
Parks	Uses external anal sphincter as point of reference: 1) Superficial 2) Intersphincteric 3) Trans-sphincteric 4) Suprasphincteric 5) Extrasphincteric	Anatomically precise. Fails to describe other perianal manifestations.
Generalized approach	Classifies on the basis of fistula tracts (low versus high) and the presence of other manifestations: 1) Simple • Low fistula • Single opening • No abscess • No anorectal stricture 2) Complex • High fistula • ± Multiple openings • ± Perianal abscess • ± Rectovaginal fistula • ± Anorectal stricture	Anatomically correct. Clinically easy to use. Addresses other perianal manifestations.

nection to an adjacent structure, and do not show any evidence of anorectal stricture. Simple fistulas tend to have a higher rate of healing and better outcomes.[12-15] Complex fistulas are high and reveal more involvement of the anal sphincters. These include high intersphincteric, high trans-sphincteric, extrasphincteric, and suprasphincteric fistulas. Complex fistulas are associated with perianal abscesses, rectovaginal fistulas, or anorectal strictures, and they may have multiple openings. Because this is an easy and clinically relevant classification scheme, it is the preferred system of many clinicians.

PATHOGENESIS

The pathogenesis of perianal fistulas in CD is largely unknown. There are, however, several proposed mechanisms (Figure 33-3). It is suspected that perianal CD may involve the development of deep penetrating anal ulcers. Further penetration of the ulcers, through fecal traffic, may lead to extension into the surrounding tissue, thereby creating a new fistulous tract.[6] Another proposed mechanism involves the anal glands located at the base of the anal crypts at the dentate line.[10] Infections of the anal glands

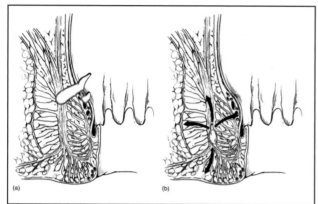

FIGURE 33-3. Proposed mechanism for fistula development. (A) Deep ulcers extend over time, as feces is forced into them by defecation pressure, resulting in fistula development. (B) Infection in an anal gland at the base of anal crypts penetrates into the intersphincteric space, resulting in fistula formation. (Modified and reprinted with permission from Schwartz DA, Herdman CR. Review article: the medical treatment of Crohn's perianal fistula. *Aliment Pharmacol Ther.* 2004;19:953-967.)

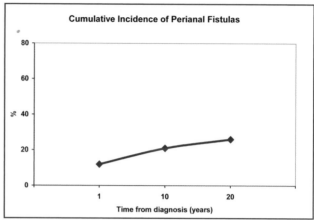

FIGURE 33-4. Cumulative incidence curve of perianal fistulas. (Reprinted from the Mayo Clinic Olmstead County, MN, USA. Adapted from Schwartz DA, Loftus EV Jr, Tremaine WJ, et al. The natural history of fistulizing Crohn's disease in Olmsted County, Minnesota. *Gastroenterology.* 2002;122:875-880.)

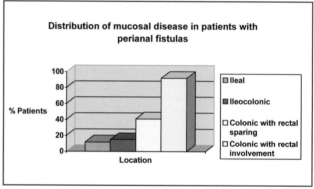

FIGURE 33-5. Risk of perianal fistulas in patients with ileal disease (12%), ileocolonic disease (15%), colonic disease with rectal sparing (41%), and colonic disease with rectal involvement (92%). (Adapted from Hellers G, Bergstrand O, Ewerth S, Holmstrom B. Occurrence and outcome after primary treatment of anal fistulae in Crohn's disease. *Gut.* 1980;21:525-527.)

may lead to penetration into the intersphincteric space. From here, a fistulous tract may form and either track downwards to the skin (intersphincteric or superficial fistula) and penetrate through the external anal sphincter (trans-sphincteric fistula) or track upwards through the intersphincteric space (suprasphincteric fistula).[16]

EPIDEMIOLOGY

Many individuals suffering from Crohn's experience perianal fistulas at some point in their disease process. Up to a quarter of patients may have perianal fistulas, according to 2 population-based studies.[17,18] Hellers et al found that 23% of a group of Swedish patients with CD had perianal fistulas.[17] Schwartz et al found a similar rate of 21% in a similar American population.[18] The cumulative incidence of perianal fistulas increases from the time of diagnosis of CD (Figure 33-4). At 1 year, the incidence is 12%. This increases to 21% at 10 years and 26% at 20 years. In addition, disease activity in the rectum is strongly associated with the development of perianal fistulas (Figure 33-5). Hellers et al found that 92% of patients who showed evidence of colonic disease activity with rectal involvement developed perianal fistulas.[17] This finding is in striking contrast to the rates seen in cases of colonic disease with rectal sparing (41%), ileocolonic disease (15%), and ileal CD (12%) (see Figure 33-5). Prediction of which patients may develop perianal fistulas can, therefore, be made on the basis of the location and extent of their luminal disease.

CLINICAL PRESENTATION

Patients may present with many different manifestations of perianal fistulas (Table 33-2), and the astute clinician looks for the development of perianal disease in all cases of CD. In up to 24% of cases, perianal manifestations may actually precede the diagnosis of luminal CD by a mean lead-time of 4 years.[19] More often, however, perianal fistulas develop later than, or concomitantly with, the symptoms associated with luminal activity. Perianal pain and discharge are the most common manifestations of a perianal fistula. Other symptoms include fever, perianal itching, and restriction of sexual activity. Because the area involved is usually a source of embarrassment for the patient, clinicians must sympathetically question patients with CD about perianal manifestations on a frequent basis.

Clinical experience suggests that people who are well-versed on Crohn's disease and its manifestations present earlier to clinicians. Thus, at the time of diagnosis, patients should be given active education pertaining to the clinical

TABLE 33-2

SYMPTOMS ASSOCIATED WITH PERIANAL FISTULAS

SYMPTOM	FREQUENCY
Perianal pain	+++
Perianal discharge	+++
Perianal itching	+
Fever	+
Restriction of sexual activity	++

TABLE 33-3

ACCURACY OF VARIOUS DIAGNOSTIC MODALITIES IN DETECTING PERIANAL FISTULA*

DIAGNOSTIC MODALITY	REPORTED ACCURACY	COMMENTS
Physical examination	62%	Inaccurate as a result of pain caused. Dependent on experience.
EUA	90%	Dependent on experience of colorectal surgeon. Allows for concomitant surgical therapy.
Fistulography	16% to 50%	Painful and unreliable. May displace septic material.
Computed tomography	24% to 60%	Poor resolution of pelvis.
EUS	56% to 100%	Operator-dependent. Access generally good.
MRI	76% to 100%	Access may be a problem.

*EUA indicates examination under anesthesia; EUS, endoscopic ultrasound; MRI, magnetic resonance imaging.

manifestations of the disease. This teaching should not just focus on luminal disease activity but should also include teaching about nutrition, extraintestinal manifestations, risks of colorectal cancer, and perianal disease possibilities and recognition.

DIAGNOSIS

PHYSICAL EXAMINATION

The diagnosis of a perianal fistula requires a combination of physical examination and, usually, radiological assessment. The sensitivities of each diagnostic modality are described in Table 33-3. Firstly, any individual who presents with perianal symptoms should be examined thoroughly. Patient comfort is paramount. Start by establishing rapport and alleviating any apprehension the individual may have. Good lighting and making sure all necessary equipment is in place prior to starting the examination are essential. An initial examination of the undergarments may reveal evidence of discharge. Next, inspect the skin with the patient in the left lateral position with the thighs and knees flexed. As the buttocks are retracted, carefully inspect the area, noting the presence of skin tags, scars, hemorrhoids, fissures, fistulas, discharge, stool, or pus. The examination then moves to palpation. Gentle pressure along the fistula tract may result in purulent material being discharged. This finding indicates an open fistula and has clinical implications (discussed later).

The physical examination continues with a formal digital rectal examination. A well-lubricated gloved finger is inserted into the anal canal. Using careful, gentle pressure, the clinician can identify the presence of fissures and fistulas. A fistulous tract feels like a cord. The internal opening of a fistula is a mound of tissue surrounded by normal smooth mucosa. Perianal pain needs to be fully taken into account by the clinician performing this examination. The heightened pain sensations in the area mean that many patients cannot undergo the formal examination just described. In that case, examination under anesthesia (EUA) should be strongly considered.

EXAMINATION UNDER ANESTHESIA

Although the previously described clinical examination can be useful, it has clear limitations: manual examination is painful for most patients, and many clinicians—even experienced colorectal surgeons—have poor accuracy.[20] Many practitioners, therefore, feel that the examination should be performed under anesthesia by an experienced surgeon. EUA has been the standard against which other diagnostic modalities are now judged. It involves the complete assessment of the perianal area through inspection, palpation, and the passing of malleable probes into fistulous tracts. To begin with, the patient is given a general anesthetic, and then the examination takes place in the operating room. The advantages of EUA include the possibility of the concomitant use of surgical procedures, if they are required, while the patient is under anesthesia. These surgical maneuvers include the placement of noncutting setons and incision and drainage of any associated abscesses.

FISTULOGRAPHY

Fistulography involves the injection of a contrast medium into the cutaneous opening of a fistulous tract via a small catheter. Accuracy is poor, ranging from 16% to 50%.[21-25] The process also causes pain to the individual during the examination and may displace septic material. Because of these problems, fistulography has a low clinical utility.

COMPUTED TOMOGRAPHY

Computed tomography also has limited clinical utility. Poor resolution of the perianal area is the primary reason. The accuracy is limited, ranging from 24% to 60%.[26-32] Because of their poor clinical utility, both fistulography and computed tomography play limited roles in the diagnosis and management of perianal fistulas. They have largely been overtaken by modalities such as MRI and EUS, described in following sections.

MAGNETIC RESONANCE IMAGING

Pelvic MRI has become a reliable tool for assessing perianal fistulas. Excellent accuracy has been reported in many studies.[33-37] Initial small studies in the mid-1990s demonstrated that the MRI has a good rate of identification of perianal fistulas and other perianal disease as compared to EUA.[35] These studies suggested the use of MRIs alone to define the extent of fistulous tracts. However, diagnostic accuracy approaches 100% when MRI is used in combination with EUA.[38] Still, a likely disadvantage involves access. Many centers have long waiting times, and a delay in diagnosis may occur as a result.

ANORECTAL ENDOSCOPIC ULTRASONOGRAPHY

Anorectal EUS has recently gained popularity among clinicians who are working on managing these fistulous tracts. Several studies have reported excellent accuracy for anorectal EUS, ranging from 56% to 100%.[39-42] The wide range in accuracy reveals that the results are clearly operator dependent. The lower results are likely those of older studies, when EUS accuracy was not as precise. A potential advantage of anorectal EUS involves the availability of, and access to, the procedure. Gastrointestinal centers are increasingly equipped with the instrument, allowing for quicker access, especially in locations where MRI is still considered a luxury. Again, when EUS is used in combination with EUA, the diagnostic accuracy consistently approaches 100%.[38]

A recent report suggests that the individual diagnostic accuracies of MRI, EUS, and EUA are similar and surpass 85%. Schwartz et al conducted a prospective triple-blinded study to formally compare the 3 diagnostic procedures.[38] None of the modalities had a greater than 91% accuracy when used in isolation. However, the accuracy increased to 100% when any 2 modalities were combined. A smaller, more recent study determined pelvic MRI and EUS to be similarly accurate.[43] These findings strongly contrast those of an earlier prospective trial. Orsoni et al reported EUS accuracy to be 82% and MRI accuracy to be 50%, in comparison to the gold standard of EUA.[40] However, the use of both linear and radial scanning instruments may account for the enhanced findings in the later studies. Pelvic MRI technique also varied. The Orsoni study used body coils for imaging, whereas the newer trials used additional local coils to enhance spatial resolution of the pelvis. The benefits of thinner slices and smaller fields of view may account for the reported differences.

Diagnostic accuracy is key in managing perianal fistulas. Pelvic MRI or anorectal EUS, alone or in combination with surgical EUA, helps in defining the extent of disease. Patients report similar discomfort with pelvic MRI and anorectal EUS and generally do not have a preference for either procedure.[44] Initial reports, which are under investigation, suggest that it might be useful to monitor response to medical therapy using serial examinations of either diagnostic method, though it is not clear whether all patients or only some might need such follow-up.[45-48] The evidence stems from recent observations of

TABLE 33-4

PERIANAL DISEASE ACTIVITY INDEX

CATEGORIES AFFECTED BY FISTULAS	SCORE
DISCHARGE	
No discharge	0
Minimal mucus discharge	1
Moderate mucus or purulent discharge	2
Substantial discharge	3
Gross fecal soiling	4
PAIN/RESTRICTION OF ACTIVITIES	
No activity restriction	0
Mild discomfort, no restriction	1
Moderate discomfort, some limitation	2
Marked discomfort, marked limitation	3
Severe pain, severe limitation	4
RESTRICTION OF SEXUAL ACTIVITY	
No restriction	0
Slight restriction	1
Moderate restriction	2
Marked restriction	3
Unable to engage in sexual activity	4
TYPE OF PERIANAL DISEASE	
No perianal disease/skin tags	0
Anal fissure or mucosal tear	1
< 3 Perianal fistulas	2
> 3 Perianal fistulas	3
Anal sphincter ulceration or fistulas with significant undermining of skin	4
DEGREE OF INDURATION	
No induration	0
Minimal induration	1
Moderate induration	2
Substantial induration	3
Gross fluctuance/abscess	4

ASSESSING DISEASE ACTIVITY

The measurement of disease activity, in order to assess clinical response to therapy, is important. The standard index used to measure overall activity of luminal CD, the Crohn's Disease Activity Index (CDAI), does not take into account morbidity in terms of perianal manifestations of Crohn's. When using the CDAI to assess the disease of patients whose main complaint is of perianal origin, a low score will inevitably and erroneously be the result. Thus, a number of index scoring systems were used in the past,[49,50] though they were not thoroughly validated and had problems with subjectivity. The Perianal Disease Activity Index (PDAI) was first introduced in 1995.[51] The evaluation focuses on 5 categories affected by fistulas: discharge, pain, restriction of sexual activity, type of perianal disease, and degree of induration (Table 33-4). Scores in each category range from a low of 0 (no symptoms) to a high of 4 (most symptomatic). The scale was first used for patients taking metronidazole for the treatment of perianal fistulas.[51] It was then used as a secondary outcome measurement in the first infliximab trial reported by Present et al.[52] Recently, it was validated in an Austrian study that prospectively evaluated antibiotics and azathioprine (AZA) for the treatment of perianal fistulas.[53]

Measuring fistula output is another method of assessing disease activity, though fistula drainage assessment is more commonly used in clinical trials (Table 33-5).[52] A fistula is considered open when purulent material can be expressed from the fistula by gently applying pressure. A clinical response to therapy is defined as the closure of at least 50% of the baseline number of fistulas for at least 4 weeks. A complete fistula closure is the closure of all fistulas for at least 4 weeks. The time to loss of fistula response and the time to loss of complete fistula closure determine the maintenance effects of therapy. Most trials report these findings as a means of assessing and comparing therapeutic regimens.

There are 2 inherent problems with using the fistula drainage assessment method. First, it does not take into account the patient's experience of morbidity; the perianal fistulas' interference in the daily activities of patients cannot be measured using this method. The PDAI score is thus more meaningful in assessing disease activity for an individual patient. Second, many completely closed fistulas are actually found to be persistently open when the matter is investigated with diagnostic imaging such as pelvic MRI or endorectal EUS. As well, after stoppage of therapy, many fistulas will begin to drain once again. Some investigators suggest using the term cessation of drainage, instead of complete closure, as a means of correctly defining the effect of therapy.[11,54]

Another method of measuring disease activity is based on diagnostic imaging. Although not in widespread use, the MRI-based score suggested by Van Assche et al is

discordance between clinical response and radiological evidence of disease.[48] The current recommendation is to follow clinical response to therapy. If a satisfactory response is not attained, a repeat examination using either MRI or anorectal EUS, in combination with surgical EUA, would be appropriate. This approach is discussed further in the treatment section.

TABLE 33-5

FISTULA DRAINAGE DISEASE ACTIVITY ASSESSMENT

ENDPOINT	DEFINITION
Improvement	Decrease in number of open draining fistulas of >50% for at least 2 consecutive visits (ie, at least 4 weeks). Closure of fistula defined as no drainage following gentle compression.
Remission	Closure of all fistulas, as defined in block above, for at least 2 consecutive visits (ie, at least 4 weeks).

TABLE 33-6

CLINICAL EVIDENCE FOR ANTIBIOTICS IN PERIANAL FISTULAS

AGENT	LEVEL OF EVIDENCE	N	DURATION OF TREATMENT	RESULTS	COMMENTS
Metronidazole	Case series[55]	3	8 weeks	100% closure	
	Prospective open-label[56]	21	6 to 8 weeks	83% closure	Later study reported high incidence of adverse events (50% paresthesias)[57]
Ciprofloxacin	Case series[58]	8	3 to 12 months	50% closure	50% required surgical intervention

quite clinically relevant.[45] Unfortunately, it also does not account for the patient's experience of morbidity. Its main attractive feature is the identification of abscesses and the detailing of fistulous tracts. The MRI-based score system is based on the number of fistulas, the presence of branching or single tracts, the location and extension of fistulas, the collections of abscesses, and the involvement of the rectal wall. It may be best suited for clearly defining fistulas if one suspects a complex type prior to therapy. This score has not been studied as a method of following patients' responses to therapy.

MEDICAL THERAPY

Once appropriate diagnostic investigations have been completed, the patient should be offered medical therapy. Agents with proven efficacy in managing perianal fistulas include antibiotics, AZA, 6-mercaptopurine (6-MP), infliximab, cyclosporine, and tacrolimus. The following section describes the advantages and disadvantages of each agent.

ANTIBIOTICS

Although antibiotics are the most commonly used therapeutic agent for the management of perianal fistulas,

there are no controlled trials showing their effectiveness (Table 33-6). The most frequently used antibiotics are metronidazole (750 to 1500 mg/day) and ciprofloxacin (1000 mg/day). The use of metronidazole was first described in 1975 in a report by Ursing and Kamme.[55] The fistulas of 3 patients were successfully closed during treatment with the drug. A later study observed the closure of fistulas for 83% of 21 patients on the antibiotic.[56] The paucity of MRI and EUS technology prevented confirmation of the clinical results, and improvement required at least 6 to 8 weeks of therapy. Two years later, a follow-up study revealed significant adverse events associated with long-term metronidazole use.[57] The occurrence of paresthesias required dosage reductions, which had detrimental effects on the management of the fistulas. Previously "healed" fistulas recurred after these dose reductions, suggesting, in fact, that metronidazole is not a long-term solution. Paresthesias were experienced by 50% of 26 patients but resolved for the majority when the drug dosage was reduced or discontinued. Onset of these neurological symptoms can occur at anytime, but the rate and likelihood increase significantly after 3 to 4 months of use. Other adverse effects of metronidazole include glossitis, metallic taste, and nausea.

Due to its relative safety, as compared to metronidazole, ciprofloxacin was proposed as an alternative form of treatment in the early 1990s. Again, most of the data are anecdotal in the form of case study series. No con-

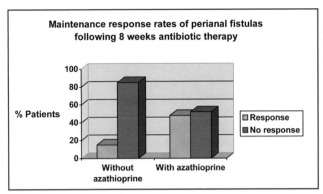

FIGURE 33-6. The effect of AZA used in conjunction with antibiotic "bridging" therapy. (Adapted from Dejaco C, Harrer M, Waldhoer T, Miehsler W, Vogelsang H, Reinisch W. Antibiotics and azathioprine for the treatment of perianal fistulas in Crohn's disease. *Aliment Pharmacol Ther.* 2003;18:1113-1120.)

TABLE 33-7

CLINICAL EVIDENCE FOR IMMUNOMODULATOR THERAPY IN PERIANAL FISTULAS*

AGENT	LEVEL OF EVIDENCE	N	DURATION OF TREATMENT	RESULTS DRUG (PLACEBO)	COMMENTS
Azathioprine	Placebo-controlled trials evaluating luminal disease[60-63]	6	2 months	33% (NA)	Evaluated perianal fistula response as secondary outcome (2 to 4 mg/kg).
		2	6 months	0% (NA)	
		10	4 months	80% (40%)	
		2	6 months	0% (NA)	
6-Mercaptopurine	Placebo-controlled trial evaluating luminal disease[64]	36	1 year	31% (6%)	Evaluated perianal fistula response as secondary outcome (1.5 mg/kg).
Both agents	Meta-analysis[67]	41	Various	54% (21%)	Pooled OR favoring fistula healing 4.44. Fistula response reported as secondary outcome. Types of fistulas not differentiated.

*NA indicates not available; OR, odds ratio.

trolled trial has been performed to assess ciprofloxacin's efficacy in managing perianal fistulas. The largest study yet reported included 8 patients.[58] Seven of the 8 had perianal fistulas; the other suffered from an enterocutaneous fistula. Patients were treated with ciprofloxacin for 3 to 12 months at dosages ranging from 1000 to 1500 mg/day. Some improvement was reported with treatment. Half of the patients, however, still had persistent discharge, and many underwent surgical intervention.

Many clinicians will use a combination of both antibiotics. Although there is no clinical evidence to support this approach, it seems a rational choice. For instance, a recent prospective trial evaluating the use of antibiotics and AZA, discussed in a following section, reported a treatment response of up to 71% following 8 weeks of ciprofloxacin and metronidazole therapy.[53] Maintenance of response, however, is not as robust, and therefore the authors of this study suggest the strategy of using of antibiotics to bridge to AZA treatment (Figure 33-6). The antibiotics control the fistula drainage and prevent further extension of the disease as a first-line treatment approach, and the AZA can be used for maintenance purposes.

AMINOSALICYLATES AND CORTICOSTEROIDS

Although used extensively in the treatment of Crohn's disease, neither aminosalicylates nor corticosteroids are used in the treatment of perianal fistulas. Steroids may prevent the healing of fistulas and lead to abscess formation, thereby complicating the clinical picture. Also, there is no evidence that supports the use of aminosalicylates, in either oral or topical form, for managing perianal fistulas.

6-MERCAPTOPURINE AND AZATHIOPRINE

Both 6-MP and AZA are antimetabolite agents. AZA is a prodrug that is converted to 6-MP. These agents interfere with nucleic acid metabolism and cell proliferation by preventing purine synthesis, resulting in impaired T cell function. Their effects on perianal fistulas are summarized in Table 33-7. AZA was first used in the treatment of CD by Brooke et al in 1969.[59] This initial study observed the healing of fistulas for patients given the drug. No randomized controlled trials have assessed these drugs solely for fistula closure rates. Much of the evidence behind their use is based on case series and secondary outcomes in controlled trials. For instance, numerous small controlled trials published in the 1970s showed improvement in fistula drainage with AZA therapy as a secondary outcome.[60-63] In the first controlled trial of 6-MP in CD, Present et al also assessed fistula response as a secondary outcome.[64] The study noted a 31% complete closure rate with 6-MP given at a dose of 1.5 mg/kg, as compared to 6% for placebo. The mean response time was 3.1 months. Similar results were reported by Korelitz and Present in an extension of the previous study.[65] In this case series, 6 of 18 patients (33%) treated with 6-MP experienced complete closure of their perianal fistulas.[65] In their study of the effectiveness and safety profile of antimetabolite agent treatment of CD, O'Brien et al report a success rate of 75% in treating perianal fistulas.[66]

To best summarize the data, a meta-analysis on the efficacy of both agents was conducted in 1995.[67] The data on fistulous disease modification were derived from 5 studies.[60-64] Overall, 24 of 41 (54%) patients receiving therapy experienced fistula response (defined as complete healing or decreased drainage), compared to 6 of 29 (21%) patients receiving placebo. The pooled odds ratio (OR) favoring fistula healing was 4.44. Although the results are favorable, there are problems with the meta-analysis. First, all studies included in the meta-analysis reported fistula response as a secondary outcome. Second, the studies are small and were mostly conducted 25 to 30 years ago. Third, the favorable OR reported does not differentiate between the types of fistulas. Although the majority of patients with CD have perianal fistulas, the studies included many patients with enterocutaneous, rectovaginal, and enteroenteric fistulas. Despite these shortcomings, this meta-analysis is the best evidence currently available for the use of AZA and 6-MP in the treatment of perianal fistula.

Further evidence for the efficacy of the use of AZA and 6-MP can be derived from the pediatric literature. In 1990, Markowitz et al reported their experience of using 6-MP to treat adolescents with CD.[68] The study was geared towards examining the intestinal effects of the drug; however,

some interesting facts were noted about perianal disease. About 40% of patients had perianal fistulas and abscesses prior to 6-MP therapy. During treatment, this number dropped to about 14%. Also, patients who previously had perianal fistulas did not develop new fistulas while on the therapy.[68] A later retrospective analysis by Jehsion et al examined the effect of these medications on perianal fistulas as a primary outcome in the case of children.[69] Twenty children were treated with AZA or 6-MP. Fifteen of these completed 6 months of treatment and were included in the final analysis. The majority of patients reported complete resolution or mild to moderate improvement in discharge, pain, fistulas, and induration. Further assessment of PDAI score showed improvement, from a mean of 7.67 ± 2.19 prior to treatment to a mean of 4.40 ± 1.72 ($P < 0.001$) after 6 months of treatment.[69]

The delay in clinical response with AZA and 6-MP combination treatment lessens its attractiveness to clinicians. Mean response time is often quoted as 3 months, although there are some reports of 8 months to achieve clinical efficacy. Many clinicians prefer to use antibiotics combined with immunosuppressives for the initial medical management of perianal fistulas.[70,71] This approach allows rapid reduction of fistula drainage with antibiotics and a bridging to AZA or 6-MP treatment to maintain remission. Evidence supporting this approach has been recently shown by an Austrian study.[53] This prospective open-label study recruited patients with perianal fistulas and assessed their clinical responses to a combination of ciprofloxacin (500 to 1000 mg/day) or metronidazole (1000 to 1500 mg/day) and AZA therapy. Antibiotic therapy was carried out for 8 weeks. Most patients began AZA therapy prior to inclusion in the study, whereas the remaining were offered the drug following 8 weeks of antibiotics. The initial response was characterized by at least a 50% reduction in the baseline number of draining fistulas, as assessed using the fistula drainage assessment. After 8 weeks of antibiotics, 50% of patients had an initial response.[53] There was no difference between those receiving antibiotics alone or in combination with AZA at the 8-week mark. Following the 8 weeks, most patients went on, either continuing with AZA (if they had been on it prior to the study) or starting it after the cessation of antibiotics. A few patients refused therapy with immunosuppressive agents. Of those who remained in the study without taking AZA therapy, only 15% experienced a maintained response after 20 weeks. In contrast, 48% of patients on AZA experienced a maintained response (see Figure 33-6).[53] The findings remained unchanged after follow-up at week 32. The study also evaluated PDAI scores and found them to be closely related to treatment response. Questions of the duration of therapy with AZA are currently unanswered in regards to perianal fistula disease. There is, however, growing evidence that supports the use of these agents for maintenance of luminal remission in CD.[67] Given these results, a reasonable approach is to initi-

TABLE 33-8

CLINICAL EVIDENCE FOR CYCLOSPORINE IN PERIANAL FISTULAS*

Reference	Level of Evidence	Year	N	Initial Response	Sustained Response	Comments
Fukushima[73]	Case report	1989	1	100%	100%	8 mg/kg oral
Lichtiger[74]	Case series	1990	10	60%	NS	4 mg/kg IV
Hanauer[75]	Case series	1993	5	100%	40%	4 mg/kg IV
Present[76]	Case series	1994	16	87%	56%	4 mg/kg IV
Abreu-Martin[77]	Case series	1996	2	100%	50%	2.5 mg/kg IV
O'Neill[78]	Case series	1997	8	87%	0%	4 mg/kg IV
Hinterleitner[79]	Case series	1997	7	100%	45%	5 mg/kg IV
Egan[80]	Case series	1998	9	78%	25%	4 mg/kg
Gurudu[81]	Case series	1999	3	66%	NS	4 mg/kg IV
Total			63	83%	38%	

*NS indicates not significant.

TABLE 33-9

CLINICAL EVIDENCE FOR TACROLIMUS IN PERIANAL FISTULAS

Reference	Level of Evidence	Year	N	Initial Response	Comments
Sandborn[86]	Case report	1997	1	100%	
Fellermann[87]	Case report	1998	1	100%	
Lowry[88]	Retrospective chart review	1999	11	100% (4 complete, 7 partial)	All patients received AZA or 6-MP
Ierardi[89]	Case series	2000	2	100%	
Sandborn[90]	Randomized, placebo-controlled trial	2003	43	43% versus 8% placebo	Oral dose (0.20 mg/kg/day) 38% experienced nephrotoxicity

ate treatment using an antibiotic (ciprofloxacin, metronidazole, or both) in combination with AZA. A controlled trial assessing this regimen in comparison to infliximab therapy would be beneficial for providing clinicians with adequate information for their patients.

Cyclosporine

Cyclosporine is a potent immunosuppressive polypeptide derived from the fungus *Tolypocladium inflatum* Gams. It decreases IL-2 secretion by T helper cells, thereby halting the differentiation and proliferation of B cells and cytotoxic T cells in response to antigenic stimulation.[72] The discussion of cyclosporine therapy is based on a few case study series.[73-81] Table 33-8 summarizes the clinical evidence for its use in perianal fistulas. Most fistulas in the studies responded to intravenous (IV) cyclosporine (4 mg/kg) and continued to experience a response when treatment was converted to the oral formulation of the drug (8 to 10 mg/kg). A response usually occurred within 1 week of starting therapy with IV cyclosporine. Once cyclosporine was withdrawn, however, a substantial proportion of patients experienced a relapse. Some studies have even shown relapse despite an attempt to bridge to AZA or 6-MP.[79-81] Due to this high relapse rate and a poor side effect profile, many clinicians only choose cyclosporine as rescue therapy for patients who have been failed by all other available treatments and are not considered good candidates for surgery. Furthermore, long-term cyclosporine therapy for luminal chronic active Crohn's disease offers little benefit, as demonstrated by Canadian and European studies.[82-84]

Adverse events associated with cyclosporine include nephrotoxicity, hypertension, paresthesias, tremor, seizures, hypertrichosis, hepatotoxicity, gingival hyperplasia, and an increased incidence of infections. Patients are at risk of developing *Pneumocystis carinii* pneumonia, and some clinicians suggest prophylactic therapy for patients on cyclosporine.

TACROLIMUS

Tacrolimus' effects on immune regulation are similar to those of cyclosporine. It also inhibits the production of IL-2 by T helper cells.[85] The advantage of tacrolimus is that it is readily absorbed by the gut mucosa. Several small case study series have been reported, and they suggest a possible role for the drug in the management of perianal fistulas.[86-89] Table 33-9 summarizes the clinical evidence. Doses between 0.1 and 0.3 mg/kg/day were shown to have some benefit for patients with CD fistulas.

A recent multicenter randomized controlled trial of 48 patients was conducted over a 10-week period to assess the efficacy of this treatment.[90] Twenty-two patients were randomized to a group receiving oral tacrolimus at a mean dose of 0.2 mg/kg/day (mean whole blood concentration of 13.7 ng/mL). The remaining 26 patients were given a placebo. Both groups were allowed to take other medications such as 5-aminosalicylic acid (5-ASA), steroids, antibiotics, AZA, and 6-MP. The rate of fistula improvement (defined as closure of ≥50% of draining fistulas) was significantly greater for the patients taking tacrolimus (9 of 21, 43%) compared with placebo (2 of 25, 8%; $P = 0.01$).[90] The OR was 8.62 in favor of fistula healing. Despite these findings, however, the study did not show a statistical difference in rates of fistula remission (10% versus 8%). Whether this failure is secondary to a weak treatment effect or due to inadequate statistical power to detect meaningful differences is uncertain. Of note is the fact that patients who had previously been treated with infliximab and were intolerant of that drug experienced fistula improvement. Of 15 patients previously treated with infliximab, 7 (47%) improved on tacrolimus, suggesting a possible role for the drug in controlling symptoms prior to surgical therapy.

A large number of patients receiving tacrolimus experienced nephrotoxicity. Eight of 21 patients (38%) experienced an increase in serum creatinine level, from baseline to a value ≥ 1.5 mg/dL (≥ 132 μmol/L), as compared to 0 of 25 (0%) of the placebo group ($P = 0.008$).[90] In a manner similar to the case of cyclosporine, the histological lesions on renal biopsy consist of striped interstitial nephritis and arteriolar alterations.[91] Because of this nephrotoxicity, some investigators have suggested an exploration of the safety and effectiveness of low-dose tacrolimus. Other adverse events include headache, insomnia, leg cramps, paresthesias, and tremor.

INFLIXIMAB

Tumor necrosis factor alpha (TNFα) plays a key role in the initiation and propagation of CD.[92] Produced by monocytes, macrophages, and T cells, TNFα is integral to the recruitment of circulating inflammatory cells to local tissue sites of inflammation. TNFα then induces local edema, activates coagulation, and plays a pivotal role in granuloma

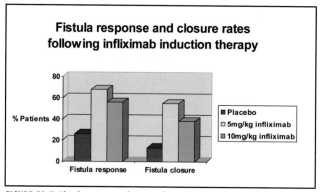

FIGURE 33-7. Fistula response (>50% of baseline draining fistulas closed) and fistula closure rates following 3 infusions of infliximab (5 mg/kg or 10 mg/kg) at weeks 0, 2, and 6 versus placebo. (Adapted from Present DH, Rutgeerts P, Targan S, et al. Infliximab for the treatment of fistulas in patients with Crohn's disease. *N Engl J Med.* 1999:1398-1405.)

formation. Several investigators began analyzing the effects of anti-TNFα on animal models of inflammatory bowel disease (IBD) in the 1990s and found positive effects.[93,94] Infliximab (formerly known as cA2) is a genetically constructed immunoglobulin (Ig) G1 murine-human chimeric monoclonal antibody that binds the soluble subunit and the membrane-bound precursor of TNFα.[95,96] Initial trials of the molecule (cA2) showed infliximab to be efficacious in the treatment of moderate-to-severe Crohn's.[97-100] During these trials, it was noted that the closure of many fistulas was associated with the treatment.

Because of the anecdotal evidence that infliximab closed fistulas, a large multicenter randomized controlled trial on the efficacy of the infliximab treatment of fistulas in CD was undertaken.[52] Again, a reduction of 50% in the number of draining fistulas at 2 consecutive visits with a minimum of 21 days in between was defined as the primary endpoint. Patients were randomized to groups receiving infliximab 5 mg/kg, infliximab 10 mg/kg, or placebo. Patients were allowed to take concomitant medications such as 5-ASA, steroids, antibiotics, AZA, and 6-MP. Treatment was given intravenously at weeks 0, 2, and 6. Patients given infliximab experienced significantly greater response rates than those who received placebo. Among the infliximab group, the 5 mg/kg achieved a response rate of 68% and the 10 mg/kg rate was 56%, as compared to the placebo's response of 26% ($P = 0.002$ and $P = 0.02$, respectively) (Figure 33-7). Response rates between the 2 infliximab groups did not differ significantly ($P = 0.35$). Complete response rates, defined as the absence of any draining fistulas for at least 4 weeks, were 55% in the 5 mg/kg infliximab group and 38% in the 10 mg/kg infliximab group, as compared to 13% in the placebo group ($P = 0.001$ and $P = 0.04$). Median time to reach a clinical response was shorter for infliximab-treated patients. Both infliximab-treated groups experienced a clinical response in a median of 14 days, as compared to 42 days for placebo.

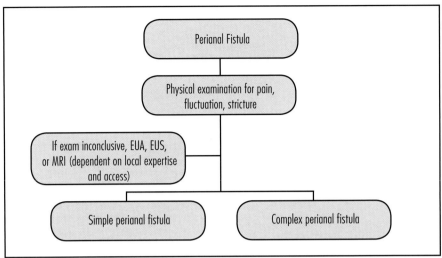

FIGURE 33-8. Algorithm for determining the classification of perianal fistulas.

The ACCENT II study has shown the benefits of maintenance infliximab therapy for perianal fistulas in CD.[101] This multicenter randomized double-blind trial demonstrated the benefits of continuing infliximab therapy for individuals whose disease initially responded to the standard infusions at weeks 0, 2, and 6. Following a response to the initial infusions, patients were randomized to continue to receive infliximab (5 mg/kg every 8 weeks through week 54) or a placebo infusion. The primary endpoint, time to loss of response, was significantly longer in the infliximab maintenance group than in the placebo group (greater than 40 weeks versus 14 weeks, *P* <0.001).[101] Further analysis also showed that at week 54, 23% of patients in the placebo maintenance group still were experiencing a response, as compared to 46% in the infliximab maintenance group (*P* = 0.001). Rates of complete response, defined as the absence of any draining fistulas, were also significantly better in the infliximab maintenance group (19% versus 36%, *P* = 0.009). In the case of patients who did not initially respond to the 3 infusions of infliximab, there was no benefit to continuing infliximab, as response rates were equal to those of placebo infusions.[101]

Although maintenance infliximab therapy is beneficial in managing perianal fistulas of CD, there are still many unanswered questions. The most important safety issues involve infusion reactions, delayed hypersensitivity reactions, formation of human anti-chimeric antibodies, formation of anti-nuclear antibodies and double-stranded DNA antibodies, and drug-induced lupus. Concomitant immunosuppressive therapy with AZA, 6-MP, or methotrexate reduces the frequency of these reactions and is therefore recommended.[102,103] Other serious adverse events include an increased propensity to infections. The largest series reported included 500 consecutive patients from the Mayo Clinic.[104] Six percent of patients experienced a serious adverse event related to infliximab, and 1% of the deaths were possibly attributable to infliximab.

Serious infections such as sepsis, tuberculosis, histoplasmosis, coccidioidomycosis, listeriosis, *Pneumocystis carinii* pneumonia, aspergillosis, cutaneous nocardiosis, and disseminated varicella have been reported.[104-115]

Durability of the response is also an important question to consider. As depicted in the ACCENT II study, an attenuated response or loss of response after a very good response often develops.[101] Much debate has been focused on the potential causes of this phenomenon. The development of antibodies to infliximab, upregulation of other cytokines, and the development of strictures have been put forward as possible major factors.[116] The best likely duration of therapy with infliximab remains unclear.

GENERAL MANAGEMENT APPROACH TO PERIANAL FISTULA

Following identification of perianal fistulas associated with CD, clear definition of the fistulous tracts should be carefully determined. Classification of fistulas into complex or simple categories helps in planning appropriate medical or surgical care. Perianal pain, tenderness, or fluctuation suggests the possibility of a perianal abscess. Confirmation via EUS, MRI, or EUA is suggested. Perianal abscesses should be surgically drained before the initiation of immunosuppressive therapy.[11] Any anal stricture found during the physical examination should also receive surgical attention.

If physical examination does not confirm tenderness, fluctuation, or stricture, then the fistulas should be classified into simple fistulas or complex fistulas. Simple fistulas are low, not associated with abscess, have 1 external opening, and do not involve rectovaginal connections or anorectal stricture. Complex fistulas, by contrast, are high and/or are associated with perianal abscess, have multiple

FIGURE 33-9. Treatment algorithm for simple perianal fistulas.

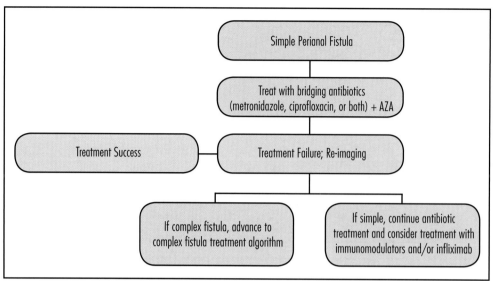

openings, and/or involve rectovaginal connection or ano-rectal stricture. The management of the fistulas often depends on this classification, so it is important to carefully investigate the matter. A suggested algorithm for the management of perianal fistulas is provided in Figure 33-8.

Not all fistulas require further diagnostic imaging or EUA. If the appearance and attributes of the fistula are simple in classification, then further treatment with antibiotics plus immunosuppressives can be considered. Some experts, however, believe that all patients who present with a perianal fistula should undergo EUS or MRI, with or without EUA.[117] One small retrospective study did find, however, that the use of EUA with seton placement as an adjunct to infliximab therapy enhanced the response rate over that of infliximab alone (100% versus 83%, P = 0.014), as well as providing a lower incidence of recurrence (44% versus 79%, P = 0.001), and a longer time to recurrence (13.5 months versus 3.6 months, P = 0.001).[13] Another small Canadian retrospective analysis found complete healing in the case of 67% of patients when selective seton placements were combined with 3 infusions of infliximab and maintenance immunosuppressives.[15] Recently, another small prospective study evaluated the treatment of complex fistulas with a combination of pretreatment surgery followed by infliximab. This combination achieved a 100% initial response, with only a 10% recurrence in 24 months. The strategy for determining course of action, therefore, should begin with delineating fistulous tracts, draining associated abscesses, and addressing surgical concerns.[118]

SIMPLE FISTULAS

These fistulas are usually the easiest to manage (Figure 33-9). Healing rates are usually higher than for other types. Patients should receive a full 8-week course of antibiot-

ics; concomitant therapy with immunosuppressive agents may be initiated at the same time.[53] Infliximab therapy should be reserved for treatment failures. If, after 8 weeks, response is limited, then the patient's disease should be treated as a complex fistula case. Further imaging to help identify factors associated with the lack of healing should be undertaken. Simple fistulas with no accompanying rectal inflammation may also be treated through surgical fistulotomy, although there is insufficient published evidence to do with postoperative morbidity. Rectal mucosal inflammation often requires strategies focused on reducing luminal activity. Although this strategy has never been formally evaluated, local therapy with 5-ASA products (such as suppositories and enemas) is used to help in achieving fistula response, as rectal inflammation is reduced. Care in the use of these therapies is necessary, as a disturbance to the fistula tract and opening may occur during their insertion.

COMPLEX FISTULAS

Clearly, these fistulas are the most difficult to treat (Figure 33-10). All complex fistulas require surgical evaluation. Associated abscesses should be drained, and non-cutting setons should usually be placed surgically prior to infliximab therapy. Failure to place a seton very often leads to closure of the fistula's opening and abscess of the internal tract. Following surgical therapy, a combination of antibiotic, immunosuppressive, and infliximab treatments may be used in an attempt to close the fistula. Clinical improvement usually occurs before complete closure is identified on diagnostic imaging. Patients should continue taking immunosuppressives and infliximab after the fistula closes, although the therapy's optimal length of time is still not fully defined. Failure of this therapy often leaves clinicians with very few options. Tacrolimus may

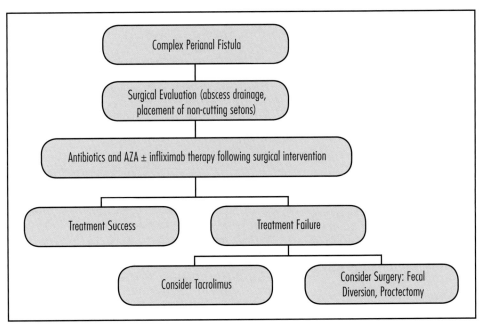

FIGURE 33-10. Treatment algorithm for complex perianal fistulas.

be used, although the adverse events and success rates are not impressive. Failure of medical treatment leads to the domain of the surgeon, who may offer fecal diversion and proctectomy in an attempt to reduce morbidity.

CONCLUSION

Perianal manifestations of Crohn's disease, including perianal fistulas, are very common. Often difficult to manage, these fistulas have a profound degree of morbidity and a deep psychological effect on many patients. Newer diagnostic imaging such as pelvic MRI and anorectal EUS are helpful in classifying types of fistulas, thus allowing prediction of response to therapy. Antibiotics and immunosuppressive therapy remain in the forefront of management of simple fistulas. Complex fistulas require evaluation by an experienced colorectal surgeon. The introduction of infliximab has revolutionized the treatment algorithm for this disease. It is used in the cases of failures in other therapies for simple fistulas and of concomitant therapy for complex fistulas. Many questions remain unanswered, however, regarding length of treatment, the development of antibodies to infliximab, and economic concerns. To this date, an approach that combines antibiotics and immunosuppressives and/or infliximab remains the best option supported by the most clinical evidence.

REFERENCES

1. Minei JP, Champine JG. Abdominal abscesses and gastrointestinal fistulas. In: Feldman M, Friedman LS, Sleisenger MH, eds. *Gastrointestinal and Liver Disease.* 7th ed. Philadelphia, PA: Saunders; 2002:431-445.

2. Jorge JMN, Wexner SD. Anatomy and physiology of the rectum and anus. *Eur J Surg.* 1997;163:723-731.

3. Keighley MRB, Williams NS. Surgical anatomy. In: *Surgery of the Anus, Rectum and Colon.* 2nd ed. Philadelphia, PA: WB Saunders; 1997:7.

4. Parks A. The pathogenesis and treatment of fistula-in-ano. *Br Med J.* 1961;1:463.

5. Goligher J. Fistula-in-ano. In: Goligher J, ed. *Surgery of the Anus, Rectum, and Colon.* 5th ed. London: Balliere Tindall; 1984:178-220.

6. Hughes LE. Surgical pathology and management of anorectal Crohn's disease. *J R Soc Med.* 1978;71:644-651.

7. Hughes LE. Clinical classification of perianal Crohn's disease. *Dis Colon Rectum.* 1992;35:928-932.

8. Francois Y, Vignal J, Descos L. Outcome of perianal fistulae in Crohn's disease—value of Hughes' pathogenic classification. *Int J Colorectal Dis.* 1993;8:39-41.

9. Pikarsky AJ, Gervaz P, Wexner SD. Perianal Crohn disease: a new scoring system to evaluate and predict outcome of surgical intervention. *Arch Surg.* 2002;137:774-777.

10. Parks AG, Gordon PH, Hardcastle JD. A classification of fistula-in-ano. *Br J Surg.* 1976;63:1-12.

11. American Gastroenterological Association. American Gastroenterological Association technical review on perianal Crohn's disease. *Gastroenterology.* 2003;125:1508-1530.

12. Bell SJ, Williams AB, Wiesel P, Wilkinson K, Cohen RC, Kamm MA. The clinical course of fistulating Crohn's disease. *Aliment Pharmacol Ther.* 2003;17:1145-1151.

13. Reguerio M, Mardini H. Treatment of perianal fistulizing Crohn's disease with infliximab alone or as an adjunct to exam under anesthesia with seton placement. *Inflamm Bowel Dis.* 2003;9:98-103.

14. Scott HJ, Northover JM. Evaluation of surgery for perianal Crohn's fistulas. *Dis Colon Rectum.* 1996;39:1039-1043.

15. Topstad DR, Panaccione R, Heine JA, Johnson DR, MacLean AR, Buie WD. Combined seton placement, infliximab infusion, and maintenance immunosuppressives improve healing rate in fistulizing anorectal Crohn's disease: a single center experience. *Dis Colon Rectum*. 2003;46:577-583.

16. Hawley PR. Anorectal fistula. *Clin Gastroenterol*. 1975;4:635-649.

17. Hellers G, Bergstrand O, Ewerth S, Holmstrom B. Occurrence and outcome after primary treatment of anal fistulae in Crohn's disease. *Gut*. 1980;21:525-527.

18. Schwartz DA, Loftus EV Jr, Tremaine WJ, et al. The natural history of fistulizing Crohn's disease in Olmsted County, Minnesota. *Gastroenterology*. 2002;122:875-880.

19. Anseline PF. Crohn's disease in the Hunter Valley region of Australia. *Austr N Z*. 1995;65:564-569.

20. Van Beers B, Grandin C, Kartheuser A. MRI of complicated anal fistulae: comparison with digital examination. *J Comput Assist Tomogr*. 1994;18:87-90.

21. Glass RE, Ritchie JK, Lennard-Jones JE, Hawley PR, Todd IP. Internal fistulas in Crohn's disease. *Dis Colon Rectum*. 1985;28:557-561.

22. Fazio VW, Wilk P, Turnbull RB Jr, Jagelman DG. The dilemma of Crohn's disease: ileosigmoidal fistula complicating Crohn's disease. *Dis Colon Rectum*. 1977;20:381-386.

23. Kuijpers HC, Schulpen T. Fistulography for fistula-in-ano. Is it useful? *Dis Colon Rectum*. 1985;28:103-104.

24. Pomerri F, Pittarello F, Dodi G, Pianon P, Muzzio PC. Radiologic diagnosis of anal fistulae with radio-opaque markers. *Radiologia Med*. 1988;75:632-637.

25. Weisman RI, Orsay CP, Pearl RK, Abcarian H. The role of fistulography in fistula-in-ano. Report of 5 cases. *Dis Colon Rectum*. 1991;34:181-184.

26. Schratter-Sehn AU, Lochs H, Vogelsang H, Schurawitzki H, Herold C, Schratter M. Endoscopic ultrasonography versus computed tomography in the differential diagnosis of peri-anorectal complications in Crohn's disease. *Endoscopy*. 1993;25:582-586.

27. Van Outryve MJ, Pelckmans PA, Michielsen PP, Van Maercke YM. Value of transrectal ultrasonography in Crohn's disease. *Gastroenterology*. 1991;101:1171-1177.

28. Fishman EK, Wolf EJ, Jones B, Bayless TM, Siegelman SS. CT evaluation of Crohn's disease: effect on patient management. *Am J Roentgenol*. 1987;148:537-540.

29. Berliner L, Redmond P, Purow E, Megna D, Sottile V. Computed tomography in Crohn's disease. *Am J Gastroenterol*. 1982;77:548-553.

30. Yousem DM, Fishman EK, Jones B. Crohn disease: perirectal and perianal findings at CT. *Radiology*. 1988;167:331-334.

31. Goldberg HI, Gore RM, Margulis AR, Moss AA, Baker EL. Computed tomography in the evaluation of Crohn's disease. *Am J Roentgenol*. 1983;140:277-282.

32. Kerber GW, Greenberg M, Rubin JM. Computed tomography evaluation of local and extraintestinal complications of Crohn's disease. *Gastrointest Radiol*. 1994;9:143-148.

33. Lunniss PJ, Barker PG, Sultan AH et al. Magnetic resonance imaging of fistula-in-ano. *Dis Colon Rectum*. 1994;37:708-718.

34. Barker PG, Lunniss PJ, Armstrong P, Reznek RH, Cottam K, Phillips RK. Magnetic resonance imaging of fistula-in-ano: technique, interpretation and accuracy. *Clin Radiol*. 1994;49:7-13.

35. Haggett PJ, Moore NR, Shearman JD, Travis SP, Jewell DP, Mortensen NJ. Pelvic and perianal complications of Crohn's disease: assessment using magnetic resonance imaging. *Gut*. 1995;36:407-410.

36. Spencer JA, Chapple K, Wilson D, Ward J, Windsor AC, Ambrose NS. Outcome after surgery for perianal fistula: predictive value of MR imaging. *Am J Roentgenol*. 1998;171:403-406.

37. Koelbel G, Schmiedl U, Majer MC, et al. Diagnosis of fistulae and sinus tracts in patients with Crohn disease: value of MR imaging. *Am J Roentgenol*. 1989;152:999-1003.

38. Schwartz DA, Wiersema MJ, Dudiak KM, et al. A comparison of endoscopic ultrasound, magnetic resonance imaging, and exam under anesthesia for evaluation of Crohn's perianal fistulas. *Gastroenterology*. 2001;121:1064-1072.

39. Tio TL, Mulder CJ, Wijers OB, Sars PR, Tytgat GN. Endosonography of peri-anal and peri-colorectal fistula and/or abscess in Crohn's disease. *Gastrointest Endosc*. 1990;36:331-336.

40. Orsoni P, Barthet M, Portier F, Panuel M, Desjeux A, Grimaud JC. Prospective comparison of endosonography, magnetic resonance imaging and surgical findings in anorectal fistula and abscess complicating Crohn's disease. *Br J Surg*. 1999;86:360-364.

41. Stewart LK, McGee J, Wilson SR. Transperineal and transvaginal sonography of perianal inflammatory disease. *Am J Roentgenol*. 2001;177:627-632.

42. Sloots CE, Felt-Bersma RJ, Poen AC, Cuesta MA, Meuwissen SG. Assessment and classification of fistula-in-ano in patients with Crohn's disease by hydrogen peroxide enhanced transanal ultrasound. *Int J Colorectal Dis*. 2001;16:292-297.

43. West RL, Zimmerman DD, Dwarkasing S, et al. Prospective comparison of hydrogen peroxide-enhanced three-dimensional endoanal ultrasonography and endoanal magnetic resonance imaging of perianal fistulas. *Dis Colon Rectum*. 2003;46:1407-1415.

44. West RL, Dwarkasing S, Felt-Bersma RJ, Schouten WR, et al. Hydrogen peroxide-enhanced three-dimensional endoanal ultrasonography and endoanal magnetic resonance imaging in evaluating perianal fistulas: agreement and patient preference. *Eur J Gastroenterol Hepatol*. 2004;16:1319-1324.

45. Van Assche G, Vanbeckevoort D, Bielen D, et al. Magnetic resonance imaging of the effects of infliximab on perianal fistulizing Crohn's disease. *Am J Gastroenterol*. 2003;98:332-339.

46. Bell SJ, Halligan S, Windsor AC, Williams AB, Wiesel P, Kamm MA. Response of fistulating Crohn's disease to infliximab treatment assessed by magnetic resonance imaging. *Aliment Pharmacol Ther*. 2003;17:387-393.

47. van Bodegraven AA, Sloots CE, Felt-Bersma RJ, Meuwissen SG. Endosonographic evidence of persistence of Crohn's disease-associated fistulas after infliximab treatment, irrespective of clinical response. *Dis Colon Rectum*. 2002;45:39-45.

48. Ardizzone S, Maconi G, Colombo E, Manzionna G, Bollani S, Porro GB. Perianal fistulae following infliximab treatment: clinical and endosonographic outcome. *Inflamm Bowel Dis*. 2004;10:91-96.

49. Present DH, Korelitz BI, Wisch N, Glass JL, Sachar DB, Pasternack BS. Treatment of Crohn's disease with 6-mercaptopurine. A long-term, randomized, double-blind study. *N Engl J Med*. 1980;302:981-987.

50. Alexander-Williams J, Hellers G, Hughes LE, Minervini S, Speranza V. Classification of perianal Crohn's disease. *Gastroenterol Int*. 1992;5:216-220.

51. Irvine EJ. Usual therapy improves perianal Crohn's disease as measured by a new disease activity index. McMaster IBD Study Group. *J Clin Gastroenterol*. 1995;20:27-32.

52. Present DH, Rutgeerts P, Targan S, et al. Infliximab for the treatment of fistulas in patients with Crohn's disease. *N Engl J Med*. 1999;1398-1405.

53. Dejaco C, Harrer M, Waldhoer T, Miehsler W, Vogelsang H, Reinisch W. Antibiotics and azathioprine for the treatment of perianal fistulas in Crohn's disease. *Aliment Pharmacol Ther*. 2003;18:1113-1120.

54. Sandborn WJ, Feagan BG, Hanauer SB, et al. A review of activity indices and efficacy endpoints for clinical trials of medical therapy in adults with Crohn's disease. *Gastroenterology*. 2002;122:512-530.

55. Ursing B, Kamme C. Metronidazole for Crohn's disease. *Lancet.* 1975;1:775-777.

56. Bernstein LH, Frank MS, Brandt LJ, Boley SJ. Healing of perineal Crohn's disease with metronidazole. *Gastroenterology.* 1980;79:357-365.

57. Brandt LJ, Bernstein LH, Boley SJ, Frank MS. Metronidazole therapy for perineal Crohn's disease: a follow-up study. *Gastroenterology.* 1982;83:383-387.

58. Turunen U, Farkkila M, Valtonen V. Long-term outcome of ciprofloxacin treatment in severe perianal or fistulous Crohn's disease [abstract]. *Gastroenterology.* 1993;104:A793.

59. Brooke BN, Hoffman DC, Swarbrick ET. Azathioprine for Crohn's disease. *Lancet.* 1969;2:612.

60. Willoughby JMT, Beckett J, Kumar PJ, Dawson AM. Controlled trial of azathioprine in Crohn's disease. *Lancet.* 1971;2:944-947.

61. Rhodes J, Beck P, Bainton D, Campbell H. Controlled trial of azathioprine in Crohn's disease. *Lancet.* 1971;2:1273-1276.

62. Klein M, Binder HJ, Mitchell M, Aaronson R, Spiro H. Treatment of Crohn's disease with azathioprine: a controlled evaluation. *Gastroenterology.* 1974;66:916-922.

63. Rosenberg JL, Levin B, Wall AJ, Kirsner JB. A controlled trial of azathioprine in Crohn's disease. *Dig Dis Sci.* 1975;20:721-726.

64. Present DH, Korelitz BI, Wisch N, Glass JL, Sachar DB, Pasternack BS. Treatment of Crohn's disease with 6-mercaptopurine. A long-term, randomized, double-blind study. *N Engl J Med.* 1980;302:981-987.

65. Korelitz BI, Present DH. Favorable effect of 6-mercaptopurine on fistulae of Crohn's disease. *Dig Dis Sci.* 1985;30:58-64.

66. O'Brien JJ, Bayless TM, Bayless JA. Use of azathioprine or 6-mercaptopurine in the treatment of Crohn's disease. *Gastroenterology.* 1991;101:39-46.

67. Pearson DC, May GR, Flick GH, Sutherland LR. Azathioprine and 6-mercaptopurine in Crohn disease. A meta-analysis. *Ann Int Med.* 1995;123:132-142.

68. Markowitz J, Rosa J, Grancher K, Aiges H, Daum F. Long term 6-mercaptopurine treatment in adolescents with Crohn's disease. *Gastroenterology.* 1990;99:1347-1351.

69. Jehsion WC, Larsen KL, Jawad AF, et al. Azathioprine and 6-mercaptopurine for the treatment of perianal Crohn's disease in children. *J Clin Gastroenterol.* 2000;30:294-298.

70. Present DH. Crohn's fistula: current concepts in management. *Gastroenterology.* 2003;124:1629-1635.

71. Lichtenstein GR, Hanauer SB, Sandborn WJ, Practice Parameters Committee of American College of Gastroenterology. Management of Crohn's disease in adults. *Am J Gastroenterol.* 2009;104(2):465-483.

72. Kahan BD. Cyclosporine. *N Engl J Med.* 1989;321:1725-1738.

73. Fukushima T, Sugita A, Masuzawa S, Yamazaki Y. Effect of cyclosporine A on active Crohn's disease. *Gastroenterol Jpn.* 1989;24:12-15.

74. Lichtiger S. Cyclosporine therapy in inflammatory bowel disease: open-label experience. *Mount Sinai J Med.* 1990;57:315-319.

75. Hanauer SB, Smith MB. Rapid closure of Crohn's disease fistulas with continuous intravenous cyclosporin A. *Am J Gastroenterol.* 1993;88:646-649.

76. Present DH, Lichtiger S. Efficacy of cyclosporine in treatment of fistula of Crohn's disease. *Dig Dis Sci.* 1994;39:374-380.

77. Abreu-Martin M, Vasiliauskas E, Gaiennie J, Voigt B, Targan SR. Continuous infusion cyclosporine is effective for severe acute Crohn's disease … But for how long? [abstract]. *Gastroenterology.* 1996;110:A851.

78. O'Neill J, Pathmakanthan S, Goh J. Cyclosporine A induces remission in fistulous Crohn's disease but relapse occurs upon cessation of treatment [abstract]. *Gastroenterology.* 1997;112:A1056.

79. Hinterleitner TA, Petritsch W, Aichbichler B, Fickert P, Ranner G, Krejs GJ. Combination of cyclosporine, azathioprine and prednisolone for perianal fistulas in Crohn's disease. *Z Gastroenterol.* 1997;35:603-608.

80. Egan LJ, Sandborn WJ, Tremaine WJ. Clinical outcome following treatment of refractory inflammatory and fistulizing Crohn's disease with intravenous cyclosporine. *Am J Gastroenterol.* 1998;93:442-448.

81. Gurudu SR, Griffel LH, Gialanella RJ, Das KM. Cyclosporine therapy in inflammatory bowel disease: short-term and long-term results. *J Clin Gastroenterol.* 1999;29:151-154.

82. Feagan BG, McDonald JWD, Rochon J, et al. Low-dose cyclosporine for the treatment of Crohn's disease. *N Engl J Med.* 1994;330:1846-1851.

83. Jewell DP, Lennard-Jones JE, The Cyclosporin Study Group of Great Britain and Ireland. Oral cyclosporin for chronic active Crohn's disease: a multicentre controlled trial. *Eur J Gastroenterol Hepatol.* 1994;6:499-505.

84. Stange EF, Modigliani R, Salvador Pena A, et al. European trial of cyclosporine in chronic active Crohn's disease: a 12 month study. *Gastroenterology.* 1995;109:774-782.

85. Liu J, Farmer JD Jr, Lane WS, Friedman J, Weissman I, Schreiber SL. Calcineurin is a common target of cyclosphilin-cyclosporin A and FKBP-FK506 complexes. *Cell.* 1991;66:807-815.

86. Sandborn WJ. Preliminary report on the use of oral tacrolimus (FK506) in the treatment of complicated proximal small bowel and fistulizing Crohn's disease. *Am J Gastroenterol.* 1997;92:876-879.

87. Fellermann K, Ludwig D, Stahl M, David-Walek T, Stange EF. Steroid-unresponsive acute attacks of inflammatory bowel disease: immunomodulation by tacrolimus (FK506). *Am J Gastroenterol.* 1998;93:1860-1866.

88. Lowry PW, Weaver AL, Tremaine WJ, Sandborn WJ. Combination therapy with oral tacrolimus (FK-506) and azathioprine or 6-mercaptopurine for treatment-refractory Crohn's disease perianal fistulae. *Inflamm Bowel Dis.* 1999;5:239-245.

89. Ierardi E, Principi M, Rendina M, et al. Oral tacrolimus (FK506) in Crohn's disease complicated by fistulae of the perineum. *J Clin Gastroenterol.* 2000;30:200-202.

90. Sandborn WJ, Present DH, Isaacs KL, et al. Tacrolimus for the treatment of fistulas in patients with Crohn's disease: a randomized, placebo-controlled trial. *Gastroenterology.* 2003;125:380-388.

91. Randhawa PS, Shapiro R, Jordan ML, Starzl TE, Demetris AJ. The histopathological changes associated with allograft rejection and drug toxicity in renal transplant recipients maintained on FK506. Clinical significance and comparison with cyclosporine. *Am J Surg Pathol.* 1993;17:60-68.

92. Van Deventer SJH. Tumour necrosis factor and Crohn's disease. *Gut.* 1997;40:443-448.

93. Kojouharoff G, Hans W, Obermeier F, et al. Neutralization of tumor necrosis factor (TNF) but not of IL-1 reduces inflammation in chronic dextran sulphate sodium-induced colitis in mice. *Clin Exp Immunol.* 1997;107:353-358.

94. Neurath MF, Fuss I, Pasparakis M, et al. Predominant pathogenic role of tumor necrosis factor in experimental colitis in mice. *Eur J Immunol.* 1997;27:1743-1750.

95. Knight DM, Trinh H, Le J, et al. Construction and initial characterization of a mouse-human chimeric anti-TNF antibody. *Mol Immunol.* 1993;30:1443-1453.

96. Scallon BJ, Moore MA, Trinh H, Knight DM, Ghrayeb J. Chimeric anti-TNF-α monoclonal antibody cA2 binds recombinant transmembrane TNF-α and activates immune effector functions. *Cytokine.* 1995;7:251-259.

97. McCabe RP, Woody J, van Deventer SJH, et al. A multicenter trial of cA2 anti-TNF chimeric monoclonal antibody in patients with active Crohn's disease [abstract]. *Gastroenterology.* 1996;110:A962.

98. van Dullemen HM, van Deventer SJH, Hommes DW, et al. Treatment of Crohn's disease with anti-tumor necrosis factor chimeric monoclonal antibody (cA2). *Gastroenterology*. 1995;109:129-135.

99. Targan SR, Hanauer SB, van Deventer SJH, et al. A short-term study of chimeric monoclonal antibody cA2 to tumor necrosis factor α for Crohn's disease. *N Engl J Med*. 1997;337:1029-1035.

100. Rutgeerts P, D'Haens G, van Deventer SJH, et al. Retreatment with anti-TNF-α chimeric antibody (cA2) effectively maintains cA2-induced remission in Crohn's disease [abstract]. *Gastroenterology*. 1997;112:A1078.

101. Sands BE, Anderson FH, Bernstein CN, et al. Infliximab maintenance therapy for fistulizing Crohn's disease. *N Engl J Med*. 2004;350:876-885.

102. Sandborn WJ, Hanauer SB. Infliximab in the treatment of Crohn's disease: a user's guide for clinicians. *Am J Gastroenterol*. 2002;97:2962-2972.

103. Panaccione R, Fedorak RN, Aumais G, et al. Canadian Association of Gastroenterology Clinical Practice Guidelines: the use of infliximab in Crohn's disease. *Can J Gastroenterol*. 2004;18:503-508.

104. Colombel JF, Loftus EV Jr, Tremaine WJ, et al. The safety profile of infliximab in patients with Crohn's disease: the Mayo clinic experience in 500 patients. *Gastroenterology*. 2004;126:19-31.

105. Sandborn WJ, Hanauer SB. Antitumor necrosis factor therapy for inflammatory bowel disease: a review of agents, pharmacology, clinical results, and safety. *Inflamm Bowel Dis*. 1999;5:119-133.

106. Schaible TF. Long term safety of infliximab. *Can J Gastroenterol*. 2000;14(suppl C):29C-32C.

107. Remicaide (infliximab) for IV injection [package insert], 2002.

108. Keane J, Gershon S, Wise RP, et al. Tuberculosis associated with infliximab, a tumor necrosis factor alpha-neutralizing agent. *N Engl J Med*. 2001;345:1098-1104.

109. Warris A, Bjorneklett A, Gaustad P. Invasive pulmonary aspergillosis associated with infliximab therapy. *N Engl J Med*. 2001;344:1099-1100.

110. Nakelchik M, Mangino JE. Reactivation of histoplasmosis after treatment with infliximab. *Am J Med*. 2002;112:78.

111. Kamath BM, Mamula P, Baldassano RN, Markowitz JE. Listeria meningitis after treatment with infliximab. *J Pediatr Gastroenterol Nutr*. 2002;34:410-412.

112. Morelli J, Wilson FA. Does administration of infliximab increase susceptibility to listeriosis? *Am J Gastroenterol*. 2000;95:841-842.

113. Leung VS, Nguyen MT, Bush TM. Disseminated primary varicella after initiation of infliximab for Crohn's disease. *Am J Gastroenterol*. 2004;99:2503-2504.

114. Velayos FS, Sandborn WJ. *Pneumocystis carinii* pneumonia during maintenance anti-tumor necrosis factor-alpha therapy with infliximab for Crohn's disease. *Inflamm Bowel Dis*. 2004;10:657-660.

115. Singh SM, Rau NV, Cohen LB, Harris H. Cutaneous nocardiosis complicating management of Crohn's disease with infliximab and prednisone. *CMAJ*. 2004;171:1063-1064.

116. Baidoo L, Lichtenstein GR. What next after infliximab? *Am J Gastroenterol*. 2005;100:80-83.

117. Schwartz DA, Herdman CR. Review article: the medical treatment of Crohn's perianal fistula. *Aliment Pharmacol Ther*. 2004;19:953-967.

118. van der Hagen SJ, Baeten CG, Soeters PB, et al. Anti-TNF-alpha (infliximab) used as induction treatment in case of active proctitis in a multistep strategy followed by definitive surgery of complex anal fistulas in Crohn's disease: a preliminary report. *Dis Colon Rectum*. 2005;48(4):758-767.

34

MEDICAL THERAPY OF DIARRHEA
FOLLOWING BOWEL RESECTION

Henry J. Binder, MD

Concepts of surgery in CD have significantly changed in the past quarter century. In a prior era, multiple intestinal resections as well as "by-pass" operations of segments of small intestine were frequently performed often resulting in short bowel syndrome and intestinal failure (see Chapter 35). More recently, because of the high rate of recurrence of CD in the operated patient (despite removal of all evidence of disease), standard surgical principles emphasize that "less is better." As a result, more limited resections are often performed with much more stringent indications.

Nonetheless, intestinal resections in patients with CD are still performed, and the clinical consequences of these operations are at times not insignificant. Although diarrhea is frequently the primary "complication" of intestinal resection, several other problems may be manifest, including gall stones and renal calculi. This chapter will summarize the problems that occur following intestinal resection, primarily emphasizing the multiple mechanisms that may be responsible for diarrhea as well as logical and practical therapeutic approaches for its treatment.

The primary determinants of the characteristics and magnitude of diarrhea that may occur following intestinal resection in patients with CD are 1) the segment of intestine that is resected, 2) the length of resection, 3) removal of the ileocecal valve, and 4) whether the residual intestinal mucosa is or is not normal (ie, is there ongoing inflammation of CD?). It is important to emphasize that following small bowel resection, the intestine undergoes adaptation that results in an increase in both structure and function that has been well studied in experimental animals and is critical to determining the extent of disability in patients

who have had a massive intestinal resection. Such adaptation is induced by several factors, but most important is oral nutrition that is required to induce the hormonal factor(s) that induce cellular and functional adaptation.[1] Further, complete adaptation may take up to 6 months to occur so that clinical evaluation immediately following an extensive small intestinal resection may not provide an accurate assessment of the patient's clinical status several months later after adaptation has been complete. Such patients are frequently referred to as *short bowel syndrome*, whose medical management is discussed in Chapter 36.

Prior to any discussion of the effects of intestinal resection, it is useful to review both normal fluid and electrolyte balance, as well as lipid digestion and absorption.

FLUID AND ELECTROLYTE MOVEMENT

Dietary fluid intake is approximately 2 L per day while normal stool output is less than 0.2 L per day on a typical Western diet. As a consequence, overall efficacy of intestinal absorption would appear to be approximately 90%. However, the total fluid load to the small intestine is substantially greater than that of dietary intake and represents the sum of salivary, gastric, pancreatic, and biliary secretion and is approximately 8 to 9 L per day. As a result, the actual efficacy of total intestinal fluid absorption is considerably greater, or approximately 98%. Thus, a relatively small reduction in fluid absorption will result in a substantial increase in stool output or diarrhea.

Lichtenstein GR, ed.
Crohn's Disease: The Complete Guide to Medical Management (pp 395-404).
© 2011 SLACK Incorporated

FIGURE 34-1. Overall model of lipid digestion and absorption. BMG = betamonoglyceride; B protein = beta protein; C = cholesterol; CE = cholesterolester; FA = fatty acid; PL = phospholipid; TG = triglyceride.

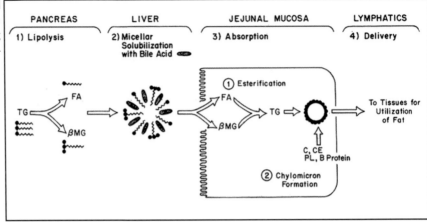

Diarrhea is discussed in terms of fluid movement, but fluid absorption and secretion are determined by solute, ie, electrolyte movement. Solute absorption in the small and large intestine differs. Fluid absorption in the small intestine is secondary to both glucose- and amino acid-stimulated Na absorption in the postprandial period and so-called electroneutral NaCl absorption in the interdigestive period. The magnitude of fluid absorption in the small intestine depends on establishing ileocecal flow that has been studied in but a handful of normal subjects and is approximately 2 L per day.[2] It should be noted that this value of ileocecal flow is substantially greater than normal ileostomy output (which is approximately 0.5 to 0.7 L per day) that is seen in patients following a total colectomy for chronic UC. This difference undoubtedly represents the adaptation that occurs in small intestinal structure and function following colectomy. As a result, the small intestine absorbs 6 to 7 L per day, which is a large volume but relatively inefficient process. Small intestinal electrolyte absorption is similar, in many ways, to that of the proximal renal tubule.

In contrast, colonic fluid absorption consists of both electroneutral NaCl absorption and so-called electrogenic Na absorption (ie, ENaC) that can be upregulated by aldosterone. The large intestine absorbs less than 2 L per day, which is a small volume but relatively efficient mechanism. Further, large intestinal ion transport has often been compared to distal renal tubular function. Although the colon absorbs 2 L per day, what is more important in any discussion of diarrhea is the *maximal* quantity of fluid that the large intestine can absorb (ie, maximal absorptive capacity that has also been determined in relatively few subjects and is estimated at between 4.5 and 5.0 L per day).[3] It is not known whether there is great variation in maximal colonic absorptive capacity in different individuals or whether patients with CD have a reduced maximal absorptive capacity. It is also important to emphasize that fluid movement in the small and large intestine is always secondary to solute movement so that to understand mechanisms of

fluid secretion, which is the basis for diarrhea, it is critical to identify the mechanism(s) responsible for changes in cellular ion transport.

Another important difference between the mechanism of fluid absorption in small and large intestine is their differing ability to absorb Na and fluid against an electro-chemical concentration gradient. Such differences can also have important consequences for patients with ileostomy following total colectomy. Net fluid absorption cannot occur in the proximal small bowel from a solution with a luminal Na concentration below 130 mEq per L or in the ileum below 75 mEq per L. In contrast, net Na absorption can occur from solutions in the colon with Na concentrations as low as 25 to 50 mEq per L. The clinical consequence of these important differences is that the patient with an ileostomy can become quickly dehydrated when placed on a low Na diet or following an acute episode of diarrhea as the ability to conserve Na is limited in the absence of a colon.

LIPID DIGESTION AND ABSORPTION

Lipid digestion and absorption involves 5 distinct processes that, if deranged, can result in an increase in stool fat excretion or steatorrhea (Figure 34-1).[4] Dietary lipid is always in the form of triglycerides, which require hydrolysis to monoglycerides and fatty acids by pancreatic lipase prior to uptake by the small intestine. Absorption of monoglycerides and fatty acids also requires a minimal concentration of conjugated bile acids (ie, critical micelle concentration, or CMC), which are needed to form mixed micelles. Different bile acids have different CMCs, with conjugated bile acids having lower CMCs than unconjugated bile acids. (The intraduodenal concentration of conjugated bile acids depends on an intact enterohepatic circulation of bile acids and will be discussed later.) Mixed micelles, water-soluble molecular aggregates of lipid material, deliver lipid across

TABLE 34-1

ONE OR MORE DEFECTS IN LIPID DIGESTION AND ABSORPTION CAN RESULT IN STEATORRHEA

	PROCESS	PATHOPHYSIOLOGIC DEFECT	DISEASE EXAMPLE
1.	Pancreatic lipolysis	Diminished lipase secretion	Chronic pancreatitis
2.	Micelle formation	Reduced intraduodenal bile acid concentration	Several (see Table 34-2)
3.	Mucosal uptake acid re-esterification	Epithelial cell dysfunction	Celiac sprue/intestinal resection
4.	Chylomicron formation	Absent betalipoproteins	Abetalipoproteinemia
5.	Exit via lymphatics	Abnormal lymphatics	Primary lymphangiectasia

the "unstirred water layer" to the apical membrane of the small intestinal epithelial cell where fatty acids and monoglycerides are absorbed most likely by a nonactive transport process. Following uptake into the intestinal epithelial cell fatty acids and monoglycerides are re-esterified by several intracellular intestinal enzymes into triglycerides that exit the epithelial cell in the form of chylomicrons via the lymphatics for delivery to the liver.

Lipid digestion and absorption is a relatively inefficient process as dietary lipid is a triglyceride and the lipid product that exists in the intestinal epithelial cell is also a triglyceride. Thus, the entire process of lipid digestion, micelle formation, uptake, and re-esterification is required as the intestinal epithelial cell does not absorb triglycerides.

Under normal circumstances, the intestine absorbs approximately 93% of dietary lipid. Defects in any of the steps in normal lipid digestion and absorption can potentially result in an increase in stool lipid or steatorrhea (Table 34-1). Thus, either a decrease in pancreatic lipolysis or a decrease in intraduodenal concentrations of conjugated bile acids may impair lipid digestion and result in steatorrhea. However, although decreased intraluminal concentrations of conjugated bile acids may occur in patients with CD (see following discussion), abnormalities in pancreatic lipolysis are not normally present in these patients.

Similarly, a reduction in intestinal epithelial function that may occur following intestinal resection can also result in a decrease in lipid absorption and steatorrhea. Very rarely abnormalities in chylomicron formation and intestinal lymphatics may produce steatorrhea and are not factors to be considered in the genesis of steatorrhea in patients with CD either before or after an intestinal resection.

The enterohepatic circulation of bile acids is critical for the maintenance of an adequate concentration of conjugated bile acids in the proximal small intestine and may be altered by intestinal resection in patients with Crohn's disease (Figure 34-2).[5] Bile acids are synthesized in the liver from cholesterol, ie, cholesterol catabolism, and are

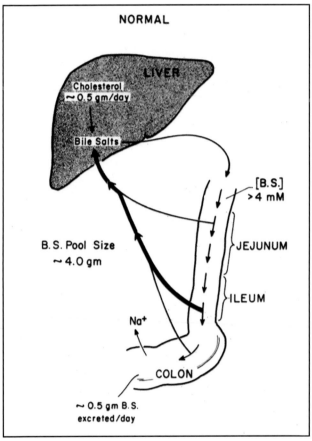

FIGURE 34-2. Model of the enterohepatic circulation of bile acids. B.S. = bile salts.

excreted into the duodenum in bile. Bile acids are absorbed via both active and nonactive transport processes and are returned to the liver, where they are excreted again into bile. Bile acids are absorbed by an active Na-dependent transport process only in the ileum, whereas bile acids can also be absorbed from the jejunum, ileum, and colon by nonactive transport processes—by either nonionic diffusion or ion diffusion. Active absorption in the ileum is the

TABLE 34-2

ONE OR MORE DEFECTS IN ENTEROHEPATIC CIRCULATION OF BILE ACIDS CAN RESULT IN DECREASED INTRADUODENAL CONCENTRATION OF BILE ACIDS

PROCESS	PATHOPHYSIOLOGIC DEFECT	DISEASE EXAMPLE
1. Synthesis	Reduced hepatic function	Cirrhosis
2. Delivery to duodenum	Abnormal canalicular function	Primary biliary cirrhosis
3. Maintenance of conjugated bile acids	Bacterial overgrowth	Jejunal diverticulosis
4. Ileal reabsorption	Ileal dysfunction	Crohn's disease

largest component of bile acid absorption. Small amounts of bile acids are lost each day in stool, and under steady-state conditions hepatic bile acid synthesis is matched by fecal bile acid losses. This enterohepatic circulation of bile acids occurs approximately twice during each meal and up to 6 to 8 times per day.

A decrease in the intraduodenal concentration of bile acids may occur whenever any 1 of the 4 steps in the enterohepatic circulation of bile acids is altered (Table 34-2). Thus, a decrease in hepatic synthesis, biliary delivery, intestinal absorption, or deconjugation of conjugated bile acids by intestinal bacteria that may occur in stagnant bowel syndrome can all potentially result in a decrease in intraluminal concentrations of conjugated bile acids in the proximal small intestine, resulting in impaired micelle formation, lipid digestion, and steatorrhea.

DIARRHEA

As noted previously, the major pathogenic mechanisms responsible for diarrhea in patients with Crohn's disease following surgery are 1) bile acids secondary to interruption of the enterohepatic circulation of bile acids, 2) steatorrhea as a result of impaired lipid digestion and absorption, 3) stasis and bacterial overgrowth, 4) inflammation in the remaining or unresected intestinal mucosa, and 5) either primary or secondary lactose intolerance. Each of these factors may be the primary mechanism or more likely to contribute, together with 1 or more other mechanisms, to the patient's diarrhea.

BILE ACID DIARRHEA

As noted previously, the primary site for bile acid absorption is the ileum. Following resection of the ileum, or in the presence of ileal inflammation, there is often a decrease in bile acid absorption with an increase in bile acids entering the large intestine.[6] To maintain the bile acid pool size, an

increase in hepatic bile acid synthesis (which also represents an increase in cholesterol catabolism) occurs, with the rate-limiting step being the regulation of 7-hydroxylase by bile acids returning to the liver. Thus, a decrease in bile acids from the ileum following ileal resection will be associated with an increase in 7-hydroxylase activity and an increase in hepatic bile acid synthesis, resulting in maintenance of the bile acid pool size and intraduodenal concentrations of conjugated bile acids that are required for micelle formation during lipid digestion and absorption. Such patients will frequently have diarrhea (but not steatorrhea). Several years ago, prior to the successes of statins in the treatment of hypercholesterolemia, ileal bypass operations were performed to reduce serum cholesterol levels by interrupting the enterohepatic circulation of bile acids and increasing cholesterol catabolism. Diarrhea was 1 of the side effects of this operation.

The observed diarrhea is a result of the effect of bile acids on colonic electrolyte transport based on experimental evidence in both normal volunteers and experimental animals. Perfusion of the colon in human volunteer subjects with concentrations of the bile acid, deoxycholic acid (as low as 3 mM) converts net fluid and electrolyte absorption to net fluid and electrolyte secretion.[7] In vitro experiments have established that conjugated and unconjugated bile acids induce active Cl secretion as well as inhibiting electroneutral NaCl absorption. Although initial studies suggested that the action of bile acids on electrolyte transport was a result of their increase in cyclic adenosine monophosphate (AMP) levels via activation of adenylate cyclase, subsequent experiments indicate that bile acids increase intracellular concentrations of Ca that lead to the observed changes in Na and Cl transport.

Therapy for so-called bile acid diarrhea or cholorrheic enteropathy is administration of an anion-binding resin, eg, cholestyramine, that binds bile acids and will frequently be very effective in the treatment of bile acid diarrhea.[6] Indications for the use of cholestyramine and predictors of its effectiveness should best be discussed only after comment is made regarding the consequences of less limited resections of small intestine (see following discussion). Nonetheless, the close relationship between bile acids and cholesterol metabolism was emphasized by the use of cholestyramine several years ago as treatment of hypercholesterolemia, which would often result in a 10% to 20% reduction in serum cholesterol levels. Cholestyramine binds bile acids, enhancing their excretion and thus increasing cholesterol catabolism (ie, bile acid synthesis).

FATTY ACID DIARRHEA

Following greater resection of the distal small intestine, both diarrhea and steatorrhea are often observed as a result of additional pathophysiologic changes in the enterohepatic circulation of bile acids. As the length of resected ileum increases, greater amounts of bile acids enter the colon, and the capacity of the liver to increase bile acid synthesis (ie, cholesterol catabolism) to maintain the bile acid pool size becomes rate limiting. It has been estimated that bile acid synthesis can maximally increase approximately 2- to 2.5-fold. As a consequence, after hepatic bile acid synthesis reaches its maximum, further fecal losses of bile acids are associated with a reduction in the bile acid pool size, which results, in turn, in reduced concentrations of intraduodenal bile acids. Intraduodenal bile acid concentrations below their CMC result in impaired micelle formation and steatorrhea. These patients have both diarrhea and steatorrhea.

The diarrhea of steatorrhea is a result of fatty acids changing net colonic fluid and electrolyte absorption to net fluid and electrolyte secretion. Similar to studies with bile acids, perfusion of the colon in normal human volunteers with an isotonic electrolyte solution containing as low as 3 mM hydroxystearic acid is associated with an inhibition of net fluid and electrolyte absorption, whereas perfusion of the jejunum with 10 mM oleic acid resulted in conversion of net fluid and electrolyte absorption to net fluid and electrolyte secretion.[8] Unlike bile acids, a specific cellular mechanism to explain fatty acid-induced net fluid secretion has not been elucidated. However, to emphasize the role of fatty acids as laxatives, it is important to recall that perfusion of the colon by ricinoleic acid, which is a hydroxyl fatty acid, and a well-known laxative (castor oil) also induces net fluid and electrolyte secretion in the colon.[9]

In general, patients with so-called fatty acid diarrhea following larger ileal resections do not respond to cholestyramine, despite persistent colonic bile acid losses. The best explanation for the failure of bile acids to contribute to the observed diarrhea is the demonstration that stool pH of such patients is relatively acidic and that bile acids precipitate in such an environment and, therefore, do not induce fluid and electrolyte secretion.[10] Thus, the important issue becomes whether there are guidelines that will predict whether cholestyramine will or will not be effective in the treatment of diarrhea following ileal resection.

The initial report describing the benefit of cholestyramine in the treatment of bile acid diarrhea more than 35 years ago provided straightforward guidelines to predict its effectiveness: length of resected ileum and amount of steatorrhea.[6] That is, patients who had less than 50 cm of ileum resected and who had less than 20 g of stool fat were likely to respond to cholestyramine, whereas those with greater than 100 cm resected and who had stool fat of more than 20 g were not likely to benefit from cholestyramine. Over time, these relatively simple criteria have not been found effective probably for several reasons:

1. These guidelines were based on 7 patients in the initial report in 1969.

2. No definition was provided for how the length of ileum resected had been measured. That is, was the length measured by the surgeon immediately prior to resection in vivo? Was the bowel length measured immediately after resection in the operating room? Or was the length of bowel resected measured in the Surgical Pathology Department after sitting in formalin overnight? There might be a 4- to 8-fold difference between these values.

3. Finally, and it is most important in patients with CD, it is critical to consider whether there is ongoing inflammation in the remaining nonresected bowel. Persistent inflammation in the ileum that was not resected will likely be associated with reduced bile acid absorption and will reduce the possibility that cholestyramine will be effective in the treatment of diarrhea that occurs following ileal resection.

In my experience, I have often predicted that some individuals should respond to cholestyramine, but found that they have not benefitted from this treatment. In contrast, I have also given cholestyramine to patients whom I suspected would not have a beneficial response to this anion-binding resin, and the patients did show a very positive effect. As a consequence, I will frequently give a 2-week therapeutic trial of cholestyramine to determine whether it will be effective. The second critical question is the dose of cholestyramine that should be prescribed. My own observations indicate that, in general, patients have an "all or none" response to cholestyramine; that is, a smaller dose does not result in a partial effect, and some patients respond to as little as 4 g/day whereas others may require 12 to 16 g/day. As a result, I usually recommend that patients take 12 or 16 g/day, with each dose being usually 4 g (4 g should be taken 30 minutes prior to each meal for 2 weeks). If there is a positive response, then the amount taken should be reduced to the lowest dose that will provide an effective therapeutic response.

Patients with intestinal resection who have not responded to cholestyramine and who have significant steatorrhea may have a beneficial response to the introduction of a reduced fat diet, with the recognition that it is often

TABLE 34-3

COMPARISON OF BILE ACID AND FATTY ACID DIARRHEA

Characteristic	Bile Acid	Fatty Acid
Length of ileal resection	Small	Large
Fecal bile acid output	↑	↑ ↑
Fecal bile acid loss compensated by hepatic synthesis	Yes	No
Bile acid pool size	Normal	↓
Duodenal (bile acid)	Normal	↓
Steatorrhea	None or mild	>20 g/24 hour
Responds to cholestyramine	Yes	No
Responds to low-fat diet	No	Yes

difficult to follow a truly low-fat diet (ie, dietary fat intake below 40 to 50 g/day) due to the wide availability of fat in most of our foods. The assistance of a well-trained dietician is often quite helpful in implementing effective dietary treatment.

The differences in the pathophysiologic events associated with "small" ileal resection (ie, bile acid-mediated diarrhea) and "large" ileal resection (ie, fatty acid-mediated diarrhea) are contrasted in Table 34-3.

STASIS AND BACTERIAL OVERGROWTH

Stasis and bacterial overgrowth syndromes are most often associated with the triad of diarrhea, steatorrhea, and macrocytic anemia, and are secondary to bacterial proliferation in an area of bowel in which there is stasis secondary to either anatomic or functional etiologies.[11,12] The clinical manifestations of diarrhea are usually thought to be directly secondary to steatorrhea, though there are a limited number of reports of patients with stasis who manifest only diarrhea and who respond to antibiotics. As a result, it has been suggested that such patients have proliferation of bacteria that are producing an enterotoxin. In the majority of patients with stasis syndromes, their diarrhea is secondary to steatorrhea (see previous text), which is due to bacterial deconjugation of conjugated bile acids to unconjugated bile acids. There are 2 distinct pathophysiologic consequences of the increase in unconjugated bile acids and the resulting decrease in conjugated bile acids that result in impaired micelle formation and then to steatorrhea:

1. Unconjugated bile acids have a higher CMC to produce micelles, and, as a consequence, higher intraduodenal concentrations of unconjugated bile acids are required to produce micelles.

2. The pKa of unconjugated bile acids is higher than those of conjugated bile acids and, as a result, a greater proportion of bile acids are non-ionized; these are more rapidly absorbed by nonionic diffusion than are ionized bile acids by ionic diffusion. The net result will be a lower effective concentration of bile acids in the proximal small intestine resulting in impaired micelle formation with the development of steatorrhea.

The macrocytic anemia in stasis syndromes is secondary to vitamin B_{12} and not to folate deficiency. Indeed, the combination of low vitamin B_{12} levels and elevated folate levels provides a very strong suggestion of the presence of a bacterial stasis and overgrowth or overgrowth syndrome. In contrast to the genesis of steatorrhea, in which bacteria are altering a normal constituent of the intestinal lumen, that of the macrocytic anemia is secondary to bacterial utilization of cobalamin (vitamin B_{12}). Folate levels are elevated as bacteria frequently produce folic acid that is then absorbed.

Stasis and bacterial overgrowth syndromes are usually divided into those associated with anatomical stasis and those with functional stasis. Examples of the former, independent of CD, are, for example, jejunal diverticulae and afferent loops; included in the latter category is scleroderma. In the unoperated patient with CD, a stasis syndrome may develop as a consequence of common complications of CD (eg, strictures and fistulae). In the operated patient with CD and, in particular, in the individual who has had a resection of the ileocecal value, increased levels of colonic-type bacteria occur proximal to the ileocolonic anastomosis. It is well known that there are both qualitative and quantitative differences in bacteria in the areas that are proximal and distal to the ileocecal value. An adequate explanation for this well-established phenomenon is not known but may be related to the higher concentrations of bile acids in the ileum (ie, proximal to the ileocecal valve as bile acids are known to have bactericidal effects). As a consequence of the removal of the ileocecal valve, bacterial proliferation ensues in the small intestine—with the result often being a bacterial stasis-like syndrome. As treatment of most stasis syndromes is cyclical administration with antibiotics (eg, tetracycline, metronidazole), patients with ileal resection that included removal of the ileocecal valve who develop diarrhea and who have not responded to cholestyramine and/or low-fat diet (see previous discussion) should try a 2- to 3-week course of an antibiotic (eg, tetracycline, metronidazole) to treat bacterial proliferation in the small intestine proximal to the ileocolonic anastomosis. Such treatment often is at least temporarily effective.

INFLAMMATION

Chronic mucosal inflammation is central to the pathogenesis of Crohn's disease and is also critical for the development of the diarrhea that is often a major symptom in many patients with CD following intestinal resection. Therefore, it is critical to remember that both prior to or following a surgical resection for CD, it is not unlikely that some component of a patient's diarrhea may be directly related to either clinical or latent mucosal inflammation.

First, it would be useful to review the effect of different proinflammatory intermediaries on ion transport in order to emphasize that many of the treatment regimens used in CD often are linked to altering the effects of one or more proinflammatory cytokines and other inflammatory agonists. Thus, the multiple inflammatory intermediates associated with this inflammation may induce diarrhea by virtue of their effects on intestinal epithelial cells, enteric neurons, lamina propria cells (eg, mast cells), and/or myofibroblasts. Most often, the common denominator of these inflammatory mediators is their ability to increase intestinal epithelial cell levels of 1 or more secondary messengers (ie, cyclic AMP [cAMP], cyclic guanosine phosphate [cGMP], and/or Ca). The result of such increases will be a decrease in neutral NaCl absorption by virtue of inhibition of Na-H exchange and Cl-HCO$_3$ exchange in villous or surface cells and/or stimulation of anion (Cl-HCO$_3$) secretion, most likely via activation or insertion of cystic fibrosis transmembrane regulator (CFTR) in the apical membrane of crypt cells.[13] The combination of these 2 events results in an increase in luminal fluid, leading to an increase in stool water excretion or diarrhea. Alterations in the integrity of the intestinal epithelial barrier and/or Na, K-ATPase may also contribute to the maintenance of normal intestinal NaCl absorption.

Studies of the inflammatory response primarily in UC but also in CD and in experimental animals have emphasized the role of 1 or more proinflammatory mediators (eg, tumor necrosis factor alpha [TNFα], interferon [IFN-γ]) as well as 1 or more secretory eicosanoids.[14-16] For example, TNFα reduces epithelial barrier function in intestinal cells, whereas down-regulated-in-adenoma (DRA), the gene that encodes Cl-HCO$_3$ exchange, is reduced in models of intestinal inflammation including UC. Other studies have shown that IFN-γ alters both Na-H exchange function and NaK-ATPase activity. Thus, it is not unlikely that inflix-imab, a monoclonal antibody to TNFα, is an important therapeutic advance in the treatment in CD at this time and may include a reversal of the changes in ion transport that occur secondary to TNFα. Similarly, evidence exists that 5-ASA and glucocorticosteroids inhibit synthesis of prostaglandins that, when released from myofibroblasts during inflammation, stimulate adenylate cyclase and increase mucosal cAMP. These studies in UC have also emphasized the importance of decreased NaCl absorption and altered mucosal barrier function and not stimulation of active anion secretion.[13] It is not known whether such phenomena also occur in patients with Crohn's disease either prior to or following intestinal resection.

The important lesion to be emphasized in the evaluation of diarrhea in any patient with CD following a surgical procedure is that it is critical not to dismiss the possibility that the patient's diarrhea might be related to persistent chronic mucosal inflammation despite a relative paucity of findings indicating ongoing inflammation. Treatment of chronic inflammation, which is always central to the treatment of CD, may well be effective in this postoperative patient whose primary symptom is diarrhea.

LACTOSE INTOLERANCE

Milk intolerance has been long linked to both CD and UC. Although initially most of the attention focused on milk-protein allergy and UC, following the identification of lactase deficiency as a clinical entity more than 45 years ago, it soon became evident that lactose intolerance is primarily responsible for the milk intolerance in patients with both CD and UC. Although extensive small intestinal involvement with CD could result in secondary lactase deficiency, most often, primary lactase deficiency is responsible for the symptoms of milk intolerance. Equally important is that there is often an increased incidence of primary lactose intolerance in some ethnic/racial groups (eg, Ashkenazi Jews) that have a high incidence of CD.

Thus, in the evaluation of patients with diarrhea that had first occurred or that had increased in severity following a surgical procedure, it is important to remember the possibility that this diarrhea may in part be related to primary lactose intolerance. Only rarely will an intestinal resection result in secondary lactase deficiency, which is discussed in the chapter on intestinal failure and short bowel syndrome (Chapter 35).

CALCULI

Both renal and gallbladder calculi are potential complications in CD, especially in patients who have had intestinal (and most often ileal) resections.[17] As the pathogenesis of these complications differ, each will be discussed separately.

RENAL URATE AND OXALATE CALCULI

There is an increase in both renal urate and oxalate calculi in patients who have had a total colectomy and an extensive small intestinal resection without a substantial colonic resection, respectively.[18,19] With regard to the development of urate calculi, there does not appear to be a defect in urate metabolism in the nonoperated patient, but an increased incidence of urate calculi has been observed following total colectomy for either Crohn's colitis or UC. The usual explanation is that the patient with a total colectomy often has chronic dehydration and a mild metabolic acidosis that leads to urate precipitation. Treatment has focused on emphasizing adequate hydration and correcting any evidence of acidosis.

An increase in the incidence of renal calculi has frequently been observed following small intestinal resection both in CD and non-CD patients, including those who had ileal bypass operations for obesity and hypercholesterolemia. Investigation of these patients resulted in the demonstration that these calculi are oxalate stones and are associated with enteric hyperoxaluria (ie, an increase in urinary excretion of dietary oxalate), which is consistent with an increase in intestinal oxalate absorption. Although a limited number of patients with calcium oxalate calculi without CD have an increase in dietary oxalate absorption, patients with CD who have not had small intestinal resection may have either calcium oxalate calculi or enteric hyperoxaluria. It is now generally accepted that the 2 critical requirements for enteric hyperoxaluria and the development of calcium oxalate calculi are steatorrhea and an intact colon. Steatorrhea leads to an increase in colonic oxalate absorption as a result of either an increase in colonic permeability by nonabsorbed fatty acids or the interaction of fatty acids, calcium, and oxalate leading to an increase in nonprecipitated oxalate in a free solution that is then absorbed either via non-ionic diffusion or via an anion exchange mechanism. Steatorrhea in the absence of a colon is not associated with either enteric hyperoxaluria or renal calcium oxalate calculi.

Treatment is directed toward reducing intestinal absorption of dietary oxalate. Dietary restriction has only limited effects as there are relatively few foods with high oxalate content (eg, spinach, rhubarb, and tea). Cholestyramine may have some effectiveness by virtue of its anion-binding capabilities by binding oxalate. Treatment of the underlying steatorrhea is most effective, but if the steatorrhea is primarily a result of an extensive intestinal resection, a low-fat diet, as discussed previously, may be the most promising therapeutic option.

GALLBLADDER CALCULI

There is also an increased incidence of gallbladder calculi in patients with ileal disease and ileal resection.[20] Such patients most often have Crohn's disease. These patients usually have cholesterol gall stones that are believed to be related to an interruption in the enterohepatic circulation of bile acids (see previous discussion of the enterohepatic circulation of bile acids) with a substantial decrease in the bile acid pool size. This latter phenomenon is associated with the development of so-called lithogenic bile and precipitation of cholesterol. However, an increase in bilirubin-containing calculi has also been identified, but a pathophysiologic explanation has been lacking. Although "garden variety" cholesterol gall stones also have lithogenic bile, these patients usually have both an increase in cholesterol excretion as well as reduced bile acid excretion to account for the generation of lithogenic bile. Although treatment with ursodeoxycholic acid may be effective in the treatment of lithogenic bile and can dissolve gall stones at times, such therapy is not effective in patients with ileal resection, as the administered ursodeoxycholic acid will not be retained as a result of the ileal resection. Therapy will only be directed toward the gallbladder disease and will frequently require cholecystectomy.

REFERENCES

1. Williamson RCN. Intestinal adaptation. Structural, function and cytokinetic changes. *N Engl J Med.* 1978;298:1393-1402, 1444-1450.
2. Phillips SF, Giller J. The contribution of the colon to electrolyte and water conservation in man. *J Lab Clin Med.* 1973;81:733-746.
3. Debongie JC, Phillips SF. Capacity of the human colon to absorb fluid. *Gastroenterology.* 1978;74:698-703.
4. Binder HJ. Disorders of absorption. In: Kasper DL, Braunwold E, Hauser S, Longo D, Jameson JL, Fauci AS, eds. *Harrison's Principles of Internal Medicine.* 16th ed. New York, NY: McGraw Hill; 2004: 1763-1776.
5. Binder HJ. Nutrient-induced diarrhea. In: Field M, ed. *Textbook of Diarrheas.* New York, NY: Elsevier; 1991:159-172.
6. Hofmann AF, Poley JR. Cholestyramine treatment of diarrhea associated with ileal resection. *N Engl J Med.* 1969;281:397-402.
7. Mekhjuan JS, Phillips SF, Hoffman AF. Colonic secretion of water electrolytes induced by bile acids: perfusion studies in man. *J Clin Invest.* 1971;50:1569-1577.
8. Ammons HV, Phillips SF. Inhibition of colonic water and electrolyte absorption by fatty acids in man. *Gastroenterology.* 1973;65:744-749.
9. Bright-Asare P, Binder, HJ. Stimulation of colonic secretion of water and electrolytes by hydroxy fatty acids. *Gastroenterology.* 1973;64:81-88.
10. McJunkin B, Fromm H, Sarva RP, Amin P. Factors in the mechanism of diarrhea in bile acid malabsorption: fecal pH—a key determinant. *Gastroenterology.* 1981;80:1454-1464.
11. Fine KD, Schiller LR. AGA technical review on the evaluation and management of chronic diarrhea. *Gastroenterology.* 1999;116:1464-1486.
12. Fine KD, Schiller LR. AGA technical review on the evaluation and management of chronic diarrhea. *Gastroenterology.* 1999;116:1464-1486.
13. Sandle GI. Pathogenesis of diarrhea in ulcerative colitis: new views on an old problem. *J Clin Gastroenterol.* 2005;39:S49-S52.

14. Barmeyer C, Harren M, Schmitz H, et al. Mechanisms of diarrhea in the interleukin-2-deficient mouse model of colonic inflammation. *Am J Physiol.* 2004;286:G244-G252.

15. Schmitz H, Fromm M, Bentzel CJ, et al. Tumor necrosis factor-alpha (TNF-α) regulates the epithelial barrier in the human intestinal cell line HT-29/B6. *J Cell Sci.* 1999;112:137-146.

16. Yang H, Jiang W, Furth E, et al. Intestinal inflammation reduces expression of DRA, a transporter responsible for congenital chloride diarrhea. *Am J Physiol.* 1998;275:G1445-G1453.

17. Kalha KS, Selling JH. Physiologic consequences of surgical treatment for inflammatory bowel disease. In: Sartor RB, Sandborn WJ, eds. *Inflammatory Bowel Diseases.* Philadelphia, PA: WB Saunders; 2004:316-332.

18. Earnest DL. Perspectives on incidence, etiology and treatment of enteric hyperoxaluria. *Am J Clin Nutr.* 1977;30:72-75.

19. Gelzayd EA, Breuer RI, Kirsner JB. Nephrolithiasis in inflammatory bowel disease. *Am J Dig Dis.* 1968;13:1027-1034.

20. Pitt HA, Lewinski MA, Muller EL. Ileal-resection induced gallstones: altered bilirubin or cholesterol metabolism. *Surgery.* 1983;96:154-162.

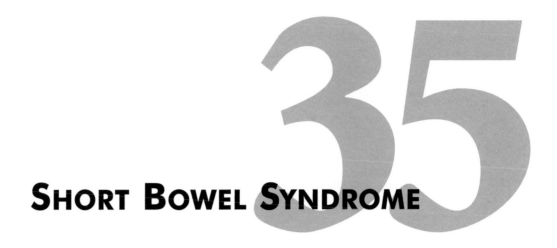

SHORT BOWEL SYNDROME

Jane E. Onken, MD, MHS

The term *short bowel syndrome* (SBS) is used to describe the clinical consequences that result from extensive intestinal resection. In some cases, SBS is defined anatomically as a small bowel length less than 200 cm.[1,2] Others prefer to define the syndrome functionally, referring to it as intestinal failure. This latter term emphasizes the fact that the remaining intestine is incapable of maintaining adequate nutritional balance without some form of supplementation.

SBS applies to a wide spectrum of nutritional compromise ranging from moderate, due to limited ileocolonic resections, to the severe compromise, associated with extensive small bowel and colonic resection. The clinical consequences are highly variable and depend on a number of factors.[3-5]

ETIOLOGY AND EPIDEMIOLOGY

Estimates of the incidence and prevalence are difficult to make, given the broad range in severity of the syndrome. Based on the number of patients with severe SBS requiring home parenteral nutrition, the incidence has been estimated at approximately 2 per million per year in the United Kingdom,[6] although a more recent European survey from 1997 suggested the incidence had increased to 3 per million.[7] In the United States, data drawn from the Oley Foundation home parenteral nutrition registry in 1992 estimated 40,000 patients per year were receiving home parenteral nutrition, of whom 26% had SBS.[8]

In adults, the 2 most common disorders leading to SBS are CD and mesenteric ischemia or infarction.[4] Typical vascular insults include thrombosis or embolism of the superior mesenteric artery and thrombosis of the superior

mesenteric vein. Risk factors for vascular insults include advanced age, severe congestive heart failure, atherosclerotic vascular disease, valvular heart disease, chronic diuretic or oral contraceptive use, and a hypercoagulable state.[4]

Other less common causes of SBS in adults include small bowel volvulus or strangulation of a small bowel hernia. Surgical procedures such as resection due to abdominal trauma or jejunoileal bypass (a procedure once performed as a treatment for morbid obesity) may lead to malabsorption.[3] Primary and secondary neoplasms of the small bowel or radiation enteropathy, although rare, may ultimately result in SBS.

In children, congenital causes of SBS include vascular accidents, intestinal atresia, gastroschisis, and mid-gut volvulus due to malfixation and malrotation.[4,9] Hirschsprung's disease of the small bowel is rare but may lead to malabsorption and nutritional compromise. The most common postnatal causes are necrotizing enterocolitis, trauma, and inflammatory bowel disease (IBD).[3]

PATHOPHYSIOLOGY

A number of factors influence the metabolic and thus nutritional consequences of intestinal resection that lead to SBS. Understanding the type and extent of malabsorption in an individual patient is aided by knowledge of normal bowel physiology and the surgical resection(s) performed. Resections can be categorized into 3 major types: limited ileal (with or without cecal resection or right hemicolectomy), extensive ileal (with or without partial colectomy), and extensive small bowel with total colectomy (resulting in a high jejunostomy).[9]

Lichtenstein GR, ed.
Crohn's Disease: The Complete Guide to Medical Management (pp 405-416).
© 2011 SLACK Incorporated

Normally, absorption occurs along the entire length of the small bowel, with each segment designed for its particular nutrient, electrolyte, mineral, or water absorptive function. The duodenum and proximal jejunum are responsible for absorption of water, electrolytes, various nutrients (fat, protein, carbohydrates), certain minerals (calcium, magnesium, iron), vitamins (B, C, folate, and the fat-soluble vitamins A, D, E, and K), and trace elements (zinc, copper).[9] The distal jejunum and colon function primarily to absorb water and electrolytes. The ileum is the site of vitamin B_{12} and bile acid absorption.

Just as functional changes occur from proximal to distal small bowel, so too does enterocyte morphology.[5] Villous height and crypt depth are significantly greater in the jejunum than in the ileum. Microvillus enzyme activity and nutrient absorptive capacity per unit length of intestine are also much higher in the proximal small bowel compared with the distal intestine.

LENGTH AND SITE OF RESECTION

In general, the more extensive the bowel resection, the greater the loss of absorptive surface area and degree of nutritional compromise. However, the normal small bowel length is quite variable, with autopsy and intraoperative measurements ranging from 3 to >10 m. These variations in intestinal length begin even before birth.[10] In addition, the average small bowel length in women is shorter than it is in men.[10-12] Given this variation, removal of the same absolute length of small bowel may represent a larger or smaller relative proportion in an individual patient. Removal of up to 50% of small bowel is usually well tolerated with respect to nutrient absorption.[5]

Although it is common for operative reports to specify the length of the intestinal segment removed at surgery, it is actually the length of the residual bowel and its function that are the more important determinants of metabolic sequelae. Measurement of the resected bowel length is usually straightforward, but intraoperative estimates of the length of remaining intestine may be technically difficult due to adhesions, spasm, etc.[12] In a study of 18 patients with a residual small bowel length measured at surgery of less than 200 cm, radiographic estimates of bowel length obtained at small bowel follow-through examination correlated well with intraoperative estimates ($r = 0.72$, $P < 0.001$).[12] Thus, when residual bowel length is not known, radiographic estimates can be made and used to assist in management decisions.

As noted previously, the degree of malabsorption is inversely proportional to the length of remaining intestine. In addition, the location of the resection and the adaptability of the intestine that remains are of critical importance in determining long-term recovery.[5] Approximately 9 L of water and electrolytes enter the proximal small bowel per day. Of this, the small intestine absorbs all but 1 L. Thus, patients who have undergone extensive small bowel and colon resection and are left with a high jejunostomy are at risk for large volume losses that may lead to hypovolemia, hyponatremia, and hypokalemia. Absorptive capacity in such patients correlates with length of residual jejunum with a minimum of 100 cm required to achieve positive water and electrolyte balance.[9]

Vitamin B_{12} and bile acid absorption is confined to the ileum. Specific transport proteins in ileal enterocytes are responsible for absorbing B_{12}-intrinsic factor complexes. The degree of B_{12} malabsorption is thus proportional to the length of resected ileum; B_{12} deficiency does not usually occur unless more than 60 cm of ileum has been resected.

Bile salt absorption also correlates with the length of the ileal resection. If less than 100 cm is resected, bile salt malabsorption is only moderate. The unabsorbed bile acids enter the colon where they induce colerrhesis (secretion of water and electrolytes by the colon) and thus diarrhea. Severe bile acid malabsorption may result from ileal resections longer than 100 cm. In addition to causing colerrhesis, the loss of bile acids may be so great that hepatic synthesis is unable to keep pace and the total bile acid pool size is decreased. If the bile acid pool is insufficient, a decrease in micellar solubilization of lipolytic products may occur, leading to fat malabsorption and worsening diarrhea (Figure 35-1).[9]

Various hormones are produced by endocrine cells located throughout the gastrointestinal tract. In the proximal gut, endocrine cells produce gastrin, cholecystokinin, secretin, gastric inhibitory peptide, and motilin.[9] These hormones are responsible for regulating intestinal motility and secretory processes. In most SBS patients, gut hormone synthesis is preserved. However, approximately 50% of patients who have undergone extensive small bowel resection develop a transient gastric hypersecretion. This subgroup of patients exhibits a temporary increase in gastric acid secretion in the early postoperative period, with documented occurrences within 24 hours of surgery.[13,14] Although the hyperacidity lessens with time and can be managed medically with proton pump inhibitors, serious peptic ulcer disease has been reported.[13] It is not clear whether jejunal or ileal resection is the more important stimulus for gastric hypersecretion;[14] nor are the mechanisms responsible known. Elevated serum gastrin concentrations or loss of inhibitory signals normally produced by the resected bowel may play a role.[13,15-17]

Endocrine cells of the ileum and proximal colon produce glucagon-like peptides 1 and 2 (GLP-1, GLP-2), neurotensin, and peptide YY.[9] GLP-1, GLP-2, neurotensin, and peptide YY are released in response to the presence of intraluminal fat and carbohydrates. Under normal circumstances, their release slows gastric emptying and intestinal transit.[18-20] In patients who have undergone jejunostomy, meal-induced release of these hormones is impaired, and rapid gastric emptying and intestinal transit result.[21,22] However, if the colon remains in continuity, plasma GLP-1 and GLP-2 concentrations increase, and gastric emptying remains normal.[23]

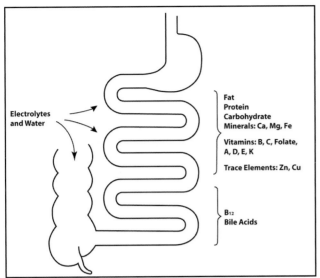

FIGURE 35-1. Specific areas of absorption of constituents of diet and secretions in the gastrointestinal tract. Macronutrients and micronutrients are predominately absorbed in the proximal jejunum. Bile acids and cobalamin (vitamin B_{12}) are only absorbed in the ileum. Electrolytes and water are absorbed in both the small and the large intestine. (Reprinted with permission from Malik A, Westergaard H. Short bowel syndrome. In: Feldman M, Friedman L, Sleisenger M, eds. *Gastrointestinal and Liver Disease*. 7th ed. Philadelphia, PA: Elsevier: 2006;1807-1816.)

PRESENCE OF ILEOCECAL VALVE

The ileocecal valve regulates passage of ileal contents into the colon and separates small bowel from colonic contents. Patients who have undergone ileocecal resection with an ileocolonic anastomosis are at increased risk of bacterial overgrowth and subsequent nutrient and vitamin B_{12} malabsorption. The bacterial overgrowth has been attributed to loss of the ileocecal valve,[13,5] although this explanation seems overly simplistic for 2 reasons. First, the ileocecal valve is not thought to be bacteriologically "competent" (ie, it cannot prevent migration of bacteria from the colon into the ileum). Second, intestinal contents likely move through too rapidly to allow retrograde movement of bacteria from the colon into the small bowel.[14]

UNDERLYING DISEASE

Survival and long-term dependence on parenteral nutrition in SBS are related to the ability of the remaining intestine to perform its functions. The underlying condition that led to intestinal resection may be important if it could recur or if it impairs the adaptive capacity of the residual bowel. Recurrence of diseases such as Crohn's or small bowel malignancy may exacerbate symptoms, worsen malabsorption, and make management even more difficult.[3] Radiation enteritis or Crohn's in the unresected bowel may impair absorptive capacity. Vascular insults leading to mesenteric infarction are likely to recur and necessitate further

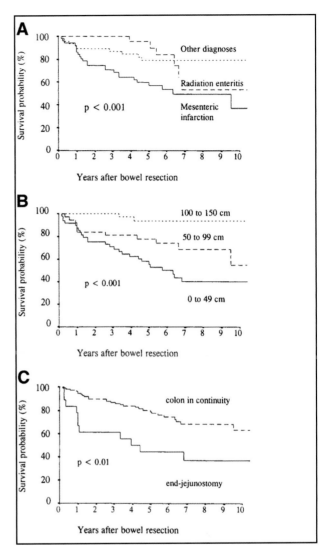

FIGURE 35-2. In a study of 124 patients with SBS, negative predictors of survival included mesenteric infarction as the underlying cause of SBS (panel A), small bowel length <50 cm (panel B), and high jejunostomy (panel C). (Reprinted with permission from Messing B, Crenn P, Beau P, et al. Long-term survival and parenteral nutrition dependence in adult patients with the short bowel syndrome. *Gastroenterology.* 1999;117:1043-1050.)

resections, which in turn diminish absorptive capacity. In a prospective study of 124 patients with SBS, Messing et al identified high jejunostomy, small bowel length less than 50 cm, and SBS due to mesenteric infarction as negative predictors of survival (Figure 35-2).[24]

DEGREE OF ADAPTATION OF REMAINING GUT

Surgical resection of bowel is one of the strongest stimuli for adaptive growth, the changes being more pronounced in the ileum than jejunum.[25] Studies in rats have demonstrated compensatory ileal hyperplasia within 3 weeks of proximal small bowel resection. A threefold increase in absorptive surface area is achieved by lengthening of villi, deepening of crypts, and accelerated proliferation of enterocytes. In addition, the rate of migration of enterocytes along the villi is doubled and enzymatic expression increased.[25]

Using calcium absorption as a marker of small bowel adaptation in humans with SBS, increases >2 years following resection have been demonstrated.[26] The same authors showed intestinal adaptation to be independent of the presence of colon in continuity, although more recent work by others directly contradicts this finding.[27] Mucosal distribution and expression of the peptide transporter PepT1 has also been used as a surrogate marker for intestinal adaptation in patients with SBS.[28] Although upregulation of PepT1 and hence selective adaptation was demonstrated in colonic tissue, in contrast to the calcium absorption data, there was no evidence that adaptation involved hyperplasia of either the small or large intestine.[28,29]

Similar adaptive changes have been identified in the small intestine of patients following bypass surgery for obesity. Solhaug and Tvete used radiological and histological studies to evaluate changes in small bowel over time in 7 patients who had undergone jejunoileal bypass.[30] Increases in diameter were identified as early as 4 months after surgery. Small bowel length increased gradually over 18 months, and ileal exceeded proximal bowel growth. Intestinal transit time was also prolonged by 12 months. Histologic measurements demonstrated increases in mean villous height in the jejunum of 14% and 55% at 6 and 12 months, respectively, compared with increases of 32% and 66% in the ileum.[30] Thus, adaptation involves both increases in intestinal absorptive surface area and prolongation of transit time.

PRESENCE OF COLON IN CONTINUITY

The colon has a reserve capacity to absorb water and electrolytes of up to 3 to 4 L per day, resulting in a normal average loss of water through stool of only 100 to 150 mL per day.[9] Thus, preservation of some or all of the colon in patients with SBS can prevent significant fecal water and electrolyte losses. In a study comparing 46 patients with jejunal length <200 cm and no colon with 38 patients with the same jejunal length but at least half of the colon in continuity, none of the patients with jejunal length >50 cm and a colon required parenteral nutrition a median of 5 years after surgery. However, in the group without a colon, 11 of 38 with a jejunal length >50 cm and 3 of 25 with a jejunal length >100 cm required some form of parenteral supplementation.[31] The authors concluded that preservation of at least half of the colon is beneficial and equivalent to approximately 50 cm of small intestinal length in terms of the need for parenteral therapy.

As discussed elsewhere in this chapter, the presence of the colon in continuity also plays an important role in absorption of calcium and nutrients, helps maintain a normal liquid gastric emptying rate, and may have a role

in stimulation of intestinal adaptation.[31] It also appears to confer a survival benefit in children with SBS.[27] Analysis of stool specimens in SBS patients whose colon remains intact has shown significant increases in fecal bacterial mass and the bacterial capacity to ferment carbohydrates, as well as an improved ability of the colon to absorb short-chain fatty acids.[32,33] Bacterial fermentation converts nonabsorbable carbohydrates to readily absorbable short chain fatty acids for use as an energy source. In normal adults, this process contributes only 5% to 10% of the energy requirements.[34] In patients with SBS and at least part of the colon intact, however, the colon can be recruited to absorb more energy.[34] This has led to the recommendation that high-carbohydrate, low-fat diets may benefit this subset of SBS patients.[32] Reduced fecal losses of energy associated with significant increases in absorption of energy from 49% to 69% have been reported in SBS patients with colon in continuity on such diets; dietary composition in SBS patients without a colon had no effect on fecal loss or absorption of energy.[35]

CLINICAL FEATURES OF SHORT BOWEL SYNDROME

POSTOPERATIVE TRENDS

The clinical course of patients with SBS typically follows 3 phases: immediate or early, intermediate, and late.[14] During the period immediately following extensive small bowel resection, the predominant symptom is diarrhea. As a result, patients are at risk of dehydration and electrolyte derangements, particularly hypokalemia, hyponatremia, hypocalcemia, and hypomagnesemia.[9] Most patients are kept fasting immediately after surgery and are fed parenterally with careful monitoring of intake and output (urinary, fecal, and stomal losses if present), weight, and volume status. Oral feeding is initiated as soon as the patient has stabilized and enteric anastomoses have healed, usually 10 to 14 days after surgery.

Oral feeding is crucial because it induces the intermediate or intestinal adaptation phase. It is during this period that malabsorption is the major threat to maintaining adequate nutrition. Initially, elemental and semi-elemental formulas are frequently recommended. Many of these contain glutamine, an amino acid thought to play a role in inducing intestinal adaptation.[36] Gradually, diet is advanced and food intake increased, with careful attention to symptoms of diarrhea, steatorrhea, bloating, etc. The adaptation phase generally occurs gradually over the course of 1 year, and it is during this time that most weaning off of parenteral nutrition occurs.[37]

The third, or late, phase is characterized by the absence of further adaptation. It is considered a state of relative equilibrium during which body weight often stabilizes and no further improvement in symptoms is expected.[3,37] Patients who still require parenteral nutrition during this phase are unlikely ever to discontinue it unless they undergo intestinal transplant (see following discussion).

DIARRHEA

Although diarrhea is an almost universal complication of extensive bowel resections, the etiologies are multifactorial, and a thorough search for the cause(s) in each patient should be undertaken. Once this has been completed, dietary and medical therapies can be tailored to meet the individual patient's needs. A number of potential explanations for diarrhea in SBS patients exist. Intestinal transit time may be reduced because of the shortened bowel length or the absence of gut hormones that normally regulate motility.[21] Malabsorption of carbohydrates, including lactose, may increase luminal osmolarity and lead to diarrhea. Stool losses may be exacerbated in patients with bacterial overgrowth. Patients who have undergone a limited ileal resection but whose colon remains in continuity may experience colerrhesis due to bile acid malabsorption (see previous discussion of this). In some, loss of ileum and right colon impairs absorption of sodium chloride[38]; this in turn reduces absorption of water and leads to diarrhea. Lastly, steatorrhea itself can induce secretion of water and electrolytes in the distal small bowel and colon.

GASTRIC ACID HYPERSECRETION

Gastric acid hypersecretion has been demonstrated as early as 24 hours after extensive small bowel resection in both experimental animals and humans.[13,14] Consequences of gastric hypersecretion include inactivation of intraluminal lipase, precipitation of bile salts, and damage to the intestinal mucosa, all of which may further impair intestinal absorption and exacerbate diarrhea in the immediate postoperative state. The fear of significant peptic ulcer disease and other sequelae of gastric acid hypersecretion led some authors to recommend vagotomy at the time of resection,[39-41] although this has been abandoned with the development of potent acid suppressive agents.

The mechanism(s) of gastric hypersecretion following intestinal resection are not known. Elevations in serum gastrin concentrations have been demonstrated by a number of investigators,[15,16,42] an effect that seems to persist up to 16 years after surgery.[16] The hypergastrinemia may be due to augmented gastrin release or to impaired breakdown following massive small bowel resection. Some have postulated the absence of a distal small bowel factor that normally inhibits gastrin release.[42] In a study designed to measure simultaneous gastric acid and gastrin production in response to a food stimulus in short bowel patients, serum gastrin levels were significantly greater compared with a control group, but associated increases in acid secretion were absent.[16] Thus, although postoperative gastrin elevations persist, the gastric acid hypersecretion seen in the immediate postoperative period seems to disappear over time.

NUTRITIONAL DEFICIENCIES

In the immediate postoperative period, water and electrolyte losses pose the greatest threat to the patient who has undergone extensive small bowel resection. Loss of significant surface area as seen in SBS overwhelms the absorptive capacity of the remaining intestine, at least initially. Fecal or stomal losses of greater than 5 to 8 L/day have been reported.[3,43] Profound hypovolemia, hyponatremia, and hypokalemia may result if fluid intake and output are not closely monitored. Patients with a high jejunostomy are particularly at risk, but some can compensate by sipping a glucose-saline solution throughout the day. This takes advantage of the coupled active transport of sodium with glucose that takes place in the jejunum.[2,9]

Malabsorption of fat in patients with SBS can lead to calcium and magnesium deficiencies.[3,9] Unabsorbed fatty acids complex can precipitate both of these divalent cations within the intestinal lumen. Magnesium deficiency may impair release of parathyroid hormone normally seen in response to low calcium.[44] In a study of 118 patients with IBD who had undergone small bowel resection, 53% had evidence of calcium malabsorption.[45] The same authors studied calcium balance and bone mineral content following small bowel resection in 83 patients. Length of resection varied from <50 cm to >150 cm; 38% had an ileostomy. An inverse correlation between net calcium absorption and length of resection was found.[46] No differences were observed between patients with an ileostomy and those with colon in continuity. Of the patients not receiving parenteral calcium supplementation, 64% were in negative calcium balance. More than half (63%) of the study subjects had evidence of bone mineral content below mean values for normal controls,[46] although concurrent or previous use of corticosteroids for treatment of chronic inflammatory bowel disease may have been a confounding factor. Both calcium and magnesium absorption respond to a low-fat diet.[47]

Absorption of the fat-soluble vitamins may also be reduced in patients who have significant steatorrhea. Malabsorption of vitamin D may worsen calcium deficiency. Vitamin A losses may be surreptitious, as serum levels may not accurately reflect vitamin stores. Assessing adaptation of the eyes to darkness may be a more useful measure of deficiency states.[44] Vitamin K deficiency, although rare, may lead to development of purpura or overt bleeding.[44]

With the exception of vitamin B_{12}, absorption of water-soluble vitamins and trace elements is usually sufficient to prevent deficiency states. As noted above, specific transport proteins confined to the ileum are responsible for absorbing B_{12}-intrinsic factor complexes. Resection of >60 cm of ileum is usually required before B_{12} deficiency occurs. Parenteral replacement is straightforward, and most patients need only a monthly intramuscular injection or a weekly nasal spray to maintain adequate stores. Zinc deficiency, when present, may present as dysgeusia.[3]

COMPLICATIONS

GALLSTONES

In addition to nutritional and vitamin deficiencies and their consequences described in the previous section, a number of other complications can arise in patients with SBS. One of these is the development of gallstones. In a study of 84 patients with SBS, the prevalence of gallstones was 44%,[31] significantly greater than the 30% prevalence observed in patients without SBS. Some of this increase may be attributed to the use of parenteral nutrition, a known risk factor for development of gallstones due to absence of enteric stimulation of bile flow and diminished gallbladder motility.[48] The higher prevalence of gallstones observed was independent of the presence or absence of a functioning colon.

One proposed mechanism for gallstone development is that interruption of the normal enterohepatic circulation of bile occurs following resection of the ileum. Malabsorption of bile acids leads to an increase in hepatic bile synthesis that, depending on the extent of bile acid losses, may or may not be able to compensate. If the bile salt pool is depleted, bile composition may be altered such that cholesterol precipitation occurs.[4,31] In turn, the supersaturation of bile with cholesterol could lead to formation of cholesterol crystals and ultimately cholesterol gallstones. Unfortunately, this theory is inconsistent with the observation that the gallstones occurring after ileal resection tend to be composed of calcium bilirubinate and not cholesterol.[31]

NEPHROLITHIASIS

Patients who have undergone ileal resections or who have extensive ileal disease are also at risk for development of nephrolithiasis. In a study comparing patients with a high jejunostomy (no functioning colon) with patients having an equivalent jejunal length in continuity with colon, 24% of those with a colon developed renal stones while none of those without a colon developed stones (P <0.001).[31] Median time to stone formation was 22 months from the last intestinal resection. Of the few stones analyzed, all were calcium oxalate.

Hyperoxaluria has frequently been observed in such patients and is presumed to result from an increase in colonic absorption of dietary oxalate.[31,49,50] At least 2 mechanisms have been proposed for the increased oxalate absorption. Under normal circumstances, oxalate in food is precipitated out as insoluble calcium oxalate in the intestinal lumen and excreted in the feces. In patients with short bowel and colon in continuity, impaired lipolysis leads to an increase in intraluminal long-chain fatty acids. The fatty acids compete with luminal oxalate for calcium and form calcium soaps. Unbound oxalate is then available for absorption in the colon and eventual renal excretion.[3,9,31]

The second mechanism involves an increase in colonic mucosal permeability to oxalate that may be caused by intraluminal bile salts and fatty acids.[3,31] Additional contributing factors for stone formation are almost certainly involved; however, other authors have reported an increased incidence of nephrolithiasis in ileostomy patients.[51] Presumably, this is due to a state of chronic dehydration and reduced urinary volumes.[4,31]

At least 1 author recommends regular monitoring of urinary oxalate excretion in SBS patients with preserved colon.[9] Treatment of hyperoxaluria includes dietary restriction of oxalate-rich foods such as chocolate, tea, colas, etc. Oral calcium citrate may also be administered to help precipitate luminal oxalate before absorption can occur.

BACTERIAL OVERGROWTH

The risk of bacterial overgrowth is increased in patients who have undergone ileocecal resection with an ileocolonic anastomosis. As noted previously, bacterial overgrowth has been attributed to loss of the ileocecal valve, although evidence supporting this explanation is weak.[14] Alterations in intestinal motility may play a more important role in the pathogenesis. In patients who have undergone bypass surgery for obesity, bacterial overgrowth is presumed due to stasis in the bypassed limb.[13] Patients with small intestinal Crohn's complicated by tight strictures or patients with anastomotic strictures may also develop stasis and bacterial overgrowth in the dilated proximal bowel.

D-LACTIC ACIDOSIS

A rare neurological syndrome associated with carbohydrate malabsorption and development of D-lactic acidosis has been reported in patients with SBS and intestinal bypass surgery.[52-54] Clinical findings associated with D-lactic acidosis include encephalopathy, nystagmus, ophthalmoplegia, slurred speech, ataxia, confusion, inability to concentrate, weakness, and inappropriate behavior.[9,55] The findings are similar in presentation to alcohol intoxication, although blood alcohol levels are normal. In addition to the neurological signs and symptoms, an anion gap metabolic acidosis is present, although serum lactate levels measured by conventional means are normal. The diagnosis is confirmed by elevations in serum D-lactic acid >3 mmol/L (normal: <0.5 mmol/L).[55]

Although the precise mechanism of the neurological syndrome is not known, the episodes of acidosis are often precipitated by ingestion of excessive carbohydrates. Carbohydrates inadequately absorbed in the small bowel are fermented by colonic bacteria and form short-chain fatty acids and lactate.[4] This leads to a reduction in colonic pH and inhibition of the growth of acid-sensitive bacteria such as *Bacteroides* species. Growth of acid-resistant bacteria, in particular the Gram-positive anaerobe *Lactobacillus*, is enhanced, leading to increased production of D-lactate. The absence of D-lactate dehydrogenase in humans means this isomer is poorly metabolized; colonic absorption and accumulation of D-lactate result in the metabolic acidosis characteristic of this syndrome.[53]

Acute management of the D-lactic acidosis syndrome involves correction of the acidosis by administration of sodium bicarbonate. Oral intake, particularly carbohydrates, should be temporarily suspended.[4,9] Successful prevention of future episodes has been reported with dietary manipulation of carbohydrates to polymeric forms,[54] use of nonabsorbable antibiotics (eg, neomycin, vancomycin, kanamycin) to suppress the abnormal intestinal flora,[55] use of probiotics to recolonize the bowel with nonpathogenic flora,[55] and administration of oral thiamine in 1 case.[53]

MANAGEMENT

MEDICAL

In addition to the necessary replacement of vitamin and mineral deficiencies, the primary goal of medical management of SBS is to control the diarrhea. The antidiarrheal agents best suited for this are narcotic derivatives that prolong intestinal transit time via their action on smooth muscle. Loperamide has the lowest potential for addiction and is a reasonable first choice.[2] More potent narcotics such as codeine or tincture of opium may be required if diarrhea is severe. For milder cases, fiber supplementation may suffice.

When symptomatic control using simple antidiarrheals fails, further investigation as to the underlying mechanism may help refine a treatment strategy. For example, in patients who have undergone limited ileal or ileocecal resections and in whom bile salt diarrhea is suspected, trial of a bile acid-binding resin is warranted. Cholestyramine is available as a powder or in more convenient tablet form (Colestid). For patients in whom bacterial overgrowth is suspected, a trial of broad-spectrum antibiotics is reasonable.[3] Depending on the time frame, recurrence of underlying diseases such as Crohn's should also be considered and treated accordingly; enteroenteric fistulas that bypass an already shortened length of bowel may exacerbate diarrhea and malabsorption. Cholylsarcosine, a synthetic conjugated bile acid resistant to bacterial degradation and lacking a cathartic effect, has been tried in SBS patients with fat malabsorption due to loss of bile acids.[56,57] Significant increases in fat absorption (40 g/day) were observed, without concomitant effects on water, carbohydrate, or protein absorption.

Octreotide, a synthetic octapeptide analog of somatostatin, has been used with varying success to control refractory diarrhea in SBS. Its mechanism of action is likely related to its ability to inhibit gastric, pancreatic, and small bowel secretions.[58] Data from randomized controlled trials are sparse, but at least 1 trial using octreotide at a subcutaneous dose of 50 mcg twice daily in 6 parenteral nutrition-dependent SBS patients without a colon demonstrated improved sodium and fluid balance. No effect on nutrient or fat balance occurred, and no patient was able to lower or discontinue parenteral nutrition.[59] An open-label trial in SBS patients with high jejunostomies using octreotide at a subcutaneous dose of 100 mcg 3 times daily showed a 30% to 40% reduction in fluid losses as well as sodium, potassium, and chloride balance.[60]

A long-acting release form of octreotide was recently investigated in an open-label study of SBS patients. After 15 weeks of treatment, no differences in stool weight, sodium, potassium, or fat losses were observed, although small bowel transit time was modestly prolonged.[61] Potential side effects include pain at the site of injection, abdominal pain, and bowel obstruction. Chronic use has been associated with development of gallstones.[62] In view of the cost, potential side effects, and limited data to support widespread use, octreotide should be reserved for the SBS patient with large volume diarrhea or ostomy output that is refractory to standard agents.[58]

Recent attention has been given to the use of agents thought to have a role in promotion of intestinal adaptation in patients with SBS. These include growth hormone, glutamine, and GLP-2. The heterogeneity of study designs, the patients studied (some dependent on parenteral nutrition, some with colons intact, some with high ostomies, etc.), as well as outcomes measured all make it difficult to compare results and to draw meaningful conclusions. In a randomized double-blind placebo-controlled trial evaluating daily low-dose growth hormone in 12 parenteral nutrition-dependent SBS patients, significant increases in intestinal absorption of energy, nitrogen, and carbohydrates was observed.[63] Increases in body weight and lean body mass were also noted. These results contradict those found previously, and until long-term data have been collected, use of growth hormone is not recommended in the treatment of SBS.[64]

Several authors have reported the use of growth hormone in conjunction with glutamine with or without a high-carbohydrate, low-fat (HCLF) diet with mixed results.[65-67] Glutamine is the most abundant nonessential amino acid in the body and serves as a nitrogen carrier between major organs.[68] It plays a role in maintaining intestinal epithelial cell function as a source of energy. It has therefore been presumed to be of critical importance in the growth of small intestinal mucosa.[68] A systematic review of published trials concluded that the benefits of administering growth hormone in combination with glutamine with or without HCLF diet were marginal, at best.[69] Interestingly, another more recent systematic review concluded that the same treatment combination, although still controversial, may be of benefit in carefully selected patients.[70] Given the mixed study results and potential side effects, which include facial edema, arthralgias, chest pain, injection site reactions, fungal infections, and vomiting,[71] use of growth hormone with glutamine in patients with SBS should not be considered standard of care.[58]

GLP-2 is a 33-amino acid peptide with intestinotrophic, antisecretory, and transit-modulating properties in rodents.[23,68,72] It is secreted from the intestinal mucosa of distal ileum and colon in response to a meal. Postprandial secretion of GLP-2 is thus impaired in SBS patients with a jejunostomy. In an open-label study of 8 such patients who received 400 mcg of GLP-2 subcutaneously twice daily for 35 days, absorption of energy and nitrogen was significantly improved, body weight increased by 1.2 kg, lean body mass increased by 2.9 kg, and gastric emptying time for solids increased without any associated change in small intestinal transit time.[73] The beneficial effects were modest, and results of larger, controlled trials are necessary before GLP-2 can be considered standard therapy in SBS.[58,74,75]

NUTRITIONAL

In the immediate postoperative period, most SBS patients are kept fasting and are given parenteral nutrition. Dehydration and electrolyte abnormalities are the greatest risks during this phase. Careful monitoring of intake and output (urinary, fecal, and stomal losses if present), weight, and volume status must be performed and adjustments in intravenous (IV) fluids and parenteral formulas made. A detailed discussion of parenteral nutrition is beyond the scope of this chapter, and the reader is referred to a number of excellent review articles on this topic,[1,76] as well as Chapter 31 of this book.

Once the patient has stabilized, usually 7 to 14 days postoperative, oral nutrition is initiated. Oral feeding in patients with SBS is crucial because it induces the intermediate or intestinal adaptation phase.[77] Elemental and semi-elemental formulas are frequently recommended.[36] These formulas are very low in fat and contain easily digestible proteins, vitamins, minerals, and carbohydrates in the form of sucrose and glucose polymers, all of which are efficiently absorbed in the proximal jejunum.[3] However, the taste of elemental and semi-elemental diets often limits their use as oral feeding, and their high osmolarity may exacerbate diarrhea. In addition, they do not appear to offer any benefit over polymeric diets.[78]

Recommendations on diet are often based on the presence or absence of colon in continuity.[58] Patients with a high jejunostomy are given an isotonic glucose-saline solution to sip slowly throughout the day. This solution takes advantage of coupled glucose-sodium absorption in the jejunum, as noted previously.[79-81] Sodium moves across the jejunal mucosa along a concentration gradient. At luminal sodium concentrations <60 mmol/L, sodium is secreted into the lumen. Sodium absorption occurs when the luminal concentration is >90 mmol/L.[80] The optimum isotonic glucose-saline solution for use in SBS patients contains sodium at a concentration of 90 to 120 mmol/L and glucose at a concentration of 50 mmol/L glucose.[4,80] Free water ingestion should be limited as it can lead to excessive stomal output of a sodium-rich effluent and result in hyponatremia.[80]

For patients in whom all or part of the colon is intact, a HCLF diet may help reduce fluid and electrolyte losses. Complex carbohydrates are preferred because they reduce the osmotic load and potentially enhance the adaptation process.[81] Lactose is usually tolerated well if the proximal jejunum is intact, so it should not be restricted unless clear evidence of intolerance is present. Concentrated sugars should be avoided due to their high osmotic load. Restricting fat to 20% to 30% of the daily caloric intake reduces steatorrhea and oxalate absorption.[81] Soluble fiber may be useful to slow gastric emptying. Gradually, diet is advanced and food intake increased, with careful attention to symptoms of diarrhea, steatorrhea, bloating, etc. The adaptation phase generally occurs gradually over the course of 1 year, and it is during this time that most weaning from parenteral nutrition occurs (Figure 35-3).[37]

SURGICAL

In addition to medical and nutritional advances in the treatment of SBS that have been made over the years, new surgical techniques have also been developed. Surgical rehabilitation is 1 option for patients who have persistent malabsorption despite maximal medical therapy and parenteral nutritional support.[82] The goals of surgical rehabilitation are to improve the function of the remaining intestine by slowing intestinal transit or increasing intestinal surface area available for absorption.[1] A number of techniques are now available to help achieve these goals.

Restoration of intestinal continuity can be performed if a suitable colonic remnant exists. This has the advantages of recruiting the colon's absorptive capacity, potentially prolonging intestinal transit time, and eliminating the need for an ostomy.[1,82] Potential disadvantages include development of bile salt diarrhea, perianal complications if diarrhea is severe enough, and formation of calcium oxalate nephrolithiasis (see previous section on nephrolithiasis). Careful patient selection is crucial, and a minimum small bowel remnant length of 3 feet is recommended to avoid perianal complications secondary to massive diarrhea.[82]

Intestinal obstruction necessitating additional surgical procedures is another potential complication that patients with SBS must face. In most cases, the obstruction is mechanical and due to stenosis at the anastomosis, adhesions, or stricture formation related to the underlying disease process (eg, Crohn's).[82] Whenever pos-

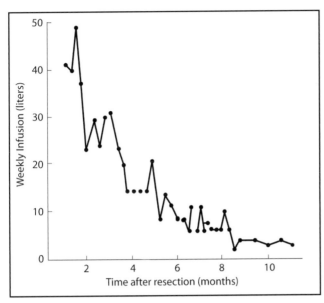

FIGURE 35-3. The decrease in weekly infusion requirements due to intestinal adaptation as a function of time after surgery in a 51-year-old man with severe short bowel syndrome after anastomosis of 25 cm of jejunum to sigmoid colon after resection for bowel infarction. (Reprinted with permission from Malik A, Westergaard H. Short bowel syndrome. In Feldman M, Friedman L, Sleisenger M, eds. *Gastrointestinal and Liver Disease.* 7th ed. Philadelphia, PA: Elsevier: 2006;1807-1816.)

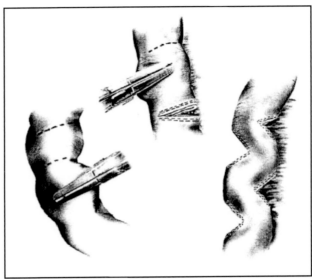

FIGURE 35-4. Preservation of small intestinal length can be achieved using Serial Transverse Enteroplasty (STEP), a technique that involves sequential stapling along the transverse plane of the intestine in a "zig-zag" fashion. (Reprinted with permission from Thompson JS. Surgical rehabilitation of intestine in short bowel syndrome. *Surgery.* 2004;135:465-470.)

sible, bowel-preserving techniques such as strictureplasty and serosal patching should be used. If resection is necessary, the length of intestine removed should be limited.

Over time, patients with chronic partial bowel obstruction can develop small bowel dilatation. The dilated segment may cause stasis and bacterial overgrowth that can further impair absorption of nutrients. Intestinal motility may also be affected. Surgical techniques to taper the dilated segments can improve motility. Clinical improvement in up to 90% of patients undergoing such procedures has been reported.[82]

Procedures to prolong intestinal transit time have been used for decades, although their efficacy has never been proven.[83] The most common procedures include segmental reversal of small bowel, colonic interposition, creation of artificial sphincters or valves, and small bowel electric pacing.[1,41,82] Segmental reversal requires a reversed intestine length of approximately 10 cm, and the segment should be inserted in the most distal portion of the small bowel to reduce the risk of obstruction.[1,41] Colonic interposition has been reported in only a dozen patients; thus, clinical experience is quite limited. Interposition of the colonic segment in the isoperistaltic direction is preferred over the antiperistaltic direction.[84]

Surgical techniques to actually lengthen the residual intestine have also been developed. These have the advantage of improving intestinal motility, increasing intestinal surface area, and reducing stasis and the risk of bacterial

overgrowth.[1,82] Potential disadvantages include interruption of normal motility in the proximal intestinal segment and altered response to gut hormones. Bianchi described the first longitudinal intestinal lengthening and tailoring procedure (LILT) in 1980.[85] Serial transverse enteroplasty (STEP) is a newer technique that involves sequential applications of a linear stapler along the transverse plane of the intestine in a "zig-zag" fashion (Figure 35-4).[82] Intestinal lengthening is the most common nontransplant procedure performed in SBS patients.[82] Short-term results suggest that up to 90% of patients demonstrate improved absorptive function and nutritional status.[82] Long-term results are not as favorable, however, with only half of the patients demonstrating sustained benefit 10 years after surgery.[86]

Intestinal transplantation is gaining momentum as a therapeutic option for patients with SBS who have developed life-threatening complications of intestinal failure or of long-term parenteral nutrition.[1] As of October 2000, Medicare approved payment for intestinal transplantation in patients who have failed parenteral nutrition. Their definition of failure includes at least 1 of the following: impending or overt liver failure, thrombosis of major central venous access, frequent line-related sepsis, and frequent severe dehydration.[1] Unfortunately, a specific reimbursement has yet to be assigned for this particular transplant; as a result, no guarantee for minimal payment level exists.[87]

SBS is the most common indication for intestinal transplantation (63%).[87] Although average waiting times for intestinal transplant are comparable to those for other organs (6 to 12 months), the mortality of those on the wait list for intestinal transplant is significantly higher than those on any other solid-organ transplant wait list.[1,88] However, nearly all of the wait list deaths have been in patients awaiting combined intestine and liver transplant. For this group of patients, organ allocation is determined by status on the liver wait list rather than status on the intestine wait list.

Patient and graft survival depend in part on whether additional organs are transplanted at the time of surgery. In a recent report, 1-year patient and graft survivals were 79% and 64%, respectively, for intestine-only transplants and 50% and 49%, respectively, in combined intestine/ liver transplants. Similar trends held true for 3- and 5-year patient and graft survivals.[1] A few cases of living related-donor intestinal transplants have been reported[89]; thus far, graft survival does not appear to differ between living and cadaveric donors.[1] Technical challenges of combined living related-donor liver and small bowel transplants have precluded widespread application.[87]

A recent report based on registry data identified the most common complications after transplant as acute rejection, chronic rejection, cytomegalovirus (CMV) infection, and posttransplant lymphoproliferative disease (PTLD).[90] Transplantation of additional organs appeared to reduce the risk of rejection, but increased the risk of viral-associated complications relative to intestine-only transplants.[90] Improvements in available immunosuppressive therapies show promise for reducing rejection rates and increasing survival.[87] Prophylactic regimens for CMV infection have led to reductions in the incidence of this complication.[87] Polymerase chain reaction has allowed the isolation of other infectious agents (eg, calicivirus) that may be pathogens unique to intestinal transplantation.[87]

QUALITY OF LIFE

The only health-related quality of life data available in patients with SBS are for those who are on parenteral nutrition or who have undergone intestinal transplant.[1,81,91] Unfortunately, subgroup analysis of the patients with SBS was not performed, although at least 1 study demonstrated that quality of life in parenteral nutrition-dependent SBS patients was no different from that of SBS patients after transplant.[91] A need therefore exists for prospective studies not only in SBS patients who require long-term parenteral nutrition but in all patients with SBS who live with its ramifications on a daily basis.

PROGNOSIS

In 1 study of 124 adults with SBS due to nonmalignant causes, the 2-year survival was 86% and at 5 years, 75%.[24] The proportion of patients dependent on parenteral nutrition was 49% at 2 years and 45% at 5 years. In multivariate analysis, survival was inversely related to end-jejunostomy,

a small bowel length <50 cm, and to arterial infarction as a cause of SBS. Dependence on parenteral nutrition was associated with residual bowel length <100 cm and absence of terminal ileum and/or colon in continuity. Small bowel length <100 cm was a significant predictor of permanent intestinal failure; lengths <50 cm also predicted decreased survival. Only 6% of patients who required parenteral nutrition for at least 2 years were ultimately able to discontinue it.[24]

In a study of 68 patients with intestinal failure, the 5-year survival was 78%; increased survival was associated with a longer length of remnant intestine, age >45 when parenteral nutrition was initiated, and eventual independence from all enteral nutrition.[92] Similar results were reported in a 25-year retrospective analysis of a cohort of 78 children with SBS who required parenteral nutrition for more than 3 months.[27] Overall survival was 73% at a median follow-up of 9 years. Improved survival was associated with residual small bowel length >38 cm, intact ileocecal valve, intact colon, takedown surgery after an initial ostomy, and primary anastomosis. Increased mortality was associated with small bowel length <15 cm and parenteral nutrition-induced cholestatic jaundice. Of the survivors, 77% showed evidence of intestinal adaptation defined as ability to maintain normal growth and fluid/electrolyte balance without parenteral support. Factors negatively associated with adaptation included small bowel length <15 cm, loss of the ileocecal valve, loss of >50% of colon, and inability to perform primary anastomosis.[27]

At least 1 retrospective study of home parenteral nutrition-dependent patients has demonstrated an overall 5-year survival of 60%; the probability of survival was dependent upon the primary, underlying diagnosis, and the age at initiation of parenteral nutrition.[93] The highest probability of survival at 5 years was associated with IBD (92%) and with age of onset of parenteral nutrition less than 40 (80%).[93] Although it appears that a high proportion (>65%) of patients with parenteral nutrition-dependent SBS are able to work, many of these shift from full-time to part-time jobs. Perhaps more meaningful, however, is the observation that the proportion of patients who are bedridden and unable to work decreases dramatically from 24% before parenteral nutrition to 9% after its initiation. This implies that parenteral nutrition improves the functional status of even the very most debilitated short bowel patient.[94]

REFERENCES

1. AGA Clinical Practice Committee. AGA technical review on short bowel syndrome and intestinal transplantation. *Gastroenterology.* 2003;124:1111-1134.

2. Lennard-Jones JE. Review article: practical management of the short bowel. *Aliment Pharmacol Ther.* 1994;8:563-577.

3. Brasitus TA, Sitrin MD. Short bowel syndrome. In: Yamada T, ed. *Textbook of Gastroenterology.* 2nd ed. Philadelphia, PA: JB Lippincott Company; 1995:1680-1696.

4. Scolapio JS, Fleming CR. Short bowel syndrome. *Clin Nutr.* 1998;27:467-479.

5. Vanderhoof JA, Langnas AN. Short-bowel syndrome in children and adults. *Gastroenterology.* 1999;113:1767-1778.

6. Mughal M, Irving M. Home parenteral nutrition in the United Kingdom and Ireland. *Lancet.* 1986;200:383-386.

7. Van Gossum A, Bakker H, Bozzetti F, et al. Home parenteral nutrition in adults: a European multicentre survey in 1997. *Clin Nutr.* 1999;18:135-140.

8. *North American Home Parenteral and Enteral Nutrition Patient Registry: Annual Report With Outcome Profiles 1985-1992.* Albany, NY: The Oley Foundation; 1994:1-23.

9. Malik A, Westergaard H. Short bowel syndrome. In: Feldman M, Friedman L, Sleisenger M, eds. *Sleisenger & Fordtran's Gastrointestinal and Liver Disease: Pathophysiology, Diagnosis, Management.* 7th ed. Philadelphia, PA: Saunders; 2002:1807-1816.

10. Bryant J. Observations upon the growth and length of the human intestine. *Am J Med Sci.* 1924;167:499-520.

11. Backman L, Hallberg D. Small-intestinal length: an intraoperative study in obesity. *Acta Chir Scand.* 1974;140:57-63.

12. Nightingale J, Bartram CI, Lennard-Jones JE. Length of residual small bowel after partial resection: correlation between radiographic and surgical measurements. *Gastrointest Radiol.* 1991;16:305-306.

13. Weser E. Short bowel syndrome. *Gastroenterology.* 1979;77:572-579.

14. Dowling RH. The short bowel syndrome. *Endoscopy Review.* 1988; 1:47-58.

15. Buxton B. Small bowel resection and gastric acid hypersecretion. *Gut.* 1974;15:229-238.

16. Williams NC, Evans P, King RFGJ. Gastric acid secretion and gastrin production in the short bowel syndrome. *Gut.* 1985;26:914-919.

17. Hyman PE, Everett SL, Harada T. Gastric acid hypersecretion in short bowel syndrome in infants: association with extent of resection and enteral feeding. *J Pediatr Gastro Nutr.* 1986;5:191-197.

18. Holgate AM, Read NW. Effect of ileal infusion of intralipid on gastrointestinal transit, ileal flow rate, and carbohydrate absorption in humans after ingestion of a liquid meal. *Gastroenterology.* 1985;88:1001-1011.

19. Spiller RC, Trotman JF, Higgins BE, et al. The ileal brake—inhibition of jejunal motility after ileal fat perfusion in man. *Gut.* 1984;25:365-374.

20. Savage AP, Adrian TE, Carolyn G, et al. Effects of peptide YY (PYY) on mouth to caecum intestinal transit time and on the rate of gastric emptying in healthy volunteers. *Gut.* 1987;28:166-170.

21. Nightingale JMD, Kamm MA, van der Sijp JRM, et al. Disturbed gastric emptying in the short bowel syndrome. Evidence for a "colonic brake." *Gut.* 1993;34:1171-1176.

22. Jeppesen PB, Hartmann B, Hansen BS, et al. Impaired meal stimulated glucagon-like peptide 2 response in ileal resected short bowel patients with intestinal failure. *Gut.* 1999;45:559-563.

23. Jeppesen PB, Hartmann B, Thulesen J, et al. Elevated plasma glucagon-like peptide 1 and 2 concentrations in ileum resected short bowel patients with a preserved colon. *Gut.* 2000;47:370-376.

24. Messing B, Crenn P, Beau P, et al. Long-term survival and parenteral nutrition dependence in adult patients with the short bowel syndrome. *Gastroenterology.* 1999;117:1043-1050.

25. Chaves M, Smith MW, Williamson RCN. Increased activity of digestive enzymes in ileal enterocytes adapting to proximal small bowel resection. *Gut.* 1987;28:981-987.

26. Gouttebel MC, Saint Aubert B, Colette C, et al. Intestinal adaptation in patients with short bowel syndrome. *Dig Dis Sci.* 1989; 34:709-715.

27. Quirós-Tejeira RE, Ament ME, Reyen L, et al. Long-term parenteral nutritional support and intestinal adaptation in children with short bowel syndrome: a 25-year experience. *J Pediatr.* 2004; 145:157-163.

28. Ziegler TR, Fernandez-Estivaris C, Gu LH, et al. Distribution of the H+/peptide transporter PepT1 in human intestine: up-regulated expression in the colonic mucosa of patients with short-bowel syndrome. *Am J Clin Nutr.* 2002;75:922-930.

29. Alpers D. How adaptable is the intestine in patients with short-bowel syndrome? *J Clin Nutr.* 2002;75:787-788.

30. Solhaug JH, Tvete S. Adaptive changes in the small intestine following bypass operation for obesity: a radiological and histological study. *Scand J Gastroent.* 1978;13:401-408.

31. Nightingale JMD, Lennard-Jones JE, Gertner DJ, et al. Colonic preservation reduces need for parenteral therapy, increases incidence of renal stones, but does not change high prevalence of gall stones in patients with a short bowel. *Gut.* 1992;33:1493-1497.

32. Briet F, Flourie B, Achour L, et al. Bacterial adaptation in patients with short bowel and colon in continuity. *Gastroenterology.* 1995; 109:1446-1453.

33. Royall D, Wolever TMS, Jeejeebhoy KN. Evidence for colonic conservation of malabsorbed carbohydrate in short bowel syndrome. *Am J Gastroenterol.* 1992;87:751-756.

34. Nordgaard I, Hansen BS, Mortensen PB. Importance of colonic support for energy absorption as small-bowel failure proceeds. *Am J Clin Nutr.* 1996;64:222-231.

35. Nordgaard I, Hansen BA, Mortensen PB. Colon as a digestive organ in patients with short bowel. *Lancet.* 1994;343:373-376.

36. Weser E. The management of patients after small bowel resection. *Gastroenterology.* 1976;71:146-150.

37. DiBaise JK, Young RY, Vanderhoof JA. Intestinal rehabilitation and the short bowel syndrome: Part 1. *Am J Gastroenterol.* 2004;99:1386-1395.

38. Arrambide KA, Santa Ana CA, Schiller LR, et al. Loss of absorptive capacity for sodium chloride as a cause of diarrhea following partial ileal and right colon resection. *Dig Dis Sci.* 1989;34:193-201.

39. Frederick PL, Craig TV. The effect of vagotomy and pyloroplasty on weight loss and survival of dogs after massive intestinal resection. *Surgery.* 1964;56:135-141.

40. Osborne MP, Frederick PL, Sizer JS, et al. Mechanism of gastric hypersecretion following massive intestinal resection: clinical and experimental observations. *Ann Surg.* 1966;164:622-632.

41. Devine RM, Kelly KA. Surgical therapy of the short bowel syndrome. *Gastro Clin N Am.* 1989;18:603-618.

42. Straus E, Gerson CD, Yalow RS. Hypersecretion of gastrin associated with the short bowel syndrome. *Gastroenterology.* 1974;66:175-180.

43. Nightingale JMD, Lennard-Jones JE, Walker ER, et al. Jejunal efflux in short bowel syndrome. *Lancet.* 1990;336:765-768.

44. Andersson H, Bosaeus I, Brummer RJ, et al. Nutritional and metabolic consequences of extensive bowel resection. *Dig Dis.* 1986;4:193-202.

45. Hylander E, Ladefoged K, Jarnum S. The importance of the colon in calcium absorption following small-intestinal resection. *Scand J Gastroenterol.* 1980;15:55-60.

46. Hylander E, Ladefoged K, Madsen S. Calcium balance and bone mineral content following small-intestinal resection. *Scand J Gastroenterol.* 1981;16:167-176.

47. Hessov I, Andersson H, Isaksson B. Effects of a low-fat diet on mineral absorption in small-bowel disease. *Scand J Gastroenterol.* 1983;18:551-554.

48. Quigley EMM, Marsh MN, Shaffer JL, et al. Hepatobiliary complications of total parenteral nutrition. *Gastroenterology.* 1993;104:286-301.

49. Earnest DL, Johnson G, Williams HE, et al. Hyperoxaluria in patients with ileal resection: an abnormality in dietary oxalate absorption. *Gastroenterology.* 1974;66:1114-1122.

50. Chadwick VS, Modha K, Dowling RH. Mechanism for hyperoxaluria in patients with ileal dysfunction. *N Engl J Med.* 1973;289:172-176.

51. Maratka Z, Nedbal J. Urolithiasis as a complication of the surgical treatment of ulcerative colitis. *Gut.* 1964;5:214-217.

52. Oh MS, Phelps KR, Traube M, et al. D-lactic acidosis in a man with the short-bowel syndrome. *N Engl J Med.* 1979;301:249-252.

53. Hudson M, Pocknee R, Mowat NAG. D-lactic acidosis in short bowel syndrome—an examination of possible mechanisms. *Q J Med.* 1990;274:157-163.

54. Mayne AJ, Handy DJ, Preece MA, et al. Dietary management of D-lactic acidosis in short bowel syndrome. *Arch Dis Child.* 1990;65:229-231.

55. Uchida H, Yamamoto H, Kisaki Y, et al. D-lactic acidosis in short-bowel syndrome managed with antibiotics and probiotics. *J Pediatr Surg.* 2004;39:634-636.

56. Heydorn S, Jeppesen PB, Mortensen PB. Bile acid replacement therapy with cholylsarcosine for short-bowel syndrome. *Scand J Gastroenterol.* 1999;34:818-823.

57. Gruy-Kapral C, Little KH, Fordtran JS, et al. Conjugated bile acid replacement therapy for short-bowel syndrome. *Gastroenterology.* 1999;116:15-21.

58. Scolapio J. Short bowel syndrome. *JPEN.* 2002;26:S11-S16.

59. Ladefoged K, Christensen KC, Hegnhoj J, et al. Effect of a long acting somatostatin analogue SMS 201-995 on jejunostomy effluents in patients with severe short bowel syndrome. *Gut.* 1989;30:943-949.

60. O'Keefe SJD, Peterson ME, Fleming CR. Octreotide as an adjunct to home parenteral nutrition in the management of permanent end-jejunostomy syndrome. *JPEN.* 1994;18:26-36.

61. Nehra V, Camilleri M, Burton D, et al. An open trial of octreotide long-acting release in the management of short bowel syndrome. *Am J Gastroenterol.* 2001;96:1494-1498.

62. Rosen GH. Somatostatin and its analogs in the short bowel syndrome. *Nutr Clin Practice.* 1992;7:81-85.

63. Seguy D, Vahedi K, Kapel N, et al. Low-dose growth hormone in adult home parenteral nutrition-dependent short bowel syndrome patients: A positive study. *Gastroenterology.* 2003;124:293-302.

64. Scolapio JS. Tales from the crypt. *Gastroenterology.* 2003;124:561-564.

65. Szkudlarek J, Jeppesen PB, Mortensen PB. Effect of high dose growth hormone with glutamine and no change in diet on intestinal absorption in short bowel patients: a randomized, double blind, crossover, placebo-controlled study. *Gut.* 2000;47:199-205.

66. Scolapio JS. Effect of growth hormone and glutamine on the short bowel: five years later. *Gut.* 2000;47:164.

67. Byrne TA, Morrissey TB, Nattakom TV, et al. Growth hormone, glutamine, and a modified diet enhance nutrient absorption in patients with severe short bowel syndrome. *JPEN.* 1995;19:296-302.

68. Botsios DS, Vasiliadis KD. Factors enhancing intestinal adaptation after bowel compensation. *Dig Dis.* 2003;21:228-236.

69. Ling L, Irving M. The effectiveness of growth hormone, glutamine and a low-fat diet containing high-carbohydrate on the enhancement of the function of remnant intestine among patients with short bowel syndrome: a review of published trials. *Clin Nutr.* 2001;20:199-204.

70. Matarese LE, Seidner DL, Steiger E. Growth hormone, glutamine, and modified diet for intestinal adaptation. *J Am Diet Assoc.* 2004; 104:1265-1272.

71. Keating GM, Wellington K. Somatropin (Zorbtive™) in short bowel syndrome. *Drugs.* 2004;64:1375-1381.

72. Jeppesen PB, Hartmann B, Thulesen J, et al. Treatment of short bowel patients with glucagon-like peptide 2 (GLP-2), a newly discovered intestinotrophic, anti-secretory, and transit modulating peptide. *Gastroenterology.* 2000;118:A178.

73. Jeppesen PB, Hartmann B, Thulesen J, et al. Glucagon-like peptide 2 improves nutrient absorption and nutritional status in short-bowel patients with no colon. *Gastroenterology.* 2001;120:806-815.

74. Warner BW. GLP-2 as therapy for the short-bowel syndrome. *Gastroenterology.* 2001;120:1041-1043.

75. Jeppesen PB. Clinical significance of GLP-2 in short-bowel syndrome. *J Nutr.* 2003;133:3721-3724.

76. Howard L, Ashley C. Management of complications in patients receiving home parenteral nutrition. *Gastroenterology.* 2003;124:1651-1661.

77. Freund HR, Beglaibter N. Total parenteral nutrition, intestinal adaptation, and short bowel syndrome. *Nutrition.* 2004;20:337.

78. Levy E, Frileux EL, Sandrucci S, et al. Continuous enteral nutrition during the early adaptive stage of the short bowel syndrome. *Br J Surg.* 1988;75:549-553.

79. Griffin GE, Fagan EF, Hodgson HJ, et al. Enteral therapy in the management of massive gut resection complicated by chronic fluid and electrolyte depletion. *Dig Dis Sci.* 1982;27:902-908.

80. Lennard-Jones JE. Indications and need for long-term parenteral nutrition: implications for intestinal transplantation. *Transplant Proc.* 1990;22:2427-2429.

81. DiBaise JK, Young RJ, Vanderhoof JA. Intestinal rehabilitation and the short bowel syndrome: part 2. *Am J Gastroenterol.* 2004;99:1823-1832.

82. Thompson JS. Surgical rehabilitation of intestine in short bowel syndrome. *Surgery.* 2004;135:465-470.

83. Thompson JS. Surgical approach to the short-bowel syndrome: procedures to slow intestinal transit. *Eur J Pediatr Surg.* 1999;9:263-266.

84. Trinkle JK, Bryant LR. Reversed colon segment in an infant with massive small bowel resection: a case report. *J Ky Med Assoc.* 1967;65:1090-1091.

85. Bianchi A. Intestinal loop lengthening—a technique for increasing small intestinal length. *J Pediatr Surg.* 1980;15:145-151.

86. Thompson JS, Pinch LW, Yound R, et al. Long-term outcome of intestinal lengthening. *Transplant Proc.* 2000;32:1242-1243.

87. Fishbein T. The current state of intestinal transplantation. *Transplantation.* 2004;79:175-178.

88. Harper AM, McBride MA, Ellison MD. The UNOS OPTN waiting list, 1988-1998. In: Cecka JM, Terasaki PI, eds. *Clinical Transplants 1998.* Los Angeles, CA: UCLA Tissue Typing Laboratory; 1999:71-82.

89. Benedetti E, Testa G, Sankary H, et al. Successful treatment of trauma-induced short bowel syndrome with early living related bowel transplantation. *J Trauma.* 2004;57:164-170.

90. Grant D. Intestinal transplantation: 1997 report of the international registry. *Transplantation.* 1999;67:1061-1064.

91. Rovera GM, DiMartini A, Schoen RE, et al. Quality of life of patients after intestinal transplantation. *Transplantation.* 1998;66:1141-1145.

92. Vantini I, Benini L, Bonfante F, et al. Survival rate and prognostic factors in patients with intestinal failure [abstract]. *Dig Liver Dis.* 2004;36:46.

93. Scolapio JS, Fleming CR, Kelly DG, et al. Survival of home parenteral nutrition-treated patients: 20 years of experience at the Mayo Clinic. *Mayo Clin Proc.* 1999;74:217-222.

94. Van Gossum A, Abdel-Malik M, Staun M, et al. Clinical, social and rehabilitation status of long-term home parenteral nutrition patients: results of a European multicentre survey. *Clin Nutr.* 2001;20:205-210.

MEDICAL MANAGEMENT OF THE PATIENT WITH AN OSTOMY

36

Aaron Brzezinski, MD, FRCP(C)

Intestinal stomas in inflammatory bowel disease (IBD) patients are used to treat complications of the disease such as obstruction, fistula, and neoplasia; in refractory disease, they protect a distal anastomosis or serve as the permanent end of the gastrointestinal tract. Stomas can be constructed either from small intestine or from the colon and are either temporary or permanent. Temporary stomas can be constructed as a loop; permanent stomas are usually an end ileostomy or a colostomy. Early complications occur within 1 month of surgery, and late complications can occur years after stoma creation. It is important to select the proper timing for surgery and define the type of surgery to prevent complications. These patients are best treated by a team of colorectal surgeons, gastroenterologists, and stoma therapists. Complications can be related to disease recurrence; extraintestinal manifestations; technical complications; or due to fluid, electrolytes, and nutrient losses. Reoperation to correct stoma problems is frequently required. In this chapter, I will discuss the most common complications related to the presence of a stoma and its management.

PRINCIPLES OF STOMA CONSTRUCTION

"An ounce of prevention…" The success of a stoma depends on proper patient selection, defining and discussing with the patient the stoma type to be constructed, surgical stages and approximate recovery time, patient education, and preoperative marking of the stoma site. A stoma therapist plays an invaluable role in this process.[1,2] Patients should be educated in regards to dietary

and lifestyle modifications that will occur after surgery, including issues related to daily life and intimacy. Patients should also be aware of the risk of postoperative sexual dysfunction including retrograde ejaculation, impotence, and dyspareunia. Stoma therapists can give invaluable advice to patients in regards to daily activities and diet. For some patients, odor or excessive gas production are a problem, and the use of chloropyllin copper complex or bismuth subgallate help decrease stool odor. To decrease gas production, patients should decrease certain foods that contain raffinose such as cabbage, beans, cauliflower, broccoli, asparagus, and Brussels sprouts, as well as starch and soluble fiber that also contribute to gas fermentation.

The optimal stoma site should be determined with the patient supine, sitting, and standing. Body habitus plays a significant role in site selection; the patient should be able to see the stoma for proper management, the stoma should be away from creases, scars, incision lines, and the umbilicus to allow for optimal pouching. Ideally, a stoma should be below the belt line, but particularly in men this may not be possible. Alternative sites are also selected, and all potential sites should be tattooed preoperatively, particularly in Crohn's disease patients where surgical findings may prevent the use of the selected site. It is important that a patient be able to see the stoma to adequately pouch it; whereas the preferred site for an ileostomy in a lean patient is in the right lower quadrant (RLQ), below the umbilicus and within the sheath of the rectus muscle on the summit of the infraumbilical fat mound, an obese patient or a wheelchair-bound patient would not be able to see that stoma, and an alternate site that is usually higher in the abdomen should be chosen. In general, the belt line is avoided, and

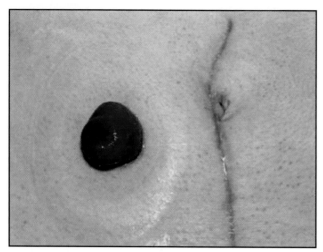

FIGURE 36-1. Ideal stoma.

there are situations in which the patient's profession has a major impact in site selection; for example, members of the police department require alternate sites for the stoma to allow them to carry their weapons. The ideal stoma (Figure 36-1) should protrude slightly (approximately 2.5 cm), be round in shape, and be away from skin folds. The color should be red, indicating viability of bowel tissue.[3]

Unfortunately, these can be accomplished only in patients undergoing elective surgery, such as in patients with dysplasia or stable disease refractory to medical treatment. In patients who undergo emergency surgery, the experience and expertise of the surgeon are crucial in determining the optimal site for stoma creation.

EARLY STOMA COMPLICATIONS

Despite all best efforts, complications of stoma creation occur. Early complications are those seen less than 1 month postoperatively and are frequently technical in nature. The most frequent complications related to stoma creation include dehydration and electrolyte imbalance, ileus obstruction, peristomal skin irritation, parastomal hernia, and ischemia with or without necrosis. Complication rates vary depending on whether the patient undergoes an elective or an emergency operation; the patient's nutritional status; whether at time of surgery there was gross peritoneal soiling, severely diseased intestine, gangrenous or perforated intestine; the segment of intestine used; the configuration of the stoma; and whether the optimal stoma site was selected a priori or during surgery.

One of the largest series published to date is from the 20 years of experience of the Cook County Hospital in Chicago. This series includes 1616 stoma creations and includes both ileostomies and colostomies. The overall complication rate was 34% (28% early, 6% late). The inde-

pendent variables that influenced the complication rate were patient age, operating team, stoma type and configuration, and preoperative marking by an enterostomal therapist (ET). In this series, only 26% of stomas were selected by an ET nurse prior to surgery; however, the incidence of postoperative stoma complications was significantly lower in these patients than in those in whom the site was not selected by an ET nurse prior to surgery. Early complications were seen with greater frequency in patients with a descending end colostomy configuration (60%), followed closely by a loop ileostomy configuration (59%). The highest overall complication rate was seen in loop colostomies (75%), and the lowest complication rate was seen with end transverse colostomies (6%).[4]

ILEUS

In the early postoperative period after an ileostomy construction, there may be a high volume of pale yellow, watery discharge containing flecks of mucous but no gas. However, neither these nor audible bowel sounds mean that adequate function has returned. Before removing the nasogastric suction or starting a diet, it is important to wait until there is passage of flatus per the stoma and the effluent becomes thicker. During this period, it is very important to replace electrolytes and maintain adequate hydration. Initially, in a distal ileostomy, the daily output is 1200 to 1500 mL; however, with adaptation over time, the ileostomy output decreases to a daily average of 600 to 800 mL. Patients with a jejunostomy or a proximal ileostomy have a higher output and are more prone to complications. Given a higher water, salt, and potassium loss in ileostomy patients, it is important to emphasize adequate water intake (particularly in hot humid weather) and teach patients early signs and symptoms of dehydration.

The ileostomy output is more caustic and liquid than the colostomy effluent because it has bile and pancreatic enzymes, whereas the contents of colostomy are firm; therefore, ileostomy patients are more susceptible to dehydration and skin irritation.[5] Ileostomy patients with persistent high output (ileostomy diarrhea) are at high risk for severe dehydration and electrolyte disturbances as well as renal failure, and kidney and gallbladder calculi. We instruct such patients to maintain adequate hydration and, when extra fluid and electrolytes are needed, to drink solutions such as the World Health Organization (WHO) rehydration formula that is used to treat patients with dysentery. Unless there is an infectious etiology, these patients should also be treated with antidiarrhea medications such as diphenoxylate, loperamide, codeine, or tincture of opium. In refractory cases, the use of octreotide, a long-acting somatostatin analogue, helps to decrease ileostomy output. The administration of a fiber supplement also helps to thicken the ileostomy output.

OBSTRUCTION

Mechanical intestinal obstruction may develop any time after surgery, from the immediate postoperative period to years after surgery. Late obstruction occurs in ~9% of patients with an ileostomy and in ~6% of patients with a colostomy.[6-8]

Common causes of obstruction include adhesions, hernias, volvulus, and food bolus. In food bolus obstruction, undigested food such as popcorn, nuts, fruit skins, olives, or fibrous vegetables block the intestinal lumen; the most common site of obstruction is in the distal segment of the intestine close to the stoma. Frequently, the patient will remember ingesting a food that is hard to digest and then suddenly experiencing obstructive symptoms. The initial management of these patients is nonoperative even when the radiographs show a complete obstruction. The treatment of these patients involves gastrointestinal decompression with a nasogastric tube, intravenous (IV) rehydration, and narcotic pain medication. If diagnosed early enough, ileostomy enemas using a Foley catheter and 100-mL aliquots of water may relieve a food bolus impaction with instant improvement in symptoms. If the obstruction does not resolve, a water-soluble retrograde contrast study should be done to identify the site and possible cause of the obstruction, and this in turn is frequently therapeutic. When an obstruction occurs in a patient with CD, it is important to exclude recurrent disease, and, depending on the degree of inflammation and stenosis, the treatment may be medical or surgical.

PERISTOMAL SKIN IRRITATION

The reported incidence of peristomal skin irritation ranges from 3% to 42%.[4,9-12] In Pearl et al's series, peristomal skin irritation was the most frequent early complication after ostomy surgery (42.1%).[9] The degree of irritation may range from mild dermatitis to full-thickness necrosis and ulceration. This complication occurs more commonly in patients with an ileostomy than in patients with a colostomy. The most common cause of skin irritation is leakage due to improper placement or inadequate fit of the appliance. Other causes of skin irritation include trauma, frequent pouch changes, or allergic reactions.

It is important to differentiate skin irritation from fungal infections (Figure 36-2), such as *Candida albicans*. This infection occurs because of excessive moisture from a leaking pouch, perspiration, or antibiotic use. The lesions in *Candida* infection are a macular and papular rash with erythema and satellite lesions extending from the ostomy site. Clinical management includes eliminating the source of moisture, using absorbent materials, and applying an antifungal powder with each pouch change.

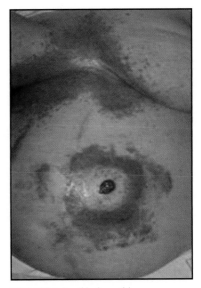

FIGURE 36-2. Candida dermatitis.

PERISTOMAL ULCERS AND PYODERMA GANGRENOSUM

Peristomal ulceration occurs more commonly in patients with a colostomy requiring irrigations or in patients with Kock pouch who require intubation. Peristomal ulcers may be due to local trauma, peristomal abscess, fistula, pyoderma gangrenosum, or CD. Ulcers that develop soon after surgery are related to surgical technique; ulcers that occur after 1 to 2 years are usually secondary to recurrent CD. When a parastomal ulcer develops, it is important to determine whether the lesion represents pyoderma gangrenosum or whether it is a traumatic lesion from improper pouching. In pyoderma gangrenosum, there is frequently a gap of normal skin separating the ulcer from the stoma. Treatment of parastomal ulcers is aimed at pain relief, prevention or treatment of secondary infection, and wound healing. Parastomal ulcers should be debrided of all infected and nonviable tissue with excision of any overhanging skin, and, depending on the size of the ulcers, the pouching system may have to be changed. Conservative treatment can take months to heal an ulcer; however, this is usually a better option than stoma relocation.

Peristomal pyoderma gangrenosum (Figure 36-3) is a complication that occurs almost exclusively in patients with IBD. Given that pyoderma gangrenosum commonly occurs at sites of trauma, a phenomenon called *pathergy*, it is difficult to manage. Whenever the patient changes the stoma appliance, there is trauma, and this is a stimulus either for ongoing ulceration or for new lesions. These lesions may extend under the skin and may communicate with the bowel.

The treatment of pyoderma gangrenosum usually requires local and systemic treatments medications. It is

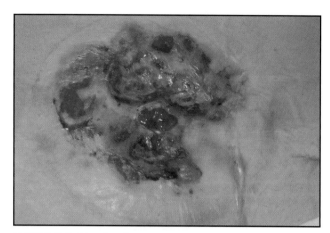

FIGURE 36-3. Peristomal pyoderma gangrenosum.

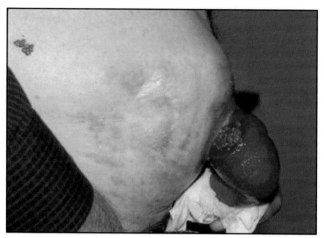

FIGURE 36-4. Parastomal hernia and prolapsed stoma.

important that a colorectal surgeon examines the lesion and debrides it, and then topical treatments can be started. Some of the topical treatments that have been used are intralesional steroids, topical steroids, or FK506 ointment. The pouching system is cut so that it does not adhere to the area of ulceration, and the ulcerated area is protected. Some of the systemic treatments that have been used include oral steroids, dapsone, and immunosuppressive therapy including cyclosporine, AZA, FK506, infliximab, and mycophenolate mofetil.[13,14]

Late peristomal ulceration may be related to trauma, abscess, fistula, pyoderma gangrenosum, or CD. These patients have pain and are at increased risk of developing abscess or other peristomal complications related to leakage. Maintaining an adequate seal to prevent leakage is difficult, and at times it is the main indication for surgery.

PARASTOMAL HERNIA

The incidence of early postoperative peristomal herniation and bowel obstruction ranges from 4.6% to 13%.[9,11,12,15] Parastomal hernia occurs more often in patients with a colostomy (1% to 58%) than in those with an ileostomy (2% to 11%). The incidence of parastomal hernias in patients with end colostomy ranges from 4% to 48%, and for a loop colostomy from 0% to 31%. The incidence of hernia in patients with an end ileostomy is 1.8% to 28.3%, and for loop ileostomy is 0% to 6.2%.[16]

Parastomal hernias have been reported to develop up to 20 years after stoma creation, and with longer follow-up, the incidences of symptomatic hernia are higher. In a retrospective study from St. Marks, the prevalence at 10 years was 36.7%, the incidence at 13 years was 51% in patients with a colostomy and 76% at 20 years for patients with an ileostomy.[7,8,17-23]

Early peristomal herniation is most commonly a technical complication because the fascial defect created for the stoma is too large to deliver the limb of intestine destined to become a stoma, poor site location, stoma fixation to

the fascia, and whether it is elective or emergency surgery. Patient risk factors that are believed to increase the risk of a parastomal hernia include obesity, an anterior abdominal wall weakened by multiple previous incisions, malnutrition, steroid use, sepsis, and raised intra-abdominal pressure.[24]

In most cases, the hernia is seen on physical exam as a palpable mass or bulge adjacent to the stoma (Figure 36-4). Occasionally a computed tomography (CT) scan may be useful, especially in obese patients.

In many cases the hernia is asymptomatic and thus no treatment is required. An abdominal wall binder decreases discomfort from the hernia and helps maintain an adequate seal. Indications for surgery include difficulty maintaining a seal, cosmesis, or symptoms such as obstruction, pain, nausea, or vomiting—particularly if these are secondary to incarceration. Depending on the duration of the hernia prior to diagnosis and the degree of vascular compromise, patients may have leukocytosis, fever, air fluid levels on upright abdominal x-ray, and if not treated promptly patients develop necrosis and an acute abdomen. Overall, only 23% to 32% of patients with a parastomal hernia require surgery.

PROLAPSED STOMA

Stoma prolapse occurs in situations similar to those resulting in parastomal herniation, such as a large opening of the abdominal wall, an inadequate surgical procedure to adhere the bowel to the abdominal wall, or increased abdominal pressure. A prolapsed stoma is the telescoping of a full-thickness segment of bowel through the stoma (see Figure 36-4). Prolapse occurs in 3% to 8% of patients with an ileostomy and in 2% to 25% of patients with a colostomy.[7,17,25-27] Risk factors include thin body habitus, redundant mesentery, a stoma located within a laparotomy incision, paraplegia, pregnancy, and transverse colostomies

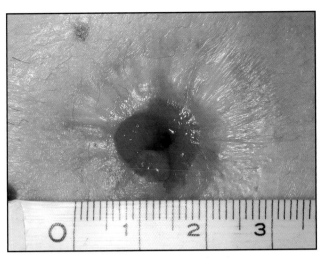

FIGURE 36-5. Stoma retraction (ruler measurement in cm).

with reported rates as high as 25%.[28-30] As in parastomal hernias, if the patient is asymptomatic, no surgery is required. To appropriately pouch this large intestinal protrusion, the clinician must compensate by using a pouch wide enough and long enough to manage the size of the protruding intestine. Repair should be done when pouch application becomes problematic, when the prolapsed segment becomes incarcerated, when the stoma is constantly injured, or when the patient's body image becomes unacceptable. During the third trimester of pregnancy, a pseudo-prolapse may be seen; however, this does not require surgical treatment and resolves after delivery.

STOMA RETRACTION

Stoma retraction is usually an early complication of surgery, although it can also present as a late complication. The reported incidence of stoma retraction is 1% to 6% for patients with a colostomy and 3% to 17% for those with an ileostomy.[7,17,26,27] Early stoma retraction is related to surgical technique; either the stoma size is inadequate or there is excess tension at the stoma site. Late stoma retraction is usually due to excessive weight gain, scar tissue that failed to fix the exiting intestine within the bowel wall, ischemia, or recurrent CD (Figure 36-5). When stoma retraction occurs in a patient with CD, recurrence of the disease must be excluded by endoscopy and contrast studies.[8] The main problem in a patient with stoma retraction is leakage of intestinal contents, which brings secondary complications. When stoma retraction occurs, alternate pouching devices including pouching systems with convexity and additional accessories (such as belts or binders) help maintain an adequate seal. As long as an adequate seal is obtained, and the patient can keep the pouch attached for 3 to 4 days, there is no need for surgical intervention.

VASCULAR COMPROMISE: ISCHEMIA AND VENOUS CONGESTION

The most serious complication of stoma creation is vascular compromise leading to stoma necrosis. When ischemia occurs during surgery, there may be the need to place the stoma at a different site; however, if the ischemia occurs postoperatively, unless there is full-thickness ischemia, it can be managed conservatively. The severity of vascular compromise varies from mild transient ischemia due to localized vasospasm and tissue trauma to infarction and necrosis. The incidence of stoma necrosis in reported series ranges from 2.3% to 17%.[4,31-33,38]

PERISTOMAL INFECTION AND ABSCESS

Peristomal skin and soft tissue infections are exceedingly rare; however, they are extremely problematic when they occur. In most patients, peristomal abscess are an early complication with a reported incidence of 2% to 14.8%.[4,9,32] Peristomal abscesses are frequently related to the presence of a fistula or an infected hematoma. Recurrent CD and trauma are causes for abscesses in mature stomas, and, in patients with a colostomy, an abscess can form secondary to perforation during irrigation. In mature stomas, folliculitis has also been reported as a cause of abscess. In the United Ostomy Association's (UOA) data registry, 5% of patients with an ileostomy and 3% of patients with a colostomy developed an abscess.[26] When an abscess develops, pouching becomes difficult because of pain and leakage. Peristomal abscesses are usually managed by the colorectal surgeons because they generally will not heal unless the abscess cavity is unroofed and adequate drainage of the abscess is achieved. Development of a fistula at an abscess site is not uncommon.

FISTULAE

Early fistulae are usually secondary to a technical surgical complication; late fistulae are usually related to recurrent CD or trauma. The incidence of fistulae at an ileostomy in patients with CD is 7% to 20%.[6,34] A fistula with an opening adjacent to the mucocutaneous junction can often be incorporated into the pouching system, avoiding the need for surgical repair. However, when fistulae interfere with pouching, the stoma should be revised and a new stoma created. The response to medical treatment with immunosuppressive medications such as azathioprine (AZA) or 6-mercaptopurine (6-MP) and infliximab is variable.

STRICTURE

ILEOSTOMY

The reported incidence of ileostomy stricture ranges from 2% to 10%.[7,26] When a stricture occurs in the early postoperative period, it is secondary to severe ischemia. In the late postoperative period, it is usually secondary to a mild degree of ischemia, which leads to fibrosis. The symptoms in patients who have a stricture at the stoma site are usually obstructive; patients feel pressure building and then a sudden passage of high-pressure intestinal contents occurs with immediate improvement in symptoms. Common causes of ileostomy stricture occurring months to years after surgery include ischemia, recurrent Crohn's disease, previous radiation therapy, or external compression (eg, constricting skin or fascial opening). Endoscopic or digital dilatation of a distal stricture at an ostomy site is rarely curative, and patients usually require surgical revision.

COLOSTOMY

When a mild colostomy stricture exists, dietary manipulation to keep the stool soft and/or colostomy irrigations may allow stool passage without surgery. Stoma dilatation, though effective initially, almost always leads to later problems. Dilatation is painful, produces bleeding, and with time causes recurrent fibrosis and scarring. Symptomatic patients should undergo surgical repair.

BLEEDING

Bleeding from either the mucosal surface, mucocutaneous junction of an ileostomy, or a colostomy commonly occurs because the mucosa with its underlying blood supply is easily traumatized. However, patients with IBD can have portal hypertension secondary to cirrhosis and portal hypertension, such as in primary sclerosing cholangitis or due to thrombosis from a hypercoagulable state, and in these patients the bleeding can be secondary to peristomal varices. Patients with portal hypertension can develop a "caput medusa"; this lesion is a painless pink- or burgundy-colored halo located around the stoma that blanches under pressure. When the bleeding is not associated with portal hypertension, simple measures such as direct pressure, cauterization with silver nitrate or injection of dilute epinephrine, and adjusting the size of the stomal appliance will solve the problem.

Bleeding from peristomal varices can be brisk but, unlike esophageal varices, is rarely life-threatening. Mortality in patients with portal hypertension is most commonly secondary to hepatic failure, not to peristomal bleeding varices. Acute bleeding is controlled by direct pressure. In 1 report, 7 of 9 patients with caput medusa were successfully treated using mucocutaneous disconnection with direct ligation of varices and repeat maturation.[35-37] Portosystemic shunts and the transjugular intrahepatic portosystemic shunt are indicated only if there is an additional indication for decompressing the portal system, such as recurrent bleeding esophageal varices.

REFERENCES

1. Bass EM, Del Pino A, Tan A, et al. Does preoperative stoma marking and education by the enterostomal therapist affect outcome? *Dis Colon Rectum.* 1997;40:440.

2. Nugent KP, Daniels P, Stewart B, et al. Quality of life in stoma patients. *Dis Colon Rectum.* 1999;42:1569.

3. Erwin-Toth P. Ostomy pearls: a concise guide to stoma sitting, pouching systems, patient education, and more. *Adv Skin Wound Care.* 2003;16(3):146-152.

4. Park JJ, Del Pino A, Orsay CP, et al. Stoma complications: the Cook County Hospital experience. *Dis Colon Rectum.* 1999;42:1575-1580.

5. Erwin-Toth P, Doughty D. Principles and procedures of stomal management. In: Hampton B, Bryant R, eds. *Ostomies and Continent Diversions: Nursing Management.* St. Louis, MO: Mosby; 1992:29.

6. Fleshman JW, Lewis MG. Complications and quality of life after stoma surgery: a review of 16,470 patients in the UOA data registry. *Semin Colon Rectal Surg.* 1991;2:66-72.

7. Leong APK, Londono-Schimmer EE, Phillips RKS. Lifetable analysis of stomal complications following ileostomy. *Br J Surg.* 1994; 81:727-729.

8. Leenen LP, Kuypers JH. Some factors influencing the outcome of stoma surgery. *Dis Colon Rectum.* 1989;32(6):500-504.

9. Pearl RK, Prasad LM, Orsay CP, et al. Early local complications from intestinal stomas. *Arch Surg.* 1985;120:1145-1147.

10. Fasth S, Hulten L. Loop ileostomy: a superior diverting stoma in colorectal surgery. *World J Surg.* 1984;8:401-407.

11. Feinberg SM, McLeod RS, Cohen Z. Complications of loop ileostomy. *Am J Surg.* 1987;153;102-107.

12. Grobler SP, Hoise KB, Keighley MRB. Randomized trial of loop ileostomy in restorative proctocolectomy. *Br J Surg.* 1992;79:903-906.

13. Daniels NH, Cullen JP. Mycophenolate mofetil is an effective treatment for peristomal pyoderma gangrenosum. *Arch Dermatol.* 2004;140:1427.

14. Regueiro M, Valentine J, Plevy S, Fleisher MR, Lichtenstein GR. Infliximab for treatment of pyoderma gangrenosum associated with inflammatory bowel disease. *Am J Gastroenterol.* 2003; 98(8):1821-1826.

15. Francois Y, Dozois RR, Kelly KA, et al. Small intestinal obstruction complicating ileal pouch-anal anastomosis. *Ann Surg.* 1989;209:46-50.

16. Carne PWG, Robertson GM, Frizelle FA. Parastomal hernia [review]. *Br J Surg.* 2003;90(7):784-793.

17. Londono-Schimmer EE, Leong AP, Phillips RK. Life-table analysis of stomal complications following colostomy. *Dis Colon Rectum.* 1994;37:916-920.

18. Pearl RK. Parastomal hernias. *World J Surg.* 1989;13:569-572.

19. Martin L, Foster G. Peristomal hernia. *Ann R Coll Surg Engl.* 1996;78(2):81-84.

20. Williams JG, Etherington R, Hayward MW, Hughes LE. Paraileostomy hernia: a clinical and radiological study. *Br J Surg.* 1990;77(12):1355-1357.

21. Rubin MS, Schoetz DJ Jr, Matthews JB. Parastomal hernia. Is stoma relocation superior to fascial repair? *Arch Surg.* 1994;129(4):413-418, discussion 418-419.

22. Carlstedt A, Fasth S, Hulten L, Nordgren S, Palselius I. Long-term ileostomy complications in patients with ulcerative colitis and Crohn's disease. *Int J Colorectal Dis.* 1987;2(1):22-25.

23. Cheung MT, Chia NH, Chiu WY. Surgical treatment of peristomal hernia complicating sigmoid colostomies. *Dis Colon Rectum.* 2001;44(2):266-270.

24. Sjodahl R, Anderberg B, Bolin T. Parastomal hernia in relation to site of the abdominal stoma. *Br J Surg.* 1988;75(4):339-341.

25. Porter JA, Salvati EP, Rubin RJ, Eisenstat TE. Complications of colostomies. *Dis Colon Rectum.* 1989;32(4):299-303.

26. Fleshman JW, Lewis MG. Complications and quality of life after stoma surgery: a review of 16,470 patients in the UOA data registry. *Semin Colon Rectal Surg.* 1991;2:66-72.

27. Shellito PC. Complications of abdominal stoma surgery. *Dis Colon Rectum.* 1998;41(12):1562-1572.

28. Edwards DP, Leppington-Clarke A, Sexton R, Heald RJ, Moran BJ. Stoma-related complications are more frequent after transverse colostomy than loop ileostomy: a prospective randomized clinical trial. *Br J Surg.* 2001;88(3):360-363.

29. Arun H, Ledgerwood A, Lucas CE. Ostomy prolapse in paraplegic patients: Etiology, prevention, and treatment. *J Am Paraplegia Soc.* 1990;13(2):7-9.

30. Chandler JG, Evans BP. Colostomy prolapse. *Surg.* 1978;84(5):577-582.

31. Birnbaum W, Ferrier P. Complications of abdominal colostomy. *Am J Surg.* 1952;83:64-67.

32. Green EW. Colostomies and their complications. *Surg Gynecol Obstet.* 1966;122:1230-1232.

33. Wara P, Sorensen K, Berg V. Proximal fecal diversion: review of ten years' experience. *Dis Colon Rectum.* 1981;24:114-119.

34. Greenstein AJ, Dicker A, Meyers S, Aufses AH Jr. Periileostomy fistulae in Crohn's disease. *Ann Surg.* 1983;197(2):179-182.

35. Beck DE, Fazio VW, Grundfest-Broniatowski S. Surgical management of bleeding stomal varices. *Dis Colon Rectum.* 1988;31(5):343-346.

36. Morris CS, Najarian KE. Transjugular intrahepatic portosystemic shunt for bleeding stomal varices associated with chronic portal vein occlusion: long-term angiographic, hemodynamic, and clinical follow-up. *Am J Gastroenterol.* 2000;95(10):2966-2968.

37. Shibata D, Brophy DP, Gordon FD, Anastopoulos HT, Sentovich SM, Bleday R. Transjugular intrahepatic portosystemic shunt for treatment of bleeding ectopic varices with portal hypertension. *Dis Colon Rectum.* 1999;42(12):1581-1585.

38. Stohert JC, Brubacher L, Simonowitz DA. Complications of emergency stoma formation. *Arch Surg.* 1982;117:307-309.

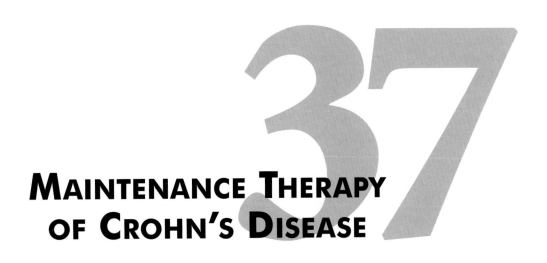

MAINTENANCE THERAPY OF CROHN'S DISEASE

Wojciech Blonski, MD, PhD; Faten Aberra, MD, MSCE; and Gary R. Lichtenstein, MD, FACP, FACG, AGAF

MEDICALLY INDUCED REMISSION

INTRODUCTION

Once a patient has achieved remission by means of medical therapy, the risk of relapse is high if treatment is not continued. Several studies have demonstrated Crohn's disease (CD) relapse rates as high as 71% to 85% after 1 year in patients who were maintained on mesalamine or placebo after treatment with corticosteroids to induce remission.[1,2]

Several medical therapies have been investigated for use in maintenance of remission of CD and include 5-aminosalicylates (5-ASA), corticosteroids, budesonide, azathioprine (AZA), 6-mercaptopurine (6-MP), methotrexate, antibiotics, probiotics, cyclosporine, biologic agents such as anti-tumor necrosis factor alpha (TNFα) antagonists (infliximab, adalimumab, certolizumab), and anti-integrin antibody natalizumab.

Several factors have been postulated to increase the risk of relapse of CD, with the strongest evidence for cigarette smoking.[3] Other potential factors with weaker evidence supporting an increase risk for relapse of CD include nonsteroidal anti-inflammatory drugs, short duration of remission (<4 years), and use of oral contraceptives.[3]

5-AMINOSALICYLIC ACID

BACKGROUND

Sulfasalazine (sulphapyridine and 5-ASA) is the first derivative of 5-ASA that was used in the treatment of patients with inflammatory bowel disease (IBD). However, this drug was associated with adverse events, limiting therapy in up to 20% of patients.[4] It was shown that 5-ASA (mesalamine) itself is the compound responsible for effectiveness of this drug whereas sulphapyridine was found to be a carrier for 5-ASA, allowing for its delivery into the colon.[5-7] The efficacy of 5-ASA is perceived to be a topical action within the lumen of the intestine.[8] Because oral administration of 5-ASA results in rapid absorption in proximal small bowel, a variety of oral formulations have been developed. The different formulations that have been developed allow release of the active moiety in different areas of the colon or small bowel. These different formulations include 5-ASA slow-release formulations (coated with an ethylcellulose), pH-dependent delayed-release formulations (coated with Eudragit L or S resins), and azo-bound prodrugs (olsalazine and balsalazide) in order to ease its delivery to more distal part of the inflamed intestine.[8,9] These formulations have different sites of release within the digestive tract. Mesalamine microgranules coated with ethylcellulose release within the duodenum, jejunum, ileum, and colon; preparations coated with Eudragit L100 resin within ileum and colon (above a pH 6); and those coated with Eudragit S resin within the terminal ileum and colon (above a pH of 7).[8,10] Azo-bound prodrugs are released by means of action of colonic bacterial azoreduction within the colon.[8] The bioavailability of these various oral preparations has ranged from 19% for release in the ileum and cecum to 75% for release in the upper gastrointestinal tract.[11] Mesalamine undergoes rapid acetylation into inactive metabolite N-acetyl-mesalamine either within the lumen of the colon by intestinal bacteria or within the wall of the colon (in that case, acetylated mesalamine is redistributed to the colonic lumen).[12,13] At least 50% of 5-ASA is excreted in the feces, and at least 25% of 5-ASA is absorbed and acetylated in the liver with subsequent excretion in the urine.[14]

CLINICAL TRIALS

There have been 9 randomized double-blind placebo-controlled multicenter trials evaluating the use of oral 5-ASA for maintenance therapy in patients with medically induced remission in CD over a 12- to 24-month period (Table 37-1). In 7 of these trials,[15-21] 1500 patients were randomized during remission, whereas in 2 trials,[2,22] 246 patients were randomized during the active phase of CD.

The first multicenter study included 248 patients who were randomly assigned to receive either oral 5-ASA at a dose of 1.5 g/day ($n = 125$) or placebo ($n = 123$) for up to 12 months.[15] Patients were eligible to enter the study if they had inactive disease defined as Crohn's Disease Activity Index (CDAI) < 150 and if their disease was controlled for 1 month before enrollment on either stable low-dose prednisolone (≤ 2.5 mg/day) or no steroids.[15] Of 248 initially randomized patients, 206 patients (101 active drug recipients and 105 placebo recipients) underwent further analysis.[15] This study has shown that the cumulative life-table relapse estimate was significantly lower in patients treated with active drug (22.4%) than those treated with placebo (36.2%, $P = 0.0395$).[15] Moreover, the cumulative annual relapse rate was significantly lower in patients with ileal involvement receiving 5-ASA (8.3% for 5-ASA versus 31% for placebo; $P = 0.0535$).[15] This was not observed in patients with colonic or ileocolonic involvement.[15] Relapse of the disease was defined as CDAI > 150 with the increase of at least 60 points from baseline score.[15]

In a randomized controlled trial (RCT) conducted by Prantera et al, oral 5-ASA (2.4 g daily) was found to be superior to placebo in preventing or delaying clinical relapse in CD, which was defined as CDAI > 150 with an increase of at least 100 points over the baseline.[19] This study evaluated 125 patients with CD in remission of duration between 3 months and 2 years (defined as CDAI < 150) who received either 5-ASA ($n = 64$) or placebo ($n = 61$) for up to 12 months.[19] The observed cumulative relapse rate at 12 months was significantly lower in patients treated with active drug (34%) than those treated with placebo (55%) ($P = 0.02$).[19] It was also demonstrated that patients with disease confined to the ileum had significantly reduced risk of relapse (0.35) over those with colonic (0.62) or ileocolonic (1.11) location of the disease.[19]

Gendre et al evaluated the efficacy of slow-release mesalamine in 161 patients with inactive disease who were randomized to treatment either with active drug ($n = 80$) given at a dose of 2 g daily or placebo ($n = 81$) for up to 2 years.[17] Patients with CDAI of < 150 with no steroids or immunosuppressive therapy for at least 1 month before study onset

and clinical remission of less than 2 years were eligible for this study.[17] The endpoints of this study were surgery for an acute complication or clinical relapse defined as CDAI > 250 or CDAI between 150 and 250 but with at least a 50-point increase from baseline.[17] This study reported that 1 patient (1.25%) receiving active drug and 2 patients (2.5%) receiving placebo required surgery for acute complications, whereas 29 mesalamine recipients (36.2%) and 34 placebo recipients (42%) experienced clinical relapse (P values not reported).[17] In addition, the participants of this trial were divided according to the duration of the disease remission.[17] Those with the duration of remission shorter than 3 months were considered the high-risk relapse group ($n = 64$) whereas subjects with remission duration between 3 months and 24 months were defined as the low-risk relapse group ($n = 97$).[17] It was observed that subjects with high relapse risk treated with placebo had significantly higher risk of relapse than those with high and low relapse risk treated with mesalamine and those with low relapse risk receiving placebo ($P < 0.003$).[17] This study has shown that mesalamine is a particularly effective maintenance therapy when given over a 2-year time to patients with short duration of remission of CD.[17]

In a study by Thomson et al, 286 patients (207 patients with CD colitis or ileocolitis and 79 patients with CD ileitis) were randomized to either oral 5-ASA at a dose of 3 g daily ($n = 138$) or placebo ($n = 148$) for 12 months.[21] The enrollment criteria included CDAI < 150 and 1 period of CDAI > 150 within 18 months of initiation of the trial.[21] The relapse of CD was considered CDAI > 150 with at least a 60-point increase from the baseline score.[21] This study did not observe any statistical difference in relapse rate between patients treated with mesalamine and placebo despite the location (colonic, ileocolonic, or ileal) of CD.[21]

In another randomized trial including only 59 patients with CD of at least 1-year duration and continuous remission for at least 6 months only on 5-ASA compounds or no therapy, mesalamine given at the 1-g daily dose was found to be significantly more effective than placebo in preventing clinical relapse over a 1-year period.[16] The clinical relapse occurred in 27% of patients treated with mesalamine and 55% receiving placebo ($P < 0.05$).[16] The benefit of mesalamine over placebo was the highest among patients older than 30 years ($P < 0.05$) and with CD confined only to small bowel ($P < 0.05$).[16]

The Canadian Study Group evaluated the 12-month maintenance therapy with mesalamine (3 g daily) in maintaining remission in RCT, including 246 patients with CD.[20] The remission was defined as CDAI < 150 with no accompanying symptoms for the preceding 30 days.[20] There were 180 patients with remission induced medically and 66 patients with remission induced surgically.[20] Among patients with medically induced remission, relapse occurred in 27 of 87 (31%) and 39 of 93 (42%) patients treated either with mesalamine and placebo, respectively

TABLE 37-1

RANDOMIZED PLACEBO-CONTROLLED TRIALS EVALUATING THE EFFICACY OF 5-ASA IN MAINTAINING REMISSION IN PATIENTS WITH CROHN'S DISEASE

Author	Preparation of Oral 5-ASA	Daily Dose of 5-ASA (g)	Number of Patients		Treatment Duration—Follow-Up	Definition of Relapse	Relapse Rates (%)		
			5-ASA	Placebo			5-ASA	Placebo	P value
International Mesalazine Study Group[15]	Eudragit L coated	1.5	125	123	12 months	CDAI >150 with an increase of at least 60 points from baseline	22.4	36.2	0.0395
Prantera et al[19]	Eudragit S coated	2.4	64	61	12 months	CDAI >150 with an increase of at least 100 points from baseline	34.0	55.0	0.02
Gendre et al[17]	Ethylcellulose coated	2.0	80	81	24 months	CDAI > 250 or CDAI between 150 and 250 with at least a 50-point increase over baseline confirmed 2 weeks after	36.2	42.0	Not reported
Thomson et al[21]	Eudragit L coated	3.0	138	148	12 months	CDAI >150 with at least a 60-point increase from baseline	22.0† 31.4‡	27.0† 23.8‡	Not reported
Arber et al[16]	Coated mesalamine similar to Eudragit L coated	1.0	28	31	12 months	Harvey-Bradshaw index > 4	27.0	55.0	< 0.05
Sutherland et al[20]	Ethylcellulose coated	3.0	87	93	48 weeks	CDAI >150 with an increase of at least 60 points from baseline	31.0	42.0	0.135
Mahmud et al[18]	Olsalazine	2.0	167	160	52 weeks	CDAI >150 with an increase of at least 60 points from baseline	48.5	45.0	Not reported
Modigliani et al[2]*	Ethylcellulose coated	4.0	65	64	1 year	CDAI >150 with at least a 100-point increase from baseline and/or need for surgery	62 ± 8	64 ±9	Not reported
de Franchis[22]*	Eudragit L coated	3.0	58	59	12 months	CDAI >150 with at least 60 points above baseline	58.3	52.2	0.26

*Patients were randomized during active phase of CD.
†Patients with CD colitis or ileocolitis.
‡Patients with CD ileitis.

(P = 0.135).[20] Although this study showed a reduced relapse rate in subjects treated with 5-ASA compound despite the location of the disease, these findings were not statistically significant.[20]

A recent randomized double-blind placebo-controlled trial by Mahmud et al studied the efficacy of another 5-ASA formulation, olsalazine, in 328 patients with inactive CD.[18] Patients were randomly allocated to either olsalazine (2 g daily) or placebo for 52 weeks.[18] The clinical relapse was defined as CDAI > 150, an increase in CDAI score of at least 60 points from baseline value, or the need for additional therapy or surgery.[18] It should be stressed that this study did not find any difference in the relapse rate between patients treated with olsalazine (48.5%) and those receiving placebo (45%; P value not reported).[18] However, the patients with ileocecal disease had significantly higher failure rates (67.9% for olsalazine versus 54.8% for placebo; P = 0.0095) than those with colonic disease (65.4% for olsalazine versus 53.6% for placebo; P = 0.0035).[18] Moreover, the rate of not completing the study was significantly higher in olsalazine (65.4%) than placebo (53.9%; P = 0.038) recipients.[18]

A recent meta-analysis of 7 aforementioned trials[15-21] did not find any evidence that 5-ASA compounds are more effective than placebo in maintaining medically induced remission in patients with CD.[23] The comparison between treatment with 5-ASA and placebo for 12 months in 6 studies (n = 1339) has shown the odds ratio of relapse of 1.00 (95% confidence interval [CI], 0.80 to 1.24)[15,16,18-21] whereas such comparison for 24-month duration of treatment in 1 study (n = 161)[17] has shown the odds ratio of relapse to be 0.98 (95% CI, 0.51 to 1.90).[23]

There have been 2 trials evaluating the efficacy of 5-ASA in maintaining remission of CD in patients randomized during the active phase of the disease, and treatment with 5-ASA was started immediately after steroid-induced remission.[2,22] In the first study, Modigliani et al evaluated 129 patients who were administered oral prednisolone at a dose of 1 mg/kg daily for 3 to 7 weeks as treatment of the active phase of CD and went into remission.[2] Clinical remission was defined as CDAI < 150 with at least a 100-point decrease from pre-inclusion to inclusion values.[2] These subjects were subsequently randomized to receive either mesalamine (n = 65) 4 g/day or placebo (n = 64) until weaning from prednisolone and for 1 year afterwards.[2] The successful weaning from prednisolone occurred in 74% (n = 48) and 58% (n = 37) of mesalamine and placebo recipients, respectively (P = 0.054).[2] Clinical relapse was defined as CDAI > 150 points with at least a 100-point increase above baseline score and/or necessity of surgical treatment.[2] The actuarial clinical relapse rates at 12 months after discontinuation of prednisolone were similar in both mesalamine (62% ± 8%) and placebo (64% ± 9%) recipients.[2] However, the relapse risk was found to be significantly lower in mesalamine (P = 0.042) recipients after adjusting for risk factors such as

high CDAI, white blood cell count > 9 x 10^9 at weaning, and use of a mesalamine in the month before study onset.[2] Overall, no significant difference was observed in time-to-failure (relapse of CD during 1-year follow-up after weaning of steroids or failure to discontinue steroids) rates between mesalamine and placebo (P = 0.144).[2]

The second trial evaluated 117 patients who were initially administered oral methylprednisolone for 4 to 8 weeks as treatment of their active CD.[22] Subjects who went into remission (CDAI < 150) were randomly assigned to either 5-ASA at a dose of 3 g daily (n = 58) or placebo (n = 59) treatment for up to 24 months with concomitant steroid-tapering.[22] Clinical relapse was defined as CDAI > 150 with at least a 60-point increase from baseline score and with concomitant increase in at least 2 acute-phase markers (erythrocyte sedimentation rate [ESR], α-1 acid glycoprotein, and α-2 globulins).[22] After 6 and 12 months, cumulative relapse rates were 34.4% and 58.3% in subjects treated with 5-ASA and 31.5% and 52.2% in placebo recipients, respectively (P = 0.26).[22] Treatment with 5-ASA was ineffective despite the location of the disease.[22]

The meta-analysis[24] of 10 RCTs,[2,15-17,19-22,25,26] including 1371 patients with medically induced remission (9 multicenter double-blind, placebo-controlled trials[2,15-17,19-22,25] and 1 single-center randomized nonspecific treatment-controlled trial[26]), failed to show a significant reduction of the risk of symptomatic CD relapse with 5-ASA. The observed pooled risk difference between 5-ASA and controls was -4.7% (95% CI, -9.6 to 2.8%).[24]

ADVERSE EVENTS

The data on safety profile of 5-ASA formulations used as a maintenance therapy in CD are limited and inconsistent between the studies evaluating its use as maintenance therapy in CD. However, the occurrence of adverse events did not differ when compared to placebo. Treatment with mesalamine may result in side effects such as nausea, dyspepsia, headache, and rare hypersensitivity reactions.[12]

FUTURE DIRECTIVES

In light of results from clinical trials, there is currently no evidence to recommend therapy with 5-ASA for maintaining medically achieved remission of CD.

CORTICOSTEROIDS

SYSTEMIC CORTICOSTEROIDS

BACKGROUND

Oral systemic corticosteroids (prednisone, methylprednisolone) have been shown to be effective in the treatment of active CD.[27,28]

Prednisone is activated by the liver into pharmacologically active prednisolone, which binds to plasma proteins

TABLE 37-2

RANDOMIZED PLACEBO-CONTROLLED TRIALS EVALUATING THE EFFICACY OF SYSTEMIC CORTICOSTEROIDS IN MAINTAINING REMISSION IN PATIENTS WITH CROHN'S DISEASE

AUTHOR	NAME OF 5-ASA	DAILY DOSE OF CORTICOSTEROID	NUMBER OF PATIENTS		FOLLOW-UP	DEFINITION OF RELAPSE	OUTCOME
			CORTICOSTEROIDS	PLACEBO			
Summers et al[27] Part I phase II NCCDS	Prednisone	0.25 mg/kg	28	20	2 years	CDAI > 150 with accompanying increase of at least 100 points from baseline, need for surgery, development of new fistula, persistent fever, or significant worsening in barium x-ray	Remission maintained (prednisone versus placebo): 1 year: 75% versus 71% (P = ns) 2 year: 64% versus 91% (P = ns)
Summers et al[27] Part II NCCDS	Prednisone	0.25 mg/kg	49	88	2 years	CDAI > 150 with accompanying increase of at least 100 points from baseline, need for surgery, development of new fistula, persistent fever, or significant worsening in barium x-ray	Results reported as outcome rank data: placebo group ranked more favorably than prednisone. P = 0.40 after 1 year and P = 0.85 after 2 years
Malchow et al ECCDS[28]	Methylprednisolone	8.0 mg	66	52	2 years	CDAI > 150	No difference between corticosteroids and placebo

in a nonlinear pattern.[13] Its distribution, concentration, and clearance depend on the dose, concentration in plasma, and time of administration.[13]

Methylprednisolone in turn binds to plasma proteins in linear fashion, and its clearance is dose independent.[13]

CLINICAL TRIALS

There were 3 randomized, double-blind, placebo-controlled trials that evaluated the efficacy of systemic corticosteroids in maintaining medically induced remission of CD (Table 37-2).[27,28]

Part I, phase 2 of the National Cooperative Crohn's Disease Study (NCCDS) assessed the efficacy of maintenance treatment of medically induced CD remission (CDAI < 150) with either prednisone (n = 28; 0.25 mg/kg daily), sulfasalazine (n = 19; up to 5 g daily), AZA (n = 19; 2.5 mg/kg), or placebo (n = 20).[27] No significant differences were observed in a proportion of patients with sustained remission after 1 year and 2 years of follow-up in any active treatment arm versus placebo.[27] Part II of the NCCDS included a different cohort of patients from that in part I with a subset of 49 patients with medically induced remission of CD (CDAI < 150) who received prednisone at a dose of 0.25 mg/kg daily and were followed for up to 2 years.[27] Other treatment arms of patients with medically induced

remission included sulfasalazine (n = 43) at a dose of 2.5 g daily, AZA (n = 46) at a dose of 1 mg/kg daily, and placebo (n = 88).[27] The treatment failure was defined as CDAI > 150 with accompanying increase of at least 100 points from baseline, need for surgery, development of new fistula, persistent fever, or significant worsening in barium x-ray.[27] Placebo-treated patients ranked insignificantly better than patients treated with prednisone or sulfasalazine, whereas patients treated with AZA ranked insignificantly better than placebo with respect to maintaining remission at 1 year and 2 years of follow-up.[27]

These data were further supported by the European Cooperative Crohn's Disease Study, which included 237 patients with inactive disease, which was defined as CDAI < 150. These patients were randomly allocated to treatment with either 6-methylprednisolone at a dose of 8 mg daily (n = 66),[28] sulfasalazine (n = 63), a combination of 6-methylprednisolone and sulfasalazine (n = 56), or placebo (n = 52) for up to 2 years.[28] There were no statistically significant differences in efficacy observed between any active treatment arm and placebo according to life table analysis for the failure and relapse.[28]

There have been 2 small studies that suggested that corticosteroids may have a beneficial effect on maintaining remission in CD.[29,30] Methylprednisolone given at a dose of 0.25 mg/kg daily for a period of 6 months was found to be more effective than placebo in maintaining remission in patients with altered laboratory tests indicating active inflammation.[29] During the 6-month study time, in the group of 9 patients treated with active drug, normalization of the laboratory tests occurred in 7, 1 patient experienced a clinical relapse while on treatment, and 5 of 7 patients with normalized laboratory tests relapsed within 1 month following the treatment discontinuation.[29] On the other hand, 7 of 9 patients not receiving corticosteroids had a clinical recurrence.[29] However, this study was not performed in a randomized double-blind placebo-controlled fashion.

In the second study, Gorard et al observed the probability of maintaining remission after treatment with prednisolone at 6 months of 0.67 and after 1 year of 0.35 in 20 patients.[30] However, this randomized study compared treatment with corticosteroids ($n = 20$) to elemental diet ($n = 22$).[30] Outcomes of patients with active disease who were treated initially with prednisolone at a dose of 0.75 mg/kg/day for 2 weeks followed by subsequent reducing doses were compared with outcomes of patients treated only with elemental diet for 4 weeks.[30]

ADVERSE EVENTS

The use of systemic corticosteroids is associated with significant dose-dependent side effects such as an increase in body weight, fat redistribution, changes in mood, osteoporosis and osteonecrosis insomnia, myopathy, development of subcapsular cataracts, hypokalemia, hypertriglyceridemia, growth retardation in children, arterial hypertension, edema of lower extremities, hyperglycemia, and acne.[12] The most common adverse events that occurred in 86 patients with active CD treated with high-dose prednisolone included "moon" face (36%), acne (23%), and swollen ankles (12%).[31] There is no sufficient information on adverse events related to treatment with systemic corticosteroids as a maintenance therapy in CD.

FUTURE DIRECTIVES

Data from clinical trials clearly demonstrate that systemic corticosteroids in low doses are not effective in maintaining remission of CD and thus should be not recommended as maintenance therapy.[32] High-dose corticosteroids have not been evaluated as a potential maintenance treatment due to an increased risk of significant side effects.

BUDESONIDE

BACKGROUND

Budesonide is a corticosteroid that demonstrates high topical activity and low systemic bioavailability (10%) and thus is associated with reduced risk of systemic complications.[13,33] Budesonide is metabolized by cytochrome P-450 in the intestinal wall and during first passage in the liver.[13] Budesonide binds to plasma proteins in 88% and demonstrates linear pharmacokinetic properties when given at doses of 3 to 15 mg/day.[33] Controlled-ileal release and pH-dependent release formulations of budesonide are used for treatment of active CD.[32]

CLINICAL TRIALS

There have been 5 randomized double-blind placebo-controlled trials evaluating the efficacy of budesonide (3 mg or 6 mg daily) as maintenance for steroid-induced remission in patients with CD (Table 37-3).[34-38]

In a study by Gross et al, 179 patients with steroid-induced remission of CD were randomly assigned to receive treatment either with budesonide (3 mg daily; $n = 84$) or placebo ($n = 95$) for 12 months.[34] Relapse of CD was defined as CDAI $\geq$ 150 points for more than 2 subsequent weeks or at the end of the study.[34] Among evaluated patients, the rates of relapse were similar in both budesonide (67%) and placebo recipients (65%) (P value not reported), demonstrating that budesonide at a dose of 3 mg daily is not effective in maintaining remission in CD.[34]

The other 4 randomized, placebo-controlled studies[35-38] were evaluated in predetermined pooled analysis.[39] These trials[35-38] included 380 patients with remission of CD (CDAI $\leq$ 150) achieved in previous induction of remission trials with either budesonide, prednisolone, or placebo.[39] Patients were randomized to receive either budesonide 6 mg ($n = 145$) or 3 mg ($n = 90$) daily or placebo ($n = 145$) for 12 months.[35-38] The primary endpoint in all 4 trials was time to relapse defined as CDAI > 150 points with accompanying increase of at least 60 points above baseline.[39] An analysis of these 4 trials[35-38] has demonstrated that relapse rates were significantly lower in patients treated with budesonide at a dose of 6 mg/daily than subjects treated with placebo after 3 months ($P < 0.001$) and after 6 months ($P < 0.05$).[39] However, after 9 and 12 months, no statistically significant differences were found between relapse rates for patients treated with budesonide (6 mg daily) and for those treated with placebo.[39] Moreover, no statistically significant difference was found in relapse rates between treatment with a lower dose of budesonide (3 mg daily) and placebo at any time during the study period.[39] Overall, the median time to relapse was 268 days in patients treated with budesonide 6 mg daily, 170 days in patients treated with budesonide 3 mg daily, and 154 days in placebo recipients ($P = 0.0072$).[39] This analysis has demonstrated that budesonide given at a dose of 6 mg daily significantly prolongs time to relapse in patients with medically induced remission of CD.[39]

There have been 3 randomized trials (1 placebo controlled) that have demonstrated the efficacy of maintenance therapy with budesonide at a dose of 6 mg daily in patients with inactive and steroid-dependent CD.[1,40,41] The first study included 118 patients (CDAI $\leq$ 200) who were randomized to receive either budesonide at a dose of 6 mg daily ($n = 59$) or placebo for 13 weeks.[41] Budesonide was found to be significantly more efficacious than placebo with relapse rates at 1 week of 17% and 41%, respectively ($P = 0.004$), and at 13 weeks of 32% and 65%, respectively ($P < 0.001$).[41] The second trial with 57 patients (CDAI < 150) receiving either budesonide ($n = 29$) or mesalamine 3 g daily ($n = 28$) for 1 year has shown that 1-year relapse rates were significantly lower in patients treated with budesonide (55%) than with mesalamine (82%; $P = 0.045$).[1] Finally, budesonide given at a dose of 9 mg daily for 2 years was found to be as effective as prednisolone given at a pre-existing dose in 90 patients with quiescent CD.[40]

It was also shown in an open-label study that treatment with pH-modified release budesonide at a dose of 9 mg daily for 6 weeks resulted in maintaining remission in 78% of patients at the end of the study. Moreover, similar efficacy for maintaining remission was observed for treatment with a flexible dose of budesonide 3 to 9 mg daily and a fixed dose of budesonide 6 mg daily for 12 months among 143 patients with CD participating in a randomized double-blind comparison.[42]

ADVERSE EVENTS

In a recent pooled analysis evaluating safety of maintenance treatment with budesonide 6 mg daily, budesonide 3 mg daily, and placebo in 376 patients with CD, the prevalence of all adverse events was lower in patients treated with budesonide 3 mg daily (67%) than those treated either with budesonide 6 mg daily (81%) or placebo (78%; P value not reported).[39]

Gastrointestinal symptoms were the most common adverse events across all studied groups and occurred in 44% of patients treated with budesonide 6 mg daily, in 41% of those treated with budesonide 3 mg daily, and in 50% of placebo recipients.[39] The majority of adverse events related to corticosteroids had similar prevalence among all patients. However, the occurrence of acne ($P = 0.045$) and moon face ($P = 0.030$) was higher in patients treated with a higher dose of budesonide when compared to placebo.[39] The MATRIX Study Group assessed the bone mineral density (BMD) among 90 corticosteroid-dependent patients with quiescent CD and 181 patients with active CD (98 corticosteroid-naïve and 83 exposed to corticosteroids in the past) who were treated for 2 years with either budesonide 9 mg/daily or prednisolone at preexisting doses and budesonide 9 mg/daily or prednisolone 40 mg/daily, respectively.[40] No significant difference in reduction in BMD was observed over a 2-year time between budesonide and prednisolone arms in corticosteroid-dependent patients (0.17 versus 0.49, $P = 0.76$) and in patients with prior exposure to corticosteroids (-1.66 versus -0.15, $P = 0.11$).[40] Among corticosteroid-naïve patients, reduction in BMD was significantly smaller in the budesonide arm compared to the prednisolone arm (-1.04 versus -3.84, $P = 0.0084$) throughout the entire treatment period.[40]

An open-label study has shown that switching from systemic corticosteroids to budesonide 9 mg daily given for 6 weeks resulted in significant reduction of corticosteroid-related side effects from 65.2% at the onset of the study to 43.3% at the end of the study.[42]

FUTURE DIRECTIVES

Current data indicate that treatment with budesonide at a dose of 6 mg daily is effective and safe in maintaining medically induced remission in CD; however, the duration may last only up to 6 months while on therapy.

AZATHIOPRINE AND 6-MERCAPTOPURINE

BACKGROUND

AZA and 6-MP are thiopurine analogues with AZA nonenzymatically metabolized to 6-MP in vivo. 6-MP is subsequently metabolized to 6-thioguanine nucleotide (6-TGN), which is perceived by some investigators to be an active metabolite that is hypothesized to lead to apoptosis of T-lymphocytes. 6-MP is also metabolized to 6-methylmercaptopurine (6-MMP) by the enzyme thiopurine methyltransferase (TPMT) and 6-thiouric acid by the enzyme xanthine oxidase (XO). Both 6-thiouric acid and 6-MMP are inactive metabolites of 6-MP. The 3 enzymes metabolizing 6-MP are in constant competition for substrate, and the concentration of the metabolites of 6-MP are based on the concentrations of these enzymes. The oral bioavailability of 6-MP and AZA has been reported to be low and a consequence of 84% of 6-MP quickly metabolized by XO found in high concentrations in enterocytes and hepatocytes, leaving only 16% to be catabolized by TPMT and hypoxanthine phosphoribosyl transferase (HPRT).[13,44] There have also been reports of lower bioavailability of generic AZA. The plasma half-life of 6-MP and AZA range from 1 to 2 hours, but 6-TGN has a plasma half-life of 3 to 13 days due to accumulation in erythrocytes.[13]

More detailed information on the metabolism of AZA and 6-MP has been provided in prior chapters.

CLINICAL TRIALS

Several trials assessed the efficacy of AZA to maintain medically achieved remission of CD. There were 6 randomized double-blind placebo-controlled trials that evaluated AZA maintenance (dose range 1 to 2.5 mg/kg) treatment of CD during a 6-month to 2-year time interval.[27,45-48] Overall, of 317 patients evaluated in these studies, 137 received AZA, and 180 received placebo.[27,45-49] Maintenance therapy with 6-MP in maintaining medically induced remission has not yet been evaluated. Many trials failed to reach statistical significance due to small sample size.

Two studies by Candy et al ($n = 63$) and O'Donoghue et al ($n = 51$) demonstrated significant benefit of AZA

TABLE 37-3

RANDOMIZED PLACEBO-CONTROLLED TRIALS EVALUATING THE EFFICACY OF BUDESONIDE IN MAINTAINING REMISSION IN PATIENTS WITH CROHN'S DISEASE

Author	Daily Dose of Budesonide (mg)	Number of Patients		Treatment Duration–Follow-Up	Definition of Relapse	Relapse Rates (%)			
		Budesonide	Placebo			Budesonide		Placebo	P value
						3 mg	6 mg		
Gross et al[34]	3	84	95	1 year	CDAI ≥ 150	66.7	–	65.3	Not reported
Ferguson et al[35]	3	26	27	1 year	CDAI >150 with an increase of at least 60 points from baseline	46.0	48.0	60.0	Not significant
	6	22							
Greenberg et al[36]	3	33	36	1 year	CDAI >150 with an increase of at least 60 points from baseline	70.0	61	67	0.75
	6	36							
Hanauer et al[37]	6	55	55	1 year	CDAI >150 with an increase of at least 60 points from baseline	–	47.3	58.2	Not significant
Lofberg et al[38]	3	31	27	1 year	CDAI >150 with an increase of at least 60 points from baseline	74.0	59.0	63.0	0.44
	6	32							

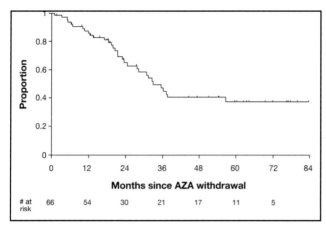

FIGURE 37-1. Cumulative probability of remaining in remission after AZA withdrawal in 66 patients. (Reprinted from Treton X, Bouhnik Y, Mary JY, et al. Azathioprine withdrawal in patients with Crohn's disease maintained on prolonged remission: a high risk of relapse. *Clin Gastroenterol Hepatol.* 2009;7(1):80-85 with permission from Elsevier.)

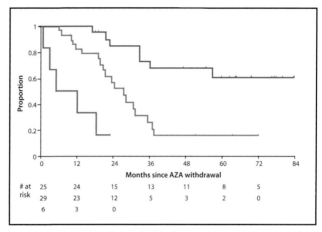

FIGURE 37-2. Relapse predicting classification according to the presence of risk factors after AZA withdrawal in 66 patients (small blue line, no risk factor, n = 25; intermediate red line, hemoglobin <12 g/dL and no other risk factor, n = 29; large green line, others, n = 6). (Reprinted from Treton X, Bouhnik Y, Mary JY, et al. Azathioprine withdrawal in patients with Crohn's disease maintained on prolonged remission: a high risk of relapse. *Clin Gastroenterol Hepatol.* 2009;7(1):80-85 with permission from Elsevier.)

in reducing clinical recurrence rates between AZA and placebo.[45,46] After 12 months of maintenance treatment, the relative protective effect of AZA (2.5 mg/kg daily) on maintaining remission was 6-fold higher compared to placebo (risk ratio [RR] = 6.84; 95% CI, 1.68 to 24.93).[45] Sustained remission rates were significantly higher in AZA than placebo-treated patients at the end of follow-up (42% versus 7%, P = 0.001).[45] Similarly, O'Donoghue et al observed significant (P < 0.01) superiority of AZA (2 mg/kg daily) over placebo in reducing cumulative probability of relapse at 6 months (0% versus 25%) and 12 months (5% versus 41%).[46]

An analysis of results of a subgroup of 10 patients with quiescent CD treated with AZA 2 mg/kg daily or placebo over 6 months observed nonsignificant superiority of AZA over placebo in maintaining remission at the end of follow-up (80% versus 40%, P = 0.5).[47] Likewise, Rosenberg et al observed clinical remission rates in an insignificantly greater proportion of patients on AZA (2 mg/kg daily) when compared to placebo (80% versus 50%, P = 0.35) over 26 weeks of treatment.[48] Both parts of NCCDS failed to show efficacy of AZA in maintaining medically achieved remission of CD over 2 years (this was discussed in the section pertaining to corticosteroid maintenance treatment).[27] Patients in part I, phase II, and part II received high (2.5 mg/kg) and low (1 mg/kg) daily doses of AZA, respectively.[27]

The successful steroid-sparing effect of AZA was observed in 2 trials that reported the use of steroids among the total of 30 patients[47,48] with pooled Peto odds ratio of 5.22 (95% CI, 1.06 to 25.68) and number needed to treat of 3.[50]

The ideal length for treatment to maintain remission of CD is not yet clear. A study by Bouhnik et al showed that after 2 years of follow-up, there was not a significant difference in relapse rates of CD patients treated with AZA for at least 4 years who then had their AZA discontinued for 2 years compared to those patients who had their AZA continued during the 2-year follow-up period.[51] Recently, a group from Greece suggested that long-term treatment (up to 8 years) with AZA was efficacious and safe in maintaining remission of steroid-dependent luminal CD.[52] Withdrawal of AZA was recently found to be associated with a high rate of clinical relapse (48%) among 66 patients with CD who were maintained on prolonged remission on AZA for at least 42 months before AZA discontinuation.[53] Cumulative probabilities of clinical relapse after 1, 3, and 5 years following AZA discontinuation were 14%, 53%, and 63%, respectively.[53] Figure 37-1 describes the cumulative probability of remaining in remission after AZA discontinuation.[53] Of note, C-reactive protein level ≥20 mg/dL, neutrophil count ≥4.0 x 10^9/L, and low hemoglobin level (<12 g/dL) were found to be independent risk factors associated with increased risk of relapse after AZA cessation (Figure 37-2).[53] On the other hand, patients presenting without any risk factors had a 61% remission rate after 5 years following AZA discontinuation.[53] Therefore, it has been suggested that temporary discontinuation of therapy with AZA might be considered in patients without such risk factors.[53]

The utility of measuring metabolites 6-TGN and 6-MMP has been evaluated to assess the likelihood of a therapeutic response, but the use of these metabolite levels for maintenance of remission is not yet clear. The sensitivity, specificity, and positive and negative predictive values of measurement of these metabolites has recently been critically analyzed. At present, measurement of these metabolites is not recommended in all patients. Therapeutic monitoring of 6-TGN might be useful in noncompliant patients and possibly patients without response to standard doses of AZA/6-M.[54] An ongoing prospective randomized trial is evaluating the efficacy of metabolite measurement and comparing this to standard weight-based titration. It was recently suggested that measurement of erythrocyte mean corpuscular volume might be a useful and inexpensive surrogate for measurement of 6-TGN concentration in patients treated with AZA/6-MP.[55]

ADVERSE EVENTS

A potential disadvantage to continuing AZA or 6-MP indefinitely is the possibility of malignancy, specifically lymphoma. The risk of lymphoma has been calculated to be approximately 4-fold (odds ratio [OR] = 4.18; 95% CI, 2.07 to 7.51) in a meta-analysis of studies assessing for risk for lymphoma with median duration of AZA use 14 months and a range of 6 to 94 months.[56] However, duration and severity of CD could not be adjusted in the analysis.[56] Additionally, duration of medication use was not completely assessed in the analysis. The risk for lymphoma has been hypothesized to be a consequence of Epstein-Barr virus infection as a consequence of immunosuppression.[57,58]

As discussed in previous chapters, potential adverse events of 6-MP/AZA use include pancreatitis, myelosuppression, nausea, infections, hair loss, and hepatotoxicity. In patients who have normal activity of the enzyme thiopurine methyltransferase, leukopenia may occur anytime during therapy and may or may not be related to elevated levels of 6-TGN.[59,60] Additionally, 6-MMP levels of >5700 pmol/8 x 10^8 is associated with hepatoxicity, but patients may have high levels with normal liver chemistries and hepatoxicity may occur at low 6-MMP levels.[61] Thus, the utility of measurement of 6-MMP is questionable when assessing hepatotoxicity. The mechanism by which 6-MP and AZA cause hepatic injury is unknown, but hepatitis, cholestasis, nodular regenerative hyperplasia, and peliosis have been observed.[51,62] Therefore, routine complete blood cell counts and periodic measurement of liver-associated chemistries are recommended for monitoring for hepatic injury and leukopenia. Patients who develop nausea on AZA may be switched to 6-MP successfully and vice versa.[63] Current Food and Drug Administration (FDA) recommendations indicate the benefit of identification of TPMT activity or genotype before the onset of therapy with AZA/6-MP.[64]

FUTURE DIRECTIVES

The main issue that remains to be answered is the optimal duration of therapy to maximize remission and minimize risk of potential complications from long-term therapy such as lymphoma. In 2000, a Markov model was performed that assumed a 3-fold risk of lymphoma in patients with CD receiving AZA as maintenance therapy compared to baseline risk among patients with CD.[65] A decision analysis model showed that maintenance therapy

of CD with AZA substantially increased quality-adjusted life expectancy.[65] The benefit of treatment with AZA could be reduced only given the 10-fold increase in risk of lymphoma in AZA-treated CD patients.[65] Because such risk has not been substantiated in the literature, the authors claimed that benefits of maintenance therapy with AZA outweigh the risk of lymphoma.[65]

METHOTREXATE

BACKGROUND

Methotrexate is a folic acid antagonist that leads to the inhibition of purine synthesis, DNA and RNA formation, and eventually inhibition of the S phase of the cell cycle. Intracellularly, methotrexate is converted to methotrexate polyglutamate. Dihydrofolate reductase, an enzyme involved in converting folate to tetrahydrofolate, is inhibited by binding to both methotrexate and the active metabolite, methotrexate polyglutmate.[66-68] Methotrexate polyglutamate is also capable of inhibiting other enzymes in the pathway of folate metabolism, leading to purine synthesis. The actual cell targets of methotrexate involved in the suppression of inflammation in chronic inflammatory conditions are not known. Potential target cells include cells within the laminal propria of the intestine, intestinal intraepithelial lymphocytes, leukocytes, monocytes-macrophages, and intestinal epithelial cells. In vitro and in vivo studies have shown increased levels of extracellular adenosine associated with methotrexate therapy; however, in a small clinical study of 10 IBD patients, plasma adenosine and rectal tissue adenosine levels were not found to be elevated after receiving methotrexate 15 or 25 mg subcutaneous per week.[69] Neutrophils, lymphocytes, and macrophages all have receptors for adenosine, which appears to suppress cytokine release from these cell lines.[70] Adenosine also appears to inhibit the production of reactive oxygen metabolites, adhesion to and injury of endothelial cells, synthesis and release of leukotriene B_4, and production of TNFα in neutrophils.[68] In macrophages/monocytes, TNFα, interleukin-6 (IL-6), and IL-8 production are inhibited and there is increased promotion of the IL-1 receptor antagonist and secretion of IL-10.[68]

Oral methotrexate is well absorbed, but this appears to be dose-dependent.[71] Lower doses are better absorbed than higher doses (>25 mg/week).[71,72] This dose effect may be related to metabolism by intestinal bacteria. Intramuscular and subcutaneous methotrexate have near complete bioavailability and have been shown to have high concentrations in intestinal mucosa.[73] It has been suggested that methotrexate is primarily delivered to the intestinal mucosa by the bloodstream rather than direct intestinal absorption into sites of inflammation due to higher concentrations of methotrexate in rectal mucosa given in the intramuscular or subcutaneous form compared to oral methotrexate. Methotrexate is primarily excreted by the kidneys.

CLINICAL TRIALS

There has been 1 controlled study assessing the effectiveness of methotrexate for maintenance of remission.[74] In this study, subjects were induced with 25 mg intramuscularly once per week of methotrexate for at least 16 weeks, then randomized to 15 mg intramuscularly once per week or placebo thereafter for 40 weeks. Sixty-five percent of those receiving methotrexate remained in remission compared to 39% in the placebo group after 40 weeks ($P = 0.04$).

ADVERSE EVENTS

Myelosuppression is a known potential side effect of methotrexate, but it is uncommon if the duration of therapy is less than 1 year.[75] Hepatoxicity is a well-known side effect of treatment. The changes in liver histology include macrovesicular steatosis, nuclear variability, chronic inflammatory infiltrates in the portal tracts, hepatocyte necrosis, fibrosis, and cirrhosis. Hepatic fibrosis and cirrhosis are the most concerning long-term potential toxicities and tend to occur with accumulated methotrexate use of >1.5 g. To avoid potential toxicities, folate supplementation is recommended, either 1 mg per mg of methotrexate divided into daily doses or 0.25 to 0.50 mg per mg of methotrexate given 4 to 24 hours after administration of weekly methotrexate.[76,77]

FUTURE DIRECTIVES

6-MP or AZA is preferred for maintenance of remission of CD rather than methotrexate due to more significant benefit, ease of administration (oral versus parenteral), and potentially fewer side effects. Optimal duration of maintenance therapy with methotrexate to minimize potential adverse events such as liver fibrosis is not yet known. Risk factors for methotrexate-related hepatotoxicity include obesity, diabetes mellitus, history of alcohol abuse, frequent dosing intervals, and cumulative dose greater than 1.5 to 2.0 g.[78-82] In a recent case series of 20 patients with IBD taking methotrexate who underwent liver biopsies (mean accumulated dose of 2633 mg over a mean of 132 weeks), only 1 patient presenting with obesity and diabetes had detected liver fibrosis.[83] This may suggest that patients with IBD may be at lower risk for liver fibrosis than psoriasis or rheumatoid patients. However, due to the limited data on methotrexate-related liver toxicity in patients with IBD, it is imperative to follow the American College of Rheumatology guidelines regarding surveillance for methotrexate-related hepatotoxicity.[84] Before treatment with methotrexate, a liver biopsy is recommended in patients with a history of alcohol abuse, persistent abnormal pretreatment values of aspartate aminotransferase, or in case of chronic hepatitis B or C.[84] During treatment with methotrexate, it is recommended that patients with elevated annual values of aspartate aminotransferase measured every 4 to 8 weeks or with decreased serum albumin levels despite reduction in methotrexate dose should undergo liver biopsy.[84] Methotrexate should be discontinued in patients with liver cirrhosis or moderate-to-severe liver fibrosis found on liver biopsy.[84]

CYCLOSPORINE

BACKGROUND

Cyclosporine is a lipophilic cyclic polypeptide that selectively inhibits IL-2 and interferon-γ production by T helper cells, IL-3, IL-4, IL-5, TNFα, and TNFβ.[13] Bioavailability ranges from 10% to 89% and can be reduced by a fat-rich meal.[85,86] Cyclosporine is primarily metabolized by CYP3A4/5 in liver and the intestine, and >90% is excreted in the bile.

CLINICAL TRIALS

There have been 2 randomized placebo-controlled trials assessing the efficacy of cyclosporine (daily dose of 5 mg/kg) as a maintenance therapy in patients with inactive CD.[87,88] There was no significant difference in aforementioned studies in the rates of patients maintaining remission between cyclosporine and placebo-treated recipients. In the first study, Feagan et al observed that more patients treated with cyclosporine when compared to placebo had experienced clinical relapse of CD (64.6% versus 50%, $P = 0.11$).[87] Similar results were obtained by Stange et al, who did not notice any significant differences in the rates of patients with inactive disease between cyclosporine and placebo recipients after 4 months (39% versus 34%) and 12 months of treatment (29% versus 26%; P values not reported).[88]

In light of the aforementioned studies, cyclosporine is not recommended for maintenance of remission of CD.

ANTIBIOTICS

BACKGROUND

Several mechanisms have been proposed to explain the mechanism of action of antibiotics for the treatment of active IBD. One theory is that changing the intestinal microbial flora prevents inhabitation of pathogenic bacteria.[89] Another potential mechanism is that there is a lack of tolerance to commensal bacteria in the gastrointestinal tract leading to activation of the gut immune system in genetically susceptible individuals. Suppression of bacterial flora may lead to downregulation of the immune system.[90] In pouchitis, reduction of inflammation can be achieved with reduction of total bacteria, aerobes, and anaerobes by antibiotics.[25,89] Antibiotics such as amoxicillin-clavulanic acid and metronidazole also may have direct anti-inflammatory effects independent of their antimicrobial activity.[91,92] For example, amoxicillin-clavulanic acid has been shown to decrease production of IL-8 and eicosanoids.[93]

Several studies have assessed the benefit of antibiotics for the treatment of active CD and ulcerative colitis.[94-100] Many studies have shown a benefit for the treatment of active CD with sparse data examining the role of antibiotics in preventing relapse of surgically induced remission of CD.[101,102]

CLINICAL TRIALS

Despite several clinical trials of metronidazole and ciprofloxacin efficacy for treatment of active CD, there are limited data on efficacy of antibiotics as maintenance therapy of nonsurgically induced remission. There continues to be speculation of an association of *Mycobacterium avium* and *Mycobacterium paratuberculosis* infections with the presence of CD. A meta-analysis of 7[103-109] randomized placebo-controlled trials in 355 patients with CD observed no beneficial effect of antituberculous therapy in maintaining remission of CD with the pooled odds ratio of 1.36 (95% CI, 0.87 to 2.13) and number needed to treat of 15.[110] However, subanalysis of 2 trials[103,104] of antituberculous therapy in 89 patients with steroid-induced remission showed significant benefit of antituberculous therapy (either monotherapy with clofazimine or combination therapy with clofazimine, ethambutol, rifampicin, and dapsone) with pooled odds ratio of 3.37 (95% CI, 1.38 to 8.24) and number needed to treat of 3.[110] A recent randomized placebo-controlled trial from Australia observed limited long-term benefit of 2-year combined therapy with clarithromycin, rifabutin, and clofazimine in maintaining remission of CD.[111] At 104 weeks of treatment, the relapse rates were 26% and 43% for antibiotic and placebo recipients, respectively, and failed to reach statistical significance ($P = 0.14$).[111] In light of available data at present, there is insufficient evidence to support use of antituberculous therapy in patients with CD.

PROBIOTICS

BACKGROUND

Probiotics have been defined as "living micro-organisms, which upon ingestion in certain numbers, exert health benefits beyond inherent basic nutrition."[112] Microbial species used as probiotics include *Lactobacilli*, *Bifidobacteria*, Gram-positive cocci, *Escherichia coli Nissle 1917*, *Saccharomyces cerevisiae*, *Saccharomyces boulardii*, fungi (*Aspergillus orizae*), or VSL #3, a combination of 8 probiotic bacterial species (4 lactobacilli, 3 bifidobacteria, and *Streptococcus salivarius* spp. Thermophilus).[113,114]

Because the role of enteric commensal bacteria in the pathogenesis of CD has been suggested, the possibility of using probiotics in altering enteric bacterial microflora has been raised.[114]

CLINICAL TRIALS

Several clinical trials evaluated the efficacy of probiotics as maintenance treatment of CD. A Cochrane review that pooled data from 3 placebo-controlled studies demonstrated similar rates of clinical relapse at the end of the study period between probiotics and placebo in patients with CD and medically or surgically induced remission (25% versus 35%, $P = 0.39$).[115-118] Overall, there was no significant difference in the risk of relapse during maintenance treatment between patients on maintenance therapy with probiotics and placebo (RR = 0.68; 95% CI, 0.34 to 1.39).[115-118] Recently, Rahimi et al published results of a meta-analysis of 8 randomized placebo-controlled trials[115-117,119-123] assessing the efficacy of probiotics in maintaining remission of CD.[124] That meta-analysis did not find the superiority of probiotics over placebo in preventing clinical (7 trials[115-117,119-122]; pooled OR = 0.92; 95% CI, 0.52 to 1.62; $P = 0.9$) or endoscopic recurrence (3 trials[116,122,123]; pooled OR = 0.97; 95% CI, 0.54 to 1.78; $P = 0.9$) of CD.[124]

In light of the aforementioned studies, probiotics are not recommended for maintenance of remission of CD.

INFLIXIMAB

BACKGROUND

Infliximab is a chimeric, mouse-human, IgG_1 monoclonal anti-TNFα antibody that consists of human constant and murine variable regions.[125] This agent has been approved by the FDA for induction and maintenance therapy in patients with moderate to severe active or fistulizing CD refractory to conventional therapies and most recently for reducing signs and symptoms, achieving remission, promoting intestinal healing, and reducing or stopping the need for steroids in patients with moderate to severe ulcerative colitis who have not responded well to other therapies.[125] Infliximab is also FDA approved for the treatment of rheumatoid arthritis, ankylosing spondylitis, and psoriatic arthritis.[125] It is administered as an intravenous infusion.

An intravenous administration of single infusions of infliximab at a dose of 5, 10, or 20 mg/kg has shown a linear and direct relationship between the dose administered, the maximum serum concentration, and the area under the curve of concentration time.[126] Its clearance rate is dose-independent.[126] The metabolism and excretion pathways of infliximab remain unknown.[127] It was shown that a single dose of infliximab 5 mg/kg had a serum half-life of 9.5 days, remaining primarily in the vascular compartment.[126]

TABLE 37-4

RANDOMIZED PLACEBO-CONTROLLED TRIALS EVALUATING THE EFFICACY OF REPEATED INFUSIONS OF INFLIXIMAB IN PATIENTS WITH NONFISTULIZING CROHN'S DISEASE WHO RESPONDED TO INITIAL DOSE OF INFLIXIMAB

		NUMBER OF PATIENTS			
AUTHOR	STUDY DESIGN	INFLIXIMAB	PLACEBO	FOLLOW-UP	COMMENTS
Rutgeerts et al[130]	Single infusion of infliximab 5, 10, or 20 mg/kg or placebo. Responders at week 8 proceeded at week 12 to infliximab 10 mg/kg or placebo every 8 weeks through week 36	37	36	48 weeks	Infliximab: • Week 12: 37.8% of patients in clinical remission • Week 44: 52.9% of patients in clinical remission Placebo: • Week 12: 44.4% of patients in clinical remission • Week 44: 35% of patients in clinical remission *P* value: 0.013 Clinical response: at least 70-point decrease in CDAI from baseline Clinical remission: CDAI < 150
Hanauer et al[131] ACCENT I	Single infusion of 5 mg/kg infliximab at week 0. Responders at week 2 proceeded to: Weeks 2 and 6 and every 8 weeks until week 46 Group I: placebo Group II: infliximab 5 mg/kg Group III: infliximab 5 mg weeks 2, 6, and infliximab 10 mg/kg every 8 weeks until week 46.	225	110	54 weeks	Patients in groups II and III had longer time to loss of response than patients in group I (*P* = 0.0002). Week 30: remission: 21% (gr. I), 39% (gr. II) and 45% (gr. III). Week 54: discontinuation of steroids: 29% of patients treated with infliximab (gr. II and gr. III) versus 9% treated with placebo (gr. I) (*P* = 0.004). Response: decrease in CDAI of at least 70 points from baseline and at least 25% reduction in total score. Loss of response: CDAI ≥ 175, increase in CDAI of at least 35%, CDAI at least 70 points more than at week 2.

CLINICAL TRIALS

Randomized placebo trials have shown that infliximab was effective in inducing remission in patients with active CD[128] and in promoting the closure of fistulas in fistulizing CD.[129] Efficacy of infliximab as maintenance therapy in patients with CD was evaluated in 3 randomized double-blind placebo-controlled trials.[130-132]

In a study by Rutgeerts et al, patients who clinically responded (reduction in CDAI ≥ 70 points from baseline) to single dose of infliximab (10 mg/kg) or placebo were randomized to receive either placebo (*n* = 36) or infliximab (*n* = 37) at a dose of 10 mg/kg at 8-week intervals for a total of 4 infusions with follow-up through week 44.[130] Fifty-three percent of patients treated with active drug maintained their remission as compared with 20% of placebo recipients (*P* = 0.013) at the end of follow-up.[130] It

was demonstrated that patients re-treated with infliximab maintained their remission of CD, whereas those receiving placebo showed gradual loss of remission.[130] There was a significant increase in the proportion of infliximab-treated patients with clinical remission (CDAI < 150) from 37.8% at initiation of retreatment to 52.9% at the end of follow-up, whereas there was a significant decrease in the proportion of placebo-treated patients with clinical remission from 44.4% at initiation of retreatment to 20% at the end of follow-up (*P* = 0.013 infliximab versus placebo).[130] After discontinuation of retreatment, patients who received infliximab had longer duration of response than those treated with placebo (>48 weeks versus 37 weeks, *P* = 0.057).[130]

The ACCENT I trial evaluated the efficacy of repeated infusions of infliximab in patients who responded to initial infusion.[131] There were 573 patients enrolled in the study

TABLE 37-5

RANDOMIZED, PLACEBO-CONTROLLED TRIAL EVALUATING THE EFFICACY OF REPEATED INFUSIONS OF INFLIXIMAB IN PATIENTS WITH FISTULIZING CROHN'S DISEASE WHO RESPONDED TO INITIAL DOSE OF INFLIXIMAB

Author	Study Design	Number of Patients		Follow-Up	Comments
		Infliximab	*Placebo*		
Sands et al[132] ACCENT II	Single infusion inflixmab 5 mg/kg at weeks 0, 2, and 6 Responders at weeks 10 and 14, proceeded to placebo or infliximab 5 mg/kg every 8 weeks through week 46	96	99	54 weeks	Maintenance of response: Week 54: • Infliximab: 46% versus placebo: 23% ($P = 0.001$). Complete response: Week 54: • Infliximab: 36% versus placebo: 19% ($P = 0.009$). • Response: reduction of at least 50% of draining fistulas from baseline. • Complete response: absence of draining fistulas. • Loss of response: recrudescence of draining fistulas, need for surgery, need for change in medication for CD or additional therapy for persistent or worsening luminal disease activity.

who received an initial infusion of infliximab at a dose of 5 mg/kg.[131] The response to treatment was defined as decrease in CDAI score of at least 70 points from baseline and at least a 25% reduction in total score.[131] Patients who responded ($n = 335$) to an induction dose were subsequently randomized to 3 groups.[131] Patients assigned to group I ($n = 110$) received infusions of placebo, whereas patients assigned to group II ($n = 113$) received infliximab 5 mg/kg at week 2 and 6 and then every 8 weeks until week 46. Those assigned to group III ($n = 112$) received infliximab 5 mg/kg at weeks 2 and 6 followed by subsequent infusions of infliximab 10 mg/kg at the same time points until week 46.[131] Study end points were to establish the proportion of patients who responded at week 2 and were in remission (CDAI < 150) at week 30 and the time to loss of response up to week 54.[131] At week 30, 21% of patients treated with placebo (group I) were in remission compared with 39% of subjects treated with infliximab 5 mg/kg ($P = 0.003$) and 45% of patients treated with infliximab 10 mg/kg ($P = 0.0002$).[131] At week 54, a clinical remission was observed in 14% of placebo patients, in 28% of recipients of infliximab 5 mg/kg ($P = 0.007$), and in 38% of patients treated with infliximab 10 mg/kg ($P < 0.0001$).[131] This study has demonstrated that re-treatment with infliximab every 8 weeks in initial responders is more effective than placebo in maintaining remission.[131] Moreover, 3 times as many patients in groups II and III combined (29%) discontinued corticosteroids and remained in clinical

remission compared with placebo (9%; $P = 0.004$), showing that maintenance treatment with infliximab may allow for effective discontinuation of corticosteroids.[131] The pooled results from 2 aforementioned trials[130,131] indicate that infliximab compared to placebo is 2.5-fold and nearly 2-fold significantly more efficacious in maintaining clinical remission and response, respectively.[133] No differences in remission rates were observed between low and high doses of infliximab.[133] Patients treated with infliximab were also more likely to successfully discontinue corticosteroids (RR = 3.13; 95% CI, 1.25 to 7.81).[133]

An ACCENT II trial assessed the efficacy of infliximab in maintaining closure of draining fistulas in patients with CD who responded to initial induction with 3 infusions of infliximab given at a dose of 5 mg/kg at weeks 0, 2, and 6.[132] Response was defined as closure of at least 50% of draining fistulas at weeks 10 and 14.[132] Of 282 patients who received induction treatment with infliximab, 195 patients who responded to induction treatment at week 14 were subsequently randomized to receive infusions of either infliximab at a dose of 5 mg/kg ($n = 96$) or placebo ($n = 99$) every 8 weeks through week 46 and were subsequently followed up to week 54.[132] A complete absence of fistulas was observed in 36% of patients treated with infliximab and 19% of patients treated with placebo at the end of follow-up ($P = 0.009$).[132] The median time to loss of response was significantly longer in patients treated with infliximab (>40 weeks) than those receiving placebo (14 weeks; $P < 0.001$).[132]

The loss of response occurred in 42% of patients treated with infliximab and in 62% of patients receiving placebo (*P* < 0.001).[132] A complete closure of fistulas was observed in 36% of patients treated with infliximab and 19% of patients treated with placebo at week 54 (*P* = 0.009).[132] Infliximab was found to be significantly more efficacious than placebo in complete healing of perianal and enterocutaneous fistulas (RR = 1.87; 95% CI, 1.15 to 3.04; *P* = 0.01).[133]

Recent preliminary 1-year data from the SONIC trial have indicated that monotherapy with infliximab or combination therapy consisting of infliximab and AZA is more likely to maintain long-term corticosteroid-free remission than monotherapy with AZA.[134] There were 508 immunomodulator-naïve patients with active CD enrolled into SONIC trial who were randomized into 3 treatment arms: monotherapy with infliximab infusions 5 mg/kg (weeks 0, 2, and 6 and then every 8 weeks), monotherapy with oral AZA 2.5 mg/kg/day, or combination therapy of both with 280 patients remaining in the maintenance phase of the study initiating at week 30.[134] Based on the assumption that patients not enrolled into the maintenance phase (*n* = 228) of the trial would not be steroid free at week 50, combination therapy and infliximab monotherapy therapy allowed for maintaining steroid-free remission in a significantly higher overall proportion of patients (46% and 35%, respectively) when compared with AZA monotherapy (24%, *P* < 0.001 versus combination therapy; *P* = 0.035 versus infliximab monotherapy) at week 50.[134]

ADVERSE EVENTS

Although overall infliximab was well tolerated in the majority of patients participating in clinical trials, some patients experienced adverse events.

Administration of infliximab may cause development of antibodies to infliximab (ATI), which increases the risk for infusion reactions. It has been observed that maintenance treatment with infliximab is associated with a lower incidence of ATI (7% to 10%)[135] than episodic treatment (30% to 61%).[135,136] The development of ATI was lower in patients receiving concomitant immunomodulators (10%) than in those treated only with infliximab (18%, *P* = 0.02).[135] It was the most significantly observed in patients receiving episodic treatment (38% versus 16%, *P* = 0.003).[135]

Infusion reactions such as headache, dizziness, nausea, irritation of injection site, flushing, chest pain, dyspnea, and pruritus occurred in 16% to 21% of patients receiving maintenance treatment and in 9% to 17% of patients who received only episodic treatment with infliximab.[131,132]

Treatment with infliximab is also associated with development of antibodies to double-stranded DNA (anti-dsDNA) and antinuclear antibodies (ANA). Clinical trials have observed higher rates of anti-dsDNA (23% to 34%) and ANA (46% to 56%) in patients receiving maintenance therapy than episodic treatment who developed anti-dsDNA in 6% to 11% and ANA in 18% to 35%.[131,132] However, the symptoms of drug-induced lupus without major organ involvement occurred in 2 (0.4%) of 524 patients on maintenance therapy (only 1 patient tested positive for anti-dsDNA and ANA).[131,132]

It was observed that, despite a 3- to 5-fold higher total mean dose of infliximab in patients on maintenance therapy, the prevalence of serious infections, infections requiring antibiotics or chemotherapeutics, complications related to CD, and malignancies was similar to those reported in patients receiving episodic treatment with infliximab.[135]

The maintenance trials have reported a total of 2 cases of lymphoma, both in patients who received episodic treatment with infliximab.[130-132] Data from TREAT registry do not indicate increased risk of serious infections in patients with CD treated with infliximab based on multivariate logistic regression analysis with odds ratio of 0.99 (95% CI, 0.64-1.54).[137] TREAT registry data from nearly 20,000 years of patient follow-up demonstrated similar incidence (per 100 patient years of follow-up) of lymphoma (0.04 versus 0.05; RR = 0.8; 95% CI, 0.22 to 2.99) and other malignancies (0.39 versus 0.53; RR = 0.74; 95% CI, 0.49 to 1.12) in patients treated and not treated with infliximab.[138]

Because of the possibility of reactivation of latent tuberculosis in patients treated with infliximab, an evaluation for latent tuberculosis with a tuberculin test (and if positive, a chest radiograph) and treatment with antituberculous therapy in case of detection of tuberculosis or a positive tuberculin test (>5 mm induration) have been strongly recommended.[139,140]

FUTURE DIRECTIVES

The recommended maintenance dose of infliximab is 5 mg/kg every 8 weeks with a possible increase to 10 mg/kg in case of loss of response. Current data clearly demonstrate that maintenance therapy with infliximab in patients with CD is superior to episodic treatment due to improved clinical response and remission rates, significant reduction in hospitalizations and surgical procedures, greater mucosal healing, faster steroid weaning, better quality of life, and reduction in antibody formation.[141,142] Because of these reasons, it was recently proposed that maintenance therapy with infliximab might be considered lifetime therapy.[141] Final data from the SONIC trial would be necessary to further assess the efficacy and safety of infliximab and AZA combination therapy versus infliximab monotherapy versus AZA monotherapy in maintaining steroid-free remission in patients with CD.

ADALIMUMAB

BACKGROUND

Adalimumab is a fully human monoclonal antibody to TNFα. This agent was approved by the FDA in 2007 as an induction and maintenance treatment of moderately to severely active CD in adult patients unresponsive to conventional therapy and in those who are intolerant to or lost response to infliximab.[143] This drug has also been FDA approved in the treatment of rheumatoid arthritis, juvenile idiopathic arthritis, psoriatic arthritis, ankylosing spondylitis, and plaque psoriasis.[143] It is administered subcutaneously. According to the manufacturer, after single subcutaneous administration of adalimumab at a dose of 40 mg to a healthy subject, the maximum serum concentration (4.7 μg/mL) was achieved after 131 hours.[143] Adalimumab has 64% average absolute bioavailability after single subcutaneous injection and displays linear pharmacokinetics after single intravenous administration within the dose range 0.5 to 10 mg/kg.[143] Adalimumab administered subcutaneously in patients with CD at the single dose of 160 mg followed by a single dose of 80 mg 2 weeks later resulted in mean trough serum concentration of 12 μg/mL measured 2 weeks after each injection.[143] Patients with CD who received adalimumab biweekly at the dose of 40 mg had mean steady trough levels of 7 μg/mL at weeks 24 and 56.[143]

CLINICAL TRIALS

Efficacy of subcutaneously administered adalimumab in maintaining remission of CD was assessed in 2 randomized double-blind placebo-controlled trials (CLASSIC II and CHARM).[144,145]

The CLASSIC II trial included patients who previously participated in the CLASSIC I[146] trial evaluating adalimumab in inducing remission of CD. All 276 patients participating in the maintenance trial received 2 injections of adalimumab 40 mg at weeks 0 and 2 in an open-label fashion, and 55 patients in clinical remission (CDAI < 150) were subsequently randomized to receive either adalimumab 40 mg (every week or every other week) and placebo through week 56.[144] At the end of the trial, significantly more patients treated with adalimumab (83% for weekly injections and 79% for injections every other week) remained in clinical remission compared to placebo recipients (44%, P < 0.05).[144] Overall, patients treated with adalimumab were nearly 2-fold more likely to remain disease free than those receiving placebo (RR = 1.82; 95% CI, 1.06 to 3.13).[133] On the other hand, no significant sparing effect of adalimumab was observed versus placebo (RR = 1.38; 95% CI, 0.68 to 2.76).[133]

A multicenter CHARM trial enrolled 854 patients with active CD who initially received open-label induction injections of adalimumab 80 mg and 40 mg at weeks 0 and 2, respectively.[145] Efficacy analysis included patients (n = 499) who responded to induction therapy (decrease in CDAI ≥ 70 points from baseline) and were randomized to receive either adalimumab (40 mg weekly or every other week) or placebo through week 56.[145] Both adalimumab treatment arms had significantly higher proportions of patients in remission than placebo recipients at week 26 (47% for adalimumab weekly, 40% for adalimumab every other week versus 17% for placebo, P < 0.001) and week 56 (41% for adalimumab weekly, 36% for adalimumab every other week versus 12% for placebo, P < 0.001).[145] Overall, patients treated with adalimumab were 3-fold more likely to remain in remission (CDAI < 150) (RR = 3.28; 95% CI, 2.13 to 5.06) and nearly 3-fold more likely to maintain clinical response than those receiving placebo (RR = 2.69; 95% CI, 1.88 to 3.86).[133] In addition, when compared to placebo-treated individuals, patients treated with adalimumab were 4-fold more likely (RR=4.25; 95% CI, 1.57 to 11.47) to discontinue corticosteroids and remain disease free at week 56.[133]

ADVERSE EVENTS

Overall, adalimumab was well tolerated as a maintenance treatment for CD. The CLASSIC II trial observed a smaller proportion of adverse events and serious adverse events in adalimumab-treated patients than in placebo-treated subjects.[144] The most common adverse events that occurred in at least 5% of patients were nasopharyngitis, deterioration of CD, and sinusitis.[144] Serious adverse events were reported in 11% of placebo recipients, 5% of patients having adalimumab administered every other week, and 0% of patients having adalimumab administered every week.[144] One case of malignancy (squamous cell carcinoma) was observed in a placebo recipient.[144] Examination of blood specimens of 269 patients exposed to adalimumab during the CLASSIC II trial detected the presence of antibodies to adalimumab in 2.6% of the patients.[144] Frequency of antibodies to adalimumab was similar among individuals receiving concomitant immunomodulators and those not receiving them (0% versus 4%). The presence of ANA was detected at baseline and the last visit in 7% and 23% of 185 patients, respectively, who were tested and exposed to adalimumab.[144] All ANA-positive patients at the last visit also had positive results for dsDNA antibodies.[144] The CHARM II trial observed similar distribution of adverse events among patients treated with adalimumab 40 mg every other week (89%) or every week (86%) or placebo (85%).[145] Safety analysis included 778 patients (ie, 499 patients included in the efficacy analysis and 279 nonresponders to induction therapy randomized to adalimumab or placebo but not included in the efficacy analysis).[145] Significantly (P < 0.05) more placebo-treated patients (13%) withdrew from the study when compared with the adalimumab weekly (5%) or biweekly arm (7%).[145] Among the most frequent adverse events that occurred in at least 5% of patients were worsening of CD, arthralgia, nasopharyngitis, headache, nausea, fatigue, abdominal pain, pyrexia, upper respiratory tract infection, injection site reaction, urinary tract infection, influenza, diarrhea, and pharyngolaryngeal pain.[145] Of those, worsening of CD was observed in a significantly (P < 0.001) higher proportion of patients receiving placebo (32%) when compared to those treated with adalimumab weekly (19%) or biweekly (20%).[145] Headache (12% versus 6%, $P < 0.05$), fatigue (8% versus 2%, $P < 0.01$), and urinary tract infection (6% versus 1.5%) were significantly more frequently reported in weekly adalimumab than placebo recipients. Injection site reactions were significantly more common in adalimumab weekly (6%, $P < 0.001$) and biweekly (4%, $P < 0.01$) than in placebo recipients (0.4%).[145] On the other hand, placebo recipients significantly ($P < 0.05$) more frequently (15%) experienced serious adverse events when compared with adalimumab given weekly (8%) or biweekly (9%).[145] Although infectious adverse events were significantly more common in patients treated with biweekly injections of adalimumab when compared to placebo (46% versus 37%, $P < 0.05$), serious infectious adverse events had similar frequency across treatment arms (3% in each adalimumab arm versus 3% in placebo arm).[145] Tuberculosis was diagnosed in 2 patients treated with adalimumab.[145] There was 1 case of malignancy (breast cancer) identified in a placebo-treated patient.[145]

Similar to infliximab, appropriate testing and clinical approach are recommended in order to rule out tuberculosis during treatment with adalimumab (see details in infliximab section above).

FUTURE DIRECTIVES

Data from 2 large trials indicate that adalimumab is efficacious in maintaining remission of CD administered at the dose of 40 mg every other week subcutaneously, but an injection given every week might be necessary in some patients to maintain remission.[144,145] A recent analysis of data from the CHARM trial suggested that continuous maintenance treatment with adalimumab is more beneficial to patients than an induction treatment followed by discontinuation and retreatment upon CD relapse.[147] Continuous treatment with adalimumab was associated with higher remission rates at week 56 (51% for biweekly injections and 49% for weekly injections) compared to the induction/retreatment approach (38%, $P < 0.05$).[147] Maintenance treatment with adalimumab also has been shown to reduce 1-year risk of hospitalizations and surgery related to relapse of CD[148] and to provide sustained improvement in health-related quality of life.[149] However, vigilance is recommended with respect to potential risk of development of lymphoma or other malignancies.

CERTOLIZUMAB PEGOL

BACKGROUND

Certolizumab pegol is a pegylated humanized Fab' fragment of anti-TNFα monoclonal antibody. Pegylation reduces the immunogenicity, increasing the circulating half-lives and solubility and improving bioavailability of the drug.[150] In 2008, this drug received FDA approval only as a treatment to reduce signs and symptoms of CD and maintain clinical response in adult patients presenting with moderately to severely active disease and inadequate response to conventional therapy.[151] It is administered subcutaneously.

Data from the manufacturer indicate that after subcutaneous administration, certolizumab pegol achieves peak plasma concentrations after 54 and 171 hours.[152] Its bioavailability is approximately 80% (ranging from 76% to 88%) after subcutaneous administration compared to intravenous administration.[152] After a fixed dose of 400 mg, certolizumab pegol has steady-state concentrations ranging from 0.5 to 90 µg/mL.[152] In patients positive for anti-certolizumab pegol antibodies, the steady-state concentrations range from 0.5 to 75 µg/m.[152] Certolizumab pegol's half-life is approximately 14 days for all doses tested.[152] This drug is eliminated with a rate of 17 mL/h, although the route of elimination of certolizumab pegol has not been assessed in human subjects.[152]

CLINICAL TRIALS

The efficacy of certolizumab pegol in maintaining remission of CD was assessed in 1 randomized double blind placebo-controlled PRECISE II trial of 428 patients with CD and clinical response (reduction in CDAI ≥ 100 points from baseline) to 3 single subcutaneous injections of 400 mg of certolizumab given every other week who were on maintenance therapy with either certolizumab 400 mg or placebo administered every 4 weeks through week 26.[153] The sustained remission (CDAI ≤ 150) rates were significantly higher in patients treated with certolizumab when compared to the placebo arm at week 26 (48% versus 29%, $P < 0.001$).[153] Likewise, maintenance of clinical response was significantly higher in patients in the certolizumab arm than in the placebo arm (63% versus 36%, $P < 0.001$) at the end of the trial.[153] Certolizumab pegol was significantly approximately 2-fold more efficacious than placebo in maintaining clinical remission (RR = 1.68; 95% CI, 1.30 to 2.16) and clinical response (RR = 1.74; 95% CI, 1.41 to 2.13) through the end of the PRECISE II trial.[133]

ADVERSE EVENTS

Certolizumab as a maintenance treatment of CD was overall tolerated very well. Safety data from the PRECISE II maintenance trial observed similar frequency of adverse events (67% versus 65%) and serious adverse events (7% versus 6%) in both the placebo and certolizumab arms.[153] The most common adverse events (≥5%) reported among 428 patients included in the maintenance trials included headache, nasopharyngitis, cough, worsening of CD, and pain at the injection site.[153] Of these, worsening of CD (12% versus 4%, $P = 0.004$) and pain at the injection site were (5% versus 0.5%, $P = 0.003$) significantly more frequent in the placebo arm than in the certolizumab arm, whereas cough (6% versus 0.9%, $P = 0.01$) was significantly more frequently observed in the certolizumab arm when compared with the placebo arm.[153] Serious infections were reported in 3% of patients receiving certolizumab and in 0.9% of placebo recipients.[153] Pulmonary tuberculosis was diagnosed in 1 patient treated with certolizumab.[153] There were no cases of malignancies identified.[153] Among 422 patients screened during maintenance treatment for antibodies to certolizumab, 18% of the placebo recipients and 8% of the certolizumab recipients had detectable levels of these antibodies.[153] Of note, all patients received 3 doses of certolizumab during the induction phase, which indicates that patients receiving episodic treatment with certolizumab are more prone to develop antibodies to certolizumab than those with scheduled treatment. Among patients receiving certolizumab and immunomodulators and those receiving placebo and immunomodulators combined, 2% and 8% developed antibodies to certolizumab, respectively.[153] On the other hand, among patients receiving monotherapy with certolizumab or placebo, 12% and 24% developed these antibodies, respectively.[153]

New ANA antibodies were detected in 8% of patients treated with certolizumab and in 1% of those receiving placebo, whereas new antibodies to dsDNA were identified in 1% of patients in each treatment arm.[153]

Similarly to infliximab, appropriate testing and clinical approach are recommended in order to rule out tuberculosis during treatment with adalimumab (see details in the infliximab section).

FUTURE DIRECTIVES

In light of the PRECISE II study, certolizumab pegol administered subcutaneously at the dose of 400 mg every 4 weeks is efficacious as maintenance therapy in patients with CD. Maintenance treatment with certolizumab has been recently shown to significantly improve the quality of the patients' lives.[154] This agent should be considered in particular in patients who lost response or were intolerant to other anti-TNFα antibodies, infliximab, and adalimumab. However, vigilance is recommended with respect to the potential risk of developing lymphoma or other malignancies.

NATALIZUMAB

BACKGROUND

Natalizumab is a humanized monoclonal antibody against α-4 integrin and belongs to a new class of biologic agents named *selective adhesion molecule inhibitors*.[155] It was approved by the FDA in 2008 as a treatment to induce and maintain clinical response and remission in adult patients with moderately to severely active CD and inflammation presenting with either an inadequate response or intolerance to conventional CD therapies and anti-TNFα agents.[156] This drug is also FDA approved for treatment of multiple sclerosis.[156] This drug is administered intravenously.

Data from the manufacturer indicate that in patients with CD who received repeat intravenous infusions of natalizumab at the dose of 300 mg, the mean maximum observed serum concentration was 101 μg/mL, and the mean steady-state trough concentration was 10 μg/mL.[156] Steady state is achieved within 16 to 24 weeks after every 4 weeks of administration.[156] Natalizumab has a half-life of 10 days, volume of distribution of 5.2 L, and rate of elimination of 22 mL/h.[156]

CLINICAL TRIALS

One randomized placebo-controlled ENACT 2 trial assessed the efficacy of natalizumab in maintaining clinical response and remission of CD in 339 patients with CD who responded to induction therapy with natalizumab 300 mg (3 intravenous infusions every 4 weeks).[157] These patients were randomized to receive a total of 12 infusions of either natalizumab 300 mg or placebo every 4 weeks through week 56 and were followed up through week 60.[157]

Rates of sustained clinical response (decrease in CDAI ≥ 70 points from baseline) were significantly higher among patients treated continuously with natalizumab when compared to placebo (61% versus 28%, $P < 0.001$) at week 36 and at week 60 (54% versus 20%, $P < 0.001$).[157] An analysis of the subgroup of 250 patients who entered the ENACT 2 trial in clinical remission (CDAI < 150) showed significantly higher rates of sustained remission in the natalizumab arm when compared to the placebo arm at week 36 (44% versus 26%) and at week 60 (39% versus 15%).[157] Patients treated with natalizumab had significantly longer median time to loss of response than placebo recipients (336 days versus 86, $P < 0.001$).[157]

Natalizumab also was superior to placebo in sustaining clinical remission in a larger proportion of patients who discontinued corticosteroids while in remission at week 36 (45% versus 22%, $P = 0.003$) and at week 60 (42% versus 15%, $P < 0.001$).[157]

ADVERSE EVENTS

After its initial FDA approval for patients with multiple sclerosis in November 2004, natalizumab was withdrawn from the market, and all ongoing clinical trials were suspended in February 2005 due to reports of progressive multifocal leukoencephalopathy (PML) associated with JC polyomavirus.[158] Among 2 patients with multiple sclerosis who were treated with natalizumab and interferon beta-1a and developed PML, 1 patient recovered[159] but the second patient died.[160] One case of fatality due to PML was also identified in an open-label extension part of the ENACT 2 trial in a patient who was exposed to therapy with natalizumab and AZA.[157] Because the evaluation of the data from all clinical trials assessing natalizumab did not identify more cases of PML, clinical trials of natalizumab resumed in February 2006, and in June 2006, the FDA reapproved natalizumab for the treatment of multiple sclerosis.[161] This drug is currently FDA approved for multiple sclerosis and CD, and it is available only to patients enrolled in the risk management program named TOUCH Prescribing Program.[161] The FDA issued a black box warning for natalizumab underlying the increased risk of PML.[161] Natalizumab is to be used only in monotherapy as 3 patients known to develop PML were also treated with either interferon beta-1a or AZA.[162]

The ENACT 2 maintenance trial assessed the safety of natalizumab based on 428 patients who responded to induction treatment with either natalizumab 300 mg ($n = 354$) or placebo ($n = 74$) and were subsequently re-randomized to maintenance treatment with natalizumab ($n = 214$) or placebo ($n = 214$).[157] Natalizumab overall was tolerated well. There was a similar frequency of adverse events in the natalizumab and placebo arms during maintenance treatment (91% versus 97%, $P < 0.05$).[157] The most frequently observed adverse events occurring in at least 10% of patients (natalizumab versus placebo) included headache (36% versus 28%), nausea (22% versus 23%), nasopharyngitis (23% versus 24%), abdominal pain (21% versus 22%), fatigue (12% versus 14%), vomiting (14% versus 14%), exacerbation of CD (14% versus 39%, $P < 0.05$), arthralgia (20% versus 21%), back pain (12% versus 9%), influenza (12% versus 5%, $P < 0.05$), influenza-like illness (11% versus 6%), pharyngitis (11% versus 10%), and diarrhea (8% versus 10%). One patient in the placebo and natalizumab maintenance arm developed skin basal-cell carcinoma.[157] Acute infusion reactions defined as any adverse event occurring within up to 2 hours after the infusion were reported in 7% and 8% of natalizumab and placebo recipients, respectively.[157] Persistent (ie, 2 positive tests at least every 6 weeks or a single positive last test) and transient (ie, not fulfilling persistent antibodies requirement) antibodies to natalizumab were detected in 6% and 3% of 390 patients tested in the ENACT 2 trial.[157]

FUTURE DIRECTIVES

Natalizumab is efficacious in maintaining remission of CD when given as an intravenous infusion over 1 hour at the dose of 300 mg every 4 weeks. This drug should be considered in patients with CD who did not succeed with prior maintenance therapy with all anti-TNFα antibodies (infliximab, adalimumab, certolizumab). Caution is recommended during treatment with this agent due to an increased risk of developing PML. Recent analysis of the ENACT 2 trial data has indicated that maintenance therapy with natalizumab is associated with increased substantial improvement in health-related quality of life.[163]

SUMMARY

Data from aforementioned trials strongly suggest that neither aminosalicylates nor systemic corticosteroids should be recommended as a maintenance therapy in patients presenting with CD. The use of budesonide is an option for maintenance, given it has demonstrated an ability to increase the time to symptomatic remission; however, it has not demonstrated a benefit for remission over placebo at the time of 1 year considered to placebo. Therapy with AZA or 6-MP seems to be a better option for maintaining remission due to higher efficacy and steroid-sparing effect in patients with CD. However, therapy with these agents may be associated with significant side effects such as a potential for lymphoma, hepatotoxicity, and myelosuppression. Methotrexate might be considered as another therapeutic option; however, further trials are needed to fully evaluate its efficacy and safety in maintenance therapy. Therapy with infliximab in repeated doses every 8 weeks seems to be very effective in patients who respond to the initial dose of infliximab. Patients, especially those with fistulizing CD, treated with infliximab are more likely to discontinue steroids and to have reduced rates of hospitalizations and surgical procedures. Patients with luminal CD who are intolerant and lost response to infliximab may benefit from treatment with adalimumab or certolizumab.

Further studies are required to assess the efficacy of adalimumab and certolizumab in fistulizing CD. Finally, patients with inadequate response, loss of response, or intolerance to all anti-TNFα antibodies may benefit from treatment with natalizumab. Current American College of Gastroenterology guidelines recommend that all FDA-approved-for-CD biologic agents (ie, infliximab, adalimumab, certolizumab, natalizumab) should be administered as monotherapy in maintenance treatment in order to maximize the risk-to-benefit ratio of treatment.[164]

SURGICALLY INDUCED REMISSION

Patients with CD presenting with disease of the terminal ileum and colon are particularly apt to undergo surgical resection due to the chronic nature of the disease, tendency for relapse, hemorrhage, bowel perforation, bowel obstruction, bowel abscess, or toxic dilation of the colon.[165] It is estimated that 75% of patients require surgery by 20 years from the onset of symptoms and 90% by 30 years.[165] It is imperative to underline that CD is a continuous process with permanent intestinal inflammation despite achievement of initial clinical remission by surgical means (radical resection).[166] Among patients who underwent ileocolic resection, 73% were found to have new ileal inflammation above the anastomosis as early as 3 months after the surgery.[166] After 1- and 3-year postresection, 73% to 93% and 85% to 100% of patients, respectively, had recurrent lesions on endoscopy.[166,167] On the other hand, lower endoscopic recurrence rates of 28%, 61%, and 77% 1, 2, and 3 years after resection, respectively, were also observed.[168] Rates of symptomatic recurrence after surgically induced remission range from 20% after 1 year and 34% after

3 years[167] to approximately 50% after 5 years[165] and 59% to 79% by 15 years.[169] Approximately 30% of patients will undergo repetitive surgery within 10 years.[170] Although some authors suggested young or older age as a risk factor predictive of early postoperative recurrence, it does not seem to be a clear predictor of relapse risk.[169,171,172] On the other hand, there is enough evidence to accept that smoking is associated with a 2.5-fold increased risk of postoperative recurrence of CD.[173]

Several medical therapies have been evaluated for use in maintenance of surgically induced remission of CD such as 5-ASA, corticosteroids, budesonide, AZA/6-MP, antibiotics, and infliximab.

5-Aminosalicylic Acid

There were 4 RCTs evaluating the efficacy of sulfasalazine in maintaining surgically induced remission of CD.[27,174-176] Only 1 study of 232 patients found significant superiority of sulfasalazine 3 g daily over placebo in maintaining remission during 2 years of follow-up.[174] Significantly lower recurrence rates were observed among patients receiving sulfasalazine compared to placebo at 1 year (16% versus 28%, $P < 0.01$) and 2 years (24% versus 38%, $P < 0.01$) postsurgery.[174] After the third year of follow-up, insignificantly lower recurrence rates were observed in patients treated with sulfasalazine versus placebo (38% versus 48%, $P = 0.09$).[174]

There were 5 RCTs that assessed the efficacy of oral mesalamine (daily dose 2.4 to 4.0 g) in 729 patients as maintenance therapy of surgically induced remission of CD.[20,177-180] A meta-analysis of these trials was published in 1997[24] and subsequently updated and published in 2000.[181] Pooled results demonstrated significant (-10%) reduction (95% CI, -16.9% to -3.2%; $P = 0.0041$) in the risk of clinical relapse in patients treated with mesalamine compared to placebo or no treatment, and the number needed to treat was 10.[181] Exclusion of 1 study comparing mesalamine versus no treatment [176] from meta-analysis resulted in an increase of the number of patients needed to treat to maintain remission to 12.[181]

Corticosteroids

Two double-blind placebo-controlled trials assessed the efficacy of prednisone as a maintenance treatment in patients with CD in surgically induced remission.[27,182]

A study by Smith et al evaluated the long-term effect of prednisone in 59 patients free from symptoms related to CD in whom there was no clinical indication for steroid treatment.[180] Patients were randomly assigned to receive either oral prednisone at a dose of 7.5 mg daily or placebo and were followed for up to 3 years.[182] There were 22 patients with previously active disease and no surgery within 1 year prior to the study and 37 patients who underwent surgery with ($n = 11$) or without ($n = 26$) residual disease.[182] Clinical

relapse was defined as the need for additional treatment with prednisolone in order to control recurrent or persistent abdominal symptoms (ie, malaise, weight loss, and colicky abdominal pain).[182] Overall, during the study period, 45% of patients treated with prednisolone and 42% of patients receiving placebo experienced either a clinical relapse, recurrence, or extension of CD.[182] There was no difference of withdrawal rate between patients treated with prednisone or placebo (30% for each treatment at 3 years).[182]

Part II of the NCCDS randomized 48 patients to receive either prednisone 0.25 mg daily ($n = 12$), sulfasalazine 2.5 g daily ($n = 15$), azathioprine 1 mg/kg daily ($n = 8$), or placebo ($n = 13$) within 1 year after surgically induced remission of CD.[27] Placebo-treated patients ranked significantly better than patients treated with prednisone ($P = 0.05$) or AZA ($P = 0.02$) and insignificantly ($P = 0.12$) better than those treated with sulfasalazine at 1 year of follow-up.[27] Analysis of outcomes during the second year of follow-up revealed insignificant superiority of placebo over treatment with prednisone, sulfasalazine, or AZA.[27]

Budesonide

Two European randomized double-blind placebo-controlled trials assessed the efficacy of 1-year treatment with low-dose (3 mg) or high daily dose (6 mg) of budesonide in maintaining surgically induced remission of CD in 213 patients.[183,184] Both studies failed to demonstrate superiority of either low-dose or high-dose budesonide over placebo in the postsurgical setting.[183,184] There was no significant difference in reduction of clinical or endoscopic recurrence in either study.[183,184] Observed endoscopic and/or clinical recurrence rates were 57% and 70% after 1 year of treatment with low-dose budesonide or placebo, respectively (P value not significant).[183] Likewise, therapy with high-dose budesonide or placebo was associated with 30% clinical recurrence rates during the trial.[184] There was no significant difference between high-dose budesonide and placebo in endoscopic recurrence at the site of anastomosis after 3 months (21% versus 47%; $P = 0.11$) and 12 months (32% versus 65%; $P = 0.047$).[184]

Azathioprine/6-MP

Efficacy of AZA/6-MP in maintaining remission of surgically induced remission of CD was evaluated in 3 double-blind, placebo-controlled trials.[27,185,186] Although the NCCDS did not observe superiority of AZA over placebo in maintaining disease-free remission,[27] 2 recent studies demonstrated otherwise.[185,186] A study by Hanauer et al compared 6-MP 50 mg daily ($n = 47$) versus mesalamine 3 g daily ($n = 44$) versus placebo ($n = 44$) administered to patients over a 2-year period.[185] Significant benefit of 6-MP versus placebo was observed in clinical (hazard ratio [HR] = 0.52, $P = 0.045$) and endoscopic (HR = 0.48, $P = 0.030$) relapse free-survival during the study interval.[185] On the other hand, mesalamine failed to show superiority over placebo in maintaining clinical (HR = 0.62, P = 0.123) and endoscopic recurrence (HR = 0.80, P = 0.458).[185] A recent study by a Belgian group studied 12-week combination therapy of AZA 100 to 150 mg/day and metronidazole 750 mg/day versus metronidazole 750 mg/day and placebo with subsequent 40-week monotherapy with AZA 100 to 150 mg/day versus placebo in 80 patients with surgically induced remission of CD.[186] Although the initial 12 weeks of combination therapy with metronidazole AZA did not show significant benefit over placebo in reducing endoscopic recurrence rates (34% versus 53%, P = 0.11), significant benefit in reduction of endoscopic recurrence was observed in the AZA arm compared with the placebo arm at the end of follow-up (44% versus 69%, P = 0.048).[186]

ANTIBIOTICS

There were 2 randomized double-blind placebo-controlled trials from Belgium that assessed maintenance therapy with oral metronidazole or ornidazole in 129 patients with surgically induced remission of CD.[101,102] Treatment was initiated within 1 week after surgery.[101,102] Among 51 patients who completed the study of metronidazole versus placebo, therapy with metronidazole at the daily dose of 20 mg/kg for 3 months was associated with significantly lower clinical relapse rates after 1 year (4% versus 25%, P = 0.044) but not after 2 (28% versus 43%, P value not significant) and 3 years (30% versus 50%, P value not significant) of follow-up when compared to placebo.[101] The significant reduction in clinical recurrence rates after 1 year were also observed after 1-year treatment with ornidazole given at the daily dose of 1 g when compared to placebo (8% versus 38%, P = 0.0046).[102] On the other hand, this therapeutic effect of ornidazole was not sustained after 2 (30% versus 45%, P = 0.17) and 3 (46% versus 48%, P = 0.53) years of follow-up when compared to placebo.[102] Endoscopic recurrence rates were significantly reduced in patients treated with ornidazole after 3 months (34% versus 59%, P = 0.047) and 1 year (54% versus 79%, P = 0.037) whereas no significant reduction was observed in metronidazole patients after 3 months (52% versus 75%, P = 0.09) compared to placebo.[101,102]

Despite the efficacy of ornidazole, significantly more patients receiving this agent stopped therapy due to side effects when compared with placebo (31% versus 13%, P = 0.041).[102] The rate of patients experiencing side effects related to ornidazole therapy was significantly higher than placebo (68% versus 30%, P = 0.0007).[102] Among patients with side effects, peripheral neuropathy was the most frequent side effect of ornidazole (31%)[100] or metronidazole (29%).[101] Although both metronidazole and ornidazole seem to be efficacious in maintaining clinical remission in the postsurgical setting for up to 1 year of follow-up, severe side effects associated with their use warrant alternate studies to establish either safe or efficacious dose of metronidazole or ornidazole or to evaluate different antibiotics.

INFLIXIMAB

There has been 1 randomized placebo-controlled trial of 24 patients that evaluated the efficacy of infliximab in maintaining remission achieved surgically.[187] Therapy with intravenous infusions of infliximab 5 mg/kg was initiated within 4 weeks of surgery and lasted for 1 year.[187] Although rates of patients with endoscopic recurrence were significantly higher compared to placebo after 1 year (85% versus 9%, P = 0.0006), no significant difference was observed for clinical recurrence rates between the infliximab and placebo arms after 1 year (80% versus 54%, P = 0.38).[187]

SUMMARY

The clinical trials have demonstrated that patients who have surgically induced remission of CD should be placed on AZA or 6-MP with metronidazole or nitroimidazole immediately after their operation. Therapy with infliximab seems to be promising in maintaining surgically induced remission. Further studies are required to assess the efficacy of anti-TNFα agents in postoperative settings.

REFERENCES

1. Mantzaris GJ, Petraki K, Sfakianakis M, et al. Budesonide versus mesalamine for maintaining remission in patients refusing other immunomodulators for steroid-dependent Crohn's disease. *Clin Gastroenterol Hepatol.* 2003;1(2):122-128.

2. Modigliani R, Colombel JF, Dupas JL, et al. Mesalamine in Crohn's disease with steroid-induced remission: effect on steroid withdrawal and remission maintenance, Groupe d'Etudes Therapeutiques des Affections Inflammatoires Digestives. *Gastroenterology.* 1996;110(3):688-693.

3. Loftus EV Jr. Clinical epidemiology of inflammatory bowel disease: incidence, prevalence, and environmental influences. *Gastroenterology.* 2004;126(6):1504-1517.

4. Martin F. Oral 5-aminosalicylic acid preparations in treatment of inflammatory bowel disease: an update. *Dig Dis Sci.* 1987;32(12 suppl):57S-63S.

5. Azad Khan AK, Piris J, Truelove SC. An experiment to determine the active therapeutic moiety of sulphasalazine. *Lancet.* 1977;2(8044):892-895.

6. Klotz U, Maier K, Fischer C, Heinkel K. Therapeutic efficacy of sulfasalazine and its metabolites in patients with ulcerative colitis and Crohn's disease. *N Engl J Med.* 1980;303(26):1499-1502.

7. van Hees PA, Bakker JH, van Tongeren JH. Effect of sulphapyridine, 5-aminosalicylic acid, and placebo in patients with idiopathic proctitis: a study to determine the active therapeutic moiety of sulphasalazine. *Gut.* 1980;21(7):632-635.

8. Clemett D, Markham A. Prolonged-release mesalazine: a review of its therapeutic potential in ulcerative colitis and Crohn's disease. *Drugs.* 2000;59(4):929-956.

9. Haagen Nielsen O, Bondesen S. Kinetics of 5-aminosalicylic acid after jejunal instillation in man. *Br J Clin Pharmacol.* 1983;16(6):738-740.

10. Christensen LA, Fallingborg J, Abildgaard K, et al. Topical and systemic availability of 5-aminosalicylate: comparisons of three controlled release preparations in man. *Aliment Pharmacol Ther.* 1990;4(5):523-533.

11. Myers B, Evans DN, Rhodes J, et al. Metabolism and urinary excretion of 5-amino salicylic acid in healthy volunteers when given intravenously or released for absorption at different sites in the gastrointestinal tract. *Gut*. 1987;28(2):196-200.

12. Stein RB, Hanauer SB. Comparative tolerability of treatments for inflammatory bowel disease. *Drug Saf*. 2000;23(5):429-448.

13. Schwab M, Klotz U. Pharmacokinetic considerations in the treatment of inflammatory bowel disease. *Clin Pharmacokinet*. 2001; 40(10):723-751.

14. Klotz U. Clinical pharmacokinetics of sulphasalazine, its metabolites and other prodrugs of 5-aminosalicylic acid. *Clin Pharmacokinet*. 1985;10(4):285-302.

15. Coated oral 5-aminosalicylic acid versus placebo in maintaining remission of inactive Crohn's disease. International Mesalazine Study Group. *Aliment Pharmacol Ther*. 1990;4(1):55-64.

16. Arber N, Odes HS, Fireman Z, et al. A controlled double blind multicenter study of the effectiveness of 5-aminosalicylic acid in patients with Crohn's disease in remission. *J Clin Gastroenterol*. 1995;20(3):203-206.

17. Gendre JP, Mary JY, Florent C, et al. Oral mesalamine (Pentasa) as maintenance treatment in Crohn's disease: a multicenter placebo-controlled study. The Groupe d'Etudes Therapeutiques des Affections Inflammatoires Digestives (GETAID). *Gastroenterology*. 1993;104(2):435-439.

18. Mahmud N, Kamm MA, Dupas JL, et al. Olsalazine is not superior to placebo in maintaining remission of inactive Crohn's colitis and ileocolitis: a double blind, parallel, randomised, multicentre study. *Gut*. 2001;49(4):552-556.

19. Prantera C, Pallone F, Brunetti G, Cottone M, Miglioli M. Oral 5-aminosalicylic acid (Asacol) in the maintenance treatment of Crohn's disease. The Italian IBD Study Group. *Gastroenterology*. 1992;103(2):363-368.

20. Sutherland LR, Martin F, Bailey RJ, et al. A randomized, placebo-controlled, double-blind trial of mesalamine in the maintenance of remission of Crohn's disease. The Canadian Mesalamine for Remission of Crohn's Disease Study Group. *Gastroenterology*. 1997; 112(4):1069-1177.

21. Thomson AB, Wright JP, Vatn M, et al. Mesalazine (Mesasal/Claversal) 1.5 g b.d. versus placebo in the maintenance of remission of patients with Crohn's disease. *Aliment Pharmacol Ther*. 1995;9(6):673-683.

22. de Franchis R, Omodei P, Ranzi T, et al. Controlled trial of oral 5-aminosalicylic acid for the prevention of early relapse in Crohn's disease. *Aliment Pharmacol Ther*. 1997;11(5):845-852.

23. Akobeng AK, Gardener E. Oral 5-aminosalicylic acid for maintenance of medically induced remission in Crohn's disease. *Cochrane Database Syst Rev*. 2005(1):CD003715.

24. Camma C, Giunta M, Rosselli M, Cottone M. Mesalamine in the maintenance treatment of Crohn's disease: a meta-analysis adjusted for confounding variables. *Gastroenterology*. 1997;113(5):1465-1473.

25. Brignola C, Iannone P, Pasquali S, et al. Placebo-controlled trial of oral 5-ASA in relapse prevention of Crohn's disease. *Dig Dis Sci*. 1992;37(1):29-32.

26. Bresci G, Parisi G, Banti S. Long-term therapy with 5-aminosalicylic acid in Crohn's disease: is it useful? Our four years experience. *Int J Clin Pharmacol Res*. 1994;14(4):133-138.

27. Summers RW, Switz DM, Sessions JT Jr, et al. National Cooperative Crohn's Disease Study: results of drug treatment. *Gastroenterology*. 1979;77(4 pt 2):847-869.

28. Malchow H, Ewe K, Brandes JW, et al. European Cooperative Crohn's Disease Study (ECCDS): results of drug treatment. *Gastroenterology*. 1984;86(2):249-266.

29. Brignola C, Campieri M, Farruggia P, et al. The possible utility of steroids in the prevention of relapses of Crohn's disease in remission: a preliminary study. *J Clin Gastroenterol*. 1988;10(6):631-634.

30. Gorard DA, Hunt JB, Payne-James JJ, et al. Initial response and subsequent course of Crohn's disease treated with elemental diet or prednisolone. *Gut*. 1993;34(9):1198-1202.

31. Rutgeerts P, Lofberg R, Malchow H, et al. A comparison of budesonide with prednisolone for active Crohn's disease. *N Engl J Med*. 1994;331(13):842-845.

32. Otley A, Steinhart A, Otley A. Budesonide for induction of remission in Crohn's disease. *Cochrane Database Syst Rev*. 2005(4): CD000296.

33. Spencer CM, McTavish D. Budesonide: a review of its pharmacological properties and therapeutic efficacy in inflammatory bowel disease. *Drugs*. 1995;50(5):854-872.

34. Gross V, Andus T, Ecker KW, et al. Low dose oral pH modified release budesonide for maintenance of steroid induced remission in Crohn's disease. The Budesonide Study Group. *Gut*. 1998;42(4):493-496.

35. Ferguson A, Campieri M, Doe W, Persson T, Nygard G. Oral budesonide as maintenance therapy in Crohn's disease: results of a 12-month study. Global Budesonide Study Group. *Aliment Pharmacol Ther*. 1998;12(2):175-183.

36. Greenberg GR, Feagan BG, Martin F, et al. Oral budesonide as maintenance treatment for Crohn's disease: a placebo-controlled, dose-ranging study. Canadian Inflammatory Bowel Disease Study Group. *Gastroenterology*. 1996;110:45-51.

37. Hanauer S, Sandborn WJ, Persson A, Persson T. Budesonide as maintenance treatment in Crohn's disease: a placebo-controlled trial. *Aliment Pharmacol Ther*. 2005;21(4):363-371.

38. Lofberg R, Rutgeerts P, Malchow H, et al. Budesonide prolongs time to relapse in ileal and ileocaecal Crohn's disease: a placebo-controlled one year study. *Gut*. 1996;39:82-86.

39. Sandborn WJ, Lofberg R, Feagan BG, Hanauer SB, Campieri M, Greenberg GR. Budesonide for maintenance of remission in patients with Crohn's disease in medically induced remission: a predetermined pooled analysis of four randomized, double blind, placebo controlled trials. *Am J Gastroenterol*. 2005;100:1780-1787.

40. Schoon EJ, Bollani S, Mills PR, et al. Bone mineral density in relation to efficacy and side effects of budesonide and prednisolone in Crohn's disease. *Clin Gastroenterol Hepatol*. 2005;3:113-121.

41. Cortot A, Colombel JF, Rutgeerts P, et al. Switch from systemic steroids to budesonide in steroid dependent patients with inactive Crohn's disease. Gut. 2001;48:186-190.

42. Andus T, Gross V, Caesar I, et al. Replacement of conventional glucocorticoids by oral pH-modified release budesonide in active and inactive Crohn's disease: results of an open, prospective, multicenter trial. *Dig Dis Sci*. 2003;48(2):373-378.

43. Green JR, Lobo AJ, Giaffer M, Travis S, Watkins IIC. Maintenance of Crohn's disease over 12 months: fixed versus flexible dosing regimen using budesonide controlled ileal release capsules. *Aliment Pharmacol Ther*. 2001;15:1331-1341.

44. Lennard L. The clinical pharmacology of 6-mercaptopurine. *Eur J Clin Pharmacol*. 1992;43:329-339.

45. Candy S, Wright J, Gerber M, Adams G, Gerig M, Goodman R. A controlled double blind study of azathioprine in the management of Crohn's disease. *Gut*. 1995;37(5):674-678.

46. O'Donoghue DP, Dawson AM, Powell-Tuck J, Bown RL, Lennard-Jones JE. Double-blind withdrawal trial of azathioprine as maintenance treatment for Crohn's disease. *Lancet*. 1978;2(8097):955-957.

47. Willoughby JM, Beckett J, Kumar PJ, Dawson AM. Controlled trial of azathioprine in Crohn's disease. *Lancet*. 1971;2(7731):944-947.

48. Rosenberg JL, Levin B, Wall AJ, Kirsner JB. A controlled trial of azathioprine in Crohn's disease. *Am J Dig Dis.* 1975;20(8):721-726.

49. Lemann M, Mary JY, Colombel JF, et al. A randomized, double-blind, controlled withdrawal trial in Crohn's disease patients in long-term remission on azathioprine. *Gastroenterology.* 2005;128(7):1812-1818.

50. Prefontaine E, Sutherland LR, Macdonald JK, Cepoiu M. Azathioprine or 6-mercaptopurine for maintenance of remission in Crohn's disease. *Cochrane Database Syst Rev.* 2009;1:CD000067.

51. Bouhnik Y, Lemann M, Mary JY, et al. Long-term follow-up of patients with Crohn's disease treated with azathioprine or 6-mercaptopurine. *Lancet.* 1996;347(8996):215-219.

52. Mantzaris G, Roussos A, Christidou A, et al. The long-term efficacy of azathioprine does not wane after four years of continuous treatment in patients with steroid-dependent luminal Crohn's disease. *Journal of Crohn's and Colitis.* 2007;1:28-34.

53. Treton X, Bouhnik Y, Mary JY, et al. Azathioprine withdrawal in patients with Crohn's disease maintained on prolonged remission: a high risk of relapse. *Clin Gastroenterol Hepatol.* 2009;7(1):80-85.

54. Aberra FN, Lichtenstein GR. Review article: monitoring of immunomodulators in inflammatory bowel disease. *Aliment Pharmacol Ther.* 2005;21(4):307-319.

55. Thomas CW Jr, Lowry PW, Franklin CL, et al. Erythrocyte mean corpuscular volume as a surrogate marker for 6-thioguanine nucleotide concentration monitoring in patients with inflammatory bowel disease treated with azathioprine or 6-mercaptopurine. *Inflamm Bowel Dis.* 2003;9(4):237-245.

56. Kandiel A, Fraser AG, Korelitz BI, Brensinger C, Lewis JD. Increased risk of lymphoma among inflammatory bowel disease patients treated with azathioprine and 6-mercaptopurine. *Gut.* 2005;54(8):1121-1125.

57. Dayharsh GA, Loftus EV Jr, Sandborn WJ, et al. Epstein-Barr virus-positive lymphoma in patients with inflammatory bowel disease treated with azathioprine or 6-mercaptopurine. *Gastroenterology.* 2002;122(1):72-77.

58. Aithal GP, Mansfield JC. Review article: the risk of lymphoma associated with inflammatory bowel disease and immunosuppressive treatment. *Aliment Pharmacol Ther.* 2001;15(8):1101-1108.

59. Connell WR, Kamm MA, Ritchie JK, Lennard-Jones JE. Bone marrow toxicity caused by azathioprine in inflammatory bowel disease: 27 years of experience. *Gut.* 1993;34(8):1081-1085.

60. Colombel JF, Ferrari N, Debuysere H, et al. Genotypic analysis of thiopurine S-methyltransferase in patients with Crohn's disease and severe myelosuppression during azathioprine therapy. *Gastroenterology.* 2000;118(6):1025-1030.

61. Dubinsky MC, Lamothe S, Yang HY, et al. Pharmacogenomics and metabolite measurement for 6-mercaptopurine therapy in inflammatory bowel disease. *Gastroenterology.* 2000;118(4):705-713.

62. Present DH, Meltzer SJ, Krumholz MP, Wolke A, Korelitz BI. 6-Mercaptopurine in the management of inflammatory bowel disease: short and long-term toxicity. *Ann Intern Med.* 1989;111(8):641-649.

63. Cheng B, Lichtenstein GR. Are individuals with Crohn's disease who are intolerant to 6-mercaptopurine able to tolerate azathioprine? *Gastroenterology.* 2000;118(4 suppl 2 part 2):A1336.

64. Lichtenstein GR, Abreu MT, Cohen R, Tremaine W. American Gastroenterological Association Institute technical review on corticosteroids, immunomodulators, and infliximab in inflammatory bowel disease. *Gastroenterology.* 2006;130(3):940-987.

65. Lewis JD, Schwartz JS, Lichtenstein GR. Azathioprine for maintenance of remission in Crohn's disease: benefits outweigh the risk of lymphoma. *Gastroenterology.* 2000;118(6):1018-1024.

66. Sandborn WJ. A review of immune modifier therapy for inflammatory bowel disease: azathioprine, 6-mercaptopurine, cyclosporine, and methotrexate. *Am J Gastroenterol.* 1996;91(3):423-433.

67. Cronstein BN. Molecular mechanism of methotrexate action in inflammation. *Inflammation.* 1992;16(5):411-423.

68. Cronstein BN. The mechanism of action of methotrexate. *Rheum Dis Clin North Am.* 1997;23(4):739-755.

69. Egan LJ, Sandborn WJ, Mays DC, Tremaine WJ, Lipsky JJ. Plasma and rectal adenosine in inflammatory bowel disease: effect of methotrexate. *Inflamm Bowel Dis.* 1999;5(3):167-173.

70. Bouma MG, Stad RK, van den Wildenberg FA, Buurman WA. Differential regulatory effects of adenosine on cytokine release by activated human monocytes. *J Immunol.* 1994;153(9):4159-4168.

71. Moshkowitz M, Oren R, Tishler M, et al. The absorption of low-dose methotrexate in patients with inflammatory bowel disease. *Aliment Pharmacol Ther.* 1997;11(3):569-573.

72. Egan LJ, Sandborn WJ. Methotrexate for inflammatory bowel disease: pharmacology and preliminary results. *Mayo Clin Proc.* 1996;71(1):69-80.

73. Shen DD, Azarnoff DL. Clinical pharmacokinetics of methotrexate. *Clin Pharmacokinet.* 1978;3(1):1-13.

74. Feagan BG, Fedorak RN, Irvine EJ, et al. A comparison of methotrexate with placebo for the maintenance of remission in Crohn's disease. North American Crohn's Study Group Investigators. *N Engl J Med.* 2000;342(22):1627-1632.

75. Cunliffe RN, Scott BB. Review article: monitoring for drug side-effects in inflammatory bowel disease. *Aliment Pharmacol Ther.* 2002;16(4):647-662.

76. Buckley LM, Vacek PM, Cooper SM. Administration of folinic acid after low dose methotrexate in patients with rheumatoid arthritis. *J Rheumatol.* 1990;17(9):1158-1161.

77. Shiroky JB, Neville C, Esdaile JM, et al. Low-dose methotrexate with leucovorin (folinic acid) in the management of rheumatoid arthritis: results of a multicenter randomized, double-blind, placebo-controlled trial. *Arthritis Rheum.* 1993;36(6):795-803.

78. Almeyda J, Barnardo D, Baker H, Levene GM, Landells JW. Structural and functional abnormalities of the liver in psoriasis before and during methotrexate therapy. *Br J Dermatol.* 1972;87(6):623-631.

79. Nyfors A. Liver biopsies from psoriatics related to methotrexate therapy: 3. Findings in post-methotrexate liver biopsies from 160 psoriatics. *Acta Pathol Microbiol Scand A.* 1977;85(4):511-518.

80. Nyfors A, Poulsen H. Liver biopsies from psoriatics related to methotrexate therapy. 1. Findings in 123 consecutive non-methotrexate treated patients. *Acta Pathol Microbiol Scand A.* 1976;84(3):253-261.

81. Roenigk HH Jr, Bergfeld WF, St Jacques R, Owens FJ, Hawk WA. Hepatotoxicity of methotrexate in the treatment of psoriasis. *Arch Dermatol.* 1971;103(3):250-261.

82. Zachariae H, Kragballe K, Sogaard H. Methotrexate induced liver cirrhosis. Studies including serial liver biopsies during continued treatment. *Br J Dermatol.* 1980;102(4):407-412.

83. Te HS, Schiano TD, Kuan SF, Hanauer SB, Conjeevaram HS, Baker AL. Hepatic effects of long-term methotrexate use in the treatment of inflammatory bowel disease. *Am J Gastroenterol.* 2000;95(11):3150-3156.

84. Kremer JM, Alarcon GS, Lightfoot RW Jr, et al. Methotrexate for rheumatoid arthritis. Suggested guidelines for monitoring liver toxicity. American College of Rheumatology. *Arthritis Rheum.* 1994;37(3):316-328.

85. Fahr A. Cyclosporin clinical pharmacokinetics. *Clin Pharmacokinet.* 1993;24(6):472-495.

86. Noble S, Markham A. Cyclosporin: a review of the pharmacokinetic properties, clinical efficacy and tolerability of a microemulsion-based formulation (Neoral). *Drugs.* 1995;50(5):924-941.

87. Feagan BG, McDonald JW, Rochon J, et al. Low-dose cyclosporine for the treatment of Crohn's disease. The Canadian Crohn's Relapse Prevention Trial Investigators. *N Engl J Med.* 1994; 330(26):1846-1851.

88. Stange EF, Modigliani R, Pena AS, Wood AJ, Feutren G, Smith PR. European trial of cyclosporine in chronic active Crohn's disease: a 12-month study. The European Study Group. *Gastroenterology.* 1995;109(3):774-782.

89. Linskens RK, Huijsdens XW, Savelkoul PH, Vandenbroucke-Grauls CM, Meuwissen SG. The bacterial flora in inflammatory bowel disease: current insights in pathogenesis and the influence of antibiotics and probiotics. *Scand J Gastroenterol.* 2001;(234 suppl):29-40.

90. Bamias G, Marini M, Moskaluk CA, et al. Down-regulation of intestinal lymphocyte activation and Th1 cytokine production by antibiotic therapy in a murine model of Crohn's disease. *J Immunol.* 2002;169(9):5308-5314.

91. Grove DI, Mahmound AA, Warren KS. Suppression of cell-mediated immunity by metronidazole. *Int Arch Allergy Appl Immunol.* 1977;54(5):422-427.

92. Arndt H, Palitzsch KD, Grisham MB, Granger DN. Metronidazole inhibits leukocyte-endothelial cell adhesion in rat mesenteric venules. *Gastroenterology.* 1994;106(5):1271-1276.

93. Casellas F, Borruel N, Papo M, et al. Antiinflammatory effects of enterically coated amoxicillin-clavulanic acid in active ulcerative colitis. *Inflamm Bowel Dis.* 1998;4(1):1-5.

94. Burke DA, Axon AT, Clayden SA, Dixon MF, Johnston D, Lacey RW. The efficacy of tobramycin in the treatment of ulcerative colitis. *Aliment Pharmacol Ther.* 1990;4(2):123-129.

95. Colombel JF, Lemann M, Cassagnou M, et al. A controlled trial comparing ciprofloxacin with mesalazine for the treatment of active Crohn's disease. Groupe d'Etudes Therapeutiques des Affections Inflammatoires Digestives (GETAID). *Am J Gastroenterol.* 1999;94(3):674-678.

96. Leiper K, Morris AI, Rhodes JM. Open label trial of oral clarithromycin in active Crohn's disease. *Aliment Pharmacol Ther.* 2000; 14(6):801-806.

97. Moss AA, Carbone JV, Kressel HY. Radiologic and clinical assessment of broad-spectrum antibiotic therapy in Crohn's disease. *AJR Am J Roentgenol.* 1978;131(5):787-790.

98. Prantera C, Zannoni F, Scribano ML, et al. An antibiotic regimen for the treatment of active Crohn's disease: a randomized, controlled clinical trial of metronidazole plus ciprofloxacin. *Am J Gastroenterol.* 1996;91(2):328-332.

99. Turunen UM, Farkkila MA, Hakala K, et al. Long-term treatment of ulcerative colitis with ciprofloxacin: a prospective, double-blind, placebo-controlled study. *Gastroenterology.* 1998;115(5):1072-1078.

100. Steinhart AH, Feagan BG, Wong CJ, et al. Combined budesonide and antibiotic therapy for active Crohn's disease: a randomized controlled trial. *Gastroenterology.* 2002;123(1):33-40.

101. Rutgeerts P, Hiele M, Geboes K, et al. Controlled trial of metronidazole treatment for prevention of Crohn's recurrence after ileal resection. *Gastroenterology.* 1995;108(6):1617-1621.

102. Rutgeerts P, Van Assche G, Vermeire S, et al. Ornidazole for prophylaxis of postoperative Crohn's disease recurrence: a randomized, double-blind, placebo-controlled trial. *Gastroenterology.* 2005;128(4):856-861.

103. Prantera C, Kohn A, Mangiarotti R, Andreoli A, Luzi C. Antimycobacterial therapy in Crohn's disease: results of a controlled, double-blind trial with a multiple antibiotic regimen. *Am J Gastroenterol.* 1994;89(4):513-518.

104. Afdhal NH, Long A, Lennon J, Crowe J, O'Donoghue DP. Controlled trial of antimycobacterial therapy in Crohn's disease: clofazimine versus placebo. *Dig Dis Sci.* 1991;36(4):449-453.

105. Elliott PR, Burnham WR, Berghouse LM, Lennard-Jones JE, Langman MJ. Sulphadoxine-pyrimethamine therapy in Crohn's disease. *Digestion.* 1982;23(2):132-134.

106. Shaffer JL, Hughes S, Linaker BD, Baker RD, Turnberg LA. Controlled trial of rifampicin and ethambutol in Crohn's disease. *Gut.* 1984;25(2):203-205.

107. Swift GL, Srivastava ED, Stone R, et al. Controlled trial of antituberculous chemotherapy for two years in Crohn's disease. *Gut.* 1994;35(3):363-368.

108. Graham D, Al-Assi M, Robinson M. Prolonged remission in Crohn's disease following therapy for *Mycobacterium paratuberculosis* infection [abstract]. *Gastroenterology.* 1995;108:A826.

109. Kelleher D, O'Brien S, Weir D. Preliminary trial of clofazimine in chronic inflammatory bowel disease [abstract]. *Gut.* 1982;23: A449.

110. Borgaonkar M, MacIntosh D, Fardy J, Simms L. Antituberculous therapy for maintaining remission of Crohn's disease. *Cochrane Database Syst Rev.* 2000;2:CD000299.

111. Selby W, Pavli P, Crotty B, et al. Two-year combination antibiotic therapy with clarithromycin, rifabutin, and clofazimine for Crohn's disease. *Gastroenterology.* 2007;132(7):2313-2319.

112. Guarner F, Schaafsma GJ. Probiotics. *Int J Food Microbiol.* 1998; 39(3):237-238.

113. Fooks LJ, Gibson GR. Probiotics as modulators of the gut flora. *Br J Nutr.* 2002;88(Suppl 1):S39-S49.

114. Sartor RB. Probiotic therapy of intestinal inflammation and infections. *Curr Opin Gastroenterol.* 2005;21(1):44-50.

115. Malchow HA. Crohn's disease and *Escherichia coli*: a new approach in therapy to maintain remission of colonic Crohn's disease? *J Clin Gastroenterol.* 1997;25(4):653-658.

116. Prantera C, Scribano ML, Falasco G, Andreoli A, Luzi C. Ineffectiveness of probiotics in preventing recurrence after curative resection for Crohn's disease: a randomised controlled trial with Lactobacillus GG. *Gut.* 2002;51(3):405-409.

117. Schultz M, Timmer A, Herfarth HH, Sartor RB, Vanderhoof JA, Rath HC. *Lactobacillus GG* in inducing and maintaining remission of Crohn's disease. *BMC Gastroenterol.* 2004;4:5.

118. Rolfe VE, Fortun PJ, Hawkey CJ, Bath-Hextall F. Probiotics for maintenance of remission in Crohn's disease. *Cochrane Database Syst Rev.* 2006;4:CD004826.

119. Guslandi M, Mezzi G, Sorghi M, Testoni PA. *Saccharomyces boulardii* in maintenance treatment of Crohn's disease. *Dig Dis Sci.* 2000;45(7):1462-1464.

120. Bousvaros A, Guandalini S, Baldassano RN, et al. A randomized, double-blind trial of *Lactobacillus* GG versus placebo in addition to standard maintenance therapy for children with Crohn's disease. *Inflamm Bowel Dis.* 2005;11(9):833-839.

121. Zocco M, Zileri Dal Verme L, Armuzzi A, et al. Comparison of *Lactobacillus* GG and mesalazine in maintaining remission of ulcerative colitis and Crohn's disease. *Gastroenterology.* 2003;124:A201.

122. Van Gossum A, Dewit O, Louis E, et al. Multicenter randomized-controlled clinical trial of probiotics (*Lactobacillus johnsonii*, LA1) on early endoscopic recurrence of Crohn's disease after ileo-caecal resection. *Inflamm Bowel Dis.* 2007;13(2):135-142.

123. Marteau P, Lemann M, Seksik P, et al. Ineffectiveness of *Lactobacillus johnsonii* LA1 for prophylaxis of postoperative recurrence in Crohn's disease: a randomised, double blind, placebo controlled GETAID trial. *Gut.* 2006;55(6):842-847.

124. Rahimi R, Nikfar S, Rahimi F, et al. A meta-analysis on the efficacy of probiotics for maintenance of remission and prevention of clinical and endoscopic relapse in Crohn's disease. *Dig Dis Sci.* 2008;53(9):2524-2531.

125. Remicade (Infliximab) [prescribing information]. *Centocor I.* 2005.

126. Wagner C, De Woody K, Zelinger D, Leone A, Schaible T, Shealy D. Infliximab treatment benefits correlate with pharmacodynamic parameters in Crohn's disease patients. *Digestion.* 1998;59(suppl 3):124-125.

127. Mouser JF, Hyams JS. Infliximab: a novel chimeric monoclonal antibody for the treatment of Crohn's disease. *Clin Ther.* 1999; 21(6):932-942; discussion 1.

128. Targan SR, Hanauer SB, van Deventer SJ, et al. A short-term study of chimeric monoclonal antibody cA2 to tumor necrosis factor alpha for Crohn's disease. Crohn's Disease cA2 Study Group. *N Engl J Med.* 1997;337(15):1029-1035.

129. Present DH, Rutgeerts P, Targan S, et al. Infliximab for the treatment of fistulas in patients with Crohn's disease. *N Engl J Med.* 1999;340(18):1398-1405.

130. Rutgeerts P, D'Haens G, Targan S, et al. Efficacy and safety of retreatment with anti-tumor necrosis factor antibody (infliximab) to maintain remission in Crohn's disease. *Gastroenterology.* 1999;117(4):761-769.

131. Hanauer SB, Feagan BG, Lichtenstein GR, et al. Maintenance infliximab for Crohn's disease: the ACCENT I randomised trial. *Lancet.* 2002;359(9317):1541-1549.

132. Sands BE, Anderson FH, Bernstein CN, et al. Infliximab maintenance therapy for fistulizing Crohn's disease. *N Engl J Med.* 2004; 350(9):876-885.

133. Behm BW, Bickston SJ. Tumor necrosis factor-alpha antibody for maintenance of remission in Crohn's disease. *Cochrane Database Syst Rev.* 2008;1:CD006893.

134. Sandborn WJ, Rutgeerts P, Reinisch W, et al. One year data from the SONIC study: a randomized, double-blind trial comparing infliximab and infliximab plus azathioprine to azathioprine in patients with Crohn's disease naive to immunomodulators and biologic therapy [abstract]. *Gastroenterology.* 2009;136:A116.

135. Rutgeerts P, Feagan BG, Lichtenstein GR, et al. Comparison of scheduled and episodic treatment strategies of infliximab in Crohn's disease. *Gastroenterology.* 2004;126(2):402-413.

136. Baert F, Noman M, Vermeire S, et al. Influence of immunogenicity on the long-term efficacy of infliximab in Crohn's disease. *N Engl J Med.* 2003;348(7):601-608.

137. Lichtenstein GR, Feagan BG, Cohen RD, et al. Serious infections and mortality in association with therapies for Crohn's disease: TREAT registry. *Clin Gastroenterol Hepatol.* 2006;4(5):621-630.

138. Lichtenstein G, Cohen R, Feagan B, et al. Safety of infliximab and other Crohn's disease therapies: TREAT™ registry data with nearly 20,000 patient-years of follow-up [abstract]. *Gastroenterology.* 2007;132:A178.

139. Rutgeerts P, Van Assche G, Vermeire S. Optimizing anti-TNF treatment in inflammatory bowel disease. *Gastroenterology.* 2004; 126(6):1593-1610.

140. Targeted tuberculin testing and treatment of latent tuberculosis infection. American Thoracic Society. *MMWR Recomm Rep.* 2000; 49(RR-6):1-51.

141. Lichtenstein GR. Infliximab: lifetime use for maintenance is appropriate in Crohn's disease. PRO: maintenance therapy is superior to episodic therapy. *Am J Gastroenterol.* 2005;100(7):1433-1435.

142. Schnitzler F, Fidder H, Ferrante M, et al. Mucosal healing predicts long-term outcome of maintenance therapy with infliximab in Crohn's disease. *Inflamm Bowel Dis.* 2009;15(9):1295-1301.

143. Humira (Adalimumab) [prescribing information]. Abbott Inc; 2008.

144. Sandborn WJ, Hanauer SB, Rutgeerts P, et al. Adalimumab for maintenance treatment of Crohn's disease: results of the CLASSIC II trial. *Gut.* 2007;56(9):1232-1239.

145. Colombel JF, Sandborn WJ, Rutgeerts P, et al. Adalimumab for maintenance of clinical response and remission in patients with Crohn's disease: the CHARM trial. *Gastroenterology.* 2007; 132(1):52-65.

146. Hanauer SB, Sandborn WJ, Rutgeerts P, et al. Human anti-tumor necrosis factor monoclonal antibody (adalimumab) in Crohn's disease: the CLASSIC-I trial. *Gastroenterology.* 2006;130(2):323-333; quiz 591.

147. Colombel JF, Sandborn WJ, Rutgeerts P, et al. Comparison of two adalimumab treatment schedule strategies for moderate-to-severe Crohn's disease: results from the CHARM trial. *Am J Gastroenterol.* 2009;104(5):1170-1179.

148. Feagan BG, Panaccione R, Sandborn WJ, et al. Effects of adalimumab therapy on incidence of hospitalization and surgery in Crohn's disease: results from the CHARM study. *Gastroenterology.* 2008;135(5):1493-1499.

149. Loftus EV, Feagan BG, Colombel JF, et al. Effects of adalimumab maintenance therapy on health-related quality of life of patients with Crohn's disease: patient-reported outcomes of the CHARM trial. *Am J Gastroenterol.* 2008;103(12):3132-3141.

150. Chapman AP. PEGylated antibodies and antibody fragments for improved therapy: a review. *Adv Drug Deliv Rev.* 2002;54(4):531-545.

151. Lang L. FDA approves Cimzia to treat Crohn's disease. *Gastroenterology.* 2008;134(7):1819.

152. Cimzia (Certolizumab pegol) [prescribing information]. UCB Inc; 2008.

153. Schreiber S, Khaliq-Kareemi M, Lawrance IC, et al. Maintenance therapy with certolizumab pegol for Crohn's disease. *N Engl J Med.* 2007;357(3):239-250.

154. Feagan BG, Coteur G, Tan S, Keininger DL, Schreiber S. Clinically meaningful improvement in health-related quality of life in a randomized controlled trial of certolizumab pegol maintenance therapy for Crohn's disease. *Am J Gastroenterol.* 2009;104(8):1976-1983.

155. Sandborn WJ, Yednock TA. Novel approaches to treating inflammatory bowel disease: targeting alpha-4 integrin. *Am J Gastroenterol.* 2003;98(11):2372-2382.

156. Tysabri (Natalizumab) [prescribing information]. Biogen Idec Inc, Elan Pharmaceuticals, Inc; 2008.

157. Sandborn WJ, Colombel JF, Enns R, et al. Natalizumab induction and maintenance therapy for Crohn's disease. *N Engl J Med.* 2005;353(18):1912-1925.

158. Adelman B, Sandrock A, Panzara MA. Natalizumab and progressive multifocal leukoencephalopathy. *N Engl J Med.* 2005;353(4):432-433.

159. Langer-Gould A, Atlas SW, Green AJ, Bollen AW, Pelletier D. Progressive multifocal leukoencephalopathy in a patient treated with natalizumab. *N Engl J Med.* 2005;353(4):375-381.

160. Kleinschmidt-DeMasters BK, Tyler KL. Progressive multifocal leukoencephalopathy complicating treatment with natalizumab and interferon beta-1a for multiple sclerosis. *N Engl J Med.* 2005; 353(4):369-374.

161. United States Food and Drug Administration. Available at: http://www.fda.gov/Drugs/DrugSafety/PostmarketDrugSafetyInformationforPatientsandProviders/ucm107188.htm Accessed July 14, 2009.

162. Honey K. The comeback kid: TYSABRI now FDA approved for Crohn's disease. *J Clin Invest.* 2008;118(3):825-826.

163. Feagan BG, Sandborn WJ, Hass S, Niecko T, White J. Health-related quality of life during natalizumab maintenance therapy for Crohn's disease. *Am J Gastroenterol.* 2007;102(12):2737-2746.

164. Lichtenstein GR, Hanauer SB, Sandborn WJ. Management of Crohn's disease in adults. *Am J Gastroenterol.* 2009;104(2):465-483.

165. Becker JM. Surgical therapy for ulcerative colitis and Crohn's disease. *Gastroenterol Clin North Am.* 1999;28(2):371-390, viii-ix.

166. Olaison G, Smedh K, Sjodahl R. Natural course of Crohn's disease after ileocolic resection: endoscopically visualised ileal ulcers preceding symptoms. *Gut.* 1992;33(3):331-335.

167. Rutgeerts P, Geboes K, Vantrappen G, Beyls J, Kerremans R, Hiele M. Predictability of the postoperative course of Crohn's disease. *Gastroenterology.* 1990;99(4):956-963.

168. McLeod RS, Wolff BG, Steinhart AH, et al. Risk and significance of endoscopic/radiological evidence of recurrent Crohn's disease. *Gastroenterology.* 1997;113(6):1823-1827.

169. Borley NR, Mortensen NJ, Jewell DP. Preventing postoperative recurrence of Crohn's disease. *Br J Surg.* 1997;84(11):1493-1502.

170. Achkar JP, Hanauer SB. Medical therapy to reduce postoperative Crohn's disease recurrence. *Am J Gastroenterol.* 2000;95(5):1139-1146.

171. De Dombal FT, Burton I, Goligher JC. Recurrence of Crohn's disease after primary excisional surgery. *Gut.* 1971;12(7):519-527.

172. Post S, Herfarth C, Bohm E, et al. The impact of disease pattern, surgical management, and individual surgeons on the risk for relaparotomy for recurrent Crohn's disease. *Ann Surg.* 1996;223(3):253-260.

173. Reese GE, Nanidis T, Borysiewicz C, Yamamoto T, Orchard T, Tekkis PP. The effect of smoking after surgery for Crohn's disease: a meta-analysis of observational studies. *Int J Colorectal Dis.* 2008;23(12):1213-1221.

174. Ewe K, Herfarth C, Malchow H, Jesdinsky HJ. Postoperative recurrence of Crohn's disease in relation to radicality of operation and sulfasalazine prophylaxis: a multicenter trial. *Digestion.* 1989;42(4):224-232.

175. Wenckert A, Kristensen M, Eklund AE, et al. The long-term prophylactic effect of salazosulphapyridine (Salazopyrin) in primarily resected patients with Crohn's disease. A controlled double-blind trial. *Scand J Gastroenterol.* 1978;13(2):161-167.

176. Bergman L, Krause U. Postoperative treatment with corticosteroids and salazosulphapyridine (Salazopyrin) after radical resection for Crohn's disease. *Scand J Gastroenterol.* 1976;11(7):651-656.

177. Brignola C, Cottone M, Pera A, et al. Mesalamine in the prevention of endoscopic recurrence after intestinal resection for Crohn's disease. Italian Cooperative Study Group. *Gastroenterology.* 1995;108(2):345-349.

178. Caprilli R, Andreoli A, Capurso L, et al. Oral mesalazine (5-aminosalicylic acid; Asacol) for the prevention of post-operative recurrence of Crohn's disease. Gruppo Italiano per lo Studio del Colon e del Retto (GISC). *Aliment Pharmacol Ther.* 1994;8(1):35-43.

179. Lochs H, Mayer M, Fleig WE, et al. Prophylaxis of postoperative relapse in Crohn's disease with mesalamine: European Cooperative Crohn's Disease Study VI. *Gastroenterology.* 2000;118(2):264-273.

180. McLeod RS, Wolff BG, Steinhart AH, et al. Prophylactic mesalamine treatment decreases postoperative recurrence of Crohn's disease. *Gastroenterology.* 1995;109(2):404-413.

181. Cottone M, Camma C. Mesalamine and relapse prevention in Crohn's disease. *Gastroenterology.* 2000;119(2):597.

182. Smith RC, Rhodes J, Heatley RV, et al. Low dose steroids and clinical relapse in Crohn's disease: a controlled trial. *Gut.* 1978;19(7):606-610.

183. Ewe K, Bottger T, Buhr HJ, Ecker KW, Otto HF. Low-dose budesonide treatment for prevention of postoperative recurrence of Crohn's disease: a multicentre randomized placebo-controlled trial. German Budesonide Study Group. *Eur J Gastroenterol Hepato.* 1999;11(3):277-282.

184. Hellers G, Cortot A, Jewell D, et al. Oral budesonide for prevention of postsurgical recurrence in Crohn's disease. The IOIBD Budesonide Study Group. *Gastroenterology.* 1999;116(2):294-300.

185. Hanauer SB, Korelitz BI, Rutgeerts P, et al. Postoperative maintenance of Crohn's disease remission with 6-mercaptopurine, mesalamine, or placebo: a 2-year trial. *Gastroenterology.* 2004;127(3):723-729.

186. D'Haens GR, Vermeire S, Van Assche G, et al. Therapy of metronidazole with azathioprine to prevent postoperative recurrence of Crohn's disease: a controlled randomized trial. *Gastroenterology.* 2008;135(4):1123-1129.

187. Regueiro M, Schraut W, Baidoo L, et al. Infliximab prevents Crohn's disease recurrence after ileal resection. *Gastroenterology.* 2009;136(2):441-450 e1; quiz 716.

APPENDIX
INFLIXIMAB TREATMENT

Lawrence W. Comerford, MD and Stephen J. Bickston, MD

TREATMENT OF INFLIXIMAB INFUSION REACTIONS

MILD REACTION

SYMPTOMS

- Hyperemia
- Hypo/hypertension
- Headache
- Dizziness

TREATMENT

- Run normal saline (NS) at 100 cc/hour throughout infusion and subsequent doses as well
- Slow rate to 10 mL/hour (4 drops/min). If symptoms do not resolve, stop infliximab
- Administer diphenhydramine 25 to 50 mg IV
- Administer acetaminophen 650 mg
- Wait 20 min then increase restart at 10 cc/hour x 15 min
- Then increase to 20 mL/hour (7 drops/min) x 15 min
- Then increase to 40 mL/hour (14 drops/min) x 15 min
- Then increase to 80 mL/hour (27 drops/min) x 15 min
- Monitor vital signs every 10 min until normal

MODERATE REACTION

SYMPTOMS

- Hypo/hypertension
- Hyperemia
- Chest discomfort (tightening)/pressure
- Shortness of breath (SOB)
- Facial flushing
- Palpitations

TREATMENT

- Stop to administer diphenhydramine 25 to 50 mg IV
- Run NS at 100 cc/hour throughout infusion and subsequent doses as well
- Administer acetaminophen 650 mg
- Wait 20 min then restart at 10 mL/hour (4 drops/min) x 15 min
- Then increase to 20 mL/hour (7 drops/min) x 15 min
- Then increase to 40 mL/hour (14 drops/min) x 15 min
- Then increase to 80 mL/hour (27 drops/min) x 15 min
- Monitor vital signs every 5 min until normal

Lichtenstein GR, ed.
Crohn's Disease: The Complete Guide to Medical Management (pp 451-454).
© 2011 SLACK Incorporated

SEVERE REACTION

PROGRESSING SYMPTOMS

- Hypo/hypertension
- Elevated temperature with rigors
- Hyperemia
- Chest discomfort (tightening)/pressure
- SOB
- Stridor—if potential to lose airway, call 911 for transport to emergency room (ER)

TREATMENT

- Stop infusion
- Infuse NS at 500 to 1000 cc/hour
- Maintain airway/O$_2$ *if available*
- Administer hydrocortisone 100 mg IV or methylprednisolone 20 to 40 mg IV
- Administer diphenhydramine 25 to 50 mg slow IV
- Administer epinephrine (1:1000) 0.1 to 0.5 subcutaneously (SQ) *(May repeat q 5 mins x 3)** (***If patient requires a second dose of epinephrine, call 911 to transfer to ER for monitoring.**)
- Administer acetaminophen 650 mg
- Meperidine 25 mg intravenous (IV), only if severe rigors or lower back pain
- Monitor vital signs every 5 min until normal
- If patient stabilizes, follow infusion rate protocol for subsequent dosing up to 80 mL/hour

SUBSEQUENT DOSES

MILD REACTION

- May wish to premedicate with acetaminophen 650 mg PO plus diphenhydramine 25 to 50 mg IV, or give a second-generation antihistamine (cetirizine/Zyrtec, fexofenadine/Allegra, loratadine/Claritin) every hour of sleep (QHS) x 5 days prior to next dose. Run NS at 100 cc/hour throughout subsequent doses.
- Test dose at 10 mL/hour (4 drops/min) x 15 min. Then increase rate to infuse over 3 hours.

MODERATE REACTION

- Premedicate with acetaminophen 650 mg PO plus diphenhydramine 25 to 50 mg IV, or give a second-generation antihistamine QHS x 5 days prior to next dose.
- Test dose at 10 mL/hour (4 drops/min) x 15 min

- Then increase to 20 mL/hour (7 drops/min) x 15 min
- Then increase to 40 mL/hour (14 drops/min) x 15 min
- Then increase to 80 mL/hour (27 drops/min) x 15 min
- Then increase to 100 mL/hour (34 drops/min) x 15 min
- Then increase to 125 mL/hour (41 drops/min) through completion

SEVERE REACTION

- Prednisone 50 mg PO BID x 3 doses prior to infusion
- Administer hydrocortisone 100 mg IV or methylprednisolone 20 to 40 mg IV as premedication 20 min prior to infusion
- Premedicate with diphenhydramine 25 to 50 mg IV plus acetaminophen 650 mg PO
- Run NS at 100 cc/hour throughout infusion
- Test dose at 10 mL/hour (4 drops/min) x 15 min
- Then increase to 20 mL/hour (7 drops/min) x 15 min
- Then increase to 40 mL/hour (14 drops/min) x 15 min
- Then increase to 80 mL/hour (27 drops/min) x 15 min
- Then increase to 100 mL/hour (34 drops/min) x 15 min

IF THE PATIENT EXPERIENCES A SECOND MODERATE-SEVERE REACTION DURING THE INFUSION

- Stop infusion
- Infuse NS at 500 to 1000 cc/hour
- Administer hydrocortisone 100 mg IV or methylprednisolone 20 to 40 mg IV
- Administer diphenhydramine 25 to 50 mg IV plus acetaminophen 650 mg PO
- Test dose at 10 mL/hour (4 drops/min) x 15 min
- Then increase to 20 mL/hour (7 drops/min) x 15 min
- Then increase to 40 mL/hour (14 drops/min) x 15 min
- Stop at the rate the patient had the reaction

UPON COMPLETION OF INFLIXIMAB, DISCHARGE PATIENT HOME ON THE FOLLOWING

- Second-generation antihistamine PO QHS x 5 days
- Have patient fill prescription for methylprednisolone (Medrol) dose pack and start this medicine if he or she experiences joint pain.

DELAYED REACTION

SYMPTOMS

- Rash/urticaria
- Muscle aches, flu-like symptoms
- Joint stiffness and pain

TREATMENT

- Instruct patient to take diphenhydramine 25 to 50 mg PO Q4-6 hours x 1 to 2 days, then a second-generation antihistamine QD x 5 days
- Acetaminophen 650 mg PO QID x 3 days
- Order a methylprednisolone dose pack to be started if patient experiences joint pain

SUBSEQUENT DOSES AFTER DELAYED REACTION

- Have patient premedicate for 4 to 5 days prior to next infliximab infusion with second-generation antihistamine
- Administer hydrocortisone 100 mg IV or methylprednisolone 20 to 40 mg IV as premedication 20 min prior to infusion

- Premedicate with diphenhydramine 25 to 50 mg IV plus acetaminophen 650 mg PO
- Run NS at 100 cc/hour throughout infusion
- Test dose at 10 mL/hour (4 drops/min) x 15 min
- Then increase to 20 mL/hour (7 drops/min) x 15 min
- Then increase to 40 mL/hour (14 drops/min) x 15 min
- Then increase to 80 mL/hour (27 drops/min) x 15 min
- Then increase to 100 mL/hour (34 drops/min) x 15 min

UPON COMPLETION OF INFLIXIMAB, DISCHARGE PATIENT HOME ON THE FOLLOWING

- Second-generation antihistamine QHS x 7 days
- Prescribe methylprednisolone dose pack to be filled and started if symptoms of joint pain or myalgia occur

Adapted with permission from Lloyd Mayer, MD, Sinai School of Medicine.

FINANCIAL DISCLOSURES

Dr. Faten Aberra has not disclosed any relevant financial relationships.

Dr. Maria T. Abreu has not disclosed any relevant financial relationships.

Dr. Pietro G. Andres has not disclosed any relevant financial relationships.

Dr. Robert N. Baldassano has not disclosed any relevant financial relationships.

Dr. Theodore M. Bayless has not disclosed any relevant financial relationships.

Dr. Charles N. Bernstein has not disclosed any relevant financial relationships.

Dr. Stephen J. Bickston has not disclosed any relevant financial relationships.

Dr. Henry J. Binder has not disclosed any relevant financial relationships.

Dr. Alain Bitton has not disclosed any relevant financial relationships.

Dr. Wojciech Blonski has no financial or proprietary interest in the materials presented herein.

Dr. Brian P. Bosworth has not disclosed any relevant financial relationships.

Dr. Aaron Brzezinski has not disclosed any relevant financial relationships.

Dr. Alan L. Buchman has not disclosed any relevant financial relationships.

Dr. Robert Burakoff has not disclosed any relevant financial relationships.

Dr. Ashish Chawlahas not disclosed any relevant financial relationships.

Dr. Adam Cheifetz has not disclosed any relevant financial relationships.

Dr. Lawrence W. Comerford has not disclosed any relevant financial relationships.

Dr. Themistocles Dassopoulos is on the speaker's bureau at Abbott and UCB.

Dr. Geert D'Haens has not disclosed any relevant financial relationships.

Dr. Iris Dotan has not disclosed any relevant financial relationships.

Dr. Francis A. Farraye has not disclosed any relevant financial relationships.

Dr. Richard N. Fedorak's research is supported by the Canadian Institute for Health Research and the Crohn's and Colitis Foundation of Canada.

Dr. Denis Franchimont has not disclosed any relevant financial relationships.

Dr. Lawrence S. Friedman has not disclosed any relevant financial relationships.

Dr. Masayuki Fukata has not disclosed any relevant financial relationships.

Lichtenstein GR, ed.
Crohn's Disease: The Complete Guide to Medical Management (pp 455-458).
© 2011 SLACK Incorporated

Dr. Louis R. Ghanem has no financial or proprietary interest in the materials presented herein.

Dr. Peter H.R. Green has not disclosed any relevant financial relationships.

Dr. Gordon R. Greenberg has not disclosed any relevant financial relationships.

Dr. Stephen B. Hanauer has not disclosed any relevant financial relationships.

Dr. Vinita Elizabeth Jacob has not disclosed any relevant financial relationships.

Dr. Sunanda Kane receives research support from and is a consultant for Shire and Proctor & Gamble.

Dr. Gilaad G. Kaplan has not disclosed any relevant financial relationships.

Dr. Arthur Kaser has not disclosed any relevant financial relationships.

Dr. Jeffry A. Katz has not disclosed any relevant financial relationships.

Dr. Joshua R. Korzenik has not disclosed any relevant financial relationships.

Dr. David Kotlyar has no financial or proprietary interest in the materials presented herein.

Dr. Harrison Lakehomer has not disclosed any relevant financial relationships.

Dr. James D. Lewis has received research funding from Centocor, Takeda, and Shire. He has served as a paid consultant for Millenium, AstraZeneca, GlaxoSmithKline, Elan, Proctor & Gamble, and Amgen.

Dr. Gary Lichtenstein is a consultant for Abbott Corporation, Alaven, Bristol-Myers Squibb, Centocor Orthobiotech, Elan, Ferring, Meda Pharmaceuticals, Millenium Pharmaceuticals, Pfizer Pharmaceuticals, Proctor and Gamble, Prometheus Laboratories Inc, Salix Pharmaceuticals, Santarus, Schering-Plough Corporation, Shire Pharmaceuticals, UCB, Warner Chilcotte, and Wyeth.

Dr. Wee-Chian Lim has no financial or proprietary interest in the materials presented herein.

Dr. Ming V. Lin has no financial or proprietary interest in the materials presented herein.

Dr. Karen L. Madsen's research is supported by the Canadian Institute for Health Research, Crohn's and Colitis Foundation of Canada and the Alberta Heritage Foundation for Medical Research.

Dr. Gerassimos J. Mantzaris has no financial or proprietary interest in the materials presented herein.

Dr. Manuel Mendizabal has no financial or proprietary interest in the materials presented herein.

Dr. Tarun Misra has not disclosed any relevant financial relationships.

Dr. David N. Moskovitz has not disclosed any relevant financial relationships.

Dr. Alan C. Moss has no financial or proprietary interest in the materials presented herein.

Dr. Pia Munkholm has not disclosed any relevant financial relationships.

Dr. Jane E. Onken has no financial or proprietary interest in the materials presented herein.

Dr. Mark T. Osterman has not disclosed any relevant financial relationships.

Dr. Jaime A. Oviedo has not disclosed any relevant financial relationships.

Dr. Remo Panaccione has not disclosed any relevant financial relationships.

Dr. Robert M. Penner's research is supported by the Canadian Institute for Health Research, Crohn's and Colitis Foundation of Canada and the Alberta Heritage Foundation for Medical Research.

Dr. Daniel Rachmilewitz has not disclosed any relevant financial relationships.

Dr. Mamoon Raza has not disclosed any relevant financial relationships.

Dr. Sarathchandra I. Reddy has not disclosed any relevant financial relationships.

Dr. Lene Riis has not disclosed any relevant financial relationships.

Dr. Ellen Scherl has not disclosed any relevant financial relationships.

Dr. Felice Schnoll-Sussman has not disclosed any relevant financial relationships.

Dr. Corey A. Siegel has not disclosed any relevant financial relationships.

Dr. Kenneth Simpson has not disclosed any relevant financial relationships.

Dr. Miles P. Sparrow has not disclosed any relevant financial relationships.

Dr. Chinyu Su is currently an employee of Pfizer, Inc. She was formerly and employee of and a stockholder in Wyeth, which was acquired by Pfizer, Inc in October 2009.

Dr. Arun Swaminath has not disclosed any relevant financial relationships.

Dr. Herbert Tilg has not disclosed any relevant financial relationships.

Dr. Ryan Urquhart Warren has not disclosed any relevant financial relationships.

Dr. Douglas M. Weine has not disclosed any relevant financial relationships.

Dr. Gary Wild has not disclosed any relevant financial relationships.

INDEX

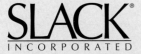